**Dictionary of Endocrinology
and Related
Biomedical Sciences**

DICTIONARY OF ENDOCRINOLOGY AND RELATED BIOMEDICAL SCIENCES

Constance R. Martin, PhD

Professor Emeritus
Hunter College and Graduate Center
City University of New York

New York ■ Oxford
OXFORD UNIVERSITY PRESS
1995

To April, Susan, Brenda, Roy, Emily
and Jesse

Oxford University Press

Oxford   New York
Athens   Auckland   Bangkok   Bombay
Calcutta   Cape Town   Dar es Salaam   Delhi
Florence   Hong Kong   Istanbul   Karachi
Kuala Lumpur   Madras   Madrid   Melbourne
Mexico City   Nairobi   Paris   Singapore
Taipei   Tokyo   Toronto

and associated companies in
Berlin   Ibadan

Copyright © 1995 by Oxford University Press, Inc.

Published by Oxford University Press, Inc.,
200 Madison Avenue, New York, New York 10016

Oxford is a registered trademark of Oxford University Press

Library of Congress Cataloging-in-Publication Data
Martin, Constance R.
Dictionary of endocrinology and related biomedical sciences
Constance Martin.
p.   cm.

ISBN 0-19-506033-4

[DNLM: 1. Endocrinology—dictionaries. 2. Endocrine Diseases—dictionaries.
WK 13 M379d 1995]
QP187.M3458 1995
612.4′03—dc20
DNLM/DLC
for Library of Congress   94-35299
                                                                                              CIP

1 3 5 7 9 8 6 4 2
Printed in the United States of America
on acid-free paper

PREFACE

Endocrinologists deal with hundreds of hormones, neurotransmitters, growth factors, pheromones, vitamins, enzymes, and other regulators, many of which are represented in the literature by acronyms. Expertise in endocrine physiology requires familiarity with the structures, biosynthesis and metabolism of those regulators, the kinds of receptors activated, the second messengers generated, the biochemical pathways and morphological features affected, the changes associated with differentiation, maturation, and aging, the interactions with other regulators (including feedback controls) and the responses to factors such as photoperiods, nutritional states, and environmental temperatures.

Clinicians are especially concerned with the causes and manifestations of endocrine system dysfunctions, diagnostic procedures, beneficial and untoward effects of therapeutic agents, and the extents to which observations on other species apply to patients.

Investigators additionally study pharmacological agents unsuitable for use in humans that mimic the actions of naturally occurring cell components or disrupt their functions. Research in various aspects of the subject requires a working knowledge of pharmacology, molecular biology, biochemistry, immunology, and genetics, or animal, plant, and cell physiology, and/or of behavioral psychology, other biological sciences, and of statistical and other procedures for analyzing data. Special expertise is also required for evaluation of possible extrapolations of conclusions drawn from one kind of study to another, since (in addition to the limited kinds on human subjects), experiments are performed on diverse vertebrate and invertebrate species, unicellular eukaryotes, prokaryotes, viruses, and non-living components of *in vitro* systems.

It has become increasingly difficult for an individual specializing in one subdivision of endocrinology to keep pace with the ever-changing terminology of distantly related, but relevant fields of inquiry, and even more difficult for investigators in different, but related biological sciences to acquire a working knowledge of the endocrine system.

This dictionary provides detailed definitions of terms used in endocrinology and related sciences, in language easily comprehended by readers unfamiliar with the specific items, and includes acronyms commonly cited in the literature. There is some emphasis on human physiology and dysfunction, but observations made on other organisms, or obtained from *in vitro* systems are presented, along with comments on species variations.

The sources of information are too numerous for detailed citation. They include *Endocrinology, Journal of Clinical Endocrinology, Endocrine Reviews, American Journal of Physiology, Molecular Endocrinology, Trends in Endocrinology and Metabolism, Trends in Biochemical Sciences, BioEssays, New England Journal of Medicine, The FASEB Journal, Proceedings of the National Academy of Sciences, Cell, Nature, Science,* and other journals, textbooks such as *Principles of Biochemistry* by E.L. Smith, R.L. Hill, I.R. Lehman,

R.J. Lefkowitz, P. Handler, and A. White, *Biochemistry*, 3rd edition by L. Stryer, *Goodman and Gilman's The Pharmacological Basis of Therapeutics*, 8th ed., edited by A.G. Gilman, T.W. Rall, A.S. Niew, and P. Taylor, *Molecular Biology of the Cell*, 2nd edition by B. Albert, D. Bray, J. Lewis, M. Raff, K. Roberts, and J.D. Watson, *Oncogenes* by G.M. Cooper, and *Immunology* by J. Kuby. Additional sources include the *Annual Review of Biochemistry*, *The Merck Index*, 11th ed., *The Dictionary of Cell Biology* by J.M. Lackie and J.A.T. Dow, *Dictionary of Immunology* by F.S. Rosen, L.A. Steiner, and E.R. Unanue, *A Dictionary of Genetics* by R.C. King and W.D. Stansfield, and several commercially prepared catalogs, among them ones provided by Research Biochemicals International, BACHEM CALIFOR-NIA, Sigma, Fluka Chemicka-Biochemika, Calbiochem, and Janssen Chemica.

The chemical structures were generated with an ISIS/Draw program (Molecular Design Ltd); and supported by the technical staff at MDI is gratefully acknowledged. Helpful suggestions for presentation of the text were also obtained from the WordPerfect staff.

The long, and at times tedious process of preparing the manuscript might never have been completed without the ever-dependable encouragement and inspiration provided by my husband, Henning R. Norbom.

A

A: (1) alanine; (2) adenine; (3) adenosine; (4) alanine type amino acid transport system; (5) absorbance; (6) argon; (7) ampere. *See* also **A blood type, A cells, A rings, A subunits**, and **mating types**.

a-: a prefix meaning absence of, as in amenorrhea. When used with acronyms, it can designate (1) acidic, as in aFGF; or (2) avian, as in aPRL (avian prolactin).

α: alpha; can designate (1) a specific member of a group, such as a cell type in a tissue or organ (*see* α **cells**), a subunit component of a dimeric or heteromeric compound (see, e.g. **integrins**), or an enzyme or receptor isoform (*see*, e.g. **adrenergic receptors**); (2) the configuration of a substitution on an asymmetric carbon atom, as α-D-glucose or 5-α-dihydrotestosterone (*see* **stereoisomerism**).

Å: angstrom.

A_1: (1) an adenosine receptor subtype; (2) the pancreatic islet cell type that secretes glucagon; (3) the predominant adult human form of hemoglobin.

A-I: angiotensin I; (2) apolipoprotein A-1.

A_2: (1) an adenosine receptor subtype; (2) a type of hemoglobin present in small amounts in the circulating blood of human adults.

A-II: angiotensin II.

A3: *N*-(2-aminoethyl)-5-chloronapthalalene-1-sulfonamide; a potent inhibitor of kinases A and G, and a weak inhibitor of kinase C and MLC kinase.

A-III: an**AIII**: angiotensin III.

A4: (1) β-A4; 4K; a 42 or 43 amino acid extracellular peptide of neuritic plaques; *see* **amyloid β-protein**.

A-4: apolipoprotein-4.

A23187: calcimycin; 6S-[(2S,3S),8βR],9β,11α]-5-(methylamino)-2-[[3,9,11-trimethyl-8-[1methyl-2-oxo-2-(1*H*-pyrrol-2-yl)ethyl]-1,7-dioxaspiro[5,5]-undec-2-yl]methyl]-4-benzoxolecarboxylic acid; a monocarboxylic lipophilic ionophore obtained from *Streptomyces chartreusensis*. It carries Ca^{2+} across plasma membranes, affects intracellular Ca^{2+} transport, and is used to study the effects of elevating cytosolic calcium ion concentrations.

A23187

iodo-Sar[1]-Ile[8]-**A-II**: a ligand used to identify angiotensin-II receptors.

AA: (1) arachidonic acid; (2) the blood type of individuals homozygous for A type erythrocyte antigens.

α-AA: α-aminoadipic acid.

A antigens: oligosaccharide components of molecules exposed on the surfaces of erythrocytes, epithelial, and endothelial cells of individuals with A (AA or AO) and AB blood types. Most are attached to glycoproteins, but small amounts bind lipids. *See* also **A, AB** and **O blood types**.

AASH: adrenal androgen stimulating hormone.

ab: antibody.

ABA: abscisic acid.

A bands: anisotropic, myosin containing thick microfilaments of skeletal muscle; *cf* **I bands**.

ABC: (1) antigen binding capacity; (2) ATP-binding casette; a motif common to members of a superfamily of proteins with six membrane-spanning segments, all of which promote ATP-dependent active transport of ions and/or molecules. *See* also **P glycoproteins.**

ABCD: avidin-biotin complex binding assay.

Abelson murine leukemia virus: A-MuLV; two closely related transforming retrovirus strains that invoke aggressive lymphomas in mice, induce conditions that closely resemble (but differ in some ways from) human chronic myelogenous leukemias, and transform B lymphocytes, γδ type T cells, plasma cells, macrophages, promyelocytes, and fibroblasts. Their actions involve formation of $p120^{gag/v-abl}$ and $p160^{gag/v-abl}$, proteins with tyrosine kinase activity that resemble interleukin-3 receptors. *See* also *abl*, **Philadelphia chromosome**, and **oncogenes**.

abetalipoproteinemias: rare diseases caused by autosomal defects that impair synthesis of apoprotein B-100, and thereby production of very low and low density lipoproteins ((VLDs and LDLs), often associated with failure to produce apoprotein B-48 and form chylomicrons. Intestinal absorption of dietary lipids (including fat-soluble vitamins and essential fatty acids as well as triacylglycerols and cholesterol) is severely compromised, as is cholesterol transport from the liver to the bloodstream. Consequently, most cells are deprived of essential nutrients, and fats accumulate in the intestine. The manifestations include neuropathy with demyelination, cerebellar ataxia, retinitis pigmentosa, abnormal erythrocyte membranes, and steatorrhea.

abl: *c-abl* is a proto-oncogene that localizes mostly to nuclei and plays essential roles in embryogenesis, and in the proliferation and differentiation of several mature cell types. It contributes to signal transduction, and is required for hematopoiesis, sperm maturation, and other functions. The protein product contains a tyrosine kinase domain, and can undergo autophosphorylation, but is present in unphosphorylated form under normal conditions. It also contains, an SH2 domain that mediates noncovalent binding of the phosphorylated form to other proteins, and an SH3 domain which exerts negative control, in part by binding to cellular inhibitory factors. When excessively activated, e.g. via phosphorylation and loss of the SH3 domain, it can transform cells and invoke leukemias and the formation of several kinds of tumors. Chromosomal translocations that replace the usual promotor with different types can stimulate overexpression; *see* **Philadelphia chromosome**. The **Abelson leukemia virus** (*q.v.*) codes for two *v-abl* products, both of which attach to a viral *gag* gene product that stimulates transcription. It can accumulate in plasma membranes and transform some cell types.

A blood type: blood in which erythrocytes express A (but no B) antigens, and the plasma contains anti-B (but no anti-A) antibodies. Individuals can be homozygous (AA) or heterozygous (AO) for the trait.

AB blood type: blood in which erythrocytes express both A and B antigens, and neither anti-A nor anti-B antibodies are present in the plasma. Individuals with this blood type have been called "universal recipients", since their plasma does not agglutinate A, B, AB, or O type erythrocytes, and the ability of antibodies in donor blood plasma to agglutinate AB erythrocytes is minimized by dilution in host plasma. However, blood typing is essential for identification of other possible incompatibilities.

ABO blood groups: a classification system for alleles on human chromosome 9, based on the kinds of antigens expressed on erythrocytes; *see* **A, B, AB**, and **O blood types**.

abortifacient: any agent that invokes expulsion of an embryo or immature fetus; *cf* **interceptive** and **contraceptive**.

abortion: spontaneous or artificially induced expulsion of an embryo or immature fetus.

ABPs: (1) androgen binding proteins; (2) actin binding proteins; (3) auxin binding proteins.

abrin: a mixture of albuminous, galactose-binding lectins obtained from the jequirity bean, *Abrus precatorius.* Abrins A, B, C, and D are monovalent 63K-67K dimeric peptides. An associated *Abrus* agglutinin is a 134.9K bivalent tetramer. Some of the lectins are toxic. Since they more effectively inhibit protein synthesis in certain cancer, than in normal cell types, they are used to arrest the growth of some neoplasms. *See* also L-**abrine**.

L-**abrine**: *N*-methyl-tryptophan; a component of *Abrus precatorius* seeds that is biologically active, but not antineoplastic.

abscisic acid: ABA; 5-(1-hydroxy-2,6,6-trimethyl-4-oxo-2-cyclohexen-1-yl)-3-methyl-2,4-pentadienoic acid; a plant growth factor initially recognized for its ability to promote separation of leaves from stems (abscision). It contributes to water balance control, in part by inhibiting opening of stomata, elevates the cytosolic pH of many plant cell types, induces the synthesis of seed proteins, and enhances adaptations to stresses. Although both plant hormones can elevate cytosol Ca^{2+} levels, ABA inhibits auxin stimulation of linear growth, and auxins oppose abscisic acid influences on stomata opening and cell pH.

absorbance: uptake of radiant energy (visible or ultraviolet light, radioactivity, or heat). Absorption at specific wave-lengths is used to identify chemical groups within molecules (*see* e.g. **cytochrome P$_{450}$**). *See* also **optical density**.

abzymes: antibodies that possess catalytic activity.

Ac, ac: acetyl.

A-CAM: a 135K cell adhesion protein related to N-cadherin, in adherens junctions of the heart and eye lens, and at some other sites. It engages in Ca^{2+}-dependent homophilic (A-CAM:A-CAM) and heterophilic (A-CAM:L-CAM) binding; *see* also **cell adhesion molecules**.

acanthosis nigricans: conditions in which the skin undergoes hyperkeratinization and accumulates brown, grey, or black pigment patches. They are commonly associated with endocrine system disorders such as Cushing's syndrome, acromegaly, or polycystic ovary disease (but in some cases with simple obesity). In a rare autoimmune form, production of antibodies directed against insulin receptors causes severe insulin resistance.

acebutolol

ACAT: cholesterol acyltransferase.

acceptors, acceptor sites: (1) DNA base sequences that bind hormone-receptor complexes and other transcription regulators; *see*, e.g. **hormone response elements**; (2) molecular components that bind electrons and/or hydrogen, amino, methyl, or other chemical groups.

accessory cells: cells that cooperate with B and T lymphocytes to achieve immune system responses. Most are monocytes or macrophages. *See* also **dendritic cells**.

accessory olfactory bulbs: AOB; bilateral components of the rhinencephalon that transmit messages from vomeronasal organs to the amygdala and neuroendocrine hypothalamus. They are not involved in conscious perception of odors. *See* also **pheromones**, and *cf* **primary olfactory bulbs**.

accessory reproductive organs: structures that do not produce gametes, but contribute to reproduction, for example by storing, transporting, and/or nurturing gametes or conceptuses. Examples include prostate glands, seminal vesicles, and Fallopian tubes. *Cf* **secondary sex characteristics**.

acclimation: adjustments to changes, especially ones externally imposed.

acclimatization: physiological adaptations to temperature, atmospheric pressure, or other environmental changes.

Accutane: a trade name for isotretinoin.

ACE: angiotensin converting enzyme.

acebutolol: N-[3-acetyl-4-hydroxy-3-[-(1-methylethyl) amino]propoxy]phenyl]butanamide; an adrenergic receptor antagonist that affects mostly β_1-type receptors, used for its effects on the heart.

aceclidine: 3-acetoxyquinuclidine; glaucostat; a muscarinic receptor agonist. It, and some derivatives are used in Europe to lower intraocular pressure in individuals with glaucoma, and to lower blood pressure.

A cells: (1) a pancreatic islet A (A_2, alpha, α) cells that secrete glucagon; (2) adrenal medulla cells that secrete epinephrine.

α cells: (1) pancreatic islet A cells; (2) adenohypophysial acidophilic cells (somatotropes, lactotropes, and mammosomatotropes).

A_1 cells: pancreatic islet delta (δ) cells that secrete somatostatin.

A_2 cells: pancreatic islet A (α) cells that secrete glucagon.

acervulus [acervuli]: calcareous concretions, present, e.g. in aging pineal glands.

acetaldehyde: a metabolite produced in the liver when large amounts of ethanol are consumed. Alcohol dehydrogenase catalyzes the reaction: ethanol + $NAD^+ \rightarrow$ acetaldehyde + NADH. Although some of the product is oxidized in a reaction that restores NADH (acetaldehyde + $NAD^+ \rightarrow$ acetic acid + NADH), the cell NAD^+:NADH ratio usually rises, and this impairs gluconeogenesis by facilitating pyruvate conversion to lactate. Acetaldehyde also forms adducts with hepatic macromolecules, some of which are neo-antigens that can invoke abnormal immune system responses.

acetaminophen: Tylenol; p-acetamidophenol; an analgesic and antipyretic agent. It lacks the anti-inflammatory potency of salicylates, possibly because it is a poor inhibitor of peripheral cyclooxygenases.

acetazolamide: Diamox; Natrionex; 5-acetamido-1,3,4-thiadiazole-2-sulfonamide; a potent, but reversible benzothiadiazine-type inhibitor of carbonic anhydrases. The most obvious effects are exerted on renal nephrons, in which it slows Na^+ reabsorption and H^+ excretion, and secondarily impairs $NaHCO_3$ reabsorption. It thereby rapidly augments urine volume, pH, and K^+ and Cl^- content. The resulting metabolic acidosis is exacerbated by influences on erythrocytes that cause CO_2 retention. Acetazolamide also affects Na^+ transport in the intestines, in the eyes, and at other sites, and it diminishes iodide uptake in thyroid glands. Many therapeutic applications have been suggested, but more desirable agents are available for most of them. It is used under some conditions as a short-term diuretic, but compensatory increases in NH_4+ production soon diminish its effectiveness. Its ability to lower aqueous humor volume has been applied to the treatment of glaucoma, but methazolamide is now preferred. The metabolic acidosis, possibly coupled with actions on neurons not related to carbonic anhydrase inhibition, can diminish epileptic seizures but also invoke drowsiness and paresthesias. Parathyroid hormone-like effects, and increased risk for formation of urinary tract calculi have been linked with diminished citrate excretion and lowering of extracellular fluid pH. Acetazolamide invokes allergic reactions in susceptible individuals, and high levels are teratogenic in laboratory animals.

acetic acid {**acetate**}: a water-soluble, short-chain fatty acid formed when acetylcholine is degraded, and in some other reactions. Plants and bacteria metabolize it to acetyl-coenzyme A or acetyl-phosphate. High concentrations are used topically to destroy warts.

$$CH_3—COOH$$

acetoacetic acid {**acetoacetate**}: 3-oxabutanoic acid; one of three **ketone bodies** *(q.v.)*. It can be converted to acetyl-coenzyme A, reduced to β-hydroxybutyrate, or decarboxylated to yield acetone.

acetoacetyl-ACP: an intermediate in the pathway for fatty acid elongation. Acetyl transacylase catalyzes the reaction: acetyl-coenzyme A + acyl carrier protein (ACP) →acetoacyl-ACP + CoA. *See also* **acyl carrier protein**.

acetoacetyl coenzyme A: acetoacetyl-CoA; a metabolite formed during fatty acid oxidation, and an intermediate in the pathway for cholesterol, fatty acid, and ketone biosynthesis. It can be made from acetoacetate + coenzyme A, and can be cleaved via reactions that yield two molecules of acetyl coenzyme A. Since the acetoacetate bonds to the sulfur atom of the coenzyme, the molecule is usually represented as shown.

acetohexamide: Dimelor; 3-cyclohexyl-1-(*p*-acetylphenyl) sulfonyl)urea; a sulfonylurea type oral hypoglycemic agent.

acetone: 2-propanone; a volatile **ketone body** *(q.v.)* excreted by the lungs. It is formed by decarboxylation of acetoacetate.

acetyl: a component of many biological molecules, including acetyl coenzyme A, acetylcholine, and melatonin. Covalent linkage to proteins and other molecules affects surface charges and other properties.

N-**acetylaspartylglutamate**: a naturally occurring acetylated dipeptide believed to function as a neurotransmitter by acting on excitatory amino acid receptors.

acetylcholine: Ach: 2-(acetyloxy)-trimethylammonia; the major neurotransmitter released by preganglionic autonomic nervous system, parasympathetic postganglionic, and some brain neurons, and by motor nerves to skeletal muscles. Choline acetyltransferase catalyzes the rate limiting reaction for its biosynthesis: choline + acetyl-CoA → acetylcholine. Choline can be obtained from the diet, or made by methylating ethanolamine. The functions affected include learning and memory, vestibular system activity, skeletal muscle contraction, contraction of some smooth muscle cells and relaxation of others, cardiac inhibition, stimulatory influences on lacrimal, sweat, salivary, sweat, gastrointestinal, and other exocrine glands, and regulation of insulin-secreting and other endocrine glands. Many effects are short-lived, because postsynaptic membranes of target organs and synaptic clefts contain acetylcholinesterases. The actions are mediated by several kinds of **muscarinic** and **nicotinic receptors** ((*q.v.*), and are modified by antagonistic regulators, and by factors that affect ligand and receptor synthesis. Most muscarinic types are linked to G proteins, and the consequences at various sites include adenylate cyclase inhibition, cGMP generation, and influences on phospholipase C isozymes that affect phosphatidylinositol hydrolysis, and on phospholipase A$_2$s that lead to eicosanoid production. Acetylcholine also acts directly on some ion channels, and it affects the functions of neurons that release other neurotransmitters. Additionally, it exerts long-range trophic effects on neurons and on skeletal muscle. It is mitogenic for some cell types, and it synergizes with other hormones at various sites (e.g with androgens in seminal vesicles). Agonists can invoke transformation in transfected fibroblasts with acetylcholine receptors.

acetylcholine receptors: *see* **muscarinic** and **nicotinic receptors**.

acetylcholinesterases: cholinesterases: enzymes in synaptic clefts and on postsynaptic membranes that rapidly catalyze hydrolysis (and thereby inactivation) of acetylcholine, via the reaction: acetylcholine + H$_2$O → choline + acetate. Pseudocholinesterases additionally act on other substrates.

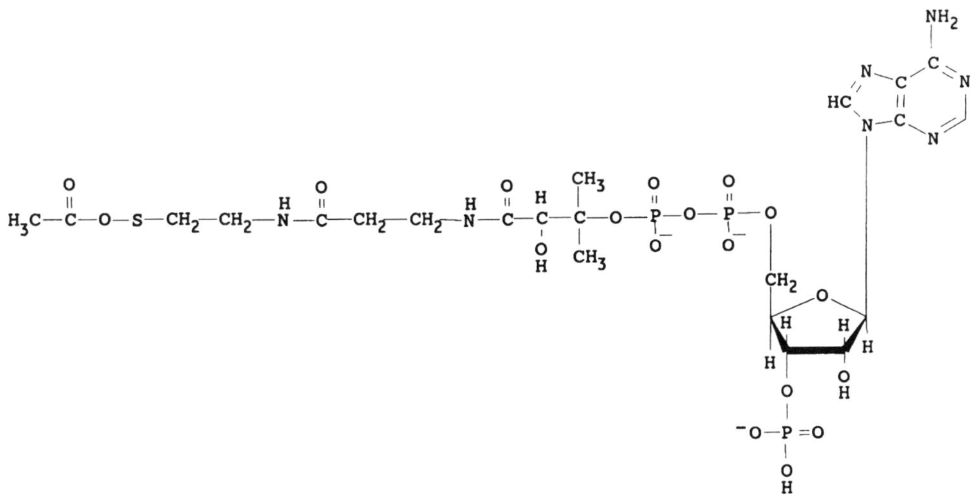

acetyl coenzyme A

acetyl-Co A: *see* **acetyl coenzyme A** for this compound, and items that follow for enzymes with names that begin with acetyl-CoA.

acetyl coenzyme A: acetyl Co-A: a major product of carbohydrate, lipid, and protein oxidation that is further metabolized via the tricarboxylic acid cycle, and is also used in the biosynthesis of cholesterol, fatty acids, ketones, and other cell components. The β-mercaptoethylamine component is linked at one end (via its S atom) to an acetyl group, and at the other end to an ATP.

acetyl coenzyme A acetyltransferases: acetyl-CoA acetyltransferases; thiolases; enzymes that catalyze transfers of acetyl groups from acetyl coenzyme A to other molecules. They require biotin cofactors.

acetyl coenzyme A acyltransferases: acetyl-CoA acyltransferases; β-ketothiolases; enzymes of the fatty acid oxidation pathway that catalyze reactions of the general type: R-CoA + CoA → X-CoA + acetyl-CoA, where R is a fatty acid moiety with n carbons, and X is a fatty acid moiety with (n-2) carbons.

acetyl coenzyme A carboxylase: acetyl-CoA carboxylase: the rate-limiting enzyme for *de novo* fatty acid synthesis. It catalyzes the reaction: acetyl coenzyme A + ATP + HCO_3^- → malonyl coenzyme A. The activity is augmented by insulin and inhibited by glucagon.

acetyl coenzyme A synthetase: acetyl-CoA synthetase; acetyl-CoA synthase; fatty acid thiokinase; an enzyme required for "activation" of fatty acids that catalyzes reactions of the general type: R-COOH + CoA + ATP → RCO-CoA + AMP + P-P, where R-COOH is a fatty acid. The product can then enter the fatty acid oxidation cycle.

N-**acetylgalactosamine**: 2-acetamido-galactose; a component of some glycosaminoglycans, glycoproteins, and glycolipids. The acetyl group can bind phosphate, sulfate, and other chemical groups, and the sugar components can form bonds with other sugar, sugar derivative, amino acid, and some lipid moieties.

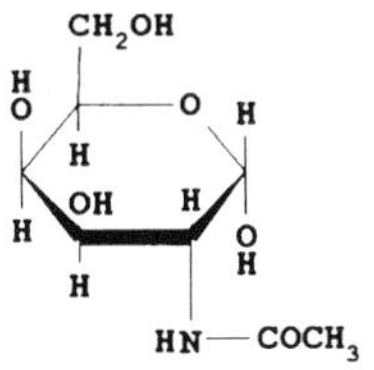

N-**acetylglucosamine**: NAG: 2-acetamido-glucose; a component of many glycosaminoglycans, proteoglycans, glycoproteins, and glycolipids. It forms linkages of the kind described for *N*-acetylgalactosamine. Chitin is a cross-linked NAG polymer. *See* also *N*-**acetylmuramic acid** and **hyaluronic acid**.

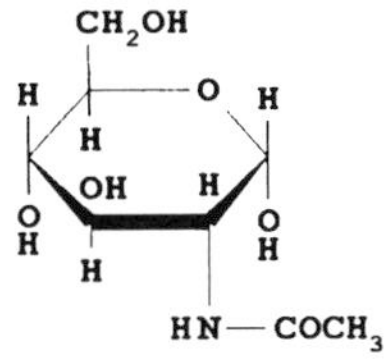

N-**acetyl-leucyl-leucyl-norleucinal**: a peptide used to inhibit calpain.

N-**acetyllactosamine**: *O*-β-D-galactopyranosyl-(14)-2-acetamido-2-deoxyglucose; a compound made from UDP-galactose + *N*-acetylgucoamine (*see* **lactose synthetase**). It is used *in vitro* to inhibit lectin-carbohydrate interactions.

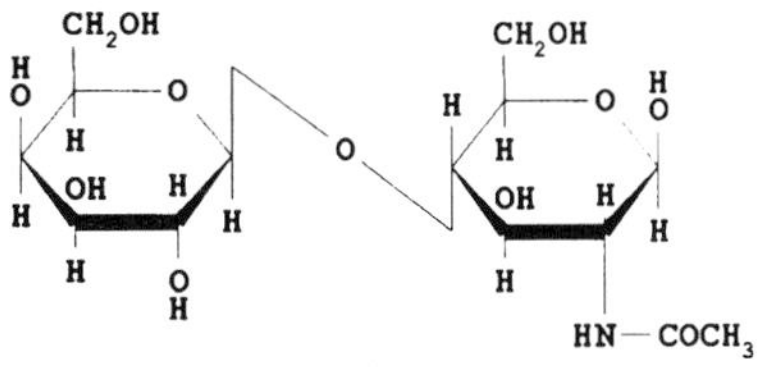

5

N-acetylmuramic acid: NAM: 2-acetamido-3-*O*-(1-carboxyethyl)-2-deoxyglucose; a component of bacterial cell wall peptidoglycans. Lysozyme catalyzes cleavage of the bond between NAM and *N*-acetylglucosamine.

N-acetylneuraminic acid: NANA; lactaminic acid; *O*-sialic acid; 5-(acetylamino)-3,5-dideoxy-D-glycero-D-galacto-2-nonulosonic acid; the most widely distributed sialic acid. It is a component of mucins, and of some glycoproteins and polysaccharides.

acetylsalicylic acid {**acetylsalicylate**}: aspirin; an agent widely used for its analgesic, anti-pyretic, and anti-inflammatory properties. The acetyl group attaches to a cyclooxygenase subunit and thereby irreversibly inhibits the synthesis of prostaglandins and related eicosanoids.

acetylserotonin: *N*-acetylserotonin; NAS: an intermediate in the pathway for biosynthesis of melatonin and related regulators from serotonin.

acetyltransacylase: an enzyme of the fatty acid synthesis cycle that catalyzes the reaction: acetyl-CoA + ACP→ acetyl-ACP + CoA.

S-acetylthiocholine iodide: (2-mercaptoethyl)trimethyl-ammonium iodide acetate; a light-sensitive acetylcholine analog, used to lower intraocular pressure in individuals with glaucoma, and as a substrate for measuring cholinesterase activity.

acetyltransferases: enzymes that catalyze addition of acetyl groups to other molecules. *N*- and *O*- types transfer them to nitrogen and oxygen moieties, respectively.

ACh: Ach: acetylcholine.

AChE: acetylcholinesterase.

AChR: acetylcholine receptor.

acid[s]: compounds that can release hydrogen ions and thereby lower pH, or donate protons to other molecules.

acid fuchsin: acid magenta; 2-amino-5-[(4-amino-3-sulfophenyl)(4-imino-3-sulfo-2,5-cyclohexadien-1-ylidine) methyl]-3-methylbenzenesulfonic acid disodium; an indicator that changes from red to colorless at pH 12. It is also used as a biological stain.

acidic amino acids: amino acids, such as aspartic and glutamic, that are negatively charged at neutral and physiological pHs.

acidic dyes: colored organic molecules that bind to (and are used to stain) negatively charged large molecules.

acidic growth factors: heparin-binding, growth-promoting, mitogenic peptides; *see* e.g. **fibroblast growth factors**.

α_1-**acidic glycoprotein**: α_1-AGP: orosomucoid; α_1M-seromucoid; immunosuppressive acidic protein; IAP; 41-50K acute phase glycoproteins (approximately 38% carbohydrate by weight, with isoelectric points of around 3.0) that inhibit mixed lymphocyte reactions and lymphoblast proliferation promoted by phytohemagglutinin. They are induced by glucocorticoids, and the levels rise up to 90-fold during inflammatory reactions. A sialic acid-deficient form is made by individuals with Hodgkin's disease, chronic myeloid leukemias and some other neoplastic diseases, and with diabetes mellitus, and rheumatoid arthritis.

acidic hydrolases: degradative enzymes with pH optima around 5.0, including acid phosphatases, proteases, glycosidases, lipases, and nucleases. Most are sequestered in lysosomes, but some are secreted (e.g. by leukocytes during inflammatory reactions).

acidic nuclear proteins: *see* **nonhistone nuclear proteins**.

acidophils: somatotropes, lactotropes, PTH-secreting parathyroid gland, and other cell types that contain granules which stain with acidic dyes such as eosin.

acidosis: acid-base imbalance associated with low blood $NaHCO_3$: $HHCO_3$ ratios. *Respiratory* acidosis is caused by CO_2 retention (which elevates $HHCO_3$ levels). In *compensated* respiratory acidosis, sodium retention raises the pH by increasing the $NaHCO_3$ concentration, so that total $NaHCO_3$ and $HHCO_3$ are high. Sodium deficiency leads to *metabolic* acidosis, in which the $NAHCO_3$ level is subnormal. The causes include sodium poor or very acid diets, aldosterone deficiency, renal dysfunction, diarrhea, and accelerated lipolysis (as in uncontrolled diabetes mellitus or starvation). In *compensated* metabolic acidosis, accelerated CO_2 loss raises the blood pH but lowers the total $HHCO_3$ and $NaHCO_3$.

acid phosphatases: enzymes with pH optima in the acidic range that catalyze hydrolysis of organic molecule phosphate bonds. Isoforms are used as markers for lysosomes in cell fractionation studies, and for identification of certain cell types (such as prethymocytes and osteoclasts). Prostate glands and some bone cancers release large amounts. *Cf* **alkaline phosphatases**, and *see* also **protein phosphatases**.

acid proteases: protein-degrading enzymes with pH optima in the acidic range. *See* also **acidic hydrolases**.

acinar glands: simple, grape-shaped (alveolar) multicellular secretory organs, for example the kinds in the exocrine pancreas that release proenzymes.

acinus [acini]: a small cavity surrounded by cells.

α configuration: *see* **stereoisomerism**.

aconitase: an enzyme of tricarboxylic acid and glyoxylate cycles that catalyzes conversion of citrate to isocitrate. *See* also *cis*-**aconitic acid**.

cis-**aconitic acid** {**aconitate**}: prop-1-ene-1,2,3-carboxylic acid; an intermediate in the tricarboxylic acid and glyoxylate cycles that remains attached to aconitase during reactions in which citrate is converted to isocitrate.

aconite: a mixture of alkaloids and other substances from *Aconitum napellus* roots, once used to reduce fever and lower blood pressure. Other names include Monkshood, wolf's bane, mouse-bane, and friar's cowl.

ACP: acyl carrier protein.

acquired immune deficiency: immune system dysfunction that is not genetically imposed.

acquired immune deficiency syndrome: AIDS; diseases attributed to HIV infection *(q.v.)*. The retroviruses bind to CD4, decrease T cell helper and inducer functions, kill T cells, and depress NK cell activity. Most symptoms are caused by opportunist infections that thrive in the environments, or from impaired ability to suppress tumor growth. However, direct toxic effects on the central nervous system have been suggested.

acquired immunity: changes in the immune system that confer ability to resist the deleterious effects of certain antigens, and/or destroy the organisms that make them. *Active humoral* immunity is initiated by antigens that are recognized by B lymphocyte subsets. The cells then proliferate and produce antibodies directed against the antigens. *Passive* humoral immunity can be achieved by administering antibodies made by other individuals of the species. *Active cellular immunity* involves antigen activated T cell subsets. In some cases, T cells from individuals previously exposed to the antigens can confer it. *See* also **humoral** and **cellular immunity** and **memory cells**.

acradinate: *see* 2,3-**quinoline dicarboxylate**.

acridine: 10-aza-anthracene; a component of several heterocyclic organic compounds that intercalate between adjacent DNA base pairs, promote insertional and deletional mutations, and cause formation of RNAs with extra bases. *See* also **acridine orange**.

acridine orange: tetramethyl acridine; an alkaline fluorescent dye used to stain nucleic acids. It is taken up by phagocytosis, and can be used to identify some cell types (e.g. macrophages and osteoclasts). When viewed under ultraviolet light, the DNA of stained cells appears green, and the RNA orange-red.

acrodynia: dermatitis, edema, and scaliness of the tail, ears, mouth and paws that develops in pyridoxine deficient rats.

acromegaly: endocrine disorders, usually caused by somatotrope-derived adenomas, in which excessive secretion of **growth hormone** *(q.v.)* in adults invokes joint enlargement, facial deformities, and metabolic defects that include insulin resistance and hyperglycemia.

acrophase: *see* **circadian rhythms**.

acrosin: a serine protease activated and released during acrosome reactions. *See* also **proacrosin**.

acrosomal membrane: a double membrane that covers the plasma membrane of a sperm head. During the acrosome reaction, the outer layer fuses with the sperm plasma membrane at several points, vesicles form, and enzymes are released.

acrosome: a sperm head organelle formed from Golgi membranes; *see* **acrosomal membrane** and **acrosome reaction**.

acrosome reaction: chemical and morphological changes in the head of a capacitated spermatozoan, with release of enzymes, that precedes and is essential for fertilization. It is initiated by mature oocytes. *See* also **acrosomal membrane** and **ZP3**.

acrosome stabilizing factor: ASF; a trimeric epididymal fluid and seminal plasma glycoprotein that reversibly inhibits the acrosome reaction, and may block fertilization by altering cholesterol:phospholipid ratios. It differs from lower molecular weight (90K, 70K, and 40K) lipid-dependent seminal vesicle and prostate gland fluid proteins that bind to spermatozoa and are lost during capacitation, and from 6K-15K inhibitors of acrosomal enzymes, antifertility factor-1, decapacitation factor, and seminalplasmin.

acrylamide: propenamide; a neurotoxin that promotes degeneration of large nerve fiber axons, and can cause paralysis. *See* also **polyacrylamide gels**.

$$H_2C=CH-NH_2$$

ACTH: adrenocorticotrophic hormone; corticotropin; *see* **adrenocorticotropic hormone**.

O-nitrophenyl sulfenyl-**ACTH**: an ACTH analog that stimulates glucocorticoid synthesis, but (unlike ACTH) does not augment cAMP production. It has been used to study the mechanisms of ACTH actions, and of other factors that control steroidogenesis.

actidione: cycloheximide.

action potentials: the electrical changes in excitable cells that follow presentation of effective stimuli which open ion channels and invoke **depolarization** (*q.v.*). Repolarization begins soon afterward. A very brief period of hyperpolarization often precedes re-establishment of the resting potential.

actin[s]: thin filament cytoskeletal proteins that affect cell shape, mediate contraction in many cell types, contribute to other forms of motility, and perform other functions. G-actins are 42K, globular monomers that polymerize to form filamentous F-actins. During pseudopod formation, the filaments establish cross-linkages in plasma membrane networks. When skeletal muscle contracts, F-actin in thin filaments forms cross-bridges with thick filament myosin. In neurons, F actin binds to synapsin I, and thereby inhibits neurotransmitter release from synaptic vesicles. Synthesis of several isoforms is developmentally regulated, and is affected by hormones and other factors. Fetal cardiac myocytes contain substantial quantities of the skeletal muscle type, but they later partially replace it with the cardiac kind. Catecholamines present in quantities sufficient to invoke cardiac hypertrophy induce the skeletal muscle type. Growth hormones stimulate synthesis in the liver. Stimuli that promote synapsin formation precipitously decrease the binding affinity.

actin binding proteins: ABPs; a very large, heterogenous group of proteins whose functions depend on binding to actin. See, e.g. α- and β-**actinins**, **fodrin**, **spectrin**, **gelsolin**, and **villin**.

α-actinin: an actin-binding 190K homodimeric protein in skeletal muscle Z lines, cardiac muscle intercalated disks, desmosomes, and stress fibers, that links actin filaments and maintains filament structure.

β-actinin: a dimeric protein composed of 37K and 36K subunits in skeletal muscle, kidney, and some other cell types that binds to, and may stabilize thin filaments.

actinomycins: the term actinomycin C (cactinomycin) refers to three antibiotics (C1, C2, and C3) made by *Streptomyces chrysomallas*, that are used to arrest the growth of some neoplasms. Actinomycin D (dactinomycin), with similar properties, is made by *Streptomyces pavullus*. Since it inhibits DNA-directed RNA synthesis in both prokaryotes and eukaryotes, by intercalating between guanine-cytidine base pairs, deforming templates, and impeding RNA polymerase progression, it is used to determine whether the effects of regulators require synthesis of new mRNA molecules.

C2: Sar = sarcosine LP = L-proline LM = L-methylvaline

LT = L-threonine DV* = D-valine DA* = D-allolysine

C3: DV* is replaced by DA*

D: DA* is replaced by DV*

activating protein-1: *see* **AP-1**.

activation energy: the energy that must be added to a system to initiate a chemical reaction. Enzymes speed reactions by lowering activation energy.

active immunity: acquisition of resistance to the effects of specific antigens, and/or the organisms that produce them, via activation of immune system cell subsets. The associated responses can include production of specific kinds of antibodies. *See* **humoral** and **cellular immunity**, and *cf* **passive immunity**.

activated cells: cells that have undergone changes in response to effective stimuli, a term applied, e.g. to leukocytes, macrophages, neutrophils, and oocytes.

activational hormones: regulators that act on differentiated cell types and exert mostly reversible effects (i.e. ones that recede if the stimulus is removed); *cf* **organizational hormones**.

active sodium transport inhibitor: ASTI; a 1.3K component of blood plasma that inhibits Na^+/K^+-ATPases, and competes with ouabain for binding sites.

active transport: movement of ions or molecules against concentration, electrical, or electrochemical gradients. Some systems involve symport or antiport mechanisms. The energy required is usually derived from ATP hydrolysis.

activins: FSH releasing peptide; FRP; 27K dimeric glycoprotein members of the transforming growth factor-β (TGF-β) superfamily, comprised of subunits similar to or identical with those of inhibins, Müllerian duct inhibitor, bone morphogenetic proteins, decapentaplegic complex protein, Vg1, and some other regulators, as well as of TGFβs; *see* also **activins A, B,** and **AB**. They are made in the gonads, by pituitary gonadotropes, and at other sites, and can exert paracrine (and possibly also autocrine) as well as endocrine effects, interact with follistatins and other regulators, and contribute to control of their own production and actions. All forms selectively stimulate follicle stimulating (but not luteinizing) hormone secretion and FSH β subunit synthesis when present in low concentrations, and may thereby be involved in protection against premature atresia of ovarian follicles and/or maturation of dominant ones. Activins can also augment gonadotropin releasing hormone-stimulated LH secretion, possibly by increasing the numbers of GnRH receptors on gonadotropes. Additionally, they contribute to control of steroidogenesis in testes as well as ovaries, stimulate insulin secretion, inhibit growth hormone secretion and somatotrope growth, inhibit adrenocorticotropic hormone and prolactin secretion, and promote erythrocyte differentiation. Several kinds of receptors that differ in affinities for activin types, and for other members of the family have been identified. All are plasma membrane spanning glycoproteins. Ligand binding leads to cAMP generation in many cell types, but phospholipase C activation has been demonstrated in some. In embryos, induction of posterior mesoderm differentiation involves binding to an ARIIB type. A different (ARII) receptor mediates the ability to prolong survival of some neurons and inhibit neural cell differentiation. It may be identical to a transmembrane receptor with serine-kinase activity in AT-20 (corticotropin secreting tumor) cells. Expression of the subunit types is developmentally and cell-type regulated, and it varies with the stages of cell differentiation. Activins generally oppose inhibins, but can synergize with or antagonize the actions of other members of the superfamily.

activin A: erythrocyte differentiation factor; a homodimeric **activin** (*q.v.*), composed of two $β_A$ 116-amino acid peptide chains identical with inhibin $β_A$ chains.

activin AB: a heterodimeric **activin** (*q.v.*), composed of one $β_A$ and one $β_B$ 112-amino acid peptide chain.

activin B: a homodimeric **activin** (*q.v.*), composed of two $β_B$ peptide chains. It has been identified in porcine follicular fluid.

actomyosin: the complex formed when actin binds to myosin.

acumentin: a 65K macrophage protein closely related to β-actinin.

acute: sharp; usually describes a reaction or effect that develops rapidly and soon subsides; *cf* **chronic**.

acute lymphocytic leukemia: ALL; *see* **leukemias**.

acute myelogenous leukemia: AML; *see* **leukemias**.

acute phase proteins: acute phase reactants; proteins synthesized in the liver and released to the bloodstream in large amounts during inflammatory reactions, following exposure to irritants, and in response to trauma and some other adverse conditions. Most are constitutively expressed in small amounts, and some are made by cancer cells. The group includes C-reactive protein, ceruloplasmin, $α_1$-MAP, and amyloid-A. Interleukin-1 is one of the known stimulants. Interleukin-6 has been included, but is additionally implicated as a stimulant for production.

A cyclase: adenylate cyclase; adenylyl cyclase.

acyclovir: 2-amino-1,9-dihydro-9[(2-hydroxyethyoxy)-methyl)]-6*H*-purin-6-one; acycloguanosine. A guanosine analog that undergoes phosphorylation to yield a metabolite which inhibits the replication of some viruses, including some *Herpes* and Epstein-Barr strains.

acylcarnitines: long-chain fatty acids covalently linked to carnitine. Their formation is essential for oxidation in mitochondria of fatty acyl-conezyme A molecules made in the cytoplasm (since the latter do not cross mitochondrial membranes). Carnitine acyltransferase I on the cytoplasmic faces of the membranes catalzyes reactions of the general type: R-coenzyme-A + carnitine → R-carnitine + coenzyme A (in which R = the fatty acid moiety). A translocase then shuttles the products across the membrane. When the carnitine is removed by mitochondrial carnitine acyl transferase II, the translocase promotes its return to the cytoplasm.

acylcarnitine transferases: carnitine acyltransferases; *see* **acylcarnitines**.

acyl carrier protein, ACP: a 77K protein with a 4-phosphopantetheine prosthetic group that binds to fatty acid moieties prior to chain elongation. The reaction: acetyl-CoA + ACP → acetyl-ACP, catalyzed by acetyltransacylase, is the first step in the pathway for biosynthesis

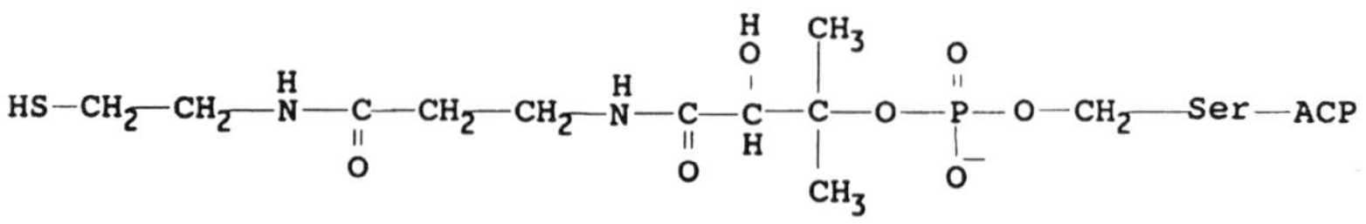

acyl carrier protein

of fatty acids from acetyl-CoA. The prosthetic group is shown.

acyl-CoA dehydrogenases: fatty acid oxidation cycle enzymes that catalyze the first reaction of the fatty acid β-oxidation cycle: R-Co-A + FAD → R-enoyl-CoA + $FADH_2$, where R is the fatty acid moiety and CoA = coenzyme A.

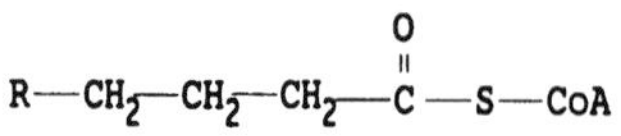

R-acyl-CoA

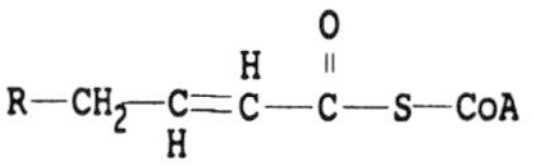

R-enoyl-CoA

acyl-CoA synthetases: acyl-CoA synthases; fatty acid thiokinases; fatty acid activating enzymes; enzymes that catalyze reactions of the general type: R-COO⁻ + ATP + HS-CoA → RCO-S-CoA + AMP + PP, where R is a fatty acid moiety, and both HS-CoA and CoA = coenzyme A. The isozymes differ in affinities for fatty acids of varying chain lengths.

acyl group: the structure shown, in which X is an organic moiety. "Activation" of fatty acids for chain elongation or degradation, and of amino acids for protein synthesis begins with formation of acyl adenylates (see **acyl-CoA synthetases**). Fatty acid products then react with co-enzyme A to form R-CO-S-CoA derivatives, and amino acid products form amino-acyl-tRNAs.

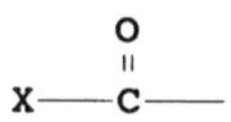

acyl 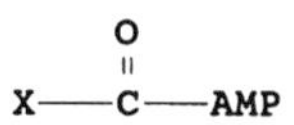   **acyl-adenylate**

ADA: adenosine deaminase.

adaptation: (1) adjustment to changes, usually of kinds imposed extracellularly. The term can refer to metabolic, structural, and/or evolutionary phenomena; (2) diminished sensitivity or responses to stimuli that are presented continuously or repeatedly at short intervals. An example is decreased conscious awareness of an environmental chemical perceived by olfactory receptors. Cf **desensitization**.

adaptins: proteins that connect clathrin molecules to the cytoplasmic tails of transmembrane proteins.

ADA-SCID: severe combined immunodeficiency syndrome caused by adenosine deaminase deficiency.

ADCC: antigen-dependent cell-mediated toxicity.

addiction: physiological and/or psychological dependence. The term usually refers to the effects of chemicals (such as narcotics or stimulants) on whole organisms. The most common manifestations include acquisition of some tolerance when the agents are continuously or repeatedly presented, as well as strong, often adverse reactions when they are withdrawn. Single cells can display comparble responses, such as gradual diminution of adenylate cyclase activity when continuously exposed to morphine, and development of supernormal levels when the alkaloid is removed from the environment.

Addison's disease: severe adrenocortical hormone deficiency; see **glucocorticoids** and **mineralocorticoids**. The causes include genetic defects that impair enzyme synthesis, autoimmune disorders, and cell destruction by some micro-organisms. See also **adrenoleukodystrophy**.

additive effects: describes responses to combinations of two (or more) agents equivalent in magnitude to the sums of responses obtained if each agent is presented alone. For different chemicals that act via identical mechanisms, low dosages summate, but maximal ones do not. The term *synergism* is more commonly applied when substances act via different mechanisms, and the responses to simultaneous presentation are more than additive. Cf **potentiation**.

addressins: selectins; plasma membrane components that mediate adhesion to specific kinds of molecules on the surfaces of other cells. They affect cell distributions within organisms, as well as cell:cell interactions. Examples include ligands for lymphocyte homing receptors.

adducin: a protein associated with the erythrocyte membrane skeleton, composed of 97K and 102K subunits. It promotes assembly of spectrin-actin complexes, binds calmodulin, and is a protein kinase C substrate.

adenine: 6-amino-purine; a nitrogenous base component of DNA, RNA, ATP, AMP, cAMP, and other biologically active substances; see also **adenosine** and **deoxyadenosine**. Although adenine nucleotides are made and used in substantial quantities by many cell types, adenine has been called vitamin B_4.

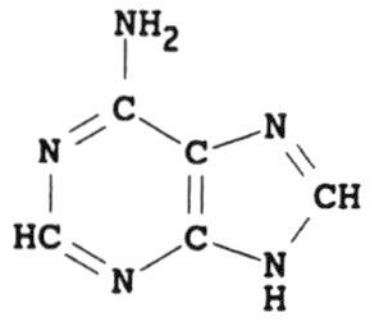

N^6-dimethyl-**adenine**: a component of some transfer RNAs.

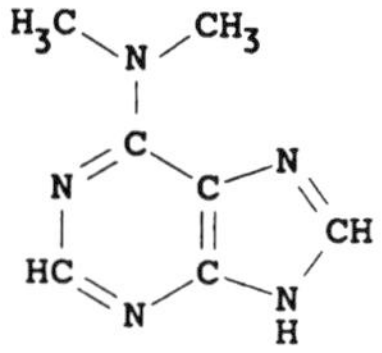

N^6-isopentyl-**adenine**: a component of some transfer RNAs.

1-methyl-**adenine**: a hormone synthesized in starfish ovarian follicles that promotes germinal vesicle breakdown.

adeno-: a prefix meaning glandular.

adenocarcinomas: gland-like epithelial cell neoplasms.

adenohypophysis: the "glandular" part of pituitary gland, derived from Rathke's pouch. The components in many species are pars distalis, pars tuberalis, and par intermedia. *See* also **anterior lobe** and **anterior pituitary**, and *cf* **neurohypophysis**.

adenohypophysial: originating in, or characteristic of the adenohypophysis.

adenosine: adenine-ribose; a neurotransmitter, neuromodulator, and hormone, and a purine nucleoside component of DNA, RNA, ATP, AMP, cAMP, and other molecules. It can be made from adenosine monophosphate (AMP), hypoxanthine, and S-adenosyl-methionine, and can undergo phosphorylation and deamination. Free adenosine acts mostly on target cells located close to the sites of synthesis. Its effects vary widely with the cell types, and with other factors. Although some (e.g. on K^+, Ca^{2+}, and Cl^- channels) may be exerted directly, others involve generation of second messengers that synergize with or oppose the release and/or actions of other regulators. At various sites, it can augment or diminish cAMP synthesis, inhibit cyclic nucleotide phosphodiesterases and phosphatidylinositol-4-kinase, modulate the effects of phospholipase C isozymes and guanylate cyclases, and lower tyrosine kinase activity. Adenosine inhibits the release of excitatory amino acids in the brain and thereby exerts sedative and anti-convulsant effects, and antagonizes thyroid stimulating hormone. It can decrease the release of acetylcholine in the vas deferens, of both acetylcholine and tachykinin in the ileum, of renin and erythropoietin in the kidney, of insulin in the pancreas, and of prolactin and growth hormone in the pituitary gland. It contributes to blood pressure control by exerting inotropic, chronotropic, and dromotropic effects on the heart, and by modulating the contraction of vascular smooth muscle (relaxation in most beds but contraction in the kidneys), renin release, and angiotensin actions. Variable influences on other smooth muscle in-

clude bronchospasm. It inhibits lipolysis in white adipose tissue and thermogenesis in brown, and exerts other influences on lipid, and on carbohydrate lipid metabolism. In the stomach, it decreases acid production. Additionally it inhibits neutrophil chemotaxis, and modulates lymphocyte functions. *See* also **adenosine receptors**.

2-chloro-**adenosine**: CADO; an adenosine receptor agonist that binds with higher affinity to A_1 than to A_2 subtypes, and can protect against ischemic damage to hippocampal neurons. *Cf* 2-chlorodeoxy-**adenosine**.

2-chlorodeoxy-**adenosine**: a nucleoside analog that, after conversion by deoxycytidine kinase to its 5′ triphosphate nucleotide derivative (CdATP), kills cells by incorporating into DNA, causing breaks in single-stranded molecules, blocking DNA polymerase II-mediated chain elongation and other DNA repair mechanisms, and depleting ATP. Lymphoid cells are especially vulnerable, even when quiescent, because of their high deoxycytidine kinase activities. CdATP is used to treating B-cell chronic lymphocytic leukemias in individuals resistant to other agents, and it can accomplish total remission in some.

2′3′-dideoxy-**adenosine**: 2′3′-DDA; an adenosine analog used to inhibit adenylate cyclases; *see* 2′,3-**dideoxy-adenosine**.

5′-*p*-fluorosulfonylbenzoyl-**adenosine**: 5′FSBA: a probe used for ADP receptors.

1-methyl-**adenosine**: a nucleoside that exerts effects on amphibian oocytes similar those of 1-methyl-adenine.

cyclic **adenosine diphosphate ribose**: *see* **cyclic adenosine diphosphate ribose**.

cyclic **adenosine-3′5′-cyclic monophosphate**: *see* **cyclic adenosine-3′5′-monophosphate** and **adenylate cyclase**.

cyclic **adenosine-3′5′-monophosphate dependent protein kinase inhibitor**: H-Thr-Thr-Tyr-Ala-Asp-Phe-Ile-Ala-Ser-Gly-Arg-Thr-Gly-Arg-Arg-Asn-Ala-Ile-His-Asp-OH; a competitive inhibitor of protein kinase A enzymes.

$N^6,O^{2'}$-dibutyryl-cyclic **adenosine-3′5′-monophosphate**; $Bu_2.cAMP$; DBcAMP; bucladesine; a cAMP analog that penetrates cell membranes, and is not rapidly hydrolyzed by cyclic nucleotide phosphodiesterases. It is used to study mechanisms of hormone and neurotransmitter actions, and the effects of high intracellular cAMP; but

slow release of butyrate can affect the responses. *See* dibutyryl-**cAMP** for structure.

adenosine deaminase: ADA; an enzyme that catalyzes irreversible conversion of adenosine to inosine, and of deoxyadenosine to deoxyinosine. The products can be oxidized to uric acid and excreted. Inherited ADA deficiency impairs immune system development and invokes neurological defects as well as severe T lymphocyte dysfunction. The problems have been variously attributed to excessive activation of adenylate cyclase by high adenosine levels, accumulation of *S*-adenosylhomocysteine (which inhibits DNA methylation), and deoxyadenosine inhibition of ribonucleotide reductase.

adenosine diphosphate: ADP; adenine-ribose-phosphate-phosphate; *see* **ADP** and **ATP**.

adenosine diphosphoryltransferase: ADPRT; an enzyme that catalyzes the reaction: NAD^+ + acceptor protein → NAM (nicotine adenine mononucleotide) + ADP-ribosylated protein. The endogenous enzyme functions physiologically in DNA synthesis and repair, cell proliferation, and cytodifferentiation. Cholera and pertussis toxins are among the agents that catalyze similar reactions which affect the functions of trimeric G proteins; *see also* **ADP-ribosylation**.

adenosine kinase: an enzyme that catalyzes the reaction adenosine + ATP → AMP + ADP.

adenosine monophosphate: AMP; adenine-ribose-phosphate; a purine nucleotide; *see* **ATP**. The term can designate either the 3′ or the 5′ form. Corresponding alternate terms are 3′- and 5′-adenylic acid.

adenosine receptors: at least three sets of molecules that bind adenosine and mediate its actions on target cells. All are members of the P_1 (purine) receptor family, and all bind 5′-*N*-ethylcarboxamidoadenosine (NEC, an agonist), and methyl-xanthines (antagonists); but *see also* **adenotin**. A_1 types, abundant in brain, heart, kidney, and adipose tissue, have high affinity for *R*-phenylisopropyl-adeonsine (*R*-PIA), and associate with pertussis toxin-sensitive G proteins (G_i and/or G_o). More selective agonists include **CPA** and **CENBA**. Highly selective antagonists include **DPCPX** (*q.v.*). Marked differences in the binding properties and potencies of pharmacological agents at various sites indicate the presence of at least two subtypes. A_{1a} predominates in brain cells believed to derive from embryonic neural tube precursors, whereas A_{1b}

adenosine-3′-monophosphate.

adenosine-5′-monophosphate.

is more abundant in autonomic system neurons of neural crest origin. The effects of receptor activation vary with location (presynaptic vs postsynaptic), and with associated influences on the actions of dopamine and other neurotransmitters. Some brain neurons express A_2 as well as A_1 type receptors, and both types are made by adipocytes, myocytes, and some other cells. All known A_2 types bind S-PIA with high affinity. They, too, are divided into subtypes (A_{2a} and A_{2b}). CGS- 21680 is one of the agents that binds specifically to the A_{2a} form. Ligand binding to A_2 receptors leads to inhibition of adenylate cyclase enzymes. This accounts for some of the negative inotropic and chronotropic actions on the heart, as well as for antilipolysis, vasodilation, and inhibition of blood platelet aggregation. Receptors at neuromuscular junctions differ from those at other sites, and are classified as A_3. They bind xanthine derivatives such as XAC with especially high affinity. *See also* **adenosine deaminase**.

adenosine triphosphate: *see* **ATP**.

adenosylmethionine: S-adenosylmethionine; SAM; a major donor of methyl groups for the biosynthesis of creatine, choline, choline-containing phospholipids, acetylcholine, melatonin, and other biologically important molecules, for DNA methylation, and for catecholamine degrading reactions catalyzed by COMT. It is synthesized via the reaction: methionine + ATP → SAM + P-P + P_i, and is converted to S-adenosylhomocysteine in the methyl transfer reactions.

adenotin: a 98K protein that binds NEC with high affinity, and interacts with adenosine receptors. It accounts for much of the binding formerly attributed to adenosine.

adenoviruses: DNA viruses that infect growth-arrested, differentiated epithelial cells in the respiratory and gastrointestinal tracts, and at some other sites. Avian, bovine, canine, equine, ovine, murine, porcine, simian, and human forms have been identified. They promote DNA synthesis, and can transform some cell types.

adenovirus early region genes: E1A genes: genes activated early during the course of adenovirus infections that promote transcription of other viral genes and modify the host transcriptional machinery. They also activate host genes that code for metastasis inhibiting proteins.

adenylate cyclases: adenyl cyclases; adenylyl cyclases; several sets of plasma membrane complexes that catalyze the reaction: ATP → cAMP + P-P. It is currently believed that there are eight G_s protein-sensitive kinds, and that these can be divided into five families. The various isozymes are distributed to most (probably all) cell types, and two or more are expressed in many of them. (The brain is known to contain at least six.) All of the enzymes share similar cytoplasmic domains, but have different transmembrane components that affect their activation and functions. Type I, a widely distributed, approximately 120K protein, is activated by Ca-calmodulin. Type II, a 120K calmodulin-insensitive form, is expressed at high levels in the brain, and in small amounts in the lungs and olfactory system. Type III resembles type I, but appears to be restricted to the olfactory system, whereas type IV resembles type II (but lacks an identifiable kinase A association site). Types V and VI closely resemble each other, and both are present in highest amounts in the heart (which also contains type IV) and brain. The activities of all isoforms are low under basal conditions, and are augmented when ligands (hormones or neurotransmitters) bind to their receptors, liberate $G_{\alpha s}$ subunits from $\beta\gamma$ types, and facilitate $G_{\alpha s}$-GTP binding to the enzymes; and they are decreased when $G_{\alpha i}$-GTP binds. However, the $\beta\gamma$ complexes decrease type I, but augment type II and type IV activities, and types V and VI are unaffected. The isozymes also differ in responses to forskolin.

adenylate kinase: a magnesium-dependent enzyme that catalyzes the reaction: ATP + AMP → ADP + ADP.

adenylation: addition of adenylate groups; *see also* **ADP-ribosylation** and **polyadenylate**.

adenyl cyclase associated protein: CAP; *see* **cyclase associated protein**.

adenylic acid: adenosine monophosphate.

5′-adenylimidodiphosphate: APP(NH)P; AMP-P-NH-P; an ATP analog that resists hydrolysis. It is used to determine whether the actions of that nucleotide on specific processes require hydrolysis to ADP (or AMP) and the release of energy.

ADF: adult T cell leukemia factor.

ADH: anti-diuretic hormone; *see* **vasopressins**.

adhesins: proteins on the surfaces of microorganisms that mediate initial binding to host target cells. Some bind with high affinities to fibronectins.

adhesion factors: *see* **cell adhesion molecules**.

adhesion plaques: focal contacts; specialized, electron-dense plasma membrane regions at sites of contact with extracellular matrices. The components include α-actinin, talin, and vinculin.

adipic acid: hexanedioic acid; a somewhat corrosive component of some vegetables that is used in industrial processes.

adipoblasts: preadipocytes; immature cells that derive from fibroblasts, and can differentiate to adipocytes. They lack the surface markers and enzymes expressed by mature fat cells.

adipocytes: fat cells; cells that differentiate from adipoblasts. They synthesize, and store large quantities of triacylglycerols, and release fatty acids and glycerol. When lipid accumulation displaces the nucleus to one side and compresses the cytoplasm to a thin rim, they are called signet-ring cells. They have receptors for insulin (which promotes lipogenesis), norepinephrine (a major regulator of lipolysis), and other hormones.

adipokinetic: fat-mobilizing.

adipokinetic hormones: hormones that promotes lipolysis. The term has been applied to β-lipotropin, but there are controversies concerning whether it functions this way under physiological conditions. Adipokinetic hormone II, obtained from *Locus migratoria* and some other insects, is believed to regulate energy metabolism during long flights. It has the amino acid sequence: pGlu-Leu-Asn-Phe-Ser-Thr-Gly-Trp-NH₂.

adipose protein-2: aP2; an adipocyte protein chemically related to myelin P2a (a Schwann cell protein induced by glucose); *cf* **adipsin**.

adipose tissue: connective tissue composed of large numbers of adipocytes, and smaller numbers of stromal and other cell types. White adipose tissue is the major site for triacylglycerol synthesis and storage, and for release of fatty acids and glycerol. *See* also **brown adipose tissue**.

adipostats: hypothetical regulatory systems that monitor body fat stores and exert controls over food intake and/or energy expenditure. The hypothalamus is the most commonly suggested locus, but sensors are also proposed to exist in other brain regions, in the liver, and elsewhere.

adipsia: failure to drink or experience thirst.

adipsin: a serine protease made in, and constitutively secreted by mature adipocytes. It is also present in Schwann cells (and possibly other cell types actively involved in lipid metabolism). Heavily glycosylated 28K circulating, and 37K and 44K intracellular forms have been identified, all of which are convertible to a non-glycosylated 25.5K protein. There are indications that adipsin regulates lipid and energy metabolism, by acting on extracellular lipoproteins, modifying lipid oxidation, invoking thermogenesis, and/or functioning as an adipostat messenger. The mRNA levels rise 2-5 fold in adipocytes during fasting. They fall in response to glucose infusion, but normal levels are maintained in animals that are overfed. Insulin appears to be a major regulator, since adipsin levels are elevated in individuals with poorly controlled insulin-dependent diabetes mellitus. Genetically obese (*ob/ob*) and diabetic obese (*db/db*) mice have regulatory defects (but no known gene mutations) that cause up to 99% reduction in adipose tissue levels of the protein. Similar impairment of a lesser degree occurs in *fa/fa* rats and in mice made obese with monosodium glutamate (MSG). Since adipsin exerts actions similar to those of complement factor D, the circulating form may contribute to the alternate pathway for complement activation.

adjuvant: an additive, usually one that nonspecifically enhances a response. Freund's adjuvant stimulates the immune system, directly or by augmenting the effects of administered antigens.

adjuvant arthritis: a T-lymphocyte dependent autoimmune disease invoked in rats with Freund's type adjuvant. It is used as a model for studying autoimmune arthritis and its associated endocrine effects.

ad lib.: *ad libitum*; as desired, a term used when test subjects take as much (or as little) of a nutrient, water, drug, or other substance as they wish.

adluminal: bordering a cavity (lumen).

ADN-138: Kyorin; an inhibitor of **aldose reductase** (*q.v.*). It is used to slow galactose conversion to sorbitol.

ADN-138

adoptive transfer: a form of passive immunity, accomplished by infusing immunocompetent cells derived from another individual.

ADP: adenine-ribose-phosphate-phosphate; a nucleotide that contributes to energy exchange via phosphorylation to **ATP** *(q.v.)* and dephosphorylation to AMP. It can be degraded to yield adenosine. When released from injured endothelial cells or erythrocytes, ADP binds to receptors on platelets (*see* **aggregin**), causes their conversion from disc-like to spiculated spherical forms by promoting phosphorylation of myosin light-chain kinase, mobilizes intracellular Ca^{2+}, initiates reversible platelet aggregation, contributes to platelet activation by collagen, thrombin, and platelet activating factor, and facilitates binding of fibrinogen. When released from α granules of activated platelets, it mediates irreversible aggregation and contributes to platelet roles in hemostasis and coagulation by inhibiting prostaglandin and adenosine mediated adenylate cyclase activation. *See* **adenosine diphosphate** for structure.

ADP-ribosylation: transfers of ADP-ribose moieties from NAD^+ to acceptor molecules. The reactions are used in DNA repair and cell differentiation. Some bacterial toxins promote promote ADP-ribose attachment to specific proteins (*see* **G proteins**, **cholera toxin**, and **pertussis toxin**). They can thereby directly alter the protein functions, and can deplete cell NAD^+.

ADP ribosylation factor: a GTP-regulated protein that affects the activities of G proteins. *See* also **cholera toxin**.

ADPRT: adenosine diphosphoribosyltransferase.

adrenal: (1) located near or on the kidney; a term sometimes used synonymously with suprarenal (above the kidney); (2) characteristic of or derived from adrenal glands.

adrenal androgen[s]: androgens secreted by adrenocortical cells of humans and some other species. *See* **adrenarche**, **adrenal androgen stimulating hormone**, **adrenogenital syndrome**, and **dehydroepiandrosterone**.

adrenal androgen stimulating hormone: AASH; cortical androgen stimulating hormone; CASH. A 60K glycoprotein in pituitary gland extracts that is reported to specifically stimulate the synthesis of adrenal androgens.

adrenal cortex: the outer region of the mammalian adrenal gland. It includes the zona glomerulosa, zona fasciculata, and zona reticularis, in which steroid hormones are made. *See* also **adrenal glands**.

adrenal demedullation: destruction of the inner, catecholamine-secreting part of the adrenal gland. It is usually performed to study adrenomedullary functions without invoking glucocorticoid or mineralocorticoid deficiencies. When all cells of the gland except a few that adhere to the capsule are scooped out, new steroid hormone-secreting tissue forms from the remnant, but the neuron-like cells of the medulla do not regenerate.

adrenal glands: suprarenal glands; endocrine organs located above the kidneys. In mammals, the steroid hormone-secreting adrenal cortex surrounds the catecholamine-secreting medulla. In some other vertebrates, steroidogenic and catecholamine secreting cells are not anatomically associated, but the term is applied to some endocrine structures that perform similar functions.

adrenal medulla: the inner region of a mammalian adrenal gland. It contains cells that secrete catecholamines and other regulators, and is surrounded by the adrenal cortex. The functions are regulated by neurotransmitters released from splanchnic nerves, and by factors supplied via small blood vessels that course through the cortex. Although epinephrine is made from norepinephrine, the two regulators are believed to be secreted by different cell types, and to be differentially controlled. Small amounts of dopamine are also released, but most dopamine outside the central nervous system originates in peripheral neurons.

adrenalectomy: removal (usually by surgery) of the adrenal glands (both cortex and medulla). The major consequences result from loss of **glucocorticoid** and **mineralocorticoid** hormones, *(q.v.)*. *See* also **adrenal demedullation**.

adrenalin: *see* **epinephrine**. The British spelling is adrenaline.

adrenarche: changes in the adrenal cortex of humans and some other species that occur shortly before pubertal maturation or coincide with its initiation, and involve increased secretion of androgens. The steroids stimulate libido in both sexes, and promote the growth of pubic and axillary hair in females.

adrenergic: neurons releasing, receptors activated by, or properties characteristic of certain catecholamines. Some authors use the term for both epinephrine and norepinephrine; others reserve it for epinephrine, and use noradrenergic for norepinephrine.

adrenergic receptor[s]: adrenoreceptors; plasma membrane-spanning compounds that bind and mediate the effects of **norepinephrine** and **epinephrine** *(q.v.)* by interacting with trimeric G proteins. The mostly commonly used classification system is based on affinities for, and responses to hormones and pharmacological agents, but terms designating locations are also used. Each group comprises subtypes, some of which bind dopamine and other regulators. The various kinds differ in amino acid composition, distribution, ligand affinities, and signal transduction mechanisms. Their synthesis is differentially regulated, and the relative numbers at any site can vary with changing conditions. Problems with classification include small differences in the properties of a subtype in one cell type as compared with another, the presence of two or more kinds in the same cell, species differences in the relative amounts at various sites, and discrepancies between the amounts of RNAs that direct their synthesis and the numbers of receptors expressed. In addition to α and β, γ types (*q.v.*), other forms have been described.

α-adrenergic receptor[s]: a class of proteins with similar seven plasma membrane spanning, and cytoplasmic regions, whose members mediate many norepinephrine and epinephrine actions. All bind to, and are inactivated by prazosin, but the subtypes differ in *N*-terminal regions, mechanisms of action, and responses to many pharmacological agents. They are abundant on smooth muscle and in the central nervous system, but are also present at many other sites. *See* subtypes.

α_1-adrenergic receptor[s]: a set of glycoproteins activated by norepinephrine and epinephrine. The α_{1A} subtypes at most sites bind the catecholamines with very high affinities, and exert most of their effects by accelerating Ca^{2+} uptake from the surrounding fluids. They are abundant on vascular and vas deferens smooth muscle, and are also distributed to the hippocampus, cerebral cortex, brain stem, heart and spleen. The α_{1B} subtypes elevate cytoplasmic Ca^{2+} levels mostly by promoting phosphatidylinositol hydrolysis and generating inositol-1,4,5-triphosphate (IP_3). They are abundant in liver, spleen, and thyroid glands. Their sensitivities to phentolamine are low, but they are easily activated by oxymetazoline and inactivated by chloroethylclonidine. Mutant forms, and ones overexpressed in transfected cells can transform some cell types. The synthesis of α_{1C} subtypes is directed by a different chromosome. Those glycoproteins are distinguishable from the first two kinds by their somewhat smaller sizes, limited distribution, and different responses to some pharmacological agents.

α_2-adrenergic receptor[s]: a class of membrane spanning proteins whose members mediate responses to norepinehrpine and epinephrine, mostly by inhibiting adenylate cyclases. At least some act on K^+ channels, or modulate ATP-mediated arachidonic acid release. The ones located presynaptically are implicated in negative feedback control over catecholamine discharge. Clonidine is an agonist, and yohimbine an antagonist. The α_{2A} subtypes on blood platelets and lung cells display high sensitivity to oxymetazoline. The α_{2B} subtypes are the only adrenergic receptors known to lack glycosylation sites. Unlike α_{2A}, but in common with α_{2C} receptors (identified in kidneys), they bind prazosin with high affinities. An α_{2D} subtype in pineal glands resembles some that also occur in platelets.

β-adrenergic receptor[s]: approximately 64K adrenergic receptor types with three-dimensional structures (including 6 membrane spanning segments) that resemble those of rhodopsin and muscarinic receptors. Isoproterenol is a nonselective agonist that acts on all subtypes. Nonselective antagonists include propranolol and pindolol. *See* β_1 and β_2 subtypes, and β-adrenergic receptor kinases.

β_1-adrenergic receptor[s]: adrenergic receptor subtypes in cardiac and some other cell types that bind norepineph-

rine and epinephrine with approximately equal affinities. Many effects of ligand binding (including stimulation of the heart) are attributed to interactions with G proteins that contain α_s subunits, and to consequent augmentation of adenylate cyclase activity. Prenalterol is a selective agonist, and atenolol is a selective antagonist.

β_2-adrenergic receptor[s]: adrenergic receptor subtypes that bind epinephrine with high affinity and mediate effects that include relaxation of bronchiolar muscle, glycogenolysis in skeletal muscle, and lipolysis. Most responses to ligand binding involve association with G proteins that containing α_s subunits, and generation of cAMP. Terbutaline and salbutamol are selective agonists. Butoxamine is a selective antagonist.

β_3 adrenergic receptor[s]: adrenergic receptors identified in brown adipose tissue with binding properties different from those of β_1 and β_2 forms. They are activated by 3-hydroxybutyrate and BRL 37344, and are believed to participate in control of fat metabolism and oxygen consumption.

γ-adrenergic receptor[s]: proteins identified at neuromuscular junctions that mediate some catecholamine effects, but display properties different from those of α and β types.

β-adrenergic receptor kinases: BARK; enzymes that catalyze serine-threonine phosphorylation of occupied β-type adrenergic receptors. Arrestins bind to phosphorylated forms, uncouple the associations with G proteins required for signal transduction, and thereby mediate homologous desensitization. Related mechanisms invoke desensitization in retinas. Rhodopsin, a rod protein, closely resembles β_2-type adrenergic receptors. When activated by light, its functions involve binding to a retinal G protein, transducin. Rhodopsin kinase catalyzes phosphorylation, and β-arrestin, which binds to the phosphorylated rhodopsin, blocks the association with transducin. Similarly, olfactory receptors for certain deodorants interact with special G proteins, and adaptation is initiated by receptor phosphorylation.

adrenochrome: 3-hydroxy-1-methyl-5,6-indolinedione; a quinone pigment formed (via a quinol intermediate) when epinephrine undergoes oxidation.

adrenocortical hormones: usually, glucocorticoids and mineralocorticoids. However, cells of the adrenal cortex additionally secrete androgens and other regulators. *See* also **adrenal androgens**.

adrenocorticotropic hormone: adrenocorticotrophic hormone; ACTH; corticotrophin; corticotropin: a hormone cleaved from POMC that promotes growth and differentiation of zona fasciculata (and to some extent also zona reticularis) cells of the adrenal cortex. It is the major stimulant for glucocorticoid synthesis under physiological conditions, and a major factor for augmenting the secretion in response to stress. The form made by humans and many other mammals is a linear peptide with the sequence: Ser-Tyr-Ser-Met-Glu-His-Phe-Arg-Trp-Gly-Lys-Pro-Val-Gly-Lys-Lys-Arg-Arg-Pro-Val-Lys-Val-Tyr-Pro-Asn-Gly-Ala-Glu-Asp-Glu-Ser-Ala-Glu-Ala-Phe-Pro-Leu-Glu-Phe. Small species variations (mostly at positions 31 or 33) are known. Nonglycosylated and gly-cosylated forms ("little" and "big" ACTHs, respectively) exert similar actions, most of which can be mimicked with synthetic $ACTH_{1-24}$ (composed of the first 24 amino acid moieties). ACTH rapidly accelerates cholesterol transport to mitochondria, augments cholesterol esterase activity, and induces *c-fos*. It more slowly increases the synthesis of proteins required for hormone production, and of other proteins; and it affects cytoskeletal structure. Many actions are mediated via cAMP, but influences on adrenal blood flow and other processes may involve different second messengers (including prostaglandins, and possibly also cGMP). Activation of phospholipase C, generation of inositol phosphates, and roles for Ca-calmodulin kinase have also been described. High levels can act via cAMP to accelerate synthesis of aldosterone in the zona glomerulosa, but the effects are short-lived and attributed to provision of steroid precursors. When presented *in vitro for* extended time periods, ACTH inhibits proliferation of those cells and causes them to modulate to fasciculata types. Circulating ACTH originates almost exclusively in adenohypophysial corticotropes (except during pregnancy, when placental cells may contribute). One extra-adrenal target organ is the liver, in which ACTH affects the synthesis of sex steroid binding globulins and some other proteins. Some ACTH is made by melanocytes, but most of it is cleaved to α-melanocyte stimulating hormone (α-MSH), corticotropin-like intermediate peptide (CLIP), and other small peptides. ACTH and/or closely related peptides are made in the central nervous system, in which they affect learning and short-term memory, but neuron ACTH probably does not contribute to the blood levels. Corticotropin releasing hormone (CRH) from the hypothalamus is the major stimulant for pars distalis cells (and a similar peptide functions in the placenta). In nonpregnant individuals, vasopressins can substantially augment the effects of CRH, and it can assume special importance during times of stress. Several other regulators (including oxytocin, serotonin, gastrin releasing peptide, epinephrine, cholecystokinin, and melatonin) modulate CRH release, corticotrope activities, or both, and contribute to fine controls. Angiotensin-II can increase ACTH release but reduce its effectiveness. Glucocorticoids exert negative feedback controls over CRH, ACTH, and vasopressin, and can affect the influences of other regulators. The cells that make them are, in turn, responsive to some direct effects of vasopressin (and also of prolactin and other hormones). Glucocorticoid levels are highest during morning hours in diurnal species (and during the early evening in nocturnal animals). The circadian rhythms are driven mostly by CRH secretion patterns, but adrenocortical cells undergo variations in sensitivities to ACTH that have been linked with changes in receptor numbers. Interactions with the immune system are complex. Some cytokines released by activated lymphocytes, including interleukins 1 and 6, can stimulate CRH and ACTH release, and some interleukin-6 is made in both pituitary glands and adrenal cortex. CRH stimulates production of opioid peptides cleaved from POMC, and both CRH and the peptides have some direct effects on lymphocytes. Moreoever, glucocorticoids exert negative feedback controls over opioid peptide synthesis and cytokine release; and some CRH is made peripherally.

adrenodoxin: a mitochondrial non-heme protein component of the cholesterol side-chain cleavage system of the adrenal cortex that accepts electrons from adrenodoxin reductase and passes them to cytochrome $P_{450\text{-scc}}$. In common with ferredoxins of other cell types, each molecule contains two iron and two sulfur atoms.

adrenodoxin reductase: an NADPH-specific flavoprotein component of the cholesterol side-chain cleavage system of the adrenal cortex that accepts electrons from NADPH and passes them to adrenodoxin.

adrenogenital syndrome: several human diseases in which adrenocortical cells secrete excessive quantities of androgens. The most common causes are mutations that impair synthesis of steroid 21-**hydroxylase** *(q.v.)*. Consequently, inadequate amounts of glucocorticoids are made, and loss of their usual negative feedback over ACTH secretion leads to production of excessive amounts of androgen precursors. Glucocorticoid administration can correct both the glucocorticoid deficiency and the overproduction of ACTH. In "salt-wasting" forms, mineralocorticoid formation is also deficient, and replacement therapy may be required. Severe conditions that begin early in life can cause total masculinization of the external genitalia of genetically female (XX) fetuses, and Wolffian duct development. Milder ones lead to partial masculinization, and XX infants are born with ambiguous genitalia. When the disorders develops postnatally, the manifestations include virilization of females and precocious puberty in males.

adrenoglomerulotropin: 1-methyl-6-methoxy-1,2,3,4-tetrahydro-2-carboline; a hypothetical pineal gland hormone that stimulates aldosterone secretion. It is believed to be an artifact formed during preparation of pineal gland extracts.

adrenoleukodystrophy: diseases in which peroxisome defects leads to the accumulation of hexacosanoate, docacosanoate, and other very long chain fatty acids. The manifestations of more severe types (Zellweger's cerebrohepatorenal syndrome, infantile Refsom's disease), caused by autosomal recessive gene mutations that affect peroxisome structure, include severe mental retardation, and vision and hearing impairments. They are progressive, and usually fatal within a few years of onset, although adrenocortical deficiency may not appear until late in the course. A milder, X-linked form, which is more common and appears during childhood or adolescence, is associated with morphologically normal peroxisomes. In some cases, severe Addison's disease precedes the onset of neurological symptoms, that can include clumsiness, and sensory, urinary and reproductive system disturbances.

adrenolutin: *N*-methyl-5,6-dihydroxyindol; a yellow pigment derived from adrenochrome.

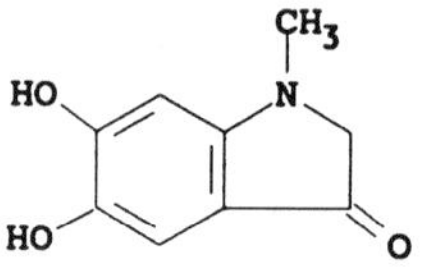

adrenomedullary: derived from or characteristic of the adrenal medulla.

adrenoreceptors: usually, adrenergic receptors.

adrenorphin: morphinamide;H_2N-Tyr-Gly-Gly-Phe-Met-Arg-Arg-Val-NH_2; a major proenkephlin A cleavage product formed in the adrenal medulla. It acts preferentially on μ (and to a lesser extent on κ) type opioid receptors.

adrenostenone: 5α-androst-16-en-3-one: a volatile steroid present in human sweat, boar saliva, and some plants that may serve as a pheromone in some species. Since some humans easily perceive the odor, whereas others do not detect it, but can learn to do so when repeatedly exposed, it is used to study olfactory functions.

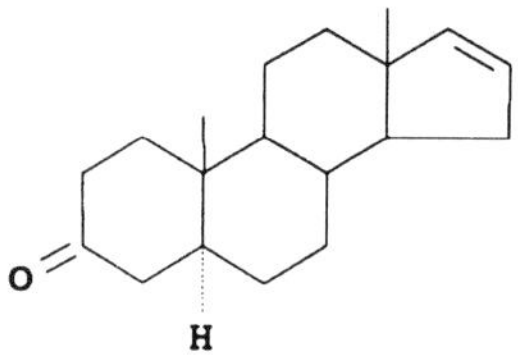

adrenosterone: androst-4-ene-3,11,17-trione; compound G; a steroid hormone metabolite. It is not biologically active in most species, but serves as a weak androgen in a few.

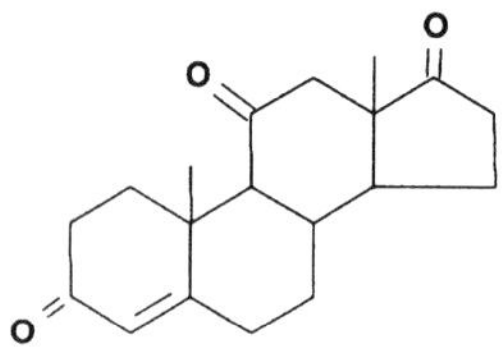

Adriamycin: doxorubicin.

ADTN: 2-amino-5,6-dihydroxy-1,2,3,4-tetrahydronaphthaline; a D_1-type dopamine receptor agonist. It is also known as A-5,6-ADTN (for α-amino-5,6-dihydroxy-1,2,3,4-tetrahydronaphthaline). The inactive 6,7 dihydro isomer (A-6,7-DTN), is administered to control animals.

adult T Cell leukemia: ATL; a malignant hemopoietic disorder that can be invoked by the HTLV-I virus, in which there is excessive expression of *c-fos*, and of the genes that direct the synthesis of interleukin-2, IL-2 receptors, and granulocyte-macrophage colony stimulating factor (GM-CSF). *See* also **leukemias**.

adult T cell leukemia factor: ATF; adult T cell leukemia derived factor; ADF: a cell surface component on $CD4^+CD8^-$ T lymphocytes of individuals infected with HTLV-I.

AEEs: excitatory amino acids; *see* **glutamate**.

aequorin: a 30K protein obtained from the jellyfish, *Aequorea aequorea*. It enters cells and fluoresces when it combines with calcium, but quin-2, fura-2, and nitra-5 are among the agents more commonly used to monitor changes in intracellular Ca^{2+} levels.

aerobes: organisms dependent on oxygen; *cf* **anaerobes**.

aerobic: using or requiring oxygen; *cf* **anaerobic**.

AEV: avian erythroblastosis virus.

AF-1: antifertility factor-1.

AFC: antibody forming cells.

AF-DX 116: a muscarinic receptor antagonist that binds with much higher affinity to cardiac M_2 than to other types, and exerts atropine-like effects on the heart. Its actions differ markedly from those of pirenzepine, which is chemically similar.

afferent: going towards; describes, for example, neurons that lead to and affect, or blood vessels that enter a structure.

affinity: binding strength, for example of receptors for ligands, or of antigens for antibodies.

affinity chromatography: *see* **chromatography**.

affinity labeling: techniques used to identify specific kinds of molecules and functions of their components. For example, TPCK, which inhibits chymotrypsin by reversibly binding to its active site, and forms covalent linkages with an adjacent site, has been used to define the functions of that enzyme. *See* also **photo-affinity labeling**.

aflatoxins: aflatoxins B, G, and M, and related mycotoxins that disrupt cell metabolism by binding to enzymes. They are metabolites of substances produced by *Aspergillus flavus* and related species. Farm animals con-

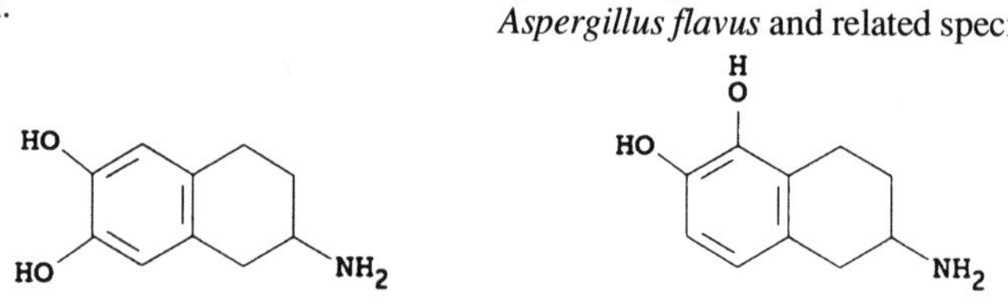

A-6,7-DTN

A-5,6-DTN

ADTN

suming nuts and grains that contain the fungi become seriously ill, and can release the poisons to milk. The toxins are believed to cause liver cancers in humans. The structure of aflatoxin B_1 is shown.

AFP: α-fetoproteins.

Ag: silver.

ω-Aga-IIIA: agatoxin-IIIA; an extremely potent component of the venom of the funnel web spider *Agelenopsis aperta* that binds to, and blocks L and N type calcium ion channels.

ω-Aga-1VA:Lys-Lys-Lys-Cys-Ile-Ala-Lys-Asp-Tyr-Gly-Arg-Cys-Lys-Trp-Gly-Gly-Thr-Pro-Cys-Cys-Arg-Gly-Arg-Gly-Cys-Ile-Cys-Ser-Ile-Met-Gly-Thr-Asn-Cys-Glu-Cys-Lys-Pro-Arg-Leu-Ile-Met-Glu-Gly-Leu-Gly-Leu-Ala; a cysteine-rich component of the venom of the funnel web spider *Agelenopsis aperta* that binds to P-type calcium ion channels.

agammaglobulinemia: severe γ globulin deficiencies, usually caused by inherited defects that impair B cell maturation. In some cases, no immunoglobulins are made, but in others only certain classes are affected. A mutation on the X chromosome causes Bruton's hypogamma-globulinemia, in which the bone marrow can contain normal numbers of pre-B cells, but mature types do not accumulate in the bloodstream or lymph nodes. In some other disorders, B cells are morphologically normal, but they do not progress to plasma cells, or plasma cells form but fail to secrete immunoglobulins. T cell functions are not necessarily affected; *cf* **severe combined immunodeficiency**.

agar: a polysaccharide complex extracted from *Rhodophyceae* seaweed. It is used as an inert support for growing bacteria and some eukaryote cells.

agarose gels: rigid, inert, neutral galactan polysaccharide gels with high water content, purified from agar. They are used as supports for separating nucleic acids and other large molecules by electrophoresis and gel chromatography. See also **sepharose**.

agatoxin: a term that usually refers specifically to ω-Aga-IVA, but is sometimes applied to other components of funnel web spider venom that act on calcium ion channels.

AGE: advanced glycosylation end products; *see* **nonenzymatic glycosylation**.

agenesis: failure to develop.

agglutination: clumping; a term usually applied to erythrocytes, viruses, bacteria, or antigens; *see also* **aggregation** and **cell adhesion**, and *cf* **coagulation**. Under normal conditions, zeta potentials cause erythrocytes to repel each other in the presence of native blood plasma. Abolition of the potentials by immunoglobulins from genetically different individuals is used in blood typing. IgMs are more effective, but IgGs are used in Rh tests. *Hemagglutination* procedures for detecting the presence of specific kinds of antibodies employ erythrocytes pretreated with agents such as tannic acid or chromium chloride that facilitate antigen attachment. Over limited concentration ranges, multivalent antibodies that bind with high affinities agglutinate the cells by forming bridges between adjacent molecules with common kinds of binding sites on the cell surfaces. (However, very high antibody concentrations interfere, since two or more epitopes can attach to the same antigen molecule.) *Agglutination inhibition* tests are based on the ability of components of serum, urine, or other fluids to prevent agglutination of latex or other particles coated with specific antigens when specific antibodies are added. The most commonly used test for pregnancy depends on displacement by hCG in test samples, of anti-hCG from hCG/anti-hCG complexes. Other applications include tests for rheumatoid factor, some viruses, and some illicit drugs.

agglutinin: an antibody, lectin, or other agent that promotes clumping (e.g. of erythrocytes or viruses). The most commonly used procedures for blood typing depend on the presence of anti-B, anti-A, and both antibodies, respectively in blood types A, B and O.

agglutinogen: an antibody or other substance that stimulates production of agglutinins.

aggregation: clumping. The term can refer to cells (as in platelet aggregation), or to complexes of molecules held together loosely; *see* **agglutination** and *cf* **coagulation**.

aggregin: a 100K glycoprotein on platelet surfaces that functions as an ADP receptor.

agonist: (1) an agent that binds to a hormone or neurotransmitter receptor and mimics the actions of endogenous ligands; *cf* **antagonist**. Some synthetic agents are more potent than native regulators because they are more resistant to degradation, or have different binding properties. *Weak* agonists may be effective only when present in high concentrations, or when the native ligand is not present. They can also function as antagonists by competing with the ligands. (Progesterone exerts mineralocorticoid activity when it binds to aldosterone receptors, and the effects are most obvious when no aldosterone is present. When present in very high concentrations, it impairs aldosterone binding.) *Partial* agonists mimic some, but not all actions of natural ligands. Some substances are mixed agonist-antagonists. (They can, for example mimic certain effects of natural ligands and oppose others, or can display activities that vary with their concentrations or change direction when certain other substances are present.) Since many receptors types exist in multiple forms, an agonist for one cell type can be an antagonist for another within the same individual. Moreover, an agonist in one species can be an antagonist for homologous cells of another; (2) a neuron or muscle that functions along with others of the same kind to accomplish a common response; (3) an animal that displays aggression towards members of the same species.

agorins: two structural plasma membrane proteins, agorin I (20K) and agorin II (40K), made in large amounts by mastocytoma cells.

agouti: (1) having fur with irregular light and dark colored bars; (2) any of several short-haired rodents species of the genus *Dasyprocta* in which the fur pattern occurs in normal individuals; (3) a term sometimes applied to chimeric mice produced by injecting DNA from animals with one kind of pigmentation into oocytes or young embryos of others with different pigmentation; (4) *See* **agouti locus**.

agouti locus: a segment on mouse chromosome 2 that controls melanin and phaeomelanin synthesis in individual hair follicles, and the distribution of the pigments throughout the fur coat, by directing generation of messengers in follicle cells that act on melanocytes. Since it additionally affects several aspects of embryonic development, and is closely linked to an *ld* locus that controls limb development, fur patterns can serve as markers for other conditions. Many alleles and pseudoalleles have been identified. Mutations, inversions, deletions, and translocations occur spontaneously, and some can be induced by radiation. Developmental defects associated with aberrant fur patterns include severe limb and kidney deformities, sterility, and high susceptibilities for development of diabetes mellitus, leukemias, and solid tumors. Some aberrations have lethal consequences during the embryonic period. Others impair the ability to acetylate α-MSH, and accumulation of unacetylated α-MSH may directly contribute to hyperphagia and development of obesity.

α₁-AGP: α_1-acidic glycoprotein.

α granules: alpha granules; *see* **blood platelets**.

agretope: an amino acid sequence that binds to major histocompatibility complex proteins and affects immune responses. It can be a T cell membrane component, or a synthetic peptide used as a vaccine.

agrin: a protein obtained from *Torpedo californica* electric organs that induces differentiation of myotubes, and the formation of neuromuscular junction type structures.

AH: anterior hypothalamus.

AHA: (1) anterior hypothalamic area; (2) autoimmune hemolytic anemia.

AHG: antihemophilic globulin.

AIH: artificial insemination of a woman with her husband's sperm.

αᵢ subunits: components of **G proteins** (*q.v.*) that mediate adenylate cyclase inhibition. Several subtypes are known.

AIB, AIBA: α-aminoisobutyric acid.

AIDS: acquired immune deficiency syndrome.

AIDS related complex: ARC; diseases caused by HIV virus infections, directly or via the devastating effects on immune system functions.

AIJ: ampullary-isthmic junction.

Al: aluminum.

Ala: alanine.

alacepril: an agent used to treat some forms of hypertension. It is converted in the liver to **captopril** (*q.v.*), which mediates the actions.

alanine: usually, L α-alanine (A; Ala; 2-amino-propionic acid); a neutral, low molecular weight component of most proteins. Although classified as essential, it can be synthesized from serine and some other amino acids. It undergoes reversible deamination, in the reaction: alanine + α-ketoglutarate $\rightleftarrows$ pyruvate + glutamate (and in others with different substrates), and is a key component of the glucose-alanine cycle which contributes to euglycemia during fasting. Other functions include stimulation of glucagon release and augmentation of glutamate actions on NMDA receptors. The D form is a component of some substances made by microorganisms, and of some pharmacological agents.

$$H_3C - \underset{\underset{H}{|}}{\overset{\overset{NH_2}{|}}{C}} - COOH$$

β-alanine: β-aminopropionic acid; a neurotransmitter that binds to glycine receptors, promotes hyperpolarization, and can block activation of some brain and spinal cord neurons.

$$H_2N - CH_2 - CH_2 - COOH$$

alanine aminotransferase: alanine transaminase; ALT; glutamic-pyruvic transaminase; GPT; an enzyme that catalyzes reversible conversion of alanine to pyruvate; *see* also **glucose-alanine cycles**. The plasma levels rise in individuals with some liver diseases, and in infectious mononucleosis.

alanine transaminase: alanine aminotransferase.

β-alanyl-histidine: carnosine.

Alaproclate hydrochloride: D,L-alanine,2-(4-chlorophenyl)-1,1-dimethylethyl ester hydrochloride; a selective serotonin uptake inhibitor, potentially useful for treating psychic depression and senile dementia.

alarmones: modified nucleotides produced in response to stress, starvation, and vitamin D deficiency.

alarm pheromones: pheromones that alert other members of the species to potential danger, and invoke defensive responses.

albinism: absence of normal pigmentation, in hair (or fur), skin, eyes, and other structures. It can be caused by mutations that block the ability to make tyrosinase, melanocyte stimulating hormones, or receptors for the hormones.

albumins: (1) the most abundant of the blood plasma proteins, made in and secreted by liver cells. They are soluble in water and dilute salt solutions, and are coagulated by heat. Circulating albumins are major factors for maintaining the oncotic pressure. Edema develops, and plasma volume declines when starvation or severe protein deprivation deplete the amino acid precursors, liver diseases impair their synthesis, or renal disorders cause loss to the urine. Plasma albumins also loosely bind to, and facilitate the transport of fatty acids and other blood components. Since they associate reversibly with many hormones and form low affinity, high capacity complexes, they can protect against sudden surges of free (active) hormone levels, and can release the regulators when the concentrations fall. They may also contribute to control of target cell uptake, and can be degraded to serve as sources of amino acids; (2) ovalbumin, lactalbumin, α-fetoprotein, and some plant seed components with similar chemical and physical properties. *See* also **bovine serum albumin**.

albuterol: salbutamol; 2-(*tert*-butylamino)-1-(4-hydroxy-3-hydroxymethyl)-phenyl)ethanol; a selective β₂-type adrenergic receptor agonist, used as a bronchodilator, and to protect against premature labor by suppressing uterine contractions.

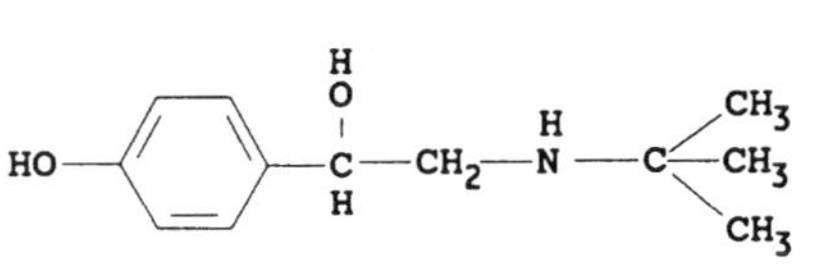

alcaptonuria: alkaptonuria: *see* **tyrosine aminotransferase**.

alcian blue: a water-soluble cationic dye used to stain polysaccharides separated by electrophoresis, to identity cells (such as gonadotropes, thyrotropes, and histiocytes) that contain large amounts of acidic glycosaminoglycan levels, and to identify polysaccharides. In the structure shown, the Xs are onium groups that split off during staining.

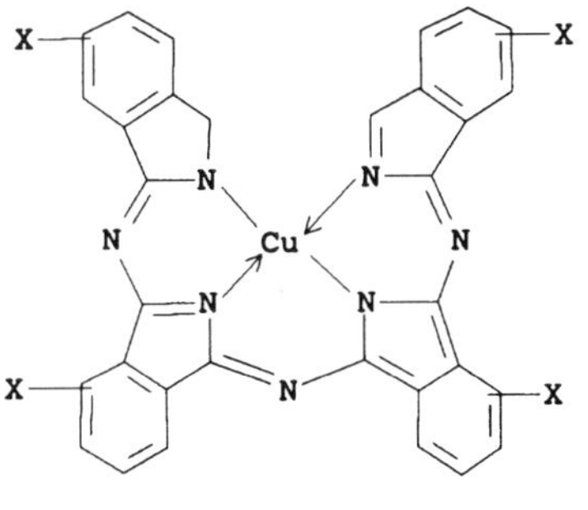

alcohol: (1) ethyl alcohol; (2) any organic compound that has one or more -C-OH groups.

aldalactone: spironolactone.

aldehyde: any compound that has a -C=O chemical group. *See*, for example, **glyceraldehyde-3-phosphate**.

aldehyde fuchsin: a dye chemically related to acid fuchsin. It is used to stain connective tissue fibers and the granules of certain cell types (such as gonadotropes and thyrotropes).

Aldomet: a trade name for α-methyldopa.

aldohexose: any 6-carbon aldose, for example glucose, galactose, or mannose.

aldose: any sugar that possesses an aldehyde group, for example glucose (an aldohexose), or ribose (an aldopentose).

aldose reductases: enzymes that catalyze conversion of aldoses to their corresponding sugar alcohols; *see* also **sorbitol**.

aldosterone: electrocortin; 11β,21-dihydroxy-3,20-dioxo-4-pregnene-18-al; the major mammalian mineralocorticoid, made in the zona glomerulosa of the adrenal cortex. The most obvious effects are exerted on the kidneys, in which it promotes Na^+ and HCO_3^- reabsorption that is associated with water retention, as well as H^+ and K^+ excretion. Aldosterone also augments Na^+/K^+-ATPase activity in muscle and at other sites, and thereby affects water and electrolyte exchange between cells and their surrounding fluids. It promotes Na^+ absorption in exchange for K^+ in the colon, and lowers $Na^+:K^+$ ratios in sweat and saliva. Although increased Na^+/K^+-ATPase activity accounts for many of the influences on sodium metabolism, it additionally stimulates Na^+/H^+ antiport, and some effects on potassium are exerted in different ways. Receptors in the brain are implicated in stimulation of salt appetite, control of cerebrospinal fluid volume and composition, and other functions. The most obvious deficiency effects include metabolic acidosis, dehydration, diminished circulating blood and interstitial fluid volumes, and abnormal intracellular and extracellular $Na^+:K^+$ ratios. In severe cases, nausea (with loss of appetite), vomiting, and diarrhea exacerbate the water and electrolyte balance. Adrenalectomized rats deprived of replacement therapy can survive if their drinking water is replaced by 1% sodium chloride. (By drinking enormous quantites, they replace sodium that is lost, and the large urine volumes carry away excess potassium.) However, although humans deficient in the hormone tend to ingest remarkable quantities of salt (and may even take it alone in handfuls or put it on foods such as ice-cream), prolonged deficiency is invariably fatal. Excess hormone can invoke edema, alkalosis, and hypertension. Since aldosterone has an OH group at position 11 that can be liberated from the hemi-acetal formed by interaction with the 18 carbon aldehyde, it has the potential for exerting glucocorticoid effects. However, it is extremely potent, in part because it does not bind with high affinity to transcortin, and the amounts present under physiological conditions are not important in this way. Angiotensin II is the major stimulant for aldosterone synthesis and secretion; *see* also **renin angiotensin system**. Supernormal extracellular K^+ concentrations can also stimulate, and extracellular Na^+ levels affect the sensitivities to regulators.

aldosterone

Atrial natriuretic peptides inhibit; *see* also **mineralocorticoid escape**. Additional regulators that may contribute to fine control include dopamine; *see* also **aldosterone stimulating hormone**. Aldosterone is a major regulator of Na^+ transport across urinary bladders in some amphibians, and appears to exert weak effects of this kind in mammals. Other structures regulated in nonmammalian vertebrates include salt and rectal glands.

aldosterone induced proteins: AIPs; several proteins made after latent periods of one or more hours, when aldoterone acts on "classical" type intracellular steroid hormone receptors. They include sodium pump and tricarboxylic acid cycle enzymes, and factors that affect ion permeabilities in plasma membranes.

aldosterone receptors: many of the actions of aldosterone are mediated via binding to intracellular "classical" type steroid hormone receptors and induction (after latent periods of one or more hours) of aldosterone induced proteins; *see* **glucocorticoid receptors**. However, in common with other steroid hormones, aldosterone also acts within minutes on plasma membranes. The early effects include activation of pre-existing Na^+/K^+-ATPases and Na^+/H^+ antiport, and changes in plasma membrane lipids.

aldosterone secretion inhibiting factor: ASIF: a 35-amino acid peptide chemically and biologically related to atrial natriuretic factor, and identical to brain natriuretic peptide, made in the brain and adrenal medulla.

aldosterone stimulating hormone: ASH; (1) a pituitary hormone different from ACTH that stimulates aldosterone secretion. An *N*-terminal "16K fragment" of POMC that augments cholesterol esterase activity exerts such effects; (2) *see* **adrenoglomerulotropin**.

alfaxalone: *see* **alphaxalone**.

ALG: anti-lymphocytic globulin.

algesia: sensitivity to pain.

Algin score: a measure of molecular homology, used mostly for polypeptides and proteins. Values of 3 or more indicate significant similarity.

alimentary: pertaining to nutrition or digestive system functions.

aliphatic: describes organic compounds with linear carbon atom chains; *cf* **aromatic**.

aliquot: a representative portion, such as one of several equivalent volume samples of test material used to perform an assay in duplicate (or triplicate), or to compare the effects of different treatments.

alkaline phosphatases: enzymes with pH optima in the alkaline range that catalyze hydrolysis of organic compound phosphate bonds; *cf* **acid phosphatases** and **phosphoprotein phosphatases**. At least four genes direct their synthesis, and most cell types make at least one isozyme. High levels are present in bone (in which the activity level provides a measure of osteoblast function), and in liver, intestine, kidney, and some leukocytes. The enzymes are used as plasma membrane markers for some cells types.

alkaloids: alkaline, bitter-tasting cyclic nitrogen-containing organic compounds obtained from plants. Most affect neuron functions, and are and toxic when taken in small amounts. Many kinds are used in pharmacological studies and therapy. Examples include atropine, morphine, cocaine, nicotine, picrotoxin, and physostigmine.

alkalosis: acid-base imbalance associated with high blood plasma $NaHCO_3:HHCO_3$ ratios; *cf* **acidosis**. Hyperventilation causes *respiratory* alkalosis, since carbon dioxide loss depletes the $HHCO_3$. In *compensated* respiratory alkalosis, accelerated urinary excretion of $NaHCO_3$ lowers the ratio. Aldosterone excess (which elevates $NaHCO_3$ levels), ingestion of very alkaline diets, and vomiting (which depletes HCl), are among the causes of *metabolic* alkalosis. In *compensated* metabolic alkalosis, increased CO_2 retention lowers the ratio.

alkaptonuria: alcaptonuria; an autosomal recessive disorder in which homogentisic acid accumulates and undergoes oxidation and polymerization to form black pigments that deposit in connective tissues. The consequences can include aortic valve stenosis and a form of arthritis. Homogentisic acid in urine slowly undergoes similar reactions that can be accelerated by adding alkali. *See* also **tyrosine aminotransferase**.

alkyl[s]: chemicals group with the general formula $-C_nH_{n+1}$.

ALL: acute lymphocytic leukemia; *see* **leukemias**.

alkylating agents: compounds that react with water, and with carbonyl, amino, imino, phosphate, and other chemical entities, and replace hydrogen atoms with alkyl groups. Examples include busulfan, nitrogen mustards, and cyclophosphamides. They are toxic, and at least potentially mutagenic, because they alter the structures of, and can cross-link proteins, nucleic acids, and other essential molecules. Their abilities to arrest cell proliferation are used to some extent in cancer therapy, since some rapidly dividing neoplastic cells are more susceptible than normal types.

allantoic acid: an end-product of purine metabolism in some fishes. Allantoicase catalyzes its conversion to urea + glyoxylate in many vertebrates.

allantoin: 5-ureidohydantion; an end-product of purine metabolism for some fishes, and for fetuses of other vertebrates. They are also made by some plants. Psoralen is a commercial preparation used to promote wound healing.

allantois: a fetal membrane derived from the hindgut that contributes to formation of the umbilical cord and placenta in eutherian mammals. It transiently performs respiratory functions in horses, goats, and a few other species, but is vestigial in most others. In developing oviparous vertebrates. it serves as a respiratory and excretory organ.

allatum hormone: *see* **juvenile hormone**.

allatostatins: peptides that inhibit the synthesis of juvenile hormones. They can be endogenous regulatory factors, substances made by other organisms, or environmental chemicals.

allatotropins: endogenous neuropeptides or environmental substances that stimulate the synthesis of juvenile hormones.

allele[s]: gene pairs on corresponding loci of homologous chromosomes that code for molecules involved in the same functions. The DNA sequences are identical in individuals homozygous for the associated traits. In heterozygotes, small differences do not always affect the phenotype in obvious ways, but they can, for example, code for different isozymes. *See* also **dominant, recessive**, and **lethal alleles**, and **multiple allelism**.

allelic exclusion: inability to express more than one of two alleles. In heterozygous individuals, all members of a B lymphocyte clone make antibodies composed of just one kind of heavy and one kind of light chain.

allelopathy: deleterious interactions between genetically different cells or organisms. The mechanisms are widely used by plants of different species that compete for a common habitat, and by some marine invertebrates.

allelotype: the frequency distribution of a set of alleles in a population.

allergens: plant pollens, food components, environmental toxins, or other agents that initiate immediate hypersensitivity reactions; *see* **allergy**.

allergoid: a chemically modified allergen that lessens allergic responses by promoting formation of IgG (rather than IgE) type immunoglobulins.

allergy: hypersensitivity; exaggerated immune system reactivity to one or more antigens (often of types that do not affect most other members of the population). Production of IgE type antibodies that attach to and cross-link Fc receptors on mast cells and basophilic leukocytes, with consequent release of histamine and eicosanoids accounts for most of the effects. Mast cells also release some cytokines, either directly or by activating T lymphocytes.

allesthesia: usually, changes in sensation caused by altered input to receptors.

allo-: a prefix meaning (1) foreign, or produced by a genetically different individual, as in allomone or allo-antigen; (2) different in chemical structure or configuration, as in allocortol. *See* also **hetero-**.

alloantigen: an agent made by some members of a species that invokes immune system responses in genetically different individuals of the same species.

alloantibody: an antibody made in response to an alloantigen.

allogamy: fertilization of an oocyte by a spermatozoan of the same species; *cf* **autogamy**.

allogeneic; allogenic; derived from a genetically different member of the same species; *cf* **heterogeneic** and **isogeneic**.

allogeneic disease: runt disease; graft vs host disease: growth retardation and other disorders that develop in response to an allograft that contains immunocompetent cells, in a host unable (because of immaturity, radiation, or immunosuppressant drugs) to reject the graft.

allogeneic effect: a generalized increase in immune system reactivity initiated by specific antigens that promote the release of cytokines and other mediators.

allograft; homograft; a tissue or organ graft from a genetically dissimilar member of the same species; *see* **graft**.

allomone: a chemical released by a member of one species that affects the behavior or physiological functions of another species, and is beneficial to the donor. The effects can (but need not) be noxious to the recipient. *Cf* **kairomone, synamone**, and **pheromone**.

allopathy: the system of medicine in which disease is treated by agents that oppose the effects of the disease processes, or of the initiating agents; *cf* **homeopathy**.

allopatric: occupying different geographic regions.

allophenic: describes (1) a characteristic not solely dependent on the genes a cell carries; (2) an individual with genetic components derived from more than one zygote, for example one that develops from fused blastocysts; (3) orderly co-existence within an organism of cells with different phenotypes.

allopregnanolone: 5α-pregnan-3α-ol,20-one; a progesterone metabolite that is excreted to the urine. It is also a **neurosteroid** (*q.v.*).

allopregnane: *see* **pregnane**.

allopurinol: 5-hydroxypyrazolopyrimidine; an agent that inhibits xanthine oxidase (which catalyzes conversion of hypoxanthine to uric acid). It is used to alleviate gout.

all-or-nothing response: an ungraded response that either does or does not occur when a stimulus is presented. A more powerful stimulus cannot invoke a greater response.

allorphine: nalorphine.

allosome: a chromosome that differs in appearance and behavior from normal autosomes. The term can refer to defective autosomes, or to healthy sex chromosomes.

allosteric: related to position; *see* **allosteric enzymes**.

allosteric enzymes: regulatory enzymes whose configurations and activities are reversibly altered by non-covalent binding of ligands to noncatalytic sites.

allotetrahydro-DOC: 3α,5α-pregna-21-ol,20-one: a **neurosteroid** (*q.v.*).

allotope: the region of an antigen that distinguishes it from other allotypes.

allotypes: genetic variants of specific kinds of molecules (such as an immunoglobulins) among members of the same species.

allotypic variation: genetic differences among members of the same species, for example of the kinds that affect blood types or histocompatibility antigens.

alloxan: 2,4,5,6-tetraoxohexapyrimidine; an agent chemically related to uric acid that preferentially destroys pancreatic islet β cells, but is also toxic to hemopoietic cells, and displays some anti-neoplastic activity. It is used to invoke experimental diabetes mellitus in laboratory animals. At least some of the effects are attributed to superoxide formation.

alloxazine mononucleotide: riboflavine phosphate.

allozymes: isoenzymes, usually ones that can be separated by electrophoresis.

allyl: the chemical group shown.

allyllysine: allysine; an aldehyde formed from lysine via a reaction catalyzed by lysine oxidase. One type of collagen cross-linking involves condensation of two allysine moieties, or of one allysine + one **hydroxyallysine** (*q.v.*).

N-**allylnormetazocine**: NANM; SKF 10,047; (2α,6α)-1,2,3,4,5,6-hexahydro-6,11-dimethyl-3-(2-propenyl)-2,6-methano-3-benzaocin-8-ol; an agent that binds selectively with high affinity to σ receptors (*see* **opioid receptors**), attaches to cell components that bind phencyclidine, antagonizes some effects of haloperidol, and exerts some μ-receptor antagonism (but does not directly affect pain perception). It can invoke schizophrenia-like symptoms that are not antagonized by naloxone. Influences on the adenohypophysis include stimulation of adrenocorticotropic hormone (ACTH) secretion and inhibition of prolactin and luteinizing hormone (LH) release. The D (+) form is more potent than the L isomer, and has been used to distinguish between σ$_1$ and σ$_2$ subtypes.

allysine: allyllysine.

alopecia: hair loss; baldness. Factors that cause abnormal hair loss include autoimmune diseases, as well as radiation, anti-neoplastic drugs, and other agents that block proliferation of cells that would otherwise rapidly divide.

alpha: *see* α, and alphabetic listings that follows α-.

alpha granules: *see* **platelets**.

alpha particle: a high energy particle emitted by some radioactive elements, equivalent in mass to a helium nucleus (2 protons plus 2 neutrons). Alpha particles travel shorter distances that beta types, but can inflict extensive tissue damage.

alpha (α) subunit: one of the peptide chains of a dimeric or oligomeric protein. Follicle stimulating, thyroid stimulating, and luteinizing hormones (FSH, TSH, and LH) and human chorionic gonadotropins (hCG) have similar or identical α subunits. (Each has a distinct beta subunit type that determines the biological activities.) Other molecules with subunit structures include activins, inhibins, and the receptors for most hormones and neurotransmitters.

alphaxalone: 3α-hydroxy, 5α-pregnane-11,20-dione; a steroid that anesthetizes by exerting non-genomic effects on neurons that involve modulation of gamma aminobutyric acid (GABA) receptors at sites different from those affected by barbiturates.

alprazolam: Xanax; 8-chloro-1-methyl-6-phenyl-4*H*-[1,2,4]triazolo[4,3a][1.4]benzo-diazepine; an agent used to relieve anxiety and avert panic attacks that does not usually promote drowsiness. Prolonged use leads to habituation. It is also a platelet activating factor (PAF) receptor antagonist.

alprenolol: 1-(*O*-allylphenoxy)-3-(isopropylamino)-2-propanol; a nonselective β-adrenergic receptor antagonist that affects both β_1 and β_2 subtypes.

ALS: (1) antilymphocytic sera; (2) amyotrophic lateral sclerosis.

ALT: alanine aminotransferase.

alternative complement pathway; properdin pathway: *see* **complement activation**.

Altrenogest: 17-hydroxy-17-(2-propenyl)estra-4,9-11-trien-3-one; a synthetic progestin.

altricial: describes species that bear hairless, immature young who require prolonged postnatal care. In most species, the litters are large, and the gestation periods are short. *Cf* **precocial**.

AluI: a restriction endonuclease made by *Arthrobacter luteus* that recognizes double stranded DNA segments with 5′ AGCT sequences, and cleaves most *Alu* TCGA 3′ sequences between C and H bases.

aluminum: Al; a metallic element (atomic number 13, atomic wt. 26.98). Only minute amounts are absorbed from food cooked in aluminum utensils, but aluminum can accumulate in biologically significant amounts in individuals with renal dysfunctions maintained on dialysis. It interacts with endothelial cell extracellular matrix molecules, and can decrease effective pore sizes. Low levels may also slowly diminish bone mass and exert other effects on calcium metabolism by inhibiting osteoblast activity and augmenting PTH secretion. Several salts are used as antiseptics and astringents.

aluminum tetrafluoride: AlF_4; an agent that attaches to guanine nucleotide binding sites of, and thereby activates some trimeric G proteins (but not small GTP binding proteins). Most of the influences on intracellular transport, endocytosis, and exocytosis are attributed to the fluoride component.

alu sequences: species-specific, repetitive, transposable, C-G rich, 150-300 base pair DNA sequences that resemble, and may have arisen via reverse transcription of 7SL RNA. The approximately 500,000 copies scattered throughout the human genome form the gram-negative bands on stained chromosomes. Most are cleaved by *Alu-1* endonuclease (*cf* **LINE-1**). Roles in initiation of DNA synthesis, and in evolutionary changes have been suggested. Although transcribed via RNA polymerase III dependent mechanisms, and present in some hnRNAs (but not mature messenger RNAs) no functions in transcription are known. The sequences are used to identify human DNA segments in transfected cells.

ALV: avian leukosis virus.

alveolar macrophages: dust cells; macrophages in lung alveoli that remove small inhaled particles and excess surfactant.

amanitins

alytesin: pGlu-Gly-Arg-Leu-Gly-Thr-Gln-Trp-Ala-Val-Gly-His-Leu-Met-NH$_2$; an amphibian peptide biologically related to gastrin releasing peptide. Thirteen of the amino acid moieties are identical with those of bombesin.

Alzheimer's disease: Alzheimer's dementia; a progressive, degenerative disease of the central nervous system that occurs in 10-20% of humans 80 years of age or older, in 1-5% at age 65, and earlier in small numbers of individuals (including ones with Down's syndrome who survive for five decades). Neurofibrillary tangles accumulate within neurons of the cerebral cortex and hippocampus, extracellular neuritic plaques form, and β-**amyloid** (*q.v.*) deposits in cerebral blood vessels. The cerebral ventricles dilate, neuroglial cells proliferate excessively, some neurons die, acetylcholine synthesis declines, and the relative numbers of acetylcholine receptor subtypes change. Degenerative changes have also been detected in the cerebellum and some other brain regions. Memory loss is the first overt symptom. Language and visuo-spatial skills then decline, and there are behavioral changes. Late manifestations include disorientation, dementia, skeletal muscle weakness, and other defects that lead to dependence on nursing care. Several kinds of indirect evidence are consistent with etiologies related to mutations of genes on chromosome 21 (the one present in an extra copy in Down's syndrome), especially in families in which early onset occurs. It has been proposed that excessive production of amyloid precursor protein (APP) leads to increased processing via lysosomal pathways, with formation of insoluble, protease-resistant fragments that then mediate the pathological changes. Alternatively, a secreted protease that normally degrades the peptides is not made in sufficient amounts. Some unsuccessful attempts to treat the condition with Tacrine and other acetylcholinesterase antagonists, or with choline precursor, have been attributed to loss of neurons that make the neurotransmitter. Cholinergic agonists (which invoke undesired side-effects) have also not yet proven beneficial. Other agents considered include substance P and estrogens. Although some observers suggest that

delivery of nerve growth factor (NGF) to specific sites should stimulate affected neurons and prolong their survival, others believe that it augments β-amyloid toxicity.

Amadori arrangement: *see* **nonenzymatic glycosylation**.

amalgam: a *Drosophila* **gene** that codes for a protein related to vertebrate cell adhesion molecule N-CAM.

amanitins: α-, β, and γ- amanitins, amatin, and related toxins made by *Amanita phalloides* that block mRNA synthesis by inhibiting RNA polymerase II enzymes. The most potent of them, α-amanitin (shown above) is used to determine whether new protein synthesis is essential for the actions of hormones and other regulators. Ingestion of the mushrooms is followed after some time by salivation, vomiting, and bloody stools. Cyanosis, convulsions and other effects lead to death within 15 hours.

amantadine: tricyclo[3.3.1.1.[3,7]]decan-1-amine; an antiviral agent effective against influenza A and some other enveloped viruses. It lowers vesicle pH, and its ability to release dopamine has been used to treat Parkinsonism.

a mating factor: *see* **mating factors**.

Amberlite: a trade name for a group of ion-exchange resins. Some are used for hemodialysis.

ambiguous genitalia: external reproductive organs not clearly recognizable as male or female. Androgens made by defective embryonic and fetal adrenal glands are major causes of masculinization in human females; *see* also **adrenogenital syndrome** and **virilization**. In males, masculinization is impaired by prenatal androgen and/or 5α-reductase deficiency, and by androgen receptor defects. The conditions can also occur in genetic mosaics and chimeras.

ambisexual: (1) having both male and female characteristics; (2) experiencing and/or displaying sexual interest in both males and females of the species.

Ambystoma mexicanum: the Mexican axolotl. Although neotenous, this salamander responds to exogenous thyroid and pituitary gland hormones, and is used to study metamorphosis and limb regeneration.

ameboid: ameba-like; *see* **ameboid movement**.

ameboid movement: cell migration that resembles the movements of *Amoeba proteus* and some other protozoa, accomplished by extending pseudopods. Neutrophilic leukocytes and other phagocytes use it to traverse narrow passageways, such as spaces between endothelial cells.

ameloblasts: enameloblasts; enamel-forming cells.

amenorrhea: failure to menstruate, a condition that occurs physiologically in female adult primates during pregnancy, after menopause, and (under certain conditions) in association with lactation. Abnormal causes include incomplete ovarian, Müllerian duct, pituitary gland, or hypothalamic maturation, ovarian dysgenesis, polycystic ovary disease, uterine cervix canal obstruction, psychogenic factors, and postnatal endocrine system dysfunctions of the hypothalamus, pituitary, thyroid, or adrenal glands. Delayed menarche, and cessation of established menstrual cycles, that are associated with malnutrition, very strenuous physical activity, or other factors that severely deplete body fat stores, have been variously attributed to inadequate extra-ovarian conversion of androgens to estrogens, excessive amounts of opioid peptides, and changes in pineal gland activities.

amensalism: *see* **symbiosis**.

amethopterin: *see* **methotrexate**.

AMF: autocrine motility factor.

amfonelic acid: 7-benzyl-1-ethyl-1,4-dihydro-4-oxo-1,8-naphthyridine-3-carboxylic acid; an agent that enhances dopamine release in response to electrical stimulation.

α-amidating peptidyl monooxygenase: PAM; *see* **peptidyl α-amidating monooxygenase**.

amidation: conversion of carboxyl (—COOH) to amide (—CONH$_2$) groups. Amidation markedly alters the biological properties of α-melanocyte stimulating and some other hormones.

amidorphin: Tyr-Gly-Gly-Phe-Met-Lys-Lys-Met-Asp-Glu-Leu-Tyr-Pro-Leu-Glu-Val-Glu-Glu-Glu-Ala-Asn-Gly-Gly-Gly-Val-Leu-NH$_2$; a *C*-terminal amidated peptide composed of amino acids 104-126 of preproenkephalin A. It is the most abundant cleavage product in the adrenal medulla, in which it can serve directly as a neurotransmitter or hormone, or undergo additional breaks to yield metenkephalins and other small, biologically active peptides. In brain, but not adrenal gland, it is cleaved to amidorphin [8-26], which lacks the *N*-terminal metenkephalin sequence and appears to be devoid of opioid type biological activity.

amiloride: 3,5-diamino-*N*-(aminoiminomethyl)-6-chloropyrzinecarboxamide; an acylguanide antibiotic that inhibits Na$^+$/Cl$^-$ cotransport and Na$^+$/H$^+$ antiport, but does not affect tetrodotoxin-sensitive Na$^+$ currents. It opposes aldosterone actions, and is used as a diuretic, but is not an antagonist for intracellular aldosterone receptors. It is also reported to inhibit kinase C isozymes, and to block T type (low threshold) Ca^{2+} channels via mechanisms unrelated to the influences on antiport.

amiloride sensitive channels: Na$^+$ ion channels on epithelial cell apical microvillar domains that can be blocked by amiloride and related agents. Polarities essential for unidirectional ion movements are maintained by associations with ankyrin, which links the channels to cytoskeletal fodrin (or spectrin).

ethylisopropyl-amiloride: an amiloride analog 100 times more potent than the parent compound.

amine: any molecule with one or more free -NH$_2$ groups. Examples include norepinephrine, dopamine, serotonin, and histamine. Melatonin and acetylcholine are substituted amines. *See* also **amino acids** and **polyamines**.

amino acids: organic compounds that contain at least one -NH$_2$, and one -COOH. The most common types are L-α- (with an amino group attached to the carbon atom adjacent to the carboxyl terminal). Proline and hydroxyproline are *imino* acids (in which -NH-replaces the -NH$_2$), but they are classified as members of the group. In the general formula shown, R = —H for glycine, and —CH$_3$ for alanine. It represents longer aliphatic chains for some, and is aromatic in tyrosine and phenylalanine. In cysteine and methionine, it contains sulfur. The major *acidic* types (proton donors in the physiological pH range) are aspartic and glutamic, with two carboxyl groups (one at each end); and the major *basic* types (proton acceptors) are lysine and arginine, which have additional amino groups. *Neutral* types are **zwitterions**. Asparagine and glutamine are amides.

Essential amino acids must be supplied by the diet. *Glucogenic* amino acids can serve as sugar precursors, and *ketogenic* types are metabolizable to acetyl coenzyme A. (Some amino acids yield both end-products.) Cystine is made from two cysteines. Peptides and proteins are amino acid chains linked by peptide bonds. Some amino acids are modified after the proteins are formed. For example, tyrosines are iodinated when thyroglobulin is synthesized in thyroid glands (and some free iodotyrosines are liberated when the proteins are degraded). Collagen processing involves conversion of substantial numbers of proline and lysine components to hydroxyprolines and hydroxylysines, respectively. The most commonly used acronyms are shown in the table. Asx can designate either asparagine or aspartic acid, and is used if either form can occupy a position of a peptide or protein, or if the form is not known.

AMINO ACID	3-Letter	1-Letter
alanine	Ala	A
arginine	Arg	R
aspartic acid	Ans	D
cysteine	Cys	C
glutamic acid	Glu	E
glutamine	Gln	Q
glycine	Gly	G
histidine	His	H
isoleucine	Ile	I
leucine	Leu	L
lysine	Lys	K
methionine	Met	M
phenylalanine	Phe	F
proline	Pro	P
serine	Ser	S
threonine	Thr	T
tryptophan	Trp	W

Small quantities of molecules with amino groups in the β position are made by both prokaryotes and eukaryotes (see, e.g. **β-alanine**). Some microorganisms make D-amino acids, and D forms are present in many antibiotics. Synthetic peptides that contain them resist degradation, and are used for metabolic and hormone studies, and for some therapeutic purposes. Glutamic acid, aspartic acid, glycine, and arginine are examples of types that directly perform biological functions, but are also incorporated into peptides and proteins. Ornithine, citrulline, and taurine function directly, but are not protein components. Tyrosine and tryptophan are major precursors of amine-type regulators. *See* also specific amino acid types.

amino acid activation: reactions of the general type: AA + ATP →aminoacyl-AMP + P-P, in which AA represents any amino acid. Aminoacyl synthetases specific for amino acid types catalyze them, and also direct the next step that must precede translation: aminoacyl-AMP + tRNA → aminoacyl-tRNA + AMP.

amino acid oxidases: flavoprotein enzymes that catalyze oxidation of amino acids in reactions that use molecular oxygen. One group is specific for D, and another for L amino acids. A *monooxygenase* (mixed function oxidase) catalyzes overall pathways of the general type: amino acid + O_2 + NADH →hydroxy-amino acid + NAD^+ + H_2O, as in conversion of phenylalanine to tyrosine. (Intermediate steps, in which biopterins serve as electron carriers are not shown.) Aromatic components of amino acids are oxidized by *dioxygenases*. Different enzymes (*aminotransferases*) catalyze oxidative deamination.

amino acid transport: active transport, supported by energy released from ATP hydrolysis, and usually associated with Na^+ symport. The processes are required because amino acid concentrations are higher in cells than in extracellular fluids. Specific carriers have been identified for *neutral* (monoamino, monocarboxylic), *basic* (lysine, arginine, ornithine, and cysteine), *dicarboxylic* (glutamic and aspartic) and *imino* (proline) types. Members of a group compete with each other for a common carrier. Some amino acids can use more than one carrier. For example, glycine binds to the first and fourth, and asparagine to the first and third.

aminoacyl-tRNAs: amino acids linked to their specific transfer RNA types. They bind to mRNA anticodons during protein synthesis. *See* also **amino acid activation** and **ribosomes**.

aminoacyl-tRNA sites: A sites; ribosome components that bind aminoacyl-tRNAs during **translation** *(q.v.)*. Cf **peptidyl sites**.

aminoacyl-tRNA synthases: enzymes that catalyze both amino acid activation and formation of aminoacyl-tRNAs.

α-**aminoadipic acid**, αAA: an NMDA receptor agonist.

3-**aminobenzamide**: a competitive inhibitor of poly(ADP-ribose) polymerase that accelerates DNA amplification responses to environmental changes and drugs, blocks NAD^+ depletion by streptozotocin and other agents, and can enhance drug resistance. It also exerts antineoplastic activity by damaging DNA and causing production of short strands.

O-**aminobenzoic acid**: 2-aminobenzoic acid; anthranilic acid; vitamin L_1; an intermediate in the pathway for bacterial synthesis of purine and pyridimine nucleotides, tryptophan, and histidine, purported to be essential for supporting lactation in mammals. It reacts with phosphoribosyl pyrophosphate to form *N*-5′-phosphoribosylanthranilate. Calcium aminobenzoate is used as an as-caricide for swine.

p-**aminobenzoic acid**: PABA; *see* **para-aminobenzoic acid**.

γ-**aminobutyric acid**: GABA; *see* **gamma aminobutyric acid**.

ε-**aminocaproic acid**: 6-amino hexanoic acid; a serine protease inhibitor used to treat menorrhagia and other conditions in which bleeding and clot formation are associated high plasmin activity. Its antifibrinolytic activity and ability to block ovulation are attributed to inhibition of tissue plasminogen (tPA).

aminocyclobutane-*cis*-1,3-dicarboxylic acid: a selective agonist for NMDA type receptors.

N-**aminodeanol chloride**: 1,1-dimethyl-1-(2-hydroxyethyl)hydrazinium chloride; a false transmitter used as a probe for cholinergic functions.

aminoglutethimide: AG; 3-(4-aminophenyl)-3-ethyl-2,6-piperidinedione; an anticonvulsant that inhibits cholesterol side-chain cleavage, and thereby cholesterol conversion to pregnenolone. High concentrations additionally inhibit $11\beta^-$, 18^-, and cholecalciferol-25 hydroxylases, and aromatases. Since its use for hormone biosynthesis is severely impaired, cholesterol accumulates in steroidogenic tissues, and the negative feedback controls those hormones normally exert on adenohypophysial cells and hypothalamic neurons are compromised. Some direct effects of AG on adrenocorticotropic hormone (ACTH) secretion have also been proposed. The agent is used in the diagnosis of glucocorticoid secretion disorders, to treat Cushing's syndrome and some forms of breast cancer, and as a laboratory tool.

α-**aminoisobutyric acid**: AIB; AIBA: 2-methylalanine; a non-metabolizable artificial amino acid that binds to alanine carriers, and is used to study amino acid uptake.

β-**aminoisobutyric acid**: a thymine degradation product.

N-methyl-**aminoisobutyric acid**: MeAIB: a non-metabolizable artificial amino acid used in transport studies. Its affinity for carriers differs somewhat from that of α-aminoisobutyric acid.

aminoguanidine: guanyl hydrazine; a diamine oxidase inhibitor that blocks putrescine conversion to gamma aminobutyric acid (GABA).

p-**aminohippuric acid**: PAH; *see* **para-amino hippuric acid**.

α-**amino-3-hydroxy-5-methylisoxazole propionic acid**: AMPA; a quisqualate receptor agonist.

δ-**aminolevulinic acid**: 5-amino-4-oxo-valeric acid; an intermediate in the pathway for biosynthesis of porphyrins and related compounds. It is made from glycine and succinyl coenzyme A.

aminooxyacetic acid: an agent used to inhibit GABA-α-oxotransaminase, which catalyzes the reaction: GABA + α-ketoglutarate → succinic semialdehyde + glutamate. Although its effects are theoretically reversible, they usually cause accumulation of GABA.

$$H_2N—O—CH_2—COOH$$

aminopeptidases: enzymes that cleave amino acids from peptide and protein *N*-terminals.

2-aminophosphobutyrate: APB; an NMDA receptor antagonist.

$$^-OOC—\underset{H}{\overset{NH_2}{C}}—CH_2—CH_2—O—PO_3H_2$$

2-D-amino-7-phosphonoheptanoate: D-AP7; 2-APH; an NMDA receptor antagonist.

$$^-OOC—\underset{H}{\overset{NH_2}{C}}—CH_2—CH_2—CH_2—CH_2—CH_2—O—PO_3H_2$$

2-D-amino-5-phosphonopropionate: an antagoist for phosphpoinositide-coupled metabotropic excitatory amino acid receptors.

$$^-OOC—\underset{H}{\overset{NH_2}{C}}—CH_2—O—PO_3H_2$$

2-D-amino-5-phosphonovalerate: D-AP5; 2-APV; a selective, competitive NMDA receptor antagonist.

$$^-OOC—\underset{H}{\overset{NH_2}{C}}—CH_2—CH_2—CH_2—O—PO_3H_2$$

aminophylline: theophylline and ethylenediamine. The combination is used as a diuretic, cardiac stimulant, vasodilator, and bronchodilator.

3-aminopropane sulfonic acid: APS; a GABA receptor agonist.

$$H_3C—\underset{H}{\overset{NH_2}{C}}—CH_2—OSO_3H$$

aminopterin: 4-aminofolic acid; 4-aminopteroylglutamic acid; an anitmetabolite used as an insecticide; *see* also **folic acid** and **methotrexate**.

2-aminopurine: 2-AP; a purine analog that can incorporate into DNA and cause transition mutations. It inhibits heme-dependent and dsRNA-dependent synthesis of eukaryote initiation factor (eIF-2α, eIF-2a) kinase, and of kinases needed for viral induction of interferon-β. It also inhibits serum-independent induction of *c-fos* and *c-myc*, and lipopolysaccharide and phorbol ester mediated induction of tumor necrosis factor-α (TNFα). In hamster (but not in human or murine) cells, it is reported to overcome the mitotic arrest caused by drugs that inhibit DNA replication.

4-aminopyridine: an agent used to block potassium channels.

9-amino-1,2,3,4-tetrahydroacridine; Tacrine; an inhibitor of cholinesterases that may exert beneficial effects in some individuals with Alzheimer's disease.

1-amino-1*H*-2,4-triazole: an agent used to inhibit catalases.

amiodarone: (2-butyl-3-benzofuranyl)[4-[2-(diethylamino) ethyoxy]3,5-diiodophenyl]methanone; an agent effective against life-threatening ventricular tachycardias. It was initially introduced for alleviating angina pectoris, but other actions preclude its use in patients who respond to safer vasodilators. It frequently invokes liver disease, and exerts deleterious influences on the corneas of the eyes. Amiodarone is structurally related to thyroxine (T_4), and many of its effects (including lowering of mysoin Ca^{2+}-ATPase activity in the heart, and stimulation of thyrotropin [TSH] synthesis in the pituitary gland) are

aminopterin

amiodarone

attributed to interactions with triiodothyronine (T_3) receptors. It also antagonizes the effects of T_3 on expression of adrenergic receptors in the heart. Additionally, it inhibits the 5'-deiodinase that catalyzes conversion of T_4 to T_3, slows deiodination of reverse T_3 (rT_3), affects cellular uptake of T_3, and lowers the circulating levels of albumin and prealbumin (but not of thyronine binding globulin). The consequences in most patients are high circulating T_4, low T_3, and small elevations of TSH and rT_3, with euthyroidism. However, it appears to exacerbate underlying autoimmune thyroid disease, and can invoke hypothyroidism in some individuals, as well as hyperthyroidism in subjects who are iodine deficient.

amitriptyline hydrochloride: Elavil; 3-(10,11-dihydryo-5-*H*-dibenzo[*a,d*]cyclohepten-5-ylidine)-*N,N*-dimethyl-1-propanamine hydrochloride; a **tricyclic antidepressant** (*q.v.*), used to treat some forms of psychic depression and compulsive behavior. At least some of the effects are attributed to inhibition of norepinephrine uptake by neurons. However, although the inhibition occurs soon after administration, therapeutic benefits are not manifested before two or more weeks of treatment. Claims that amitriptyline exerts fewer "side-effects" than imipramine on histaminergic and cholinergic functions have not been universally accepted.

ammonia: NH_3; a volatile compound released when amino acids are deaminated. It rapidly combines with H^+ to form NH_4^+ ions which are neurotoxic. In the liver (the major site for gluconeogenesis), most of the ions are rapidly converted to urea. Ammonium ions generated in the kidneys are directly excreted to the urine. Renal production accelerates in response to acidosis, and it ameliorates the conditions, since excretion in association with Cl^-, phosphates, and other anions facilitates Na^+ conservation. *See also* **ammonium chloride**.

ammonium chloride: NH_4Cl; a salt that transiently invokes diuresis, and is sometimes used for short time periods to alleviate edema. The liver rapidly converts the ammonium ions to urea. The chloride ions are then excreted with Na^+ and other cations, and water is osmotically drawn to the urine; and the urea produced may contribute to the water loss. Urine acidity increases (in part because less bicarbonate enters). Sodium depletion soon leads to development of metabolic acidosis, which additionally facilitates water loss. However, the effects are transient, because metabolic acidosis soon stimulates NH_4^+ production in the kidneys (*see also* **ammonia**), and

the Na^+ depletion and the associated water loss can increase renin release and aldosterone secretion.

amnioblasts: embryonic cells derived from ectoderm that form the amnion.

amniocentesis: insertion of a needle through the maternal abdomen into amniotic fluid, usually to draw fluid and cells for analysis, infuse dyes for radiographic studies, or induce abortion.

amnion: the thin, tough, transparent innermost embryonic/fetal membrane, derived from ectoderm and backed with mesoderm. It lines the fluid filled cavity that surrounds the conceptus. *See also* **amniotic fluid**.

amniotes: mammals, some reptiles (e.g. turtles, crocodilians, and squamates) and other species in which an amnion develops.

amniotic fluid: the fluid secreted by amnioblasts that accumulates in the amnion. It provides mechanical protection and a site for fetal:maternal exchange of regulators, nutrients, and metabolic wastes.

amobarbital: *see* **Amytal**.

amoeboid movement: ameboid movement.

amorphic: describes genes that do not code for proteins; *cf* **amorphous**.

amorphous: without definite form; describes, for example, non-crystalline matter.

amoxapine: 2-chloro-11-(1-piperazinyl)dibenz[b,f][1,4]-oxazepine; a **tricyclic antidepressant** (*q.v.*) that inhibits neuronal norepinephrine uptake.

AMP: adenine-ribose-phosphate; *see* **adenosine monophosphate** and **ATP**.

AMPA: *see* **α-amino-3-hydroxy-5-methylisoxazole-propionic acid**.

amphenone-B: 3,3-bis(*p*-aminophenyl)-2-butanone; an agent that invokes necrosis of the zona fasciculata and zona fasciculata of the adrenal cortex, and inhibits several enzymes required for steroidogenesis (including 11β-, 17α-, and 21- hydroxylases and $\Delta^{4,5}$-ketoisomerase). It is used to study steroid hormone synthesis, and (to a limited extent) to treat Cushing's syndrome. It also exerts some anti-estrogen effects.

amphetamine: racemic β-aminopropylbenzene; deoxynorephedrine; orally effective drugs, chemically related to catecholamines. Although both forms are powerful central nervous system stimulants, the D isomer (dexedrine) is more potent, whereas the L form (benzedrine) exerts greater cardiovascular effects. Both transiently elevate mood, improve mental and physical performance, and can invoke euphoria. The effects are usually followed by psychic depression and physical fatigue; and repeated use can lead to addiction. (The street term is "speed".) High doses elevate systolic and diastolic blood pressures, and can cause headache, dizziness, tremors, restlessness, insomnia, and agitation in humans, and stereotyped behavior in laboratory animals. "Psychotic" symptoms, including disorientation, hallucinations and delusions, persist in some individuals who have taken repeated high doses, even after the drugs are withdrawn. Paradoxically, amphetamines can abolish seizures in some forms of epilepsy. They have also been reported to relieve restlessness and improve attention span in hyerpactive children (but ritalin is more commonly used). Their ability to stimulate urinary bladder sphincter muscle can alleviate enuresis and urinary incontinence. Since they suppress appetite (probably via influences on the ventromedial hypothalamus), elevate the metabolic rate, and inhibit gastrointestinal tract functions, they were at one time used to treat some forms of obesity. Their long-range effectiveness has been questioned (since tolerance develops), and the drugs are usually considered too toxic for this purpose. Amphetamines transiently prolong the effects of endogenous catecholamines by inhibiting their uptake across neuronal membranes, but can slowly deplete the regulators by accelerating their degradation. Many effects are attributed to elevation of norepinephrine levels, but amphetamines also promote dopamine release, and large doses additionally release serotonin. Some actions may involve binding to adrenergic and serotonin receptors, but others appear to be mediated via different types which may be identical with phenylethanolamine sites.

amphi-: a prefix meaning two, both, or either, as in amphibian or amphipathic.

amphibian: (1) capable of living both on land and in water; (2) an animal that spends part of its time on land and part in water, or lives in water during some phases of its life-span and on land at other times; (3) an animal of the class *Amphibia*, which includes frogs, toads, and salamanders. Most are aquatic during larval stages, and later develop lungs; but some (for example mudpuppies) retain gills throughout life. With few exceptions, land-living adults return to water for mating.

amphidiploid: allotetraploid; describes a tetraploid organism that possesses a complete set of diploid genes derived from one parental species plus another complete set from a different species.

amphimixis: sexual reproduction.

amphipathic: having both hydrophilic and hydrophobic chemical groups. Phospholipids and most proteins are amphipathic.

amphiphenazole: *see* **DAPT**.

amphiregulin: AR; a secreted 78-amino acid heparin binding growth factor initially identified in a human breast cancer cell line, and subsequently shown to accumulate in most colorectal cancers. Small amounts are made by some epithelial cells, but the levels in gastrointestinal mucosa are very low. AR shares homology with epidermal and transforming growth factors (EGF and TGFα), binds to 170K EGF receptors, and activates the receptor tyrosine kinases. In common with EGF and TGFα, it stimulates the growth of keratinocytes and some other normal epithelial cell types, and of some epidermal cancer cells. However, it is less potent than EGF on the kidney, and does not promote anchorage-independent growth in the presence of transforming growth factor-β (TGF-β). It also binds to ERRB3, but its primary receptor seems to be ERBB2; *cf* **heregulin**. Since AR can inhibit the growth of MCF-7 breast cancer and some other malignant cell types, and abrogate the effects of TGFα on growth of cells that over-express the EGF receptor, it may protect against the development of some kinds of neoplasms.

ampholytes: substances that carry both positive and negative charges.

amphoteric: describes compounds that accept protons at low pHs and donate them at higher ones.

amphotericin B: a polyene antifungal agent made by *Streptomyces nodosus*. It exerts some aldosterone-like effects by accelerating passive transport of Na^+ across cell membranes.

amplexus: clasping, a form of behavior used to accomplish fertilization. Male frogs use large thumbs to maintain their hold on and squeeze the abdomens of females. When the females release eggs, the males release sperm. (The frogs also clasp small rocks and other objects during the mating season if no females are present.)

amplification: *see* **gene amplification**.

AMP-PNP: an ATP analog in which a nitrogen atom replaces the β phosphate. Since it resists hydrolysis by ATPases, it can be used to determine whether ATP re-

amphotericin B

quirements for some processes depend on the release of energy and inorganic phosphate.

amprotropin phosphate: Syntropan; α-(hydroxymethyl)-benzeneactic acid 3-(diethylamino)-2,2-dimethylpropyl ester phosphate; an agent used to relieve smooth muscle spasm, mostly by acting as a muscarinic type acetylcholine receptor antagonist.

ampulla: a small, sac-like dilation of a tube or canal, usually located near its origin or termination.

ampullary-isthmic junction: AIJ; the constricted region of the Fallopian tube that serves as the major site for fertilization in mammals.

amrinone: 5-amino-(3,4'-bipyridin)-6-(1H)-one; a non-glycosidic agent with selective inotropic properties that is used as a cardiac stimulant.

AMV: avian myeloblastosis virus.

amygdala: paired neuron clusters in the dorsomedial regions of the temporal lobes of the brain. Although regarded by some authors as basal ganglia complexes, they are limbic system components that contribute to the control of growth hormone and glucocorticoid secretion rhythms and other endocrine functions, and to initiation of behavioral responses to olfactory and other signals. Roles in learning and memory have also been described.

amygdalin: laetrile; [[6-O-β-D-glucopyranosyl-β-D-glucopryanosyl)oxy]-benzeneacetonitrile; a toxic substance obtained from the seeds of bitter almonds that is also present in peach and apricot seeds. It has been called vitamin B_{17} (although there is no evidence that it functions as a vitamin). Its purported beneficial effects in individuals with cancers have not been substantiated. (See structure on p. 34.)

amygdaloid: almond-shaped.

amylases: enzymes that catalyze cleavage of α1 → 4 glucosidic linkages of starch, glycogen, and their degradation products. They are secreted by pancreatic acinar cells and salivary glands, and are also made by microorganisms and plants. The α- types are endoamylases that act on polysaccharides and oligosaccharides. Exoamylases (from plants and microorganisms) include β- types that cleave maltose units from the ends of carbohydrate chains, and γ-amylases (glucoamylases) which release glucose.

amylins: diabetes associated peptides; DAPs; peptides chemically similar to calcitonin gene related peptide (CGRP) that inhibit basal and insulin-stimulated glycogenesis in skeletal muscle, and accelerate Cori cycle reactions. They are major components of normal intracellular pancreatic islet amyloid. The levels rise in many individuals with diabetes mellitus, and some peptide is released to extracellular fluid. The human type has the amino acid sequence: H₂N-Lys-Cys-Asn-Thr-Ala-Thr-Cys-Ala-Thr-Gln-Arg-Leu-Ala-Asn-Phe-Leu-Val-His-Ser-Ser-Asn-Asn-Phe-Gly-Ala-Ile-Leu-Ser-Ser-Thr-Asn-Val-Gly-Ser-Asn-Thr-Tyr-NH₂.

amyloid: starch-like, a term applied to some proteins and other opalescent substances that physically resemble starches. *See* also **amyloidosis**, **β-amyloid protein**, and **acute phase proteins**.

amygdalin

amyloidosis: diseases in which extracellular hyaline (amyloid) fibrils form around, and can can constrict and damage the liver, heart, kidney, spleen, gastrointestinal tract, joints, blood vessels, and/or brain. In primary (AL) types, B lymphocyte or plasma cell dyscrasias lead to release of immunoglobulin light chain fragments that form the fibrils. In secondary, reactive (AA) types, the fibril protein derives from amyloid A (an acute phase lipoprotein that accumulates in individuals with chronic inflammatory diseases). All of the deposits additionally contain serum amyloid P (SAP), a normal blood component.

amyloid precursor protein: APP; several closely related sulfated glycoproteins whose synthesis is directed by a gene in the q21 band on the long arm of human chromosome 21. Alternate mRNA splicings lead to production of APPs 770, 751, 714, and 695, all of which contain the amino acid sequence for β-amyloid protein, the major component of neurofibrillary tangles that accumulate in individuals with Down's and Alzheimer's diseases, and of APP 563 which does not. They are made in all embryonic and mature tissues, but the types display differential distributions and change with development. Whereas the amounts of APPs 770 and 751 are similar in the central nervous system and peripheral tissues, APP 695 predominates in brain neurons (which also make AP 563). In humans, the relative amounts of the 751 form increase with age. The promoters contain components that bind translation factor AP-1, and ones that recognize heat-shock factors. APPs insert into plasma membranes, in which most are cleaved by a secretase. Some of the products are released to cerebrospinal fluid and blood, and are substrates for extracellular enzymes that catalyze formation of soluble 4K and 3K fragments. However, the proteins additionally contain an amino acid sequence required for incorporation into clathrin-coated vesicles, and cleavage by lysosomal enzymes releases different products. Proteins 770, 751, and 563 have a Kunitz protease-inhibitor domain, and the secreted form of APP 751 is identical to protein nexin II, which acts extracellularly. The enzymes they inhibit include trypsin, chymotrypsin, blood coagulation factor XIa, a protease associated with the γ subunit of nerve growth factor, and a protease that cleaves EGF-BP (epidermal growth factor binding protein). The APPs that accumulate in blood platelet α granules are believed to function in coagulation control. Abnormal platelet membranes may expose sites for activation that lead to excessive release to the bloodstream. The proteins also display growth-promoting activity and may contribute to tissue repair and wound healing. Individuals with Down's syndrome have an extra copy of chromosome 21; and unusually high APP751:APP695 ratios, and mutations in the region that directs APP synthesis have been detected in some families with Alzheimer's disease. Suggested causes of β-amyloid deposition in the brains include overproduction of APPs, which consequent acceleration of lysosomal processing, formation of abnormal proteins that undergo cleavages at unusual sites, and inability to make sufficient secretase.

β-amyloid peptide: A-4; β-A4; a 4K protein that accumulates in neurofibrillary tangles in the cerebral cortex and hippocampus of individuals with Alzheimer's disease and Down's syndrome. Substantial amounts are also found in the brains of normal infants and elderly persons. Nerve growth factor stimulates its production. Neurotropic effects similar to those exerted by epidermal growth factor, and roles in central nervous system regeneration have been proposed, but A-4 is also implicated in neuron deterioration and apoptosis. The amino acid sequence for β-amyloid [1-28] is: H$_2$-N-Asp-Ala-Glu-Phe-Arg-His-Asp-Ser-Gly-Tyr-Gln-Val-His-His-Gln-Lys-Leu-Val-Phe-Phe-Ala-Glu-Asp-Val-Gly-Ser-Asn-Lys-OH. Smaller fragments, including β-amyloid [12-28], have been identified.

amyotrophic lateral sclerosis: ALS; a progressive disorder in which skeletal muscle degeneration is attributed to neuron dysfunction. It may be caused by glutamate toxicity.

Amytal: amobarbital: 5-ethyl-5-isopentylbarbituric acid; an agent used clinically as a sedative, and in the laboratory to block transfer of electrons from FAD to ubiquinone in mitochondria.

ANA: anti-nuclear antibodies.

Anabolex: a trade name for stanolone.

anabolic: building up; growth-promoting.

anabolic steroids: androgen analogs designed to achieve greater protein synthesizing effects than the naturally occurring gonadal steroids. They are used clinically to some extent to accelerate growth in premature infants, hasten convalescence following debilitating illnesses in adults, accelerate bone fracture healing in older individuals, and treat osteoporosis. Their androgenic and anti-estrogen actions have also been used to treat endometriosis, and some forms of breast cancer. Some kinds are taken illegally by athletes to augment skeletal muscle mass and strength, and to improve endurance. The effects are attributed in part to increased motivation and ability to participate in demanding training. Prolonged use of large amounts can invoke liver dysfunction (with increased susceptibility for developing liver cancer), atherosclerosis, sterility, gynecomastia in males, virilization in females, mood disturbances such as uncontrolled rage and aggression, and "psychotic" symptoms.

anabolism: building up; metabolic pathways in which amino acids and other small molecules are used to synthesize larger ones. *Cf* **catabolism**.

Anadrol: a trade name for oxymetholone.

ANAE: α-naphthylesterase.

anaerobic: without air; describes organisms, chemical reactions, or metabolic pathways (such as glycolysis) that do not require molecular oxygen.

anagen: the growth phase of a hair cycle; *cf* **catagen** and **telogen**.

analgesics: agents that block pain sensations but not other forms of sensory perception; *cf* **anesthetics**.

analog; analogue; a substance chemically related to a another, usually one designed to achieve special properties such water solubility, resistance to degradation, ability to cross membranes, or high affinity for cell components. Some analogs are more potent than the orginal compounds, exert more sustained actions, and are effective when administered orally. Others are potent antagonists.

analogous structures: body components that perform the same kinds of functions in different species, but do not necessarily develop in the same way, for example the wings of bats and the wings of birds; *cf* **homologous**.

analysis of variance: ANOVA; statistical procedures that permit partitioning of the total **variance** (*q.v.*) of a population, to separate out the effects of two or more independent factors. For example, when sham operations are performed, the hormonal and metabolic consequences of surgically removing an endocrine gland can be separated from the effects of the anesthesia, stress, and trauma.

anamnesis: memory.

anamnestic responses: responses that depend on previous experience, for example secondary immune responses.

anandamide: arachidonylethanolamide; an arachidonic acid metabolite identified in brain that binds to cannabinoid receptors.

anandamide

anandron: nilutamide; 5,5-dimethyl-3-[4-nitro-3-(trifluoromethyl)phenyl]-2,4-imidazolidinedione; a nonsteroidal androgen receptor antagonist under investigation for use in the treatment of prostate gland cancers.

anaphase: the stage of mitosis or meiosis during which chromosomes move to opposite poles of the cell. It is preceded by metaphase and followed by telophase.

anaphase lag: slow or delayed movement of one or more chromosomes during anaphase. Sex chromosomes display this, and are are sometimes extruded.

anaphylatoxins: anaphylactins: small peptides (C3a and C5a) generated in the alternate pathway for complement activation. They bind to mast cells and basophilic leukocytes, promote release of histamine and other mediators, and can invoke immediate sensitivity reactions. The term was initially applied to antigens that bind IgE.

anaphylaxis: acute, systemic, antigen-specific immune system responses invoked by exposure to foreign substances, mediated primarily by IgE and consequent release of mediators. They can be initiated in sensitized individuals by plant allergens, bee-stings and other chemicals, and by transfusion of incompatible blood. The manifestations can include bronchospasm, edema, diarrhea, vomiting, and circulatory shock.

anaplasia: de-differentiation; loss of normal cell morphology and functions.

anaplerosis: filling up; repair; restoration; describes chemical reactions that reestablish adequate levels of crucial metabolic intermediates, for example ones that normalize tricarboxylic acid cycle functions by promoting pyruvate conversion to oxaloacetate.

Anapolon: a trade name for oxymetholone.

anatoxin A: ANTX-a; 1-(9-azabicyclo[4.2.1]non-2-en-2-yl)-ethanone; a nicotonic receptor antagonist that acts on neuromuscular junctions.

Anavar: a trade name for oxandrolone.

ancestral genes: DNA components of organisms that lived a long time ago (and may now be extinct) which have undergone duplications, mutations, and/or rearrangements and are progenitors of molecules made by modern species. For example, the genes that direct the synthesis of growth hormones and prolactins share sequence homologies, and are believed to derive from a common ancestral DNA segment.

anchorage dependence: the requirement for cells to attach to a substrate to achieve growth and proliferation. Many kinds of tumor cells become anchorage-independent, and can be grown in suspensions.

androgen[s]: 5α-dihydrotestosterone, testosterone, related steroid hormones, and synthetic analogs that direct male-type differentiation and maturation of accessory reproductive structures and secondary sex characteristics, maintain the associated functions, and support spermatogenesis. They also exert anabolic effects (for example on skeletal muscle), augment erythropoiesis, contribute to negative feedback controls over luteinizing and gonadotropin releasing hormone (LH and GnRH) secretion, promote bone maturation, induce liver and kidney enzymes, affect mood, appetite and behavior, and perform other functions. Naturally occurring types are 19-carbon steroids with oxy groups attached to carbons 3 and 17. The interstitial cells of the testes are the major sources of circulating androgens in males. Adrenal glands of humans and some other species make "weak" androgens that are converted to more potent regulators. They are important in females (but aromatases convert androgens to estrogens in ovaries, skin, adipose tissue, some neurons, and elsewhere). Testosterone induces 5α-reductase, which catalzyes conversion of testosterone to dihydrotestosterone (DHT). Although testosterone acts directly on some cell types, and different metabolites perform special functions, DHT is the primary ligand for androgen receptors in most target cells.

androgen binding proteins: ABPs; 90K dimeric glycoproteins, different from androgen receptors, that bind androgens with high affinities. They are made by Sertoli cells of humans and other species, secreted to testicular fluid, and concentrated in the epididymis. Follicle stimulating hormone (FSH) stimulates their synthesis, and testosterone indirectly maintains high levels. The livers of adult humans, rabbits, and many other species (and of fetal rats) secrete testosterone-estrogen binding proteins with similar or identical amino acid sequences, but different oligosaccharides.

androgenesis: development of a haploid embryo whose genome derives exclusively from paternal chromosomes, accomplished when the maternal nucleus of a fertilized ovum degenerates. This form of development occurs in a few species, but is not possible in mammals.

androgenic: invoking masculinization or virilization.

androgenous: (1) preferentially producing male offspring; *cf* **androgynous**; (2) in nonscientific discussions and publications, it can mean male-like.

androgen receptors; ARs; molecules that bind androgens with high affinity and mediate their actions. The term usually refers to intracellular "classical" types (*see* also **steroid hormone receptors**). These are species-specific glycoproteins whose synthesis is directed by X chromosome genes. 5-α-dihydrotestosterone (DHT) is the major ligand for most cell types, but testosterone can bind when present in high concentrations. In humans, a 917 amino acid precursor yields 76K and 110 forms. Both 76K and N-terminal extended 94K types are made by rats. Ligand binding leads to temperature-dependent "activation" that confers high affinity for **androgen response elements** *(q.v.)* that regulate gene transcription. Some androgen actions involve binding to other kinds of receptors which have not been characterized.

androgen response elements: AREs; DNA base sequences that bind components of dimerized, ligand-bound androgen receptors, and regulate the expression of specific genes. The base sequences are of the general type GGTACAnnnTGTTCT, where n represents undefined components. Similar (but not identical) DNA base sequences bind occupied estrogen, progesterone, glucocorticoid, mineralocorticoid, triiodothyronine, and retinoic acid receptors. *See* also **steroid response elements**.

androgynous: having both male and female characteristics.

Androlone: a trade name for stanolone.

androstane: a 19-carbon "parent" compound used for nomenclature of androgens and related steroids. Androstane steroids have saturated A rings, with hydrogen atoms on carbon 5 in either α or β configurations. *Androstanediols* have alcoholic groups, usually at positions 3 and 17, and *androstanediones* have two ketone groups. *Androstenes* (including androstenediols and androstenediones) have unsaturated A rings. The positions of double bonds are indicated by superscript numbers that follow triangles (as in Δ^4), or by numbers of the first followed by a dash (as 4-ene). Some naturally occurring steroids related to androstane are biologically active, whereas others are degradation products. *See* also **steroids** and specific molecular types, and *cf* **pregnane** and **estrane**.

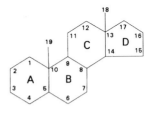

N,N-dimethyl-4-methyl-3-oxo-4-aza-5α-**androstane-17β-carboxamide**: DMAA; a 5α-reductase inhibitor, used mostly to block testosterone conversion to 5α-dihydrotestosterone. *See* 4-**MA**.

androstanediols: 19-carbon steroids with saturated A rings and two alcohol groups. *See* specific types and **androstane**.

5α-androstane-3α,17β-diol: a steroid hormone made from testosterone and 17α-hydroxypregnenolone that can be converted to DHT, but is not an aromatase substrate. It is implicated as a regulator of gonadotropin secretion, hair growth, and some prostate gland functions, and may be an autocrine growth factor for tumor cells. The amounts secreted by testicular, ovarian, and adrenocortical cells vary with the species.

5α-androstane-3α,17β-diol glucuronide: a conjugate of 5α-androstane-3α,17β-diol and glucuronic acid, excreted in urine. Large amounts can accumulate in the skins of hirsute women. Blood levels are used as indicators of dihydrotestosterone production.

5β-androstane-3α,17β-diol: an androgen metabolite that does not bind to dihydrotestosterone receptors.

androstanediones: steroids with saturated A rings and two ketone groups, usually on carbons 3 and 17. *See* **androstane** and **5α-androstane-3,17-dione**.

5α-androstane-3,17-dione: a metabolite derived from, and convertible to 5α-dihydrotes-tosterone.

5α-androstane-17β-ol-3-one: dihydrotestosterone.

1,4,6-androstatriene 3,17 dione; ATD; a steroid hormone analog used to inhibit aromatase enzymes.

androstenes: 19-carbon steroids with unsaturated rings. The most common sites for double bonds are between carbons 4 and 5 or 5 and 6. *See* **androstane** and **androstene-3,17-dione**.

Δ^4-**androstene-3,17-dione**: a major secretory product of immature Leydig cells, released in moderate amounts by adrenocortical cells of some species, and in smaller ones by ovaries. It can be made from testosterone, but progesterone is the major precursor. Many effects are attributed to conversion to testosterone or estrogens, but its ability to decrease inhibin levels in the immature testis does not seem to be mediated via receptors for those hormones.

Δ^5-**androstene-3,17-dione**: a steroid made from 17α-hydroxyprogesterone in the testis, ovary, and adrenal cortex of many species (including humans). At least some of the actions are attributed to conversion to testosterone and dihydrotestosterone.

Δ^5-**androstene-3-β-ol-17-one**: *see* **dehydroepiandrosterone**.

Δ^4-**androstene-3,16,17 trione**: a suicide inhibitor of aromatase enzymes.

Δ^4-**androstene-3-one,20-carboxylic acid**: a synthetic inhibitor of testosterone 5α-reductase.

6α-bromo-**androstene-3,17-dione**: a competitive inhibitor of aromatase enzymes.

6ß-bromo-**androstene-3,17-dione**: a suicide inhibitor of aromatases.

4-hydroxy-**androstenedione**: a potent aromatase inhibitor that exerts weak androgen-like effects.

19-hydroxy-**androstenedione**: a steroid secreted by adrenal glands that inhibits aromatase enzymes and raises blood pressure.

androstenone: 5α-androst-16-en-3-one; a volatile pheromone made by boars from testosterone, and secreted by kidneys and salivary glands. It stimulates reproductive behavior in sows. Small amounts are also made by androgen regulated human sweat glands. Most humans detect a somewhat unpleasant, musty odor. However, since a few do not when it is first presented, but can learn to do so after repeated exposure, it is used in studies of olfaction.

androsterone: 3α-hydroxy-5α-androstan-17-one; an androgen metabolite that is excreted to the urine. Its ability to exert testosterone-like effects is generally weak, and varies with the species.

anecdysis: the stage of the arthropod molting cycle during which newly formed shells harden.

anemia: conditions in which the blood contains subnormal quantities of hemoglobin and/or insufficient numbers of erythrocytes. In *microcytic* types (most commonly related to protein deficiencies), the cells are small but the total numbers can be in the normal range. Iron deficiency can lead to development of *hypochromic* types, in which the cells contain too little hemoglobin, and appear pale on blood smears. In *hemorrhagic* types, blood loss (often from internal vessels) invokes compensatory changes that include accelerated erythropoiesis and reticulocytosis. Similar changes can occur in response to *hemolytic* types, caused by phagocyte dysfunctions, pharmacological agents, or parasites. In *pernicious* anemias, there are too few cells, and the ones made are large, fragile, and misshapen. The major initiating factor is intrinsic factor deficiency that impairs absorption of vitamin B_{12} (which is essential for erythrocyte maturation). Other causes of anemia include deficiencies of folic acid and other vitamins, autoimmune diseases that destroy bone marrow cells, mutations that affect globin synthesis (*see* **sickle cell** and **Cooley's anemias**), and leukemias.

anergy: failure to mount immune responses to antigens that are usually effective stimulants for other members of the species.

anesthetics: agents that block perception of all sensory stimuli; *cf* **analgesics**. *General* anesthetics affect both central and peripheral nervous systems. *Local* ones act close to the sites of administration. They are often administered in combination with vasoconstrictors, to retard absorption into the systemic bloodstream.

anestrus: absence of estrous cycles, conditions that occur physiologically in most nonprimate female mammals of reproductively competent ages during pregnancy, and during reproductively quiescent phases in seasonal breeders. Progressively longer and more frequent periods of anestrus usually precede age-associated cessation of ovarian functions. In younger females, the major causes are ovarian, pituitary gland, or hypothalamic dysfunctions.

aneucentric: describes a chromosome with more than one centromere.

aneuploid: describes cells or individuals with abnormal chromosome numbers. The causes include deletions, duplications, and translocations. *See* also **nondisjunction**, **polyspermy**, **monosomy**, **trisomy**, **triploid**, and **tetraploid**.

aneurysm: a weakened, bulging region of an artery that forms when pressure is exerted against a site of injury or deterioration. Severely damaged regions, and ones subjected to high pressures can rupture.

ANF: atrial natriuretic factor; *see* **atrial natriuretic peptides**.

angiectasis: enlargement or lengthening of blood vessels.

angiectomy: removal of part or all of a blood vessel.

angina: usually (1) *angina pectoris*, in which pain and strangling sensations are caused by coronary vessel stenosis; (2) sore throat, tonsil infections, and some other painful conditions.

angio-: a prefix meaning blood vessel.

angioblasts: embryonic cells that give rise to blood vessels. Mesodermal cells in the visceral wall of the yolk sac first aggregate to form angiogenetic clusters. Blood islands appear when the inner cells differentiate to primitive hematopoietic types, and the outer ones to epithelium. Neighboring walls of the blood islands then fuse to form capillaries.

angiodystrophy: a vascular disorder attributed to nutritional deficiency.

angioedema: swelling caused by leakage of fluid from damaged blood vessels. An inherited form is caused by deficiency of a complement system C1 esterase inhibitor.

angiogenic factors: endogenous regulators that promote blood vessel formation. Various types can directly stimulate endothelial cell proliferation and/or migration, mobilize and/or activate macrophages and other cells that produce growth factors, or antagonize naturally occurring inhibitors. They perform physiological roles in growth, development, maturation, wound healing, inflammation, and functional hypertrophy. Some support tumor growth and metastasis, and/or contribute to non-neoplastic vascular diseases. The group includes epidermal, fibroblast, transforming, platelet derived, and vascular endothelium growth factors (EGF, FGFs TGFs, PDGFs and VEGF), and angiogenins. Prostaglandins E_1 and E_2 (but not F), polar lipids made by adipocytes, and angiotensins also stimulate. Heparin, and heparin fragments that do not affect blood coagulation, can promote endothelial cell migration by exerting some stimulatory and some inhibitory influences on growth factor functions. Copper enhances heparin-stimulated movement, supports the actions of Gly-His-Lys, and is needed for the angiogenic effects of ceruloplasmin. The inhibitors include glucocorticoids and other steroids, and protamines; *see* also **angiostatic steroids**.

angiogenesis: neovascularization; formation of new blood vessels. The processes, which involve growth of new capillaries from venule sprouts, endothelial cell migration and proliferation, and localized basement membrane degradation, are essential for normal tissue growth and repair. They can also contribute to pathological changes in blood vessels, tumor growth and metastasis.

angiogenins: a term applied to some angiogenic factors. One is a 14.4K protein made by hepatocytes and some adenocarcinoma cells that is chemically related to pancreatic ribonuclease. (However, that protein lacks the catalytic potency; and pancreatic ribonuclease is not angiogenic.) Others include partially characterized low molecular weight peptides released by some tumor cells, a high molecular weight protein made by thymocytes, and some epithelial cell mitogens identified in ovary, placenta, kidney, and thyroid glands. Additional uncharacterized peptides from wound fluids and monocytes are chemotaxins for macrophages (which release growth factors).

angiomas: benign blood or lymph vessels tumors.

angioneurotic: involving nerves and blood or lymph vessels.

angiostatic: inhibiting angiogenesis.

angiostatic agents: protamine, heparin, pentosan polysulfate, angiostatic steroids, and other substances that inhibit formation of new blood vessels.

angiostatic steroids: glucocorticoid metabolites that interact with heparin or heparin fragments to inhibit angiogenesis via mechanisms unrelated to glucocorticoid or mineralocorticoid activities. Tetrahydro-11-deoxycortisol is highly potent. Corticosterone, cortisol and 17α-hydroxy-progesterone display some activity, but dexamethsone is totally ineffective.

angiotensin I: A-I; decapeptides cleaved from renin substrates and related peptides and proteins. The type made by humans and many other species is H-Asp-Arg-Val-Tyr-Ile-His-Leu-Pro-Phe-His-Leu-OH. The bovine form has a valine moiety at position 5. Most circulating A-I is formed in the bloodstream from renin substrates secreted by the liver; *see* **renin angiotensin system**. Smaller amounts are made locally at many sites. Although specific A-I receptors that contribute to control of blood flow through the inner renal cortex and medulla have been described, A-I has limited biological potency. It functions primarily as the precursor of **angiotensin II** (*q.v.*)

angiotensin II: A-II; H-Asp-Arg-Val-Tyr-Ile-His-Leu-Pro-OH, made by most species (including humans), and closely related octapeptides of bovines and some others. Almost all of the circulating hormone is cleaved from plasma **angiotensin I** (*q.v.*) via reactions catalzyed by angiotensin converting enzymes in the lungs; *see* also **renin angiotensin system**. Under normal conditions, it exerts some negative feedback control over renin release. A biologically less important enzyme, tonin, directly releases small amounts from some proteins. The octapeptide is also generated at many other sites, where it exerts mostly paracrine and/or autocrine effects, some of which involve interactions with adenosine receptors. Many target organs respond to peptides from both sources. In the central nervous system, some neurons possess renin-like activity, glial cells make angiotensin substrate, and converting enzymes are extracellular. Other sites for synthesis include the intimal epithelium and smooth muscle of blood vessel walls, components of pituitary gland, uterus, ovary, testis, kidney, and reproductive tracts, polymorphonuclear leukocytes, monocytes, and macrophages. In brain, A-II functions as a neurotransmitter and neuromodulator involved in regulation of blood pressure, salt appetite, glial cell functions, pituitary hormone secretion, circadian rhythms, learning, and memory. Its ability to invoke thirst and drinking is attributed to interactions with receptors on subfornical organs and related regions. A-II also stimulates catecholamine release from nerve endings (and also from adrenomedullary cells), and it potentiates their actions. Some of its effects are accomplished in this way. For example, norepinephrine contributes centrally to vasopressin release, and peripherally to vasoconstriction and myocardial stimulation. Dopamine dampens prolactin responses to stress, but augments luteinizing hormone (LH) release around the time of ovulation. Circulating A-II is the major stimulant for zona glomerulosa cells of the adrenal cortex, in which it promotes aldosterone secretion by rapidly accelerating cholesterol conversion to pregneonolone and more slowly promoting cortisol conversion to its 18-hydroxy derivative. The effects are accomplished with very low concentrations, especially when sodium levels in extracellular fluids are low; and they can contribute to blood pressure elevation. A-II is also a direct and potent stimulant for vascular smooth muscle (an effect sometimes enhanced by vasopressin as well as norepinephrine). It modulates blood flow through the kidney, and additionally acts directly on the myocardium. It also antagonizes several atrial natriuretic peptide functions. Hypertensive individuals have high tendencies to develop **atherosclerosis** (*q.v.*), and several other A-II actions are implicated. The circulating peptide potentiates blood platelet activation and aggregation, inhibits plasmin, and is chemotactic for monocytic leukocytes. Locally produced peptide stimulates intimal cell proliferation when arterial walls are injured, and it promotes growth and migration of smooth muscle cells. It also enhances superoxide anion production by polymorphonuclear leukocytes, and it binds to and augments macrophage-mediated peroxidation of low density lipoprotein (LDL) phospholipids. Other functions include synergisms with gonadotropins to promote ovulation and possibly also spermatogenesis, acceleration of steroidogenesis in gonads, stimulation of smooth muscle contraction in the uterus and gastrointestinal tract, and contributions to gluconeogenesis in the liver. It is a growth stimulant for some cell types, and is implicated as a promotor of angiogenesis and liver regeneration, and a stimulant for skeletal muscle in fetuses. In some nonmammalian vertebrates, it acts on salt glands. Older terms for A-II include angiotonin and hypertensin.

angiotensin III, A-III: heptapeptides formed when aminopeptidases cleave the *N*-terminal amino acid moieties of angiotensin-IIs. They are less potent vasoconstrictors than A-IIs, but bind with high affinity to one class of angiotensin receptors. There is limited support for the concept that they are more potent than A-II for stimulation of aldosterone secretion.

angiotensin converting enzymes: ACE: peptidyl dipeptidases (carboxypeptidases), similar to or identical with enkephalin convertases that catalyze conversion of an-

giotensin-I to **angiotensin II** (*q.v.*). Other substrates include **kallidin** (*q.v.*) and other kinins. Although widely distributed, the highest levels are in the lungs.

angiotensinases: nonspecific enzymes that cleave angiotensins to inactive fragments.

angiotensinogen: renin substrate.

angiotensin receptors: three classes of plasma membrane spanning proteins that bind angiotensins with high affinity have been identified with pharmacological agents. AT_1 types are widely distributed, and appear to mediate most of the early effects (some of which become apparent within 15 seconds after presentation of the peptide). They bind specific antagonists (such as losartan, DuP753), in a manner inhibited by low concentrations of dithiothreitol, and have greater affinity for angiotensin-II (A-II) than for angiotensin III (A-III). Ligand binding is followed by influences on steroidogenesis, vasoconstriction, vasopressin and catecholamine release, water intake, uterine muscle contraction, and other functions. Various influences are mediated via coupling with trimeric G proteins, followed by phospholipase C activation, phosphatidylinositol hydrolysis, and/or increased Ca^{2+} uptake from surrounding fluids, and (in some cases) inhibition of adenylate cyclases. Two subtypes are known, AT_{1A}, a 359-amino acid, 41K protein which predominates in vascular smooth muscle, and a chemically similar AT_{1B} which is more abundant in the zona glomerulosa. AT_2 receptors bind different antagonists (such as PD123177) in a manner unaffected by dithiothreitol, display equal affinities for A-II and A-III, and have been observed to activate phosphotyrosine phosphatases and inhibit particulate guanylate cyclases. They have been identified in mesenchymal tissues, and are implicated as mediators of the growth-promoting effects in fetuses. However, although they predominate in adrenal medulla, their postnatal functions have not been defined. In cells of the adrenal gland, heart, brain, and uterus which contain both A_1 and A_2 forms, most rapidly induced actions seem to be mediated by the former. A third kind of receptor, AT_3, with no affinity for A-III, and the ability to activate soluble gunaylate cyclases, is made by some neuroblastoma cells.

angstrom: Å; 10^{-10} meter; a unit of length used for electromagnetic radiation wavelengths, atomic dimensions, and (less commonly) for the diameters or lengths of structures in electron micrographs.

ANH: atrial natriuretic hormone; *see* **atrial natriuretic peptides**.

animal hemisphere: the region of a young embryo that gives rise to cells of the nervous system and skin epidermis. *See* also **animal pole**, and *cf* **vegetal hemisphere**.

animal pole: the end (pole) of an oocyte that contains the most cytoplasm and the least yolk, from which polar bodies are extruded. The nucleus migrates to this region when the zygote prepares for cleavage. *See* also **animal hemisphere**, and *cf* **vegetal pole**.

anions: negatively charged ions.

anionic detergents: amphipathic substances with negatively charged hydrophilic components.

aniracetam: 1-(4-methoxybenzoyl)-2-pyrrolidine; an agent that acts on quisqualate receptors, and affects learning and memory in rodents.

anisogamy: sexual reproduction that involves fertilization of large, immobile oocytes by smaller, mobile spermatozoa.

anisomycin: 2-*p*-methoxyphenylmethyl-3-acetoxy-4-hydroxypyrrolidine; an antibiotic that reversibly inhibits protein synthesis. It is used to treat some protozoal infestations and control the growth of fungi. Its effects on RNA polymerase II are more specific than those of cycloheximide, and it is less toxic when used to inhibit protein synthesis in laboratory animals.

anisotropy: having a crystalline or fibrillar structure which is not the same in all directions. Anisotropic substances therefore display birefringence when viewed under polarized light.

ankylosing spondylitis: a joint disease in which vertebrae fuse. Histocompatibility antigen HLA-B2 increases the susceptibility.

ankylosis: fusion of bones across a joint, usually in response to damage invoked by chronic inflammation.

ankyrin: a globular 200K protein that anchors cytoskeletons to plasma membranes by binding fodrin, spectrin, erythrocyte band-3, and/or other proteins. It restricts lateral movements of membrane proteins, and thereby maintains Na^+ channel polarities and differences in Na^+ transport along axonal membrane regions.

anlagen: a component (usually a cell cluster) of an embryo from which a specific part of the mature organism develops.

annealing: pairing of DNA strands (from the same molecule after heat separation, or of segments from two different single stranded ones with complementary base sequences).

annelids: earthworms and other segmented worms of the phylum *Annelida*. Laboratory tools and clinically useful substances derived from them include nereistoxin (an insecticide made by marine worms and used for defense), and hirudin, which is made by leeches.

annexins: at least nine structurally related proteins with similar 70-amino acid cores that display calcium-dependent binding to membrane phospholipids. All inhibit phospholipase A-2 (and consequent generation of eicosanoids), but some effects are related to their abilities to serve as tyrosine kinase substrates. They are implicated as regulators of stimulus-response coupling, exocytosis, and cytoskeletal functions, and they affect inflammation, immune system responses, and cell morphology. Some inhibit blood coagulation. Most are known by other names:

> annexin I: lipocortin I; calpactin II; chromobindin 9; GIF; p35.
>
> annexin II: lipocortin II; calpactin I; chromobindin 8; PAP-14, protein I; p36.
>
> annexin III: lipocortin III; 35α calcimedin; PAP-III.
>
> annexin IV: lipocortin IV; 35β calcimedin; 32.5K calectrin; chromobindin 4; protein II; PP4-X; PAP-II; endonexin.
>
> annexin V: lipocortin V; 35K calectrin; 35γ calcimedin; calphobindin I; anchorin C11; PAP-I; PP4; VAC-α; IBC; endonexin II.
>
> annexin VI: lipocortin VI; 67K calectrin; 67K calcimedin; chromobindin 20; protein III; calphobindin II; p68; p70; 73K.
>
> annexin VII: synexin.
>
> annexin VIII: VAC-β.

annulus: a ring-shaped structure.

anode: a positively charged electrode.

anodyne: a substance that can relieve pain but is less potent than an analgesic.

anodynin: an uncharacterized peptide, cleaved from pro-opiomelanocortin (POMC) and released by pituitary glands, that diminishes the sense of pain.

anomaly: usually, a malformed structure, or an abnormal function.

anomers: isomers of sugars and related molecules that are identical except for the positions of alcohol groups attached to hemiacetal carbon atoms. Examples of anomer pairs include α-D-glucose and β-D-glucose. The two forms are interconvertible, via an enol intermediate. The optical activity of a solution that initially contains one type changes as an equilibrium mixture of the two is established; *see* also **mutarotases**.

anorchism: congenital absence of one or both testes in a genetic male.

anorectic: (1) lacking appetite; (2) an agent that depresses appetite; (3) an individual who lacks appetite.

anorectin: the C-terminal peptide of the prohormone for growth hormone releasing hormone (GRH), so named because it can diminish appetite.

anorexia: (1) refusal of, or aversion to food; (2) severely diminished appetite.

anorexia nervosa: self-inflicted starvation; *cf* **bulimia**. The disorder is most prevalent in adolescent girls and young women. Preoccupation with thoughts of food, its caloric content, and its preparation, distorted body images, and (in early stages) with tendencies to engage in strenuous exercise are often manifested. The consequences of chronic nutrient deprivation, which can be fatal, include emaciation, electrolyte imbalances and cardiac dysrhythmias. Although commonly attributed to psychological factors such as fear of obesity, or of acquiring mature secondary sex characteristics, and desire to exert control over oneself or other persons, hypothalamic dysfunction that includes decreased gonadotropin releasing hormone (GnRH) and increased corticotropin releasing hormone (CRH) secretion can often be detected before overt symptoms develop.

anosmia: inability to perceive odors. Congenital conditions, often associated with hypothalamic dysfunction, and especially with gonadotropin deficiency, are attributed to impaired development of olfactory system anlagen; *see* also **Kallmann syndrome**. They can be caused later in life by head injuries. Hyposmia commonly develops in elderly persons, and in some it progresses to anosmia.

ANOVA: analysis of variance.

anovulatory: failing to accomplish ovulation, usually because oocytes and their follicles do not mature, or mechanisms for mounting LH surges are impaired.

anoxia: absence of oxygen, a term often used when hypoxia would be more appropriate.

ANP: atrial natriuretic peptides.

ANS: (1) autonomic nervous system; (2) 8-anilo-1-naphthalene sulfonic acid, a probe for hydrophobic binding sites, and for detection of small structural changes in proteins.

antagonists: agents that block or oppose the actions of hormones, neurotransmitters, or other regulators; *cf* **agonists**. *Competitive* types can form non-functional, high-affinity (but dissociable) complexes with receptors and thereby impair binding of the usual ligands. The effects can be minimized by increasing the ligand concentrations. *Noncompetitive* types render the receptors nonfunctional by irreversibly altering their properties. Antagonists can also work indirectly, for example by affecting enzymes and/or substrates involved in the responses, or by stimulating processes that oppose those of the ligands. Because of differences in receptor structures and microenvironments, some pharmacological agents are antagonists at certain sites and agonists at others.

antegrade: anterograde; proceeding in the usual direction; *cf* **retrograde**.

antenatal: before birth or during pregnancy.

anterior: towards the head or front end; *cf* **posterior**.

anterior lobe: usually, the most anterior part of the hypophysis, a term sometimes used synonymously with pars distalis or adenohypophysis. *See* also **anterior pituitary**.

anterior pituitary: the part of the hypophysis of some species (for example laboratory rodents) that is most easily removed when the ventral surface is exposed. It comprises pars distalis and some of the pars tuberalis (but no pars intermedia). The term is sometimes used synonymously with pars distalis, or with adenohypophysis.

anterior pituitary protein of the pig, AAPG: *see* **peptide 7B2**.

anterograde: antegrade.

Anthopleura elegantissima: the sea anenome. In common with other coelenterates, it makes *N*-terminal amidated neurotransmitters, including anotho-K-amide (L-3-Phenyllactyl-Phe-Lys-Ala-NH$_2$), anotho-RF amide (*p*-Glu-Gly-Arg-Phe- NH$_2$), and related longer peptides (antho-RI- and antho-RN- amides).

anthracene-9-carboxylic acid: an agent used to inhibit chloride excretion in laboratory animals.

anthranilate: *o*-aminobenzoate; an intermediate in pathways used by bacteria for biosynthesis of tryptophan, histidine, purine nucleotides, and pyrimidine nucleotides. It reacts with phosphoribosyl pyrophosphate to form *N*-5′-phosphoribosylanthranilate.

2′-*o*-anthraniloyl cAMP: a fluorescent cAMP analog, used as a cyclic nucleotide phosphodiesterase (PDE) substrate.

2′-o-anthraniloyl cGMP: a fluorescent cGMP analog used as a substrate for calmodulin-dependent cyclic phosphodiesterase isozymes. *See also* **2′-o-anthraniloyl cAMP**.

anthropoid: (1) resembling humans; (2) ape-like; (3) a member of the *Pongidae* (tailless ape) family, which includes chimpanzees, gorillas, orangutans, and gibbons.

anthropomorphism: attribution of human characteristics to nonhuman entities (other species, or inanimate objects).

anti-androgens: agents that oppose the effects of male type gonadal steroid hormones. Most form non-functional associations with androgen receptors that do not interact with hormone response elements, and block the binding of natural ligands; *see*, for example, **flutamide**.

antibiotic: originally, an agent produced by one type of microorganism that inhibits the growth of, or kills another type. The term now additionally applies to substances derived from those agents, and to synthetic ones that exert similar effects. Most inhibit the activities of essential enzymes of the microorganisms. The least toxic types have minimal effects on the host counterparts.

antibodies: specific proteins produced in response to antigens that bind the antigens with high affinity. The term usually refers to immunoglobulins made by plasma cells. They contribute to body defenses by attaching to microorganisms and/or their toxins; but ones that interact with host molecules can disrupt normal functions (*see* **autoimmune diseases**). Since each type binds tightly to just one (or a few related) molecular species, antibodies are used to identify receptors, enzymes, and other substances within cells and body fluids, to isolate specific substances, and to block the their actions. *Monoclonal* types are especially useful for such purposes. Antibodies with more than one binding site can promote receptor aggregation, and thereby mimic some hormone actions.

antibody-dependent cell-mediated cytotoxicity, ADCC: destruction of antibody coated cells via mechanisms that involve Fc receptors on natural killer cells, killer cells, T lymphocytes, or eosinophils.

anticipatory control: regulation that averts (rather than corrects) imbalances. For example, insulin released just prior to or during food ingestion protects against prandial hyperglycemia; and vasopressin released in response to warm environments protects against loss of water to the urine before sweating can invoke dehydration.

anticodons: *see* **transfer RNAs**.

Antide: *N*-acetyl-Dβ-Nal-*p*-Cl-D-Phe-D-3-pyridyl-D-Ala-Ser, *N*-ε-nicotinyl-D-Lys-Leu-*N*-ε-isopropyl-Lys-Pro-D-Ala-NH₂; a highly potent, long-acting, orally effective gonadotropin releasing hormone (GnRH) antagonist that is almost devoid of histamine-releasing activity. It is used to inhibit ovulation, testosterone biosynthesis, and other luteinizing hormone (LH) dependent processes.

antidiuretics: agents that diminish urine volume; *cf* **diuretics**.

antidiuretic hormone: ADH; *see* **vasopressins**.

antidromic: proceeding in a direction opposite to the usual or expected one, for example passage of a nerve impulse, or uptake of a growth factor, from an axon terminal to the cell body.

anti-enzyme: usually, an antibody directed against an enzyme that blocks the activity.

anti-estrogens: agents that block estrogen actions. Most form nonfunctional associations with estrogen receptors. A widely used type is **tamoxifen** (*q.v.*).

antifertility factor-1: AF-1; a 200K glycoprotein that impairs the ability of capacitated sperm to penetrate the corona radiata. It does not inhibit acrosin, hyaluronidase, or acrosome reactions.

antifertilizins: approximately 10K acidic proteins on the surfaces of spermatozoa of animal types that utilize external fertilization. They bind with high affinities and specificities to fertilizins on oocyte coats of the same species. Proposed functions include assistance in fertilization, prevention of fertilization by sperm of other species, and (since there are limited numbers of fertilizin molecules) protection against polyspermy.

antifibrinolytics: agents that inhibit fibrin degradation. Some are used to control bleeding.

antigalactics: agents that diminish milk production.

antigen[s]: substances that promote production of specific kinds of antibodies by stimulating the immune system. *See also* **B lymphocytes**, **plasma cells**, **T-dependent** and **T-independent antigens**.

antigen binding sites: immunoglobulin molecule domains that bind tightly to specific kinds of antigens.

antigen bridges: complexes formed when antigens attach to two different antibody molecules. They can promote aggregation when the antigens are on cell surfaces.

antigen-dependent cell cytotoxicity: ADCC; destruction of cells (usually foreign, virus infected, or tumor types) by antigen-activated immune system cells.

antigenic competition: suppression of immune system responses to specific antigens, by presenting closely relateds ones that compete for limited numbers of binding sites.

antigenic determinants: the sites on antigen molecules that define the immunological specificities; *see* also **epitope** and **paratope**.

antigenic modulation: configurational changes in antigens that follow binding to antibodies.

antigen presenting cells: APC; cells that take up antigens, process them, and present them (in combination with major histocompatibility complex proteins) to T or B lymphocytes. Most are macrophages. Others types include Langerhans, dendritic, or interdigitating cells. B lymphocytes also present under some conditions.

antigen processing: modification of an antigen made by one cell type that renders it recognizable by another. Antigen presenting cells take up the molecules by endocytosis, and use intracellular proteases to cleave them to smaller fragments.

antiglobulin test: *see* **Coomb's test**.

antihemorrhagic factor: vitamin K.

anti-idiotypic antibody: an antibody formed in response to a different antibody (which functions as an antigen). It can closely resemble the antigen that promoted formation of the first antibody, and invoke tolerance to it; and can also, in turn, act as an antigen that stimulates formation of a third antibody type (with high affinity for the second). For example, thryoid stimulating hormone (TSH) directs formation of anti-TSH which can, in turn, promote production of an anti-anti-TSH that resembles TSH. *See* also **immune networks**, and **idiotypes**.

anti-inflammatory agents: glucocorticoids, nonsteroidal anti-inflammatory agents (NSIAs), and other substances that suppresses inflammatory reactions. They are used to alleviate pain, reduce swelling, counteract fever, and protect against damage. Most types interfere with the synthesis and/or release of eicosanoids and other mediators.

antilymphocytic serum: ALS; blood serum that contains antibodies directed against T lymphocytes. The antibodies can slow or block thymus gland regeneration following radiation, protect against graft rejection, or attenuate autoimmune processes.

anti-metabolite: a chemical that resembles an intermediate of a biosynthetic pathway, and competes with it as a substrate for the same enzyme. Many antibiotics act in this way.

antimony, Sb: an element (atomic number 51, atomic weight 121.75). Some antimony salts are used to combat parasitic infections, but they are toxic and can invoke vomiting.

anti-Müllerian hormone: AMH; *see* **Müllerian duct inhibitor**.

antimycin A: antibiotics made by *Streptomyces* species that inhibit oxidative phosphorylation by blocking electron transfers from ubiquinones to cytochrome C. They are used as fungicides, miticides, and insecticides, and to study mitochondrial functions. The structure of antimycin A_3, 3-methylbutanoic acid 8-butyl-3-[[3-(formyl-amino)-2-hydroxybenzoyl]amino]-2,6-dimethyl-4,9-dioxo-1,5-dioxonan-7-yl ester, is shown.

anti-oncogenes: DNA segments that protect against tumorigenesis by suppressing the effects of oncogenes, and/or opposing excessive activities of proto-oncogenes. *See*, for example, **p53** and *Rb*.

antioxidants: vitamin E, ascorbic acid, glutathione, bilirubin, urates, and other substances that retard oxidation. They protect against free radical formation, and against conversion of fatty acids, phospholipids, and other molecules to toxic compounds.

antipain: [(*S*)-1-ethoxycarbonyl-2-phenylethyl]-carbamoyl-Arg-Val-Arg-al; a serine-thiol type protease inhibitor made by *Actinomycetes*, with properties similar to those of leupeptin.

antiparallel: parallel in position but running in the opposite direction. The two strands of DNA molecules, and the subunits of some proteins are arranged in this way.

antipellagra vitamin: niacinamide.

α_2-**antiplasmin**: the major endogenous plasmin inhibitor. It is a single-chain 70K plasma glycoprotein that stabilizes blood clots, and is used to study coagulation mechanisms. Deficiencies cause bleeding disorders.

antipodal: describes entities located on opposite ends or sides of a structure.

antiport: countertransport; transport of one substance across a membrane that is coupled to transport of another in the opposite direction; *cf* **symport**.

antipsychotic agents: neuroleptics; pharmacological agents used to alleviate symptoms of schizophrenia and other mental disorders. Many are dopamine receptor antagonists.

antipyrine: phenazone.

antirachitic vitamin: vitamin D.

antiscorbutic vitamin: vitamin C; *see* **ascorbic acid**.

antiseminalplasmin: a 39K seminal fluid protein that opposes the anti-fertility effects of seminalplasmin.

anti-sense DNA: a DNA strand complementary to one that usually directs RNA synthesis. It can be used to identify coding sequences, and to block the transcription of specific genes. Some types are transcribed.

anti-sense RNAs: RNAs with base sequences complementary to those transcribed from DNA sense strands. They can base pair with, and affect the functions of conventional RNAs. Synthetic mRNA types made from anti-sense DNAs are used to direct formation of proteins that oppose the effects of naturally occurring gene products.

antiserum: usually, blood serum that contains antibodies generated in response to specific antigens. Preparations are used to block specific kinds of responses, and in some assay procedures.

antisterility vitamin: vitamin E.

anti-Tac: monoclonal antibodies directed against interleukin-2 receptors.

antithrombins: Antithrombin III, a 68K α-antitrypsin-like glycoprotein, is a potent inactivator of thrombin and some other enzymes, and a weaker one for coagulation factors IX, X, XI, and XII. Antithrombin I enhances adsorption of thrombin by fibrin. Antithrombin II is a cofactor for the anti-thrombin effects of heparin.

antitoxins: usually, antibodies that combine with and alter the properties of bacterial toxins.

α-antitrypsin: α_1-AT; α_1-proteinase inhibitor; 3.5S α_1-glycoprotein: a 52K acute phase protein whose levels rise in response to inflammation, hepatic disease, trauma, and the presence of neoplasms, and also during pregnancy and oral contraceptive use. It is the most abundant plasma anti-protease, and the major endogenous inhibitor of plasminogen activator. It also degrades trypsin, chymotrypsin, plasmin, elastase, and other proteins, and is believed to retard development of emphysema and protect against the potentially damaging effects of inflammatory mediators.

antrum: (1) a closed cavity, for example the fluid-filled vesicle of a preovulatory follicle; (2) the dilated part of the pyloric region of the stomach.

anxiogenic: anxiety-invoking.

anxiolytics: agents used to decrease anxiety.

AOAA: aminooxyacetic acid.

AOB: accessory olfactory bulbs.

AP: anterior pituitary.

α_2-AP: α_2-antiplasmin.

4-AP: 4-aminopyridine.

AP-1: activating protein-1; transcription factor complexes composed of proteins with leucine zipper domains encoded by *ap-1* genes. They form dimers that bind to promoter/enhancer regions of genes with TGAC/GTCA and closely related DNA base sequences (*see also c-jun* and *c-fos*), and mediate the transcriptional effects of tumor necrosis factor-α (TNFα), interleukin-1 (IL-1), epidermal growth factor (EGF) transforming growth factor-β (TGFβ), and other endogenous regulators, of tumor-promoting phorbol esters and other non-native protein kinase C activators, of several protoncogenes (including *c-Ha-ras*, *c-mos*, and *c-src*), and of some oncogenes. The affected proteins include collagenases, metallothioneins, and some SV40 components. Cell depolarization, cAMP, several growth factors, and other signals enhance AP-1 production. Glucocorticoids oppose the effects on most genes that contain glucocorticoid response elements. JunD is one of the translation factors that normally protects against overactivity. Deregulated expression of

proteins normally made, and some mutant forms can invoke cell transformation.

ap-1: a gene that directs the formation of Jun proteins (including Jun-1, Jun B, and Jun D). Although some expression is constitutive, the transcription of specific types is closely regulated. C-jun protein activates the *c-jun* gene via mechanisms that can be antagonized by JunB. *See also* **AP-1**.

aP2: adipocyte protein-2.

AP-5: 2-amino-5-phosphonopentanoic acid; an NMDA receptor antagonist.

$$HO-\overset{\overset{O}{\|}}{\underset{\underset{H}{\overset{|}{O}}}{P}}-CH_2-CH_2-CH_2-\overset{\overset{NH_2}{|}}{\underset{\underset{COOH}{}}{CH}}$$

13-APA : 13-azaprostanoic acid.

apamin: a neurotoxin in the venom of the honey bee, *Apis mellifera* that blocks calcium-activated potassium channels, and decreases after-polarization, possibly by acting on receptors for endogenous apamin-like peptides. It is a peptide with the amino acid sequence Cys-Asn-Cys-Lys-Ala-Pro-Glu-Thr-Ala-Leu-Cys-Ala-Arg-Arg-Cys-Gln-Gln-His-NH₂, in which the cysteine moieties at positions 1 → 11 and 1 → 15 are joined. *See also* **ATP**.

APB: 2-amino-4-phosphobutyrate.

APC: antigen presenting cells.

2-APH: 2-aminophosphohexanoate.

aphagia: refusal of food, or inability to eat.

aphidicolin: tetradecahydro-3,9-dihydroxy-4,11b-dimethyl-8,11a-methano-11a*H*-cyclohepta-naphthalene-4,9-dimethanol; an antibiotic made by *Cephalosporium aphidocola* that blocks the synthesis of double-stranded DNAs in eukaryotes and some viruses by inhibiting DNA polymerase α enzymes, and causes accumulation of unreplicated DNA (which interrupts cell cycle S → M progression). It also impairs actin filament organization, uncouples centrosome:nucleus interactions, and affects cell migration during embryogenesis (but does not affect the activities of polyermases β and γ).

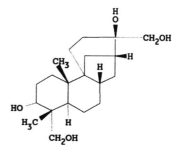

aphrodisiacs: agents that stimulate sexual desire. Although numerous pheromones capable of stimulating mating behavior are known, and androgens can restore functions in hormone deficient subjects, most substances purported to exert such effects in humans appear to lack pharmacological activity of this kind.

aphrodisin: an acidic, water-soluble 17K protein in hamster vaginal secretions that acts on vomeronasal organ receptors of conspecific males and stimulates copulatory behavior.

apical: describes the narrow surfaces of conical cells, or the parts of cells that border lumens.

Apis: the honey-bee genus. *Apis mellifera* is the species most widely studied, and from which some biologically potent venoms are extracted.

aplasia: incomplete development of a structure.

APL: acute promyelocytic leukemia; *see* **leukemias**.

Aplysia californica: the sea-hare, a marine gastropod with large neurons, in which the effects of lipoxygenase metabolites and other agents that affect synaptic transmission are easily monitored. It is used for studies of neuron functions, reflex responses, and learning.

p-**APMSF**: amidinophenylmethanesulfonyl fluoride: a specific, irreversible inhibitor of serine proteases, effective against trypsin, thrombin and some other blood coagulation factors, and some complement components.

apo-: a prefix meaning removed or derived from. It usually describes a protein separated from an essential component or co-factor; *see* **apoenzymes and apolipoproteins**.

APO: a 52K protein expressed on the surfaces of activated T and B lymphocytes, and on some leukemia cells. Monoclonal antibodies directed against it invoke apoptosis. APO-1 (Fas) is the same, or a closely related cell surface protein that mediates the anti-proliferative effects of p53.

Apo-A, Apo-B, Apo-C, Apo-D, Apo-E: apolipoproteins A, B, C, D, and E. *See* **lipoproteins** and specific apoprotein types.

apocrine: describes (1) exocrine glands whose secretions contain cytoplasmic components (vesicles or granules) as well as fluid. Most are coiled tubules; (2) the secretions produced by those glands. *Cf* **merocrine** and **holocrine**.

apoenzyme: the protein part a holoenzyme that does not function (or has very low activity) when separated from a coenzyme or other factor with which it usually associates.

apoferritins: metal-free major iron transporting proteins; *cf* **ferritins**. A 460K horse spleen type is used in laboratory studies.

apolipoproteins: lipid-free apoprotein components of lipoproteins. For most of them, upper case Roman letters designate the families, and numbers the subtypes. The various kinds can be separated by electrophoresis; and most of the Greek letters used refer to the mobilities. *See* **lipoproteins**, and specific types (such **apoproteins A, B**, and **C**).

apolysis: during molting, the first stage of proecdysis, during which the epidermis separates from the exoskeleton that will be discarded.

apomorphine: 5,6,6a,7-tetrahydro-6-methyl-4*H*-dibenzoquinoline-10,11-diol; a morphine derivative that acts both pre- and postsynaptically as a dopamine receptor antagonist. It can elevate brain serotonin levels, and is sometimes used in veterinary medicine to invoke vomiting.

apomyxis: apomixis; asexual reproduction from a single gamete, a process that occurs in many plants. *See* also **parthenogenesis**.

apoprotein: a protein from which other factors (such as metallic or lipid substances) required for its function have been removed; *see*, for example, **apoenzyme**. Terms such as Apo-A and Apo-B refer to specific kinds of apolipoproteins.

apoprotein (a): Apo (a); apolipoprotein (a): a 300-800K plasminogen-like glycoprotein that binds via disulfide groups to apoprotein B-100 in lipoprotein(a) particles of species (including humans) that do not synthesize ascorbic acid. It displays serine-protease (but no plasmin) activity. Its anti-fibrinolytic effects are attributed to competition with plasminogen for binding to both fibrin and endothelial plasminogen receptors. Associations with fibrinogen and fibrin probably contribute to roles in wound healing. The particles do not appear to be cleared by LDL receptors. When present in excessive amounts, Apo(a) deposits in arterial walls; and high levels are regarded as a risk factors for development of atherosclerosis. It has been suggested that ascorbic acid deficiency leads to Apo(a) accumulation, and thereby facilitates cancer cell progression.

apoprotein A-I: Apo A-I; A-1; apolipoprotein A-1; a single-chain, nonglycosylated 28.3K protein component of high density lipoproteins (HDLs), made in the small intestine, incorporated into chylomicrons, and taken up by the liver (in which it binds to receptors on both hepatocytes and macrophages). It is present in higher concentrations in lymph than in blood plasma, and is a minor component of bile. Estrogens stimulate its production. By serving as a co-factor for lecithin:cholesterol acyltransferase (LCAT), Apo-A1 facilitates cholesterol ester accumulation in HDLs. It also binds triodothyronine (T_3) and thyroxine (T_4), and contributes to the intestinal absorption of thyroid hormones. T_3, in turn, augments

LCAT activity. APO-A1 additionally acts in the placenta to facilitate prolactin release.

apoprotein AII: Apo A-II; A-2; apolipoprotein A-II; a homodimeric protein component of high density lipoproteins (HDLs), composed of 17.4K subunits. In common with Apo A-I, it is made in the intestine, incorporated into chylomicrons, and taken up by hepatocyte and macrophage receptors. A-2 binds phospholipids, cholesterol and triacylglycerols, and activates hepatic lipases, but may inhibit LCAT.

apoprotein A-IV: Apo A-IV; A-4; apolipoprotein A-IV; a protein component of chylomicrons.

apoprotein B: apo-B; apolipoprotein B; *see* **Apoprotein B-48** and **apoprotein B-100**.

apoprotein B-48: apo-B-48; apolipoprotein B-48: a 210K protein, identical to the *N*-terminal region of apoprotein B-100, that facilitates transport of dietary lipids. It is essential for chylomicron formation in the intestine; and diets rich in fats and cholesterol augment its synthesis. When lipoprotein lipases catalyze removal of chylomicron triacylglycerols, it remains associated with the remnants and is taken up by hepatic receptors.

apoprotein B-100:, Apo-B-100; the largest (550K) of the protein components of lipoprotein particles, composed of 4536 amino acid moieties. It is made in the liver, and is incorporated into, and essential for the assembly of very low density lipoproteins (VLDLs); *see* **lipoproteins**. It mediates transport of lipids from the liver to the bloodstream. VLDLs are converted to low density lipoproteins (LDLs), which bind to receptors on many cell types and deliver cholesterol to them. They are recognized by LDL receptors (which also bind apo-E). Apo-B-100 additionally binds heparin, and it participates in other functions such as wound healing. In some particles, it is linked via disulfide bonds to Apo(a).

apoprotein-CI: Apo-CI; a 6.5K component of very low density lipoproteins (VLDLs) that activates lecithin:cholesterol acyltransferase (LCAT). Small amounts are also present in high density lipoproteins (HDLs).

apoprotein C-II: Apo C-II; an 8.8K component of very low density lipoproteins (VLDLs) that facilitates chylomicron uptake by liver cells. Small amounts are also present in high density lipoproteins (HDLs). It activates lipoprotein lipases, and cell type-specific regulation of its secretion facilitates selective delivery of fatty acids. Its biosynthesis is augmented in adipocytes by carbohydrates, and decreased by fasting and insulin deficiency. Fasting increases levels in heart, and also in mammary glands soon after parturition.

apoprotein C-III: Apo C-III; an 8.75K component of very low density lipoproteins (VLDLs). Small amounts are also present in high density lipoproteins (HDLs). It appears to block Apo C-II mediated activation of lipoprotein lipase, and may contribute to cell uptake of triacylglycerols.

apoprotein D: Apo-D; apolipoprotein-D; a 22K member of the α_2 microglobulin superfamily, present in low concentrations in chylomicrons, and in very low and high density lipoproteins (VLDLs and HDLs). It facilitates transfers of lipids from one type of lipoprotein particle to another. Apo-D is also present in some tissues in which the levels are increased by glucocorticoids and decreased by estrogens. Since the concentrations vary inversely with cell proliferation rates in cystic breast tissue and prostate glands, roles in limitation of cell proliferation have been suggested.

apoprotein E: Apo-E; 34-37K proteins synthesized in liver, spleen, kidney, brain, and other organs. They are components of chylomicrons and very low density lipoproteins (VLDLs); and small amounts occur in a subclass of high density lipoproteins (HDLs). They bind to very low density lipoprotein (LDL) receptors, facilitate hepatic uptake of chylomicron remnants, and thereby contribute to removal of excess circulating cholesterol. Macrophages also contain them; and the amounts are increased by high cholesterol levels and by endotoxin. Apo-E binds heparin, and is implicated as a mediator of interactions between cell surfaces and extracellular matrices, and as a factor that contributes to the development of atherosclerosis. It facilitates tissue repair, is neurotropic, can inhibit lymphocyte proliferation, and plays roles in the regulation of growth and differentiation of some cell types. APO-E-Є4 is a variant form that may contribute to the development of Alzheimer's disease, possibly by encouraging deposition of, and/or interfering with the removal of amyloid β protein.

apoprotein H: apolipoprotein H; β_2-glycophorin I; β_2-GPIl; a 50K (326-amino acid) proline-rich plasma β_2-globulin that binds to lipoproteins, anionic phospholipids (such as cardiolipins), blood platelets, heparin, DNA, mitochondria, and some infectious microorganisms. It inhibits ADP-mediated platelet aggregation and the intrinsic pathway for blood coagulation, and may provide protection against intravascular clotting.

apoprotein J: APO-J; a plasma protein that mediates cholesterol transport, mostly from cells to extracellular fluids. *See* also **clusterin**.

apoptosis: "programmed" cell death, which involves chromatin condensation, nuclear membrane constriction, endonuclease-mediated DNA degradation to nucleosome sized fragments, cell shrinkage (cytoplasmic condensation), and plasma membrane blebbing. It requires the synthesis of special proteins, can be blocked with cycloheximide, and differs in other ways from necrosis (which begins with plasma membrane damage and cell swelling). In various cell types, it can be initiated by tumor necrosis factors α and β (TGF-α and TGF-β) and other cytokines, glucocorticoids, antibodies directed against certain cell surface components, and some intracellular factors, and also by nutrient and/or growth factor deprivation. Under physiological conditions, selective cell destruction contributes to hematopoiesis, implantation, embryogenesis, metamorphosis, T-lymphocyte selection in the thymus gland, involution of organs that no longer perform special functions (such as the enlarged uterus after parturition, or the mammary glands when lactation is terminated), and other processes. It also provides mechanisms for eliminating some senescent cell types (including polymorphonuclear leukocytes) as well as virus-infected and transformed cells. Under pathological conditions, it can cause atrophy of useful tissues.

α position: if a steroid, prostaglandin, sugar, or other molecule with one or more ring structures is visualized as lying flat against a plane, chemical groups attached to the ring that project above the plane are said to be in the α position, and are represented by a broken line; *cf* β **position**.

apotransferrins: proteins involved in iron transport; *see* **ferritin**. Human 80K and bovine 77K forms have been identified.

APP: amyloid precursor protein.

APP563: a 563-amino acid protein whose synthesis is directed by the mRNA for amyloid precursor protein. It does not contain an A4 sequence of β-**amyloid peptide** (*q.v.*). *See* also **APP695**.

APP695, APP751, APP770: proteins with A-4 sequences, composed, respectively of 695, 751, and 770 amino moieties, that can serve as precursors of β-**amyloid peptide** (*q.v.*). A single premessenger RNA type undergoes alternate splicing, and its products direct the synthesis of all three (and also of APP563).

APP(NH)P: *see* **5-adenylimidodiphosphate**.

APPP: acute phase plasma proteins.

apposition: describes growth accomplished by deposition of new tissue along the peripheries of existing structures; *cf* **intersusception**.

A-PPT: α-PPT; *see* **preprotachykinin**.

apresoline: *see* **hydralazine**.

A protein: galactosyltransferase. *See* also **lactose synthetase**.

aprotinin; Trasylol: a competitive serine protease inhibitor, effective against trypsin, chymotrypsin, kallikrein, plasmin, some leukocytic, blood coagulation, and other proteolytic enzymes, and also against some esterases. The highest concentrations occur in parotid gland, lung, and pancreas; and lower levels circulate. Aprotinin can lessen inflammation, and protect against stress-associated cardiovascular failure by decreasing the production of toxic plasma protein derivatives. It is used clinically to treat pancreatitis and carcinoid syndrome, and to block protein degradation during radioimmunoassays. Disulfide bonds link the cysteine moieties at positions 5-50, 14-38, and 30-51 of the sequence shown: Arg-Pro-Asp-Phe-Cys-Leu-Glu-Pro-Pro-Tyr-Thr-Gly-Pro-Cys-Lys-Ala-Arg-Ile-Ile-Arg-Tyr-Phe-Tyr-Asn-Ala-Lys-Ala-Gly-Leu-Cys-Gln-Thr-Phe-Val-Tyr-Gly-Gly-Cys-Arg-Ala-Lys-Arg-Asn-Asn-Phe-Lys-Ser-Ala-Glu-Asp-Cys-Gly-Gly-Ala.

APSAC: anisolated plasminogen streptokinase activator complex; a modified streptokinase preparation used for its thrombolytic activity.

APUD: an acronym for amine precursor uptake and decarboxylation; *see* **APUD cells**.

APUD cells: cells that pass through a developmental stage during which they can take up amino acids and convert them to catecholamines, serotonin, melatonin, histamine, or other biologically active amines. Some types retain the characteristics when they mature. Others acquire the ability to make peptide-type hormones such as neurotensin, vasoactive intestinal peptide (VIP), cholecystokinins (CCK), gastrins, calcitonin, glucagons, insulins, and hypophysial hormones. *See* also **APUD hypothesis** and **APUDoma**.

APUD hypothesis: a concept for explaining similarities among secretory cells of the nervous system, gut, and other structures. It was proposed that APUD progenitor cells originate in embryonic neural crests and associated neuroectoderm, migrate to and colonize the gastrointestinal tract, pancreatic islets, adrenal medulla, thyroid, pineal, pituitary, and thymus glands, and other organs, undergo differentiation (which includes acquisition of abilities to make peptide and protein type hormones and other molecules), and establish a diffuse neuroendocrine system. A neural crest origin for calcitonin-secreting, adrenomedullary, melanocyte, thymus epithelium, and some other cell types has been established. However, most observers now believe that gastrointestinal tract secretory cells originate in endoderm. They may pass through an APUD-like stage.

APUDomas: neuroendocrine tumors said to originate from APUD cells, including insulinomas, glucagonomas, VIPomas, gastrinomas, and thyroid gland medullary carcinomas. Some secrete large quantities of hormones.

2-APV: 2-aminophosphovalerate.

aqueous humor: the fluid in the anterior and posterior chambers of the eye, secreted by ciliary body cells. It performs cleansing and nutrient functions, and is drained by the Canal of Schlemm. *See* also **glaucoma**.

AR: androgen receptor.

α-AR: alpha-type adrenergic receptor.

β-AR: beta-type adrenergic receptor.

ara-A: vidarabine.

arabinose: an aldopentose sugar component of complex polysaccharides made by many plants, and by mycobacteria and other organisms. It is used in some culture media, and some derivatives are antiviral and antineoplastic agents. *See* also **vidarabine**.

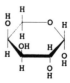

ARA-C: *see* **cytosine arabinoside**.

arachidonic acid {**arachidonate**}: AA; 5,8,11,14-eicosatetraenoic acid; an essential fatty acid obtained directly from food or made from other essential fatty acids. It is a component of phospholipids, cholesterol esters, and other lipids, and the major precursor of prostaglandins, prostacyclins,

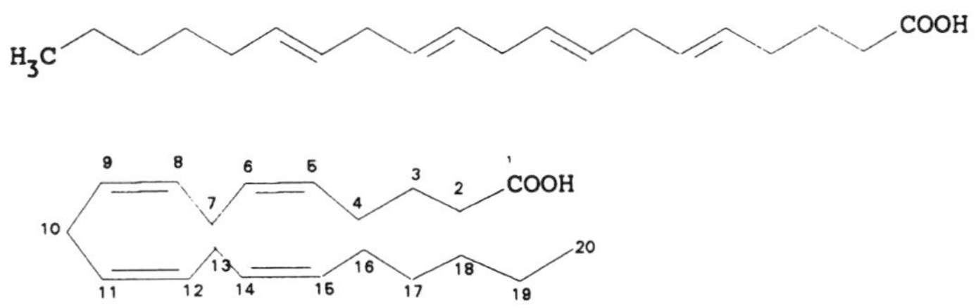

arachidonate

thromboxanes, leukotrienes, and other eicosanoids. Many regulators liberate it from those compounds by activating phospholipase A_2 isozymes, cholesterol esterases, or lipases. AA exerts some direct effects, for example on plasma membrane fluidity and enzyme microenvironments, and it contributes to long-term potentiation in the brain. It inhibits glutamate uptake by glial cells, and may decrease the time courses for currents through NMDA regulated ion channels by binding to receptors sites different from ones that bind glutamate. Hypoxia leads to accumulation of high levels in the brain; and neuron death can result from excessive effects on glutamate receptors. However, most influences are accomplished via conversion to eicosanoids. The rate limiting step for their formation is liberation of AA in free form. The folded structure shows the relationship to those molecules. See also **cyclooxygenase**, **lipoxygenases**, and **epoxygenases**.

ARAT: acyl-CoA retinol acyltransferase.

ARC: (1) arcuate nucleus: (2) AIDS related complex.

archencephalon: (1) the primitive brain; (2) the component of the embryonic neural tube that gives rise to the rhinencephalon and some other brain components.

archenteron: the embryonic cavity that forms during gastrulation and becomes the primitive gut.

arcuate nucleus: infundibular nucleus; ARC: a neuron cluster in the medial basal hypothalamus near the floor of the third ventricle that controls tonic gonadotropin secretion, contributes to the regulation of prolactin, growth hormone, and somatostatin release, and exerts other influences on the endocrine system. Some of the neurons make gonadotropin releasing hormone (GnRH). Other regulators in the nucleus include dopamine and norepinephrine.

ARE: androgen response element.

area postrema: a circumventricular organ that borders the fourth ventricle of the brain. It is a site for regulated exchange of substances between blood and cerebrospinal fluid.

α_1, α_2 **receptors**: *see* **adrenergic receptors**.

arecoline: *N*-methyltetrahydronicotinate; the major alkaloid of betel nuts. It is a nonspecific muscarinic-type acetylcholine receptor agonist that enters the brain, and exerts central, as well as peripheral effects. For example, it invokes euphoria, and stimulates the gut. High doses additionally exert some nicotinic actions. Arecoline is

also used to treat some parasitic infections, and in veterinary medicine as a cathartic.

ARF: ADP-ribosylation factor.

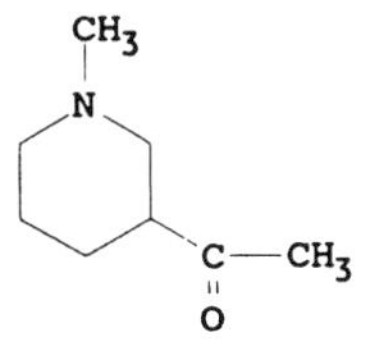

Arg: arginine.

arg: a gene of the *abl* family that directs formation of a protein with a nonreceptor type tyrosine kinase domain.

argentaffin cells: cells that stain directly with silver salts; *see* **chromaffin cells**.

Arg-Gly-Asp: RGD; an amino acid sequence present in one or more copies in fibronectin, fibrinogen, laminin, vitronectin, thrombospondin, type I collagen, osteopontin, von Willebrand factor, and other extracellular matrix glycoproteins. It is a recognition site (receptor) for many cell adhesion molecules (*see* **integrins**), and for some growth factors, and contributes to cell adherence, inflammation, immune system responses, and other functions.

arginase: an enzyme of the urea cycle and of pathways for polyamine biosynthesis. It catalyzes the reaction: arginine + $H_2O \rightarrow$ ornithine + urea.

arginine: Arg; R; a basic essential amino acid and a component of many peptides and proteins. It directly stimulates release of glucagon, insulin, and growth hormone, is a precursor for endothelium derived relaxation factor (EDRF, nitric oxide), creatine and polyamines, a growth stimulant for some species, and a component of the urea cycle. *See* also **arginosuccinate synthetase**, **arginase**, and **Arg-Gly-Asp**.

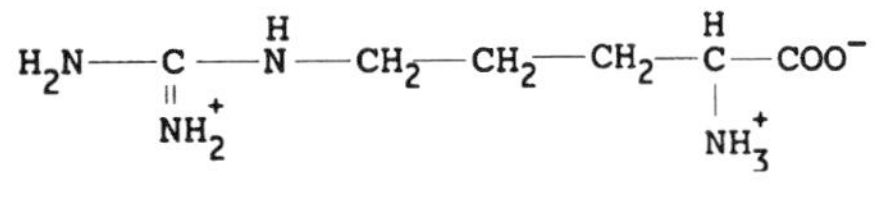

arginine vasopressin: AVP; antidiuretic hormone; ADH; the major neurohypophysial hormone for promoting water conservation in mammals (but *see* also **lysine vasopressin**). It accelerates osmotic reabsorption across collecting duct cells of the kidney by promoting translocation of water channels to apical plasma membranes, an effect dependent on microtubules, mediated via cAMP, and antagonized by prostaglandin $F_{2\alpha}$. Deficiency leads to the development of diabetes insipidus. Most of the circulating peptide is synthesized (along with arginine neurophysin) in hypothalamic magnocellular neurons, and is transported via hypothalamo-hypophyseal nerve tracts to the neural lobe, in which it is stored, and from which its is released to systemic blood capillaries. Osmo-, baro-, thermo-, and nociceptors communicate directly with the magnocellular neurons; and more of the hormone is during some forms of stress. AVP released to hypothalamo-hypophysial blood vessels markedly potentiates the effects of corticotropin releasing hormone (CRH) on adrenocorticotropic hormone (ACTH) secretion, but exerts only minor influences when presented alone. Peripherally, it directly stimulates vascular smooth muscle (especially in skin, skeletal muscle and mesenteric regions), can elevate blood pressure, and reduce sweating, and is used to treat circulatory shock. High concentrations additionally stimulate the smooth muscle of the gut and uterus, promote glycogenolysis in the liver, and accelerate the growth of some cell types. AVP is also made at several other sites. Small amounts in suprachiasmatic nuclei contribute to the control of circadian rhythms. In the extrahypothalamic brain, it (or fragments derived from it) facilitate learning and long-term memory. In the adrenal cortex and gonads, it augments steroidogenesis. Angiotensin-II stimulates AVP secretion, whereas atrial natriuretic peptides and glucocorticoids exert inhibitory influences.

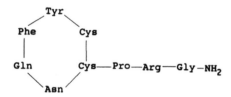

arginine vasopressin receptors: *see* **vasopressin receptors.**

arginine vasotocin: AVT: a peptide structurally related to **arginine vasopressin** *(q.v.),* but with the amino acid composition Cys-Tyr-Ile-Gln-Asn-Cys-Pro-Arg-Gly-NH_2. It is a neurohypophysial hormone, made by all nonmammalian vertebrates, that promotes water transport across the skin of some amphibians, and across urinary bladders of amphibians and reptiles, and additionally affects water balance by decreasing renal blood flow and glomerular filtration rates. Other effects include stimulation of the smooth muscle of oviducts and some other structures. AVT is made by mammalian fetuses, in which it affects water transport across amniotic membranes. Postnatally, small amounts in pineal glands and suprachiasmatic nuclei may contribute to the control of circadian rhythms.

arginosuccinate lyase: *see* **arginosuccinate synthetase** and **urea cycle.**

arginosuccinate synthetase: an enzyme that catalyzes the reaction: citrulline + aspartate + ATP → argininosuccinate + AMP + P-P. Arginosuccinate lyase then catalyzes cleavage of arginosuccinate to arginine + fumarate. The reactions are components of the urea cycle. Fumarate can enter the tricarboxylic acid cycle, or be used for gluconeogenesis. Arginine is a precursor of nitric oxide (NO), and of polyamines. Glutamine inhibits the synthetase, and thereby NO production.

A ring: the first of the four ring structures of a steroid or chemically related compound. In steroids, it is formed by carbons 1,2,3,4,5, and 10, and shares the last two with with the B ring. The 3 position is oxygenated in cholesterol and steroid hormones. Most adrenocortical and some gonadal hormones have a 4:5 double bond and a methyl group attached to carbon 10. Estrogens lack that methyl group and have aromatic A rings.

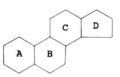

aromatase: usually, an enzyme complex that catalyzes desaturation of steroid A-rings. Enzyme systems that include a cytochrome P-450$_{aromatase}$, a flavoprotein (NADPH-cytochrome reductase) and an iron-sulfur protein catalyze conversion of Δ^4-androstenedione to estrone and of testosterone to estradiol in ovary, testis, adipose tissue stromal cells, skin, and some brain regions. A related system in syncytiotrophoblast converts 16α-hydroxy-androsterone to estriol. The reactions use three molecules of oxygen and two of NADPH for each steroid. See also **steroidogenic factor 1**.

aromatase hypothesis: a widely supported concept that androgens must be converted to estrogens before acting on certain target cells, including some within the hypothalamus that affect reproductive system functions.

aromatic: usually (1) describes compounds with benzene rings. Aromatic amino acids include phenylalanine, tyrosine, and tryptophan. Estrogens are aromatic steroids; (2) fragrant.

arrestins: α-arrestin is a 48K protein in retina rod cells that is chemically related to transducin, competes with it for binding to the phosphorylated form of rhodopsin, and thereby blocks transducin effects on a phosphodiesterase. It can also bind to β-adrenergic receptors (which are similar to rhodopsin). β-Arrestin is a widely distributed substrate for the β-adrenergic receptor kinase (BARK) that binds to ligand bound β-adrenergic receptors and blocks their interactions with G proteins. *Drosophila* photoreceptors contain a related 49K protein that undergoes phosphorylation when activated by light.

ARS: automatic replicating sequence.

arsenic: As; an element (atomic number 33, atomic weight 74.92). Although it has been suggested that minute amounts are essential for growth, arsenic compounds are toxic, in part because they interfere with oxidative phosphorylation and other reactions that use phosphate. Some compounds are insecticides.

arsenoazo-III: *o*-(1,8-dihydroxy-3,6-disulfonaphthylene-2,7-*bis*azo)-*bis*benzene arsinic acid; a calcium-sensitive dye.

aresenoazo-III

arteriole: a small, resistance-type blood vessel, composed of tunicas intima, media, and adventitia, that branches from an artery (or larger arteriole) and delivers blood to a smaller arteriole, precapillary, or capillary. Arteriolar smooth muscle contracts or dilates in response to several regulators, and thereby affects blood distribution to specific body regions. Agents that simultaneously affect many arterioles can elevate or lower diastolic blood pressure.

arteriosclerosis: "hardening of the arteries". In the most common type, *atherosclerosis* (*q.v.*), lipid deposits narrow the lumens, and thereby restrict blood flow to cells fed by the vessels. Diastolic blood pressure rises when many arteries are affected. A less common form, caused by calcium salt deposition in the tunica media, blunts the stretch and retraction that normally occur during systole and diastole, respectively. Consequently, systolic and pulse pressures are elevated, and diastolic pressure can be subnormal.

arteriosclerotic: pertaining to arteriosclerosis.

artery: a large vessel that receives blood from the heart or a larger artery and delivers it to a smaller artery or an arteriole. Pulmonary arteries carry deoxygenated blood to the lungs, whereas systemic vessels deliver oxygenated blood.

arthritis: any joint inflammation; see **rheumatoid arthritis** and **osteoarthritis**.

arthropods: animals of the phylum *Arthropoda*, which includes insects, spiders and related *Arachnids*, and crustaceans. All have exoskeletons, jointed appendages, ventrally located nervous systems, compound eyes, and open circulatory systems.

Arthus phenomenon: Arthus reaction; a localized necrotic lesion that forms rapidly following intradermal or subcutaneous injection of an antigen against which the individual has previously made antibodies. Localized antigen-antibody complexes initiate inflammation; activated complement, fibrin, platelets and neutrophilic leukocytes accumulate at the site; and thrombi occlude blood vessels.

artificial insemination: intravaginal or intracervical injection of spermatozoa to achieve fertilization. In some cases, a husband's sperm is with those of a donor. The procedure is also used to inseminate female farm animals, race horses, pure-bred dogs and other animals with sperm from specially selected stud males, and to achieve fertilization in members of endangered species.

As: arsenic.

Aschheim-Zondek test: A-Z test; "mouse test"; a pregnancy test used before more modern methods were developed, based on the ability of urine that contains human chorionic gonadotropin (hCG) to promote intrafollicular hemorrhages and luteal cell development in the ovaries of immature mice. The procedure is expensive, requires facilities to house mice, and involves killing several animals. The long time periods required for responses to develop preclude repetition with the same urine specimen. Moreover, since the responses are affected by many factors, both false positive and false negative results are often obtained. *See* also **pregnancy tests**.

Aschoff bodies: small granulomas formed in response to inflammation, composed of macrophages and lymphocytes that surround hyaline (acellular) collagenous matter.

ascites: fluid accumulation in the peritoneal cavity. The causes include myocardial insufficiency and consequent back-pressure on veins that drain the region, high pressure in hepatic portal system vessels (a common complication of cirrhosis), subnormal plasma albumin levels, infections, and severe irritation.

ascites tumors: tumors composed of cells that can grow when suspended in liquid media. Antibodies can be collected from ascites fluids of animals when hybridomas are cultured in peritoneal cavities.

ascorbic acid: vitamin C; 3-ketothreohexuronic acid; an essential dietary component for humans, other primates, guinea pigs, and other species that cannot synthesized the vitamin. It is a major water-soluble physiological antioxidant and reducing agent that protects lipids and many enzymes (including lysine hydroxylase, dopamine-β-hydroxylase, peptidyl glycine α-amidating monooxygenase, HMG-CoA reductase, a hydroxylase needed for carnitine synthesis, some types required for steroidogenesis, and hepatic types that affect drug metabolism) against oxidative degradation. It also protects tissues against damage by free radicals. Additionally, it is a cofactor for several monooxygenases, and a regulator of copper and iron metabolism. Dehydroascorbic acid is the reduced form. Deficiency leads to the development of scurvy, in which loss of the ability to stabilize prolyl hydroxylase in its active form impairs collagen cross-linking. The adrenal cortex accumulates large amounts, and a bioassay procedure for adrenocorticotropic hormone (ACTH) depends on the ability of that hormone to deplete the stores. Ascorbate may impose physiological limitations on glucocorticoid production. Even higher concentrations are found in the adrenal medulla, and uptake from the cortex can augment catecholamine production in times of stress. Claims that ingestion of large amounts protects humans against common colds and other infections, and against development of cancers have not been substantiated.

asexual reproduction: formation of new cells in which all genetic components are derived from single parent cells. Mitosis, a major form, is used during growth, and to replace worn out cells with new ones of the same kinds (for example in the intestine, skin, and bone marrow). *Cf* **sexual reproduction**.

ASH: aldosterone stimulating hormone.

asialoglycoprotein[s]: glycoproteins that do not contain sialic acid. When neuraminidases catalyze degradation of sialoproteins, they usually leave a galactose moiety on the exposed surface that can be recognized by asialoglycoprotein receptors. Most of the naturally occurring enzymes are on endothelial cell surfaces. Neuraminidases are used to study the roles of oligosaccharides in hormone binding and actions. Although clearance rates vary with protein structures, removal of sialic acid groups usually leads to more rapid removal of proteins from the bloodstream, and to more rapid degradation.

asialoglycoprotein receptors: receptors on the plasma membranes of hepatic cells that recognize asialoglycoproteins and internalize them via endocytosis.

ASIF: aldosterone secretion inhibiting factor; a 35-amino acid peptide in the adrenal medulla with homology to atrial natriuretic peptides, that is reported to inhibit aldosterone synthesis.

A site: *see* **aminoacyl-tRNA site**.

Asn: asparagine.

asolectin: a wheat germ agglutinin that binds, and is used as a marker for Golgi apparatus components.

Asp: aspartate; aspartic acid.

asparagine: Asn; P; α-amino-succinic acid; a non-essential amino acid that can be synthesized from oxaloacetate. It is a component of many proteins, and a common site for attachment of carbohydrate groups. Asparaginase catalyzes it conversion to aspartic acid.

aspargtocin: AST; a peptide structurally similar to arginine vasopressin, with the amino acid sequence Cys-Tyr-Ile-Asn-Asn-Cys-Pro-Leu-Gly-NH$_2$. It is an elasmobranch neurohypophysial peptide chemically related to oxytocin, believed to promote smooth muscle contraction and affect blood pressure in fishes. It lowers blood pressure in birds, and stimulates both uterine smooth muscle and mammary gland myoepithelial cells in mammals. (It is not related to aspartocin, an antibiotic made by *Streptomyces griseus* that is effective against gram positive bacteria.)

Aspartame: NutraSweet; Equal; α-aspartyl-phenylalanine-1-methyl ester; a low-calorie artificial sweetening agent, approximately 100 times as potent as sucrose. When metabolized, it releases phenylalanine (which is toxic to individuals with phenylketonuria) and aspartate. Ordinary amounts are well tolerated by healthy persons, but

very high aspartate levels can cause injury by acting on receptors for excitatory amino acids.

aspartate: *see* **aspartic acid**.

N-methyl-D-**aspartate**: NMDA; a specific agonist for one class of **glutamate/aspartate receptors** (*q.v.*). It competes more strongly with aspartate than with glutamate.

aspartate aminotransferase: glutamate oxaloacetate transaminase; a pyridoxal phosphate dependent enzyme that catalyzes the reaction: aspartate + α-ketoglutarate $\rightleftarrows$ oxaloacetate + glutamate. Since it leaks from injured heart and liver tissues, the levels in serum (SGOT) are used in diagnosis.

aspartate transcarbamoylase: a CAD component, used for pyrimidine biosynthesis, that catalyzes the reaction: carbamoyl phosphate + aspartate → N'-carbamoyl aspartate.

aspartic acid {**aspartate**}: Asp; D: an acidic amino acid, classified as nonessential, but a physiological ligand for aspartate/glutamate receptors in the brain, and a component of many peptides and proteins, including several enzymes. Since it is interconvertible with oxaloacetate (*see* **aspartate aminotransferase**), it can both derive from and enter the tricarboxylic acid cycle. It is also an arginine precursor (*see* **arginosuccinate synthetase**), and an intermediate in several metabolic pathways including gluconeogenesis and ureagenesis. Bacteria use it to make threonine, methionine, lysine, and pyrimidines (*see* **aspartate transcarbamoylase**).

aspartic proteases: pepsins, renins, cathepsins D and E, and other 30K-40K enzymes whose active sites contain aspartate. They preferentially cleave peptide bonds flanked by hydrophobic moieties, and are inhibited by pepstatins.

aspartocin: an antibiotic, made by *Streptomyces griseus spiralis*, that is effective against gram positive bacteria.

asperlicin: a potent, long-acting agent isolated from the fungus, *Aspergillus alliaceus*. It binds peripheral type cholecytokinin receptors with high affinity and specificity.

aspidin: acellular bone.

asperlicin

aspirin: acetylsalicylic acid (*q.v.*); an analgesic, antipyretic, anti-inflammatory agent that irreversibly inhibits cyclooxygenases.

astemizole: Hismanal; 1-(*p*-fluorobenzyl)-2-[[1-*p*-methoxyphenylethyl)-4-piperidyl]amino]-benzimidazole; an H_1-type histamine receptor antagonist that does not invoke drowsiness, and is used to treat some respiratory system disorders.

asters: star-like structures; usually, the microtubule arrays that surround animal cell centromeres during mitosis and meiosis.

asthenia: weakness; loss of strength and energy.

ASTI: active sodium transport inhibitor.

ASTP: ATP-stimulated translocation promotor.

astrocytes: neuroglia cells that attach neurons to blood vessels, exert influences on blood capillaries and cerebral blood flow, are components of blood brain barriers, and play important roles in development of the corpus callosum and other brain structures. They contain glutamine synthetase, and metabolize gamma-aminobutyric acid (GABA) and glutamate, contribute to synaptic reorganization, remove debris, release growth factors, and stimulate cytokine release by microglial cells. Although responses to NMDA and glycine have not been observed, they generate inositol-1,4,5-triphosphate (IP_3) and mobilize Ca^{2+} from intracellular sources when exposed to quisqualate. Kainate promotes depolarization and activates Ca^{2+}-dependent voltage gated channels that facilitate Ca^{2+} uptake from the environment. The cells also take up K^+, and are implicated as regulators of cerebrospinal fluid electrolyte levels. Responses to other regulators, including epidermal growth factor (EGF), and catecholamines acting on β-adrenergic receptors, have been described. *Fibrous* types predominate in central nervous system white matter, and *protoplasmic* types in the gray. Glial fibrillary acidic protein (GFAP) is present in the intermediate filaments, and is used as a marker for the cells. Other components include scatter factor and clusterin.

astroglial growth factors: nervous tissue peptides that promote proliferation and differentiation of astrocytes, oligodendrocytes, and pheochromocytoma cells, prolong the survival of some neurons, and augment choline acetyltransferase activity in the central and peripheral nervous systems. Astroglial growth factor-1 may be identical with acidic fibroblast growth factor (α-FGF), and astroglial growth factor 2 with a basic fibroblast growth factor (β-FGF).

A (α, alpha) subunit: a peptide chain of a dimeric or oligomeric protein. *See*, for example, **glycoprotein hormones**, **G proteins**, and **activins**.

ASV: avian sarcoma virus.

Asx: B; asparagine or aspartic acid, an acronym used when the molecule can contain either form at a specific locus, or it is not known which of the forms is present.

asymmetric carbon atom: a carbon atom linked to four other atoms, at least one of which differs from the others. Two compounds identical except for the spatial arrangements of those groups are enantiomers; *see*, for example, 5α- and 5β-dihydrotestosterone. Most enzymes and receptors recognize just one member of the pair.

AT-10: dihydrotachysterol.

AT-20: a cell line derived from adenohypophysial corticotropes that secretes adrenocorticotropic hormone, and is used to study ACTH synthesis.

Atabrine: a trade name for quinacrine hydrochloride.

ataractics: tranquilizers.

atavism: reversion to an earlier evolutionary type; reappearance of a hereditary trait that has not been expressed for several generations.

ataxia: impaired muscle coordination, usually caused by deterioration of cerebellar components.

ataxia telangiectasia: an autosomal recessive disorder attributed to diminished ability to repair damaged DNA. Impaired coordination associated with cerebellar deterioration, immune systems dysfunctions with poor resistance to infection, and susceptibility to development of lymphatic system cancers are characteristic findings.

ATD: *see* 1,4,6-**androstatriene 3,17 dione**.

ATF: Hela cell transformation factor; a 45-47K protein similar to CREB that interacts with cAMP response elements and invokes cell transformation.

atherosclerosis: the most common form of arteriosclerosis, in which cholesterol-containing plaques deposit in the intimal layers of large and medium sized arteries,

astemizole

partially (or totally) occlude the lumens, and present roughened surfaces to blood cells. It can invoke ischemia, stroke, myocardial infarction, thrombosis, and/or hypertension. The initiating factors include disruption of endothelium integrity, with consequent exposure of cells to collagen and other connective tissue components, and activation of macrophages. Progression of the lesions involves abnormal proliferation of vascular smooth muscle, fibrosis, and calcification. **Angiotensin-II** (*q.v.*) may be a major contributing factor, since it exerts several influences on blood vessels. It is reported to attach to receptors on macrophages and accelerate peroxidation of low density lipoprotein (LDL) phospholipids. The products attach to scavenerger receptors on the macrophages, and can convert them to foam cells. *See* also **apoprotein (a)**. Predisposing factors include diets that lower HDL:LDL ratios, androgens in the amounts made by normal males, some hormone imbalances, and inherited lipid metabolism defects. Estrogens and exercise appear to confer protection. Some atherosclerotic changes occur in the vessels of most elderly individuals.

athymic mice: nude mice: animals with genetic defects that impair thymus gland development and cellular immunity. They accept transplants rejected by normal counterparts, and are used to grow some kinds of tumors, and to study thymus gland functions.

ATL: adult T cell leukemia; *see* **leukemias**.

ATL-derived factor: ADF; adult T cell leukemia factor.

atomic force microscopy: techniques in which nanogram-sized diamond probes mechanically scan surfaces, and deflections are monitored by optical systems. For hard materials, the probes provide information on spatial arrangements of atoms with resolutions of 1-2 Å without damaging the specimens. They do injure soft surfaces, but some biological materials can be analyzed at resolutions of approximately 50 Å if frozen. When combined with computer simulation and tunneling microscopy, the techniques can be used to study contact formation, adhesion, and deformation.

atopy: inherited abnormal tendencies to develop immediate hypersensitivity, usually associated with excessive production of IgE type antibodies.

ATP: adenosine-5'-triphosphate; adenine-ribose-P-P-P; a ubiquitous nucleotide that releases the major direct source of energy for cell functions when it is undergoes hydrolysis (ATP → ADP + Pi or ATP → AMP + P-P). Its synthesis from ADP + P is accomplished via both substrate-linked and oxidative phosphorylations. ATP is the direct precursor of cAMP, the donor of phosphate groups for many molecules, including large numbers of protein kinase substrates, and an allosteric regulator of fructose-biphosphate and other enzymes. Several functions are unrelated to energy release, and can be mimicked with non-hydrolyzable analogs. Some are mediated via binding to P_2 type purine receptors (which are more sensitive to it than to adenosine). ATP directly opens some Ca^{2+} channels, augments plasma membrane permeability in macrophages, mast and some other cell types, and inhibits and K^+ channels in cardiac, smooth and skeletal muscle cells and pancreatic islet β cells. It is also a neurotransmitter at certain sites (for example for gastrointestinal tract cells that secrete vasoactive intestinal peptide). Apamin directly opposes the effects on VIP release

but does not influence hydrolysis. Fertilization is believed to be involve ATP release from sperm, followed by ATP binding to oocyte membrane ATP receptors, with consequent augmentation of oocyte Na^+ permeabilty. *See* also **ATPases**.

ATPases: enzymes that catalyze formation of ATP from ADP + P in mitochondria, and the reverse reaction at most other sites. (They can also catalyze the reverse the reaction in mitochondria under some conditions.) Various types in which energy released by ATP is coupled to ion exchanges are named for the kinds of ions moved; *see*, for example, Na^+/K^-, Na^+/H^+-, K^+/H^+-, and Ca^{2+}/Mg^{2+}-**ATPases**. The enzymes are classified on the basis of structures (and associated locations, functions, and responses to pharmacological agents). P types (E_1E_2-ATPases) are plasma membrane proteins that facilitate ion translocations. All are inhibited by vanadate, and many also by fluorescein isothiocyanate and *N*-ethylmaleimide. Most Na^+/K^--ATPases are inhibited by ouabain. F types (F_1F_2-ATPases) are on inner mitochondrial (and on chloroplast thylakoid and bacterial) membranes. They use proton (or Na^+) gradients to synthesize, and can also hydrolyze ATP; and they are inhibited by azide (and by oligomycin in mitochondria). V types (vacuolar ATPases) are on coated vesicles and some secretory granules. They use proton gradients to acidify cellular compartments, and are strongly inhibited by bafilomycin A_1.

ATPγS: adenosine-5'(thio)-triphosphate; adenosine 5'o-thiophosphate; an ATP analog that resists hydrolysis, and is used to study the mechanisms whereby ATP affects specific functions.

ATP-stimulated translocation promotor: ASTP; a 93K homodimeric protein that augments the affinities of glucocorticoid receptors for chromatin via ATP-dependent mechanisms that do not involve ASTP binding to steroids.

ATP synthase: *see* F_oF_1**-ATPase**.

atractyloside: atracyclin: $(2\beta,4\alpha,15\alpha)$-15-hydroxy-2-[[2-$O$-(3-methyl-1-oxobutyl)-3,4-di-O-sulfo-β-D-gluco-pyranosyl]oxy]-19-*nor*-kaur-16-en-18-oic acid dipotassium salt; a glycoside obtained from the *Atractylis gummifera* thistles that blocks oxidative phosphorylation by binding to and inhibiting mitochondrial ATP-ADP translocase when the nucleotide site faces the cytoplasm. *See* also **bongkrekic acid**.

atracyclin: atractyloside.

atresia: (1) collapse of, or failure to develop a lumen or orifice; (2) degeneration of ovarian follicles and their oocytes. Large numbers of ovarian follicles deteriorate during fetal life in normal female mammals. The processes continue throughout juvenile and later periods; and total depletion of oocytes occurs in elderly females. Atresia seems to be essential for attaining fertility, possibly because it establishes appropriate balances between germinal and other cell types and decreases competition for limited amounts of gonadotropins. Thymectomy performed soon after birth is reported to impair the processes in laboratory rodents, and to adversely affect ovarian function when the animals mature. During normal ovarian cycles, cohort follicles undergo atresia shortly before the time of ovulation (when they are no longer needed). High androgen and low estrogen levels, and fewer gonadotropin receptors distinguish them from the ones that proceed to preovulatory stages.

atrial glands: exocrine glands believed to contribute to egg-laying behavior in the marine mollusc *Aplasia*, possibly in part by releasing a pheromone. *See* also **egg laying hormone**.

atrial natriuretic factors: ANFs; *see* **atrial natriuretic peptides**.

atrial natriuretic hormones: ANH: *see* **atrial natriuretic peptides**,

atrial natriuretic peptides: ANPs; atrial natriuretic factors; ANFs; peptides initially identified in cardiac myocytes that contribute to the control of blood pressure, water and electrolyte excretion, and other functions. The major circulating human, bovine and canine form (also known as hANF, α-ANP, and ANP-28) has the amino acid sequence Ser-Leu-Arg-Arg-Ser-Ser-Cys-Phe-Gly-Gly-Arg-Met-Asp-Arg-Ile-Gly-Ala-Gln-Ser-Gly-Leu-Gly-Cys-Asn-Ser-Phe-Arg-Tyr, with a bond connecting the two cysteine components. One type made by rats, mice, and rabbits differs by a single amino acid moiety. Some smaller circulating forms may be degradation products. ANPαs are *C*-terminal cleavage products of a 126-amino acid prohormone storage form (proANP-126), and some numbering systems are based on it. (Thus, ANP-28 is also ANF 99-126). Urodilantin contains an additional *N*-terminal Thr-Ala-Pro-Arg sequence. Related peptides made by rats and named on the basis of their relationships to the rat 28 amino acid form include atriopeptins I, II, and III (atrial natriuretic peptides [5-25, 5-27, and 5-28], respectively, and auriculins A and B (atrial natriuretic peptides [4-27] and [4-28]). The major sources of circulating ANPs are atrial myocytes. Salt deprivation and fluid depletion promote prohormone storage in myocyte granules, whereas increases in blood volume and other factors that stretch cardiac muscle stimulate processing and release. Endothelin-1 accelerates prohormone synthesis and hormone release via mechanisms that involve protein kinase C activation. Catecholamines acting on α_1 type receptors inhibit by acting on L type Ca^{2+} channels and promoting Ca^{2+} uptake; and negative feedback control by ANP has also been suggested. **Brain natriuretic peptides** (*q.v.*) are related hormones initially identified in the central nervous system that are now called B-type ANFs, BNFs, and BNPs. In contrast with the A types, considerable species variations are known. Human, bovine, and rat types isolated contain, respectively, 32, 35, and 45 amino acid moieties. Although prevalent in the paraventricular nuclei and periventricular regions, they are no longer believed to be the primary central nervous system types (*see* **atrial natriuretic peptide receptors**). BNPs are also made by ventricular cardiac myocytes and adrenomedullary cells. A third peptide, C-ANP, appears to be limited to central nervous system neurons and pituitary glands, to be highly conserved among mammalian species, and to exist in both 22 and 53 amino acid forms. Catecholamines acting on α_2 adrenergic receptors facilitate release of the brain types. ANP is very rapidly cleared from the bloodstream, in part because of degradation by nonspecific neutral proteases that are most abundant in the kidneys, but also via uptake and sequestration by more widely distributed "clearance receptors". (The half lives in rats and humans are approximately 0.5 and 2.5 seconds, respectively). The receptors are widely distributed, and the effects of ligand binding include relaxation of smooth muscle in most vascular beds (but reduction of hepatic blood flow), cardiac inhibition, diuresis and natriuresis via actions on renal tubules as well as inhibition of renin, aldosterone, and vasopressin secretion. ANPs also decrease progesterone, POMC-derived peptide, and growth hormone secretion, relax intestinal smooth muscle, activate lung fibroblasts, and augment testosterone secretion. Receptors on bone marrow and thymus gland stromal cells are consistent with participation in immune system functions; and receptors on choroid epithelium are believed to mediate influences on the blood brain barrier, and on the production of cerebrospinal fluid. Centrally produced ANPs act within the brain to control blood pressure and cardiac functions, salt and water intake, and water balance in the brain. They also decrease the release of both aldosterone and glucocorticoids, but have little or no direct diuretic or natriuretic potency.

atrial natriuretic peptide receptors: at least three kinds of proteins that bind **atrial natriuretic peptides** (*q.v.*) with high affinity and specificity, and a fourth that binds with high capacity. A 120-130K type isolated from PCP12 (adrenomedullary derived) and endothelial cells binds ANP with high affinity, also binds some BNP, but has little affinity for CNP. It is variously called A receptor, ANP-A receptor, and GC-A (because it associates with a G protein that activates a guanylate cyclase). It mediates most of the peripheral actions of ANF-A, and has been identified on cardiac muscle, vascular and intestinal smooth muscle, zona glomerulosa, glomerular, juxtaglomerular and Henle loop kidney cells, lung fibroblasts, hypothalamic and other brain neurons, and stromal cells of the bone marrow and thymus gland. A second receptor type was initially named B receptor when it was believed to be the major mediator of BNP actions. It, too promotes guanylate cyclase activation, and is therefore also known as GC-B. It is abundant in the vicinity of the AV3V region of the brain, and is also made in aortic, mesangial cells and other cells types. In some, it co-exists with the GC-A types. It appears to be the primary receptor for CNP (rather than BCP), and the mediator of centrally controlled effects on blood pressure, salt and water intake, and adrenocortical steroid secretion. It is also present in bone marrow and thymus. Since neither GC-A nor GC-B binds BNP with the affinity displayed for the other ligands, yet a different receptor type for BNF may exist. Atrial natriuretic peptides inhibit adenylate cyclases in some cell types, but the kinds of receptors involved are not known. The possibility that other mechanisms contribute to the overall effects has been suggested, but no influences on phosphatidylinositol hydrolysis are known. The fourth receptor type is a 60-70K protein initially called type C, but now known as the clearance receptor. It is expressed on vascular cells, and it binds ANFs with low affinity but high capacity. It also binds limited amounts of BNP, and this may account for the longer half-life of BNP in the bloodstream. The clearance receptor does not couple to G proteins, but rapidly takes up circulating ANPs. Its major function appears to be protection against excessive build-up of peptide levels in the bloodstream. It may also serve as a reserve source, from which the regulators can be rapidly released in response to sudden changes in blood pressure or volume.

atriopeptides: atriopeptins; *see* **atrial natriuretic hormones**.

atrophy: wasting or shrinking of a structure after it has developed; *cf* **agenesis**. The term can refer to both pathological processes and reversible changes that occur when a structure is underused, deprived of stimulants and/or nutrients, or exposed to inhibitors. *See also* **involution, atresia, apoptosis**, and **necrosis**.

atropine: α-(hydroxymethyl)benzeneacetic acid 8-methyl-8-azabicyclo-octy-3-yl ester; a highly potent alkaloid made by *Atropa belladonna*, *Datura stramonium* and related plants, most often administered as a sulfate salt. Low concentrations block actions mediated by muscarinic type acetylcholine receptors on parasympathetic system target cells. High levels additionally inhibit neurotransmission in autonomic ganglia (but do not affect skeletal muscle neuromuscular junctions). Atropine has been used to relax intestinal smooth muscle and thereby control diarrhea, to facilitate examination of the eyes by dilating the pupils, and to decrease salivary and bronchial secretions in preparation for surgery. It has been replaced for many purposes by more specific and/or less toxic agents. High concentrations can invoke disorientation, hallucinations, hyperthermia, tachycardia, and circulatory failure.

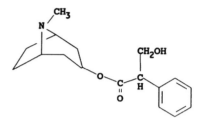

At-T cells: a corticotrope-like tumor cell line used to study adrenocorticotropic hormone (ACTH) secretion.

attenuate: weaken; in immunology, render less virulent.

attenuation: gene expression control by an attenuator.

attenuator: a termination site that regulates gene expression in bacteria, located between an operator and a gene that codes for the first enzyme of a metabolic pathway for amino acid synthesis. High levels of the amino acid terminate transcription by altering its structure.

atrotoxin: a high molecular weight, heat labile component of the venom of the rattlesnake, *Crotalus atrox*, that rapidly and reversibly binds specifically to cardiac Ca^{2+} channel proteins, and augments voltage dependent Ca^{2+}currents. It acts extracellularly, and affects the protein configurations, but does not (in effective concentrations) display phospholipase or protease activity, or change Na^+ or K^+ conductances. Its actions are dose-related, and are opposed by nitrendipine, cobalt, and other Ca^{2+} channel agonists, but not by α or β adrenergic receptor antagonists. Atrotoxin also binds dihydroyopyridines. The venom additionally contains other components that affect Ca^{2+} currents, some of which display phospholipase activity.

atroxin: a purified extract of *Bothrops atrox* venom that contains enzymes used to assay fibrinogen to fibrin conversion.

Au: gold.

AUG: the RNA base sequence that codes for methionine and directs initiation of translation on ribosomes; *see* also **initiation complex**.

aureomycin: chlortetracycline.

auriculin: *see* **atrial peptides**.

aurin: *p*-rosolic acid; 4-[*bis*(4-hydroxyphenyl)methylene]-2,5-cyclohexadien-1-one; an organic compound used to make aurintricarboxylic acid and other dyes.

aurin

aurintricarboxylic acid: a dye made from aurin that inhibits protein synthesis by binding to templates, and to some proteins that interact with nucleic acids.

aurothioglucose: *see* **gold**.

auranofin: *see* **gold**.

autism: thinking and behavior linked to self-preoccupation, with little or no relationship to other individuals or environmental factors.

autocatalytic: usually describes reactions catalzyed by a substrate cleavage product. For example, when trypsinogen cleavage yields small quantities of trypsin, trypsinogen becomes a trypsin substrate.

autacoids: regulators that act locally (close to their sites of production), a term applied to prostaglandins, histamine, growth factors, and other regulators that act via autocrine, paracrine, and/or intracrine mechanisms.

autocrine control: describes systems in which a regulator secreted by a cell acts on neighboring cells of the same kind, and/or returns to act on the cell that made it. For example, norepinephrine released from noradrenergic neuron terminals acts on presynaptic receptors to inhibit tyrosine hydroxylase (the rate-limiting enzyme for norepinephrine biosynthesis). Similarly, high levels of glucocorticoids inhibit additional glucocorticoid production. In these cases, protection against release of excessive amounts of the regulators is conferred. In contrast, many growth factors are autocrine stimulants. Some tumors grow rapidly because the cells have acquired the ability to synthesize stimulants not made by the normal counterparts. *Cf* **intracrine** and **paracrine controls**.

autocrine motility factor: AMF; a heat-stable, 55K protein initially isolated from melanoma conditioned media and subsequently identified in some individuals with familial type breast cancers. It acts via a G protein to promote cell dispersion (possibly by affecting hyaluronic acid synthesis), and may contribute to metastasis.

autogamy: self-fertilization by fusion of two nuclei within the same cell, or by fusion of nuclei from two daughter cells that derive from the same parent cell.

autoimmune disease: dysfunctions caused by immune system aberrations that lead to destruction of normal body components. They can involve excessive stimulation by T_H cells, and/or impaired ability to terminate responses no longer required to combat infections or suppress tumor growth. The causes include genetic defects, loss of normal mechanisms for maintaining self-tolerance, injuries that lead to release of antigenic molecules that are usually sequestered, and cross-reactivities invoked by antigens on infecting microorganisms that resemble endogenous types.

autoimmunity: immune system responses to endogenous antigens; *see* also **autoimmune disease**.

autoinduction: usually describes processes in which substances made by cells stimulate production of more molecules of the same kind. For example, transforming growth factor-α promotes TGFα synthesis in skin cells.

autologous: usually, (1) from the same individual, as in autologous graft; (2) describes a neoplasm derived from cell types that normally reside within the tissue that bears the tumor.

autolysis: self-destruction; usually cell or organelle rupture associated with release of lysosomal enzymes. By lowering cell pH, oxygen and nutrient deprivation can facilitate release of lysosomal enzymes and provide conditions under which they become more active. *Cf* **apoptosis** and **necrosis**.

automatic replicating sequence: ARS; automatic replicating segment; a DNA segment that supports independent replication of a plasmid in a host cell.

automatism: reflex or other behavior that is involuntary.

automixis: *see* **autogamy**.

autonomic: not under voluntary control; *see* **autonomic nervous system**.

autonomic nervous system: ANS; the part of the nervous system that regulates involuntary functions, such as blood pressure, digestion, secretion, and urine formation (but *see* **biofeedback**). Preganglionic neurons with cell bodies in the central nervous system extend axons that synapse in ganglia with postganglionic types whose axons travel to the target organs. Acetylcholine is the major neurotransmitter released by preganglionic neurons, and also by postganglionic neurons of the parasympathetic division. Since most parasympathetic ganglia are located close to the target organs, one kind of response can be accomplished with little effect on the others. In contrast, most sympathetic ganglia are close to the spinal cord, and messages can pass from one to another. Norepinephrine is the major transmitter for postganglionic sympathetic neurons.

autonomous: controlled by endogenous factors; capable of proceeding without externally delivered regulators.

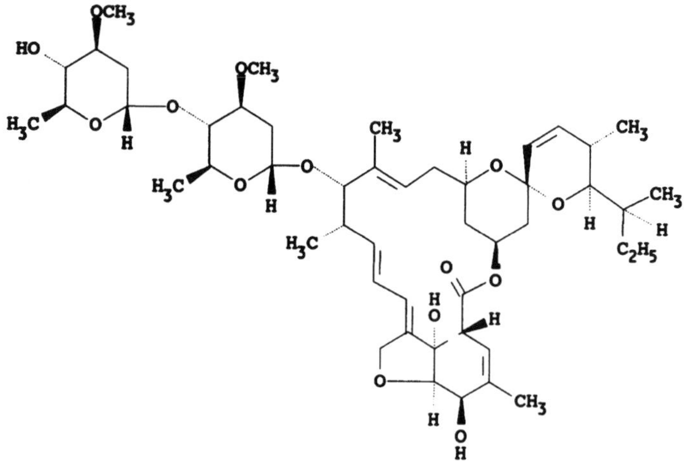

avermectin

autoxidation: usually, oxidation that is not catalyzed by enzymes.

autophagosomes: membrane-enclosed vesicles (usually phagolysosomes) in which cell components undergo digestion.

autophagy: intracellular degradation, usually in phagolysosomes. It can occur under physiological conditions, for example during embryogenesis, and in lactotropes after weaning. *See* also **lysosomes** and *cf* **apoptosis**.

autophosphorylation: covalent addition of phosphate groups, directed by components of the affected substrates. Receptors for many hormones undergo autophosphorylation when they bind their ligands.

autoploid: having two or more chromosomes or chromosome sets derived from the same haploid precursor.

autoradiography: radioautography; techniques for localizing specific molecular species (such as hormone receptors or enzymes). Preparations treated with radioactive ligands are fixed to slides or plates and covered with photographic emulsions. When developed, the radioactive sites appear as black spots.

autosensitization: processes that augment reactivity to self-antigens.

autosomes: chromosomes other than **sex chromosomes** (*q.v.*). Human cells have 22 homologous pairs whose members are similar in appearance, and control the same kinds of functions. They have somewhat different base sequences in heterozygotes (*see* **alleles**). Although structurally identical in males and females, many autososomes contribute to reproductive system functions (for example by directing the synthesis of gonadal hormones).

autotrophs: organisms that synthesize their organic nutrients form inorganic matter, and are therefore not dependent of other organisms for growth and survival. Examples include most green plants and many microorganisms.

autozygous: homozygous at a specified genetic locus.

auxins: plant growth hormones that facilitate linear growth. The best known type is indoleacetic acid (IAA), which induces specific proteins and promotes root and vascular bundle formation. Some effects are attributed to plasma membrane hyperpolarization, changes in cell wall space pH, activation of pH-sensitive hydrolases, and rupture of calcium cross-bridges. The resulting decreases in cell wall rigidity facilitate turgor-driven expansion. Other auxins include indole-3-methane sulfonate and naphthalene acetic acid. Ethylene slows IAA uptake and transport at some sites, and stimulates growth of lateral shoots. Auxin binding proteins that may be specific receptors include 65K plasma membrane and 40K intracellular types.

auxological: affecting body growth.

Ava I: a restriction endonuclease from *Anabaena variabilis* blue-green algae that cleaves DNA at the sites shown. Py represents any pyrimidine base, and Pu any purine type.

$$\downarrow$$
$$5'\ C\ \ Py\ C\ G\ Pu\ \ G\ \ 3'$$
$$3'\ G\ \ Pu\ G\ C\ Py\ \ C\ \ 3'$$
$$\uparrow$$

avermectins: the term can refer to several related compounds obtained from *Streptomyces avermitilis* (including types A_{1a}, A_{2a}, B_{1a}, and B_{2a}), or specifically to the B_{1a} form (shown below), from which ivermectin is made. The compounds are used to kill larval and adult nematodes. Some of the actions are attributed to influences on $GABA_A$ type receptors, since they can be mimicked with muscimol and antagonized with picrotoxin.

aversion: turning away; dislike; a term applied to spontaneous responses (for example to unpleasant substances or excessive amounts of food, and to manipulations, such as stimulation of certain brain regions). Some authors regard aversion as an exaggerated form of **satiety** (*q.v.*).

aversion "centers": brain regions said to mediate unpleasant sensations; *cf* **pleasure "centers"**.

avian: derived from, or characteristic of birds.

avian erythroblastosis virus: AEV; an acute transforming avian leukemia virus that carries *v-erbA* and *v-erbB* genes, and can invoke fibrosarcomas as well as leukemia in birds.

avian leukemia viruses: avian erythroblastosis, avian myeloblastosis, and some other RNA replication-defective tumor viruses that require helper viruses to invoke acute leukemias and tumor growth in birds.

avian leukosis virus: *see* **avian lymphatic leukemia virus**.

avian lymphatic leukemia virus: ALV; a replication-competent RNA tumor virus that causes slowly developing leukemias (but not fibrosarcomas) in birds.

avian myeloblastosis virus: AMV; an avian leukemia virus that carries the *v-myb* transforming gene.

avian myelocytomatosis virus: an avian leukemia virus that carries the *v-myc* transforming gene.

avian sarcoma virus: ASV; *see* **Rous sarcoma virus**.

avidin: an egg-white protein secreted by avian oviducts. Since it production is enhanced in cells exposed first to estrogen and then to progesterone, it is used to study steroid hormone actions. High levels invoke biotin deficiency by binding to the vitamin.

avidin-biotin complex DNA-binding assays: ABCD; techniques used for DNA analysis, based on the high binding affinities of the components.

avidity: usually (1) the total binding strength of a complex system that contains antigens and antibodies. The value depends on both the numbers of binding sites and the affinities; (2) eagerness or greediness.

Avogadro's number: Avogadro's constant; 6.03×10^{23}; the number of atoms in one gram molecular weight of an element.

A vitamin: *see* **vitamin A**.

avitaminosis: vitamin deficiency.

AVP: arginine vasopressin; *see* **vasopressins**.

d(CH_2)-Tyr(Met)-**AVP**: a V_1-type vasopressin receptor antagonist.

d-Phe-Tyr(Met)-**AVP**: a V_2-type vasopressin receptor antagonist.

AVT: arginine vasotocin.

AV$_3$V: the anterolateral ventral region of the third ventricle of the brain. It is a major site for central nervous system regulation of blood pressure, and of water and electrolyte balance.

axenic: germ free; free of contaminating cells or organisms.

axial filaments: *see* **axoneme**.

Axid: a trade name for Nizatidine.

axo-axonic: contact (usually synaptic) between the axon of one neuron and the axon of another.

axodendrite: a dendrite that is a side-branch of an axon.

axokinin: a 56K protein that reactivates axonemes when it is phosphorylated by a protein kinase A catalyzed reaction.

axolemma: the plasma membrane of an axon; *cf* **neurolemma**.

axolotl: the salamander, *Ambystoma mexicana*. It is usually neotenous, but undergoes metamorphosis when treated with thyroid hormones.

axon[s]: nerve cell processes that usually conduct impulses away from cell bodies. A typical neuron has a single long axon that receives vesicle-enclosed neurotransmitters synthesized in the cell body, transports the vesicles to terminals for storage, and releases the neurotransmitters to a synaptic cleft or neuromuscular junction when the neuron is stimulated. *Cf* **dendrite**, and *see* also **antidromic** and **axon-axon transmission**.

axon-axon transmission: although most neurons release their transmitters from axon terminals to synpatic clefts, some have axons that communicate with those of other neurons.

axoneme: (1) axial filament; the central microtubule complex of a eukaryote cilium or flagellum (which is composed of 2 centrally located and 9 concentrically arranged pairs of tubules). In a spermatozoan, the filament extends from the neck region to the tip of the tail; (2) the axial core of a chromosome.

axopetal: in the direction of the axon.

axoplasm: the cytoplasm of an axon.

5-azacytidine: 4-amino-1-β-D-ribofuranosyl-1,3,5-triazine-1(1*H*)-one; a cytidine analog that incorporates into DNA molecules, but does not undergo methylation. It blocks inactivation of differentiation promoting genes, but can activate genes otherwise quiescent in the cell type, and thereby invoke changes such as production of fetal type hemoglobin and other substances not usually made by the differentiated cell type. It is used to treat some neoplasms, and as a laboratory tool to invoke mutagenesis.

5-azacytosine: 4-amino-triazin-2(1*H*)-one; a cytosine analog that is converted to azacytidine.

8-azaguanine: 5-amino-1,4-dihydro-7*H*-1,2,3-triazolo [4,5-d]pyrimidin-7-one; a purine antimetabolite that incor-

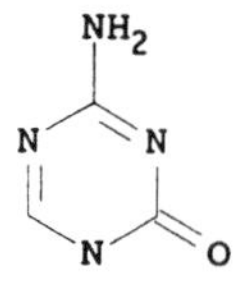

5-azacytosine

porates into nucleic acids. It is used to inhibit the growth of some kinds of tumor cells.

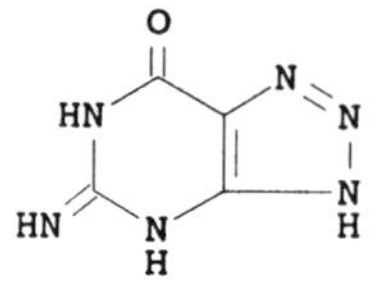

azamethonium bromide: Pentamin; 2,2'-(methylimino) bis-[*N*-ethyl-*N*,*N*-dimethylethanamin-ium]dibromide; a ganglion blocking agent used to lower blood pressure, and to diminish bleeding during surgery.

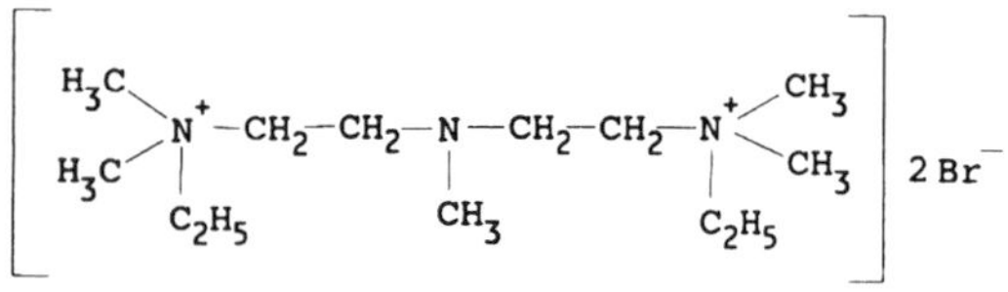

azapetine: 6,7-dihydro-6-(2-propenyl)-5*H*-dibenzazepine. The phosphate (Ilidar) is an α₁-type adrenergic receptor antagonist. It is used to lower blood pressure, and as a tranquilizer.

azaprostanoic acids: anti-inflammatory agents that inhibit the synthesis and/or block responses to thromboxanes, prostaglandins, and related regulators. 9,11-azaprost-13-enoate inhibits the synthesis of thromboxanes, and 13-azaprostanoic acid is a TXA₂/PGH₂ receptor antagonist.

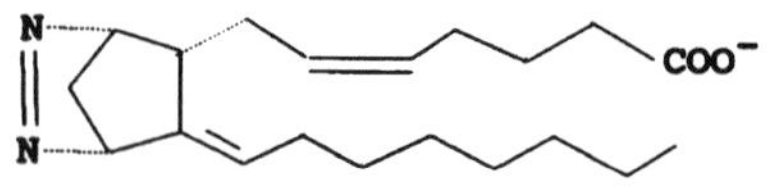

9,11-azaprost-13-eonate

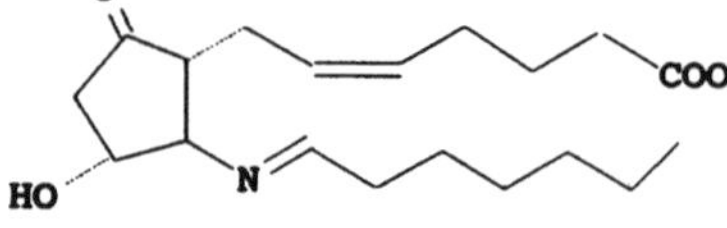

13-azaprostanoic acid

azaserine: *O*-diazo-acetylserine; an antibiotic obtained from *Streptomyces* species that inhibits purine (and therefore nucleotide) synthesis by blocking transfers of amino groups to acceptor molecules. It is used to treat fungus infections and some neoplasms, but can cause formation of abnormal chromosomes.

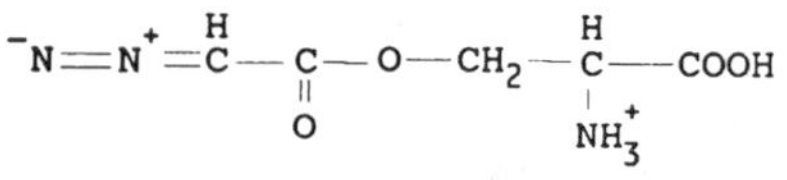

azaserine

azatidine: 6,11,-dihydro-11-(1-methyl-4-piperidinylidene)-5*H*-benzo[5,6]-cycloheptal[1,2-*b*]-pyridine; an H₁ type histamine receptor antagonist.

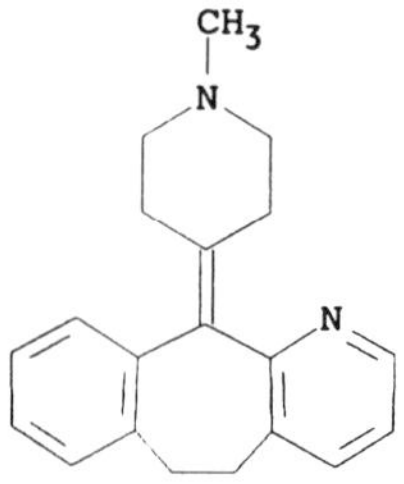

azathioprine: Imuran; 6-[1-methyl-4-nitroimidazol-5-yl) thio]purine; a 6-mercaptopurine analog that invokes long-term immunosuppression. It is under investigation for the treatment of systemic lupus erythematosus, rheumatoid arthritis, and some forms of leukemia, but is potentially carcinogenic.

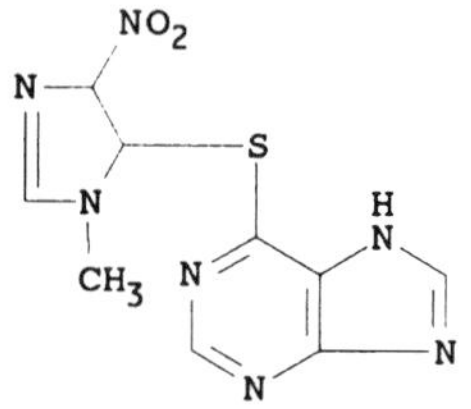

6-azauridine: 2-β-D-ribofuranosyl-1,2,4-triazine-3,5(2*H*, 4*H*)-dione: a pyrimidine antimetabolite that blocks nucleic acid synthesis. It is used to treat psoriasis, polycythemia, some fungus infections, and some neoplastic diseases.

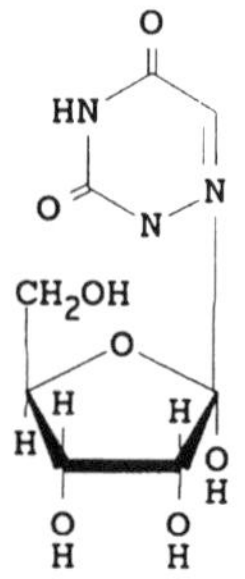

L-**azetidine-2-carboxylic acid**: a specific inhibitor that incorporates into, and modifies the properties of proline-containing proteins.

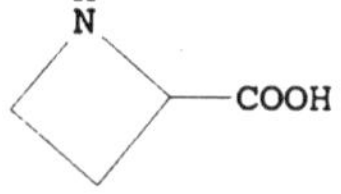

azide: (1) N₃-, or compounds that contain the chemical group -N₃; (2) NaN₃, an agent used to study mitochondrial functions, and to inhibit bacterial growth in reagents and culture media. By binding to the ferric form of cytochrome oxidase heme groups, it blocks transport of electrons to molecular oxygen.

3′azido-3-deoxythymidine; AZT; Retrovir; zidovudine; an inhibitor of retroviral reverse transcriptases. It is used to prolong survival in patients with AIDS, but the toxic effects include bone marrow suppression.

azo: describes compounds of the general type: R-N=N-R; azo- in the name of a compound indicates that a nitrogen atom has replaced a carbon atom.

azoic: lifeless.

azoles: compounds that contains five-membered heterocyclic rings with at least one nitrogen atom. Pyrroles, diazoles (such as imidazole), triazoles, and tetrazoles, have, respectively, 1, 2, 3, and 4 nitrogens per ring.

azoospermia: inability or failure to produce spermatozoa.

azotemia: abnormally high circulating levels of nitrogen compounds, and especially of urea. The major cause is renal dysfunction.

AZT: 3-azido-3′deoxythymidine.

A-Z test: Aschheim-Zondek test.

azurophils: cells that stain with blue aniline dyes.

B

B: (1) boron; (2) an antigen on the surfaces of erythrocytes of individuals with B and AB blood types. *See also* **B subunits**.

b: (1) bovine, as in bGH (bovine growth hormone); (2) basic, as in bFGF (basic fibroblast growth factor).

β: *see* **β subunits**, **β position**, **β cells**, and β-type **adrenergic receptors**.

B.: bacillus, as in *B. subtilis*.

B_1, B_2, B_3: *see* **backcross**.

B-7: an antigen on the surfaces of macrophages, dendritic cells, and activated B lymphocytes that interacts with CD28 on T lymphocytes and directly stimulates interleukin-2 production. It appears to be an essential costimulant (along with processed foreign antigens and class 2 major histocompatibility proteins that are recognized by T cell receptors) for T_C toxicity directed against at least some cell types. It is believed that tumor cells which express MHC antigens can escape killing if they do not also express B-7.

B-48, B-100: *see* **apoproteins**.

7B2: *see* **protein 7B2**.

Ba: barium.

bacalovirus: a retrovirus whose genome directs formation of the $p21^{v-ras}$ oncogene.

backcross: techniques used to study inheritance, usually performed on plants, fruit flies, or other organisms with short generation times, in which all individuals are mated with an initial set of parents (or with genetically identical organisms). The first backcross produces the B_1 generation; *cf* **testcross**. The second backcross (B_1 mating with the original parental type), produces the B_2 generation. A third backcross, B_2 mating with the same parental type, yields the B_3 generation.

bacillus [bacilli]: (1) any rod-shaped bacterium; (2) any member of the *Bacillus* genus.

Bacillus: a genus of aerobic, spore-forming, rod-shaped bacilli. Most are 0.5-1μm long.

Bacillus Calmette-Guérin: BCG; attenuated *Mycobacterium tuberculosis* organisms. They are potent leukocyte stimulants, used in vaccines to protect against tuberculosis and leprosy, and as adjuvants to enhance immune system responses to other antigens.

bacitracins: antibiotics obtained from *Bacillus subtilis* and *Bacillus licheniformins* that inhibit glycosylation reactions. They are used topically to combat bacterial and fungal infections, and as laboratory tools that block glycosylation of hormones and other molecules.

baclofen: β-(4-chlorophenyl)-γ-aminobutyric acid; a $GABA_B$ type receptor agonist that additionally exerts some antagonistic effects unrelated to interactions with that receptor. It is used as a muscle relaxant.

bacteria: a major class of prokaryote microorganisms. A typical bacterium has a single, circular chromosome that is not enclosed within a nucleus, and 70S ribosomes whose responses to antibiotics and other agents differ from those of eukaryote cell 80S forms.

bacteriocins: exogosins secreted by bacteria that kill closely related strains. The best known types include *Escherichia coli* colicins and *Pseudomonas aeruginosa* pyocins.

bacitracins

bafilomycin A₁

bacteriophages: viruses that infect bacteria, each composed of a protein (capsid) that encloses a DNA or RNA molecule. The genetic material is injected into the host, in which it replicates. *Temperate* types (such as bacteriophage λ, a coliphage that infects *E. coli*) integrate into host genomes but do not kill the cells. *Virulent* ones usurp the host transcriptional and translational machinery, self-assemble to form new phage particles, and escape when they cause host cell wall rupture. Some phages are used as vectors for DNA studies.

bacterium: a single organism of the bacteria group.

bacteroid: small bacteria that colonize nitrogen-fixing plant root nodules. Most are irregular rods.

bafilomycins: macrolide antibiotics made by *Streptomyces* species that inhibit the growth of gram positive bacteria and some fungi. Bafilomycin A₁ specifically inhibits vacuolar ATPases.

bag cell neurons: clusters of approximately 800 electrically-coupled abdominal ganglion neurons in *Aplysia* species that release several hormones (and possibly also pheromones) which act in conjunction with atrial glands to control egg laying. Four similar, coordinately controlled genes direct formation of prohormones, each of which is cleaved to yield multiple active peptide fragments; *see* **bag cell peptides**.

bag cell peptides: BCPs; peptides secreted by bag cell neurons that promote egg-laying. A 34K (242 amino acid) prohormone is cleaved to at least nine fragments, including egg laying hormone (ELH), and bag cell peptides α, β, and γ. A second, closely related gene product yields peptides A and A-ELH, and a third provides other regulators. The highly basic *Aplysia californica* ELH has the amino acid sequence: H-Ile-Ser-Ile-Asn-Gln-Asp-Leu-Lys-Ala-Ile-Thr-Asp-Met-Leu-Leu-Thr-Glu-Gln-Ile-Arg-Glu-Arg-Gln-Arg-Tyr-Leu-Ala-Asp-Leu-Arg-Gln-Arg-Leu-Leu-Glu-Lys-OH. Most of the activity of BCP-α is contained within its first nine amino acids: H₂N-Ala-Pro-Arg-Leu-Arg-Phe-Tyr-Ser-Leu-OH. The γ-peptide factor is H₂N-Arg-Leu-Arg-Phe-Asp-OH. The β peptide factor lacks the Asp of the γ-type. Peptide A is H-Ala-Val-Lys-Leu-Ser-Ser-Asp-Gly-Asn-Tyr-Pro-Phe-Asp-Leu-Ser-Lys-Glu-Asp-Gly-Ala-Gln-Pro-Tyr-Phe-Met-Thr-Pro-Arg-Leu-Arg-Phe-Tyr-Pro-Ile-OH. The first nine amino acids of peptide B are Ala-Val-Lys-Ser-Ser-Ser-Tyr-Glu-Lys-, and amino acids 10 through 34 are identical with those of peptide A.

baicalein: 5,6,7-trihydroxyflavone; a component of *Scutellaria baicalensis* roots that inhibits 12-lipoxygenase, and thereby the biosynthesis of some leukotrienes. It also inhibits the release of liposome enzymes, and has astringent properties.

BAL: dimercaprol; British antilewisite; 2,3-dimercapto-1-propanol. It chelates heavy metals, and is used to treat mercury poisoning.

BAL-31: a nuclease made by *Alteromonas espejiana* BAL-31 bacteria that cleaves double-stranded DNAs at both ends, and can progressively shorten restriction fragments. It is used to create deletion mutants.

Balb mice: highly inbred mouse strains used in immunology and genetic studies because of special characteristics such as coat color, and histocompatibility antigen patterns.

Balbiani rings: puffs on the giant chromosomes of some insects that contain large quantities of transcriptionally active DNA.

ballooning: usually, the preovulatory uterine swelling in rats and other species caused by estrogen-stimulated fluid production and cervical constriction.

BAM HI: a type II restriction endonuclease from *Bacillus amyloliquefaciens H* that cleaves DNAs at the sites shown.

```
      ↓
5' G  G A T C  C 3'
3' C  C T A G  G 5'
              ↑
```

band III: band 3 protein: an abundant 103K dimeric integral transmembrane glycoprotein that forms erythrocyte anion exchange channels, mediates HCO_3^-/Cl^- counterport, is essential for control of CO_2 movement, and has binding sites for ankyrin and other proteins.

band 4.1 protein: *see* **protein 4.1**.

band cells: immature neutrophilic leukocytes with spherical nuclei.

banding patterns: transverse stripes on stained chromosomes. G bands appear when warmed chromosomes are stained with Giemsa dye, and A bands (reverse of G bands) when they are pretreated with hot alkaline solutions before Giemsa staining. Quinacrine intercalates into DNA helices, and yields Q bands. Although it has been widely assumed that the patterns relate directly to gene types, regional differences in transcription activities can affect the staining reactions.

bank: gene bank.

bantam syndrome: Seabright bantam syndrome; a form of pseudohypoparathyroidism that is associated with insensitivity to androgens.

BAP: bacterial alkaline phosphatase; an enzyme made by *Escherichia coli* that catalyzes removal of 5′ terminal phosphate groups from DNA chains. It is used to prevent recircularization of vector molecules during gene cloning.

BAPTA: 1,2 *bis*-(2-amniophenoxy)-ethene-*N,N, N′N*-tetraacetic acid; an aromatic buffer that rapidly and selectively chelates calcium (with little affinity for magnesium), is pH insensitive, and undergoes changes in fluorescence and ultraviolet absorption that can be monitored. The acetoxymethyl ester (BAPTA/AM) penetrates cell membranes and is cleaved by cytoplasmic esterases to free BAPTA.

barbiturates: amobarbital (Amytal), hexobarbital, pentobarbital (Nembutal), phenobarbital, secobarbital (Seconal), and other 2,4,6-trioxohexahydropyrimidine derivatives. They are central nervous system depressants, used clinically as sedatives and hypnotics. They exert GABA-like actions and inhibit catecholamine and serotonin turnover; and some also enhance 5α-reductase activity. Barbiturates additionally slow hepatic degradation of steroid hormones and many drugs, and affect other liver functions. In laboratory animals, low doses are used to block central nervous system mediated release of gonadotropins and some other hormones. Pentobarbital is also used in larger amounts for anesthesia and euthanasia.

barium: Ba; a metallic element (atomic number 56, atomic weight 137.33). Since they are electron dense, the salts are used in radiology. The divalent ions inhibit ATP-sensitive K^+ channels. Although toxic, the properties they share with Ca^{2+} are applied in calcium transport and metabolism studies. Several isotopes are available.

BARK: β-ARK: β-adrenergic receptor kinase.

baroreceptors: pressoreceptors; structures that respond to changes in stretch or pressure. Most are in the vascular system.

Barr bodies: densely staining chromatin masses near the peripheries of nuclei in neutrophilic leukocytes, and in superficial epithelial and other cells that contain inactivated X chromosomes. Individuals in which they can be demonstrated are said to be chromatin positive. Since the number per cell is one less than the number of X chromosomes, they can be used to detect abnormal sex chromosome patterns. Normal (XX) females and XXY males have one, and XXX females have two. Normal (XY) male mammals have none, and are said to be chromatin negative.

barrier contraceptives: condoms, diaphragms, spermicidal vaginal suppositories, and other devices that block sperm entry into the uterus.

barrow: a castrated hog, boar, or other male swine.

Bartter's syndrome: conditions in which juxtaglomerular cell hyperplasia and excessive renin secretion cause secondary hyperaldosteronism. The common manifestations are hypokalemia and alkalosis. However, although the levels of angiotensin-II are high, blood pressure is often within the normal range.

basal activity: usually, the level of enzyme or other activity in "resting" cells (ones not exposed to external stimulants or inhibitors).

basal bodies: kinetosomes; cylindrical intracellular structures at the bases of cilia and flagella, similar to or identical with centrioles, each composed of nine sets of microtubule triplets held together by proteinaceous fibers. They are nucleation centers from which microtubules grow (for example during mitosis), and are believed to be self-replicating.

basal cells: usually, epithelial cells that divide by mitosis, renew populations within a tissue, and give rise to more differentiated cell types.

basal ganglia: large bilateral masses of gray matter (neuron clusters) at the bases of the cerebral hemispheres that regulate extrapyramidal tract functions. The corpus striatum is the major component, but some authors include the subthalamic and amygdaloid nuclei. Dopamine is a major neurotransmitter.

basal laminae: thin sheets of specialized extracellular matrix that underlie basal surfaces of epithelia, and surround tubes, muscle, fat, and Schwann cells, composed mostly of type IV collagen, proteoglycans and laminin. They are secreted by the overlying cells, and are components of basement membranes. The laminae organize proteins in adjacent plasma membranes, serve as highly selective filters, provide highways that both facilitate and limit cell migration, affect cell differentiation and metabolism, and can, at some sites, determine cell polarities.

basal metabolic rate, BMR: the heat production rate in a resting, postabsorptive subject (or in cells or tissues taken from such an individual), usually expressed as Calories/square meter body surface/hour (or as a per cent of the normal value) for whole organisms, and as Calories (or calories) per unit time per unit mass for tissues. The values are usually obtained indirectly by measuring oxygen consumption rates under standardized conditions and calculating the heat equivalents.

basal surface: the surface (1) farthest from the lumen of a follicle or other cavity; (2) on the wider part of a conical cell.

base: (1) alkali; a substance that can accept protons; (2) a purine or pyrimidine component of a nucleic acid, oligonucleotide, nucleotide, or nucleoside; (3) the main ingredient or the binding component of a mixture.

Basedow's Disease: an old term for Graves' Disease; *see* also **goiter**.

basement membrane: the extracellular matrix of an epithelial tissue, composed of the basal lamina secreted by the epithelium, plus a reticular layer made by underlying connective tissue. The components include collagen (some of which forms fiber networks), glycosaminoglycans, fibronectin, laminins, entactin, and nidogen. They affect cell differentiation and proliferation, adhesion, motility and shape.

base pair: a set of two complementary nitrogenous bases, usually on two different nucleotide strands. The major ones in DNAs are adenine:thymine and guanine:cytosine, linked by hydrogen bonds in double-stranded molecules. The bonds are severed prior to DNA replication, and each of the bases on the separated strands pairs with a new one of the complementary type. RNA synthesis, which proceeds along one DNA strand, involves transient formation of mostly adenine:uracil and guanine:cytosine bonds. During translation, transfer RNA (tRNA) anti-codon bases pair with messenger RNA (mRNA) codon bases.

base-pair ratio: the ratio of (adenine + thymine) to (guanine + cytosine) in a DNA molecule.

basket cells: cerebellar cortex molecular layer neurons with long, multibranched axons that extend toward and surround Purkinje cells.

basolateral surface: the plasma membrane surface closest to the basal lamina. In many cell types, it holds receptors for hormones and other regulators, and/or enzymes used to actively extrude ions. *Cf* **apical surface**.

basophils: (1) cells with granules that take up alkaline dyes; examples include thyrotropes and gonadotropes; (2) basophilic leukocytes.

basophilia: abnormally high levels of circulating basophilic leukocytes. Whooping cough, measles, tuberculosis, and hepatitis are among the infectious diseases in which it occurs.

basophilic leukocytes: basophils; the least numerous of the circulating white blood cells, similar in appearance to mast cells. They derive from myelocytes, have IgE receptors, and contribute to allergic reactions, inflammation, and the control of blood coagulation; *see* also **basophilia**. The cells are nonpolymorphic and nonphagocytic. Their basophilic secretory granules contain histamine bound to a heparin-like matrix. Those components are separated and released, along with proteases, platelet activating factor (PAF), and other regulators when the cells are activated.

BAT: brown adipose tissue.

batrachotoxins: steroidal alkaloid neurotoxins made in the skin of frogs of the genus *Phyllobates* that have been used as arrow poisons. They accelerate Na^+ entry into cells by binding to opened sodium channels. The most potent type is batrachotoxin A, 20-(2,4-dimethyl-1-*H*-pyrrole-3-carboxylate.

BAY-K 8644: 1,4-dihydro-2,6-dimethyl-3-nitro-4-(2-trifluormethylphenyl)-pyridine-5-carboxylate; an agonist for L-type calcium channels that prolongs the open state and thereby facilitates Ca^{2+} entry.

B/B rats: homozygotes of a mutant strain that are lymphopenic and display T cell deficiencies. They have exaggerated tendencies to develop autoimmune diseases

batrachotoxin A

which affect thyroid glands and pancreatic islet β-cells, and are used as animal models for diabetes mellitus.

BBB: blood brain barrier.

B blood type: blood characterized by the expression of B (but not A type) antigens on erythrocyte surfaces, and the presence of anti-A antibody in the plasma. Homozygotes have two alleles that code for the antigen and are classified as BB; heterozygotes have one, and are BO.

BCDF: B cell differentiation factor; *see* **interleukin-6**.

BCECF: 2′,7′*bis*-(2-carboxyethyl)-5,6-carboxyfluorescein; an agent used to measure cell acidity. It is administered as the acetoxymethyl ester (BCECF-AM), which penetrates cell membranes and is converted by intracellular enzymes to free BCECF.

B cell[s]: (1) B lymphocytes; (2) β cells, definition 1.

β cell[s]: (1) insulin-secreting pancreatic islet cells; (2) basophilic cells of the adenohypophysis (for example thyrotropes and gonadotropes).

B cell activating factor: BAF; an old term for interleukin-1.

B cell differentiation factor: BCDF; B cell stimulatory factor 2; BSF-2; BSF II; a 26K, 184-amino acid lymphokine secreted by antigen-activated helper type T lymphocytes, now called **interleukin-6** (*q.v.*)

B cell growth factor I: BCGFI; B cell stimulatory factor I; BSFI; *see* **interleukin-4**.

B cell growth factor II: BCGF II: *see* **interleukin-5**.

BCG: Bacillus Calmette Guérin.

BCGFs: B cell growth factors I and II, now known, respectively, as **interleukin-4** and **interleukin-5** (*q.v.*).

bcl-1: proto-oncogenes that regulate lymphocyte survival, located at chromosomal sites susceptible to breakage. The human *BCL1* (B cell lymphoma 1) region on chromosome 11 (11q13) is close to the *PRAD1* (parathyroid adenomatosis) locus that codes for a cyclin; and *BCL1* translocations are believed to cause overexpression of *PRAD1* in parathyroid adenomas by affecting the regulatory elements. *BCL1* translocations that involve attachments to promoters of different genes and cause overexpression of the proto-oncogene are common in intermediate differentiation type lymphocytic lymphomas, and have been detected in some individuals with plasma cell myelomas, B-cell chronic lymphocytic leukemias and related diseases.

bcl-2: proto-oncogenes initially identified in a B cell lymphoma, and expressed by B lymphocytes, apparently after negative selection (which eliminates cells that either do not display antigen receptors, or have receptors that recognize self-antigens) has been completed. The genes are located at sites susceptible to chromosome breakage; and translocations that permit fusion with immunoglobulin promoters lead to overexpression and the formation of follicular lymphomas. In transgenic mice, overexpression of the messenger RNA and protein do not block lymphocyte selection processes or affect T cell survival, but do prolong the survival of mature resting B cells (including memory types) and plasma cells, even after exposure to radiation. They also protect against the apoptosis of pro-B and promyelocyte cell lines that otherwise occurs when interleukin-3 is withdrawn. The ap-

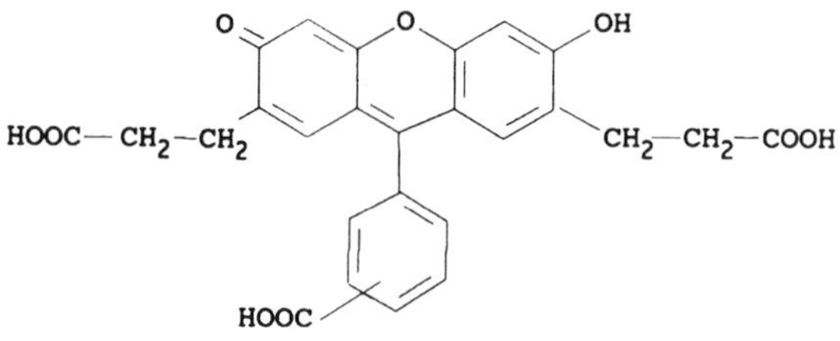

BCECF

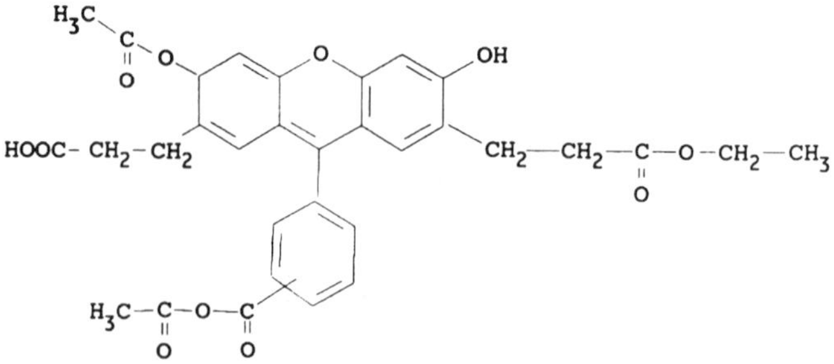

BCECF-AM

proximately 25K integral membrane protein products localize to inner mitochondrial membranes and nuclear envelopes of many proliferating cell types, but are also present in the dendrites of some neurons. They are widely distributed, for example in thymus glands (with highest levels in the medulla), tonsil follicular mantles, bone marrow hematopoietic precursor, promyelocyte and myelocyte cells (but not mature progeny), exocrine and endocrine pancreas, and the epithelium of thyroid follicles, breast ducts, prostate glands, intestinal crypts, and epidermis basal layers. However, the are not detectable in muscle cells or fibroblasts. The proteins inhibit the apoptosis that otherwise follows growth factor withdrawal, mediate the mitogenic effects of *c-myc* products, and are important regulators of central nervous system development. Their influences are normally controlled by tumor suppressor genes. When deregulated, *bcl-2* products support the growth of cancer cells, and can increase the survival of cells infected with Epstein-Barr and some other viruses. The *C. elegans* gene, *ced-9*, similarly opposes apoptosis, and is antagonized by *ced-3*, *ced-4*, and other genes that trigger DNA disintegration.

BCPs: bag cell peptides.

bcr: break-point cluster region; *see* **Philadelphia chromosome.**

bcr-abl: *see* **Philadelphia chromosome** and **leukemias.**

BCNU: carmustine; 1,3-bis (2-chloroethyl)-1-nitrosourea: an alkyl sulfonate that inhibits glutathione-*S*-transferases. It is used to arrest the growth of some neoplasms.

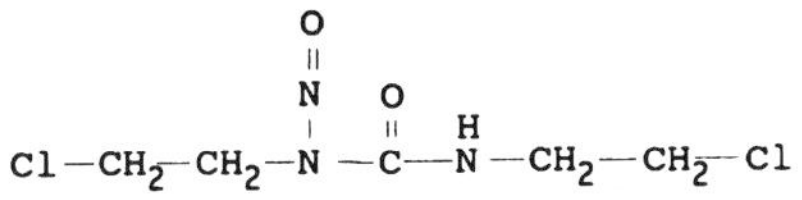

$$Cl-CH_2-CH_2-\underset{\underset{N}{\overset{O}{\|}}}{N}-\overset{O}{\overset{\|}{C}}-\overset{H}{N}-CH_2-CH_2-Cl$$

BCRF-1: an Epstein-Barr virus protein; *see* **interleukin-10.**

bcy-1: a mutated yeast gene whose product invokes constitutive activation of adenylate cyclase by affecting the enzyme regulatory subunit.

BDGF: bone-derived growth factor.

B-DNA: the most common (Crick-Watson) form of **DNA** *(q.v.).*

BDNF: brain derived neurotrophic factor.

beclomethasone: 9α-chloro-16β-methylprednisolone; a topically effective synthetic glucocorticoid.

becquerel: Bq: a radioactivity unit equal to 1 disintegration per second, and approximately equivalent to 2.7 x 10^{-11} Curie.

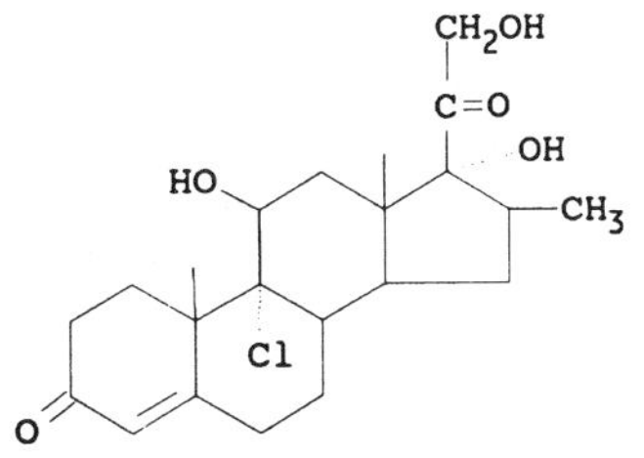

beclomethasone

Beer-Lambert Law: describes the relationship between the amount of monochromatic light (or other electromagnetic radiation) absorbed by a solution and the solute concentration, expressed as $Log_{10}I_0/I = kcb$, where I_0 = incident light intensity, I = transmitted light intensity, c = solute concentration in moles/liter, b = path length in cm, and k is a constant determined by the nature of the solvent.

BEI: butanol extractable iodine; *see* **protein bound iodine.**

beige mice: a mouse strain in which beige colored fur is associated with impaired resistance to infections, tendencies to develop lymphadenopathies and reticulum cell neoplasms, and the presence of giant lysosomal granules in leukocytes.

bek: a mouse oncogene that codes for a protein kinase similar to a fibroblast growth factor (FGF) receptor.

benanserin hydrochloride: 1-benzyl-2-methyl-5-methoxytryptamine hydrochloride; a potent, broad-spectrum serotonin receptor antagonist.

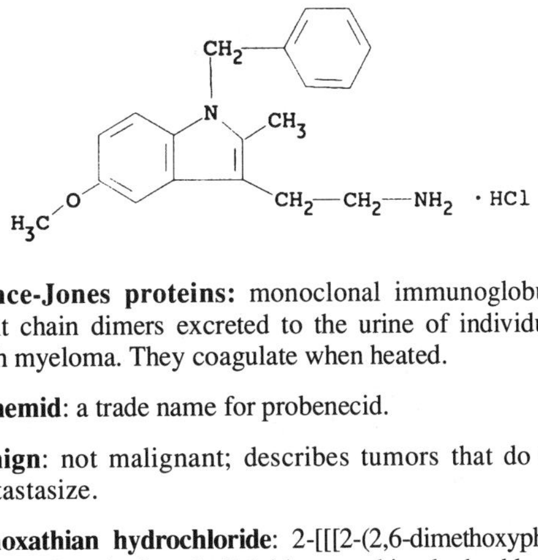

Bence-Jones proteins: monoclonal immunoglobulin light chain dimers excreted to the urine of individuals with myeloma. They coagulate when heated.

Benemid: a trade name for probenecid.

benign: not malignant; describes tumors that do not metastasize.

benoxathian hydrochloride: 2-[[[2-(2,6-dimethoxyphenoxy)ethyl]-amino]-methyl]-1,4-benzoxathian hydrochloride; a selective α_1-type adrenoreceptor antagonist.

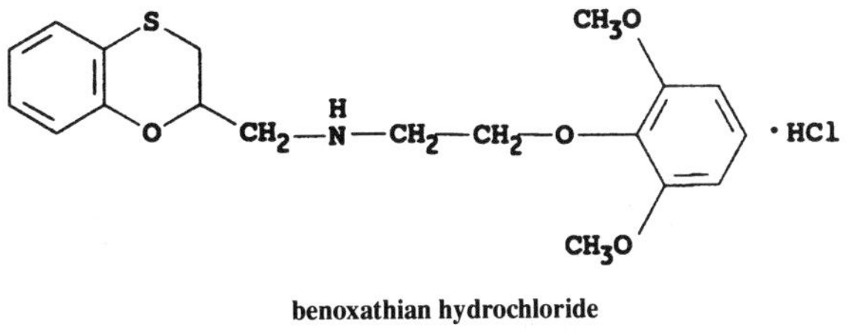

benoxathian hydrochloride

benserazide: serine-2-[2,3,4-trihydroxyphenyl)methyl hydrazide; an agent used to inhibit DOPA decarboxylase, and thereby peripheral conversion of DOPA to dopamine. Since it does not cross the blood brain barrier, it is used to increase the amount of systemically administered DOPA that enters the brain.

benzamidine: a selective serine protease inhibitor, effective against trypsin but not chymotrypsin.

benzamil: 3,5-diamino-[amino-(benzylamino)methylene]-6-chloro-pyrazinecarboxamide; a potent Na^+ channel inhibitor derived from amiloride.

benzidine: *p*-diaminodiphenyl; an analytical reagent for determination of sulfates and metals. It forms a blue derivative when it attaches to heme groups, and has been used to detect blood, but has been largely replaced by other agents because its carcinogenic properties endanger the users.

benzodiazepines: diazepam, chlordiazepoxide hydrochloride, oxazepam, lorazepam, triazolam, and related agents that are used as tranquilizers, muscle relaxants, anticonvulsants, sedatives, hypnotics, and/or anxiolytics. They attach to $GABA_A$ receptors at sites different from ones that bind GABA, and facilitate GABA neurotransmission. Most additionally act via different mechanisms to modify central nervous system turnover of several other neurotransmitters; and some directly bind peripheral receptors.

benzodioxans: dibozane, idoxazane, piperoxan, and related α-type adrenergic receptor antagonists. They also affect the functions of other neurotransmitters. *See* also **guanoxan**.

benzoic acid: phenylformic acid; an agent that can be extracted from some plant gums, but is synthesized for most purposes. It is an orally effective antiseptic, diuretic and expectorant. Small amounts are rapidly metabolized to hippuric acid, but large ones are toxic. It arrests the growth of some fungi when administered topically, and is also used as an analytical reagent and food preservative.

benzomorphans: pentazocine, phenazocine, and other synthetic agents related to morphine that have lower analgesic potency, but are far less addictive and invoke fewer side-effects. Most are mixed agonist-antagonists for μ type opioid receptors, and most additionally interact with κ-type receptors. 6,7-benzomorphan-11-ol is shown.

benzoquinonium hydrochloride: Mytolon; 2,5-*bis*(3-diethylaminopropylamino)-benzoquinone-*bis*(benzyl chloride); a nicotinic type acetylcholine receptor antagonist. It is used as a muscle relaxant.

benzothiadiazides: chlorothiazide, acetazolamide, and chemically related agents that are used as diuretics. They inhibit Na^+ reabsorption in distal nephrons, and secondarily augment water, K^+ and Cl^- excretion; and they augment Mg^{2+}, but retard Ca^{2+} excretion. *See* individual agents, and *cf* **loop diuretics**.

benzothiazepines: diltiazem and related agents used to block voltage gated Ca^{2+} channels. They also inhibit Na^+-dependent Ca^{2+} extrusion from mitochondria.

benzoquinonium hydrochloride

benzotript: *N*-(4-chlorobenzoyl)-L-tryptophan; a selective cholecytokinin antagonist that acts on gastrin receptors.

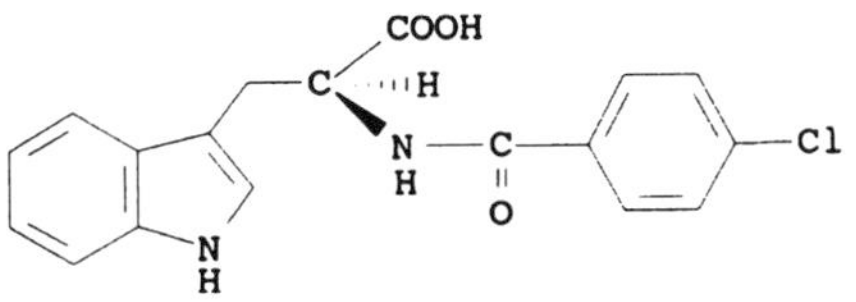

benztropine mesylate: Cogenin; 3-(diphenylmethoxy)-8-methyl-8-azabicyclo[3.2.1]octane methanesulfonate; an orally effective antagonist for muscarinic type acetylcholine receptors that also displays anti-histamine and local anesthetic properties, and affects behavior in laboratory animals. When used to treat some individuals with Parkinson's disease, the side-effects can include mood changes, tachycardia, drowsiness or insomnia, constipation, blurred vision, dryness of the mouth, nose and throat, and skin rashes. Excessive amounts can invoke hallucinations, breathing difficulties, and/or seizures.

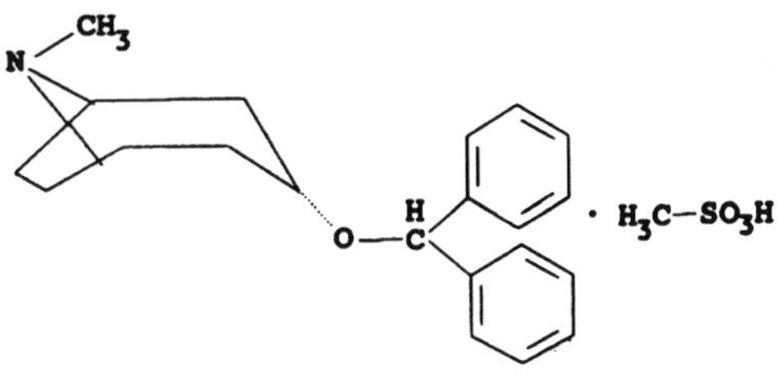

benzylpenicillin: Bicillin; penicillin G; *see* **penicillins**.

bepirone: a buspirone analog. It is a selective serotonin 5HT$_{1A}$ type receptor antagonist.

bepridil: 1-isobutoxy-2-pyrrolidino-3-*N*-benzylanilinopropane; a calmodulin antagonist that blocks voltage-gated Ca^{2+} channels, and is used to treat angina pectoris.

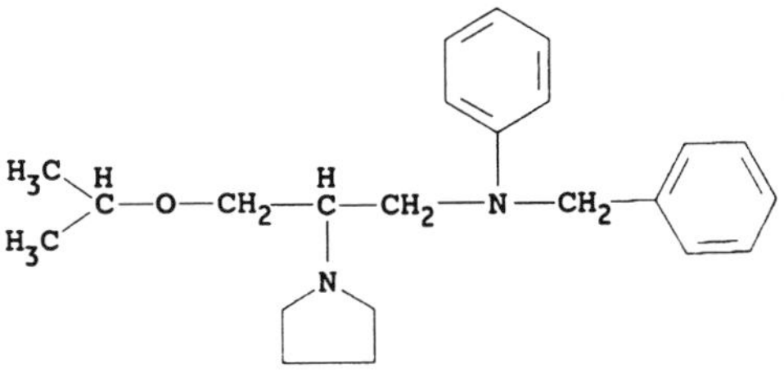

beriberi: a thiamine deficiency disease. The manifestations include skeletal muscle weakness, cardiovascular dysfunction, edema, polyneuritis associated with sensory defects and burning sensations, and encephalopathy that can lead to convulsions.

bestatin: ubenimex; [(2*S*-3*R*)-3-amino 2-hydroxy-1-oxo-4-phenylbutyl)]-L-leucine; an antibiotic, immunomodulator, and anti-cancer agent made by *Streptomyces olivoreticuli* that competitively inhibits aminopeptidase B and leucine aminopeptidase. It enhances blastogenesis, activates macrophages and T lymphocytes, and affects delayed hypersensitivity reactions.

beta (β) cells: (1) insulin-secreting pancreatic islet cells; (2) basophilic adenohypophysial cells.

beta-endorphin: *see* β-**endorphin**.

betaine: trimethylglycine; oxyneurine; a metabolite made from choline in reactions that transfer hydrogen atoms to FAD and NAD$^+$, and from glycine by transmethylation. It donates methyl groups for the biosynthesis of methionine and other molecules, can correct methionine deficiency effects, and also inhibits some peptidases. The chloride salt is used to increase gastric acidity, and as a lipotropic agent.

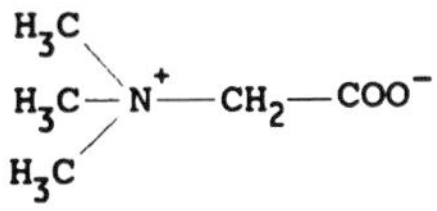

betamethasone: 9α-fluoro-16α-methylprednisolone; a slowly degraded, topically and orally effective glucocorticoid receptor agonist with virtually no mineralocorticoid potency, used for its anti-inflammatory properties.

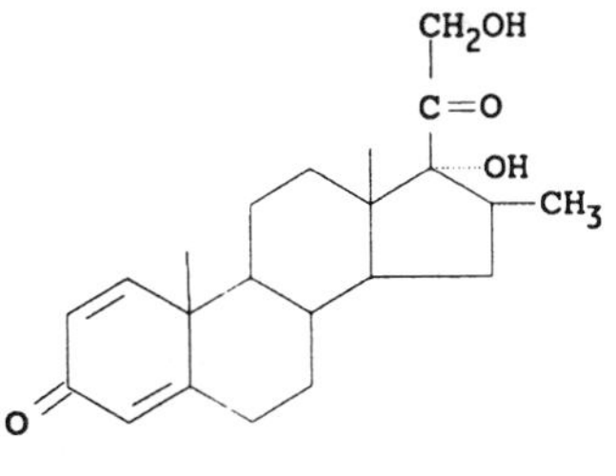

beta-*N*-methylamino-L-alanine: BMAA: a neurotoxic component of some plant seeds that activates NMDA receptors, and exerts lesser effects on quisqualate and kainic acid types.

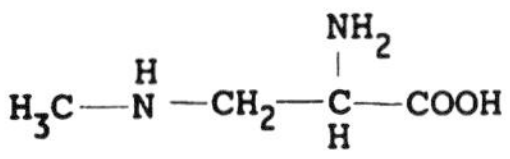

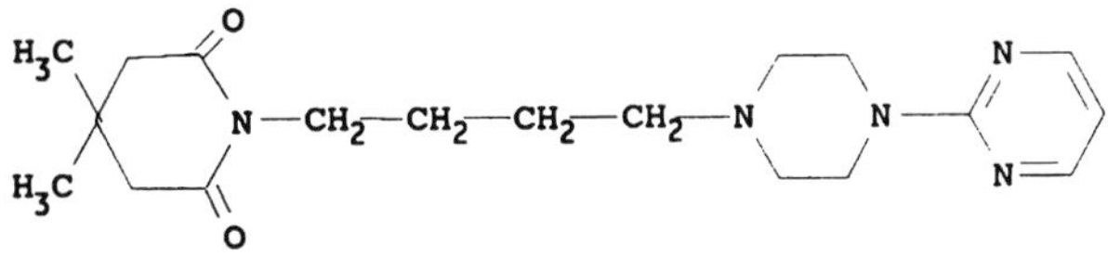

bepirone

69

[chemical structure diagram]

betaxolol

beta-*N*-oxylamino-L-alanine: a neurotoxin in chick-peas that activates quisqualate and kainic acid receptors, and is a weak agonist for NMDA types.

[chemical structure diagram]

betaferon: a preparation used to treat multiple sclerosis; *see* **interferons**.

beta particles: high energy electrons emitted during the decay of many radioactive elements. Their ability to penetrate biological tissues is intermediate between those of γ rays and alpha particles.

beta subunit: a peptide chain of a dimeric or oligomeric peptide or protein.

betaxolol: 1-(isoproplyamino)-3-[*p*-(cyclopropylmethoxyethyl)phenoxy]-2-propanol; a β_1-type adrenergic receptor antagonist used to treat hypertension.

bethanechol chloride: 2-carbamoylpropyltrimethylammonium chloride; an orally effective muscarinic acetylcholine receptor agonist that does not affect nicotinic types, and is not degraded by acetylcholinesterases. It stimulates gastrointestinal tract, ureter, and urinary bladder smooth muscle, but is less potent than carbachol on M_1 and M_2 receptors.

[chemical structure diagram]

bezafibrate: α-4[-(benzoylaminoethyl)phenoxy]isobutyric acid; an agent used to lower blood cholesterol levels in patients with hypercholesterolemia, by accelerating receptor-mediated LDL clearance.

[chemical structure diagram]

bFGF: basic fibroblast growth factor.

BFU: burst forming unit.

BFU-E: burst forming unity, erythrocyte.

Bgl II: a *bacillus globigii* restriction endonuclease that cleaves at the sites shown, and generates sticky ends that can anneal to fragments cleaved by several other endonucleases.

$$\downarrow$$
$$5'\,A\,G\,A\,T\,C\,T\,3'$$
$$3'\,T\,C\,T\,A\,G\,A\,5'$$
$$\uparrow$$

BGA: bone growth promoting activity.

BGP: bone gla protein; *see* **osteocalcin**.

BHK: baby hamster kidney; a cell line with fibroblast and smooth muscle cell characteristics. It is used to study cell differentiation and transformation.

bicuculline: 6-(5,6,7,8-tetrahydro-6-methyl-1,3-dioxolo-[4,5-*g*]-isoquinolin-5yl)-furol[3,4,*e*]-1,3-benzodioxol-8-(6*H*)-one; a $GABA_A$ type γ-aminobutyric acid receptor antagonist.

b.i.d: twice a day.

bifid: split; divided.

bifunctional vector: bifunctional plasmid; DNA that can replicate in two different organisms.

bifurcate: two-pronged; branching.

big: describes high molecular weight forms of peptide and protein hormones. In most cases, glycosylation accounts for the greater weight, but some forms have more amino acids.

big big: describes much larger entities than small and big hormone types, for example regulators complexed with other proteins.

biguanides: derivatives of the compound shown; *see* **oral hypoglycemic agents**.

[chemical structure diagram]

bihydropteridine: *see* **pteridines**.

bile: an alkaline fluid produced in the liver, stored in the gall bladder, and secreted to the duodenum. Its components include **bile salts** (*q.v.*), cholesterol, some hormones and hormone metabolites, and metabolic wastes such as bilirubin and drug degradation products. Lipids in the small intestine promote its release. Secretin augments the salt and water content, and augments bile flow. Cholecystokinin (CCK) promotes bile release from the gall bladder by stimulating the smooth muscle of the walls and relaxing the sphincter of Oddi. *See* also **biliribin**.

bile salts: salts of taurocholic, deoxycholic, and other acidic cholesterol derivatives, made in the liver, stored in the gall bladder, and secreted in bile. They emulsify dietary lipids, activate pancreatic lipases, and are essential for intestinal absorption of lipids (including fat-soluble vitamins).

bilirubin: 2,17-diethenyl-1,10,19,22,23,24-hexahydro-3,7,13,18-tetramethyl-1,19-dioxo-21H-biline-8,12-dipropanoic acid; an orange to reddish brown pigment formed by the reaction: biliverdin + NADH + H$^+$ → bilirubin + NAD$^+$. It is the major hemoglobin degradation product in mammals. Liver cells conjugate it with glucuronic acid; and water-soluble digluconate is the most abundant bile pigment. Under normal conditions, small amounts circulate complexed with albumin, and minute quantities of conjugated bilirubin are excreted to the urine. Bilirubin functions physiologically as an anti-oxidant via conversion to biliverdin, and is implicated as an important hydroperoxide scavenger. Cirrhosis of the liver, bile duct obstruction, and excessively rapid hemoglobin degradation lead to the accumulation of high blood levels which account for the coloration in jaundice; and high concentrations of conjugates impart dark brown coloration to urine. In infants, high blood levels retard growth and cause brain damage.

biliverdin: 2,17-diethenyl-1,19,23,24-tetrahydro-3,7,13,18-tetramethyl-1,19-dioxo-21H-biline-8,12-dipropanoic acid; a green pigment derived from the pathway: heme + O$_2$ + NADPH → biliverdin + Fe^{3+} + NADP$^+$ + CO + H$_2$O. It is the major hemoglobin degradation product in birds and amphibians. In mammals, most is normally converted to bilirubin (*q.v.*), but biliverdin accumulates under pathological conditions such as liver cancer, hepatic cirrhosis, and bile duct obstruction.

nor-**binaltorphimine dihydrochloride**: a highly selective κ-type opioid receptor antagonist.

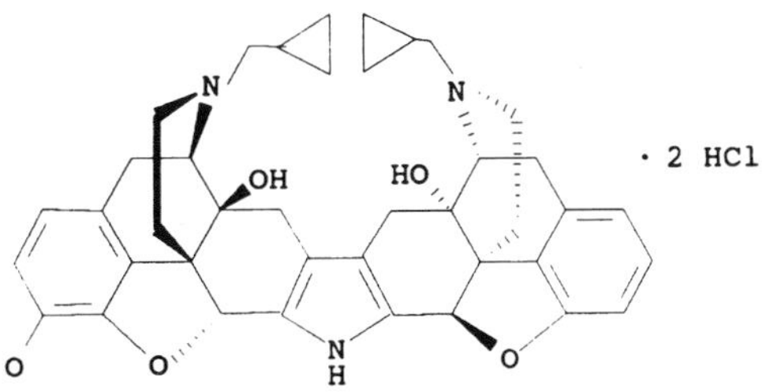

bindin: a 30K protein of sea urchin acrosomes that mediates species-specific gamete adhesion by binding to oocyte vitelline layers.

binucleation: formation of two nuclei with no division of the cytoplasm.

binovular: biovular: derived from two ova. *See* also **twins**.

bioassays: procedures for determining the biological potencies of hormones and other substances, based on responses of cell components, cells, tissues, organs, or whole organisms to a series of concentrations of test materials. Many kinds are sensitive and specific; and most do not require extensive purification of the test materials or knowledge of the chemical structures. The limitations can include subjectivity, poor reproducibility which may relate to undefined variations in the experimental conditions, and effects brought about indirectly by other components of the test preparations. The data can be affected by species and/or sex differences in either the individuals from which the preparations were obtained or the responding components, and by factors such as nutritional or endocrine histories, time of day, and/or the season of the year. Since the values usually depend on interactions with receptors, they can differ from those measured via radioimmunoassays or other procedures that involve different sites on the molecules. In some cases, bioassay: immunoassay ratios provide information on chemical heterogeneities.

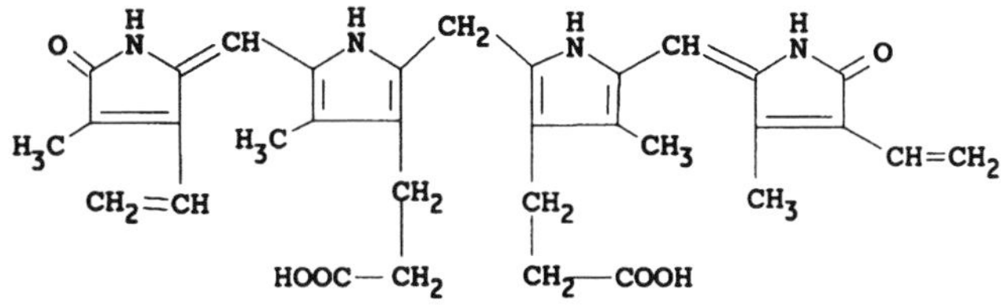

bilirubin

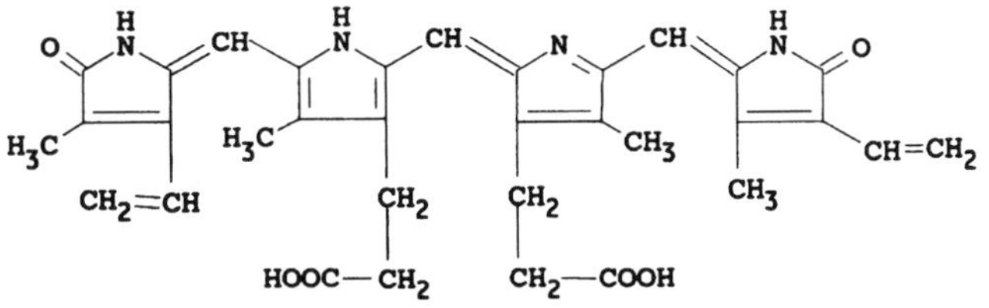

biliverdin

biocytin

biocytin: -N-biotinyl-lysine; a biotin source for most organisms (but not for some bacteria).

biofeedback: processes used to gain voluntary control over autonomic functions such as blood pressure, heart rate, or skin temperature. Changes in the parameters are monitored, and associated visual, auditory or other signals are presented to the subject. The subject then learns ways to control the signals that can be perceived.

bioflavonoids: vitamin P complex; permeability vitamin; widely distributed components of fruits and other plant entities. They are implicated as physiological regulators of plasma membrane permeability, and are used to treat capillary fragility. See **flavonoids**.

biogenic amines: a term loosely applied to choline, acetylcholine, catecholamines, tryptamine, serotonin, histamine, spermine, and other naturally occurring amines that exert regulatory functions.

biological clocks: internal oscillators that spontaneously undergo rhythmic changes and drive associated rhythms in other structures. The activities can be synchronized with external factors such as photoperiods (*see*, for example, **suprachiasmatic nuclei**) or feeding rhythms.

bioluminescence: light emission by living organisms. Preparations made from the compounds involved are used for assay procedures; *see*, for example, **firefly luciferin**.

biomass: all of the living organisms (including animals, plants, and bacteria) of a region.

biopterin: 2-amino-4-hydroxy-6-(1,2-dihydroxypropyl)-pteridine; a widely distributed pteridine, implicated as a growth factor for insects.

biotin: hexahydro-2-oxo-1*H*-thieno[3,4-*d*]imidazole-4-pentanoic acid; vitamin H; anti-egg white factor; coenzyme R; factor S; factor W; factor X; a vitamin B complex component essential for normal lipid metabolism. It is a cofactor for acetyl-Co-A carboxylase, pyruvate carboxylase, and other enzymes that catalyze carboxylation, decarboxylation, and transcarboxylation reactions. Avidin binds biotin with high affinity; and large amounts invoke deficiency by blocking its absorption from the small intestine. The symptoms include dry skin, anemia, growth retardation, and hypercholesterolemia. Since the vitamin binds to many other proteins at sites different from the ones that bind avidin, columns loaded with radioactive biotin are used to extract and identify those proteins in solutions. Cellular proteins can be identified with biotin linked to enzymes that react with those molecules, or with antibodies directed against the vitamin. See also **biotinylated DNA**.

biotinylated DNA: DNA that has incorporated biotin labeled deoxyuridine triphosphate. It can be detected with streptavidin-biotin-horseradish peroxidase complexes, and used as a non-radioactive probe for hybridization studies.

biotinylated proteins: proteins linked to **biotin** (*q.v.*).

biovular: binovular.

BiP: Grp78; Hsp78; an immunoglobulin made by pre-B lymphocytes and other cells. It is a glucose-regulated heat shock protein chemically related to hsp70s, believed to function as an endoplasmic reticulum protein folding factor. It binds to and promotes hydrolysis of ATP when it associates and dissociates from proteins and peptides. Agents that block the secretion of some proteins cause accumulation of complexes composed of those proteins plus BiP.

biphasic responses: (1) responses that change direction when an agent is presented for an extended time period. For example, stimulation can be followed by inhibition. The factors involved can include accumulation of cellular components that alter the binding properties and/or actions a regulator, increased production of antagonists, and changes in the numbers of receptors for synergists or antagonists; (2) stimulation at low concentrations and inhibition at higher ones (or inhibition at low and stimulation at high levels). Low concentrations bind preferentially to high-affinity receptors. In some cases, higher ones additionally attach to low-affinity sites that mediate different effects. Concentrations also influence the tendencies of regulators to dimerize, and the relative amounts of monomers as compared with dimers that interact with receptors.

bipotential: capable of acting or developing in two different ways, a term applied, for example, to an undifferentiated gonad that can develop into either an ovary or a testis.

Birbeck granules: rod-shaped organelles with faint striations and dense central regions in Langerhans epidermal cells.

birefringence: double diffraction, a term applied to entities that split light into two perpendicular waves which travel at different speeds. *Crystalline* (intrinsic) b. is caused by asymmetric arrangements of bonds between ions or molecules, and *form* b. by the presence of rods or other submicroscopic structures, or when the light transmitting properties of objects differ from those of the surrounding media. *Flow* (streaming) b. is related to the orientation of anisotropic particles moving in a suspension. *Strain* b. is caused by pressure or tension exerted on otherwise isotropic substances or tissues.

bisexual: (1) having anatomic or behavioral characteristics of both genders; (2) experiencing and/or expressing sexual interest in members of both genders of a species.

bivalent: describes (1) an ion with a double postive or negative charge (for example Ca^{2+} or HPO_4^{2-}); (2) a compound with two reactive components, for example an antibody with two antigen-binding sites.

BK: bradykinin.

BK 8644: Bay K 8644.

blanching: paling, for example of tadpole skin in response to melatonin.

blast cells: (1) immature proliferating cells (such as erythroblasts or lymphoblasts) that give rise to more mature types; (2) cells that make special products, for example osteoblasts or fibroblasts.

blastema: a cell cluster capable of giving rise to a differentiated tissue, organ, or individual.

blastocoele: blastocele; the cavity of a **blastocyst** (*q.v.*).

blastocyst: a hollow, fluid-filled spherical structure that develops from a morula within a few days after conception in eutherian mammals. The outer wall is formed by a single layer of small trophoblast cells that secrete chorionic gonadotropins, soon engage in implantation, and are progenitors of the chorion. Several larger, internally located cells (inner cell mass, embryoblast) give rise to the developing individual and to some extraembryonic tissues.

blastocytes: undifferentiated embryonic cells; *cf* **blastomeres**.

blastocytomas: blastomas; neoplasms that develop from undifferentiated cells.

blastoderm: (1) in mammals, when unqualifed, the outer layer of a **blastocyst** (*q.v.*). The term *extra-embryonic* blastoderm refers to cells that give rise to embryonic and fetal membranes, and related entities that will be discarded, and *embryonic* b. to the inner cell mass. The *trilaminar* b. is the structure formed when all three embryonic germ layers have been laid down; (2) in birds, amphibians, insects, and other species that produce egg cells with large quantities of yolk, the layer of embryonic cells in which mitosis proceeds; *cf* **blastodisc**, definition 2.

blastodisc: (1) in young mammalian embryos, the bilaminar structure formed by ectoderm and endoderm; (2) in oviparous species, the blastomere layer that borders the yolk, in which cells undergo incomplete mitosis.

blastokinins: uteroglobins.

blastomas: blastocytomas: neoplasms derived from undifferentiated embryonic cells.

blastomere: (1) one of the two cells formed when a zygote completes its first mitotic division; (2) any cell formed during early cleavage stages.

blastopore: (1) in mammals, the opening or pit formed during gastrulation, located at the cephalic extremity of Hensen's node; (2) in many nonmammalian species, the opening formed where ectoderm becomes continuous with invaginating endoderm.

bleomycins: copper-chelating glycopeptide antibiotics made by *Streptomyces verticillus* that differ from each other at terminal amine groups (*see* R^* in the structure shown). Their anti-tumor activities involve interactions with ferrous ions and oxygen that lead to DNA fragmentation.

blk: a gene of the *src* family, expressed by B lymphocytes. It directs synthesis of a 55K protein with tyrosine kinase activity.

blocking antibody: an antibody that invokes desensitization by competing with another kind for cell surface receptors.

blood: in vertebrates, the fluid that circulates in blood vessels, composed of blood plasma plus the formed elements (erythrocytes, leukocytes, and platelets). *See* specific components. The term is also applied to some extracellular fluids that perform comparble functions in invertebrates.

blood brain barrier: BBB; layers formed by astrocytes wrapped around blood capillaries that impede free exchange of hydrophilic substances between blood and cerebrospinal fluid. The barrier contributes to the maintenance of cerebrospinal fluid volume and composition, and protects central nervous system neurons against sudden variations in their microenvironments when blood concentrations of regulators and osmotically active substances change rapidly. It limits simple diffusion, but not facilitated transport or endocytosis. *See* also **circumventricular organs**.

blood coagulation: *see* **coagulation** and **coagulation factors**.

blood groups: phenotypes defined by the kinds of antigens expressed on erythrocytes. The ABO classification is the most widely used (*see* **A**, **B**, **AB** and **O blood types**); but several other antigens (including M, N, and P types) can sometimes affect responses to transfusion. *See* also **Rh factor**.

blood plasma: the fluid component of blood, obtained by centrifuging whole blood that has been treated with an anticoagulant, and removing the formed elements; *cf* **blood serum**. The composition in healthy human adults is approximately 91.5% water, 8.5% protein (*see* **albumin**, **globulins**, and **coagulation factors**) and 1% small

bleomycins

solutes (including inorganic ions, nutrients, nitrogenous wastes, enzymes, and hormones).

blood platelets: *see* **platelets**.

blood serum: the fluid released when blood clots. It lacks several factors present in blood plasma, including coagulation types and some others derived from blood platelets, but contains immunoglobulins and other proteins. Diluted sera are widely used to support the growth of cultured cells. Fetal preparations are especially rich in growth stimulants.

blood testis barrier: the tight junctions betweem adjacemt Sertoli cells impede free exchange (via simple diffusion) between testicular lymph and the special compartments of seminiferous tubules in which germinal cells undergo differentiation and maturation. The term "lymph testis barrier" may therefore be more appropriate.

Bloom's syndrome: a recessive disorder in humans, in which increased risk for development of cancers is attributed to a DNA ligase deficiency.

B lymphocytes: B cells; the major cell types involved in humoral immunity. The members of each clone express many copies of their special kinds of antibody on their plasma membranes. When activated by specific antigens, most B cells enlarge and proliferate, and the progeny undergo terminal differentiation to plasma cells that synthesize and secrete large quantities of the same kind of antibody; but limited numbers become memory cells. Activated B lymphocytes can also provide stimulants for T cells; *see* **B-7**. In mammals, B lymphocyte precursors originate in bone marrow and are believed to undergo early maturational stages there in or gut-associated lymphatic tissues (*see* **Peyer's patches**, and *see* also **bursa of Fabricius**). They circulate in the bloodstream, enter and leave body tissues, and accumulate in specific regions of the lymph nodes, spleen, and other lymphatic organs. New cells are made in lym-

phatic tissue germinal centers. *See* also **humoral immunity**, and *cf* **T lymphocytes**.

blunt ends: describes DNA fragment termini that lack single-stranded extensions; *cf* **cohesive ends**.

β-2m: β_2-microglobulin.

BM 13505: daltroban.

BMAA: β-methyl-α,β-diaminopropionic acid hydrochloride; beta-N-methylamine alanine; a neurotoxin made by tropical *Circas circinalis* plants that acts on metabotropic glutamate receptors, and is believed to cause a form of amyotrophic lateral sclerosis. A synthetic hydrochloride preparation is used to study the receptors.

BMI: bicuculline methyl iodide; *see* **bicuculline**.

BMP, BMP-1, BMP-2A, BMP-2B, BMP-3: *see* **bone morphogenetic proteins**.

BMR: basal metabolic rate.

BN 52021: an agent obtained from *Ginkgo bilbua* tress that blocks the effects of platelet activating factor (PAF).

BNI: binaltorphimine.

BNP: brain natriuretic peptide.

BNTX hydrochloride: benzilidinealtrexone hydrochloride; (5α)-17-(cyclopropylmethyl)-4,5-epoxy-3,14-dihydroxy-7-(phenylmethylene)-morphinan-6-one hydrochloride; a selective δ_1-type opioid receptor antagonist.

L-BOAA: (S)-β-oxalyl-α,β-diaminopropionic acid; a neurotroxin made by *Lathyrus sativus* that may contribute to

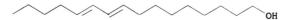

BNTX hydrochloride

the development of Lathyrism in individuals who ingest the beans (but is probably not the major offending ingredient).

boc-: butyloxycarbonyl-; *see* **butyloxycarbonyl amino acids**.

body mass index: body weight in kilograms divided by body height in centimeters.

BOH: β-hydroxy-butyric acid; *see* **ketone bodies**.

BOL: bromo-LSD.

bolandiol: estra-4-ene-3β,17β-diol; an anabolic steroid. Trade names for the dipropionate ester include Anabiol and Storinal.

bolasterone: Myagen; 7α,17-dimethyltestosterone; a synthetic anabolic steroid.

boldenone: 17-hdyroxyandrosta-1,4-diene-3-one; a synthetic anabolic steroid.

bombesin: *p*Glu-Gln-Arg-Leu-Gly-Asn-Gln-Trp-Ala-Val-Gly-His-Leu-Met-NH_2; a peptide initially identified in the skins of *Bombina bombina* and *Bombina variegata*, and later found in the gastrointestinal tracts and brains of these, and also of other frogs (including ones that make different but related skin peptides, such as the ranatensin of *Rana pipiens*). Mammalian brains may make small amounts; but gastrin releasing peptide (GRP) appears to be the primary mammalian homolog that acts on the same receptors and exerts the same kinds of actions. The peptides function as neurotransmitters, neuromodulators, and hormones. They are mitogenic for bronchial epithelial, some lung, and some other cell types (and certain kinds of lung cancer cells release large amounts). Although they directly stimulate the release of growth hormone, glucagon, somatostatin and several gastrointestinal cell regulators, slowly developing effects on gastrin secretion are attributed to mitogenesis. They also stimulate the smooth muscle of the urinary tract, and of blood vessels, and promote gall bladder contraction (along with relaxation of the sphincter of Oddi). Additionally, they can invoke hypothermia, and have been implicated as physiological appetite depressants.

[D-Phe[12]]-bombesin: one of several bombesin analogs used as bombesin/GRP receptor antagonists.

Bombus: an insect genus that includes the bumblebee.

bombykol: 10,12-decaheptenol; a silk worm pheromone.

Bombyx mori: the silk moth, an insect used in genetics and protein structure studies.

bond energy: the energy required to break a chemical bond.

bone: the major connective tissue of most vertebrate skeletons, composed mostly of rigid extracellular matrix. It supports body structures, houses hematopoietic tissue, encloses and protects the brain and spinal cord, makes up most of the rib cage, and provides levers for movement. It also holds around 99% of the body calcium and 85% of the phosphorus, and is a major contributor to calcium and phosphorus homeostasis. Bone cells account for only 1% of the total weight, but the tissue is metabolically active, innervated, and richly supplied with blood vessels. *See* **bone matrix**, **bone marrow**, **bone types**, and specific bone cell types. Some fish species have acellular bone. In elasmobranchs, the skeleton is composed mostly of cartilage.

bone cells: the cells in the skeletons of most vertebrates that make and resorb bone matrix, and contribute to mineral homeotasis; *see* **osteoprogenitor cells**, **osteoblasts**, **osteocytes**, and **osteoclasts**.

bone-derived growth factor: BDGF; a term that usually refers to an approximately 10K mitogen initially identified in conditioned media of fetal rat calvariae, that appears to be identical with $β_2$-microglobulin. Many endocrine and paracrine factors regulate bone growth, differentiation, and functions.

bone fluid: the specialized extracellular fluid that surrounds osteoblasts and osteocytes. It derives from bulk

bombykol

extracellular fluid, but the calcium, magnesium, and sodium concentrations are lower. The potassium levels vary with the physiological status (but not directly with plasma levels). The concentration is approximately 25 mM in mature bone, and can exceed 100 mM during rapid skeletal growth.

bone gla protein: *see* **osteocalcin**.

bone ground substance; ossoemucin: a semi-fluid component of bone matrix that accounts for approximately 1% of the weight. It contains several noncollagenous proteins (including osteocalcin and osteonectin), sialoglycoproteins, glycosaminoglycans, phospholipids, and other substances that support bone growth, bone remodeling, and mineral metabolism.

bone marrow: the tissue contained within endosteum-lined bone cavities. Red marrow has an abundant blood supply, and is the major postnatal site for hematopoiesis. In adults, most of it resides in trabecular bone; but the cavities of long bones contain substantial amounts in children. In addition to stem cells, and committed types in various stages of differentiation, it contains stroma which supplies numerous growth factors. Yellow (white, fatty) marrow is metabolically less active, but can be converted to the red type when the need for additional hematopoiesis arises (for example after hemorrhages).

bone matrix: the non-living, extracellular component of bone that accounts for around 99% of the tissue weight in most species. Approximately one-third is collagen, the major organic constituent. It provides the framework, into which minerals are deposited. Most of the remainder (65% in most bone) is inorganic, initially laid down as calcium phosphate but later converted to hydroxyapatite. Other constituents include noncollagenous proteins, along with small amounts of ground substance and bone fluid.

bone morphogenetic proteins: BMPs: proteins initially identified in conditioned media of cultured fetal calvariae and osteosarcoma cells. They support bone and bone marrow formation by promoting mesenchymal cell differentiation. BMP-1, with 730 amino acid moieties, contains a protease domain, and an epidermal growth factor (EGF)-like sequence. BMP-2A, BMP-2B, and BMP-3 comprised, respectively of 396, 408, and 472 amino acid moieties, are related to (but biologically distinguishable from) transforming growth factor-β (TGF-β) and inhibin.

bone remodeling: new bone formation coupled to destruction of older tissue. It proceeds continuously under physiological conditions, and is essential for mineral homeostasis, bone growth and repair, and skeletal system adaptations to changing needs. The relative rates of osteogenesis and osteolysis determine whether bone mass increases, remains constant, or decreases. Coupling factors released by osteoblasts affect the activities of osteoclasts; and osteoclasts, in turn, affect osteoblast functions. Circulating parathyroid hormone (PTH), calciferols, gonadal steroids, and growth hormone are among the endocrine regulators of bone cell functions. The numerous, locally made paracrine factors include insulin-like growth factor-1 (IGF-I) and eicosanoids.

bone types: *cancellous* (trabecular, spongy) bone, which is found in metaphyses, epiphyses of young individuals, around marrow cavities, in vertebrae, pelvis, ribs, and sternum, is characterized by the presence of bone spicules (trabeculae). It is lighter, mechanically weaker, and metabolically more active than the *cortical* (dense, compact) tissue of long bone diaphyses, and it contains more red marrow in adults. *Woven* bone, which forms first in cortical regions (and also later during repair of injuries) is loosely organized. Much of it is replaced by the dense, lamellar type, which contains Haversian systems. *See* also **ossification**.

bongkrekik acid: 3-carboxymethyl-17-methoxy-6,18,21-trimethyldocosa-2,4,8,12,14,18,20-heptanedioic acid; an antibiotic made by *Pseudomonas cocovenenans* that inhibits mitochondrial ATP translocases by binding to the enzymes when their nucleotide sites face the mitochondrial matrix; *cf* **atractyloside**.

Bordetella pertussis: a gram negative bacillus that makes **pertussis toxin** (*q.v.*), endotoxin, and other poisons, and is the infectious agent that causes whooping cough.

boron: B: an element (atomic number 5, atomic weight 10.81). It is used to label organic molecules, in antiseptic preparations, and as a neutron absorber. Analogs of some biologically active compounds (such as acetylcholine), in which a boron atom replaces a carbon, retain the activities of the parent compounds, but resist degradation by endogenous enzymes.

Bothropsinase: a trade name for an enzyme obtained from the venom of *Bothrops atrox* snakes that catalyzes conversion of fibrinogen to fibrin. The activity is not affected by heparin.

botulism: a paralytic, often fatal disease caused by *Clostridium botulinum* strains in spoiled food or infected wounds. Botulinum neurotoxin type A promotes ADP-

bongkrekik acid

76

ribosylation of G protein α_i-subunits, and thereby blocks inactivation of adenylate cyclases. It acts presynaptically to inhibit acetylcholine release from motor nerves. Minute amounts are used to treat muscle spasms caused by excessive neurotransmitter release.

bovine: derived from or characteristic of cattle.

bovine serum albumin: BSA; the most abundant protein in cattle blood serum. Aseptic preparations are purified in various ways for special purposes. They are used, for example, as nutrients in cell culture media, to maintain isotonicity for serological studies, and to stabilize assay systems for enzymes, vitamins, and other biological components. For physiological functions, *see* **albumins**.

Bowman's capsule: the part of a renal corpuscle that surrounds the glomerular capillaries, receives the glomerular filtrate, and sends it to the proximal convoluted tubule. The outer (parietal) layer is composed of squamous epithelium. Visceral layer cells (podocytes) extend pedicels that interdigitate with those of other podocytes, and thereby cover most of the endothelium basement membrane. The filtrate passes through mintue spaces between the pedicels that are called slit pores.

Bowman's glands: mucus-producing glands in the connective tissue that underlies olfactory epithelium.

bp: (1) boiling point; (2) base pair.

BPA: burst promoting activity.

β position: a position in space occupied by a chemical group attached to an asymmetric carbon atom. If a sugar, steroid, prostaglandin, or other molecule with one or more ring structures is visualized as lying flat against a plane, chemical groups attached to it and projecting below the plane are said to be in the β position, and the bonds are represented by solid lines; *cf* α **position**.

BPP23: *see* **calbindins**.

B-PPT: β-preprotachykinin.

B protein: *see* **lactose synthetase**.

Bq: becquerel.

brachionectin: a large extracellular matrix protein chemically and biologically related to cytotactin.

brady-: a prefix meaning slow, as in bradycardia.

bradykinin: BK; Arg-Pro-Pro-Gly-Phe-Ser-Pro-Phe-Arg, a nonapeptide chemically related to kallidin and T-kinin that is cleaved from kininogens by kinin catalyzed reactions, and is inactivated by angiotensin converting enzyme (kinase II). It dilates blood vessels, lowers blood pressure, increases capillary permeability, stimulates nonvascular smooth muscle, augments the secretion of saliva, and is a potent mediator of inflammation-associated pain. The name derives from slowly developing effects on guinea pig ileum. Some actions are mediated via phospholipase-A_2 activation, and consequent prostaglandin synthesis, but vasodilation has been linked with generation of nitric oxide. Large amounts of BK accumulate in individuals with Bartter's and carcinoid syndromes.

brain derived neurotrophic factor: BDNF: a 112 amino acid basic (pI = 9.9) peptide chemically related to nerve growth factor (NGF) and neurotropic factor-3 (NT-3). It is made in and secreted by central nervous system neurons. The levels are higher than those of NGF in the hippocampus; and substantial amounts are present in the superior colliculi and spinal cord. BDNF prolongs the survival of certain neuron populations, and is believed to play essential roles in their development. Its targets include sensory neurons (derived from neural crests), nodose ganglion cells (from ectodermal placodes), and retinal ganglion cells. Although some of those neurons also respond to NGF and/or NT-3, BDGF does not affect sympathetic ganglion cells, and little or none of the peptide is found in peripheral tissues.

brain hormone: prothoracicotropic hormone.

brain natriuretic peptide: BNP: a peptide chemically and biologically related to atrial natriuretic peptides, and possibly identical to aldosterone secretion inhibiting factor. It contributes to central nervous system control of blood pressure, blood volume, and electrolyte balance, and is also made by adrenomedullary cells and cardiac myocytes. The human type has the amino acid sequence: H_2-N-Ser-Pro-Lys-Met-Val-Gln-Gly-Ser-Gly-Cys-Phe-Gly-Arg-Lys-Met-Asp-Arg-Ile-Ser-Ser-Ser-Gly-Leu-Gly-Cys-Lys-Val-Leu-Arg-Arg-His-OH.

brainstem: the central core of the brain. Some authors limit use of the term to midbrain, pons, and medulla oblongata, but others additionally include the diencephalon.

branchial: pertaining to or resembling gills.

branchial pouches: gill pouches; paired, serially arranged embryonic structures that contain precursor cells for thymus glands in all jawed vertebrates, parathyroid glands in amphibians, reptiles, birds, and mammals, and carotid and aortic bodies. The calcitonin cell precursors migrate to ultimobranchial bodies in fishes, amphibians, birds, and reptiles, but become thyroid gland parafollicular cells in mammals. Most species have seven pairs. *See* also **DiGeorge syndrome**.

Brattleboro rats: a mutant strain of rats developed in Vermont, in which the messenger RNA for arginine vasopressin is made, but a genetic defect blocks its processing to the active hormone in the hypothalamus. (Vasopressin is, however, made at some other sites). The animals develop diabetes insipidus, and are used to study antidiuretic hormone functions.

breakage and reunion: a process essential for crossing over during meiosis, in which chromatids of homologous chromosomes break, DNA segments from one strand exchange with corresponding segments of the other, and fusion restores the normal lengths.

breast: *see* **mammary gland**.

breast cancers: carcinomas that originate in mammary gland tissues. Various types differ from each other in hormone requirements and responses to pharmacological agents. Since normal breast tissues are regulated by many growth factors and proto-oncogenes, mammary gland cancers can be induced in laboratory animals by viruses, chemical carcinogens, and excessive amounts of some naturally occurring regulators; but some animal models (for example types that are highly dependent on prolactin) do not mimic typical human conditions. Estrogens are potent mitogens for some of the cells, and both tamoxifen (an antiestrogen), and oophorectomy promote tumor regression in some premenopausal women. They seem to be most effective when estrogen receptors and responses to estrogen (including induction of progesterone receptors) can be demonstrated. There are controversies concerning the mechanisms whereby very large (pharmacological) doses of synthetic estrogens confer benefits in limited numbers of postmenopausal women, including some with tumors that do not express the receptors. Epidermal growth factor (EGF) is a potent mitogen that can activate estrogen receptors (and estrogens regulate the numbers of EGF receptors in some cell types). Transforming growth factor-α (TGFα) acts on EGF receptors, and excessive production has been implicated in some cases (whereas TGF-β isoforms may confer protection); *see* also *neu*. Progestins and androgens counteract some estrogen effects, and are effective in some cases, but progestins can also stimulate. In addition to providing glucocorticoids, the adrenal cortex is a major source of estrogen precursors after menopause. Glucocorticoid administration has proven beneficial in some women, and adrenalectomy in others. The side-effects of hormone manipulations are better tolerated than those of radiation and chemotherapy, but some breast cancer cells do not respond.

breast feeding: *see* **lactation** and **milk**.

brefeldin A: ascotoxin; γ4-dihydroxy-2-(6-hydroxy-1-heptenyl)-4-cyclopentane-crotonic acid λ-lactone; a neurotoxin made by *Penicillium brefeldianum* that inhibits secretion, and causes rapid and massive, but reversible disassembly of Golgi apparatus complexes, with redistribution of Golgi enzymes to the endoplasmic reticulum and fusion of *trans* components with endosomes. The effects are associated with loss of β-COP, an adaptin-like protein that covers non-clathrin coated vesicles and plays roles in vesicle formation and disassembly, and probably also masks binding sites for microtubule proteins. Brefeldin A inhibits egress from endoplasmic reticulum of both integral membrane and secreted proteins, including newly synthesized Class I types. It also exerts some influences on lysosomes, and inhibits intracellular release of Ca^{2+} ions.

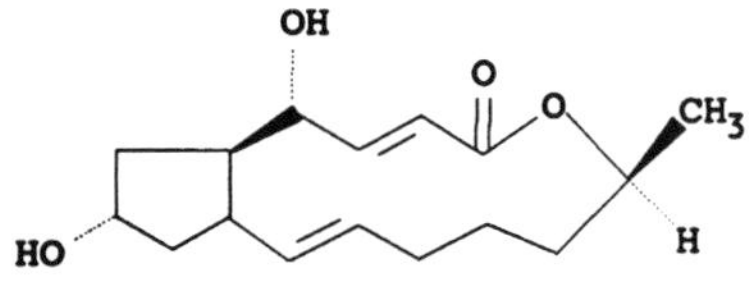

brefeldin A

bremazocine: 6-ethyl-1,2,3,4,5,6-hexahydro-3-[(1-hydroxycyclopropyl)methyl]-11,11-dimethyl-2,6-methano-3-benzazocin-8-ol; a potent κ-type opioid receptor agonist.

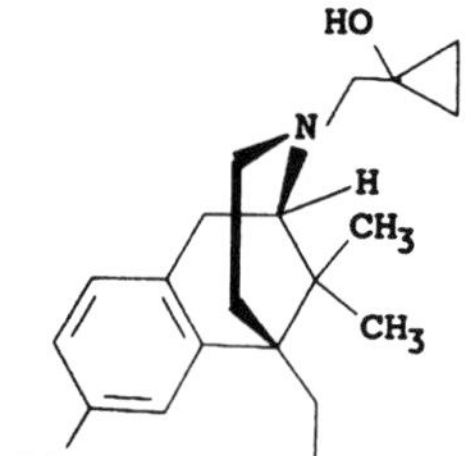

bretylium tosylate: 2-bromo-N-ethyl-N,N′-dimethylbenzenemethanaminium-4-methylbenzene sulfonate; a β₁-type adrenergic receptor antagonist used to treat hypertension and cardiac dysrhythmias.

brevetoxins: BTXs; lipid-soluble neurotoxins made by the "red tide" dinoflagellate *Ptychodiscus brevis* that cause food poisoning by activating Na^+ channels. In the structure shown, R^* is the side chain that defines types A, B, and C.

B ring: the second ring of a heterocyclic compound. In steroids, it is formed by carbon atoms 5 through 10. Numbers 5 and 10 are shared with the A ring, and 8 and 9 with the C ring. Cholesterol, most calciferols, pregnenolone, and dehydroepiandrosterone (DHA) have 5:6 double bonds, whereas progesterone, glucocorticoids, and most androgens have them at 4:5. *Cf* **A ring** (*q.v.* for structure).

BRL 34915: cromokalin.

BRL 37344: an agent that acts selectively on β₃-type adrenergic receptors of brown adipose tissue and stimulates lipolysis and thermogenesis, but has little effect on β₁ or β₂ types.

bromconduritol: an agent used to inhibit N-linked glycosylation of newly formed proteins in the endoplasmic reticulum. It blocks removal of glucose moieties in the step: glucose₂-mannose₉-N-acetylglucos-

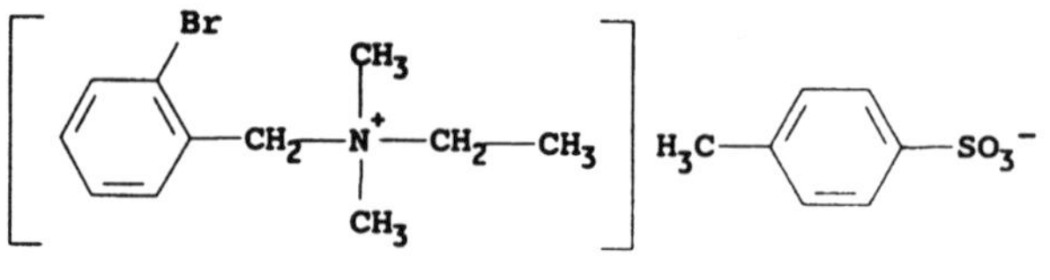

bretylium tosylate

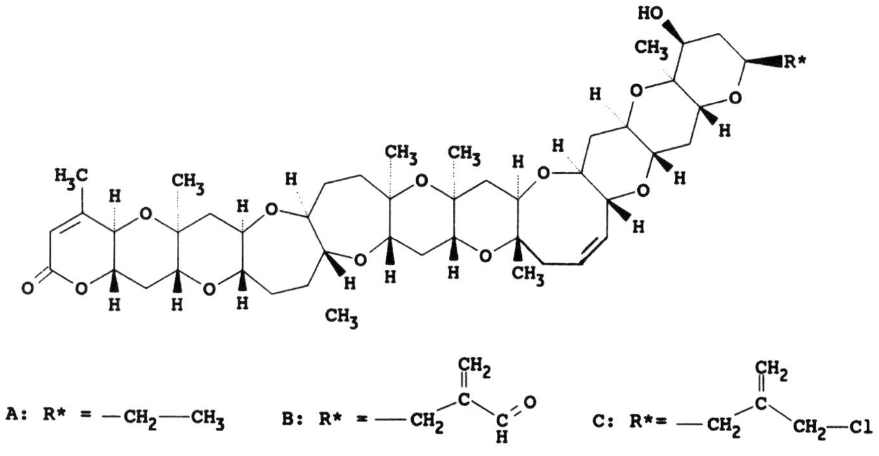

A: R* = —CH$_2$—CH$_3$ B: R* = —CH$_2$—C(=CH$_2$)—C(=O)H   C: R* = —CH$_2$—C(=CH$_2$)—CH$_2$—Cl

brevetoxins

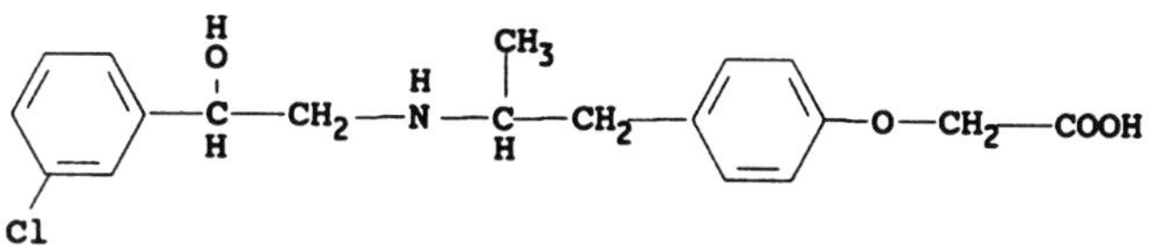

BRL 37344

amine-asparagine → mannose$_9$-N-acetylglucosamine-asparagine.

bromelain: bromelin; approximately 30K glycoprotein thiol proteases, obtained from pineapples. They also act on amides and esters, and are used clinically to reduce inflammation and promote wound repair. Commercial applications include meat tenderizing and preparation of protein hydrolysates.

bromocriptine; CB-154; 2-bromo-12′-hydroxy-2′-(2-methylethyl)-5′-(2-methylpropyl)ergotaman-3′,6′,18-trione; an ergot derivative used as a dopamine receptor agonist to inhibit prolactin secretion. It also inhibits growth hormone secretion in some individuals with acromegaly (but not in healthy subjects), alleviates some forms of Cushing's syndrome, promotes regression of some breast cancers, and affects prolactin influences on immune system cells. Unlike several other ergot derivatives, it does not stimulate uterine smooth muscle. Parlodel is a trade name for bromocriptine mesylate.

5-bromodeoxyuridine: BUDR; a thymidine analog in which the methyl group is replaced by a bromine atom. It incorporates into DNA molecules and, by competing for thymidine, selectively inhibits transcription of a class of regulatory genes, including some that code for factors required by skeletal muscle and erythrocytes. High concentrations cause chromosome breakage. BUDR also affects DNA staining properties, and can therefore be used for crossing over studies.

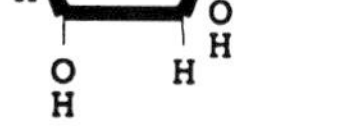

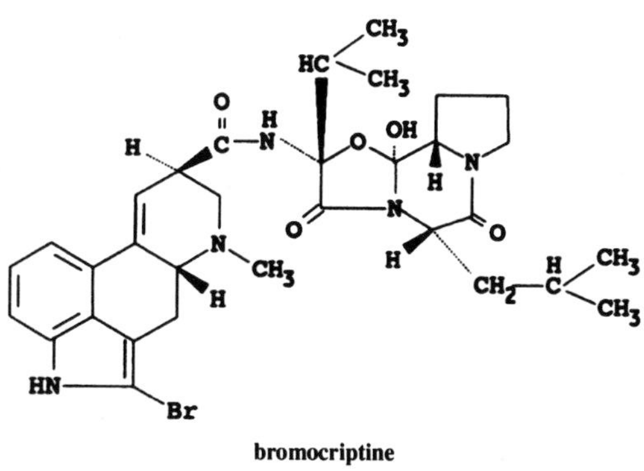

bromocriptine

bromohomibotenic acid: α-amino-4-bromo-2,3-dihydro-3-oxo-5-isoxazolepropanoic acid; a potent agonist for AMPA type excitatory amino acid receptors.

bromo-LSD: BOL; BOL-148; bromolysergic acid; 2-bromo-*N,N*-diethyl-*D*-lysergamide; a serotonin receptor antagonist that does not invoke LSD-type hallucinosis.

p-**bromophenylacyl bromide**: 2′,4′ dibromoacetophenone; a phospholipase A_2 inhibitor that binds to carboxylic acids. It is used to identify the acids, and to inhibit prostaglandin synthesis.

5-**bromouracil**: a mutagenic pyrimidine analog that incorporates into, and is used as a marker for newly synthesized DNA.

bromphenol blue: 3′,3″,5′,5″-tetrabromophenolsulfonephthalein; an indicator that changes from yellow at pH 3.0 to blue at pH 4.6. It binds to, stains, and, can be used to identify protein amino groups.

Bromsulphalein: BSP: a trade name for sulfobromophthalein sodium.

bromthymol blue: 3′,3″-dibromothymolsulfonephthalein; a vital dye, and an indicator that is green at neutral pH, and changes from yellow to blue over the pH range 6.0 to 7.6.

bromthymol blue

bronchioles: fine subdivisions of bronchial trees, with walls that are not supported by cartilage. A *terminal bronchiole* has a complete circle of smooth muscle that responds to vasoconstrictors (such as leukotrienes) and to epinephrine and some other vasodilators. Its branches are respiratory bronchioles, each of which communicates with two or more alveolar ducts.

broodiness: egg-incubating behavior in birds. Prolactin is the major stimulant.

brown adipose tissue: BAT; pigmented adipose tissue that is abundant in neonatal and hibernating mammals. It is the major site for accelerated calorigenesis in response to cold environments, and during rewarming following torpor or hibernation. Mature, nonhibernating species have only small amounts, but food intake associated elevation of the metabolic rate may depend on it. It is claimed that the tissue is more abundant in individuals who tend to be lean, and that locally applied β_3 type receptor agonists can diminish fat stores at specific sites. The functions depend on specialized mitochondria, and on thermogenin which facilitates uncoupling of oxidative phosphorylation.

Bruce effect: pregnancy interruption in mice and some other rodents, invoked by exposure to a pheromone released by alien (non-stud) males of the same species.

Brunn effect: body swelling caused by excessive uptake and retention of water, invoked in frogs and other amphibians by vasopressin injection.

Brünner's glands: tubulo-alveolar glands in the submucosal layer of the duodenum. Their secretory products include urogastrone.

brush borders: apical cell surfaces with large numbers of closely-packed microvilli, present, for example, in the small intestine and the proximal convoluted tubules of the kidney. Microvilli facilitate absorption by increasing surface areas.

brushite: the readily recruitable mineral first deposited in bone matrix, composed mostly of $CaHPO_4 \cdot 2H_2O$. It is slowly converted to hydroxyapatite.

Bruton's disease: congenital agammaglobulinemia; a recessive, sex-linked disease in which B lymphocytes fail to mature from pre-B cell precursors. Maternally-derived immunoglobulins protect afflicted infants against fatal infections during the first few postnatal months.

bryostatins: several macrocyclic lactones made by the marine bryozoan *Bugula neritina*. All are potent neoplastic agents, but differences in their side chains affect other biological properties. For example, bryostatin 1 additionally activates neutrophilic leukocytes and exerts granulocyte-macrophage colony stimulating factor (GM-CSF)-like influences on bone marrow hematopoietic cells, whereas bryostatin 13 does not. Some effects have been linked with activation of protein kinase C isozymes.

BSA: bovine serum albumin.

BSF-1: B cell stimulating factor 1: *see* **interleukin-4**.

BSF-2: B cell stimulating factor 2; B cell differentiating factor; *see* **interleukin-6**.

BSO: buthionine sulfoximine.

BSP: Bromsulphalein; *see* **sulfobromophthalein sodium**.

BTCP: *N*-[1-(1-benzo[b]thien-2-yl-cyclohexyl)]piperidine; a neurotoxin that selectively inhibits dopamine uptake. It has little affinity for PCP sites.

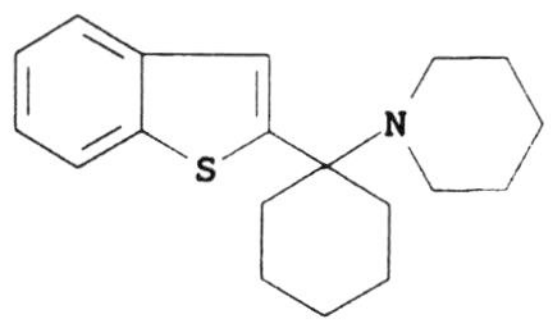

BTX: brevetoxins.

buccal: (1) pertaining to the mouth; (2) towards the cheek.

buccalin: H-Gly-Met-Asp-Ser-Leu-Ala-Phe-Ser-Gly-Gly-Leu-NH$_2$: a neuropeptide made in *Aplysia* motor neurons that relaxes muscles used for feeding, by acting

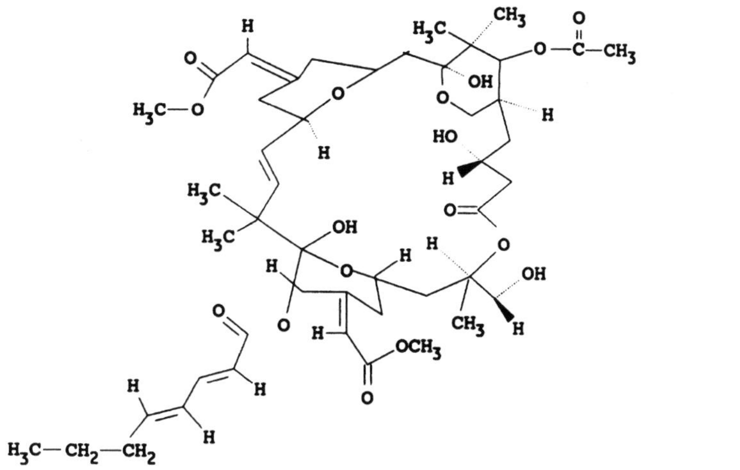

bryostatin 1

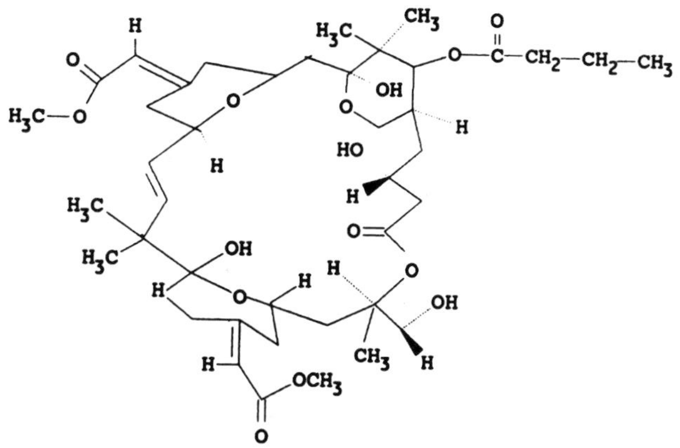

bryostatin 13

bryostatins

presynaptically to inhibit acetylcholine release. It does not antagonize the stimulatory effects of exogenous acetylcholine.

buck: a term applied to adult males of many vertebrate species, including deer, rabbits, rats, and mice.

bucillamine: *N*-(2-mercapto-2-methyl-1-oxopropyl-L-cysteine; an immunomodulator that acts on macrophages and lymphocytes. It is under investigation for the treatment of rheumatoid arthritis.

bucladesine: a cAMP analog that penetrates cell membranes, and is used as a cardiac stimulant. *See N[6],2-dibutyryl*-**adenosine-3′5′-cyclic monophosphate** and dibutyryl-**cAMP**.

budesonide: 16,17-butylidine-*bis*(oxy)-11,21-dihydroxy-pregna-1,4-diene-3,20-dione; a synthetic glucocorticoid receptor agonist, used as an anti-inflammatory agent.

BUdR: 5-bromo-deoxyuridine.

bufalin: 3,14-dihydroxybufa-20,22-dienolide; a component of the venom of the Chinese toad *Bufo Bufo gargarizans*. It is used as a cardiac stimulant.

buffalo hump: accumulation of fat on the back of the neck, a common manifestation of glucocorticoid excess in humans.

buffers: stabilizers; agents that diminish the effects of external factors. In biological and chemical systems, the term usually refers to substances that protect against large changes in pH when acids or alkalies are added. Amino acids can stabilize pH by functioning as **zwitterions** (*q.v.*). Commonly used buffers for *in vitro* systems are combinations of weak acids and their ionized salts. They are effective because addition of a strong acid suppresses ionization of the weak acid of the buffer, but increases ionization of the salt; and strong alkalies exert the opposite effects. For example, if hydrochloric acid is added to a solution that contains acetic acid and sodium acetate, much of it is neutralized by the salt. (The sodium ions associate with the chloride, as the liberated hydrogen atoms are sequestered in unionized acetic acid.) If sodium hydroxide is added, much of it is neutralized by the weak acid of the buffer. (The hydroxyl ions combine with the liberated protons to form water, and more poorly ionized sodium acetate is formed.) The major blood buffer system, carbonic acid plus sodium bicarbonate, is especially effective for protecting against a fall in pH, since carbonic acid can be rapidly converted to water plus carbon dioxide (which is eliminated by the lungs). Chelators can protect against large changes in in the concentrations of certain kinds of free ions, by binding them in inactive forms.

Bufo: a toad genus.

buformin: *N*-butylimidocarbonimidic diamide; a biguanide type oral hypoglycemic agent.

bufotalin: 16-(acetoxy)-3,14-dihyroxybufa-20,22-dienolide; a toxin in the venom of the European toad *Bufo vulgaris* that stimulates the heart.

bufotenine: 5-hydroxy-*N,N*-dimethyltryptamine; a serotonin metabolite made by toads, and a component of cahoe beans and some mushrooms (such as *Psilocybe mexicana*) that causes hallucinations. It is used in some aboriginee rites, and in studies of chemically induced psychic effects. Small amounts are made by humans, and it has been suggested that overproduction contributes to some manifestations of psychoses.

budesonide

bufotenine

bufotoxin: the major cardiostimulatory component of the venom of the European toad, *Bufo vulgaris*.

bulbocapnine: 10-methoxy-1,2-(methylenedioxy)-6aα-aporphin-11-ol; an alkaloid chemically related to apomorphine, isolated from the tubers of *Corydalis cava* (a member of the "Dutchman's breeches" family), and from some other plants. It is a dopamine receptor antagonist that invokes narcosis and a form of plastic rigidity (catatonia) that can be prolonged with scopolamine and opposed by amphetamines. Small amounts were once used to alleviate the tremors of Parkinson's disease. Bulbocapnine also lowers blood pressure, stimulates the uterus, and can invoke convulsions.

bulbogastrone: a factor of unknown chemical composition, different from secretin, that inhibits gastrin release and diminishes meal-associated hydrochloric acid production. Its status as a hormone has not been established.

bulbourethral glands: bulbocavernosus glands; Cowper's glands: small lobulated organs that flank the male urethra and secrete lubricants.

bulimia: (1) hyperphagia; (2) an eating disorder in which recurrent episodes of "binge" eating (during which enormous quantities of food are ingested) are followed by induced vomiting or purging. It is associated with fear of obesity, and with varying degrees of psychic depression and low self-esteem. Typically, the behavior is conducted in private, with efforts to avoid detection by family members and others. The individual recognizes that the behavior is abnormal, but feels out of control. Repeated contact with gastric acid can damage the teeth and esophagus, purgatives can injure the lower gastrointestinal tract, and electrolyte imbalances are created by both the vomiting and the purging. There are controversies concerning whether neurotransmitter and/or hormonal dysfunctions contribute to the etiology. Tricyclic antidepressants often confer beneficial effects; and subnormal cholecystokinin levels have been detected in some cases.

bulk extracellular fluid: the interstitial fluid that derives from blood plasma and surrounds most body cells. The relative concentrations of various ions resemble those of the plasma, but the protein content is much lower; and no cells are present under normal conditions. The amounts stored in areolar connective tissues are related to total body sodium content, but are also affected by plasma proteins (*see* **albumins**), and by hormones that control ion transport across cell membranes. The composition differs somewhat from those of cerebrospinal, bone, eye, and ear extracellular fluids.

bull: the adult male of various animal types, such as cattle, elephants, and moose.

BUN: blood urea nitrogen. Elevated levels are usually associated with renal dysfunction.

α-bungarotoxin: a 74-amino acid neurotoxin in the venom of *Bulgarus multicinctus* snakes that invokes curare-like skeletal muscle paralysis by binding irreversibly to neuromuscular junction type nicotinic acetylcholine receptors. It is used to identify, isolate, and study those receptors. It also binds to brain neuron components that may be thymopoietin receptors. Different kinds of receptors may mediate inhibition of luteinizing hormone (LH) release when the toxin is injected into cerebral ventricles.

β-bungarotoxin: a peptide composed of 13.5K and 7K subunits in the venom of *Bulgarus multicinctus* that blocks transmission in neuromuscular junctions. It acts presynaptically to block acetylcholine release. Some effects on nerve terminals are attributed to phospholipase A$_2$ activation, but direct influences on potassium ion channels have been suggested.

buprenorphine: [5,7α(S)]-17-(cyclopropylmethyl)-α-(1,1-dimethylethyl)-4,5,-epoxy-18,19-dihydro-3-hydroxy-6-methoxy-α-methyl-6,14-enthoanmorphinan-7-methanol; a semi-synthetic opioid derived from thebaine. When used as an analgesic, it is less addictive than morphine, invokes less euphoria, and is associated with shorter withdrawal periods; but it can cause respiratory depression and miosis. It is a mixed agonist/antagonist that acts mostly on μ-type opioid receptors. Although it can suppress withdrawal effects in morphine-dependent laboratory animals, it invokes them in humans who have taken morphine for long time periods.

bupropion: 1-(3-chlorophenyl)-2-[(1,1-dimethylethyl)-amino]-1-propane; an agent with activities similar to those of tricyclic antidepressants, but claimed to exert fewer side-effects. Its use in hyperactivity-attention defect syndromes is under investigation. Wellbutrin is a trade name for the hydrochloride.

burimamide: 4-butylnitrosourea-imidazole; an H_2-type histamine receptor antagonist. It has been used to treat peptic ulcers, but, because of low potency, has largely been replaced by cimetidine and metiamide.

Burkitt's lymphoma: a disease attributed to Epstein Barr virus infections, in which malignant, B-cell derived lymphoblast tumors develop at multiple sites. It occurs mostly in tropical countries, probably because of the immunosuppressant effects of concomitant malaria infections. Reciprocal translocations of portions of human chromosome 8 with chromosomes 2, 14, or 22 bring *c-myc* genes under the control of immunoglobulin promoters, and thereby cause overexpression of the proto-oncogene.

bursa of Fabricius: a gland on the posterodorsal wall of the avian cloaca, composed predominantly of lymphoid follicles in which pre-B cells proliferate and undergo maturation. It is essential for establishing and maintaining humoral immunity in birds (*see* **bursin**), and has receptors for glucocorticoids, testosterone, and estrogens (and for progesterone after exposure to estrogens). High doses of testosterone can totally destroy the gland, but low levels stimulate. The functional equivalent in mammals has not been established; but *see* **Peyer's patches**.

bursicon: an insect hormone that promotes cuticle maturation after molting.

bursin: Lys-His-Gly-NH$_2$; a hormone made in the bursa of Fabricius, formerly known as bursopoietin. It stimulates cAMP and cGMP generation, and promotes maturation of pre-B lymphocytes that includes commitment to production of a single type of antibody. *Cf* **thymopentin**.

bursopoietin: *see* **bursin**.

burst forming units: BFUs: clusters of undifferentiated bone marrow cells, identified by their abilities to respond to certain growth factors and differentiate into specific kinds of more mature hemopoietic cell types. At the next stage, they are called colony forming units (CFUs). Burst forming unit-E types (BFU-E) are composed of stem cells of erythroid lineage that respond to erythropoietin and form CFU-Es.

burst promoting activity: an old term for interleukin-3 that relates to its function as a growth factor for erythroid progenitor cells.

buserelin: *p*Glu-His-Trp-Ser-Tyr-D-Ser-(tBu)-Leu-Arg-Pro-Gly-NH-Et; a potent gonadotropin releasing hormone (GnRH) analog that suppresses the secretion of follicle stimulating and luteinizing hormones (FSH and LH) by desensitizing gonadotrope cells. It is used to treat precocious puberty, endometriosis, prostate cancers, uterine leiomyomas, and some forms of breast cancer.

buspirone: BuSpar; 8-[4-[4-(2-pyrmidinyl)-1-piperazinyl]butyl]8-azaspiro[4,5]-decane-7,9-dione; an anxiolytic agent that does not invoke sedation, psychomotor impairment, or habituation. It is a partial agonist for $5HT_{1A}$-type serotonin receptors. It also interacts weakly with D_2-type dopamine receptors, but does not affect gamma aminobutyric acid (GABA) types.

busulfan: Myleran; 1,4-butanediol dimethanesulfonate; an alkylating agent that destroys rapidly proliferating cells, including germinal cells in the ovaries and testes and T lymphocytes. It is used clinically to treat chronic granulocytic leukemia, myeloid metaplasia, and polycythemia vera, and to transiently suppress cellular immunity, but is potentially teratogenic. It is also used to study the effects of germ cell removal on gonadal development, and as an insecticide.

butaclamol: 3-(1,1-dimethylethyl)-2,3,4,4a,8,9,13b,14-octahydro-1*H*-benzo[6,7]cyclo-hepta[1,2,3-de]pyrido[2,1-a]isoquinolin-3-ol; a tranquilizer. The (+) form binds to D_2-type dopamine receptors, and the (-) isomer to σ sites (*see* **opioid receptors**).

2,3-butanedione: an agent used to identify guanine groups in peptides and proteins. It promotes persistent activation of protein kinases, but does not affect cyclic nucleotide binding to the enzymes.

butanol-extractable iodine, BEI: *see* **protein bound iodine.**

butazolamide: Butamide; 5-butyramido-1,3,4-thiadiazole-2-sulfonamide; a carbonic anhydrase inhibitor that is used as a diuretic.

buthionine sulfoximine, L-buthione-*S,R*-sulfoximine; BSO: a specific inhibitor of γ-glutamylcysteine synthase (an enzyme essential for glutathione biosynthesis) that augments the effects of radiation and chemotherapeutic agents on cancer cells. It is used to block the GSH redox cycle, and to study the effects of glutathione depletion.

butorphanol: 17-(cyclobutylmethyl)morphinan-3,4-diol; an agent chemically related to morphine, and believed to act mostly on *k* and σ-type receptors (*see* **opioid receptors**). It is used to control coughing. Analgesic doses invoke less severe respiratory depression and psychotomimetic effects than morphine. Although withdrawal symptoms follow abrupt cessation of medication when large doses are used for extended time periods, butorphanol neither invokes nor relieves morphine withdrawal symptoms.

butoxamine: α-1[[(1,1-dimethylethyl)amino]ethyl]-2,5-dimethoxybenzenemethanol; a β$_2$-type adrenergic receptor antagonist that blocks epinephrine inhibition of smooth (but not cardiac) muscle. It also inhibits fatty acid mobilization, and is used as a hypolipemic agent.

butyloxycarbonyl amino acids: t-BOC amino acids; compounds used for solid phase protein synthesis. Tertiary butoxylcarbonyl (t-BOC) groups are attached to amino acids before the carboxyl groups are prepared for peptide bond formation with agents such as dicyclohexylcarbodiimide (DCC), because free amino groups can interfere with the reactions. After the peptide bond is formed, the DCC is released as dicyclohexylurea, and the t-Boc is removed with dilute acid. An amino acid linked to both t-Boc and DCC is shown.

butyric acid: butanoic acid; a short-chain fatty acid product of carbohydrate fermentation in ruminants that is released in substantial amounts to milk (and accounts for much of the flavor of table butter). It is also formed (in these and other species) when long-chain fatty acids are degraded, and is a minor component of sweat. Since it affects transcription by inhibiting histone acetylation, it is used to study gene expression. Arginine butyrate can promote production of fetal type hemoglobin in individuals with sickle cell anemia. Butyrate is also a potent stimulant for insulin secretion. Some effects of dibutyryl-cAMP are attributed to the butyrate released by cell enzymes.

β-hydroxy-**butyric acid:** β-OH-butyric acid: *see* **ketone bodies.**

γ-hydroxy-**butyric acid:** 3-hydroxybutyrate: a metabolite made in the brain that blocks transmission in dopaminergic neurons, and decreases food intake in laboratory animals.

butyryl-ACP: butyric acid linked to acyl carrier protein. It is an intermediate in the pathway for fatty acid biosynthesis.

butyrophenones: haloperidol and related agents that affect dopamine functions, and are used for their tranquilizing and anti-psychotic effects.

butyrophilin: an intermediate filament protein made in mammary glands that covers milk fat globules.

C

C: (1) carbon; (2) cysteine; (3) cytosine; (4) cytidine; (5) Calorie; (6) Centigrade; (7) catalytic subunit; (8) Curie; (9) coulomb; (10) capacitance.

c: (1) calorie; (2) canine, as in cLH; (3) complementary, as in cDNA.

c-: cellular, used for protooncogenes, as in *c-abl*. *Cf v-*.

C1, C2, C3...C9: (1) complement factors 1-9; (2) designates the positions of carbon atoms at specific loci in compounds. When two numbers are used, as in C17-C20-lyase, it indicates an enzyme cleavage site.

CA: catecholamine.

Ca: calcium.

CA antigen: epitectin; a glycoprotein expressed on the surfaces of sweat gland, pneumocyte, urinary bladder epithelial, and some tumor cells. It is a differentiation antigen. Small amounts of the glycoprotein are excreted in urine.

CAAT boxes: components of many gene promoters, with base sequences of the general type GGNCAATCT. Their contributions to transcription efficiency are regulated by binding numerous transcription factors. *See also* C/EBP.

CAAT box enhancer binding protein: *see* C/EBP.

Ca^{2+}-ATPases: approximately 100K enzymes that use energy released by ATP hydrolysis for active transport of calcium ions. They are present in all plasma membranes, cell nuclei, and endoplasmic reticula (with especially high levels in sarcoplasmic reticula), and are essential for maintaining subcellular compartment Ca^{2+} levels. The actions involve binding of two calcium ions, consequent phosphorylation of an aspartate moiety, and subsequent dephosphorylation.

C-banding: procedures for staining chromosomes; *see* banding patterns.

cabergoline: FCE 21336: 1-ethyl-3-(3′-dimethylaminopropyl)-3-(6′-allylergoline-8′,β-carbonyl)urea; an orally effective dopamine receptor antagonist, used clinically to inhibit prolactin secretion. It is chemically related to metergoline, but has a much longer duration of action.

c-abl: *see* abl, Abelson murine leukemia virus, and Philadelphia chromosome.

CaBPs: calcium binding proteins.

Ca-calmodulin: Ca-CaM; *see* calmodulins.

cachectin: tumor necrosis factor-α (TNFα).

cachexia: debilitation and tissue wasting. The causes include malnutrition, some kinds of hormone deficiencies

(*see*, for example Addison's and Simmonds's disease), psychological factors, severe infections, and products formed in individuals with malignant tumors. *See also* tumor necrosis factor-α.

caclicmycin: A23187.

caco-: a prefix meaning bad, as in cacogenic.

cacodylic acid: hydroxymethylarsine oxide; a component of buffers used to fix specimens for electron microscopy.

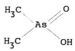

cacogenetic: describes deterioration in species caused by disadvantageous sexual selection.

cactinomycin: toxic antibiotics made by *Streptomyces chrysomallus*. *See* actinomycins.

CAD: a 240K eukaryote multi-enzyme complex used for pyrimidine biosynthesis, composed of covalently linked carbamoyl phosphate synthase, aspartate transcarbamoylase, and dihydroorotase.

Ca^{2+}-dependent hydrophobic-interaction chromatography: techniques for isolating proteins that display calcium-dependent binding to phospholipids.

cadaverine: 1,5-pentanediamine; a lysine degradation product in decaying organic matter that is made by bacteria.

$$H_2N-CH_2-CH_2-CH_2-CH_2-CH_2-NH_2$$

cadherins: a family of cell adhesion molecules (*q.v.*), whose members mediate calcium-dependent binding to molecules of the same kind, other cadherins, catenins, and certain other proteins. They are transmembrane glycoproteins with common LDREXXXXXXL and other amino acid sequences, but different N-termini; *cf* integrins. They mediate homotypic cell:cell and/or cell:-extracellular matrix adhesions, colocalize with actin filaments, and contribute to the formation of intermediate junctions. The functions affected include cytokinesis, embryonic tissue compaction and invagination, and fertilization. Additionally, they contribute to the maintenance of cell shape and polarization, and to control of intercellular tension. The *ret* gene product, and some others display tyrosine kinase activity. All vertebrates have characteristic combinations of the various types; and related glycoproteins have been identified in *Drosophila* and other organisms. In mammals, they are expressed in preimplantation embryos, and the relative amounts of each type change during development. (Some disappear when new types are expressed.) There is indirect evidence that loss of E-cadherin (and possibly of other types) contributes to tumor cell metastasis. *See* individual types.

A-cadherin: a glycoprotein identical to **N-cadherin** (*q.v.*).

E-cadherin: E-CAM: a 120-125K cell adhesion molecule identical with uvomorulin (identified in intestinal epithelium and trophectoderm), and with L-CAM and cell CAM 120/80, that mediates embryonic cell compaction, epithelial cell aggregation, cytoskeletal rearrangements, and the formation of tight and gap junctions. It appears to engage in mostly homophilic (E-cadherin to E-cadherin) binding, but the existence of different kinds of E-cadherin receptors has been suggested. High levels are present in epithelial tissues that line surfaces, and in mammalian preimplantation embryos.

L-cadherin: L-CAM; a cadherin in liver which appears to be identical with E-cadherin (E-CAM), uvomorulin, and cell CAM 120/80, and has also been called Arc-1.

N-cadherin: N-CAM; a 135K cadherin prevalent in neuronal, neuroepithelial, and muscle tissues, and in eye lens. It is expressed in all three embryonic germ layers, and may be identical with A-cadherin (A-CAM) of cardiac intercalated disks and eye lens, and with a neural retina adhesion molecule. The functions are strongly affected by glycosylation. In embryos and young fetuses, polysialylated forms contribute to cell migration, whereas at later times unsialyated molecules play roles in cell differentiation and tissue organization. Embryonic types occur in glucagonomas and some other tumors.

P-cadherin: P-CAM; a 130K cadherin initially identified in placenta, but also present in epidermis and other tissues. It is believed to mediate some aspects of morphogenesis.

cadmium: Cd; an element (atomic number 48, atomic weight 112.41). Low levels exert zinc-like effects; and Cd replaces zinc in some metalloenzymes of marine algae. However, high levels impair zinc metabolism, close voltage gated calcium channels, cause irritation, and exert deleterious effects on the skin and its appendages. Chronic exposure can damage the lungs, kidneys, heart, liver, and gonads, and invoke a form of osteomalacia. High concentrations also impair DNA deletion processes, and block repair (but can protect against deletional mutations). Rat fetuses that develop in mothers given high doses during pregnancy have serious developmental defects attributed mostly to interference with zinc utilization. Metallothionein provides some protection by binding Cd, and is also induced by Cd. The salts are used to study metal metabolism, ion channels, and DNA processing, and to treat worm infestations.

CADO: *see* 2-chloro-**adenosine**.

cADPR: cyclic adenosine diphosphate ribose.

caecum: cecum.

caeno-: ceno-.

Caenorhabditis elegans; *C. elegans*: a nematode, uniquely useful for the study gametogenesis, development, apoptosis, and genetics. The adult male has only 970 somatic cells, and the adult, self-fertilizing hermaphrodite 810. All are visible under light microscopy, and a cell by cell analysis of development of 500-cell larvae has been achieved. Extensive genetic maps have been compiled, and mutations are easily detected. *See* also unc-86.

caerulein: cerulein:
5-oxo-Pro-Gln-Asp-Tyr-Thr-Gly-Trp-Met-Asp-Phe-NH$_2$;

$$SO_3H$$

a decapeptide initially identified in the skin of the tree frog *Hyla caerulea*. It, and related peptides, are made in the brains and gastrointestinal tracts of all vertebrates studied, and in invertebrates. The terminal pentapeptide is identical to that of cholecystokinins and gastrins; and the biological properties overlap with those hormones. Caerulein promotes secretion of gastrin and hydrochloric acid in the stomach, and of pancreatic enzymes and bile. It stimulates contraction of gall bladder wall smooth muscle, and of the pyloric sphincter, and increases intestinal motility, but relaxes the lower esophageal sphincter and the sphincter of Oddi. The ability to decrease food intake may depend in part on its ability to slow gastric emptying (but *see* **cholecystokinin**). The effects on vascular smooth muscle vary with the species; in most cases, the blood pressure is elevated. The peptide also inhibits fatty acid synthesis and the myristoylation of proteins. Some effects are secondary to release of substance P, acetylcholine, and other regulators.

caerulein related peptides: phyllocaerulein, Asn^2-Leu^6-cerulein, and other amphibian skin peptides that are chemically and biologically similar to cerulean.

caeruloplasmin: ceruloplasmin.

CAF-1: a protein that promotes nucleosome assembly of replicating DNA.

cafeteria diet: supermarket diet: assortments of highly palatable nutrients, usually rich in carbohydrate and/or fat content, and sometimes referred to as "junk food". Most laboratory animal species that maintain normal body weights on standard chow rations rapidly accumulate body fat when given free access to them. The diets are used to study obesity development, associated metabolic problems, and factors that affect food intake.

caffeic acid: 3,4-dihydroxycinnamic acid; a glycoside component of several plants, isolated from green coffee. It is used to inhibit lipoxygenases.

caffeine: 1,3,7-trimethylxanthine; an alkaloid in coffee, tea, cola nuts, chocolate, and some other commonly ingested plant derivatives. In the amounts usually taken, it can lessen fatigue, shorten reaction time, improve mental functions, raise metabolic rate, and elevate mood. Although some tolerance develops, and withdrawal can lead to headache, fatigue, and other symptoms, caffeine is said to be habituating rather than addictive. Excessive amounts invoke restlessness, insomnia, fine tremors, and hyperesthesias; and stimulation of intestinal smooth muscle can cause nausea, vomiting, and diarrhea. Since caffeine augments the sensitivity of the respiratory center of the medulla oblongata to carbon dioxide, facilitates arousal, and stimulates the heart, it has been used to counteract the effects of hypnotics and other pharmacological depressants, and as a cardiac stimulant; but overdosage invokes convulsions. It is incorporated into several analgesic preparations, presumably to elevate mood, but its effectiveness for such purposes is questioned. Caffeine also augments glomerular filtration rates, and is sometimes used as a diuretic. Other effects include relaxation of coronary and renal vascular smooth muscle; but potentiation of the stimulatory effects of ergot alkaloids on cerebral vessels is beneficial in some individuals with migraine headaches. Relaxation of respiratory tract smooth muscle can be useful in cases of bronchial asthma. The ability to increase gastric acidity may be indirect. Some effects, including potentiation of certain norepinephrine and epinephrine actions, and some influences on dopaminergic functions are attributed to inhibition of cAMP phosphodiesterase activity. Although now largely replaced by isobutylmethylxanithine (IBMX), it has been used to study cAMP functions. Caffeine also promotes intracellular Ca^{2+} translocation, and it is reported to overcome mitosis arrest caused by agents that block DNA synthesis in the cells of hamsters and some other species (but not in humans or mice). Coffee opposes some effects of A_2 type adenosine receptor activation, but decaffeination does not diminish the responses.

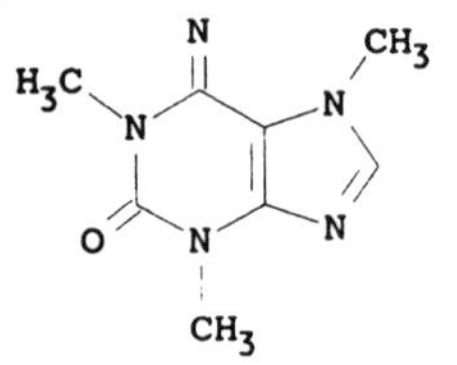

caged molecules: compounds enclosed in hydrophobic, photolabile "cages" that protect the active components from extracellular degradation, but permit them to enter cells. Subsequent exposure to short pulses of light or other forms of radiation releases the active components. Some caged molecules are labeled with radioactive markers, such as [32]P. The structures of caged ATP [(adenosine-5'-triphosphate, P-1-(2-nitrophenyl)ethyl ester sodium salt], and caged cGMP [guanosine-3'5'-cyclic monophosphate-P-1-(2-nitrophenyl) ethyl ester] are shown.

CAH: congenital adrenal hyperplasia.

Cajal cells: (1) astrocytes; (2) neuroglial cells arranged horizontally in the molecular layer of the cerebral cortex.

Cajal method: gold chloride staining of astrocytes for microscopy.

cal: calorie.

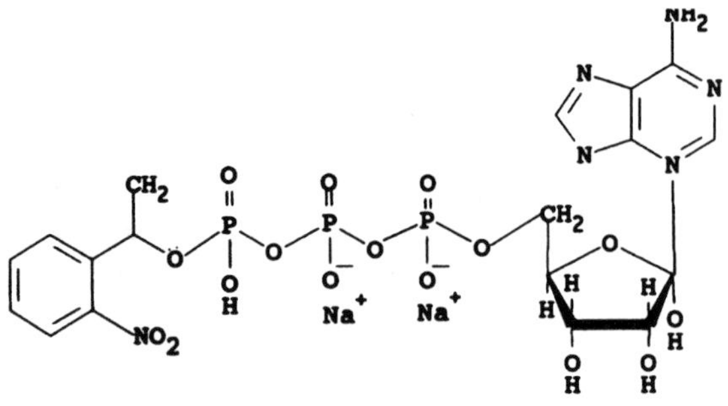

caged ATP

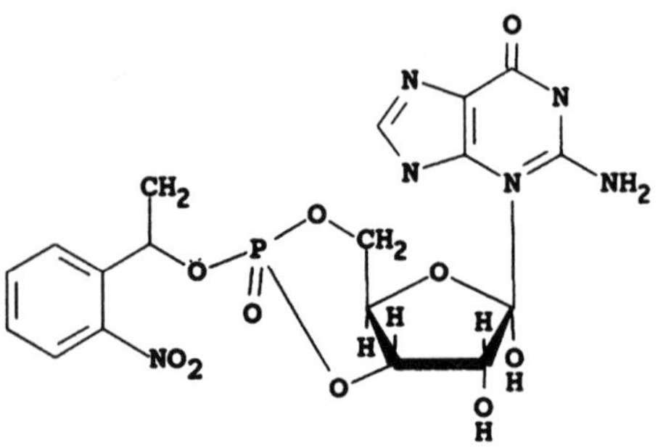

caged cGMP

Cal: Calorie; kilocalorie.

calbindins: soluble proteins chemically and structurally related to calmodulins, parvalbumin, S-100, troponin-C, and oncomodulin, all of which bind two Ca^{2+} ions per molecule. Calbindin-D_{28K} predominates in avian tissues responsive to calciferols, and is also present in mammalian kidney. In mammalian brain, the highest concentrations of the 28K form are in cerebellar Purkinje cells, one of the few sites where induction by 1,25-dihydroxyvitamin D cannot be demonstrated. Some neuronal types contribute to sensory functions in the eyes and ears. Calbindin$_{29K}$ (protein 10, which may be identical with calretinin and BPP23) is concentrated in cochlear nuclei, and 9-10K forms have been described for visual cortex and hippocampus. Calbindin D_{9K}, an 8.5K, 75-amino acid protein, is the major type in mammalian intestine, in which it contributes to absorption of dietary calcium. The amounts made there are directly related to calciferol levels. It is also found in ameloblasts, chondrocytes, extracellular matrix vesicles of calcifying cartilage, and embryonic yolk sac. Estrogens stimulate, and progesterone inhibits its synthesis in endometrium and myometrium during the third trimester of pregnancy. Since they facilitate calcium transport to fetuses, endometrial types may be essential for mineralization of fetal skeletons. Other sites in which calbindins occur include insulin-secreting pancreatic cells and eggshell glands. In at least some cell types, the proteins are short-term calcium buffers that protect against excessive elevation of intracellular Ca^{2+}, by binding the ions and facilitating their movements.

calcein: fluroexon; *bis[N,N-bis*(carboxymethyl)aminomethyl]fluorescein; a fluorescent indicator used for calcium and magnesium determinations.

calcidiol: calcifediol; 25-hydroxyvitamin D_3; *see* 25-hydroxy-**cholecalciferol**.

calcifediol: calcidiol: 25-hydroxyvitamin D_3; *see* 25-hydroxy-**cholecalciferol**.

calciferols: vitamin D and related secosteroids; *see.* **cholecalciferol**, 25-hydroxy-**cholecalciferol**, and 1,25-dihydroxy-**cholecalciferol**.

Calcimar: a trade name for a salmon calcitonin preparation that is used to treat Paget's disease.

calcimedins: calmedins; calcium mediator proteins: proteins that interact with Ca^{2+} to regulate cAMP-dependent phosphorylation of inositol triphosphate receptors, and thereby decrease receptor sensitivity. The 67K form is similar to or identical with 67K calelectrin. Although not chemically related to calmodulins, they bind phenothiazine type calmodulin inhibitors.

calcineurins: proteins homologous to protein phosphatases 1 and 2A, in skeletal muscle, and in neural and other tissues. They are composed of 61K A subunits plus Ca^{2+}-binding B types. The multiple forms may arise from alternate splicing of a common mRNA. The dimers bind calmodulins, promote dephosphorylation of Ca^{2+} channels that are phosphorylated by protein kinase A and Ca-calmodulin activated kinases, and antagonize other Ca-calmodulin effects, for example on cyclic nucleotide phosphodiesterases. One isozyme is a rate-limiting determinant for T lymphocyte activation via its TCR receptor, and for induction of transcription factors (including NF-AT and NF-IL2A) that promote the synthesis of interleukin-2 and some other cytokines. It is also the major target for immunosuppression mediated by FK506-FKBP (but not rapamycin-FKBP) complexes; *see* also **immunophilins**. Roles for other isozymes in control of sperm motility have been suggested.

calciseptin: a 60-amino acid toxin in the venom of the black mamba spider, *Dendroapsis polyepsis polyepsis*, with eight cysteines that form four disulfide bonds. It lowers blood pressure by specifically inhibiting L Ca^{2+} channel subtypes in blood vessels and cardiac muscle, and exerts lesser effects on neurons, but does not affect skeletal muscle L subtypes, N or P Ca^{2+} channels, or voltage sensitive Na^+ and K^+ ion channels.

calciosomes: cell organelles that accumulate and release calcium, and are implicated as major regulators of intracellular Ca^{2+} levels. They contain a protein similar to or identical with calsequestrin. There are controversies concerning whether they the primary targets for inositol 1,4,5-triphosphate (IP_3).

calciphorin: a mitochondrial protein implicated in the control of calcium transport.

calciphylaxis: deposition of calcium salts in soft tissues, induced by administration of antigens to sensitized individuals, or of large quantities of calcium and phosphate salts.

calcitonin[s]: CT; 32-amino acid, species-specific peptides secreted by thyroid gland parafollicular cells in mammals, by ultimobranchial bodies of all other vertebrates except cyclostomes, and in large amounts by thyroid gland medullary carcinomas. Identical or closely related peptides are made by some other cell types. The cysteine moities at positions 1 and 6 are joined in the sequence for human CT: H_2N-Cys-Gly-Asn-Ser-Thr-Cys-Met-Leu-Gly-Thr-Tyr-Thr-Gln-Asp-Phe-Asn-Lys-

calcein

Phe-His-Thr-Phe-Pro-Gln-Thr-Ala-Ile-Gly-Val-Gly-Ala-Pro-NH$_2$. Salmon CTs have similar three-dimensional configurations. Although they share only 16 of the amino acid moieties, they are approximately 10 times as potent in mammals because of long half-lives and high affinities for mammalian receptors. The messenger RNA that codes for CT prohormone undergoes alternate splicing in neurons and some other cell types, and directs the synthesis of **calcitonin gene related peptide** (*q.v.*) and other peptides. Hypercalcemia promotes calcitonin secretion, and CT corrects the condition, mostly by inhibiting osteoclast activity and osteocytic osteolysis, and thereby slowing bone resorption. However, high levels rarely invoke hypocalcemia. CT also accelerates urinary excretion of calcium and phosphate, regulates calcium and phosphate uptake by many cell types, lowers blood phosphate levels, and can inhibit intestinal absorption of calcium. Stimulatory effects on osteoblasts have been suggested, but they may be mediated by other peptides derived from the same mRNAs. Although inhibition of new bone formation has been described, it may be accomplished via release of paracrine mediators. The effects on bone cells are transient, in part because sustained receptor occupancy leads to down regulation of receptor numbers. Moreover, high levels stimulate parathyroid hormone secretion (which exerts opposing effects). Calcitonins are used to treat Paget's disease, in which the main problem is excessively rapid remodeling. Although they transiently alleviate the hypercalcemia of malignancy, they can augment release of **parathyroid hormone related protein** (*q.v.*). The peptides are not effective when used alone for slowing bone loss in postmenopausal osteoporosis, but intermittent administration, with other agents presented during the withdrawal periods, may be beneficial. Plasma CT concentrations rise shortly before the usual times of meal ingestion, and additional release is stimulated by some gastrointestinal tract hormones (gastrin in some species, and cholecystokinin in others). By averting postprandial hypercalcemia, and consequent mineral loss to the urine, dietary calcium is conserved, and this may be the major function in non-pregnant adult mammals. (CT deficient mammals are not hypercalcemic, but they do slowly lose some bone mineral.) The hormone that is released to milk may contribute to calcium conservation in infants, but it also delays gastric emptying and suppresses appetite; and high levels inhibit prolactin secretion. During pregnancy, CT protects maternal skeletons against excessive mineral depletion. Other calcitonin effects include acceleration of urinary sodium, chloride, and water excretion, and this may be a major function in non-mammalian vertebrates in which it exerts little or no influences on blood calcium levels. CT also dilates some blood vessels, and facial flushing is a common side effect of CT injection. The peptides bind to some heat shock proteins and affect their configurations, and they slow sperm motility. Additional target cells are in the lungs, gonads, and lymphocytes. In non-mammalian vertebrates, CT promotes calcium accumulation in egg shells and vertebral lime sacs. Most actions have been linked with cAMP generation.

N^α-propionyl Di-Ala^{1,7},des-Leu-**calcitonin**: CTR: RG 12851: a noncyclic calcitonin analog developed for treatment of Paget's disease and hypercalcemia of malignancy. It is equipotent with calcitonin for effects on bone and kidney, but invokes fewer side-effects such as anorexia, nausea, and facial flushing.

calcitonin/CGRP genes: genes with 6 exons that undergo alternate splicings, and direct the synthesis of 13-14K preprocalcitonins. 12K procalcitonins, from exons A, B, C, and D, predominate in mammalian thyroid parafollicular cells. In addition to calcitonins, the prohormone cleavage products include 7K, 57-amino acid *N*-terminal peptides (N-CAP, N-proCT), and 2K *C*-terminal peptides (C-CAP, katacalcin). N-ProCT, which is co-secreted in equimolecular amounts with calcitonin, is mitogenic, and a stimulant for osteoblasts and their precursors. A different protein, derived from exons A, B, C, E, and F, predominates in nervous tissues, adrenal medulla and hypophysis, but is also made in small amounts in thyroid glands, and in larger ones in medullary carcinomas. Its best known product is calcitonin gene related peptide-α (C-GRPα).

calcitonin gene related peptide: CGRP;: CGRP-αs are species specific peptide products of calcitonin/CGRP genes. They are chemically related to amylin, can accumulate in pancreatic islets, and can inhibit insulin secretion and insulin-stimulated glycogenesis. The human type is H$_2$N-Ala-Cys-Asp-Thr-Ala-Thr-Cys-Val-Thr-His-Arg-Leu-Ala-Gly-Leu-Leu-Ser-Arg-Ser-Gly-Gly-Val-Val-Lys-Asn-Asn-Phe-Val-Pro-Thr-Asn-Val-Gly-Ser-Lys-Ala-Phe-NH$_2$. CGRP-βs are closely related peptides derived from different genes that are normally made in largest amounts in neural tissue, adrenal medulla and adenohypophysis. Small amounts are secreted by thyroid glands, and much larger ones by medullary carcinomas. In other organs, including the heart, they probably originate in peripheral nerves. CGRPs circulate, and are extremely potent, persistent vasodilators. The effects are attributed to opening of ATP-sensitive K$^+$ channels that are not affected by Ca^{2+}, but may involve interactions with G proteins. The responses are not modified by cholinergic or adrenergic agents, or by prostaglandin synthesis inhibitors. In contrast, chronotropic effects on the heart are accomplished by augmenting catecholamine regulated Ca^{2+} currents, and are opposed by isoproterenol. CGRPs co-localize with substance P in sensory neurons, and may be co-mediators or co-modulators of synaptic functions, but can invoke analgesia. They promote differentiation (but not survival) of olfactory epithelium sensory neurons that synapse with dopaminergic types in olfactory bulbs, induce tyrosine hydroxylase, increase the numbers of acetylcholine receptors, and may function as trophic factors for skeletal muscle. They also exert weak calcitonin-like effects on calcium metabolism, affect the secretion of iodinated thyroid hormones, inhibit the secretion of gastrin, HCl, pepsin, glucose dependent insulinotropic peptide (GIP), and enteroglucagon, but augment somatostatin secretion.

calcitriol: 1,25-dihydroxyvitamin D$_3$; *see* 1α,25-dihydroxy-**cholecalciferol**.

calcitroic acid: 1α-hydroxy-24,25,26,27-tetranor-3-carboxy-vitamin D_3, a major degradation product of 1α,25-dihydroxycholecalciferol (1,25-dihydroxyvitamin D).

calcitropic hormones: parathyroid hormone, 1,25-dihydroxyvitamin D, and other calcium mobilizing hormones.

calcium: Ca; an element (atomic number 20, atomic weight 40.08). It is a major regulator of virtually all biological functions, including plasma membrane permeability and cell excitability, cell shape, motility, deformability and fragility, skeletal, cardiac, and smooth muscle contraction, cell adhesion, agglutination and aggregation. It participates in blood coagulation, complement activation, exocytosis and phagocytosis, ATP generation, fertilization, zona reactions, and photoreception, and it affects cell proliferation, morphology, differentiation, and transformation. Some effects on enzymes are exerted directly. Others involve interactions with calmodulins and other proteins. Ca is also a major component of bone and dentin. "Resting" cells maintain cytoplasmic concentrations of free Ca^{2+} ion concentrations in the general range of 1×10^{-8} to 1×10^{-7} M, while surrounded by extracellular calcium levels that are closer to 1×10^{-3}M. Closed plasma membrane Ca^{2+} channels limit uptake, Ca^{2+}-ATPases extrude some excess ion, and intracellular organelles sequester substantial amounts. Many hormones and neurotransmitters rapidly raise the levels to 10^{-5}-10^{-4} M by opening the channels and/or mobilizing Ca^{2+} from intracellular sites. Since binding to proteins, phospholipids, and other molecules that mediate the effects proceeds rapidly, a sustained Ca^{2+} rise is not essential for maintaining many responses; and most cells display oscillatory changes for extended time periods following stimulation. Secondary influences on channels for K^+ and other ions can contribute to the effects. Depending on the conditions, activation of Na^+/Ca^{2+} exchange mechanisms can either raise or lower the concentrations. *See* also **parathyroid hormone**, **calcitonin**, and 1,25-dihydroxy-**cholecalciferol**.

calcium binding proteins: CaBPs; (1) calmodulins, synexin, S-100, calcyclins, vitamin K-dependent proteins, and other proteins that bind calcium with high affinity; (2) calbindins and other calcium-binding proteins induced by 1,25-dihydroxyvitamin D.

calcium channels: several kinds of membrane components that regulate Ca^{2+} ion movements into and out of cells, or across intracellular membranes. A single cell can have several types, some of which admit Ba^{2+} and other cations when Ca^{2+} levels are low. *Voltage-dependent* channels open in response to depolarization. The opening of plasma membrane *T* (transient), low threshold, rapidly inactivated subtypes in fibroblasts, cardiac and smooth muscle, and some other cells can be blocked by phenylalkylamines such as verapamil, but not by dihydropyridines. Verapamil also blocks the widely distributed *L* (long-term), high threshold, non-inactivating subtypes that remain open for extended time periods following depolarization; but those channels are additionally sensitive to dihydropyridines. Their activities are affected by kinase A mediated phosphorylation, by glucose in pancreatic islets, and by other regulators. G proteins augment the effects of depolarization, both directly (without second messengers) and via adenylate cyclase activation. Bay K 8644 increases, and nitrendipine decreases Ca^{2+} entry across K^+ sensitive subtypes. *N*, high-threshold inactivating channels in neurons, which function in neurotransmitter release, are blocked by ω-conotoxin and cadmium, and by norepinephrine acting on α_1-type adrenergic receptors. Purkinje cell *P* channels share some properties with N types, but differ in their responses to pharmacological agents. *Receptor operated* calcium channels (ROCC) are controlled by hormones, neurotransmitters, and/or other ligands (some of which additionaly modify the functions of voltage-dependent types). Endoplasmic reticulum stores Ca^{2+} that can be recruited to the cytoplasm by several kinds of regulators. Sarcoplasmic reticulum Ca^{2+} channels in skeletal muscle are essential for excitation-contraction coupling, and myocardium contains these as well as other types. *See* also **calciosomes**, **inositol phosphates**, **ryanodine**, and **cyclic adenosine diphosphate ribose**.

calcium dependent regulator protein: CDRP; an obsolete term for calmodulins.

calcyclin: a calcium-binding protein induced by platelet-derived growth factor (PDGF), epidermal growth factor (EGF), and other growth stimulants (and by vinblastine). It forms homodimers and also binds to calpactins, and is believed to contribute to tumor metastasis.

caldesmons: calcium and calmodulin binding proteins that affect cell adhesion, morphology, motility, and contractility, and are believed to play essential roles in cytoskeletal reorganization during mitosis. They exist as monomers, dimers, and oligomers that can assume elongated or globular forms. In nonmuscle cells, an 83K type predominates, but 135K and 140K amino acid chains, as well as 150K types and 150K/147K dimers have been identified in stress fibers. Oligomers bind F-actin, form cross-links, and thereby contribute to the organization of filament bundles. They are substrates for cdc2 kinases; and a mitosis specific kinase promotes dissociation from microfilaments. Transformation of several cell types correlates with low caldesmon concentrations. A 77-K cleavage product has been found in fibroblasts, platelets, aorta, and uterus, and also in the adrenal medulla (in which it affects catecholamine secretion). In smooth muscle, caldesmons are contractile apparatus components that promote formation of noncycling or slowly cycling "latch bridges". In the absence of Ca^{2+}, they bind to and promote myosin aggregation and inhibit actin-activated

Mg^{2+}-ATPase; but in its presence they bind calmodulin and promote actomyosin formation. Phosphorylation, catalyzed by Ca^{2+}-calmodulin kinase, decreases the affinities for both actin and calmodulin, and dissociation from actin abolishes the inhibitory effects on ATPases.

calelectrins: several proteins that display reversible, calcium-dependent binding to cell membranes and phospholipids. The largest, 67K form is similar to or identical with 67K calcimedin, lymphocyte membrane-associated Ca^{2+}-binding protein, a chromobindin, and some other calcium-binding proteins. It is also structurally related to lipocortins I and II and to some other oncogene and growth factor tyrosine kinase substrates.

calhibin: a calcium-binding protein that reversibly inhibits angiotensin-II and arginine vasopressin binding to hepatocyte membranes.

γ$_1$-calichemicin: a highly potent anti-tumor agent that specifically cleaves double stranded DNA TCCT/AGGA base sequences.

calmedins: calcimedins.

calmidazolium: [(1-*bis*-p-chlorophenyl)methyl]-3-[2,4-dichloro-β-(2,4-dichlorobenzyloxy)-phenyl]-imidazolium chloride; a potent, phenothiazine type inhibitor of calmodulin-dependent enzymes.

calmodulin[s]: CaM; calcium dependent regulator protein: 17K intracellular proteins chemically and biologically related to troponin-C, S-100, calbindins, and parvalbumin. They are constitutively expressed in all eukaryote cell types, with similar structures in all species. Some are subunits of muscle glycogen phosphorylases or other enzymes, whereas others attach to enzymes when activated. CaMs are said to function as calcium sensors and molecular switches. Each molecule can bind one to four Ca^{2+} ions to form Ca-calmodulin complexes (Ca-CMs) whose conformations are directly related to the numbers bound. The complexes then change the configurations of the proteins with which they associate. Since the binding is concentration-dependent, Ca-CMs can mediate graded responses when cell activation leads to elevation of cytoplasmic Ca^{2+}. Although the binding is reversible, the effects on the proteins are sustained because the associations persist for some time after the cytoplasmic Ca^{2+} returns to resting levels. Moreover, the activation is accomplished in some cases by augmentation of the enzyme affinities for phosphate ions; and phosphorylation can convert the enzymes to forms no longer dependent on high Ca^{2+} levels. There are also at least two Ca^{2+}-dependent calmodulin dependent kinases (CaM kinase I and CaM kinase II). The regulatory enzymes activated by Ca-CaMs including adenylate cyclases, cyclic nucleotide phosphodiesterases, plasma membrane and nuclear Ca^{2+}/Mg^{2+}-ATPases, endonucleases, myosin light chain kinase, microtubule proteins, and some phosphatases. The processes affected include neurotransmitter release, glucose metabolism, immune system responses, and cell proliferation. Several hormones regulate calmodulin translocation within cells, but few (if any) affect its synthesis.

calmodulin binding proteins: proteins whose functions are modulated by binding calcium-calmodulin (Ca-CaM) complexes. Most have phosphorylation sites affected by the binding; and most contain a PEST (*p*Glu-Asp-Ser-Thr-) sequence that confers sensitivity to calpains.

calorie: c; cal; (1) the amount of heat required to raise the temperature of one gram of water from 14.5° to 15.5°

γ1-calcichemicin

Celsius at a pressure of 1 atmosphere; (2) in nutrition studies, c is sometimes used for kilocalorie.

Calorie: C: Cal; kilocalorie; one thousand calories; the amount of heat required to raise one kilogram of water from 14.5° to 15.5° Celsius at a pressure of 1 atmosphere; but *see* **calorie**.

calorigenesis: heat production.

calpactins: calcium dependent cysteine proteases chemically related to endonexin, 32.5K calelectrin, and protein II. They are tetramers, with two heavy (35-36K) and two light (10K) peptide chains. The heavy chain of calpactin I is identical to lipocortin II and similar to the intestinal brush border p36 protein; and the heavy chain of calpactin II (p35) is identical to lipocortin I. Calpactins bind to F-actin, spectrin, and anionic phospholipids, and are substrates for some oncogene and growth factor receptor tyrosine kinases, including $pp60^{src}$ and the epidermal growth factor (EGF) receptors. Phosphorylation affects the binding, and phosphatidylserine increases the calcium sensitivity. (Phosphatidylcholine is ineffective). Calpactins contribute to control of actin filament bundles, and the maintenance of plasma membrane structure (including linkages to the cytoskeleton). They participate in inflammatory reactions, and appear to be essential for exocytosis. Their ability to inhibit phospholipase A_2s is attributed to nonspecific substrate binding. Annexins are competitive antagonists.

calpain[s]: calcium activated neutral proteinases; CANPs; dimeric cysteine proteases with 80K and 27-30K subunits, present in high levels in cardiac muscle, liver, blood platelets and adenohypophysial gonadotropes, lactotropes, and thyrotropes (but not corticotropes), and in smaller amounts in other cell types. They differ from each other in Ca^{2+} requirements for activation (micromolar and millimolar levels for calpains I and II, respectively.) The subunits contain domains homologous with those of calmodulin and papain, and share properties with transglutaminases. Both calpain types mediate intracellular protein degradation, contribute to excitation-secretion coupling, and activate plasma type transglutaminase. They catalyze degradation of fodrin, α-actinin, talin, and other proteins, and also conversion of membrane-bound protein kinase C to a soluble, persistently activated form. Influences on microtubules may account for facilitation of granule movement to plasma membranes, neutrophil degranulation, mitotic spindle dissolution, and redistribution of calcium-binding proteins during mitosis. They associate with chromosomes from prometaphase through anaphase, and with plasma membranes during telophase and interphase. Inhibitors include calpastatin and leupeptin.

calpain inhibitor peptide: Asp-Pro-Met-Ser-Ser-Thr-Tyr-Ile-Glu-Glu-Leu-Gly-Lys-Arg-Glu-Val-Thr-Ile-Pro-Pro-Lys-Tyr-Arg-Glu-Leu-Leu-Ala; a potent, selective inhibitor of calpains I and II.

calpastatin: an endogenous calpain inhibitor. High levels in adenohypophysial corticotropes are believed to protect against intracellular protein degradation (although the cells contain little or no calpain).

calphostin C: a potent specific inhibitor of kinase C isozymes, made by *Cladosporium cladosporides*, that acts on the regulatory domains but does not compete for calcium or phospholipid binding.

calretinin: a neuronal protein that may be identical with calbindin$_{29K}$.

calsequestrin: CS; a 44K skeletal muscle sarcoplasmic reticulum protein that terminates contraction by binding Ca^{2+}.

caltrin: a 47-amino acid, basic seminal fluid protein that adheres to the acrosome and tail regions of ejaculated spermatozoa, decreases motility and protects against premature activation within the epididymis by inhibiting Ca^{2+} uptake (possibly via interaction with citrate). The oviduct environment facilitates its transformation to a protein that promotes calcium uptake during capacitation.

calvaria: the part of the skull that covers and protects the frontal, parietal, and occipital brain lobes. Fetal calvariae are used to study factors that regulate bone growth and development.

Calvin cycle: Calvin-Benson cycle; the metabolic pathway for carbon dioxide fixation during the "dark" phase of photosynthesis in plants and some bacteria. It begins with conversion of ribulose 1,5-biphosphate to an enediol intermediate. Ribulose carboxylase then catalyzes a reaction in which the sugar phosphate takes up CO_2 to form 2'-carboxy-3-keto-D-arabinotol-1,5-biphosphate. Each product molecule then yields two 3-phosphoglycerates. The pathway from 3-phosphoglycerate to fructose-6-phosphate is identical with gluconeogenesis reactions in mammals, except that the photosynthetic glyceraldehyde-3-phosphate dehydrogenase uses NADPH.

calphostin C

calyculin A: a protein phosphatase inhibitor made by the marine sponge, *Discodermia calyx*, that is much more potent than okadaic acid, but acts indiscriminately on both 1 and 2A types (with little or no effects on most other phosphatases). Its ability to invoke inflammation compares with that of phorbol esters, but (in common with okadaic acid) it is a relatively weak promotor of tumor growth.

CAMs: *see* **cell adhesion molecules**.

CAM 120/80: *see* E-**cadherin**.

Ca^{2+}-Mg^{2+}-ATPases: enzymes that catalyze the use of energy derived from ATP hydrolysis to drive active transport of Ca^{2+} in exchange for Mg^{2+}. *See also* **Ca^{2+}-ATPases**.

cAMP: *see* **cyclic 3′5′-adenosine monophosphate**.

8-bromo-cAMP: 8-Br-CAMP; a lipophilic cyclic adenosine monophosphate analog that crosses plasma membranes and resists hydrolysis by cyclic nucleotide phosphodiesterases. It is especially useful for studying the effects of prolonged elevation of cAMP levels when butyrate (released from some other cAMP analogs) can complicate interpretations.

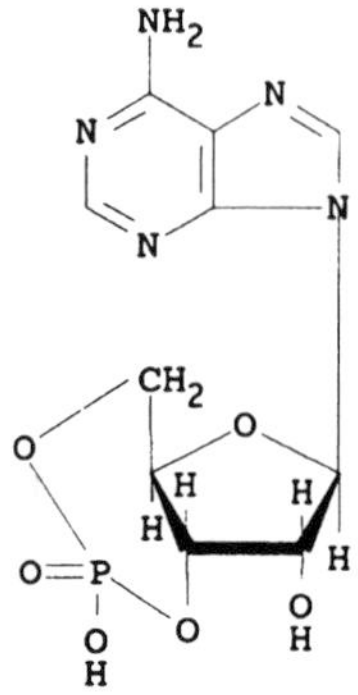

N^6,O-2′dibutyryl-cAMP

N^6,O-2′dibutyryl-**cAMP**: (Bu)$_2$cAMP; bucladesine; a long-acting, lipophilic cAMP analog that rapidly enters cells and is only slowly degraded by cyclic nucleotide phosphodiesterases. Although widely used to study cAMP functions, some effects are attributed to release of butyrate; *see* 8-bromo-**cAMP**.

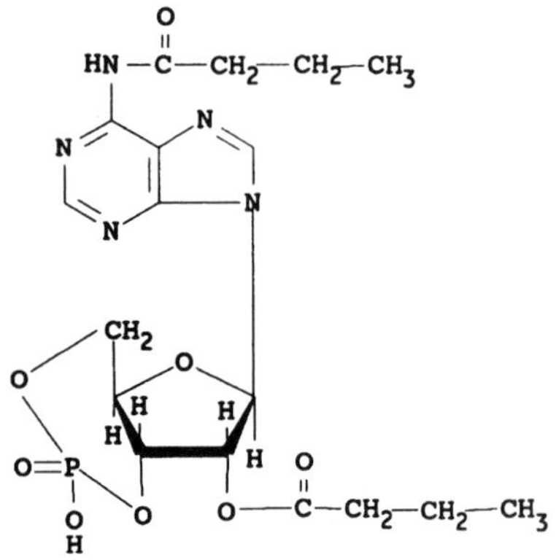

cAMP-dependent protein kinases: *see* **kinase A**.

campesterol: (24R)-ergost-5-3n-3β-ol; a steroid in soybean, rape-seed and wheat germ oils, and in some other plant preparations, that blocks cholesterol metabolism and arrests the growth of some tumor cells.

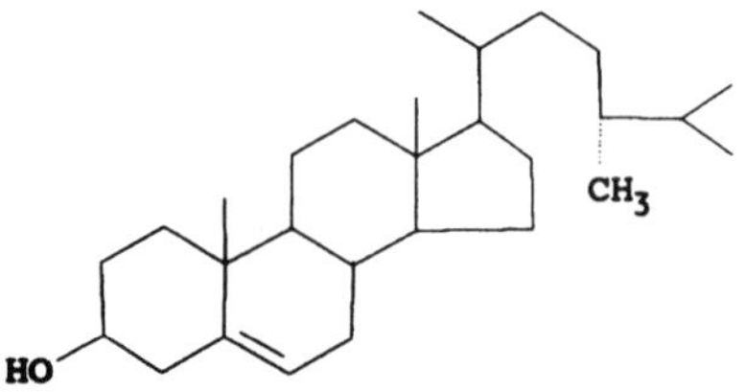

campothecin: 4-ethyl-4-hydroxy-1H-pyrano-[3′,4′6,7] indolizino[1,2b]quinoline-3,14-(4H,12H)-dione; an alkaloid obtained from rape-seed (*Campotheca acuminata*) that is also present in wheat-germ, soybean, and some other plant oils. It blocks DNA topoisomerase catalyzed breakage and reunion of DNA strands, and is used to treat colon cancer and some forms of leukemia, but can invoke leukopenia.

cAMP response element: *see* **CRE**.

cAMP response element binding protein: *see* **CREBP**.

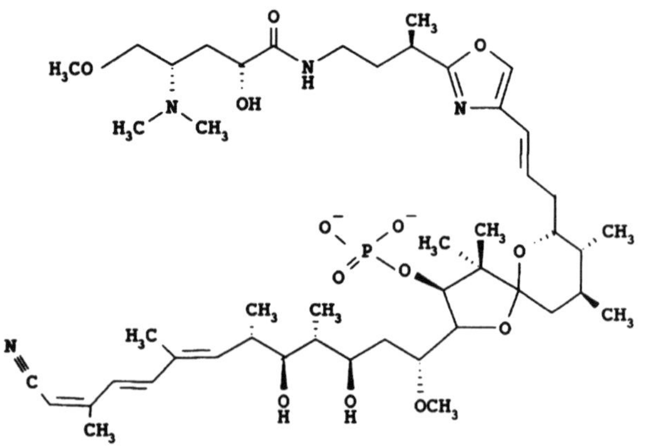

calyculin A

campothecin

canaliculus: a small channel. Some bone cells communicate with each other via caniculi, and small channels in the liver transport bile.

canavanine: 2-amino-4-(guanidoxy)-butyric acid; a basic amino acid from the jack bean, *Canavalia ensiformis*, and from alfalfa seeds and sprouts, that inhibits the growth of some microorganisms by interfering with arginine metabolism. It also blocks nitric oxide production by macrophages (but not endothelial cells). In mammals, it can invoke systemic lupus erythematosus-like hematological and serological abnormalities.

cancer: any malignant neoplasm; *see*, for example, **sarcoma**, and *cf* **adenoma**.

cancellous: spongy; *see* **bone types**.

canine: c; derived from, or characteristic of dogs and related species of the *Canus* genus. The term also describes cuspid teeth.

cannabinol: 6,6,9-trimethyl-3-pentyl-6*H*-dibenzo[*b,d*] pyran: a cannabis component with actions similar to those of tetrahydro-cannabinol, but much less potent.

tetrahydro-cannabinols: several isomeric cannabis components, the most potent of which is Δ⁹-THC, tetrahydro-6,6,9-trimethyl-l3-pentyl-6*H*-dibenzo[*b,d*]pyran-1-ol. They are sedatives that invoke euphoria, and can relieve some unpleasant effects of chemotherapeutic agents without blocking their actions on malignant cells. It is claimed that therapeutic use does not lead to addiction. Cannabinols also lower intra-ocular pressure in individuals with glaucoma. However, when used in large amounts to promote euphoria, they impair short-term memory and sense of time, affect sensory perception, and exert other effects on brain functions. Large doses can invoke anxiety, hallucinations, delusions, and paranoia, and nerve deterioration. Peripherally, cannabinols accelerate cardiac rate, elevate blood pressure (but dilate some blood vessels), and weaken skeletal muscle. Chronic use compromises reproductive and immune system functions, and damages respiratory system organs.

cannabis: Indian hemp; marijuana; the dried, flowering tops of *Cannabis sativa*. Tetrahydro-**cannabinols** (*q.v.*) are the most active components. Others include cannabinol, and cannabidiol.

CANP: calcium-activated neutral proteinase; *see* **calpain**.

canrenone: 17-hydroxy-3-oxo-17-pregna-4,6-diene-21-carboxylic acid γ-lactone; an aldosterone receptor antagonist. It is the active metabolite of spironolactone, used directly as a diuretic in some countries (but not the United States).

CAP: (1) cAMP activated protein; *see* **catabolite gene activator protein**; (2) adenylate cyclase associated protein; *see* **cyclase associated protein**.

capacitance: (1) ability to store an electrical charge; (2) the charge stored by a condenser for a given potential difference across its terminals; (3) the ratio of charging current magnitude to rate of change in voltage. In a circuit of unit capacitance, one ampere of current flows for each volt per second change. In cell membranes, capacitance varies directly with surface area; (3) a measure of the amount of something that can be held by a vessel, compound, or other entity.

capacitance vessel: vessels (mostly large veins) that hold considerable quantities of blood under most conditions; *cf* **resistance vessels**.

capacitation: the final steps that prepare spermatozoa for acrosome reactions. They normally proceed in the uterus or Fallopian tube, and involve changes in the head that lead to the release of enzymes (including ones required to penetrate the zona pellucida). Estrogens create favorable environments for capacitation during periovulatory phases of ovarian cycles, whereas the progestins of luteal phases exert opposing influences. Although sperm can be capacitated *in vitro* and then used to fertilize oocytes, the processes may not mimic the kinds that occur under physiological conditions.

cap binding protein: a 24K protein (different from capping protein) that binds to 5′ ends of messenger RNAs and accelerates translation, possibly by facilitating mRNA binding to 40S ribosome subunits.

capillary:(1) hair-like; (2) *see* **capillaries**.

capillaries: the smallest vessels of the cardiovascular system. Most *blood* capillaries connect small arterioles with venules (but *see* **portal systems**). They are composed of single layers of endothelium supported by basement membranes that permit free diffusion of oxygen, carbon dioxide, nitrogen, nitric oxide, and other gases, and of water and small solutes. Transient opening and closing, regulated by precapillary sphincters, preferentially shunts blood to specific regions. Higher pressure at the arteriolar ends favors filtration, and thereby transfer of water and small solutes (including nutrients) to extracellular fluids. Lower pressure at the venule ends facilitates reabsorption of water, wastes, and other substances. Limited numbers of capillaries are specialized for specfic functions; *see*, for example **blood brain barrier**. *Lymph* capillaries, composed mostly of endothelium, have valve-like arrangements that permit uptake (but not egress) of water, proteins, and other substances from extracellular fluids, and their passage to larger lymphatic vessels.

capillarity: changes in the configuration of liquid surfaces, caused by physical interactions with the walls of narrow tubes.

capping: (1) addition of cap binding protein to messenger RNAs; (2) aggregation of cell surface molecules, initiated by the binding of ligands, antibodies, or other molecules. It is energy-dependent, involves microfilaments (*cf* **patching**), and can lead to cell activation or agglutination. In many cell types, hormone receptor aggregation is essential for initiating responses to ligands; (3) binding of proteins to the ends of F-actin molecules or other linear polymers. It usually blocks addition of more subunits.

capping proteins: heterodimers composed of 32-36K α, and 28-32K β subunits that attach to the barbed ends of actin subunits and thereby affect filament elongation.

capsaicin: (4-hydroxy-3-methoxyphenyl)-8-methyl-6-nonenamide; a neurotoxin from several species of *Capricum* (red peppers and pimento) that selectively destroys C type nerve processes (including some vagal efferents when applied locally), but does not damage nerve cell bodies. It is used as a laboratory tool to selectively destroy innervation at specific sites. Capsaicin acts on sensory neurons that release substance P, substance K, and other peptidergic neurotransmitters, and it depletes neuronal substance P and calcitonin gene related peptide (CGRP), but not vasoactive intestinal peptide (VIP), which it releases. It also blocks retrograde uptake of nerve growth factor (NGF), and antagonizes CGRP effects on cardioacceleratory nerves. Since it is a counterirritant that raises thresholds for perception of pain and heat, but does not interfere with tactile sense, it is used to treat peripheral neuropathies, and to relieve peripheral pain in individuals with diabetes mellitus and some other diseases.

capsazepine: *N*-[2-(4-chlorophenyl)ethyl]-1,3,4,5-tetrahydro-7,8-dihydroxy-2*H*-2-benzaepine-2-carbothiamide; a specific capsaicin antagonist.

capsids: protein shells that cover the nucleoproteins of virus and virion nucleic acid cores. Most are composed of layers of multimeric proteins. Some viruses are additionally enclosed by more superficial lipid bilayers that con-

capsazepine

tain other proteins which they acquire during budding from host cell plasma membranes.

captopril: 1-(3-mercapto-2-methyl-1-oxopropyl)-l-proline; an agent that inhibits angiotensin converting enzymes, and thereby slows degradation of kallidin and related kinins, as well as conversion of angiotensin I to angiotensin II. It is administered to lower blood pressure. Although usually effective, it can increase the numbers of cells that make renin, and the amounts of renin released.

carbachol: carbamylcholine chloride; 2-[(aminocarbonyl)oxyl]-*N,N,N*-trimethylethanaminium chloride; a clinically useful acetylcholine analog that is not degraded by acetylcholinesterases. It is a potent agonist for M_2-type muscarinic receptors of the cardiovascular system, gastrointestinal tract, urinary tract, and eye, and is used to treat glaucoma. High levels also act on other muscarinic, and on ganglionic nicotinic receptors.

5′*N*-ethyl-**carbamoxamidoadenosine**; NECA; a nonspecific agonist for **adenosine receptors** (*q.v.*). It relaxes smooth muscle, and it antagonizes the effects of oxytocin by diminishing the ability of that hormone to elevate cytosolic Ca^{2+} levels.

carbamoyl phosphate: an intermediate in the vertebrate urea cycle, synthesized via the reaction: $CO_2 + NH_4^+ + 2ATP + H_2O \rightarrow$ carbamoyl phosphate $+ 2$ ADP $+$ Pi $+ 3H^+$. It combines with ornithine to yield citrulline. In bacteria, it is synthesized from glutamine and CO_2, and reacts with aspartate to form carbamoylaspartate, an intermediate in the pathway for pyridine biosynthesis.

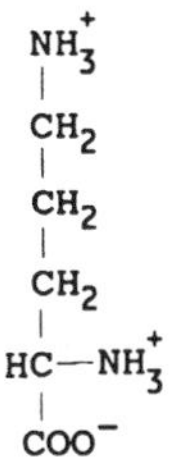

ornithine

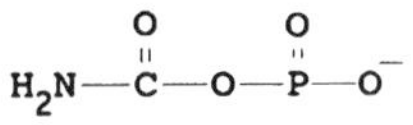

carbamoyl phosphate

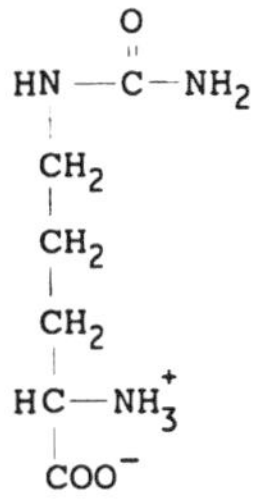

citrulline

carbidopa

carbamoyl phosphate synthase: carbamoyl phosphate synthetase; enzymes that catalyze the biosythesis of **carbamoyl phosphate** *(q.v.)*.

carbamylcholine chloride: carbachol.

carbenoxolone: 18β-glycyrrhetic acid hydrogen succinate; 3-O-(β-hydroxypropionyl)-11-oxo-18β-olean-12-en-3O-oic acid; an ester of glycyrrhetinic acid (GE, 3β-hydroxy-11-oxo-18β-olean-12-en-30-oic acid). It exerts some glucocorticoid-like anti-inflammatory effects by inhibiting prostaglandin $F_{2\alpha}$ synthesis, and can protect mucosal membranes and promote healing of gastric and duodenal ulcers by coating the surfaces. Large amounts of this compound (and of licorice, which contains GE) can cause life-threatening hyperaldosteronism (with manifestations that include edema, hypertension, and hypokalemia) by inhibiting renal and hepatic 11-β-dehydrogenases that catalyze oxidation of cortisol to cortisone. Cortisol then accumulates in the kidney and acts on mineralocorticoid receptors (which are not activated by cortisone). The 11β-oxidorectase that catalyzes cortisone reduction is not affected.

carbidopa: S-α-hydrazino-3,4-dihydroxy-α-methylbenzenepropanoic acid monohydrate; an orally effective dopamine analog that inhibits dopamine-β-decarboxylase, and thereby DOPA conversion to dopamine. Since it does not cross blood brain barriers, it increases the amount of systemically administered L-DOPA that enters the brain, and is used in conjunction with L-DOPA to treat Parkinson's disease. Carbidopa additionally inhibits tryptophan conversion to 5-hydroxytryptophan.

carbimazole: 2,3-dihydro-3-methyl-2-thioxo-1*H*-imidazole-1-carboxylic acid ethyl ester; an agent that inhibits iodine oxidation and incorporation into thyroglobulin. It is used to treat some forms of hyperthyroidism.

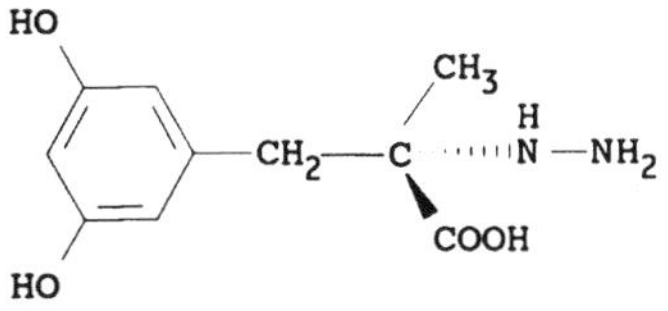

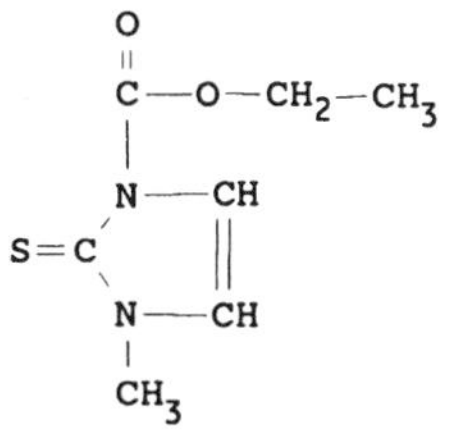

carbodiimide: cyanamide; $HN=C=NH \rightleftarrows H2N-C\equiv N$; an agent used to form peptide bonds *in vitro*. See *N,N'-dicyclohexylcarbodiimide*.

carbohydrate[s]: sugars, sugar polymers, and closely related compounds; see glucose, fructose, glycogen, starches, cellulose, and other specific types.

carbohydrate recognition domains: CRD; components of proteins and other compounds that bind to specific kinds of sugar moieties.

β-carbolines: compounds with fused benzene, indole and pyridine rings. β-Carboline-3-carboxylic acid (βCCB, shown) and some others are anxiogenic agents that block

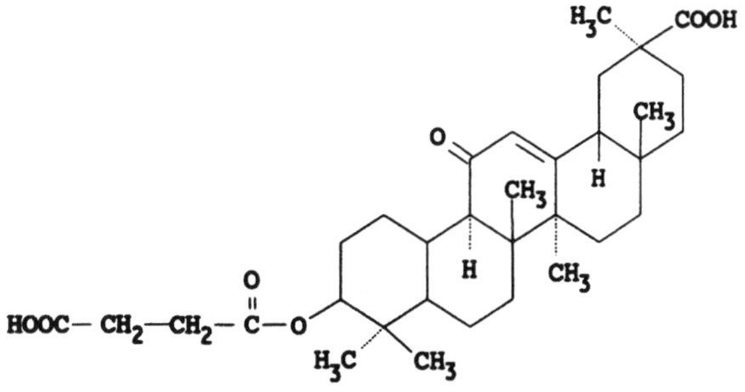

carbenoxolone

γ-aminobutyric acid access to GABA$_A$-type receptors by binding to their α subunits.

$$S=C \begin{array}{c} \\ N-CH \\ \\ N-CH \\ | \\ CH_3 \end{array} \quad \begin{array}{c} O \\ || \\ C-O-CH_2-CH_3 \\ | \\ \end{array}$$

carbon: an element (atomic number 6, atomic weight 12.011), present in all organic compounds. Each atom can form single covalent bonds with four others, as well as double and triple covalent bonds. Carbon isotopes are used to label molecules in metabolism studies. Since ^{14}C decays very slowly (with a half-life of 5760 years), comparisons of the amounts present with those of ^{12}C can provide information on the ages of organic substances that have been around for as long as 40,000 years.

carbonic anhydrases: CA; enzymes that accelerate the reaction: $CO2 + H_2O \rightleftarrows HHCO_3$. $HHCO_3$ dissociates spontaneously to $H^+ + HCO_3^-$. The erythrocyte enzyme is essential for efficient CO_2 transport from tissues to blood, and from blood to expired air (see **chloride shift**). The gastric enzyme provides H^+ ions for hydrochloric acid, and exocrine pancreas CA provides HCO_3^- ions that neutralize chyme. Since the renal enzyme facilitates HCO_3^-. H^+ and Na^+ transport, and contributes to acid-base balance, inhibitors are used to some extent as diuretics. Small amounts of CA are also made in salivary glands. Kinase A catalyzes CA phosphorylation, and thereby increase its activity.

carbon monoxide: C=O; a colorless, odorless gas, initially known as an environmental pollutant (generated by oxidation of fuels and other compounds, and a component of tobacco smoke) that binds irreversibly to hemoglobin to form a cherry-red product, and thereby blocks oxygenation. However, a type-1 heme oxygenase in liver and spleen, which catalyzes hemoglobin conversion to biliverdin, generates small amounts. Although minute quantities of CO form in glial cells and certain neurons during heat shock, that enzyme is not usually made in the brain in detectable amounts. In contrast, heme oxygenase-2 is distributed to discrete brain regions (where little or no hemoglobin is degraded). It associates there with δ-aminolevulinate synthetase (an enzyme that promotes porphyrin synthesis), cytochrome P-450 reductase (which provides electrons for heme oxygenase), and guanylate cyclase. The distribution differs from that of nitric oxide. High heme oxygenase-2 levels are also present in the olfactory epithelium, the neuronal and granular layers of the olfactory bulbs, and the olfactory bulbs; and substantial ones are in the pyramidal cell layer and dentate gyrus of the hippocampus, and in the granule and Purkinje layers of the cerebellum. CO activates guanylate cyclases, and is now believed to mediate some effects formerly attributed to nitric oxide (including contributions to long-term potentiation and memory, as well as to olfaction). CO can additionally act via cGMP to promote vasodilation and block blood platelet aggregation.

carbon tetrachloride: a hydrocarbon avidly taken up by hepatic cells. It is an industrial toxin, and is used to invoke liver injury in laboratory animals.

$$Cl-\underset{\underset{Cl}{|}}{\overset{\overset{Cl}{|}}{C}}-Cl$$

carbonylcyanide-*p*-trifluoromethoxyphenylhydrazone: FCCP; a potent protonophore that uncouples oxidative phosphorylation by transporting H^+ ions across inner mitochondrial membranes.

carbonylimidazole: an agent used to cross-link proteins, and to transfer imidazole groups.

carboxyfluoresceins: CFs; fluorescent dye indicators used to study cell:cell, cell:liposome, and liposome:liposome interactions, and also actions of enzymes on liposomes and effects of lipoproteins and apolipoproteins on lipid bilayers. The diacetates (5-CFDA and 6-CFDA) penetrate cell membranes, and release the corresponding carboxyfluoresceins.

γ-carboxyglutamate: Gla; 3-amino-1,1,3-propane tricarboxylic acid; an *N*-terminal component of osteocalcin, prothrombin, coagulation factors VII, IX, and X, protein C, and some other biologically active calcium binding molecules. Vitamin K-mediated carboxylation of glutamate moieties is accomplished posttranslationally.

$$H_3N^+ - \underset{\underset{\underset{\underset{-OOC}{\diagup} \diagdown COO^-}{CH}}{CH_2}}{\overset{\overset{COO^-}{|}}{C}} - H$$

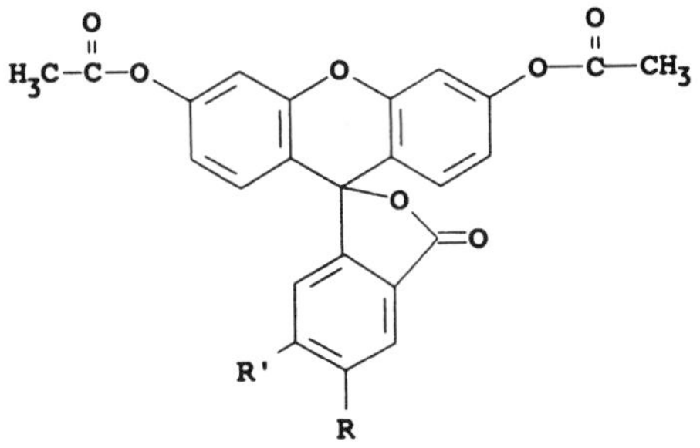

carboxyfluorescein
diacetates

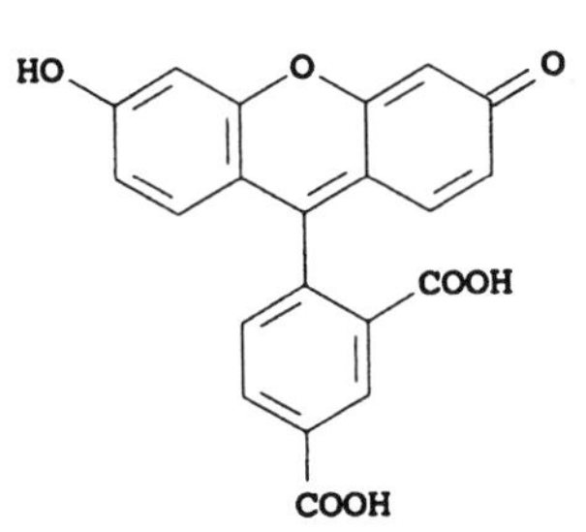

5-CF

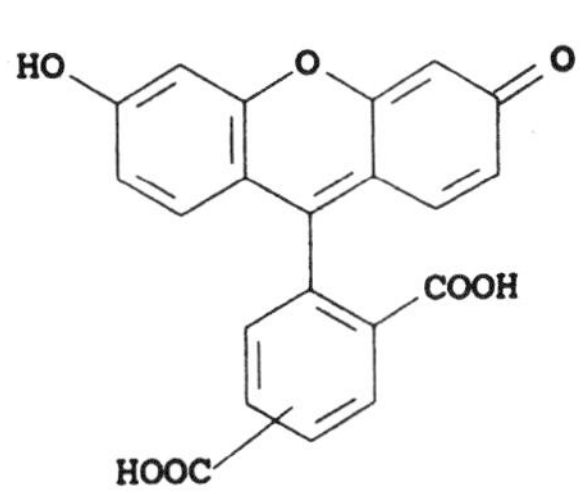

5,6-CF

carboxyfluoresceins

carboxypeptidases: exopeptidases that catalyze cleavage of peptide bonds closest to the *C*-terminals of peptides or proteins; *cf* **aminopeptidases** and **endopeptidases**. The enzymes made in exocrine pancreas and intestine release amino acids during food digestion, and are used *in vitro* to define amino acid sequences. *Carboxypeptidase A*, purified from bovine pancreas, is a 34.5K zinc metalloproteinase that preferentially releases tryptophan. *Carboxypeptidase B* is a similar protein from porcine pancreas that releases basic amino acids. The P type is a 51K serine protease made by *Penicillium janthinellum* that releases proline as well as other amino acids at low pHs, whereas the Y (a 51K yeast serine proteinase) releases basic amino acids at neutral pH, but requires lower pHs for basic amino acids. It does not cleave dipeptides.

3-(2-**carboxypiperazine-4-yl)-propyl-1-phosphonic acid:** CPPP; an NMDA receptor antagonist, more potent than AP5 and AP7.

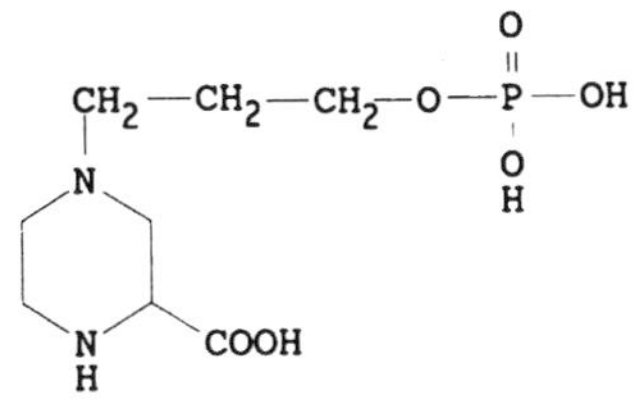

carbutamide: 1-butyl-3-sulfanyl urea; an oral hypoglycemic agent.

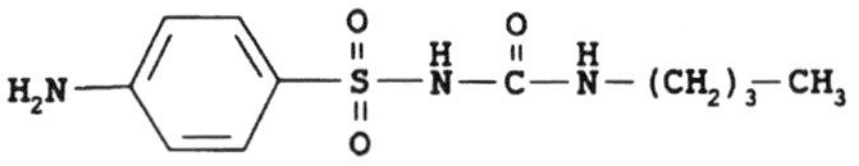

carcinoembryonic antigen: CEA; a 200K cell surface glycoprotein, chemically related to immunoglobulins and N-CAM, that functions as a cell adhesion molecule. It is made by gastrointestinal epithelia of normal embryos and fetuses, in which it is believed to play roles in development, and in minute amounts postnatally. Since high levels are expressed by colorectal adenocarcinomas, and lower ones by breast, lung, ovary, pancreas, and prostate gland tumors, it is a useful marker for some malignant cell types.

carcinogens: chemical or physical agents that invoke cell transformation and cancer growth.

carcinogenic: capable of causing cancers.

carcinoids: malignant tumors derived from endocrine cells, also called argentaffinomas (because the cells stain with silver dyes). Although most originate in the appendix or small intestine, some occur in the cecum, stomach, pancreas, thymus or thyroid glands, respiratory tract, or urinary tract. They usually grow slowly and have limited tendencies to metastasize. Many secrete two or more amines (mostly commonly serotonin, histamine, and bradykinin). Gastrinoma types secrete large quantities of gastrin, and vipomas make vasoactive intestinal peptide (VIP). At least 20 other regulators, including adrenocorticotropic hormone (ACTH), growth hormone, insulin, glucagon, dopamine, norepinephrine, pancreatic polypeptide, parathyroid hormone, and vasopressin, are made by some cell types.

carcinoid syndrome: argentaffinosis; manifestations associated with carcinoid tumors. Skin flushing and itching, diarrhea, cardiac murmurs, and bronchoconstriction were initially attributed to excess serotonin, but bradykinin (formed when tumors release kallikrein), histamine, and/or gastrin account for some. In many cases, control is achieved with somatostatin analogs.

carcinomas: epitheliomas; malignant tumors that originate in epithelial tissue. *Adenocarcinomas* derive from glandular types, and *embryonal* tumors from testicular or ovarian germinal cells.

cardiac: (1) pertaining to the heart; (2) pertaining to the part of the stomach closest to the esophagus.

cardiodepressant factors: cardioinhibitory factors: peptides released during stress or shock that depress myocardial functions, including myocardial depressant factor (MDF) from pancreatic cells, passively transferred lethal factor (PTLF) from erythrocytes, and larger peptides that originate in the small intestine. They are cleaved from cellular and circulating proteins by lysosomal enzymes released when the intracellular pH falls in visceral tissue damaged by vasoconstriction-invoked ischemia. Glucocorticoids can confer protection by stabilizing lysosomal membranes.

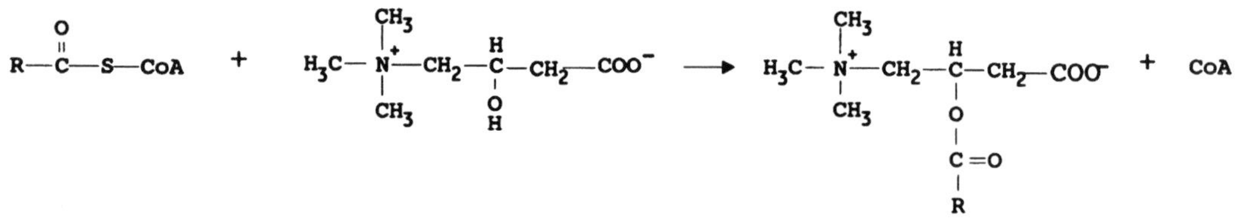

acyl-CoA   carnitine   acylcarnitine

cardiolipins: diphosphatidyl glycerols of inner mitochondrial and bacterial membranes that diminish permeability. In the structure shown, R and R′ are fatty acid moieties. The antigen in the Wassermann test for syphilis is a cardiolipin. Other types are used for diacylglycerol assays.

cardiotoxin: (1) any agent that damages the heart; (2) a 60-amino acid peptide in cobra venom that promotes irreversible depolarization of cardiac and smooth muscle plasma membranes, and phospholipase A-mediated cell lysis.

carminatives: agents used to alleviate gastrointestinal pain and/or decrease production and release of gastrointestinal tract gas.

carmustine: *see* **BCNU.**

carnitine: γ-amino-β-hydroxybutyric acid trimethylbetaine; vitamin B_t. It is essential for transporting activated fatty acids (acyl-CoAs) across mitochondrial membranes, and therefore for fatty acid oxidation. A carnitine acyltransferase I on the cytosolic face of the membrane catalyzes a reaction in which acyl-coenzyme A and carinitine combine to form **acylcarnitine** (*q.v.*). A translocase then shuttles the product across the membrane, and a carnityl acyltransferase II promotes its transfer to acetyl coenzyme A within the mitochondrion. Carnitine then returns to the cytoplasm. Deficiency is associated with high plasma triacylglycerol and free fatty acid levels, lipid deposition in liver and muscle, impaired ketogenesis, and muscle weakness. Prolonged, severe deficiency can impair growth, and invoke neurological disturbances. It may additionally cause congestive heart failure and hepatic coma.

Carnitor: a trade name for levo-carnitine.

carnityl transferases I and **II:** CAT 1 and 2; closely related enzymes essential for fatty acid oxidation; *see* **carnitine.** They differ in affinities for specific kinds of activated fatty acids. The levels are raised by excess glucagon, and in insulin deficiency states.

carnivores: (1) members of the mammalian order Carnivora, that includes dogs, cats, foxes, wolves, hyenas, bears, otters, minks, weasels, skunks, badgers, seals, walruses, and sea-lions. All have sharp-pointed premolar (canine) teeth and shearing molars; and all eat meat; (2) meat-eating organisms, a term usually applied to animals, but also to a few plants.

carnivorous: meat-eating; *see* **carnivores,** definition 2.

carnosine: β-alanyl-histidine; a putative neurotransmitter for primary olfactory neurons. It is also made in mammalian skeletal muscles, in which it may play some role in contraction, and is additionally implicated in wound healing.

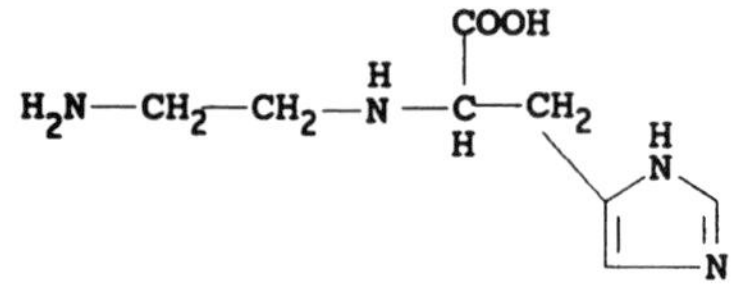

carotenes: several terpene pigments with ionone rings, made by plants and microorganisms. Two molecules of geranylgeranyl pyrophosphate combine in reactions that remove the phosphate groups and two hydrogen atoms to form phytoene, a linear terpene that is dehydrogenated to lycopene. Formation of the first ring yields γ-carotene, the direct precursor of β-carotene which can, in turn, be converted to α-carotene. Animals take up the pigments from food, store, and metabolize them. Two molecules of vitamin A are obtained from each of the β-type (the major source of the vitamin), but only one from each α or γ type. Metabolic defects in individuals with diabetes mellitus and hypothyroidism can lead to accumulation of excessive amounts of carotenes. *See* also **carotenoids.**

carotenoids: carotenes, xanthophylls, and related lipophilic yellow to red terpene plant pigments that absorb light, pass energy to chlorophyll, and protect chlorophyll

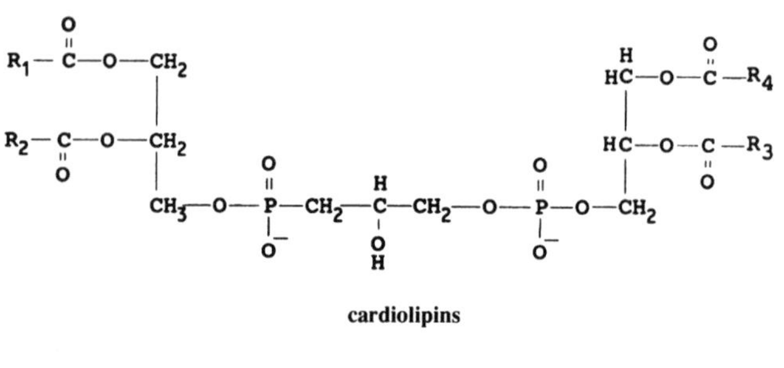

cardiolipins

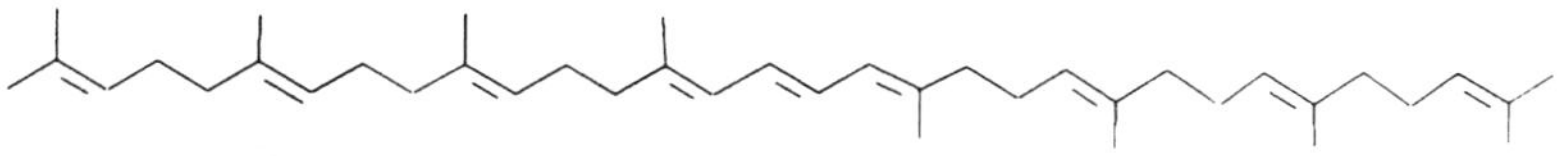

phytoene

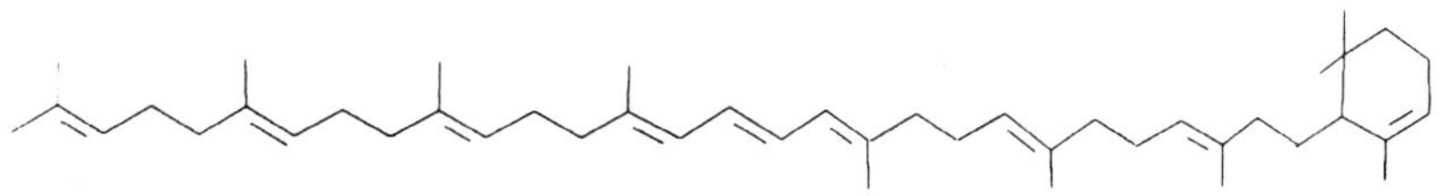

γ-carotene

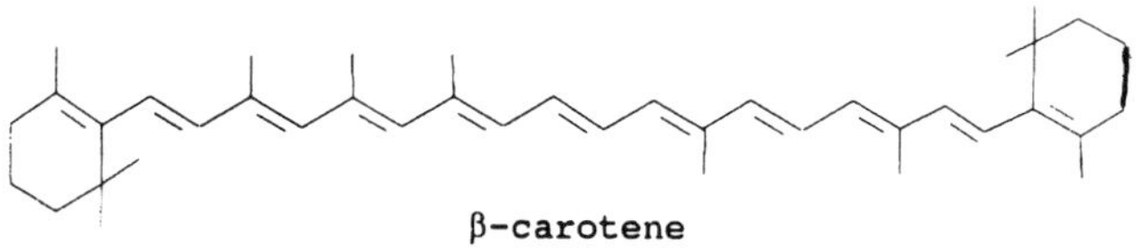

β-carotene

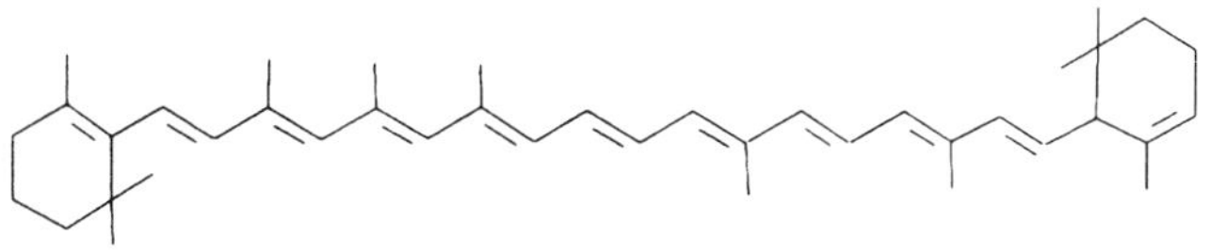

α-carotene

carotenes

against photo-oxidation. When eaten by animals, they can accumulate in, and impart color to skin, feathers, and adipose tissue.

carotid bodies: bilateral clusters of neural crest derived cells, located near the carotid sinuses. They sense decreases in blood oxygen levels, and communicate with the respiratory center in the medulla oblongata via glossopharyngeal nerves.

carotid sinuses: bilateral dilated regions of the internal carotid arteries, located close to the sites of bifurcation from the common carotid arteries, and innervated by carotid nerve branches of the glossopharyngeal nerves. They contain baroreceptors that contribute to blood pressure control.

carrageenins: carrageen; carragheen; carragheenin: structural polysaccharides composed of alternating copolymers of β(1→3)-D-galactose and (1→4) anhydro-D or L-galactose, some of which have attached sugar acid sulfates and their salts. They are extracted from red seaweed members of the genus *Rhodophycae*, and are used in foods and other products as gelling, emulsifying, and stabilizing agents, and to invoke inflammatory reactions (probably via complement activation) in laboratory animals.

carriers: (1) cell components that facilitate the transport of sugars, amino acids, and other small solutes across plasma membranes; (2) proteins or other substances that bind to hormones and other substances and facilitate their transport through body fluids; (3) coenzymes, such as nicotine adenine dinucleotide, and other compounds that accept electrons and chemically reactive groups from one compound and donate them to another; (4) proteins and other large molecules that bind haptens and thereby render them immunogenic; (5) individuals heterozygous for recessive genes who are phenotypically normal but can transmit genes that cause diseases; (6) individuals who harbor and can transmit infectious agents, but display no signs of infection.

carrier mediated transport: movement of molecules or ions across membranes that is facilitated by carriers (including facilitated diffusion and active transport).

cartilage: a connective tissue type composed mostly of an extracellular semi-rigid matrix that is secreted by chondrocytes. The major constituent is type II collagen. Small amounts of ground substance contain chondroitin sulfate and other compounds. During early stages of development, a surrounding perichondrium forms, in which new chondrobasts originate. The cells grow, divide by mitosis, and mature to chondrocytes. After secreting the matrix components, they reside in lacunae. (Most lacunae contain a single cell, but some have two or three). Since the matrix is avascular, chondrocytes take up nutrients and release wastes via diffusion. Differences in appearance and properties of the subtypes are related to the composition and arrangements of matrix fibers, some of which contain type V collagen. *Hyaline* cartilage, which appears clear under light microscopy but contains fibers, is the most abundant type. The symphysis pubis and the intervertebral discs contain *fibrocartilage*, which is stronger and more rigid. *Elastic* cartilage, with networks of elastic fibers, maintains the shapes of some organs that require both rigidity and flexibility (epiglottis, Eustachian tubes, and ear pinnae). Since hylaine cartilage is lighter and more flexible than bone, grows faster, and requires less calcium, it is well suited for formation of most of the fetal skeleton. Although replaced by bone at most sites, it is retained in the nose and ears, vertebral disks, and the ends of moveable bones. Growth hormone promotes cell differentiation and production of insulin-like growth factor-I (IGF-I), the major growth stimulant. 1,25-dihydroxyvitamin D, other circulating hormones, and numerous paracrine and/or autocrine factors contribute to growth and remodelling. *See also* **ascorbic acid**. Androgens promote maturation as well as growth. Other maturation factors include estrogens and triiodothyronine. Low levels of glucocorticoid stimulate, but higher ones exert mostly inhibitory influences.

cartilage-derived growth factor-1: CDGF: a growth factor for cartilage now known to be identical with a form of β-fibroblast growth factor (β-FGF).

cartilage inducing factors: CIF-A and CIF-B, peptides chemically related to transforming growth factors β_1 and β_2 (TGF$_{\beta1}$ and TFG$_{\beta1}$), that contribute to chondroblast differentiation.

caryo-: karyo-; a prefix that refers to the nucleus.

cascade: a series of events, each of which each invokes the one that succeeds it. Amplification at various steps can lead rapidly to final responses of considerable magnitudes. For example, it has been estimated that a single glucagon molecule can promote formation of one million of free glucose in less than one minute when the hormone is released in response to hypoglycemia. The responses involve activation, by small numbers of hormone molecules, of many more adenylate cyclase types in the liver. Each cyclase then generates considerable quantities of cAMP, each of which activates one of protein kinase A. Each kinase A molecule, in turn, converts many molecules of glycogen phosphorylase kinase *b* to glycogen phosphorylase kinase *a* (the active form whose substrate is glycogen phosphorylase *b*). Consequently, many glycogen phosphorylase *b* enzymes are converted to glycogen phoshorylase *a*, which catalyzes glycogen degradation. Finally, the glucose-1-phosphate generated is soon converted to glucose-6-phosphate by a substrate-controlled reaction, and glucose-6-phosphatase (which is also controlled by glucagon) provides free glucose. Cascades are essential for blood coagulation, complement activation, and other processes; and ones involving specific protein kinases regulate cell proliferation. The sequences can be complex, involve more than two initiators, and yield multiple products. *See* also **domino effect** and *cf* **sustained action model**.

casein[s]: several chemically related, calcium binding 20-30K phosphoproteins (α, β, γ, and *k* types). They are the major proteins of milk, and are substrates for matura-

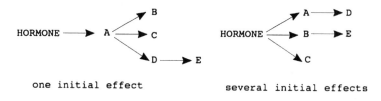

one initial effect   several initial effects

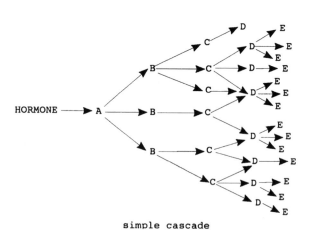

simple cascade

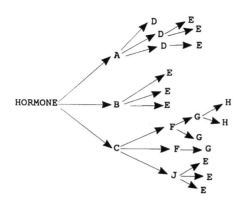

complex cascade

castanospermine: CSP; 1,6,7,8-tetrahydroxy-octahydro-indolizine; an alkaloid obtained from the Australian chestnut tree, *Castanospermum australe*, that inhibits α-glycosidase I catalyzed removal of glucose moieties from asparagine N-linked oligosaccharides. It is used to study oligosaccharide functions and glycosylation processes. In thyroid glands, it blocks thyroglobulin exocytosis. Its anti-viral properties are attributed to influences on envelope glycoproteins.

castration: gonadectomy; removal of the testes or ovaries. When unqualified, the term refers to surgical excision; but *see* chemical castration. The procedure is performed in humans with gonadal tumors, and to terminate production of gonadal steroids that promote growth of breast, prostate gland and other steroid hormone-responsive cancers. Bilateral gonadectomy is used to study the functions of gonadal hormones, or to eliminate their influences on other processes; and unilateral gonadectomy to investigate compensatory hypertrophy and the effects of limited hormone deficiency.

castration cells: enlarged gonadotropes that appear in the adenohypophysis when gonadal steroid deficiency severely limits negative feedback control over gonadotropin secretion. They develop in adults that cannot synthesize adequate amounts of hormones, in ones with androgen receptors defects, and following castration.

CAT: (1) choline acetyltransferase; (2) chloramphenicol acetyltransferase; (3) computer assisted tomography.

CAT 1, CAT 2: *see* carnitine acyltransferases.

catabolic: promoting catabolism (*q.v.*).

catabolin: a synovial fluid protein that promotes nonenzymatic cartilage proteoglycan degradation. It may be identical with interleukin-1.

catabolites: products formed during catabolism.

catabolism: degradation of organic molecules, for example proteolysis, lipolysis, or glycolysis. Some of the reactions release energy for ATP synthesis and other cell processes. *Cf* anabolism.

catabolite activating protein: *see* catabolite gene activating protein.

catabolite gene activating protein: catabolite activating protein; CAP; CRP; cAMP regulator protein; a 22K homodimeric bacterial protein that binds to both cAMP and the promoters for several genes. CAP-cAMP facilitates transcription by augmenting RNA polymerase binding; *see* also catabolite repression. (In eukaryotes,

tion promoting factor (MPF) and some other protein kinases. Prolactin promotes β-casein gene expression in mature mammary glands. In its presence, insulin, glucocorticoids, and other hormones enhance production of the protein by affecting transcription and/or stabilizing the messenger RNA. Legumins are related proteins in beans and nuts.

casein kinases: at least three enzyme components (CKs I, II, and III) of cascades that catalyze nucleotide-dependent phosphorylation of serine and threonine moieties of casein, phosvitin, and other acidic proteins, and contribute to cell growth. They differ from each other in size, amino acid make-up, substrate preferences, modes of activation, and abilities to use GTP as well as ATP. CKI (KI) is a widely distributed 37K monomer that undergoes autophosphorylation, and predominates in cytosol but is also present in microsomes, mitochondria, and nuclei, with highest levels in muscle and adipose tissue. Its substrates include phosphorylase kinase and poly A polymerases (both of which are activated by phosphorylation), as well as muscle glycogen synthase and aminoacyl-tRNA synthases (inhibited by phosphorylation). CKII (PKII) exists in several forms. In higher eukaryotes it has two 37-44K α subunits (which are identical at some sites) and two β subunits (24-28K for most forms), with highest levels in spleen and testis. Its activity is augmented by polyamines, decreased by heparin, and affected by epidermal growth factor (EGF), insulin, and other growth stimulants. Its substrates include eukaryote initiation factors, RNA polymerase II, kinase A, heat shock protein 90, nucleolin, non-histone nuclear proteins, topoisomerase II, some oncogene proteins (including the *c-myb* product whose affinity for DNA is diminished by phosphorylation), the insulin receptor β-subunit, and possibly also CREB protein. *See* also clathrin.

casomorphins: species-specific opioid peptides in milk casein fractions. Human β-casomorphin is H_2N-Tyr-Pro-Phe-Val-Glu-Pro-Ile-OH.

cAMP functions mostly as an activator of protein kinase A.) *Cf* **cyclase activating protein**.

catabolite repression: decreased production of catabolic enzymes, invoked by high levels of substances generated by the same enzymes, or by alternate sources of energy. For example, high concentrations of glucose (which provide energy) inhibit galactosidase and galactokinase synthesis in bacteria. They lower cAMP levels, and thereby inhibit RNA polymerase binding (*see* **catabolite activating protein**). cAMP overcomes the inhibition.

catacalcin: katacalcin.

catagen: the involutional phase of hair growth cycles; *cf* **anagen** and **telogen**.

catalases: heme-containing enzymes that catalyze conversion of hydrogen peroxide (H_2O_2) to $H_2O + O_2$; *cf* **peroxidases**. Most are in peroxisomes, but secreted forms protect against some potentially deleterious effects of neutrophil products during inflammatory reactions.

cataplexy: sudden loss of muscle tone.

catecholamines: norepinephrine, epinephrine, dopamine, and chemically related amines with the general structure shown; *see* also specific types. The major rate-limiting step for biosynthesis is tyrosine hydroxylase catalyzed conversion of tyrosine to dihydroxyphenylalanine (DOPA). Decarboxylation, catalyzed by dopa decarboxylase (DDC) then yields dopamine, which is directly released by some cell types. Where present, dopamine β-hydroxylase promotes dopamine hydroxylation to norepinephrine. In some cell types, phenylethanolamine-*N*-methyltransferase (PNMT) then methylates the nitrogen atom to yield epinephrine: Tyrosine → DOPA → dopamine → norepinephrine → epinephrine. Since the enzymes can act on alternate substrates, small amounts of epinine, *N*-methyl epinephrine, and other compounds are formed. Although not true catecholamines, octopamine and synephrine (derived from phenylalanine) are sometimes included. *See* also **false transmitters**.

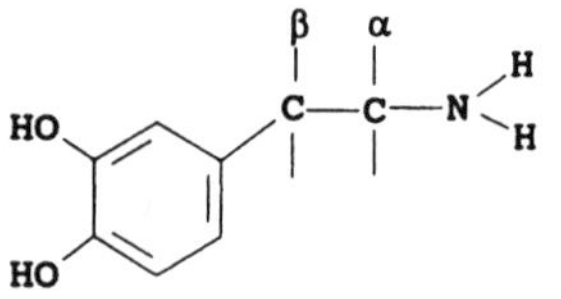

catecholamine-*O*-methyltransferase: COMT; an enzyme that catalyzes replacement of a hydrogen atom with a methyl group on catecholamines, estrogens, and other phenolic compounds. It converts dopamine, epinephrine and norepinephrine to 3-hydroxy-dopamine, metanephrine and normetanephrine, respectively. All the products are biologically inactive, and are monoamine oxidase substrates.

catechol estrogens: estrogens oxygenated at carbons 2, 4, or both; examples include 2-hydroxy-estrone, 4-hydroxy-estradiol, and 2,4-dihydroxy-estradiol. Their formation is catalyzed by peroxidases in adenohypophysis, hypothalamus, adrenal cortex, ovary, and other estrogen target organs, in which they may perform special functions by binding to their own, or to estrogen and/or catecholamine receptors, or by competing with catecholamines as catecholamine-*O*-methyltransferase substrates. Antagonism of kinase C activated Ca^{2+} uptake, possibly via activation of proteases that catalyze conversion of kinase C to kinase M, has also been suggested. Some effects may be exerted on brain regions that lack estrogen receptors. Roles in enhancing uterine blood flow during pregnancy that cannot be mimicked with estradiol have been described for gilts.

catenins: cytoplasmic proteins similar to plakoglobin (and to the product of the *Drosophila* polarity gene *Armadillo*) that bind to the cytoplasmic tails of E-cadherin, interact with actins, and are required for cadherin-mediated cell to cell adhesion. Three types have been described, including an α form which resembles vinculin, and a 92K β identified in *Xenopus* that seems to be important for development.

cathepsins: large proteases present in high concentrations in liver, kidney, and spleen. A, B, C, D, E, G, H, L, and N types have been described, but some categories may include more than one molecular species or be identical with others. Most are lysosomal enzymes that degrade a variety of macromolecules; but a few that are active at cytoplasmic pH levels are secreted. Special functions are performed by isozymes in immune system cells, endocrine glands, uterus, and elsewhere. Some are needed for prohormone and proenzyme processing, and others mediate apoptosis and tissue restructuring. A 27.5K hepatic cathepsin B is a lysosomal cysteine protease that differs from cathepsin L (a 29K cysteine protease of liver lysosomes), but is similar to enzymes in other tissues. The same, or a closely related enzyme degrades parathyroid hormone. It is induced by relaxin in the symphysis pubis, where it contributes to preparations

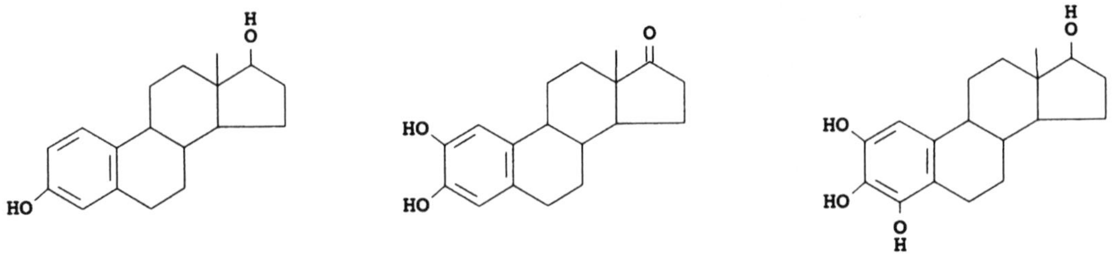

17β-estradiol

2-hydroxyestrone

2,4-dihydroxyestradiol

catechol estrogens

for parturition. Cathepsins B and D are implicated as autocrine growth factors, and as agents that facilitate metastasis by degrading extracellular matrices. Cathepsin C is a 210K thiol proteinase extractable from spleen that catalyzes successive removal of *N*-terminal dipeptides, and also acts on dipeptidyl amides or esters with free α amino or imino groups. It converts prothrombin to thrombin, and also catalyzes amidations and peptide polymerization. Cathepsin D is a pepsin-like aspartic protease that promotes cleavage of angiotensin I from its substrate, thyroglobulin processing, and breakdown of collagen and proteoglycans. It is induced by growth hormone in some cell types, and by estradiol in others (including breast cancer cells), and its mitogenic precursor is implicated in transformation and metastasis. In endometrium, a cathepsin induced by progesterone contributes to implantation. Cathepsin G is a chymotrypsin-like enzyme made by neutrophilic leukocytes and other cell types, needed for protein processing in antigen presenting cells. It degrades collagens and proteoglycans, and may contribute to rheumatoid arthritis, emphysema, and other diseases. Cathepsin H is a 29K cysteine protease obtained from kidneys, that, in common with cathepsin N, also functions as an aminopeptidase.

cations: positively charged ions, such as Na^+ and Ca^{2+}; *cf* **anions**.

catron: pheniprazine; 1-phenyl-2-hydrazinopropane; a selective inhibitor of B type monoamine oxidases. It can protect against orthostatic hypotension by slowing norepinephrine inactivation, but effects on epinephrine may account for its ability to lower blood pressure in some forms of hypertension.

caudal: relating to the tail, or towards the tail end (*cf* **posterior** and **cephalad**).

caudate nuclei: bilateral, elongated, arch shaped neuron clusters within the cerebral cortex that border the brain lateral ventricles, composed of head, body and tail regions. The nucleus on each side is separated from the putamen by the internal capsule. The two sets of gray matter make up the neostriatum of the basal ganglia. The corpus striatum, which additionally includes the lentiform nuclei, is the major control site for extrapyramidal motor functions. The neurons receive afferent inputs from the cerebral cortex, thalamus, and midbrain, and they send efferents to the putamen and globus pallidus. The region is richly supplied with multiple dopamine receptors types, and with receptors for nerve growth factor (NGF) and other regulators.

benzoyl chlorocarbonate

Cavia porcellus: the guinea pig.

CB-154: bromocriptine.

CBG: corticosteroid binding globulin.

cbl: an oncogene made by the mouse Cas *N-1* virus that directs the synthesis of p100^{gagcbl}.

CBP: cholesterol binding protein.

CBP35: carbohydrate binding protein; *see* **mac-2**.

p-**CB-PzDA**: *p*-chlorobenzoyl-2,3-kynurenic acid; a broad-spectrum excitatory amino acid receptor antagonist, more potent for NMDA than for kainate and quisqualate types.

CBZ compounds: benzoylcarbonyl (carbobenzoxy) amine, amino acid, and peptide derivatives, formed by reactions with benzyl chlorocarbonate. CBZ protects the compounds against degradation during peptide and protein synthesis, and in other reactions.

CCAAT: DNA components of all MHC class II genes in humans, and related genes of other mammals, usually located 40-120 base pairs upstream from the start site, that contribute to optimal promoter function. *See* also **CCAAT binding proteins**.

CCAAT binding proteins: proteins that bind to CCAAT DNA bases sequences, and regulate expression of *HLA-DRA* and other MHC class II proteins. They also affect transcription of heat shock 70 proteins via mechanisms antagonized by p53, and interact with several transcription factors to affect other genes. A murine type (YEBP) activates thymidine kinase promoters.

βCCB: β-carboline.

C3-convertase: C5-convertase: *see* **complement**.

CCCP: carbonyl cyanide *m*-chlorophenylhydrazone; a proton ionophore used to uncouple oxidative phosphorylation, and to study the functions of organelles in which acidification occurs.

C cells: clear cells: thyroid gland parafollicular cells that secrete calcitonin.

CBZ-amino acid

CBZ compounds

CCFs: chromatin condensation factors.

CCK: cholecystokinin.

CCK-8: cholecystokinin octapeptide; cholecystokinin [26-33]; *see* **cholecystokinins**.

CCK-PZ: cholecystokinin-pancreozymin; *see* **cholecystokinins**.

cCMP: cyclic cytidine monophosphate.

CD antigens: cluster of differentiation antigens; cluster determinant antigens; cluster designation antigens; proteins expressed by immune system, hematopoietic, and some other cell types that have been identified with monoclonal antibodies. Most are glycosylated, and several are members of the immunoglobulin superfamily. The expression of diverse combinations varies with the cell type, the developmental stage, and in some cases with state of activation. Functions have been established for only some of the molecules, and it is likely that additional roles (and new subtypes) will be identified. Although devised for human cells, the CD system is also used for other species. An older (T) system has been used for molecules on T lymphocytes and their precursors. Leu, Ly, and Lyt refer to antigens on mouse cells. A w after the number indicates a working designation.

CD1: approximately 36K single-chain plasma membrane proteins (43-49K after glycosylation), structurally related to class I major histocompatibility complex proteins, and similar to the "nonclassical" MHC-like molecules recognized by T cells with $\gamma\delta$ type receptors. Their synthesis in humans is directed by five genes clustered on chromosome # 1. CD1.1 (CD1a, 49K), CD1.2 (CD1b, 45K), and CD1.3 (CD1c, 43K) are subtypes. All associate non-covalently with β_2-microglobulin. Limited amounts are expressed on the surfaces of cortical thymocytes during an intermediate stage of differentiation, on some medullary thymocytes, on a subpopulation of peripheral B cells, and on dermal dendritic (Langerhans) and intermediate cells. Larger amounts on intestinal crypts and in hepatocyte cytoplasm, as well as CD1a and CD1c recognition by CD4$^-$8$^-$ cytolytic T cells with $\gamma\delta$ type receptors (and some with $\alpha\beta$ types), suggest major roles in epithelial cell immunity, and possibly in gastrointestinal localization of intraepithelial lymphocytes. In antigen-activated Langerhans cells, CD1s co-internalize with HLA-DR. In developing thymocytes, they interact with newly rearranged CD3 receptors, and provide signals for both surface expression of those receptors and continued cell maturation. CD1a (T6, Leu6, OKT6) also forms disulfide-linked heterodimers with CD8 in the thymus gland cortex. Abnormal responses to CD1 antigens (or interactions with closely related viral products) may contribute to the pathogenesis of rheumatoid arthritis, systemic lupus erythematosus, and some other autoimmune diseases.

CD2: LFA-2; T11; 45-58K single chain glycoproteins of the immunoglobulin superfamily whose production in humans is directed by chromosome 1. They are expressed on some bone marrow precursor cells, and on prethymocytes before the appearance of T cell receptor-CD3 complexes. They are retained during subsequent development, and provide proliferation signals associated with acquisition of MHC restriction and self-tolerance. When resting T lymphocytes are stimulated, subtypes CD2$_1$ (T11$_1$) and CD2$_2$ (T11$_2$ Leu5) synergize with antigen receptor complexes to achieve signalling via inositol phosphate mediated pathways (functions dependent on CD45 activated protein phosphatase). A third (CD2$_3$, T11$_3$) type appears after cell activation and elevation of intracellular Ca^{2+}, is associated with expression of interleukin-2 receptors, and is found in highest levels on memory cells. CD2 proteins synergize with and/or modify signals initiated by T cell antigen receptor-CD3 complexes, in part by interacting with accessory factors. T11 was initially identified as the E (sheep red blood cell, SRBC) receptor on T lymphocytes that attaches to erythrocytes and forms E rosettes. The erythrocyte acceptor (CD59) is also expressed on most leukocytes, and contributes to T cell activation. CD2 binding to lymphocyte function-associated antigen-3 (LFA-3, CD58) mediates T cell adhesion to antigen presenting cells. It also promotes the adhesion to target cells essential for accomplishing cytotoxicity (and evidently performs comparable functions for natural killer cells). The binding sites for CD58 and CD59 differ, but overlap. Antibodies directed against both (but not against either alone) block activation mediated IL-2 production (but *see* also **CD28**). The possibility that CD2 is involved in additional functions is suggested by observations that a soluble T cell component can invoke CD2 mediated antigen-independent activation.

CD3: T3; Leu4; OKT3; complexes of at least five polypeptides (25Kγ, 20Kδ, 20Kϵ, 16Kζ which forms dimers, and 22Kη) that associate closely (but non-covalently) with mature T lymphocyte antigen receptors, are essential for membrane expression of $\alpha\beta$ and $\gamma\delta$ receptor dimers, stabilize receptor mediated interactions with class 2 proteins and other molecules, are phosphorylated following activation, and appear to be essential for signal transduction. The ϵ and ζ types are not glycosylated. A 28K ω type is synthesized but is not expressed on the cell surfaces.

CD4: T4; Leu3; L3T4; 55-60K glycoproteins on the surfaces of most helper and inducer type T lymphocytes, some thymocytes, some macrophages, a subset of B lymphocytes, and some brain cells. Immature cells can express both CD4 and CD8 (are CD4$^+$8$^+$), but mature helper and inducer types are CD8-negative. At least some T cells with receptors bearing $\delta\gamma$ subunits lack both CD4 and CD8. CD4 antigens are essential for T cell adhesion to target cell class 2 proteins, and are believed to play roles in T cell differentiation. They also bind immunoglobulin Fab regions. CD4 is also a receptor for the gp120 envelope protein of the AIDS virus. Although coupled to a protein kinase (P56^{lck}) that phosphorylates the CD3 complex, it may not be directly involved in signal transduction.

CD5: T1; Leu1; Ly1; a 65K-67K membrane glycoprotein on all human T lymphocytes (with higher levels expressed on helper types), and on a subset of rapidly renewing peritoneal and pleural B lymphocytes. It may be involved in antigen-independent activation, and in proliferation of activated cells.

CD6: T12; a 100-120K glycoprotein on some T and B lymphocyte populations that functions as a receptor for some immunoglobulin Fc components.

CD7: TP-40; Leu9; a 40K membrane glycoprotein on T cells, thymocytes, prothymocytes, and some leukemia cells that binds some Fc receptors.

CD8: T8; Leu2; Ly2,3; 30-38K glycoproteins expressed as homo- or heterodimers, or as multimers, on cytotoxic T lymphocytes and some thymocytes. The α chain is identical with Ly2. CD8 stabilizes T cell receptor-mediated interactions with class 1 proteins, is coupled to a protein kinase (p56^{lck}) that phosphorylates the CD3 complex, and is believed to be essential for cytotoxicity. Within the thymus gland, it acts via mechanisms that do not involve CD3 complexes to confer tolerance to self-antigens. Although immature cells can express both CD4 and CD8, mature cytotoxic lymphocytes are usually CD4-negative. At least some T cells bearing receptors with δγ subunits lack both CD4 and CD8. The immunosuppressive effects of estrogens appear to be related to influences on CD8 molecules.

CD9: p54; a 24K membrane glycoprotein on monocytes, immature B cells, and blood platelets that functions as a transferrin receptor.

CD10: J5; CALLA; BA-3; neutral endopeptidase; a 100K glycoprotein on B cell precursors, and on acute lymphoblastic leukemia cells (but not on mature B lymphocytes). It is also an ectoenzyme expressed on renal glomeruli and tubular cells, and on endometrial stromal and epithelial cells. The substrates include enkephalins, bradykinin, oxytocin, substance P, neurotensin, FMLP, gastrin, IL-1, IL-2, and atrial natriuretic peptides. *See also* **CD13**.

CD11a: LFA-1 α chain; integrin subunit α$_L$; a 177K cell surface glycoprotein that forms dimers with CD18 and related 95K β subunits. It is present on all leukocytes, and on mast cells, and it mediates leukocyte:leukocyte and leukocyte:endothelium adhesion by binding to intercellular adhesion molecules adhesion molecules 1 and 2 (ICAM-1 and ICAM-2). *N-myc* regulates its expression in B cells. *See also* **lymphocyte function associated antigen-1**.

CD11b: CR3 α chain; Mac-1 α chain; MO-1; integrin subunit α$_M$; Leu15; 165K proteins on the surfaces of monocytes, granulocytes, and natural killer cells. They dimerize with **CD18** (*q.v.*) and related 95K β subunits to form integrins that mediate cell:cell adhesion, affect phagocytosis and blood clotting, and function as receptors for complement factor iC3b. They bind lipopolysaccharide, intercellular adhesion molecule-1 (ICAM-1), fibrinogen, and coagulation factor X.

CD11c: CR4 α chain; integrin α$_X$ subunit; Leu M5; a 150K protein that forms dimers with **CD18** (*q.v.*) and related β subunits, expressed on monocytes, natural killer

cells, and granulocytes. It mediates adhesion and serves as an iC3b complement receptor.

CD12: an incompletely characterized plasma membrane molecule on monocytes, blood platelets, and cells of myeloid lineage (including mature granulocytes).

CD13: a single-chain 150K surface protein of monocytes and granulocytes. It is an aminopeptidase N ectoenzyme on intestinal and kidney brush border membranes that acts on kallidin and metenkephalin. The levels in the endometrium rise after decidualization, as the those of CD10 decline.

CD14: LeuM3; Mo-2; lipopolysaccharide binding protein; LBP; 55K phosphatidylinositol-glycan linked surface glycoproteins on monocytes, macrophages, activated granulocytes and dendritic cells of spleen germinal follicles, believed essential for differentiation of cells of myelocyte and monocyte lineages. Their synthesis is directed by genes on human chromosome 5, which also bears genes for interleukin-3, granulocyte-macrophage colony stimulating factor (GM-CSF), colony stimulating factor-1 (CSF-1), monocyte stimulating factor, endothelial cell growth factor (ECGF), platelet derived growth factor (PDGF) and other stimulants. In addition to receptor functions, CD14 is believed to play essential roles in disposal of gram negative bacteria; and the levels increase during acute phase responses. When macrophage CD14 binds lipopolysaccharide, large amounts of tumor necrosis factor-α (TNFα) are released, and uncontrolled activity can lead to endotoxic shock. However, CD14 can be shed in a soluble form that binds lipopolysaccharide (LPS) and protects against its deleterious effects. Failure to express CD14 has been linked with malignancy in individuals with acute nonlymphocytic leukemias.

CD15: a cell surface marker for granulocytes and some tumor cells. It includes a Lewis x component (Le^x) that mediates low-affinity binding of neutrophilic leukocytes to platelets, is recognized by **CD62** (*q.v.*) and endothelial cell adhesion molecule-1 (ELAM-1), and may contribute to diapedesis. CD15 also inhibits CD18 mediated neutrophilic leukocyte adhesion to endothelium.

CD16: FcRγIII; Leu11; oligomeric glycoproteins with at least three peptide chains on granulocytes, eosinophils, natural killer cells, large lymphocytes, and tissue macrophages (but not on circulating monocytes), that bind with low affinity to immunoglobulins IgG1 and IgG3 and mediate antigen-antibody complex initiated cytotoxicity. At least two genes (*CD16 I* and *II*) direct CD16 synthesis in humans, and granulocytes have two or more alleles. Natural killer cell CD16s are 36-38K transmembrane forms that trigger NK mediated killing, and can stimulate lymphokine production and expression of interleukin-2 receptors. Granulocytes have 30K glycoproteins that do not display such activities. They are anchored to cell membranes by phosphatidylinositol glycans, but can be released by phosphatidylinositol phosphate phospholipases.

CD17: a lipid on granulocytes, macrophages, and blood platelets.

CD18: LFA-1 β chain; 95K proteins on leukocytes that combine with α subunits to form integrins; *see* **CD18 complexes**. Although not expressed on endothelium, the dimers promote diapedesis and augment the effects of other regulators that promote leukocyte attachment to inflamed venules. They also mediate leukocyte to leukocyte adhesion, contribute in other ways to inflammatory responses, initiate coagulation cascades by promoting adherence of activated neutrophilic leukocytes to fibrinogen, and are implicated in the etiology of atherogenesis. Additionally, they are receptors for *Herpes simplex* viruses. The oncogenic effects of *c-myc* are associated with down regulation of LFA-1, impaired B cell adhesion to natural killer cells and vascular endothelium, and resistance to T cell cytotoxicity.

CD18 complexes: dimers composed of CD11 α, and CD18 β subunits. LFA-1 is formed with CD11a, CR3 (Mac-1, Leu 15, OKM1) with CD11b, and gp150,95 with CD11c.

CD19: B4; B-cell specific 90-95K members of the immunoglobulin superfamily, expressed on mature B cells and their precursors, but not on plasma cells. They associate with antigen receptors, stabilizes antigen binding in a manner comparable to CD4 and CD8 effects in T cells, and augment B cell proliferative and antibody responses to the antigens. The functions involve activation of a tyrosine kinase that promotes phosphorylation of phospholipase Cγ-1. CD19 also contributes to myeloid lineage differentiation, and may be a receptor for a low molecular weight (12K) B cell growth factor required for proliferation. Additionally, it associates with CD21 (CR2) and contributes to the immunopotentiating effects of complement. The mechanisms may be different from ones initiated by antigen binding to B cell surface immunoglobulins, since the tyrosine kinase affected does not act on the phospholipase. The complexes are also *Epstein-Barr* virus receptors.

CD20: B1; a 35-37K surface protein on circulating B lymphocytes, and on dendritic cells of spleen germinal centers, but not on T lymphocytes. It may be a Ca^{2+} channel component.

CD21: CR2; C3d receptor; TAPA-1; a 140K protein on B lymphocytes and spleen germinal center dendritic cells that directly binds complement fragments iC3b and C3dg, and augments complement system stimulation of antibody production. It also forms complexes with CD19 that bind *Epstein-Barr* virus.

CD22: a 135K protein in the cytoplasm of B lymphocyte precursors (but not mature B cells), implicated as a director of B cell maturation. It binds to sialotransferase dependent epitopes, and association with CD75 mediates some cell to cell interactions.

CD23: BLAST-2; FcRIIb; Lyb-2; 45-59K transmembrane proteins of B lymphocytes, monocytes, and eosinophils that bind immunoglobulin IgE with low affinity, and may be receptors for a low molecular weight B cell growth factor. Interleukin-5 enhances their synthesis. A 17K CD23 modulating protein (a component of the

suppressive factor of allergy) decreases the affinity for IgE.

CD24: gp45/55/65: a phosphatidylinositol glycan anchored protein on granulocytes and B lymphocyte precursors, but not on mature B cells. It associates with p56^{lck}, and is believed to contribute to signal transduction.

CD25: Tac antigen; the low-affinity (55K) interleukin-2 receptor on subsets of activated T lymphocytes, some activated B cells, and some activated macrophages.

CD26: dipeptidyl peptidase IV; DPP IV; a 120K serine peptidase of some activated T cell subsets, B cells, and macrophages that binds to collagen, and probably also to fibronectin.

CD27: a 55K protein of undetermined function, expressed by T cells and plasma cells.

CD28: Tp44; a 44K glycoprotein homodimer on the surfaces of 80% of circulating human T lymphocytes (possibly limited to T$_H$ subsets), involved in antigen-independent activation. It synergizes with other factors that promote secretion of interleukin-2, tumor necrosis factors α and β (TNFα and TNFβ), interferon γ, and granulocyte-macrophage colony stimulating factor (GM-CSF), by stabilizing the associated messenger RNAs, and possibly also by serving as a co-receptor for some. The pathways do not affect cell proliferation or expression of interleukin-2 receptors, and are not inhibited by cyclosporine. *See* also **B7**.

CD29: VLA β chain; 4B4; a 130K adhesion molecule expressed on leukocytes that associates with **CD49** subtypes (*q.v.*) to form the VLA integrins. Memory T lymphocytes have much higher levels than naive cells. The *c-myc* gene exerts inhibitory controls over its synthesis.

CD30: a 120K protein recognized by antibodies Ki-1 and Hefi-1 that is expressed on the surfaces of some activated T and B cells, and by Reed-Sternberg cells. Although used as a marker for Hodgkin's lymphoma neoplastic cells, it is also present on subsets of Burkitt's lymphoma cells and on cells transformed by certain viruses (including human Epstein Barr and T cell lymphotrophic viruses I and II). It can be induced on normal types by lectins, and is believed to play roles in normal cell activation, proliferation, and apoptosis. It is a member of the tumor necrosis factor/nerve growth factor (TNF/NGF) receptor family. A ligand obtained with a chimeric probe composed of the extracellular domain plus truncated immunoglobulin heavy chains is a cytokine with homology to tumor necrosis factors α and β, and to a ligand for CD40.

CD31: platelet-endothelial cell adhesion molecule-1; PECAM-1; gpIIa; endoCAM; a 130-140K glycoprotein on monocytes, granulocytes, blood platelets, endothelial cells, and some T cells. It is structurally related to carcinoembryonic antigen, cell adhesion molecules N-CAM and I-CAM, and fasciculin II. CD31 is implicated as a differentiation factor for myelocytic and monocytic hematopoietic cells, and as a cell recognition factor. It promotes adhesion to injured vascular endothelium, and may play roles in initiation of inflammation and wound healing. Additionally, it binds some viruses and may protect them against immune system attack.

CD32: FCRII; a 40K glycoprotein on monocytes, granulocytes, blood platelets, and B lymphocytes that binds Fc regions of IgG immunoglobulins.

CD33: a 67K protein expressed by cells of myeloid lineage that contributes to differentiation.

CD34: 105-120K proteins expressed on primitive hematopoietic stem cells that may be involved in commitment to myeloid differentiation.

CD35: CR1; C3b receptor; 160-250K proteins on granulocytes, macrophages, dendritic cells of spleen germinal follicles, and erythrocytes that contribute to complement system functions. They are receptors for C4b as well as C3b.

CD36: gpIIIb; platelet glycoprotein IV; GPIV; an 88K leukocyte differentiation antigen on blood platelets, monocytes, and some melanoma cells. It associates with protein kinases encoded by *fyn*, *lyn*, and *yes* genes, contributes to platelet adhesion, and binds erythrocytes infected with the malaria parasite, *Plasmodium falciparum*.

CD37: 40-52K B lymphocyte antigens whose functions have not as yet been determined.

CD38: T10; a 45K antigen on B cells, thymocytes, and activated T cells.

CD39: 70-100K antigens on mature B cells.

CD40: Bp50; 44-50K B lymphocyte proteins that resemble the type II tumor necrosis factor receptor, participate in proliferation, differentiation, and activation, and may contribute to memory acquisition. They are also expressed on interdigitating cells of thymus glands, and on some malignant cell types.

CD41: gpIIb/IIIa; a blood platelet glycoprotein. It is an integrin receptor for fibrinogen, fibronectin, and von Willebrand factor that contributes to platelet aggregation.

CD42: gpIX; gpIIb; blood platelet glycoproteins that contribute to adhesion. 23K (CD42a) and 135K (CD42b) forms have been described.

CD43: sialophorin; leukosialin; gp L115; a heavily glycosylated transmembrane protein on leukocytes and blood platelets, composed of 115K and 135K subunits. It is first expressed at an early stage of thymocyte differentiation, and is implicated in acquisition of antigen specificity. It then maintains the morphology and prolongs the survival of circulating T cells, and mediates activation via a pathway independent of the T cell receptor-CD3 complexes, in part by serving as a kinase C substrate. The Wiskott-Aldrich syndrome is attributed to CD43 deficiency.

CD44: phagocytic glycoprotein-1; Hermes lymphocyte homing receptor; Hermes-1 antigen (H-CAM in humans and Pgp-1 in mice); extracellular matrix receptor III; ECMR III; Ly24; erythrocyte antigen In(Lu); fibroblast extracellular matrix receptor III; hyaluronic acid receptor; Hutch-1; 90K transmembrane glycoproteins related to cartilage link proteins, expressed on thymocytes, lymphocytes, monocytes, granulocytes, fibroblasts, erythrocytes, epithelial, glial, and other cell types. They are extracellular matrix receptors that bind hyaluronic acid, collagen types I and IV, and probably also fibronectin, link cytoskeletons to extracellular matrices, modulate CD2-dependent adhesion, contribute to T cell signal transduction, and promote release of tumor necrosis factor-α and interleukin-1β. They also inhibit macrophage migration, promote leukocyte adhesion to high endothelium cells of lymphatic organ postcapillary venules patches, and mediate homing of lymphocytes and monocytes to lymph nodes and sites of inflammation. (L-PAM is a related molecule that promotes homing to Peyer's patches.) Some effects have been linked with phosphotyrosine phosphatase activity. Since they can trigger T_C cell lytic activity even when the T cell receptor is unoccupied, and can redirect the lysis to antigen-negative, Fc positive cells, they are believed to cause nonspecific damage at sites of Tc-mediated inflammation. gp90^{MEL} is a different, mouse type lymphocyte receptor. gp100^{MEL}, on neutrophilic leukocytes, mediates adhesion to endothelial cells adjacent to inflammation sites.

CD45: leukocyte common antigen; Ly5; L-CA; T200; B220; a major family of heavily glycosylated 180K-220K transmembrane proteins on all nucleated cells of hematopoietic origin. Similar proteins whose biosynthesis is directed by a single gene are present in spleen, thymus gland, placenta, and brain. The diverse functions in various cell types are attributed to marked differences in carbohydrate components. The tyrosine phosphatase activity is essential for coupling antigen receptor and CD2 activation to phosphatidylinositol pathways, probably via dephosphorylation and thereby activation of pp56^{lck} and other protein kinases. CD45s associate with CD4, CD8 and antigen receptors of T cells (and with Thy-1), contribute to interferon-α and interleukin-1β release, and are required for antigen-stimulated T cell entry into cell cycles. They also mediate both B cell activation and natural killer (NK) cell cytotoxicity. CD45RA (2H4, UCHL-1), which predominates on unstimulated T cells, is believed to be involved in establishment of tolerance to self-antigens. Impaired ability to synthesize it has been linked with multiple sclerosis, systemic lupus erythematosus, and other autoimmune diseases. It predominates on T memory cells, whereas CD45RB is expressed on B cells.

CD46: membrane cofactor protein; MCP; 55-66K leukocyte and epithelial cell proteins that activate the complement cascade.

CD47: an incompletely characterized 47-52K leukocyte protein of unknown function.

CD48: a 41K leukocyte protein that associates closely with, and may activate p56^{lck}.

CD49a: VLA-1 α chain; integrin α_1 subunit; a phosphatidylinositol-glycan anchored glycoprotein of T cells and monocytes that associates with CD29 to form the

VLA-1 integrin. The complex mediates interactions with extracellular matrices by binding collagens and laminins.

CD49b: VLA-2 α chain; gpIa; integrin α_2 subunit; a 165K glycoprotein on platelets, monocytes, and activated T cells that associates with CD29 to form the VLA-2 integrin (which is also known as extracellular matrix receptor II, ECMRII). The complex binds collagens and laminins.

CD49c: VLA-3 α chain; gpIIc; integrin α_3 subunit; a 135K glycoprotein on B and some T cells that associates with CD29 to form the VLA-3 integrin (extracellular matrix receptor I, ECMRI). The complex binds collagens, laminins, and fibronectin.

CD49d: VLA-4 α chain; integrin α_4 subunit: a 250K glycoprotein on monocytes, T and B cells that associates with CD29 to form the VLA-4 integrin. The levels are three to four fold greater in memory than in unstimulated T cells. The complex mediates interactions with extracellular matrices by binding fibronectin, and is also a major receptor for vascular cell adhesion molecule (V-CAM).

CD49e: VLA-5 α chain; gpIc*; integrin α_5 subunit; a glycoprotein made by monocytes, T, and some B cells that associates with CD29 to form the integrin VLA-5 (fibronectin receptor, FNR, extracellular matrix receptor VI, ECRVI). The levels are three to four fold greater in memory than in unstimulated T cells. The complex mediates interactions with extracellular matrices by binding fibronectin.

CD49f: VLA-6 α chain; gpIc; integrin α_6 subunit; a platelet glycoprotein that associates with CD29 to form the integrin VLA-6. The levels are three to four fold greater in memory than in unstimulated T cells. The complex binds laminins, and appears to be critical for lymphocyte migration.

CD50: 104-108K leukocyte proteins whose functions have not been established.

CD51: the 140K vitronectin α chain on blood platelets.

CD52: 21-28K leukocyte proteins whose functions have not been established.

CD53: 32-40K leukocyte proteins whose functions have not been established.

CD54: intercellular adhesion molecule-1; ICAM-1; a 90K integral membrane glycoprotein of the immunoglobulin superfamily, made by vascular endothelial cells, thymus epithelium, fibroblasts, and some other cell types that binds LFA-1 and mediates homotypic adhesion. Its synthesis is promoted by tumor necrosis factor-α and interferon-γ.

CD55: decay accelerating factor; a widely distributed 70K complement system regulator that has also been identified in some colon carcinoma cells. It associates closely with p56^{lck} and may contribute to signal transduction.

CD56: Leu-19; NKH⁺; 135-220K glycoproteins used as natural killer (NK) cell markers that mediate intercellular adhesion and perform other functions.

CD57: HNK-1; a 110K protein made by natural killer cells, and by some T and B lymphocytes, that contributes to cytotoxicity.

CD58: LFA-3; 40-65K adhesion glycoproteins on T lymphocytes, granulocytes, blood platelets, and epithelial cells (but not on thymocytes), anchored to the plasma membranes by phosphatidylinositol glycans. They bind CD2 (LFA-2), and are believed to contribute to memory acquisition. They contribute to both cell activation and suppression of T_C cell cytotoxicity.

CD59: MIRL; homologous restriction factor 20; HRF 20; H 19; MEM 43; an 18-20K phosphatidylinositol glycan anchored glycoprotein on most leukocytes that binds **CD2** (*q.v.*), associates closely with p56^{lck}, and regulates the formation of membrane attack complexes. It is also made by, and is essential for maintaining the integrity of erythrocytes. CD59 deficiency can cause paroxysmal nocturnal hemoglobinuria.

CD60: a protein made by blood platelets and some T cells.

CD61: gpIIIa; vitronectin β chain; a 110K blood platelet adhesion receptor that binds to **CD31** (*q.v.*) to form gpIIb/IIIa.

CD62: GMP-140; PADGEM; a 140K blood platelet, endothelial cell, and monocyte selectin stored in blood platelet α granules, and in vascular endothelial cell granules. Mediators of hemostasis and inflammation promote its migration to cell surfaces, where it mediates the rolling of marginated leukocytes along vessel walls and migration of those cells to postcapillary venules at sites of injury. CD62 then facilitates chemoattractant-stimulated interaction of neutrophilic leukocyte integrins with intercellular adhesion molecules (I-CAMs), arrests migration, and strengthens adhesion to the injury sites.

CD63: a 53K lysosome-associated protein on activated blood platelets, monocytes, and macrophages.

CD64: FC$_\gamma$R1; a 72-75K monocyte and macrophage protein that contributes to phagocytosis, macrophage activation, and antigen dependent cell mediated toxicity.

CD65: a granulocyte protein believed to contribute to the activation of neutrophilic leukocytes.

CD66: 180-200K proteins on granulocytes whose functions have not been determined.

CD67: a 100K protein on granulocytes whose functions have not been determined.

CD68: a 110K monocyte and macrophage protein of undetermined function.

CD69: a 60K dimeric protein identified on activated B and T cells, and on macrophages and NK cells.

CD70: a protein on activated T and B cells.

CD71: T9; a dimeric 190K protein composed of two 95K subunits. It is the transferrin receptor on activated macrophages, T and B lymphocytes, some other proliferating cells types, and nucleated erythrocytes.

CD72: a dimeric protein with 43K and 39K subunits, made by B lymphocytes.

CD73: ECTO-5-NT; a 69-70K surface glycoprotein made by CD8$^+$ T and some B lymphocytes that binds fibronectin and laminin, and contributes to T cell proliferation. It is an ectoenzyme 5′-nucleotidase, linked to plasma membranes by fatty acid glycosyl phosphatidylinositols.

CD74: 53K MHC class II v chains.

CD75: a 53K protein on mature B lymphocytes and some T cell subsets that associates with **CD22** (*q.v.*).

CD76: an 85K/67K dimeric glycolipid identified on mature B lymphocytes, and on some T cells.

CD77: a protein identified on follicular center B cells.

CD78: Ba; a B lymphocyte protein of unknown function.

cdc: cell division cycle; *cdc* genes code for proteins that regulate entry into and/or passage through the various stages of mitosis and/or meiosis. They direct the synthesis of proteins whose concentrations and/or activities vary with cell cycle events. Some species differences in their products and functions are known. In some cases, genes designated by certain numbers in one species differ from genes of other species assigned similar numbers. *See* specific *cdc* gene types and **cdc kinases**.

cdc1: a *Schizosaccharomyces pombe* (fission yeast) gene that is in some way essential for mitosis, but is not related to *cdc2* or other genes for which specific roles in cell cycles have been established.

cdc2: a cell division cycle gene of fission yeast that codes for p34^{cdc}, a protein kinase that attachs to cyclins and, in association with other gene products, is essential for S → G$_2$ transitions in meiotic and mitotic cell cycles. (Temperature sensitive [*ts*] fission yeast mutants grow into long rods, but cannot divide at restrictive temperatures.) The protein functions at start and again during mitosis in those cells. Its activity is controlled mostly by protein kinases and phosphoprotein phosphatases. Addition of phosphate to some serine-threonine loci augments, whereas phosphorylation at specific tyrosyl moieties decreases the activity (and different serine-threonine loci can also contribute to inactivation). The major regulators are a *cdc25* gene-directed protein (which is not related to the *CDC25* product of budding yeast), and the *wee-1* product. The **CDC28** gene of budding yeast (*q.v.*) codes for a similar product that controls S → G$_2$ transitions. Related genes have been identified in eukarote cells of humans and other species. *See also* **cdc2 kinases**.

cdc2 kinases: when unqualified, the term cdc2 kinase designates a cell division cycle enzyme, p34^{cdc2}, encoded by *cdc2*, that (when activated) catalyzes serine-threonine phosphorylation of certain cell division cycle proteins. It complexes with B cyclins as an essential component of **MPF** (maturation promoting factor, *q.v.*). The enzyme made by fission yeasts is both chemically and biologically related to 34K *CDC2* kinases of other species. Some assay procedures are based on close similarities to H1

kinase. A different, but similar p33^{cdc2} kinase that associates with proliferating nuclear cell antigen (PCNA, a 36K nuclear A cyclin) is required for DNA polymerase δ-mediated DNA chain elongation.

cdc3: a protein identified in budding yeast believed to direct the synthesis of profilin.

CDC3: a fission yeast protein required for cytokinesis.

CDC7: 56K and 58K protein kinases made by budding yeast that are required for G$_1$ → S transitions of cell division cycles. They appear to be involved in initiation of DNA replication, and are known to promote DNA repair and premeiotic recombination. The concentrations do not vary with the cell cycle phases, but the activities are affected by phosphorylations at specific sites, and possibly also by cytoplasmic to nuclear translocation.

cdc10: a fission yeast gene whose product, p85^{cdc10}, acts in conjunction with the *cdc2* product to accomplish cell cycle G$_1$ → S transitions. p85^{cdc10} shares amino acid sequence homology with two proteins (SW14 and SW16) that control DNA synthesis in budding yeast.

cdc13: a *Schizosaccharomyces pombe* cell division cycle gene that directs cyclin synthesis; *see* **MPF**.

cdc22: a *S. pombe* gene that directs the synthesis of the large subunit of ribonucleotide reductase. It is expressed during the S phases of cell cycles, and is required for DNA synthesis.

cdc25: a *Schizosaccharomyces pombe* cell division cycle gene (different from the *CDC25* of budding yeast) that directs the synthesis of an 88K phosphoprotein phosphatase. The enzyme catalzyes dephosphorylation of a specific tyrosyl moiety on p34^{cdc}, and is essential for activation of **MPF** (*q.v.*). The *wee1* gene product catalyzes phosphorylation at the same site. Its effects are sustained until the cells have acquired sizes and nucleus: cytoplasmic ratios suitable for entering the M phases of the cell cycles.

CDC25: an *S. cerevisiae* gene that directs the synthesis of a guanine nucleotide exchange protein which acts on Ras. Cells with non-functioning mutations do not grow and enter cell cycles. *Cf* **cdc25**.

CDC28: a budding yeast (*S. cerevisiae*) gene that performs functions comparable to those of fission yeast *cdc2*. The cells of other eukaryotes (including humans) have similar genes, all of which direct the synthesis of p34^{cdc}.

CDC42: G25K; a geranylgeranylated, GTP-binding protein made by yeasts, homologous with Rho proteins, that contributes to budding and the establishment of cell polarities. Related proteins in complex animals may contribute to cell polarity and secretory processes.

CDC43: an enzyme that catalyzes transfers of geranylgeranyl groups from geranylgeranyl-pyrophosphate to cdc42.

p34^{cdc}: 34K cell division cycle proteins essential for meiosis and mitosis. Their synthesis is directed by *cdc2*,

choline

phosphorylcholine

CDP-choline

phosphatidylcholine

CDC2, CD28 and related genes in various species. Although affected by some proto-oncogenes, the concentrations do not change in normal cells throughout cell cycles. However, the activities rise to highest levels at the metaphase/anaphase transition, and they decline rapidly thereafter. The proteins display serine/threonine protein kinase activity when they combine with cyclins (*see* **MPF**) and undergo the necessary phosphorylations and dephosphorylations on specific amino acid moieties. The yeast *cdc25* gene product is a protein phosphatase that activates by catalyzing $p34^{cdc}$ dephosphorylation at a specific tyrosine locus. Its effects are antagonized by the *wee1* product (which catalyzes tyrosine phoshorylation); and *Nim1* proteins are negative regulators of *wee1*. Several other enzymes can affect the properties by catalyzing phosphorylations or dephosphorylations at different sites. Numerous cell proteins are $p34^{cdc2}$ substrates, including histones H1, H2B and H5, lamins, nucleolin, myosin light chain kinase, $pp60^{src}$, and microtubule components. Many of them contain a (Zaa)-Ser/Thr-Pro-(Xaa)-Zaa sequence (in which Z is Arg or Lys, X is a polar amino acid, and a is any amino acid). A few undergo changes in affinity for DNA. The consequences of $p34^{cdc}$ activation include chromosome condensation, nuclear envelope disintegration, and spindle formation. *See* also **GVMD, cyclins, MPFs, SPFs,** *c-mos*, and **cell cycles**.

CDE: chlordiazepoxide.

CDFs: cytotoxic lymphocyte differentiation factors; a general term for regulators that promote differentiation of T_C lymphocytes.

CDGF: cartilage-derived growth factor; *see* β-**fibroblast growth factor**.

CD kinases: enzymes that catalyze phoshorylation of proteins involved in the control of cell cycles. CDK1 (cdck1) is closely related to the protein encoded by the yeast *cdc2* gene. It binds B cyclins, and regulates S → G_2 phase transitions. CDK2 may be the human homolog of amphibian Eg1. It associates with D cyclins around the time of the restriction point, with cyclin E in the late G_1 phase, and with cyclin A during S, appears to be essential for cell cycle G_1 → S transitions, and plays essential roles

in the control of DNA synthesis. The functions of CDK3 have not been elucidated. CDK4-D cyclins and CDK5-D cyclins accumulate around the time of the restriction point, and are implicated in cell cycle controls by growth factors and oncogenes.

cDNA: complementary DNA; single-stranded DNA molecules synthesized from messenger RNAs via reactions catalyzed by reverse transcriptases. A hybrid molecule composed of the mRNA plus a DNA strand with complementary base sequences is formed first (when a primer and the four deoxyribonucleoside triphosphates are provided). The mRNA is then removed by hydrolysis. cDNAs are used as gene probes in hybridization studies. When employed as templates for formation of double-stranded DNAs, the products contain all of the gene exons that code for mRNAs, but no introns. They can be inserted into vectors to direct bacterial synthesis of new RNAs and proteins. Human growth hormone, insulin, and other regulators that cannot otherwise be obtained in large quantities are made in this way. cDNA (rather than native DNA) is used because bacteria lack the enzymes for intron excision.

C domains: *see* **constant domains**.

CDP: cytidine-5'-diphosphate; *see* also **CDP-choline**.

CDP-choline: cytidine-diphosphate choline; an intermediate in the pathway for biosynthesis of phosphatidylcholine from dietary choline via three reactions: choline + ATP → phosphorylcholine + ADP, followed by phosphorylcholine + CTP → CDP-choline + P-P, and then CDP-choline + diacylglycerol → phosphatidylcholine + CMP.

CDP-diacylglycerol: an intermediate in one pathway for phospholipid biosynthesis, formed from phosphatidic acid (phosphatidate) + CTP. The product then reacts with serine, choline, ethanolamine, inositols, or other alcoholic compounds.

CDR: (1) calcium-dependent regulator: *see* **calmodulins**; (2) complementarity determining region.

CEA: carcinoembryonic antigen.

phosphatidate

CDP-diacylglycerol

C/EBP: CAAT box enhancer binding protein; a term initially applied to all proteins that bind specific DNA base sequences (*see* **CAAT box**) and function as *trans* activators of gene expression, but now restricted to a special type that forms homodimers, positively regulates its own production, initiates and directs differentiation genes in adipocytes and some other cell types, rises to high levels in fully differentiated cells, and maintains the differentiated states. It also forms heterodimers with a CAAT binding protein that regulates albumin synthesis. *See* also **CCAAT binding proteins**.

cecropins: species specific, basic, cysteine-free peptides that contribute to defenses against bacterial infections, initially found in and named for silkworm moths, and later identified in porcine intestine. Cecropin A is Lys-Trp-Lys-Leu-Phe-Lys-Lys-Ile-Glu-Lys-Val-Gly-Gln-Asn-Ile-Arg-Asp-Gly-Ile-Ile-Lys-Ala-Gly-Pro-Ala-Val-Ala-Val-Val-Gly-Gln-Ala-Thr-Gln-Ile-Ala-Lys-NH₂. Cecropin B is Lys-Trp-Lys-Val-Phe-Lys-Lys-Ile-Glu-Lys-Met-Gly-Arg-Asn-Ile-Arg-Asn-Gly-Ile-Val-Lys-Ala-Gly-Pro-Ala-Ile-Ala-Val-Leu-Gly-Glu-Ala-Lys-Ala-Leu-NH₂.

C. elegans: *Caenorhabditis elegans*.

cell adhesion molecules: CAMs; plasma membrane glycoproteins that mediate specific kinds of noncovalent cell:cell and cell:extracellular matrix contacts. Many are known under two or more names that relate to the cell types on which they are expressed, or to their functions; *see* **cadherins**, **integrins**, **CD antigens**, and **ELAM-1**. A few are membrane bound hormones, prohormones, or hormone receptors. LEC-CAM (lectin-EGF-complement-CAM) is a type whose binding properties depend in part on carbohydrate components. The contacts established by cell adhesion molecules can initiate massive redistributions of integral membrane proteins, including clustering and capping, establish junctions for intercellular exchanges of ions and small molecules and cell synchronizations, and/or influence cytoskeletons and intracellular transport. Various types change cell shapes, influence entry into cell cycles, and, by stimulating or inhibiting cell motility, support or oppose processes such as inflammation and metastasis. The contacts can promote two-way cell signalling, or activate just one cell type, via mechanisms that involve changes in the properties of proteases and other enzymes and the generation of second messengers. In addition to strengthening tissues, cell adhesions at various sites play essential roles in embryonic development, histogenesis, wound healing, hemostasis, leukocyte recirculation and homing, phago-

cytosis, and the direct killing of virus infected and cancer cells. A-CAM is identical to N-CAM, A-cadherin, and N-cadherin. E-CAM is also known as CAM 120/80, L-CAM, E-cadherin, L-cadherin, and uvomorulin. H-CAM is a homing receptor; *see* **CD44**. INCAM-10 is inducible cell adhesion molecule-110. Leu-CAM is a term applied to some leukocyte cell adhesion molecules. Ng-CAM mediates neuroglial cell:neuron attachments. P-CAM is P-cadherin. PADGEM (granulocyte membrane protein 140, GMP140) is expressed on blood platelets and monocytes as well as on polymorphonuclear leukocytes. PECAM-1 is CD31. V-CAM-1 is vascular cell adhesion molecule-1.

cell culture: cell growth *in vitro*. Large numbers of cells of a single type can be obtained for detailed studies of their compositions and functions, and of the factors required for survival, growth, differentiation, proliferation, and in some cases transformation. However, since the cells are not organized into the tissues in which they would otherwise reside, they are deprived of paracrine regulators, heterotypic adhesions, and other physiological factors. Tumor cells are often used because they are more easily maintained in proliferative states, but they can display properties very different from those of normal counterparts.

cell cycles the changes cells undergo as they prepare for, and then accomplish orderly gene replication and separation. The four stages usually cited for eukaryotetypes are: G₁ (first growth phase), S (DNA replication), G₂ (second growth phase), and M (mitosis); but subdivisions are useful for some kinds of studies. Entry into G₁, and the G₁ → S and G₂ → M transitions are major control points, which are associated with changes in the concentrations and/or activities of specific molecular species (*see cdc* **genes** and **MPF**). Some regulators prolong growth phases until a suitable cell size and nuclear:cytoplasmic mass ratio is attained. Others promote progression by antagonizing those factors and/or stimulating processes such as DNA replication and entry into mitosis or meiosis. Factors that affect the various phases include hormones and nutrients. Cytokinesis usually begins during telophase, but is not an essential component of the cycle. A cell that completes division can proceed directly to the next G₁, or pause in a "resting" (G₀) phase.

cell cycle genes: *see cdc* **genes**.

cell death: cells can be killed by exogenous toxins, radiation, trauma, and other external factors, but large numbers die under physiological conditions. Normal development involves production of more cells of a given type than are needed, and selective destruction (which depends in part on localized deprivation of tropic factors) is essential for establishing and maintaining healthy mature tissue. Cyclical changes in ovaries, endometrial preparations for implantation, pregnancy, and lactation are among the processes in which substantial numbers of certain kinds are needed for limited time periods and must later be discarded. Thymocyte maturation involves selective destruction of cells that can damage normal tissue. Defenses against virus infections and tumorigenesis are accomplished by direct killing of abnormal types. Erythrocytes have limited life spans because they are subjected to mechanical stress and lack the machinery for repair; and dying as well as dead cells are removed by phagocytosis. In epidermis, superficial cells undergo keratinization and other changes as they are pushed away from the blood supply by others that originate in basal layers, and both dying cells and dead cell remnants protect the underlying tissue against dehydration and other environmental dangers. Similarly, short-lived superficial gastrointestinal tract cells protect the ones below against digestive system enzymes and food chemicals, and are sloughed off. *See* also **apoptosis, autophagy, necrosis,** and **cell senescence.**

cell determination: the processes by which undifferentiated cells become committed to specific developmental pathways, and lose their potential to mature into other cell types.

cell differentiation: *see* **differentiation.**

cell electrophoresis: separation of cells by subjecting them to electrical fields. The movements depend on cell surface charges, and are affected by the pH and other properties of the media in which they are suspended. Electrophoresis is used to study cell surface properties, and to obtain homogenous populations of specific cell types.

cell fractionation: (1) preparation of **cell fractions** (*q.v.*); (2) separation of the various cell types of a heterogenous population, usually by flow cytometry.

cell fractions: cell components obtained by homogenizing tissues and employing techniques for separating various types from each other. Ultracentrifugation separates layers of different densities, and is used to obtain nuclear, mitochondrial, microsomal, and cytosolic fractions. It is used to define intracellular localizations of enzymes, receptors, and other cell components, and to study their functions. Enzymes and other substances whose localizations are known can be used as markers of contamination with other fractions.

cell-free extract: fluid obtained by rupturing cells and subjecting the products to centrifugation for removal of particulate material and remaining cells. *See* **cell free synthesis.**

cell free synthesis: the use of cell preparations that contain enzymes, substrates, co-factors, and sometimes organelles, to synthesize large molecules, to study enzyme functions, biosynthetic pathways, and factors that affect them, or to obtain preprohormones and other molecular species that cannot be recovered from intact cells (*see* **signal sequences**). Reticulocyte lysates are among the most commonly used preparations.

cell fusion: union of previously distinct cells. It occurs under phsyiological conditions, for example during fertilization, establishment of the syncytiotrophoblast, development of skeletal muscle, and formation of macrophages. Artificial fusion can be accomplished with chemical agents that such as polyethylene glycol, with some viruses, and with high-frequency electrical fields, all of which alter plasma membrane properties. Heterokaryons can divide, and generate progeny with single nuclei that contain genetic elements from both sources. Usually, some chromosomes are lost, and hybrids with just one or a few chromosomes from one of the original species are convenient tools for gene mapping. Some hybrid types produce large quantities of specific kinds of messenger RNAs and proteins; and some can be used to study the effects of cytoplasmic components of one cell type on genetic components introduced from another.

cell line: usually, the cultured progeny of a single parent cell. Some types retain the properties of the parent cell, and can therefore be used to study differentiation, enzyme functions, and control mechanisms, or as sources of specific kinds of molecules; and cancer-derived types can provide information on factors that lead to malignancy. However, many cell types change under culture conditions. Lines derived from cells in which specific kinds of mutations have been induced are used to investigate gene functions.

cell lineage: the immature cell type or tissue from which differentiated types derive.

cell lysis: disruption of cell plasma membranes, and consequent dissolution of the components. It can be initiated by toxins or substances generated following activation of immune system processes, and can be invoked artificially with detergents, enzymes, hypo-osmotic environments, and other factors.

cell mediated immunity: CMI: *see* **cellular immunity.**

cell memory: retention of a change invoked by a regulator after the regulator has been removed. It occurs, for example, in the immune system (*see* **memory cells**), and in the central nervous system (*see* **long term potentiation**).

cell migration: cell movement, for example during embryogenesis, inflammatory reactions, or immune system responses.

cell motility factors: cytokines that selectively stimulate cell movements, but do not affect cell proliferation. Many growth factors affect both processes.

cell movement: (1) cell migration; (2) changes in cell shapes and/or arrangements of cell components.

cell polarity: specializations that make one surface (or end) of a cell different from another, including differences in enzyme, receptor, or carrier content, or the kinds of

cellulose

associations with neighboring cells. Polarity is essential for processes such as directed transport and selective enzymatic degradation.

cell renewal: replacement of cells with others of the same type, for example in hematopoietic tissue, epidermis, and mucous membranes.

cell specificity: the characteristics that make one cell type different from another. Within an organism, most differences are related to selective augmentation and/or suppresion of the activities of specific genes types.

cell strain: cells of a single type, derived from a primary cell culture or cell line by selection and cloning of progeny with specific properties or markers.

cell surface marker: a substance (usually a glycoprotein) expressed on a plasma membrane surface that can be used to identify a specific cell type (or a group of closely related ones), or the stage of maturation.

cell synchronization: conditions in which all cells of a given population are in the same phase of activity (usually, the same stage of the cell cycle). It can be artificially imposed with reversible inhibitors of microtubule and/or enzyme functions.

cellular immunity: cell mediated immunity; CMI; immune system responses that involve direct cell-to-cell interactions, usually initiated by antigens, and usually mediated by T lymphocytes or natural killer cells; *cf* **humoral immunity**. It is used under physiological conditions to destroy cells that are foreign to the body (such as mutated types and ones altered by viral infections), but can also destroy grafted tissue and cause autoimmune disease.

cellular respiration: glycolysis, oxidative phosphorylation, and other metabolic reactions involved in nutrient catabolism and energy exchange.

cellularity: the proportion of a tissue mass composed of cells (as opposed to extracellular components).

cellulases: enzymes that catalyze hydrolysis of β 1→4 glycoside linkages (for example of cellulose). They are made by plants, some microorganisms, and some invertebrates. Higher animals do not make them, but the gastrointestinal tracts of termites, ruminants and some others house microorganisms that do.

cellulose: a complex structural polysaccharide in cell walls of plants, some bacteria, and some fungi. The predominant component is a β-D-glucose polymer (see structure), but some types additionally contain lignin and peptidoglycans. Since it does not dissolve in biological fluids, and cannot be digested by most animals, dietary cellulose is called insoluble fiber.

Celsius: Centigrade; °C; a unit of temperature equivalent to 1/100 the difference between the temperatures of melting ice (0°C) and boiling water (100°C) at 1 atmosphere of pressure. 0°C = 32° Fahrenheit and 373° on the Kelvin scale. The Fahrenheit equivalent is approximated by multiplying the degrees C by 9/5 and adding 32.

CENBA: 5′chloro-N^6-(2-*endo*-norbonyl)-adenosine; an adenosine receptor antagonist that is highly selective for A_1 subtypes.

ceno-; caeno-: a prefix meaning (1) new or recent; (2) empty; (3) common or shared.

Centigrade: *see* **Celsius**.

centi-: a prefix meaning 1/100, as in centiliter or centimeter.

centiliter: cl; 1/100 liter; 10 milliliters.

centimorgan: centiMorgan; cM; a unit of distance between genes on a chromosome. The probability that crossing over will occur during meiosis varies directly with the distance, and is 1% for genes separated by 1 centimorgan.

central nervous system: the brain, spinal cord, and their associated components; *cf* **peripheral nervous system**.

centrifugal: (1) moving away from the center; (2) conducting away from the central nervous system or from some other entity.

centrifugation: separation of components of a mixture or suspension on the basis of density differences, by applying gravitational forces that are generated by rapid rotation. Low speed centrifugation can separate entities with very large density differences (for example blood cells from blood plasma, or suspended particles from surrounding fluids). **Ultracentrifugation** *(q.v.)* is used for mixtures of proteins, lipoproteins, and other macromolecules, and for determination of molecular weights.

centrioles: organelles of animal (and some lower plant) cells, usually located close to nuclear envelopes. They are pairs of hollow, orthogonally arranged cylinders, approximately 0.4 μm long and 0.15-.20 μm in diameter. Each cylinder has a wall of nine microtubule triplets (one complete A, fused to two incomplete B and C types) embedded in a gelatinous matrix. A resting cell has one centriole (two cylinders). When it prepares for division, the centrioles replicate, and one organelle travels to each of the poles. The basal body of a cilium or flagellum has the same structure. *See* also **centrosomes**.

centripetal: (1) moving toward the center; (2) conducting toward the central nervous system or other structure; *cf* **centrifugal**.

centrolecithal: describes egg cells in which the centrally located yolk is surrounded by a peripheral layer of protoplasm. Most insects have eggs of this kind. *Cf* **telolecithal**.

centromere: the constricted region of a chromosome, visible at metaphase, that contains base sequences required for chromosome segregation, and is the site for kinetochore formation. The DNA is less condensed than in other parts of the chromosome.

centrosome: the amorphous region that surrounds a centriole. It is a microtubule organizing center (nucleation center for microtubule polymerization). In proliferating cells, it replicates and organizes the two poles of the mitotic spindle.

cephalic: pertaining to the head.

cephalic phase of secretion: release of small quantities of hormones or other regulators in response to environmental stimuli, or to messages originating in other ways that descend from the cerebral cortex. It is a major mechanism for **anticipatory control** (*q.v.*). For example, the sight, aroma, or thought of food invokes the release of small quantities of insulin and gastrin. The insulin protects against development of prandial hyperglycemia, and the gastrin prepares the stomach for digestion. If food is then ingested, additional secretion is stimulated by gastrointestinal factors.

cephalins: an obsolete term for nervous tissue phosphatidylserine, phosphatidylethanolamine, and other phospholipids with primary amine groups. Since flocculation occurs when a cephalin-cholesterol emulsion is added to serum with abnormally low albumin or abnormally high globulin concentrations, cephalin-cholesterol flocculation tests are sometimes used to assess liver functions.

cephalization: (1) progressive development of the head regions of an embryo; (2) in comparative anatomy, the tendency for complex structures to concentrate in the head region.

ceramides: *N*-acyl-sphingosines; lipids formed in reactions of the general type: sphingosine + fatty acyl-coenzyme A → ceramide + coenzyme A. The various types differ from each other in the kinds of fatty acid moieties (all of which are long chain). Ceramides react with UDP-glucose or UDP-galactose to yield cerebrosides, and with CDP-choline to yield sphingomyelins.

ceramides

cerebellin: H_2N-Ser-Gly-Ser-Ala-Lys-Val-Ala-Phe-Ser-Ala-Ile-Arg-Ser-Thr-Asn-His-OH; a peptide used as a specific marker for cerebellum in studies of development. A second peptide identified in that brain region, [Des-Ser^1]-cerebellin, is identical with amino acids 2-16.

cerebellum: a major component of the hindbrain, composed of two hemispheres and a connecting vermis. It contains Purkinje cells whose activities are controlled by excitatory amino acids, γ-aminobutyric acid (GABA), and other regulators, and is an important site for controlling balance, coordination, and fine muscular movements.

cerebrosides: glycolipids in which glucose or galactose moieties replace the hydrogen atoms on the terminal alcoholic groups of ceramide sphingosine components, and related compounds that contain dihydrosphingosine. The highest concentrations are in nervous tissue, and especially in myelin sheaths. Cerebrosides are metabolized by lysosomal hydrolases (*see* also **saponins**). Fabry, Gaucher's, Niemann-Pick, and Tay-Sachs diseases, and leukodystrophies, are inherited disorders attributed to impaired production of those enzymes.

cerebrospinal fluid; CSF; the fluid made by choroid plexuses that fills cerebral ventricles, circulates around the spinal cord, provides an environment essential for neuron functions, and serves as a shock absorber. In addition to oxygen and nutrients, it contains numerous hormones and other regulators. Although derived from blood, normal CSF contains no erythrocytes, fewer leukocytes, less protein, and somewhat different relative concentrations of electrolytes, glucose, and other solutes. Blood brain barriers protect against sudden fluctuations in the composition when the concentrations of blood plasma components change rapidly; and they block the entry of many endogenous substances and pharmacological agents. However, circumventricular organs and ependymal cells provide avenues of communication.

cero-: a prefix meaning wax.

cerulein: caerulein.

cerulenin: 3-(1-oxo-4,7-nonadienyl)-oxiranecarboxamide; an antibiotic made by *Cephalosporium caerulens* that inhibits glycoprotein acylation and *de novo* synthesis of fatty acids and sterols. It is used to treat fungus infections.

cerulenin

ceruloplasmin: 120-160K acute phase glycoproteins secreted by the liver, and named for their blue color. They are major copper binding and transporting proteins, and they protect against copper deposition in tissues. They also display ferroxidase, amine oxidase, and superoxide dismutase activities, contribute to iron mobilization, and are implicated as mediators of inflammation. In electrical fields, they migrate with plasma α_2-globulins.

cervical: pertaining to the (1) neck; (2) uterine cervix.

cervix: *see* **uterine cervix.**

cesium: Cs; caesium; an element (atomic number 55, atomic weight 132.9). It is a silver-white metal, liquid at room temperatures, that is used in photocells and as a catalyst for hydrogenation reactions. Macromolecules are suspended in high density solutions of the chloride salts for some ultracentrigation procedures, and the ions are used in the laboratory as potassium channel blockers.

cetiedil: α-cyclohexyl-3-thiophenacetic acid; a calmodulin antagonist that blocks voltage-gated calcium channels, and is used to promote vasodilation.

cf: compare with.

CF: (1) cystic fibrosis; (2) citrovorum factor; (3) complement fixation; (4) Christmas factor.

6-CF: 6-carbonyl fluorescin; a fluorophore that does not cross plasma membranes. It is used as a marker for endocytosis. *See* **carboxyfluoresceins.**

CFA: (1) complete Freund's adjuvant; (2) complement fixation antibody.

CF Ag: cystic fibrosis antigen.

CF-ICA: complement fixing islet cell antibodies; *see* **diabetes mellitus.**

c-fos: a proto-oncogene that affects the functions of many other genes, and is a major regulator of cell proliferation. Its protein product, Fos, forms heterodimers with *c-jun* products that bind to specific DNA base sequences. The levels are low in most "resting" cells. They rise rapidly within minutes after exposure to numerous growth factors and tumor promotors, and usually peak within half an hour. Environmental light induces Fos in the suprachiasmatic nuclei, in which it contributes to the control of circadian rhythms. *V-fos* is an oncogene made by mouse FBJ osteosarcoma cells.

CFS: chronic fatigue syndrome.

CFT napthalene sulfonate: -(-)-2β-carbomethoxy-3-β-(4-fluorophenyl)tropane 1,5-naphthalenedisulfonate; a cocaine receptor agonist that inhibits dopamine transport.

CFU-E: colony forming unit-erythrocyte.

CFU-S: colony form unit-spleen.

CG: chorionic gonadotropin.

CGA: Cga; chromogranin A.

C genes: DNA regions that code for antibody constant domains (*see* **immunoglobulins**), and for T lymphocyte antigen receptor α and β chains.

CGL: chronic granulocytic leukemia.

cGMP: cyclic guanosine 3′5′-monophosphate.

cGMP-dependent kinase: kinase G; *see* **protein kinases.**

CGN: *cis*-Golgi network.

CGP-12177A: 4-[c-[(1,1-dimethyl)amino]-2-hydroxy-propoxyl]-1,3-dihydro-2*H*-benzimidazol-2-one; a non-specific β-type adrenergic agonist that binds with high affinity to central nervous system and pineal gland receptors, and a partial agonist for brown adipose tissue types.

CGRP: calcitonin gene related peptide.

CGS-12066B: 7-trifluoromethyl-4-(4-methyl-1-piperazinyl)-pyrrolo[1,2-alquinoxaline: a serotonin receptor agonist selective for 5HT$_{1B}$ subtypes.

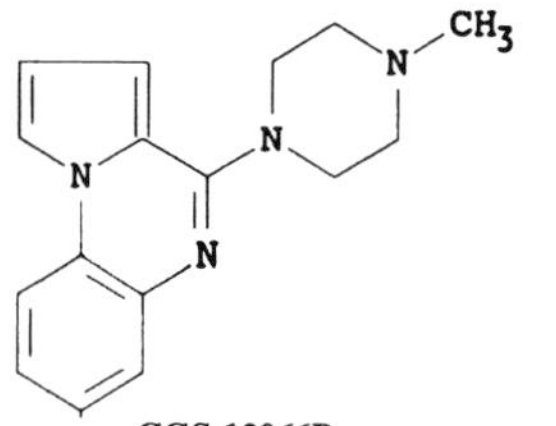

CGS-12066B

CGS 19755: 3-(2-carboxypiperazin-4-yl)methyl-1-phosphonic acid; a competitive NMDA receptor agonist.

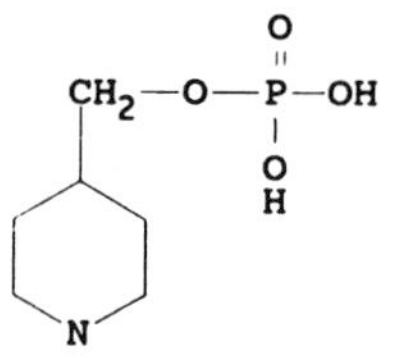

CGS 16949A: 4-(5,6,7,8-tetrahydroimidazo)-[15a]-pyridine-5-yl-benzonitrile monochloride; an inhibitor of aromatase enzymes.

CGS 21680: 2-[p-(2-carbonylethyl)phenylethylamino-5-N-ethylcarboxadmino]-adenosine; an excitatory amino acid receptor agonist, highly specific for A_{2a} subtypes. An I^{125} derivative, PAPA-APEC, is used for photo-affinity labeling.

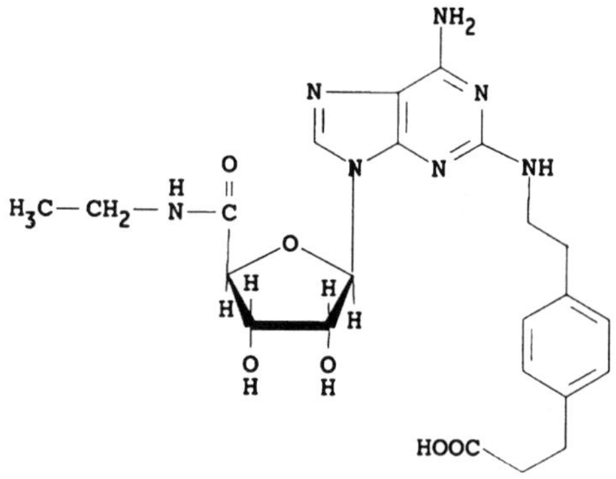

C_H: immunoglobulin heavy chain.

Chaikoff effect: *see* **Wolf-Chaikoff effect**.

chalone: a term that usually refers specifically to epidermal mitosis inhibiting peptide, pGlu-Glu-Asp-Ser-Gly-OH; but *see* **chalones**.

chalones: although initially applied to hormones that exert inhibitory effects on their target organs, the term now describes non-cytotoxic autocrine regulators released by proliferating cells that reversibly inhibit mitosis of the same cell types, and thereby protect against hyperplasia. The amounts that accumulate in cells and their environments vary directly with the cell numbers. Tissue-specific (but not species-specific) peptides for epidermal and kidney cells, hepatocytes, melanocytes, fibroblasts, lymphocytes, granulocytes, and erythrocyte precursors have been described; and a different type may limit spermatogenesis. Tumor necrosis factor-β (TNFβ) and other cytokines may account for some of the activities. Epidermal mitosis inhibiting pentapeptide is one of the few that have been characterized. *See* also **colyones**.

channel proteins: multimeric proteins that form hydrophilic pores in lipid membranes which permit passage of small ions and water-soluble molecules.

chaotropic: describes agents that increase the solubility of hydrophobic substances in aqueous media by dissolving in and disrupting the physical structure of water. Examples include arylamines, thiocyanate ions, perchlorate ions, and 6M alkaline urea solutions.

chaperonins: molecular chaperones; proteins that promote, preserve, and/or correct the folding of polypeptides and proteins, and the assembly of multimeric molecules. They bind reversibly to their targets during translation, intracellular transport, and/or posttranslational processing. Some are stress proteins.

CHAPS: [3-(3-cholamidopropyl)-dimethylammonio]-1-propane sulfonate; a zwitterion detergent, used to release integral membrane proteins from lipid bilayers, to promote disaggregation of membrane-associated enzyme complexes, and in electrophoresis. It does not denature proteins.

CHAPSO: [3-(3-cholamidopropyl)-dimethylammonio]-2-hydroxy-1-propane sulfonate; a hydroxylated CHAPS derivative that is more polar, but otherwise displays properties similar to those of the parent compound.

charybdotoxin: Glu-Phe-Thr-Asn-Val-Ser-Cys-Thr-Thr-Ser-Lys-Glu-Cys-Trp-Ser-Val-Cys-Gln-Arg-Leu-His-Asn-

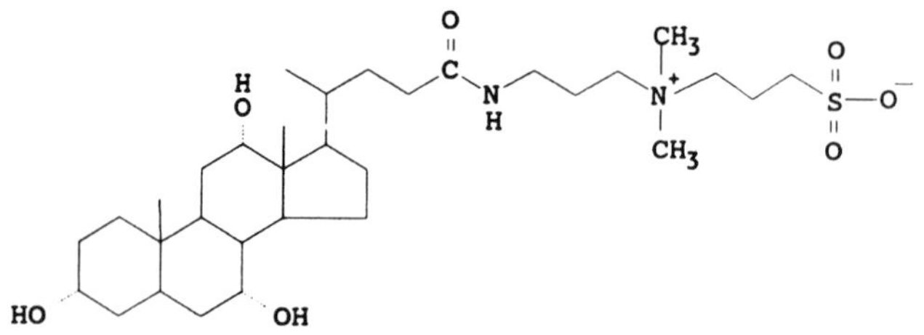

CHAPS

Thr-Ser-Arg-Gly-Lys-Cys-Met-Asn-Lys-Lys-Cys-Arg-Cys-Tyr-Ser; a toxin in the venom of the scorpion, *Leirus quinquestriatus* that binds to, and is a selective inhibitor of calcium activated potassium channels.

chase: *see* **pulse chase**.

chelators: "claw-like" molecules that bind divalent cations and form stable, water-soluble complexes (*see*, for example **EDTA**, **EGTA**, and **DTPA**). They vary in ion selectivities. Calcium chelators added to extracellular fluids block cell Ca^{2+} uptake. They are used to treat some forms of hypertension, and to provide information on the mechanisms of cell excitation and hormone actions. These and other types are also used to treat heavy metal poisoning.

chemical castration: disruption of gonadal functions by agents that block receptor functions, inhibit steroidogenic enzymes, or interfere with the secretion of trophic factors. It is used to temporarily arrest precocious puberty, treat some cancers, and study hormone functions. *See* also **gonadotropin releasing hormone**.

chemical potential: the amount of energy released when one gram molecular weight of a dissolved solute is transferred to a solution with a lower concentration of the same solute (or the amount of work required to move it in the opposite direction). *See* also **electrochemical potential**.

chemical sympathectomy: disruption of sympathetic system functions with agents that destroy neurons, inhibit catecholamine synthesizing enzymes, or block neuron development. *See* 6-hydroxy-**DOPA** and **immunosympathectomy**.

chemical synapse: communication between a presynaptic and a postsynaptic neuron, or between a neuron and a muscle or gland cell, accomplished via release of a neurotransmitter that travels across a synaptic space and acts on target cell receptors.

chemiluminescence: light emission invoked by chemical reactions. Bioluminescence (light production by living organisms) provides signals by which by some insects and deep sea organisms communicate with other members of the species. Firefly luciferase is used with suitable substrates (luciferins) to assay ATP and the generation of free radicals by phagocytic cells.

chemiosmotic hypothesis: a widely accepted concept for explaining oxidative phosphorylation. It states that electrochemical gradients across the two sides of inner mitochondrial membranes are created by transport of protons (from reduced coenzymes in the matrix) to the outer surfaces (and/or by transport of electrons in the opposite direction). The energy released by spontaneous dissipation of the gradients then drives the synthesis of ATP from ADP + Pi.

chemoattractants: agents that promote positive **chemotaxis** (*q.v.*).

chemokines: agents that increase generalized cell motility in any direction; *cf* **chemoattractants**.

chemokinesis: accelerated random cell movement in response to chemokines; *cf* **chemotaxis**.

chemoreceptor: a cell or organ specialized for sensing changes in the concentrations of one or more chemicals, and for communicating the effects (to other cells, or to components of the same cell.) Examples include carotid body oxygen receptors, hypothalamic sodium sensors, and pancreatic islet glucoreceptors.

chemosurgery: destruction of cells or tissues by chemical means. *See* **chemical castration**, **chemical sympathectomy**, and **capsaicin**.

chemotactic: promoting chemotaxis.

chemotaxins: agents that promote directed cell movement; *see*, for example *f*-**Met-Leu-Phe**, **thymotaxin**, **PAF**, and **chemotaxis**; and *cf* **chemokines**.

chemotaxis: directed cell migration, usually in response to a chemical gradient. It can be *positive* (towards the highest concentration of a chemoattractant) or *negative* (away from a chemical). *Cf* **chemokinesis**.

chemotherapy: (1) use of chemicals to kill cancer cells; (2) treatment of disease with antibiotics, toxins, or other agents that affect the release or actions of noxious factors.

chenodeoxycholic acid: 3,7-dihydroxycholan-24-oic acid; a major bile acid, usually secreted as the sodium salt of a glycine or taurine conjugate.

CHH: crustacean hyperglycemic hormone.

Chiari-Frommel syndrome: persistent postpartum galactorrhea and amenorrhea, usually caused by a prolactin-secreting pituitary gland microadenoma.

chiasma [chiasmata]: (1) a site of crossing, for example of nerves or other anatomical entities, as in optic chiasma; (2) during meiosis, the regions of contact between non-sister chromatids of homologous chromosomes. *See* **crossing over**.

chick embryo fibroblasts: CEF; immature fibroblasts that are easily maintained in culture. They respond to numerous regulators, and are used to study differentiation.

chief cells: (1) PTH-secreting parathyroid gland cells; (2) pepsinogen-secreting gastric cells.

chimera: usually (1) an individual with genetic components derived from two or more parent cells. The abnormality can arise spontaneously if an oocyte is fertilized by more than one spermatozoan, a polar body adheres to a fertilized oocyte, two zygotes fuse, or dizygotic twin fetuses exchange cells; (2) an individual with some cells of one genetic type and some of another,

chitin

caused, for example by spontaneous or environmentally induced mutations of limited numbers of cells, viral infections, injections of heterologous bone marrow cells, or grafts from compatible but genetically different individuals. Chimeras can be produced artificially by joining two blastocysts, grafting embryonic tissue from one organism onto another, or injecting foreign DNA into oocytes; (3) a ratfish; (4) a monster; a term originally applied to a mythical, fire spouting animal with a lion's head, goat's body, and serpent's tail.

chimeric DNA: recombinant DNA that contains segments different from the ones in the original source. The alien components can derive from other species.

chimeric proteins: proteins that contain some amino acid sequences different from the ones present in native molecules. They can be obtained by injecting artificial DNAs or messenger RNAs into cells, and are used to investigate the functions of specific domains, or to study processes involved in acquisition of tertiary or quaternary structures.

Chinese hamster ovary cells: CHO; a fibroblast cell line widely used in transfection studies.

chiral: describes molecules that are optically active when dissolved, with structures that cannot be superimposed on their mirror images. See **asymmetric carbon atoms** and **stereoisomerism**.

chirality: "handedness"; molecular asymmetry; see **stereoisomerism**.

chi square: χ^2; a statistical measure of how closely a set of observed values fits expectations for that parameter. For example, if a hypothesis predicts that half the offspring of a mating will express a specific trait, then the theoretical frequency (F) for its appearance in a given set of observations is determined by dividing the total numbers of observations by 2. If A = the number of offspring that do, in fact, express the trait, and B the number that do not, then $\chi^2 = (A\text{-}F)^2/F + (B\text{-}F)^2/F$. A very low χ^2 value supports the hypothesis (whereas a high one is cause for rejection). The statistical significance is determined from tables that relate the numbers of determinations to the probabilities of obtaining values as great (or greater) when all variations are random.

chitin: semi-rigid structural polysaccharides composed mostly of unbranched N-acetyl-D-glucosamine polymer chains. They are the major components of crustacean and insect skeletons, and are also made by some fungi, marine invertebrates, and plants. Three of the repeating units are shown. Chitins are used as weak ion exchange

resins, to treat contaminated water, to immobilze α-amylase, and for *in vitro* synthesis of oligosaccharides. Sulfated derivatives are weak anticoagulants. *See also* **chitosans**.

chitinases: enzymes that degrade chitins and chitosans. Commercial types are obtained from *Streptomyces griseus*.

chitosans: polymers composed mostly of 2-amino-2-deoxy-$(1\rightarrow4)$-β-D-glucopyran subunits, made by deacylating chitins. Low molecular weight types lower blood and liver cholesterol levels in laboratory animals fed large quantities of sterols, and somewhat counteract sterol mediated depression of hepatic 3-hydroxy-3-methyl-glutaryl coenzyme A (HMG-CoA) activity. The effects are dose-related, and attributed to binding, via the glucosamine groups, to bile acids and/or cholesterol. Since chitosans do not appear to invoke the pathological effects of cholestyramine on the liver, and (unlike that resin) do not seem to increase the risk for developing colon cancers, they may prove useful for treating some forms of hypercholesterolemia. Chitins dissolve in acids to form viscous solutions that can accelerate wound healing, and are also used as components of photographic emulsions. Their abilities to function as weak basic ion exchange resins at pH levels of 6 or lower are applied in water treatment systems. Additionally, they are good substrates for chitinase determinations. The repeating unit is shown.

Chlamydia: a genus of minute prokaryote parasites, with genomes smaller than those of most bacteria, that use host-derived ATP for metabolic processes, but can be grown in culture. *C. psittaci* infects birds, and can cause ornithosis in humans. *C. trachomatis* infects human eyes and genital tracts and can inflict serious damage.

Chlamydomonas: a genus of unicellular algae used to study cytoplasmic inheritance, circadian rhythms, flagellar architecture, and other biological phenomena.

chloasma: patchy skin pigmentation. High estrogen levels during pregnancy, or steroids taken for therapeutic purposes or contraception, invoke the condition in some women.

chlorambucil: 3-amino-2,5-dichlorobenzoic acid; an alkylating agent that acts on DNA and kills cells during mitosis. It is used to treat some forms of leukemia, but can cause deletion mutations.

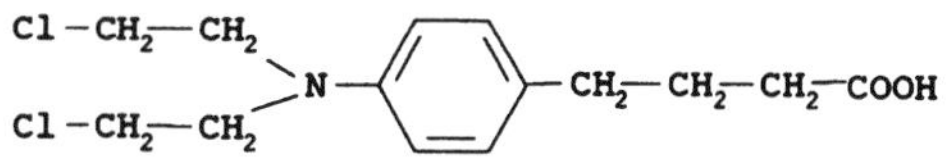

$$Cl-CH_2-CH_2$$
$$Cl-CH_2-CH_2$$ N—⟨ ⟩—$CH_2-CH_2-CH_2-COOH$

chloramines: *N*-chloro substituted amines, amides, or imides. They are oxidizing and chlorinating agents, effective as topical antiseptics. Chloramine T (the sodium salt of *N*-chloro-*p*-toluene sulfonamide) converts iodine ions to forms (I^o or I^+) that bind to tyrosine moieties. Although used to label molecules with radioactive iodine, it denatures some proteins.

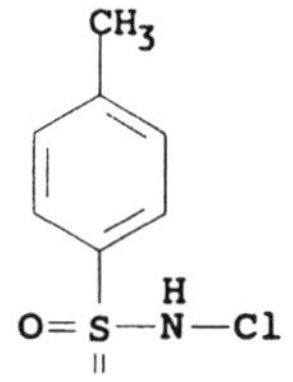

CH_3

$O=\overset{\text{H}}{\underset{O}{S}}-N-Cl$

chloramphenicol: Chloromycetin; 2,2-dichloro-*N*-[2-hydroxy-1-(hydroxymethyl)-2-(4-nitrophenyl)ethyl]acetamide; an antibiotic made by *Streptomyces venezuelae* that inhibits protein synthesis in bacteria and in eukaryote mitochondria, by attaching to 50S ribosome subunits, but does not disrupt the functions of eukaryote cytoplasmic (60S) ribosome subunits. Although effective against rickettsia and many bacteria species, it is usually prescribed only when other antibiotics prove inadequate, since the side effects include hypersivitity reactions, bone marrow aplasia, and deleterious influences on several liver enzymes. *See* also **chloramphenicol acetyltransferase**.

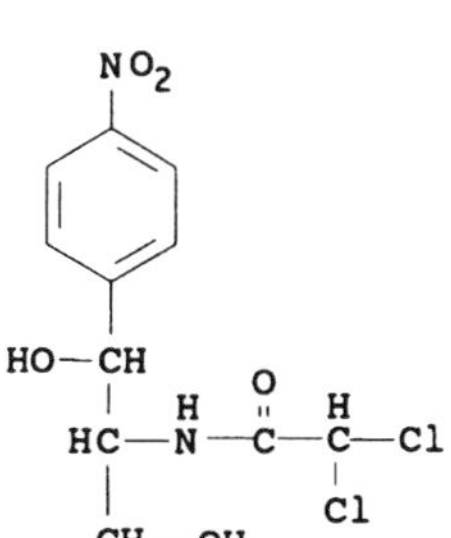

NO_2

$HO-CH$
$HC-\overset{H}{N}-\overset{O}{\overset{\|}{C}}-\overset{H}{\overset{}{C}}-Cl$
CH_2-OH Cl

chloramphenicol acetyltransferase: CAT; an enzyme made by bacteria that catalyzes acetylation of chloramphenicol. The DNA that directs its synthesis is a useful reporter gene for transfection studies, since it is stable in transfected mammalian cells when fused to eukaryote promoters; and the rate of enzyme synthesis directly reflects the transcriptional activity of the promoter. The acetylation products are easily measured, and the amounts formed are directly related to the enzyme levels when excess coenzyme A is presented. CAT is used to

investigate cell-specific gene expression, *trans*-acting factors, and other aspects of promoter functions.

chlordiazepoxide: CDE; 7-chloro-*N*-methyl-5-phenyl-3*H*-1,4-benzodiazepin-2-amine-4-oxide; a benzodiazepine that antagonizes some central effects of cholecystokinin. The chloride (Librium) is a widely used, orally effective anxiolytic.

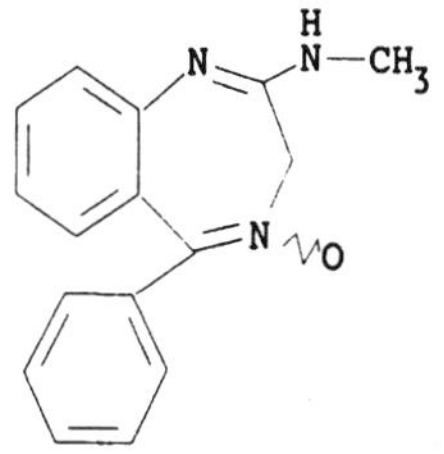

$N=\overset{H}{\overset{}{N}}-CH_3$

chloride: Cl^-; the most abundant anion of extracellular fluids and bile, an important contributor to intracellular negative charge, and an activator of kallikreins and some other enzymes. Its levels and movements are influenced by Na^+ concentrations at most sites, but some cell types exchange it for HCO_3^-. The ion is actively secreted to gastric juice, and into the fluid that surrounds long Henle loops and renal collecting ducts. γ-aminobutyric acid (GABA) and some other regulators that promote cell hyperpolarization accelerate Cl^- extrusion by opening chloride channels. *See* also **chlorine**.

chloride cells: cells that actively transport large quantities of chloride, for example in the integuments of some fishes.

chloride shift: *see* **erythrocytes**.

chlorine: an element (atomic number 17, atomic weight 35.45); *see* **chloride**.

2-chloroadenosine: *see* 2-chloro-**adenosine**.

chlorisondamine-HCl: *N*-[(2-dimethylammonium)ethyl]-4,5,6,7-tetrachloroisoindolium-dimethylchloride; a hexamethonium type ganglionic blocking agent. It is used to treat some forms of hypertension and edema.

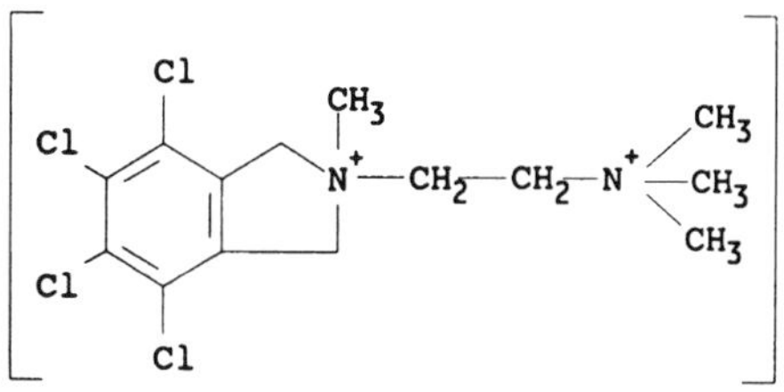

Cl CH_3 CH_3
Cl N^+—CH_2—CH_2—N^+ CH_3
Cl CH_3
Cl

chlormadinone acetate: Lorman; Luteran; 6-chloro-17-hydroxypregna-4,6-diene-3,29-dione acetate; a synthetic progestin used to treat some ovarian dysfunctions, and a component of Menova, C-quens, and some other oral contraceptives.

2-chloroadenosine triphosphate: a highly potent agonist for P_2 purine receptors that mediates relaxation of smooth muscle.

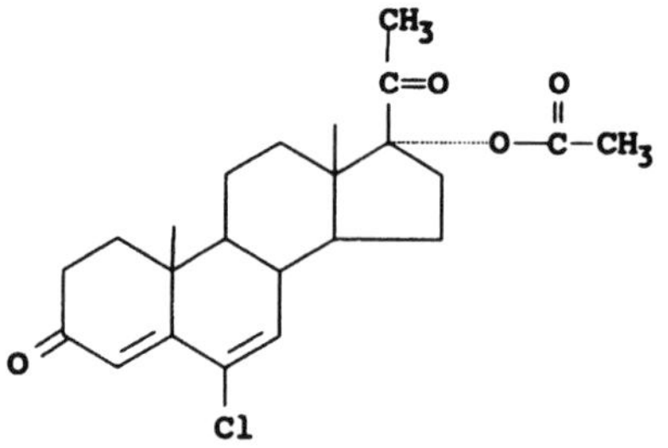

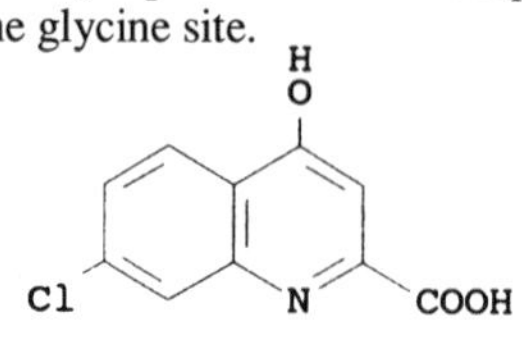

Chloromycetin: a trade name for chloramphenicol.

4-chloro-1-naphthol: a chromogen used in immunoperoxidase studies.

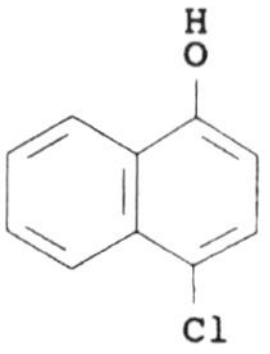

chlormadinone acetate

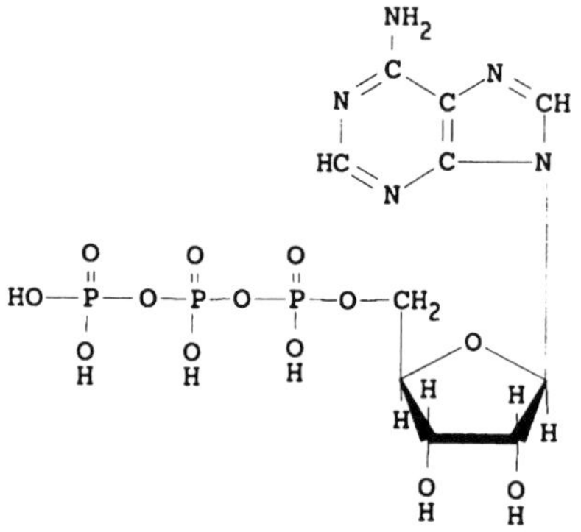

2-chloroadenosine triphosphate

4′-chlorodiazepam: 7-chloro-5-(4-chlorophenyl)-1,3-dihydro-1-methyl-2*H*-1,4-benzodiazepin-2-one; a ligand that binds to peripheral type benzodiazepine receptors and is used to distinguish them from central types.

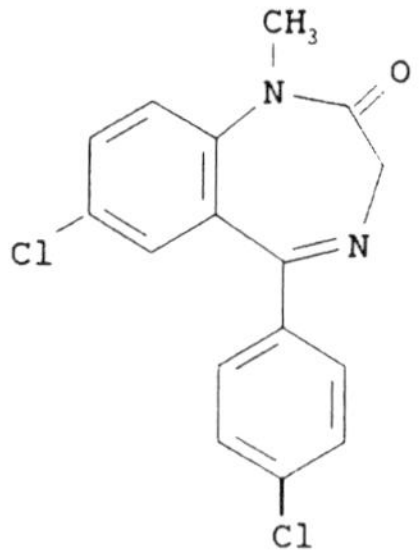

chloroethylclonidine dihdyrochloride3: CEC; a clonidine derivative that irreversibly blocks α$_1$ type adrenergic receptors.

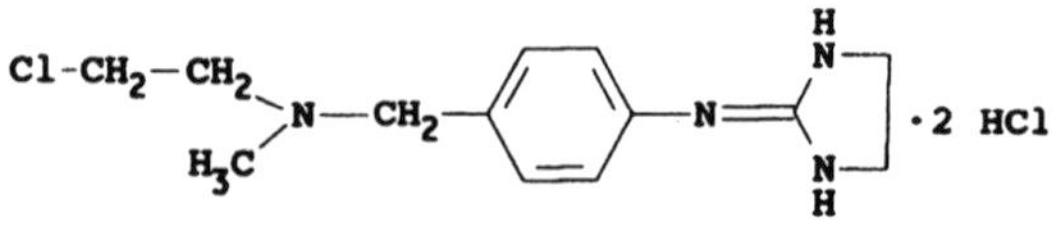

7-chlorokynurenic acid: 7-chloro-4-hydroxyquinoline-2-carboxylic acid; a potent NMDA receptor antagonist that acts on the glycine site.

p-**chlorophenylalanine**: *p*-CPA; an agent that binds irreversibly to tryptophan hydroxylase in the brain, and thereby blocks serotonin biosynthesis.

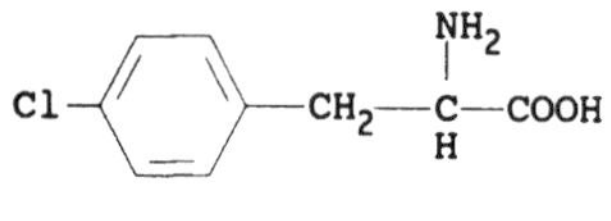

1-(*m*-chlorophenyl)-biguanide hydrochloride: *m*-CPBG hydrochloride; a potent and highly selective agonist for 5-HT$_3$ type serotonin receptors.

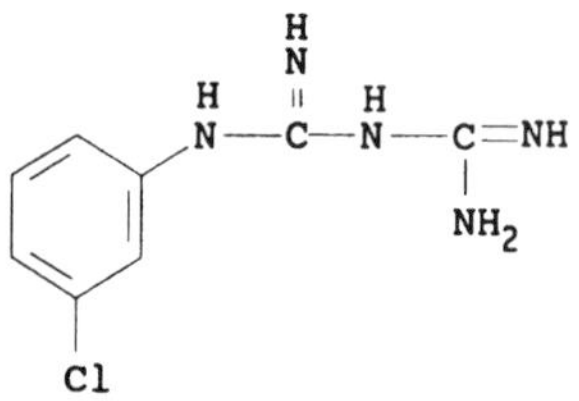

m-**chlorophenylpiperazine**: an agent that stimulates appetite in laboratory animals.

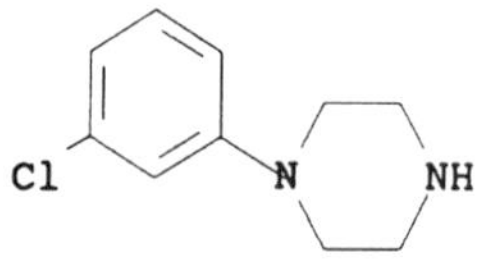

chlorophylls: light-absorbing pigments made by organisms that engage in **photosynthesis** (*q.v.*), composed of a porphyrin (pheophytin, which resembles the erythrocyte porphyrin but has different side-chains on the rings, and holds magnesium rather than iron), plus a phytol side-chain. Green plants, algae, diatoms, dinoflagellates, and some bacteria make chlorophyll a (in which the asterisk in the structure shown represents a methyl group). Green plants and green (but not red) algae also make chlorophyll b (which absorbs at different wave lengths, and in which the asterisk represents a formyl group). In brown algae, diatoms, and dinoflagellates, the a type is associated with a third kind, chlorophyll c. Different, but related pigments (bacteriochlorophylls) are made by prokaryotes that do not release oxygen to the environment. *See* also **grana**.

chloroplasts: complex organelles of higher plants, in which photosynthesis is accomplished. A typical cell contains 50-200, each 5-2.0 μm long and 3-10 μm in diameter. The bilipid layer outer membrane, which resembles endoplasmic reticulum, is freely permeable to small ions

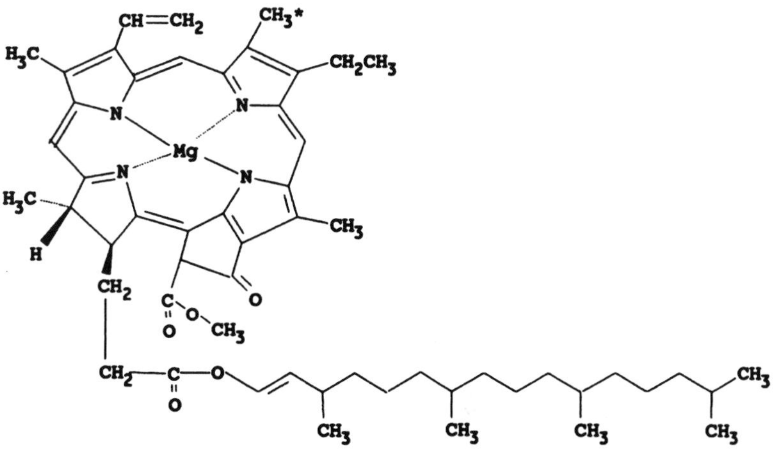

chlorophylls

and molecules, and to some larger ones. The inner membrane surrounds the stroma (matrix), which contains many enzymes, most of which are used for the dark reactions of photosynthesis. It permits diffusion of water and respiratory gases, but is impermeable to protons, hydroxyl ions, most charged molecules, and many small uncharged types. Selective transport across it requires an adenine nucleotide translocase (which mediates ADP entry, but not ATP egress), a dicarboxylate translocase (for bidirectional movements of dicarboxylic acids), and a phosphate translocase that facilitates phosphate entry in exchange for dihydroxyacetate or 3-phosphoglycerate. The interior of a chloroplast contains 10-100 grana (stacks) of flattened membranous disks (thylakoids), connected to each other by membranes, that surround thylakoid spaces. The chlorophyll resides in both disks and membranes. Chloroplasts also contain circular DNA which directs formation of messenger RNAs that code for some of the organelle proteins.

chloroquine: 7-chloro-4-(4- diethylamino-1-methylbutyl-amino)quinoline; an agent that inhibits ATP-dependent lysosome and receptosome proton pumps, and thereby blocks acidification of the vesicle contents. It is used in the laboratory to study intracellular transport, and the degradation of hormone receptors and other molecules taken up by endocytosis; and clincially to treat malaria, amoeba infestations, and lupus erythematosus. The phosphate salt ameliorates some forms of hypercalcemia by inhibiting 25-hydroxyvitamin D conversion to 1,25-di-hydroxyvitamin D.

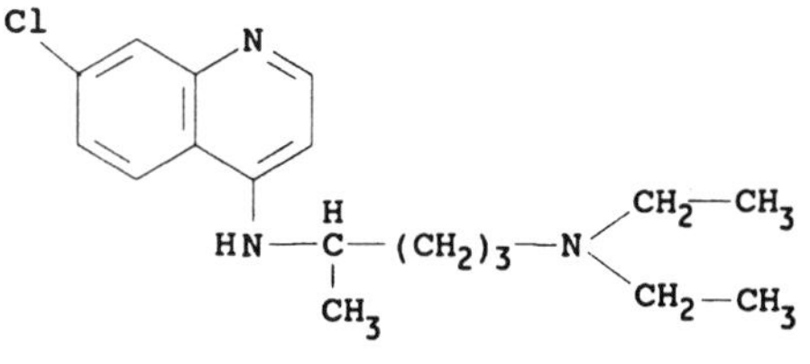

chlorosis: paling (or yellowing) of green plant components, because of impaired synthesis of chlorophyll, and/

or loss of pigments already made. It is caused by light deprivation, and by some pathogens.

chlorothiazide: Diuril; 6-chloro-$2H$-1,2,4-benzothiadiazine-7-1,1-dioxide; a loop diuretic that inhibits Cl^- (and thereby Na^+) transport in distal regions of nephrons, and additionally inhibits carbonic anhydrase activity. It is used to treat edema and hypertension, but can invoke hypokalemia.

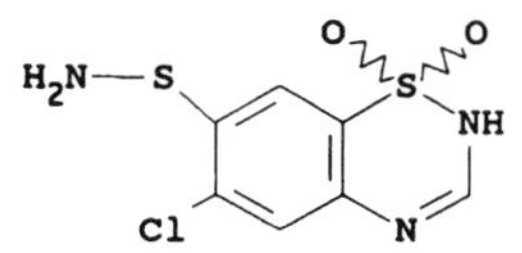

chlorotrianisene, TACE: chlor-*tris*(*p*-methoxyphenyl) ethylene; a non-steroid estrogen receptor agonist.

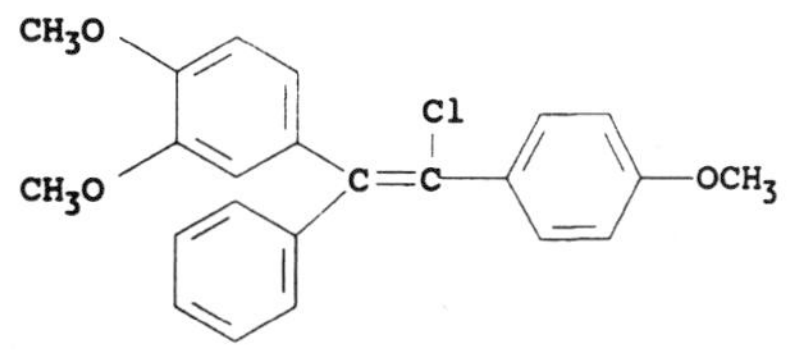

chlorpheniramine: 1-(*p*-chlorophenyl)-1-(2-pyridyl)-3-dimethylaminopropane; an H_1 type histamine receptor antagonist used to treat allergies.

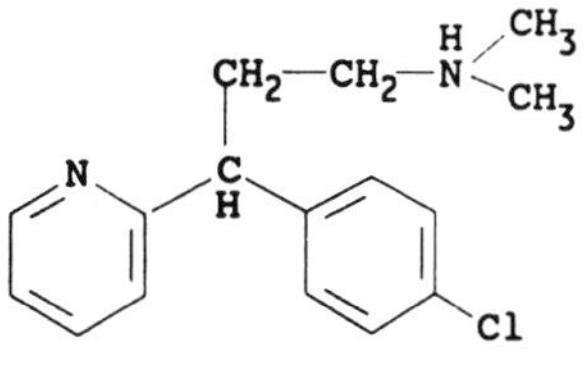

chlorpromazine: *N*-(3-dimethylaminopropyl)-3-chlorophenothiazine; a tranquilizer and sedative used for its "anti-psychotic" effects, to alleviate nausea and control emesis (caused, for example by radiation or chemotherapy), and to potentiate the effects of analgesics. Most of the clinical effects are attributed to dopamine receptor

123

antagonism, but influences are also exerted on α_1-type adrenergic, H_1-type histamine, muscarinic, and serotonin receptors. It additionally lowers blood pressure, possibly by antagonizing calmodulin. Laboratory use for calmodulin antagonism is limited by additional effects exerted on plasma membranes.

chlorpropamide: 1-(p-chlorobenzenesulfonyl)-3-propylurea; Diabinese, Melitase; Stabinol; an oral hypoglycemic agent. It also promotes vasopressin release and enhances its anti-diuretic effects, and can exacerbate the hyponatremia invoked by some diuretics.

chlorprothixene: 3-(2-chloro-9H-thioanthen-9-ylidine)-N,N-dimethyl-1-propanamine: a tranquilizer with properties generally similar to those of chlorpromazine, but lower hypotensive potency.

chlortetracycline: Aureomycin; 7-chlorotetracylin; a broad spectrum antibiotic, effective against gram-negative bacteria and some protozoa. It inhibits protein synthesis in bacteria by binding to ribosome 30S subunits and blocking transfer RNA access to acceptor sites. Low doses do not act on mammalian cells, because of low affinity for mammalian ribosome subunits, and because those cells lack plasma membrane pumps that facilitate uptake of the drug.

chlorthalidone: 2-chloro-5-(2,3-dihydro-1-hydroxy-3-oxo-1H-isoindol-1-yl)benzenesulfonamide; a thiazide type diuretic that acts directly on renal tubules and accelerates the excretion of sodium, chloride, and water. It is used to treat edema caused by myocardial insufficiency, and to decrease urine volume in individuals with

diabetes insipidus. Concentrations greater than the ones usually prescribed also inhibit carbonic anhydrases.

chlorthion: O,O-dimethyl O-(3-chloro-4-nitrophenyl) thionophosphate; a cholinesterase inhibitor used as an insecticide.

Chlor-trimeton: a trade name for chlorpheniramine maleate.

cholanic acid: 5β-cholan-24-oic acid; a compound used for bile salt nomenclature.

chole-: a prefix meaning bile.

cholecalciferol: vitamin D_3; 9,10-secacholesta-5,7,10 (19)-trien-3-ol; a secosteroid synthesized from 7-dehydrocholesterol in skin exposed to ultraviolet radiation, or obtained from fish oils and a few other lipid-rich foods. It does not appear to be biologically active, but serves as the precursor of 1,25-dihydroxy-**cholecalciferol** (q.v.) and other hormones, and can be stored in lipid-rich tissues. The most obvious deficiency effects are rickets and osteomalacia.

25-hydroxy-**cholecalciferol**; calcifediol; 25-hydroxy-vitamin D_3; 25(OH)D_3: the major circulating vitamin D_3 metabolite, made mostly in the liver from cholecalciferol, and stored in lipid-rich tissues. Severe hepatic disease impairs its production. Physiological amounts are not

124

biologically active, but serve as precursors of 1,25-dihydroxy-cholecalciferol and other hormones. Blood levels rise during the summer months in individuals exposed to seasonal variations in ultraviolet radiation.

1,25-dihydroxy-cholecalciferol: 1,25-dihydroxyvitamin D$_3$; 1,25(OH)$_2$D$_3$; 1,25-D; calcitriol; the major hormone made from vitamin D, via the reaction catalyzed by 25-hydroxycholecalciferol-1α-hydroxylase. It is essential for efficient intestinal absorption of dietary calcium, which begins in the duodenum but is accomplished mostly in the jejunum. Non-genomic effects on brush border membrane phospholipids augment Ca^{2+} permeability within 20 minutes, but the quantitatively most important actions, which involve induction of a serosal surface Ca^{2+}-ATPase that pumps the ions to extracellular fluids for uptake by the bloodstream, are first detected after one hour. Although the hormone also induces an intracellular calcium binding protein in a dose-related manner, that protein does not directly promote absorption. Rather, it is believed to sequester cytosolic Ca^{2+} (and thereby protect intestinal cells against excessively high levels). It may additionally aid in transport of the ions to the serosal surfaces. 1,25-D accelerates phosphate absorption over most of the length of the small intestine. Some effects on bone are exerted indirectly, via influences on mineral levels in extracellular fluids; but the hormone induces osteocalcin in osteoblasts, affects collagen synthesis, and contributes to mineralization; and it stimulates osteoclasts. The actions on kidneys include negative feedback control over cholecalciferol 1α-hydroxylase, as well as influences on electrolyte excretion. Indirect controls over blood mineral levels include stimulation of calcitonin release and inhibition of parathyroid hormone secretion. Some effects on skeletal muscle, pancreatic islets, and other target cells have been linked with the regulation of cytosolic Ca^{2+} levels. In skeletal muscle, 1,25-D enhances ATP synthesis and Ca^{2+} storage; and deficiency causes weakness. It is a stimulant for thymus glands, activates T lymphocytes, and contributes to hematopoiesis, but also exerts some antiproliferative effects, possibly by inhibiting the release of interleukin-2 and interferon-γ. In skin, it augments tyrosinase responses to ultraviolet radiation. Direct effects on some neurons, some gonadal cells, and other targets have also been described. Since the amounts made are rigidly controlled under physiological conditions, plasma levels do not undergo seasonal variations. 1,25-D directly inhibits its own formation from 25-hydroxycholecalciferol; and inhibitory controls over the same 1α-hydroxylase en-

zyme are also exerted by high calcium and high phosphate levels. The hormone additionally induces the renal cholecalciferol-24-hydroxylase that diverts the 25-hydroxy precursor to 24,25-dihydroxycholecalciferol. A different form of protection is conferred by conversion to 1,24,25-trihydroxy-cholecalciferol in target organs, and to several degradation products in the liver. However, repeated ingestion (or injection) of pharmacological amounts of vitamin D, or administration of large doses of 1,25-D or of 1α-hydroxycholecalciferol, can overwhelm the protective mechanisms, accelerate bone resorption, elevate circulating calcium and phosphorus levels, and promote metastatic calcification.

24,25-dihydroxy-cholecalciferol: 24,25-dihydroxyvitamin D$_3$; 24,25(OH)$_2$D$_3$; 24,25-D; a secosteroid synthesized from 25-hydroxy-cholecalciferol via a reaction catalyzed by 25-hydroxy-cholecalciferol 24-hydroxylase. The circulating levels are highest during the summer months in individuals exposed to seasonal variations in ultraviolet radiation, since sunlight promotes conversion of 7-dehdyhyrocholesterol to vitamin D (the substrate precursor). 1,25-dihydroxycholesterol (1,25-D) induces the enzyme in the kidneys (the major site for synthesis). That hormone also raises the calcium and phosphorus levels; and high concentrations of the ions inhibit the 1α-hydroxylase which converts the substrate to 1,25-D. Since 24,25-D binds to receptors on several kinds of target cells that respond to 1,25-D, but does not stimulate intestinal absorption of calcium, it has been suggested that it maintains some 1,25-D actions without invoking hypercalcemia. There are controversies concerning whether it performs special functions of its own that differ from those of 1,25-D, for example in fetal development, bone formation, and suppression of parathyroid hormone secretion. However, alternative hypoptheses have been offered. For example, observations that avian embryos require vitamin D, but do not undergo normal development when 1,25-D is substituted, have been explained on the basis of poor penetration of the hormone (which is more polar than the vitamin). 24,25-D is metabolized to 1,24,25-trihydroxy-cholecalciferol and other products.

1,24,25-trihydroxy-cholecalciferol: 1,24,25-trihydroxy-vitamin D$_3$; 1,24,25(OH$_3$)D$_3$; a metabolite of both 1,25-and 24,25-dihydroxy-cholecalciferols. It exerts some 1,25(OH)$_2$-D-like actions but is less potent. Its formation protects against accumulation of excessive amounts of 1,25-D.

24,25-dihydroxy-cholecalciferol

1,24,25-trihydroxy-cholecalciferol

25,26-dihydroxy-**cholecalciferol**: a vitamin D metabolite made in the kidneys. Its functions have not been established.

25-hydroxy-**cholecalciferol-23,26 lactone**: a vitamin D degradation product, made in the liver via a pathway in which 23,25-dihydroxycholecalciferol is an intermediate.

cholecalciferol 25-hydroxylase: an enzyme, most abundant in liver but also made by some 1,25-dihydroxycholecalciferol target cells, that catalyzes conversion of cholecalciferol (vitamin D_3) to 25-hydroxy-cholecalciferol. Some negative feedback control is exerted over its activity, but the same reaction can be catalyzed by a less specific cholesterol-25-hydroxylase when toxic amounts of vitamin D are ingested or injected.

25-hydroxy-**cholecalciferol 1α-hydroxylase**: an enzyme most abundant in the kidney (but also made in placenta and elsewhere) that catalyzes conversion 25-hydroxycholecalciferol to 1,25-dihydroxycholecalciferol, and of 1,24-dihydroxy-cholecalciferol to the 1,24,25-trihydroxy derivative. The activity is augmented by parathyroid hormone, and is inhibited by high levels of calcium, phosphorus, and 1,25-dihydroxy-cholecalciferol.

25-hydroxy-**cholecalciferol 24-hydroxylase**: an enzyme present in highest concentrations in the kidneys that catalyzes conversion of 25-hydroxy-cholecalciferol to 24,25-dihydroxy-cholecalciferol, and thereby diverts the substrate away from the 1α hydroxylase pathway. Lower concentrations in bone and other calciferol targets may protect against 1,25-dihydroxy-cholecalciferol toxicity by converting the hormone to 1,24,25-trihydroxy-cholecalciferol. The enzymes additionally act on other metabolites and contribute to their degradation. 1,25-dihydyroxy-cholecalciferol promotes its synthesis, and high calcium and phosphorus levels augment its activity. Parathyroid hormone is a major inhibitor.

1,25-dihydyroxy-**cholecalciferol receptors**: the major types are glycoprotein members of the steroid receptor superfamily. *See* **vitamin D receptors**.

cholecalcin: *see* **calbindins**.

cholecystagogues: agents that promote bile release to the intestine. Most stimulate contraction of gall bladder wall smooth muscle, and relax the sphincters.

cholecystokinins: CCK; cholecystokinin-pancreozymin; CCK-PZ; pancreozymin; widely distributed amidated peptides with common *C*-terminal amino acid sequences and sulfated tyrosyl moieties. CCK was named for its ability to stimulate contraction of gall bladder wall smooth muscle, and to relax the sphincter of Oddi when released by cells of the duodenum and jejunum in response to fatty acids and chyme. It was subsequently shown to be identical with pancreozymin, which stimulates the secretion of exocrine pancreas enzymes and of pancreatic polypeptide, and was therefore for a time called cholecystokinin-pancreozymin (CCK-PZ). CCK-58 (with 58 amino acids) and CCK-39 may be precursors that are cleaved to yield the others. CCK-33 predominates in the gut, whereas CCK-8 is most prevalent in the nervous system, in which it serves as a neurotransmitter and/or neuromodulator. Large amounts are made in the cerebral cortex, and substantial ones in the limbic system. In some parts of the brain, CCK co-localizes with, and promotes the release of γ-aminobutyric acid, whereas GABA tonically inhibits CCK release. In some paraventricular nuclei neurons, it co-localizes with corticotropin releasing hormone, and is a highly potent stimulant for CRH release. Some effects are direct, but others are secondary to stimulation of fine, unmyelinated sensory subdiaphragmatic vagal afferent fibers that communicate with nucleus solitarius neurons (which, in turn, send projections to the PVN). In the neurohypophysis, it stimulates the release of vasopressin and oxytocin. CCK additionally co-localizes at some sites with dopamine, and it elevates dopamine levels in the PVN. Most central effects appear to be mediated via A type receptors, which localize to discrete brain regions. The N-terminal segment is similar to metenkephalin; and CCK is degraded by enkephalinase. Although it can directly promote analgesia, it opposes analgesic and other actions of enkephalins and endorphins. Its anxiogenic effects are exerted on the limbic system; and injection into susceptible human volunteers precipitates panic attacks. The effects are antagonized by agents that act on opioid receptors, and are attenuated by lesions that interrupt CRH release pathways. CCK also contributes to memory; and it acts on estrogen-controlled sexually dimorphic olfactory pathways that affect reproductive system functions. It can also promote prolactin release via its influences on vasoactive intestinal peptide (VIP) neurons, and has been identified in corticotropes. CCK-33 can be cleaved peripherally to peptides CCK-12 and CCK-8 in the gut, and CCK-4 is the predominant form in pancreatic neurons. Most direct gastrointestinal effects are attributed to actions on B type receptors (which are similar to or identical with peripheral gastrin receptors). The ability to antagonize some gastrin effects is probably related to its similarity to the gastrin C-terminal Ala-Tyr-Gly-Trp-Met-Asp-Phe-NH$_2$ sequences, some of which have sulfated Tyr moieties. The CCK C-terminal heptapeptide, (Tyr) SO$_4$-Met-Gly-Trp-Met-Asp-Phe-NH$_2$, displays similar activity. Appetite suppression appears to be exerted at several levels. Brain CCK levels are low in individuals with some forms of obesity, and many bulimics fail to display normal increments in both CCK and adrenocorticotropic hormone (ACTH) following meal intake. In anorexia nervosa, the systems are overactive. Delayed gastric emptying and consequent gastric distention contribute. CCK also stimulates intestinal motility, and it promotes the release of insulin, glucagon, pancreatic polypeptide, and calcitonin. Other effects may include contributions to fertilization, since CCK is present in acrosomes, binds to receptors on oocytes, and can stimulate sperm motility.

cholera toxin: CT; CTX; an 87K multimeric toxin made by *Vibrio cholerae*, an organism that causes severe diarrhea with loss of sodium and water. The 23K A$_1$ component of the dimeric A subunit promotes ADP-ribosylation of G protein α_{1s} subunits, and thereby loss of GTP-ase activity. This leads to persistent activation of adenylate cyclases. The effects appear to be enhanced by cellular ADP-ribosylation factors. The B subunit, composed of five peptide chains, interacts with a plasma membrane GM$_1$ ganglioside and facilitates A chain entry into cells. CTX is used to study the effects of high cAMP levels, and to identify G protein types involved in signal transduction (since it does not act on G$_i$ or G$_o$ forms). However, it does affect some processes that are inhibited by cAMP, and it can elevate inositol phosphate and Ca^{2+} levels (with or without concomitant effects on phospholipases). Moreover, ADP-ribosylation of esterases, channel proteins, and other cell components may contribute to its effects.

choleragen: cholera toxin.

choleretics: agents that stimulate bile secretion.

cholestane: a 27-carbon saturated steroid used as the "parent" structure for nomenclature of cholesterol, calciferols, and related substances. Letters A, B, C, and D are assigned to the ring structures, and numbers to each of the carbon atoms.

cholestanol: dihydrocholesterol; 3β-hydroxy cholesterol; a cholesterol metabolite in feces and gallstones. It is also present in egg yolks.

cholestatics: agent that diminish bile flow.

cholesterol: cholest-5-en-3β-ol; a sterol in all eukaryote cells (in which it affects membrane fluidity), and the primary precursor of steroid hormones and bile acids. Some cholesterol is obtained from food, packaged into chylomicrons in the small intestine, and delivered to the bloodstream via large lymphatic vessels. Under most conditions, intestinal absorption is limited, and hepatocytes make substantial amounts from acetyl coenzyme A. (The quantities synthesized vary inversely with the dietary intake.) Hepatocytes take up cholesterol from chylomicrons (and from other lipoprotein particles), and package it, along with synthesized molecules, into low density lipoprotein particles (LDLs), which are released to the bloodstream. Although circulating LDLs are major sources of cholesterol for most cell types, the sterol is also synthesized locally for internal use, especially when LDL levels are low. The rate-limiting step is catalyzed by hydroxymethylglutaryl coenzyme A reductase (HMG-CoA reductase). Cholesterol metabolites exert negative feedback control over the enzyme, and they also slow formation of LDL receptors. High density lipoproteins (HDLs) take up excessive amounts and carry them to the liver for disposal. Some is secreted to the bile and stored in the gall bladder. Subsequent delivery to the small intestine facilitates removal of excessive amounts, and provides a lubricant that facilitates egestion of feces. Hormones that contribute to the closely controlled metabolism of cholesterol include insulin, gonadal steroids, and triiodothyronine. Several kinds of genetic defects impair the processes; and dysregulation can have serious consequences. Cholesterol is a major component of most gall stones, and of atherosclerotic plaques. Accumulation in the bloodstream (especially in LDLs) is associated with high risk for myocardial infarction; but agents used to lower the levels do not always confer beneficial effects; and most have serious drawbacks. *See* also **apoprotein (a)** and **apoprotein E**.

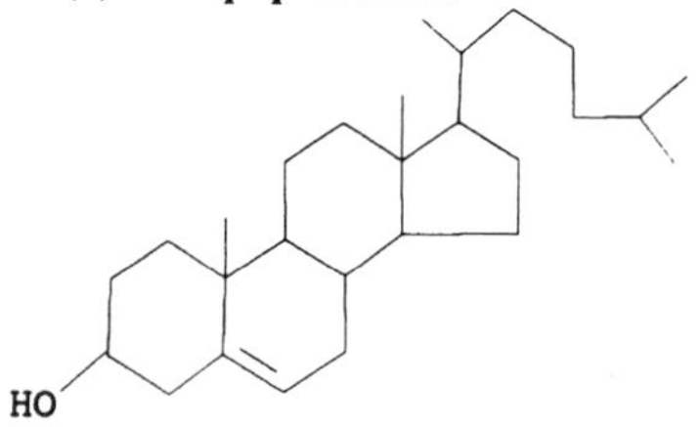

7-dehydro-cholesterol: provitamin D; a sterol made in the liver, and also formed from cholesterol in the intestine, via a reaction catalyzed by cholesterol-7-dehydrogenase. It accumulates in skin and is converted by ultraviolet radiation to cholecalciferol. *Cf* **pre-vitamin D**.

cholesterol acyltransferase: ACAT; an enzyme that catalyzes the generalized reaction: cholesterol + fatty acyl-CoA → cholesterol ester + coenzyme A. The esters accumulate in lipoprotein particles, and are stored in the lipid droplets of cells that make steroid hormones. Cholesteryl esterases release free cholesterol from the esters.

cholesterol binding proteins: CBPs; sterol carrier proteins that facilitate cholesterol transport, especially to mitochondria of cells that synthesize steroid hormones.

cholesterol-7-dehydrogenase: an enzyme most abundant in the intestine that converts cholesterol to 7-dehydro-cholesterol, the direct precursor of cholecalciferol.

cholesterol ester[s]: cholesterol covalently linked to fatty acid moieties. They are stored in lipoprotein particles, and in cytoplasmic droplets of steroid hormone secreting cells.

cholesterol esterases: enzymes that catalyze cleavage of cholesterol esters to free cholesterol and fatty acids. Their activities are augmented by adrenocorticotropic hormone (ACTH) in the adrenal cortex, and by luteinizing hormone (LH) in gonads. Prolactin and γ-melanocyte stimulating hormone (γ-MSH) are additional stimulants for steroid hormone synthesizing cells.

cholesterol 25-hydroxylases: enzymes that catalyze conversion of cholesterol to 25-hydroxy-cholesterol. They are most abundant in the liver, where they are required for bile acid formation. They also act on other substrates, and can promote conversion of cholecalciferol to its 25-hydroxy derivative when cholecalciferol levels are very high.

cholesterol side-chain cleavage: SCC; a set of reactions in which cholesterol is converted to pregnenolone (the major precursor of all steroid hormones). *See* **cholesterol side-chain cleavage system**.

cholesterol side-chain cleavage system: pregnenolone synthase; desmolase; a mixed function oxidase enzyme complex on the surfaces of inner mitochondrial membranes of all steroid hormone producing cells, and in liver

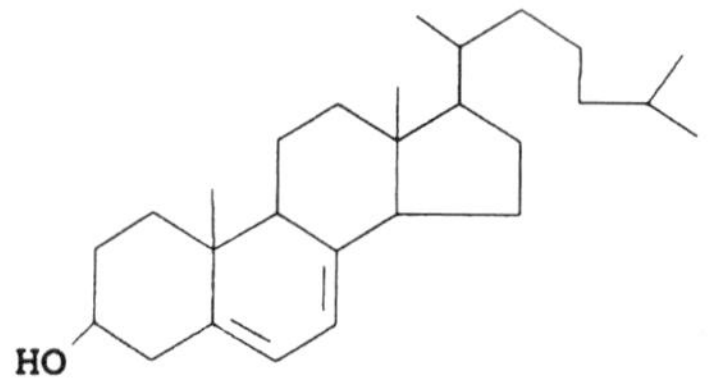

7-dehydro-cholesterol

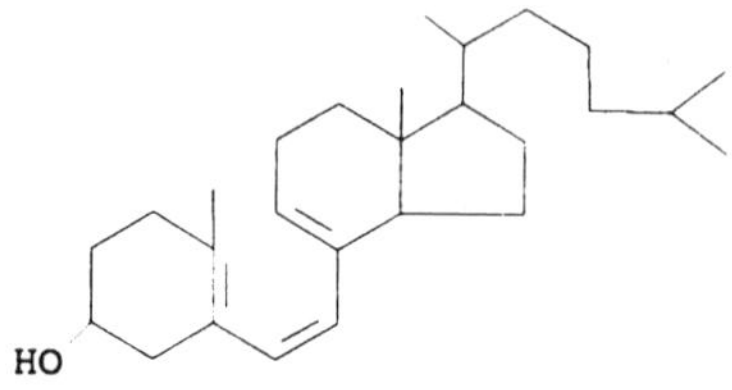

pre-vitamin D$_3$

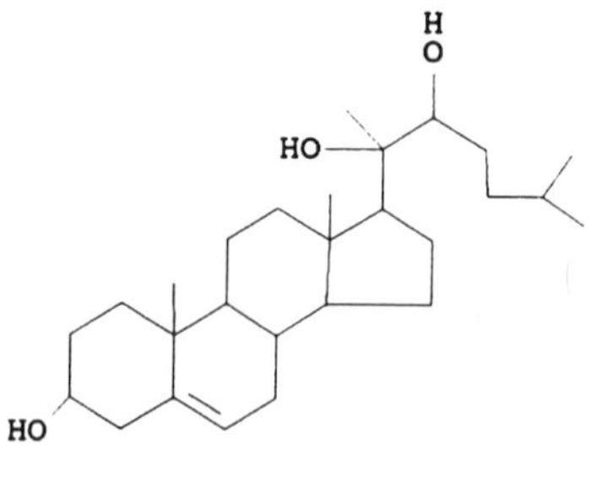

20.22-dihydroxycholesterol

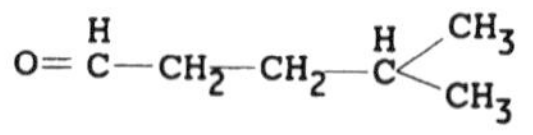

isocaproaldehyde

cholesterol side-chain cleavage system

and some other cell types. It catalyzes conversion of cholesterol to pregnenolone by promoting oxidation at positions 20 and 22, and subsequent release of isocapro-aldehyde (which is rapidly oxidized to isocaproic acid). The system includes a non-heme iron-sulfur protein (adrenodoxin in adrenocortical cells), an NADPH-dependent flavoprotein (such as adrenodoxin reductase), and a substrate-specific heme protein, cytochrome P-450$_{SCC}$. The rate limiting step is cholesterol delivery to the cytochrome component. The activity is augmented by adrenocorticotropic hormone (ACTH) in the adrenal cortex, and by luteinizing hormone (LH) in the gonads, via cAMP-dependent activation of proteins that promote sterol transport.

cholesterol sulfates: cholesterol derivatives in which a sulfate group replaces a hydrogen atom, most commonly on carbon 3. They are direct precursor of some sulfated steroid hormones. Sulfatases act on both cholesterol sulfates and their metabolites.

cholesterol-3-sulfate

cholestyramine: Questran; a strongly basic anion exchange resin with quaternary ammonium groups linked to styrene-divinylbenzene copolymers. By chelating bile salts, it slows delivery of food lipids to the liver, and accelerates bile salt and lipid loss to the feces. Bile salt depletion stimulates conversion of hepatic cholesterol to new bile salts, and cholesterol depletion decreases low density lipoprotein (LDL) receptor expression on hepatic membranes. Cholestyramine is used to treat some forms of hypercholesterolemia, but it blocks absorption of fat soluble vitamins, folic acid, thyroxine, some mediators, and other substances, elevates circulating very low density lipoprotein (VLDL) and triacylglycerol levels, and can cause nausea and constipation. Large amounts invoke fatty degeneration of the liver in laboratory animals; and human use may increase susceptibility for development of liver cancers.

cholic acid: $3\alpha,7\alpha12\alpha$-trihydroxy-5β-cholanic acid; a major bile salt component, made in the liver from cholesterol, and usually excreted as the sodium salt of a taurine or glycine conjugate. When administered, it accelerates bile flow, provides some protection against gallstone formation, improves lipid absorption by intestinal cells, and can alleviate some forms of constipation. The sodium salt is also used as a detergent.

choline: (β-hydroxyethyl)trimethylammonium; a vitamin B complex component that can also be made from serine and S-adenosylmethionine. It is required for the biosynthesis of acetylcholine, phosphatidylcholines, and sphingolipids. Severe deficiencies can cause fatty degeneration of liver cells.

choline acetyltransferase: CAT; an enzyme made by all cholinergic neurons that catalyzes the reaction: choline + acetyl-CoA $\rightarrow$ acetylcholine + coenzyme A. The acronym, CAT is also used for chlorampehiccol acyltransferase.

cholinergic: describes (1) neurons that synthesize and release acetylcholine; (2) the associated receptors; and (3) responses to that neurotransmitter.

cholinergic neuron differentiation factors: CDNFs; several glycoproteins in nervous tissue, and in cardiac and skeletal muscle, that promote neuronal morphogenesis and neurite elongation (but not growth or survival), enhance the ability to synthesize acetylcholine (and in some cases also substance P), and suppress formation of enzymes used to make catecholamines. Four forms have been described: 27K in spinal cord, 29K in sympathetic ganglia, 45K in cardiac muscle, and 50K in brain. One or more of the types may additionally regulate growth and differentiation of embryonic hematopoietic stem and myeloid cells. They may be identical with differentiation inducing factors.

cholinesterases: enzymes that catalyze hydrolysis of choline esters. Acetylcholinesterases cleave mostly acetylcholine, whereas pseudocholinesterases additionally act on related substrates.

cholinomimetics: acetylcholine receptor agonists. The term usually refers to kinds that act on muscarinic receptors.

chondro-: a prefix meaning cartilage.

chondroblasts: immature cells that differentiate from perichondrial fibroblasts, and mature to chondrocytes. *See* **cartilage**.

chondrocytes: mature cartilage cells that develop from chondroblasts. After secreting matrix components, they become trapped in lacunae (most of which contain single cells). *See* **cartilage** and **endochondral ossification**.

chondroitin[s]: highly viscous glycosaminoglycan components of corneas, eye lenses, and some connective tissues, composed of alternating *N*-acetyl-β-galactosamine and β-glucuronic acid moieties. Small amounts are also stored in the secretory granules of some cell types; and activated natural killer (NK) cells release them. Most of the molecules are sulfated. In the A type, which predominates in mammals and most other vertebrates, *N*-acetylgalactosamine moieties are sulfated at 4 positions. Chondroitin sulfate C, sulfated at 6 positions, is the major component of shark cartilage. It can inhibit angiogenesis, and is under investigation for clinical use to arrest the growth of neoplasms. *Cf* **chondroitin sulfate B**.

chondroitin sulfate B: glycosaminoglycans composed of mostly of repeating β-iduronic and *N*-acetyl-β-galactosamine subunits, now more commonly called **dermatan sulfates** (*q.v.*), or, in some cases, β-heparins. They are most abundant in skin, but are also present in arterial walls, heart valves, and other non-rigid connective tissues. *See also* **proteoglycans** and **chondroitins**.

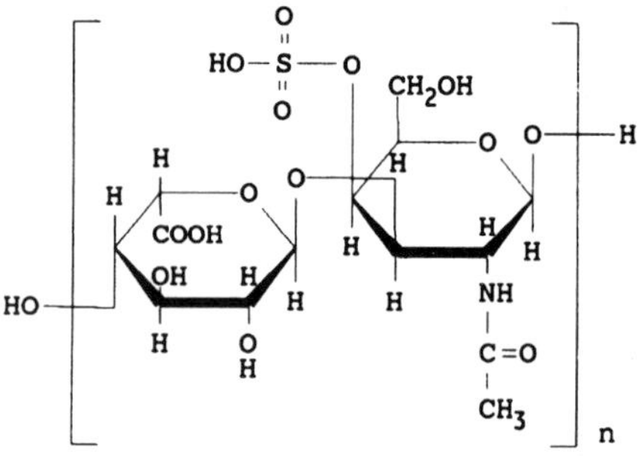

chondrosamine: galactosamine.

chondrosarcomas: malignant tumors composed mostly of cartilage synthesizing cells. The cartilage can become calcified, but it is not replaced by bone.

Chordata: chordates; a phylum that includes all animals that form a notochord, a dorsal hollow nerve cord, and gill slits or gill pouches at some stage of development. The major subphylum is vertebrata (craniata), which includes cyclostomes, fishes, amphibians, birds, and mammals. Acorn worms, sea squirts, and *Amphioxus* are members, respectively of the Hemichordata, Urochordata and Cephalochordata subphyla.

choriocarcinomas: highly malignant neoplasms derived from trophoblast tissue that secrete chorionic gonadotropin (hCG in humans). The uterus is the most common site of origin; but some develop in testes or ovaries.

chorioid plexus: choroid plexus.

chorion: usually (1) the outermost mammalian fetal membrane, formed from trophoblast and extra-embryonic mesoderm cells that associate with the endometrium and are incorporated into the placenta. It develops villi across which substances are exchanged between the mother and the conceptus; (2) the shell of an insect.

chorionic corticotropin: cACTH; an adrenocorticotropic hormone-like peptide made in the placenta, and implicated as a regulator of glucocorticoid synthesis during pregnancy.

chorionic gonadotropins: CGs; glycoprotein hormones secreted in large amounts by trophectoderm, syncytiotrophoblast, and some tumor cells, and in smaller ones by other cell types. The kinds and functions vary with the species, but all are essential for establishing and/or maintaining pregnancy. *See* **hCG**.

chorionic growth hormone-prolactin: *see* **chorionic somatomammotropin**.

chorionic luteinizing hormone release factor: cLRF; a peptide identical with adenohypophysial gonadotropin releasing hormone (GnRH, LRH), made by cytotrophoblast cells and implicated as a regulator of chorionic gonadotropin (hCG) secretion.

chorionic somatomammotropin: hCS; chorionic growth hormone-prolactin: placental lactogen; hPL; a hormone made by human placentas that is chemically related to human prolactin, and (to a lesser extent) to human growth hormone. Production by trophoblast cells begins several

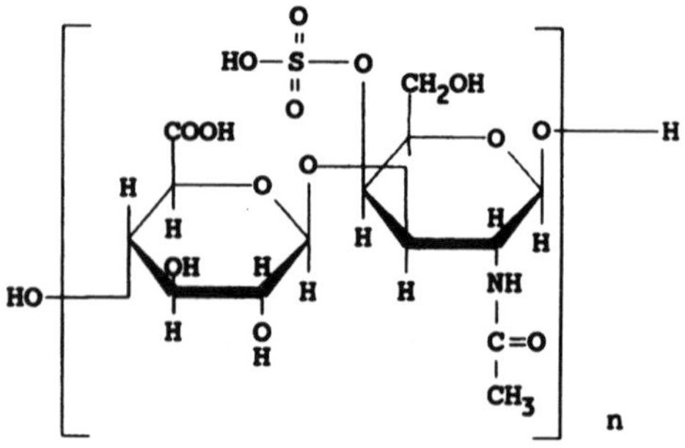

chondroitin sulfate A

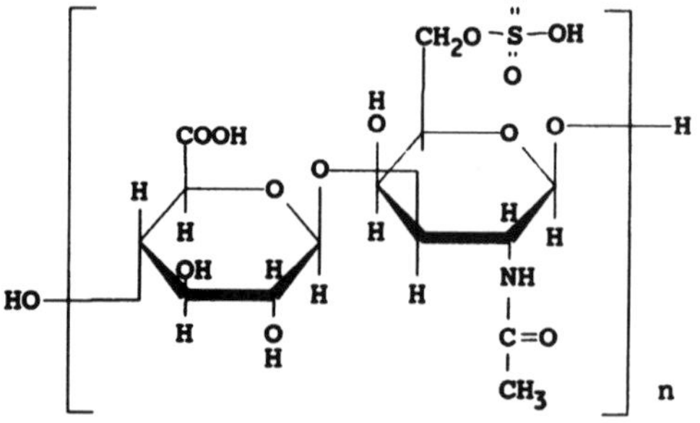

chondroitin sulfate C

days after implantation, and the rate increases as the syncytiotrophoblast develops. Since the amounts made correlate with placental size they have been used to estimate fetal age; but the levels are low when fetuses are small for age. Some hCS enters amniotic fluid, but most is secreted to the maternal system, in which it regulates pancreatic B cells. Maternal plasma levels rise during fasting, and the hormone then decreases glucose oxidation, enhances lipolysis, and can cause ketosis. Following food intake, it promotes lipogenesis. It has been proposed that hCS augments the glucose supply to conceptuses when the mother is fasting or undernourished, and facilitates maternal accumulation of energy reserves for use during pregnancy and lactation when food intake is adequate. It may also contribute to mammary gland maturation during pregnancy, but is proposed to inhibit milk synthesis by competing for prolactin receptors. High levels are implicated in the etiology of the transient diabetes mellitus-like syndrome that develops in some women during pregnancy. According to some observers, the hormone performs no useful function in well-nourished pregnant women.

chorionic thyrotropin: cTSH: a glycoprotein hormone made by human placentas that is chemically and biologically related to adenohypophysial thyroid stimulating hormone.

chorionic villus sampling: techniques for detecting genetic defects in conceptuses, in which uterine cannulas are used to collect extra-embryonic cells. They can be performed in women as early as the ninth week post-conception.

choroid plexus: chorioid plexus: a network of ependymal cells and blood vessels that lines the cerebral ventricles. It secretes, absorbs, and regulates the volume and composition of cerebrospinal fluid, and mediates transfer of hormones and other regulators to and from the bloodstream. It may additionally synthesize hormones and transport substances to and from the pineal gland.

Christmas factor: *see* **factor IX**. *Hemophilia B* is caused by an X-linked genetic defect that impairs its production.

chromaffin bodies: chromaffin cell aggregates.

chromaffin cells: cells that originate in neural ectoderm, store catecholamines, stain brown when treated with aqueous potassium chromate (which oxidizes the amines), and release their products when their nicotinic type acetylcholine receptors are activated. Most additionally make enkephalins and other peptides. In fetuses, clumps of cells form chromaffin bodies, including the organs of Zuckerkandl that migrate to the para-aortic bodies, or accumulate near the inferior mesenteric arteries. Ones that originate in the neural crest are progenitors of adrenomedullary cells. Many of the fetal cells die, but small numbers persist in mature skin, gonads, and prostate glands, and around sympathetic ganglia. Postnatally, they occur predominantly in the adrenal medulla. Postganglionic sympathetic neurons are not usually included in the category, because they contain only small quantities of the amines; but some authors suggest that the enterochromaffin cells of the gut, and other cells outside the adrenal gland with similar staining properties that do not receive preganglionic innervation should be included.

chromatids: the structures formed when chromosomes undergo longitudinal duplication in preparation for mitosis or meiosis. Sister chromatids, which are identical to each other, are initially joined by centromeres. They separate at mitotic metaphase, and one complete set travels to each pole during anaphase. During the synapsis stage of meiosis, they associate with the chromatids of homologous chromosomes to form tetrads.

chromatin: heavily staining components of cell nuclei, composed of mostly of nucleic acids and proteins. During interphase, they appear granular or thread-like. *See* also **euchromatin, heterochromatin**, and **chromosomes**.

chromatin bodies: Barr bodies.

chromatin condensation factors: nuclear components that promote highly ordered chromosome coiling. The levels rise during cell cycle M phases.

chromatin negative: *see* **Barr bodies**.

chromatin positive: *see* **Barr bodies**.

chromatocytes: cells that synthesize and/or contain large quantities of pigments.

chromatography: techniques for separating, purifying, and identifying mixture components, based on differences in partition coefficients between solid-liquid, liquid-liquid or liquid-gas phases. In *paper c.*, paper serves as a stationary support, through which test materials in immiscible solvents travel via capillarity. In *thin layer c.* (TLC), the support is cellulose or some other inert material spread over a glass plate. For *two-dimensional c.*, separation is made with one solvent, the support is rotated 90°, and the process is repeated with a different solvent. Electrophoresis (which separates on the basis of differences in isoelectric points) can be used instead of chromatography for the second process. *Ion exchange c.* is especially useful for amino acids. The stationary phase is an anionic or cationic resin that binds oppositely charged molecules, but the separation can depend in part on hydrophobic and other nonionic forces. For *affinity c.*, the stationary phase holds antigens, antibodies, or other (naturally occurring or synthetic) components that bind specifically to test material domains. Solid phases composed of gel particles that separate on the basis of molecular size are the supports for *gel c.* In *gas c.*, which is used mostly for lipids, the moving phase is an inert gas, and separation is based on differences in volatility. The specimens can be held on solid supports. *High pressure (high performance) liquid chromatography*, HPLC, employs high pressures to achieve fine resolution.

chromatolysis: disintegration of strongly staining entities, a term that usually refers to the changes in neuron Nissl bodies that follow axon injury.

chromatophores: cells that contain moveable pigment granules, such as melanophores or iridophores. They occur in the skins of fishes, amphibians, and some reptiles, and in the irises of birds.

chromomycin A₃

chrome hematoxylin: hematoxylin with a chromium salt mordant. It is used to stain myelin.

chromium: Cr; an element (atomic number 24, atomic weight 51.996). It is an essential nutrient, required in trace amounts. The deficiency effects include impaired glucose tolerance which appears to be related to insulin resistance, cholesterol metabolism defects, subnormal high density, and elevated low density lipoprotein numbers in blood plasma, and neuropathies. Cr may function at some sites as a coenzyme. Both synergistic and antagonistic interactions with vanadium have been suggested. A radioactive isotope (^{51}Cr) is used to label erythrocytes.

chromobindins: proteins in chromaffin cell granules, chemically related to calectrins, that display calcium-dependent binding to phospholipids. They are believed to contribute to exocytosis.

chromogen: any color-forming agent.

chromogranins: calcium binding glycoproteins in the secretory granules of all endocrine and neuroendocrine (but not exocrine) cells, and in hormone-secreting tumor cells. They undergo tissue specific cleavage to several biologically active peptides. Both the glycoproteins and their products co-localize with hormones and neurotransmitters. They can be co-released, but the amounts of the two kinds of molecules do not necessarily vary in parallel. Although some chromogranins and their products may stimulate hormone and/or neurotransmitter release, others appear to inhibit exocytosis by binding Ca^{2+} and promoting granule condensation. Chromogranin A (secretory protein I, SP-1) is a 450-amino acid acidic glycoprotein. 74K and 60K molecules may be precursors. The term *pancreastatin* has been applied to at least two

carboxyamidated peptides that inhibit glucose stimulated insulin release, one composed of chromogranin A amino acids 243-294, and the other of amino acids 240-288. *Parastatin*, which inhibits parathyroid hormone release, is composed of amino acids 251-294. *Chromostatin*, which inhibits catecholamine release, is an *N*-terminal peptide composed of amino acids 5-24. The functions of chromogranins B and C are not known.

chromomembrins: protein components of secretory granule membranes that are not released with the secretory products.

chromomycin A₃: 3β-*O*-(4-*O*-acetyl-2,6-dideoxy-3-*C*-methyl-α-arabino-hexopyranosyl)-7-methylolivomycin D; an antibiotic made by *Streptomyces griseus* that inhibits both DNA and RNA polymerases by intercalating between G and C nucleotides. It is used to treat some forms of cancer.

chromophils: cells with granules that stain with dyes. Examples include thyrotropes, gonadotropes, somatotropes, and lactotropes. *Cf* **chromophobes**.

chromotropism: movement or orientation towards, or other responses to a specific color or pigment.

chromophobes: cells devoid of granules that stain with dyes; *cf* **chromophils**. The ones in the adenohypophysis may be degranulated or degenerating cells, ones that contain granules too small to be visible under light microscopy, nonsecretory types, or immature secretory cell precursors.

chromosomal sex: genetic sex; the kinds of sex chromosomes possessed by an individual. Most normal male mammals have one X and one Y type, and most normal females two of the X type. Certain kinds of mutations and/or deletions disrupt the usual relationships to **phenotypic sex** (*q.v.*).

chromosome[s]: units composed of DNA, some RNA, and some proteins, that replicate during cell cycle interphase and carry the genetic information to daughter cells. In quiescent (nondividing) eukaryote cells, they are suspended in nucleoplasm, which is surrounded by a double nuclear membrane. A typical "resting" somatic cell is said to be diploid, because its chromosomes occur in homologous pairs whose numbers vary with the species. Most are autosomes with common characteristics in males and females. The two members of a homologous pair are morphologically identical, and they carry the same kinds of genes. Corresponding types (alleles) perform similar functions, and can be either identical, or slightly different in DNA make-up. (For example, two related genes can code for eye color, but one for blue and the other for brown.) The typical cell also contains a pair of sex chromosomes, so named because they differ in males as compared with females. Human types have 22 pairs of autosomes, plus two X type sex chromosomes in females, and one X type plus one smaller Y in males. When a somatic cell prepares for division, all chromosomes replicate, and the two identical sister chromatids of a pair are joined by a centromere. During mitosis, the chromatids separate, and each daughter cell receives one complete set. Germinal cells (primary spermatocytes and primary oocytes) divide by meiosis, which proceeds in two stages. Replicated homologous chromosomes pair, and the first division yields two cells, each of which contains two copies of a single set of alleles (but *see* **crossing over**). The second division leads to the formation of haploid cells, each of which contains a single copy of one set of alleles. The diploid number is restored by fertilization. *See* also **nucleosomes, histones, nonhistone proteins**, and **mitochondrial chromosomes**. Prokaryote cells do not have nuclear membranes. Most have a single circular chromosome suspended in the cytoplasm.

chromosome banding: *see* **banding patterns**.

chromosome jumping: *see* **chromosome walking**.

chromosome map: *see* **genetic map**.

chromosome puffs: swollen (decondensed) regions of chromosomes that are actively engaged in DNA replication or transcription. They are prominent in the giant chromosomes of insect salivary gland cells.

chromosome walking: a laborious, but effective technique for locating a specific DNA segment on a gene bank chromosome. If D is the desired segment, K is a gene known to be present, and letters C through L represent contiguous DNA segments known to include K, the search can begin with construction of a K segment probe that hybridizes with, and thereby identifies fragments KLM, JKL, and IJK (none of which contain D). Next, an IJK probe is obtained and used to identify fragments

JKL, HIJ, and GHI. The "walk" is continued with a GHI probe that identifies GHI, FGH, and EFG. Finally, probe EFG identifies fragments DEF and CDE. A more recently developed, less time-consuming technique, chromosome *jumping*, uses larger fragments and takes advantage of chromosomal aberrations that serve as markers.

chromostatin: a peptide cleaved from chromogranin A in catecholamine secreting cells that inhibits release of the regulator. It is composed of amino acids 5-24 of the precursor. The human type has the amino acid sequence: Ser-Asp-Glu-Asp-Ser-Asp-Gly-Asp-Arg-Pro-Gln-Ala-Ser-Pro-Gly-Leu-Gly-Pro-Gly-Pro.

chronaxie: chronaxy; the minimum time period required to invoke a response when a stimulus two times the threshold intensity is presented.

chronic: of extended duration; the term usually refers to a condition that develops slowly and persists, or to an agent that is presented over an extended time period; *cf* **acute**.

chrono-: a prefix meaning time.

chronobiology: the study in living organisms of time-related phenomena, such as life-spans or aging processes.

chronotropic: affecting the rates of rhythmic processes (such as cardiac cycles).

chrysalis: an insect pupa with a relatively rigid integument but no cocoon.

chryso-: chrys-; a prefix meaning gold.

chrysotherapy: treatment of diseases with gold preparations.

CHTX: charybdotoxin.

Chvostek's sign: facial muscle spasms invoked by a tap on the facial nerve. It is used as a preliminary test for hypocalcemia, but small numbers of healthy subjects display the response.

CHX: cycloheximide.

chyle: the fluid in intestinal lymph vessels. The vessels are called lacteals, because chyle looks like milk when it contains large quantities of lipids.

chylomicrons: globules 80-1000 nm in diameter, composed mostly of triacylglycerols. They also contain some phospholipids, specific kinds of proteins (mostly apoproteins B-48, C-I, C-II, C-III and E), small amounts of cholesterol and cholesterol esters, and traces of fat-soluble vitamins and other dietary lipids. Chylomicrons are synthesized by epithelial cells of the small intestine when food-derived lipids are absorbed, and are largest when the diet is rich in fats. They are taken up by lacteals, transported via larger lymphatic vessels, and delivered to the bloodstream, in which they are visible under light microscopy. Most of the triacylglycerol is hydrolyzed and released by lipoprotein lipases for uptake by adipocytes and other cells. The liver removes the resulting chylomicron remnants and some chylomicrons, and repackages some of the components into different lipoprotein particles.

chylomicron remnants: the particles that remain when most of the lipids have been removed from **chylomicrons** (*q.v.*).

chymodenin: an approximately 5K gastrointestinal tract peptide, implicated as a hormone that stimulates exocrine pancreas cells to secrete pancreatic juice rich in chymotrypsin.

chyme: a semi-liquid mixture of partially digested food and gastrointestinal tract secretions, formed in the stomach and delivered to the small intestine.

chymosin: a pepsin-like enzyme in the stomachs of young ruminants that curdles milk and initiates casein digestion. It was formerly known as rennin, a term still applied to preparations used to make puddings; *cf* **renins**.

chymotrypsins: pancreatic juice endopeptidases that catalyze hydrolysis of peptide bonds formed with carbonyl groups of phenylalanine, tryptophan, or tyrosine. Chymotrypsin A_4 is a 25K serine protease that acts preferentially on bonds formed by aromatic amino acids, but it also hydrolyzes some amides and amino acid esters. *See* also **chymotrypsinogen**.

chymotrypsinogen: a 245-amino acid, single chain proenzyme held together by 5 disulfide bonds. It is made by pancreatic acinar cells, stored in granules, and then secreted. Since it is catalytically inactive, it does not digest proteins in the cells that make it. In the intestinal lumen, trypsin catalyzes cleavage of the bonds between amino acids 15 and 16 to yield π-chymotrypsin, which is active. π-chymotrypsin then acts autocatalytically to remove two dipeptides (amino acid moieties 14-15, and 147-148) to yield α-chymotrypsin, which displays similar activity but is more stable.

Ci: Curie.

CI: (1) color index; (2) coronary insufficiency.

CI-988: [R-(R*,R*,R*]-4-[[3-(1*H*-indol-3-yl)-2-methyl-1-oxo-2-[[(tricyclo[3,3,1,1]dec-2-yloxy)carbonyl]amino]-propyl]amino]-1-phenylethyl]amino]-4-oxobutanate *N*-

methyl-D-glucamine; a selective B type CCK receptor antagonist that blocks the anxiogenic effects.

Cibacalcin: a trade name for a preparation of human calcitonin.

cibracon blue F3GA: procion blue H-B; reactive blue-2; a sulfonated tetrazine dye used to probe nucleotide binding sites on proteins, in affinity chromatography of steroid receptors and nicotine adenine nucleotide-dependent enzymes, and to purify immunotoxins.

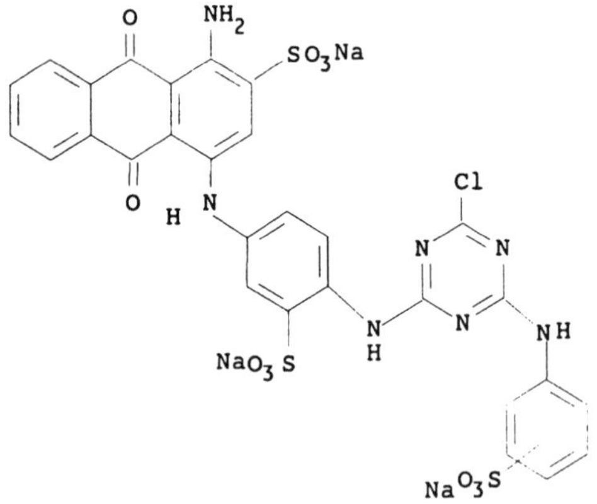

CIF: cytosolic inhibitory factor: a component of estrogen target cells that inhibits the binding of estrogen-receptor complexes to DNA.

CIF-A, **CIF-B**: cartilage inducing factors A and B.

CIG: cold insoluble globulin; a bovine fibronectin preparation.

ciglitazone: 5-[4-(1-methyl-cyclohexo-methoxy)-benzil]-thiazolidine-2,4-dione; an agent that stimulates glucose metabolism, lipogenesis, insulin receptor synthesis, and postreceptor actions of the hormone in laboratory animals with insulin-resistant diabetes mellitus.

cilia: (1) slender motile processes, approximately 0.25u in diameter, that extend outward from cell surfaces. In the respiratory tract, they move mucus and trapped debris toward the mouth, and in the oviduct they facilitate oocyte transport. The appendages some microorganisms use to trap food, and/or propel themselves through liquid

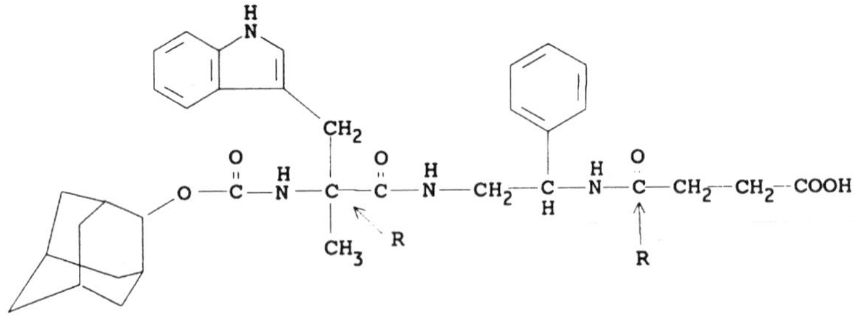

CI-988

134

media, and sperm flagella are longer but have similar structures; *see also* **centrioles**. The axoneme (filament), which is anchored by a basal body, is a membrane-enclosed core of longitudinally arranged microtubules. Nine doublets along the circumference, held together by nexins, extend radial spokes inward toward a central sheath that encloses two singlet A type tubules. Each doublet is composed of a complete (A type) plus an incomplete B type tubule with dynein "arms" that interact with adjacent A tubules to accomplish bending; (2) eyelashes.

ciliary: hair-like; the term can refer to cilia, or describe anatomical structures, as in ciliary ganglia.

ciliary body: a component of the vascular tunic of the eye, innervated by the oculomotor (third cranial) nerve. It contains cells that secrete aqueous humor, and intrinsic muscles that mediate accommodation for near vision. By loosening the suspensory ligament, muscle contraction permits the lens to assume a more globular form.

ciliary ganglion: a parasympathetic ganglion that innervates the ciliary body and the circular muscles of the iris.

ciliary neurotropic factor: CNTF; a 199-amino acid growth factor initially isolated from sciatic nerves that prolongs survival of the embryonic neuron precursors of parasympathetic, sympathetic, and sensory ganglia, promotes differentiation of sympathetic neuroblasts and astrocytes, and induces enzymes for neurotensin synthesis. It is not homologous to nerve growth factor, fibroblast growth factors, or other known neurotropic agents.

Ciliata: ciliates; a class of protozoa whose members use cilia for locomotion. It includes *Paramecia* and some parasites that live in the intestines of vertebrates.

cilium: singular of cilia.

cilostamide: an inhibitor of particulate (but not soluble) phosphodiesterases that catalyze cAMP conversion to AMP.

cimetidine: Tagamet: *N*-cyano-*N′*-methyl-*N″*-[2-[[(5-methyl-1*H*-imidazol-4-yl)methyl]thio]ethyl]-guanidine; an H_2 type histamine receptor antagonist that reduces gastric acidity, and is used to treat peptic and duodenal ulcers. It ameliorates some immune system deficiencies, possibly by inhibiting the activities of suppressor type T lymphocytes.

cimoxatone: a competitive inhibitor of monoamine oxidases, more effective on the A types. It is chemically related to toloxatone, and exerts similar effects.

cinanserin: *N*-[2-[[3-(dimethylamino)propyl]thio] phenyl]-3-phenyl-2-propenamide; a mixed agonist/antagonist for serotonin receptors. It stimulates the sympathetic system by acting on central nervous system $5HT_{1A}$ subtypes, and promotes vasopressin release via $5HT_{1c}$ and $5HT_2$ subtypes.

cinchona: the dried roots and stem barks of cinchona trees. It contains substantial quantities of quinine, some cinchonine, and several other alkaloids used for medicinal purposes.

cinchonine: cinchona-9-ol; an alkaloid made by *Cinchona micrantha* and related species, with quinine-like properties. It is used to protect against, and to treat malaria.

cinchophen: 2-phenyl-4-quinolinecarboxylic acid; a synthetic anti-inflammatory agent with aspirin-like properties, no longer used for its analgesic and antipyretic activities, or to treat gout, because it is hepatotoxic.

cingulate gyri: bilateral limbic system components of the cerebral hemispheres that border the corpus callosum.

cingulin: a 22K tight junction protein.

cinnamic acid: 3-phenyl-2-propenoic acid; a component of coca leaves, made in plants via a pathway catalyzed by phenylalanine ammonia lyase, and converted to salicylic acid.

$$HC=\overset{H}{C}-COOH$$

ciprofibrate: 2-[4-(2,2-dichlorocyclopropyl)phenoxy]-2-methylpropanoic acid; an agent with actions similar to those of clofibrate, but more potent. It enhances receptor-mediated clearance of low density lipoproteins (LDLs), and is used to lower plasma cholesterol levels.

$$Cl_2\text{-cyclopropyl}-\text{phenyl}-O-\overset{CH_3}{\underset{CH_3}{C}}-COOH$$

circadian: describes biological rhythms with periodicities of around one day. Some types are generated by environmental signals. Endogenous types usually have 23-26 hour cycles when free running, but can be entrained to 24 by environmental light/dark cycles or other regularly recurring cues. Many are superimposed on shorter cycles with smaller amplitudes.

circannual: circumannual.

circatrigintan: describes biological rhythms (for example human menstrual cycles) with periodicities of approximately 30 days.

circhoral: describes biological rhythms with approximately one hour cycles.

Circle of Willis: a channel of anastomosing blood vessels at the base of the brain that includes the anterior and posterior communicating arteries. It encircles the hypophysial and chiasmatic regions and receives blood from the right and left internal carotid, and the anterior, middle, and posterior cerebral arteries.

circumannual: circannual; describes biological rhythms (for example some seasonal reproductive system patterns) that recur yearly.

circular dichroism: *see* **dichroism**.

circumventricular organs: CVO; vascular and ependymal cell complexes in the brain that facilitate communication between blood and cerebrospinal fluid, and provide entry sites for substances that circulate in the bloodstream. They have receptors for hormones and neurotransmitters, and at least some secrete hormones. *See*, for example **subfornical organs** and **OVLT**. The neurohypophysis, pineal gland, and area postrema contain such complexes.

cirrhosis: chronic disease characterized by diffuse fibrosis and nodular regeneration. The term usually refers to liver disorders (some of which are caused by alcoholism or exposure to volatile environmental toxins), but is also applied to some lung diseases.

cis: describes (1) a configuration in which two chemical groups of a compound attached to different carbon atoms are on the same side of the molecule; (2) a transcription factor or other agent that binds to a molecule and affects another part of the same molecule; (3) the occurrence of two alleles on the same chromosome. *Cf trans*.

cis **activation**: describes the stimulatory effects of one part of a complex molecule (such as a DNA) on other components of the same molecule, or of factors that bind to one part of that molecule and affect another. *Cf trans* **activation**.

cis **dominance**: the control exerted by a genetic locus over the activity of one or more adjacent loci on the same chromosome.

cisplatin: Platinol; *cis*-diamminodichloroplatinum; an agent that cross-links DNA strands by binding to guanine bases, impairs methionine transport, and antagonizes folic acid actions. The therapeutic effects are attributed to specific recognition by HMG1 (a high mobility group protein essential for DNA repair), and possibly also by other cellular factors essential for survival, of cisplatin-modified DNA. Although it is a potent inhibitor of DNA replication, effective for retarding the growth of some ovarian and other cancers resistant to other chemotherapeutic agents, its use is limited by its nephrotoxic, ototoxic, mutagenic, and teratogenic properties.

$$\begin{array}{c} Cl^- \\ \\ Cl^- \end{array} Pt^{++} \begin{array}{c} NH_3 \\ \\ NH_3 \end{array}$$

cistern: cisterna [cisternae]: a membrane-enclosed, fluid-filled cavity, for example an endoplasmic reticulum compartment, or a brain region filled with cerebrospinal fluid.

cis-trans **isomerization**: conversion from a *cis* (definition 1) to a *trans* configuration, usually catalyzed by an isomerase. Reactions of this kind occur, for example, during fatty acid oxidation and visual excitation. Most enzymes that act on one isomeric form do not affect its counterpart.

cistron: a DNA segment that codes for a specific protein, plus adjacent regions that control its expression. Cistron is a more restricted term than gene (which can include DNA regions that exert influences on other genes).

citrate: citric acid ion; a key intermediate in the tricarboxylic acid cycle, a participant in several other metabolic pathways (*see*, for example **citrate lyase**), and a regulator of several enzymes (including acetyl-CoA carboxylase and phosphofructokinase). Some properties are linked with its ability to combine with Ca^{2+} to form poorly ionized salts, and thereby lower free Ca^{2+} concentrations. Seminal fluid citrate retards semen coagulation; and sodium citrate is added to drawn blood to prevent clotting. Parathyroid hormone promotes citrate accumulation in bone cells by inhibiting isocitric dehydrogenase, and this partially explains PTH-mediated elevation of extracellular fluid calcium:phosphorus ratios. Calcium citrate diffuses out of bone (without phosphate) and is taken up by the bloodstream. Some calcium then accumulates in the bloodstream, as the citrate is excreted to urine, or is oxidized by cells. Sodium citrate administration can invoke alkalosis, since the anion is oxidized, and some of the Na^+ liberated associates with bicarbonate to raise $NaHCO_3$:$HHCO_3$ ratios. *See also* **citric acid.**

citrate lyase: an enzyme that catalyzes cleavage of citrate to oxaloacetate + acetate. Oxaloacetate is used in the tricarboxylic acid cycle, for biosynthesis of some amino acids, and in other metabolic pathways.

citrate synthase: citrate synthetase; citrogenase: an enzyme that catalyzes the reaction: oxaloacetate + acetyl coenzyme A → citryl-coenzyme A. The product is rapidly hydrolyzed to free citrate; *see* **tricarboxylic acid cycle.** Glucocorticoids augment synthesis of the enzyme. Insulin indirectly accelerates citrate formation in the liver, but it activates citrate lyase.

citric acid: 2-hydroxy-1,2,3-propane tricarboxylic acid; The acid and its salts are components of grapefruit, oranges, lemons, pineapples and other fruits. Preparations extracted from them or made by mycological fermentation of sugars, are used as flavoring agents, diuretics, and anti-oxidants, in analytical reagents, and for many industrial purposes that include the manufacture of resins and of some inks. *See also* **citrate.**

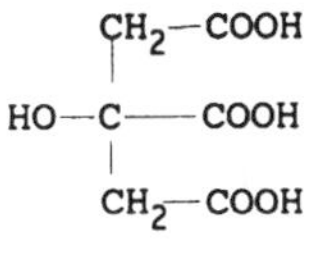

$$CH_2-COOH$$
$$HO-C-COOH$$
$$CH_2-COOH$$

citric acid cycle: Krebs cycle: *see* **tricarboxylic acid cycle.**

citrinin: (3R-*trans*)-4,6-dihydro-8-hydroxy-3,4,5-trimethyl-6-oxo-3H-benzopyran-7-carboxylic acid; a miticide chemically related to antimycin, made by *Aspergillus niveus*, and in small amounts by *Penicillium citrinum*.

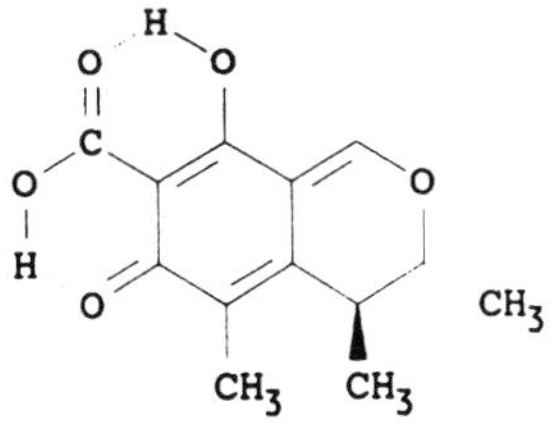

citrogenase: an old term for citrate synthase.

citronellal: 3,7-dimethyl-6-octenol; a component of many volatile plant oils, perceived by insects as an alarm pheromone, and used as an insect repellant.

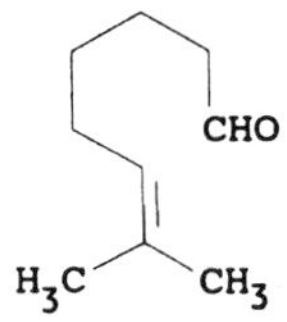

citrovorum factor: CF; folinic acid; FH_4; 5-formyl-5,6,7,8-tetrahydroptyl glutamic acid; a widely distributed folic acid metabolite, identical to **leucovorum** (*q.v.*), and an essential growth factor for some microorganisms. It is used to counteract some of the toxic effects of methotrexate, 5-fluorouracil, and some other chemotherapeutic agents.

citrulline: α-amino-δ-ureidovaleric acid; an amino acid made from ornithine and carbamoyl phosphate in the urea cycle. It combines with aspartate to yield arginosuccinate.

civetone: 9-cycloheptadecen-1-one; a pheromone component of civet musk.

c-jun: *see* **jun.**

C_K: immunoglobulin kappa chain.

CKI, CKII, CKII: casein kinases I, II, and III.

C kinase: kinase C; *see* **protein kinases.**

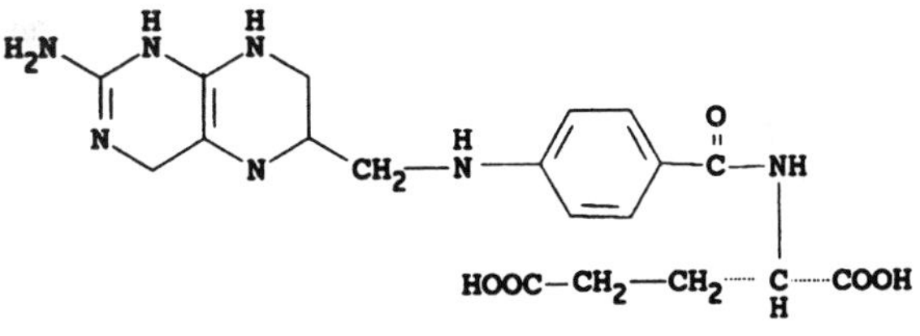

citrovorum factor

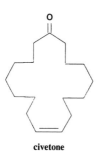

citrulline

civetone

c-kit: a protooncogene that codes for the stem cell factor receptor; *see* **W locus**. Ligand binding activates its tyrosine kinase component.

cl: centiliter; 100 milliliters.

C_L: immunoglobulin light chain constant domain.

cladistics: a system for classifying organisms, in which ancestral types are divided into phyla, and branching trees represent the relationships to more recent species.

class: (1) a set of molecules whose members share some chemical, physical, and/or immunological properties, or perform related functions, or whose synthesis is directed by related genes; (2) a subdivision of a phylum or subphylum. It can be partitioned, successively into subclasses, orders, families, genera, and species. For example, the vertebrate subphylum comprises mammal, bird, reptile, amphibian and other classes. Eutherian mammals form a *subclass*, one order of which includes all primates. Modern humans are members of the hominoid family, the *Homo* genus, and *sapiens* species. (3) an interval arbitrarily selected for statistical analysis. For example, in a study of temperature-related variables, all values obtained for each five degree range could be assigned to a class.

classic complement pathway: *see* **complement**.

class 1 proteins: class I histocompatibility antigens: species-specific 44K glycoproteins whose synthesis is directed by major histocompatibility complex loci (A, B, and C in humans, D and K in mice). They bind noncovalently to β_2-microglobulins, and are expressed on the surfaces of most cell types, including erythrocytes, but not on corneal epithelium, exocrine pancreas cells, central nervous system neurons, villus trophoblast, or spermatozoa. Normal endocrine cells have limited numbers, but large amounts can be made following autoimmune attacks. Cytotoxic type T lymphocytes that mediate graft rejection and destroy cells altered by mutations or viral infections recognize processed foreign antigens when they are presented in association with self type class I proteins.

class 2 proteins: class II histocompatibility antigens; Ia antigens; species specific glycoproteins whose synthesis is directed by major histocompatibility complex loci (mostly DR in humans, and I in mice). They are composed of 30-40K α (heavy) chains noncovalently linked to 27-29K β (light) chains, and are expressed on the surfaces of B lymphocytes, antigen-presenting cells, and some endothelial cells (but not on brain capillaries or placenta). Under pathological conditions, they are also expressed on some other cell types (for example in thyroid glands and pancreatic islets). Helper type T lymphocytes recognize processed foreign antigens that are presented in association with native class II molecules.

class 3 proteins: C4c and B components of the complement system whose synthesis is directed by components of the major histocompatibility complex that do not code for class 1 or class 2 proteins.

class restriction: Cytotoxic T lymphocytes are activated by processed antigens when they are presented in association with class 1 proteins, whereas helper and suppressor types respond when they are presented with class 2 types.

class switching: a change from production of one form of antibody to another, usually from IgM to IgG.

clathrin: a fibrous protein that forms three-legged triskelions, each composed of 3 heavy (180K) and 3 noncovalently linked lighter (30-40K) peptide chains. The molecular complexes polymerize and form flexible basket-like shells around coated pits and vesicles. The pits contain specific kinds of receptors, for example for low density lipoproteins (LDLs), or for compounds with mannose-6-phosphate groups; and ligand binding initiates endocytosis of the occupied receptors. Some pits also contain casein kinase II. Kinase-mediated phosphorylation may facilitate anchoring of receptors to the pits, or endocytosis. It has been proposed that clathrin serves as a "molecular sieve" that admits or excludes specific substances. Alternatively, or in addition, it may facilitate transport of substances between the endoplasmic reticulum and the Golgi apparatus, through the Golgi compartments, or between the Golgi apparatus and lysosomes. Clathrin coated vesicles traverse intracellular pathways different from the ones taken by uncoated vesicles. An ATP-dependent enzyme that catalyzes clathrin removal converts them to endosomes.

clearance: usually, the rate of removal of an entity from the bloodstream, via endocytosis, excretion, or other processes. For substances eliminated mostly by the kidneys, the volume of blood cleared by a single passage through that organ is determined by $C = (U \times V)/P$, where C is the clearance rate in ml/min, U the concentration of the substance in the urine in mg, and V its concentration (mg/ml) in blood.

cleavage: (1) the cell divisions that follow fertilization; (2) the splitting of complex molecules into smaller units; (3) a skin furrow in a region between underlying dermal fiber bundles. *See also* **segmentation**.

Cleland's reagent: dithiothreitol.

CLI: complement cytolysis inhibitor; *see* **clusterin**.

climacteric: in women, the symptoms (psychological as well as physical) and the endocrine events associated with cessation of ovarian cycles, manifested during the time period that begins shortly before, and continues through completion of menopause. Male climacteric is a less well defined entity, related to the changes associated with aging and decreasing androgen production rates. Sensitivity to the steroids may also decline; but the blood levels may not change markedly because hormone clearance rates also decline.

climax: peak; (1) the highest point of sexual excitement; (2) events associated with the brief time period during which the most severe effects of a disease are manifested.

clindamycin: 7-(*S*)-chloro-7-deoxylincomycin; a semi-synthetic antibiotic made from lincomycin that inhibits protein synthesis in bacteria but not in eukaryotes.

CLIP: corticotropin-like intermediate peptide.

clitoris: the female homolog of a part of the penis. It is an erectile sensory organ that develops from the genital tubercle.

clitoromegaly: enlargement of the clitoris, usually caused by of exposure to high androgen levels. *See also* **pseudohermaphroditism**.

CLL: chronic myelogenous leukemia; *see* **leukemias**.

cloaca: a structure that receives the terminations of the reproductive, urinary, and gastrointestinal tracts, through which products are removed from the body. In the females of some species, it also serves as the site for sperm entry. A rudimentary cloaca forms in all vertebrate embryos. It persists in members of most classes; but in eutherian mammalian embryos, it is soon divided into a rectum and urogenital sinus, and the latter undergoes further development.

cloacal gland: (1) an organ in bony fish that contributes to the control of water and electrolyte metabolism by secreting salts; (2) a gland in some mammals that secretes pheromones.

clock: *see* **biological clocks**.

clock mutants: organisms with gene mutations that disrupt, or change the timing of biological rhythms.

clofibrate: Atromid-S; Amotril; ethyl 2-*p*-chlorophenoxyisobutyrate; an agent that accelerates low density lipoprotein (LDL) mediated clearance of circulating cholesterol, and may additionally slow cholesterol synthesis in the liver, accelerate cholesterol degradation, and promote biliary excretion. It lowers plasma cholesterol and very low density lipoprotein (VLDL) levels, and mobilizes cholesterol stores in individuals with dysbetalipoproteinemia, but is not effective for treating most other conditions caused by faulty cholesterol metabolism. It also diminishes blood platelet adhesiveness. Its anti-diuretic effects are attributed to stimulation of vasopressin release and augmentation of the hormone actions on the kidneys. The side effects can include flu-like symptoms, exaggerated appetite, and impotence.

Clomid: clomiphene citrate: *see* **clomiphene**.

clomiphene: 2-[*p*-(2-chloro-1,2-diphenylvinly)phenoxy]triethylamine; a non-steroidal agent that exerts mostly antagonistic effects on hypothalamic estrogen receptors, but can display weak agonist activity. It promotes gonadotropin release by augmenting the secretion of gonadotropin releasing hormone (GnRH, LRH). The citrate salt is used to determine the causes of low gonadotropin levels, to overcome some forms of infertility in men and women, and to treat polycystic ovary disease. The incidence of multiple births in women treated with clomiphene to achieve conception is lower than in those receiving gonadotropins.

clomipramine: chloripramine; 3-chloro-10,11-dihydro-5-(3-dimethylamino)propyl-5*H*-dibenzazepine: a tricyclic antidepressant reported to be more effective than aminotryptiline for treating compulsive-obsessive disorders.

clonal anergy: failure to mount B lymphocyte responses to an antigen (or to a group of closely related ones). *See* **clonal selection theory**.

clonal deletion: loss (usually during fetal life) of B lymphocytes capable of reacting against self-antigens; *see* **clonal selection theory**.

clonal selection theory: an almost universally accepted hypothesis for explaining the specificity of immune system responses. All mature B lymphocytes derived from a single parent type make just one kind of immunoglobulin (antibody) and can respond to a specific kind of antigen (or to a group of very closely related ones); and **T lymphocytes** (*q.v.*) display related forms of specificity. Under normal conditions, B cells are activated mostly by foreign molecules, for example the kinds expressed on the surfaces of infectious organisms. Cytotoxic T cells respond to abnormal cell types within the body, for example ones that have been altered by viral infections. Lymphocyte progenitors that recognize normal body components are destroyed if they encounter them during early stages of differentiation (but *see* **autoimmunity**.) When B lymphocytes that have completed maturation encounter their specific antigen types, they undergo activation and proliferation, and form clones of cells identical to the parent types. Most develop into plasma cells that secrete large quantities of the antibodies, but small numbers become memory cells.

clonazepam: 5-(*o*-chlorophenyl)-1,3-dihydro-7-nitro-2H-1, 4-benzodiazepin-2-one; a benzothiazepine type tranquilizer that acts mostly on γ-aminobutyric acid (GABA) receptors. When used to prevent convulsions, the undesirable effects can include drowsiness, muscular incoordination, cardiovascular and respiratory depression, excessive salivary and bronchial secretion, disturbances in mental functions, and habituation.

clone: (1) genetically identical progeny of a single parent cell; (2) genetically identical organisms derived asexually from one parent.

clonidine hydrochloride: 2-(2,6-dichloroanilino)-2-imidazoline hydrochloride; an α$_2$ type adrenergic receptor agonist with weak, transient effects on peripheral α$_1$ types. Its potent inhibition of presynapthic central nervous and sympathetic system neurons is used to lower blood pressure, and to alleviate migraine headaches in some individuals. Clonidine also augments growth hormone secretion, probably via influences on neurons that make growth hormone releasing hormone (GRH). Its ability to invoke lordosis in female rodents is attributed to actions on peripheral receptors.

cloning vectors: *see* **plasmids**.

clonus: repetitive rhythmic contraction and relaxation. It occurs during convulsions, and can be invoked in a spastic limb by stretching a muscle. It is elicited in nerve-muscle preparations by administering repetitive stimuli at intervals too short to permit complete relaxation (but too long to invoke tetanic contraction).

clopamide: 3-(aminosulfonyl)-4-chloro-*N*-(2,6-dimethyl-1-piperidinyl)benzamide; an orally effective agent with actions on renal tubules similar to those of chlorothiazide. It is used to lower blood pressure and promote diuresis.

clorgiline: *N*-methyl-*N*-propargyl-3-(2,4-dichlorophenoxy)-propylamine; a specific inhibitor of A type monoamine oxidases. It is used as an antidepressant.

closed mitosis: cell division in which the nuclear membrane is retained throughout mitosis, and the spindle forms inside the membrane. When cytokinesis follows, that membrane constricts at its center, and two new nuclei form.

closed reading frame: an RNA segment that contains one or more termination codons. *cf* **open reading frame**.

clotrimazole: 1-(*o*-chlorotrityl)imidazole; an agent that inhibits cholesterol side-chain cleavage, and is used to treat bacterial and fungus infections.

clotting: *see* **coagulation**.

clotrimazole

clozapine: Clozaril; Loptex; 8-chloro-11-(4-methyl-1-piperazinyl)-5*H*-dibenzo[b,e][1,4]diazepine; an atypical tricyclic antidepressant with greater affinity for D_4, than for other dopamine receptor types, used to treat schizophrenia that does not respond to more commonly used agents. It does not increase prolactin secretion, and is not known to invoke tardive dyskinesia (possibly because of preferential binding to limbic rather than extrapyramidal system neurons), but displays anti-adrenergic, anti-cholinergic, and antihistamine properties. The numerous potential side-effects include agranulocytosis, orthostatic hypotension, cardiac dysrhythmias, seizures, fever, vomiting, salivation, and urinary incontinence.

cLRF: chorionic luteinizing hormone release factor.

hCLRF: human chorionic luteinizing hormone release factor.

cluster determination antigens: *see* **CD antigens**.

clusterin: sulfated glycoprotein-2; SGP-2; testosterone regulated repressed messenger-2; TRPM-2; CMB-1; compounds initially identified as factors secreted in large amounts by Sertoli cells that promote aggregation of Sertoli, erythrocyte, and some other cell types, and suggested to function in cell to cell interactions. The best known form is a 70-73K dimer composed of disulfide linked 43K α and 35K β chains. The levels rise in prostate glands and some other reproductive system structures, just prior to the onset of the apoptosis that follows androgen withdrawal. Since it is also secreted by other cell types in response to injury, more generalized roles in apoptosis have been suggested. High levels have been found in the brains of individuals with Alzheimer's, Pick's and other degenerative diseases, and in malignant gliomas and epileptic foci. A very similar messenger RNA is made in scrapie-infected hamster brains, and in Rous sarcoma virus infected quail neuroretinal cells. Clusterin appears to be identical with gp80, which is secreted by kidney epithelial cells. SP-40,40 (CLI), a human homolog, is a potent inhibitor of complement mediated cytolysis that attaches to components assembled from factors C5-C9; and clusterin-complement complexes deposit in the kidneys of individuals with some forms of nephritis. However, roles in neuron differentiation and other physiologcial processes, and in protection of proteins against degradation have also been suggested. Clusterin is similar to or identical with an astrocyte glycoprotein, and to one made by neuroendocrine cell secretory granules called secretogranin IV (glycoprotein III in cattle). Large amounts are synthesized by adrenomedullary, pituitary, ovarian, testicular, and gut endocrine cells, and by thyroid gland C-cells and melanocytes. Lower levels are found in the thymus gland, spleen, kidney, lung, heart, and uterus, and in lactating mammary gland. A second, nonallelic gene that is regulated differently codes for a lower molecular weight type, and most cell types express both genes. Roles for the 70K protein in spermatogenesis and sperm maturation are suggested by observations that it is also made by Leydig cells, and is taken up from seminiferous fluid by spermatid plasma membranes. Cells of the caput epididymis remove it via endocytosis, destroy it in lysosomes, and replace it with the low molecular weight type (which is lost as the sperm complete their journey through the epididymis). Clusterin also appears to be identical to apoprotein-J (Apo-J), a plasma protein that mediates cholesterol transport from cells to extracellular fluids. It forms high density complexes with apoprotein-A-1, and is proposed to function in lipid transport and local lipid redistribution.

cM: centimorgan.

c-mas: a protooncogene that codes for a protein which is similar to or identical with an angiotensin receptor; *see* **mas**.

c-met: a protooncogene that codes for a 145K protein with protein kinase activity. It is closely related to an oncogene identified in some gastric tumors and osteosarcomas; *see* **met**.

CMB-1: clusterin.

CMF: cyclophosphamide-methotrexate-fluoracil; a combination of agents used to arrest the growth of some kinds of breast cancers.

CMK: chloromethylketone.

CMI: cell mediated immunity.

CMOs: corticosterone methyl oxidases.

c-mos: a protooncogene that directs the synthesis of phosphoprotein p39^{mos}, a serine-threonine kinase that plays major roles in meiosis, mitosis, and cell differentiation. *See* **mos**.

CMP: cytidine 5-monophosphate.

c-myb: a protooncogene whose messenger RNA undergoes alternate splicing and directs formation of several related 3.4-4.5K helix-turn-helix type DNA-binding nuclear transcription factors. *See* **myb**.

c-myc: a protooncogene that exerts major influences on cell differentiation, proliferation, and functions by directing production of Myc, a nuclear protein with leucine zipper domains. *See* **myc**.

CNDF: cholinergic neuron differentiation factors.

CNQX: 6,7-dinitroquinoxaline-2,3-dione; a selective antagonist for quisqualate type excitatory amino acid receptors.

CNS: central nervous system.

CNTF: ciliary neurotropic factor.

CO: carbon monoxide.

CoA: Co-A; Co-ASH; coenzyme A.

coagulating glands: accessory reproductive organs of rats and other species, adjacent to the seminal vesicles. They secrete factors that coagulate semen and promote formation of vaginal plugs.

coagulation: sol to gel transformation; clotting, for example of blood, semen, milk, or albumin. Blood clots (thrombi) are composed mostly of fibrin and trapped cells. Their formation involves at least 30 factors, most of which are secreted by the liver. Other regulators protect against intravascular coagulation, or promote dissolution of clots that are no longer needed. When tissue thromboplastin (factor III), a protein-phospholipid component of all plasma membranes, is released by injured cells, it initiates *extrinsic cascades* by activating factor VII (proconvertin) and, in conjunction with it, factor IX (Christmas factor, antihemophilia factor B). Activated factor VII, along with factor VIII (anti-hemophilic factor A), Ca^{2+} ions (factor IV), and factor IX convert factor X (Stuart factor, Stuart-Prower factor) to factor X_a. In the presence of a platelet phospholipid (platelet thromboplastic factor, platelet factor III), Ca^{2+} ions, and factor V (accelerin, accelerator globulin, platelet factor I), factor X_a catalyzes conversion of prothrombin (factor II) to thrombin. Thrombin, in turn, catalyzes conversion of fibrinogen (factor I) to fibrin monomers, and additionally exerts positive feedback control over its own formation. Finally, factor XIII (fibrin stabilizing factor) and Ca^{2+} ions promote polymerization of fibrin and cross-linking of fibrin filaments to form dense networks. The *intrinsic pathway* begins with blood platelet injury or activation (usually because of exposure to collagen), and consequent activation of factor XII (Hageman factor). The pathway can also be initiated by a kinin (formed when circulating kallikrein catalyzes proteolysis of a high molecular weight kininogen). The kinin activates factor XII, a second catalyst for the kininogen. The next step is activation of factor XI (plasma thromboplastin antecedent). Factor XI then activates factor IX and reactions described for the extrinsic pathway follow. Kallikrein, factors XII, XI, X, IX, VII and thrombin, are serine proteases. Factors X, IX, VII and prothrombin are proteins whose synthesis requires vitamin K. Hemophilia A (classical hemophilia) is an X-linked genetic disorder caused by inability to make factor VIII, whereas hemophilia B (Christmas disease) results from factor IX deficiency. *See* also **anti-thrombins, fibrinolysis, plas-**

min, thrombomodulin, thrombospondin, heparin, platelets and **syneresis**.

coagulation factors: *see* **coagulation** for functions of **blood** factors I-V and VII-XIII. Factor VI is no longer regarded as a separate entity.

Number	Alternate Names
I	fibrinogen
II	thrombin
III	thromboplastin; platelet thromboplastic factor III
IV	Ca^{2+}
V	accelerin; accelerator globulin; platelet factor I
VI	——
VII	proconvertin
VIII	anti-hemophilic factor A
IX	Christmas factor; anti-hemophilic factor B
X	Stuart factor; Stuart-Prower factor
XI	plasma thromboplastin antecedent
XII	Hageman factor
XIII	fibrin stabilizing factor

coatomers: COPs; coat proteins; high molecular weight protein complexes that cycle between the cytoplasm and Golgi apparatus, and bind reversibly to Golgi membrane cytoplasmic faces. They are components of non-clathrin coated vesicles that mediate bulk trafficking of large molecules. Four high molecular weight types chemically related to adaptins (170K α-, 110K β-, 98K γ-, and 61K δ-COPs) are associated with several smaller types, two of which are ADP-ribosylation factors (ARF). One ARF seems to be directly involved in regulation of vesicle assembly and disassembly. The binding of at least one type, β-COP (110K) is regulated by a small GTP-binding protein, and is inhibited by brefeldin A. COPs have domains for phosphorylation by kinases A and C; and vesicle dissolution associated with meiosis and mitosis may be related to hyperphosphorylation by p34^{cdc2} kinase.

coated pits: clathrin covered invaginated plasma membrane regions involved in endocytosis. They contain receptors for specific nutrients and regulators. *See* **clathrins**.

coat proteins: coatomers.

CoA-SH: CoA; coenzyme A, represented in this way because its sulfhydryl group combines with other compounds, for example to form acetyl-coenzyme A.

cobalamin: a form of vitamin B_{12}; **cyanocobalamin** (*q.v.*) minus the cyano group that attaches to the cobalt atom. It reacts with deoxyadenosine triphosphate to form coenzyme B_{12} (5′-deoxycobalamin).

cobalamin enzymes: enzymes that require coenzyme B_{12} to function. They catalyze intramolecular rearrangements, methylation reactions, and reduction of ribonucleotides to deoxyribonucleotides. *See* **cyanocobalamin**.

cobalt: Co; an element (atomic number 27, atomic weight 58.933), required in trace amounts. Since it is a component of cyanocobalamin and related cofactors, deficiency causes a rare form of pernicious anemia. High concentrations of cobalt chloride are used in the laboratory to selectively destroy pancreatic α cells, and to inhibit heme synthesis (usually for the purpose of accelerating erythropoietin production). The ions also block Ca^{2+} ion channels via mechanisms that differ from those of nifedipine and related agents. [60]Co is a radioactive isotope used to kill some kinds of cancer cells.

cobralysins: phospholipase A enzymes and other components of cobra venom that promote red blood cell lysis.

cobratoxin: *see* α-**cobrotoxin**.

cobra venoms: poisons secreted by the salivary glands of snakes of the *Naja* genus. Various types lyse erythrocytes and cause other damage by degrading phospholipids or blocking neurotransmission. Some are directly cardiotoxic. *See* also α-**cobrotoxin**.

α-cobrotoxin: a 62-amino acid protein obtained from the venom of the Thailand cobra, *Naja naja kaouthia* that blocks neurotransmission by binding to acetylcholine receptors with lower affinity than α-bungarotoxin. It is used to collect and purify the receptors.

cocaine: 2β-carbomethoxy-3β-benzoxytropane; an alkaloid from *Erythoxolon* leaves that potentiates the effects of catecholamines, mostly by inhibiting neuronal uptake. It is a potent central nervous system stimulant that can invoke dysphoria, mydriasis, emesis, convulsions, and body temperature elevation. The euphoria is attributed mostly to inhibition of dopamine uptake in the limbic system. Addiction develops rapidly, and is often associated with severe personality disorders. It appears to be related to dopamine stimulation of frontal cortex and nucleus accumbens neurons. The stimulation is followed by depression which can lead to respiratory failure. Central effects on the vagus system, and peripheral ones on the sympathetic system, initially slow the heart rate. However, direct, early influences on the myocardium,

cobalamin

and delayed ones that lead to infarction, can cause cardiac arrest. Cocaine also blocks transmission in peripheral nerves and is a potent local anesthetic, but is no longer used for that purpose because it damages tissues.

cockerel: a male chicken less than one year old.

cocarboxylase: an old term for thiamine pyrophosphate.

cocarcinogen: an agent that does not directly cause cancer when presented alone, but facilitates or is essential for the actions of one that does.

co-culture: use of a second cell type (S) when culturing a desired kind (D), to facilitate growth of the D type, or to provide information on D:S interactions. Proliferation of the S types can be prevented by irradiating them before addition.

code: usually, information (for example in the form of nucleotide triplets) that cells or other systems use to direct synthesis of specific substances; *see* **genetic code**.

codeine: methylmorphine; an alkaloid prepared from opium poppies, and used in the form of phosphates and other salts. Its analgesic potency is less than that of morphine, but it synergizes with salicylates, is orally effective and less addictive, and does not invoke respiratory depression. Low doses are used to control coughing.

coding strand: the component of double-stranded DNA that directs transcription; but *see* **complementary strand** and **anti-sense DNA**.

codominance: a pattern of inheritance in which both alleles for a trait contribute to the phenotype; *cf* **dominance**.

codon: a set of three messenger RNA (mRNA) nucleotides that imparts a specific kind of information required for protein synthesis. Most codons hydrogen bond to just one kind of transfer RNA (tRNA) anticodon, and thereby facilitate correct positioning of the associated amino acids on ribosomes. A few are said to be degenerate, because they can pair with two or more anticodon types. Messenger RNAs also contain start codons for initiating, and stop codons for terminating translation. "Nonsense" codons are triplets that do not pair with specific tRNA types. Some do not seem to affect mRNA functions, but mutations or insertions of others can cause premature termination of peptide chain elongation, or accelerate mRNA degradation.

coel-: cel-; a prefix meaning hollow or cavity, as in coelom or Coelenterata.

-coele: a suffix used for hollow cavities, as in blastocoele.

Coelenterata: a phylum of marine invertebrates that includes jellyfish, corals, hydras, and sea anenomes. All have diploblastic bodies composed of a layer of ectoderm, separated by a thin mesoglia from a layer of endoderm that surrounds a central cavity. Coordination is achieved with simple nerve networks.

coelom: the cavity of annelids and of animals higher on the evolutionary scale that develops between two layers of embryonic mesoderm. In mammals, it gives rise to the pleural, pericardial, and peritoneal cavities.

coenzyme: an organic molecule or chemical group that binds to an enzyme and affects (or is essential for) its activity. Many coenzymes are carriers for electrons, hydrogen atoms, or other reaction intermediates. Most are derived from B-complex vitamins. *Cf* **cofactor**.

coenzyme I: an obsolete term for NAD.

coenzyme II: an obsolete term for NADP.

coenzyme A: CoA; CoA-SH: a coenzyme synthesized from pantothenic acid, cysteamine, adenosine and phosphate, that catalyzes acetyl transfer reactions; *see* also **acetyl coenzyme A**, and enzymes that follow that listing

coenzyme A

(such as acetyl Co-A acyltransferases, acetyl-CoA carboxylase, and acetyl-CoA synthetase).

coenzyme B$_{12}$: *see* **cobalamin**.

coenzyme Q: *see* **ubiquinones**.

cofactor: (1) a metallic ion or other substance that augments the activity of, or is essential for actions of an enzyme; (2) an inorganic ion, coenzyme, growth factor, or other agent that contributes to, and/or may be essential for a process, but does not by itself promote the effects.

cofilin: a 21K protein in nuclei and cytoplasm that binds F-actin and contributes to cytoskeleton organization. In muscle cells, it is one of the factors that blocks tropomyosin interactions with myosin.

coherin: a 4K neurohypophysial peptide implicated as a hormone that stimulates intestinal motility.

cohesive end: sticky end; a 5′terminal of a single stranded DNA fragment released by an endonuclease, that hydrogen bonds to a complementary 3′ strand of another fragment released by the same enzyme. The property permits splicing of genes from different species for transfection studies.

cohort follicles: ovarian follicles that accomplish partial maturation during the follicular phases of ovarian cycles, and contribute to reproduction by secreting estrogens. They then undergo atresia, as one or more dominant follicles prepare for ovulation. They are smaller than dominant follicles, produce less estrogen (and probably more androgen) and have fewer luteinizing hormone (LH) receptors.

Cohn fraction II: a serum protein fraction, composed mostly of γ-globulins, obtained by an ethanol centrifugation procedure.

coitus: sexual intercourse. In males of most vertebrate species, both motivation and performance are androgen-dependent. Androgens also stimulate libido in females, but in mammals with estrous cycles, receptivity is regulated by estrogens and other hormones. In induced ovulators, the associated stimulation of nerve endings is essential for mounting the luteinizing hormone (LH) surges that invoke ovulation.

colcemid: demecolcine; *N*-deacetyl-*N*-methylcolchicine; a colchicine derivative used to treat some forms of cancer, and as a laboratory tool that promotes microtubule depolymerization.

colchicine: *N*-(5,6,7,9-tetrahydro-1,2,3,10-tetramethoxy-9-oxobenzo-[a]heptalen-7-yl)acetamide; an alkaloid made by the Autumn crocus, *Colchicum autumnale*, that binds to tubulin polymers and blocks addition of subunits to the growing ends of microtubules (but does not interfere with depolymerization). Since it reversibly arrests cells in mitotic metaphase (by inhibiting spindle formation), it is used to prepare chromosomes for microscopy, and to synchronize cell cycles. By impairing microtubule-dependent vesicle movement, it blocks transport of secretory vesicles to plasma membranes, and thereby exocytosis. The influences on granulocyte migration and histamine release from mast cells can alleviate gouty arthritis. Colchicine also inhibits the secretion of insulin and other hormones, and melanin granule movement in melanophores. It blocks neurotransmitter transport to axon endings and causes accumulation of the molecules in storage vesicles. In some brain regions, it inhibits the synthesis of choline acetyltransferase, but accelerates *c-fos* expression and formation of the p75 nerve growth factor (NGF) receptor component. It can also increase galanin formation. Its use for arresting the growth of some neoplasms is limited by side effects, such as bone marrow dysfunctions, fever, vasoconstriction, vascular damage, and diarrhea.

cold antibodies: cold agglutinins; IgM type immunoglobulins that react with specific blood groups and agglutinate erythrocytes at temperatures lower than 37°C.

cold insoluble globulins: *see* **cryoglobulins**. CSI is a commercial preparation of fibronectin.

cold nodule: usually (1) a thyroid gland protuberance composed of cells that do not take up radioactive iodine, and therefore, presumably, do not synthesizing thyroxine. (Cool nodules take up subnormal amounts.); (2) any cell cluster that does not take up radioactive markers.

colestipol-hydrochloride; Colestid; *N*-(2-aminoethyl)-1,2-ethanediamine polymer with chloromethyloxirane; an ion exchange resin with properties similar to those of cholestyramine.

colicins: proteins made by some strains of *Escherichia coli* and related species that kill other organisms by inserting into plasma membranes and forming ion channels. They are used to study nonspecific defenses against infection, and cellular mechanisms for inserting proteins into membranes.

coliphage: a bacteriophage that attacks *Escherichia coli*.

collagens: extracellular fibrous proteins that collectively account for almost a quarter of the total body protein in mammals. Bone contains the largest amounts, but collagen is also a major component of cartilage, dentin and

145

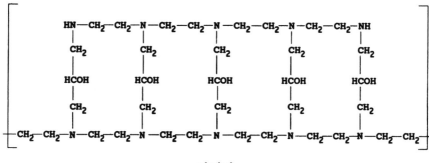

colestipol

dermis, and it is present around blood vessels and between cells of the liver, kidneys, and other organs. Formation of at least 13 types (I-XIII) is directed by at least 25 genes. All are composed of sets of three approximately 1000-amino acid α peptide chains that wind around each other to form triple helices. Every third moiety is glycine, and there are substantial amounts of proline, alanine, and lysine, along with small numbers of other amino acid components (but no cysteine in most types). Pro-α chains undergo extensive intracellular posttranslational processing that includes glycosylation, and proline and lysine hydroxylation, to form *procollagens*, which are secreted. The chains are then shortened by selective proteolysis, and cross-linked; *see* **hydroxylysine**. Some types are assembled into fibrils. Roman numerals designate the kinds of α chains (which differ from each other in amino acid composition, glycosylation, and distribution). For example $\alpha_1(I)_2 \alpha_2(II)$ contains two type I α_1 chains, and one type II α_2. The genes have corresponding names, such as *COL1A2* for type I α_2 chains. Types I, II, III, V, and XI are fibrillar (have long arrays of overlapping, cross-linked helices). Fibroblasts, chondrocytes, and osteoblasts are the major sources. Type I, which is low in hydroxylysine, predominates in bone, dentin, tendon, skin, and fascia, whereas Type II (heavily glycosylated and rich in hydroxylysine) predominates in cartilage. Type III, the major collagen of reticular fibrils, is low in hydroxylysine. Type IV is found in kidney glomeruli, eye lens capsules, and the basal laminae of epithelial and endothelial tissues. Type V is widely distributed in small amounts, especially in the basal laminae of smooth and striated muscle. Other collagens form networks of shorter units; and type IX has sulfated glycosaminoglycan side-chains. In addition to providing strength, mechanical protection, and varying amounts of rigidity, collagens contribute to cell differentiation and maintenance of phenotype and polarity, blood coagulation, and inflammation. Specific receptors (for example VLA-2 on blood platelets and fibroblasts) have been identified. Some interactions may involve Arg-Gly-Asp (RGD) sequences on the α chains. The collagen in small blood vessel walls is exposed when the endothelial linings are injured, and blood platelets that adhere to it contribute to hemostasis.

Exposed collagen also initiates formation of atherosclerotic plaques, in part by activating macrophages. Under pathological conditions (such as rheumatoid arthritis), collagens act as antigens that activate subpopulations of cytotoxic T lymphocytes. Many cell types make specific kinds of **collagenases** (*q.v.*).

collagenases: enzymes that degrade specific collagen types. They contribute to morphogenesis, bone remodeling, ovulation, wound healing, tissue reorganization, metastasis, and tissue destruction during inflammatory reactions. Stromelysin, TIMP (thioinosinic acid), and other somewhat specific physiological inhibitors limit the activities at various sites. Zinc metalloproteinases purified from microorganisms are used for special purposes. Collagenase H, a 105K enzyme from *Clostridium histolyticum* degrades helical regions of collagen, preferentially at X-Gly bonds (where X is usually a neutral amino acid component of the sequence: -Pro-X-Gly-Pro-), and is used to disperse cells for *in vitro* studies. A 70K enzyme from *Achromobacter iophagus* cleaves bonds close to propyl moieties that resist the effects of other proteases, and is used in to study protein structure.

collecting ducts: tubules in mammalian kidneys that receive processed glomerular filtrate from the distal ends of several nephrons, and send it on to the renal papilla. The cells have vasopressin receptors, and are major sites for urine concentration.

collecting tubules: small segments of the nephrons of some species that receive processed glomerular filtrate from distal convoluted tubules and send it to collecting ducts. They are major sites for aldosterone regulation of Na^+ and K^+ excretion.

colloid: (1) a mixture that contains solute particles intermediate in size between those of suspensions and true solutions. Since light rays pass through them, but are scattered by the solute particles, colloidal solutions are translucent; (2) the substance that collects in thyroid gland follicle lumens, composed mostly of thyroglobulin; (3) matter that physically resembles thyroid gland colloid.

colloid goiters: enlarged thyroid glands that contain large quantities of colloid (definition 2). Under normal conditions, thyroxine exerts negative feedback control over adenohypophysial thyrotropes, decreases thyroid stimulating hormone (TSH) secretion, and thereby limits the amounts of thyroglobulin-rich colloid synthesized. When the diet contains inadequate amounts of iodine, more TSH is secreted, and thyroid gland follicular cells enlarge and become overactive. They produce large quantities of poorly iodinated thyroglobulin, which is rapidly taken up by the cells and degraded (but make very little thyroxine). At this stage, the condition can be corrected by administering iodine. However, chronic iodine deficiency leads to severe hypothyroidism, formation of colloid goiters, and loss of sensitivity to iodine.

colon: the part of the large intestine that extends from the cecum to the rectum, and comprises ascending, transverse, descending, and sigmoid segments. Since it is a major site for absorption of water delivered by more anterior regions of the gut, and engages in selective, glucocorticoid regulated ion transport, it is a major contributor to water and electrolyte balance. The motility is controlled by physical factors, as well as by hormones and neurotransmitters. Bacteria that normally colonize the region degrade some undigested food remnants and bile components, synthesize several vitamins, and protect against invasion by pathogenic microorganisms.

colony forming units: CFUs; hemopoietic stem cells that respond to specific growth factors and form colonies composed of one (or a group of related) somewhat more differentiated cell types. CFU-Es (erythrocyte colony forming units) contain primitive cells committed to differentiation along pathways that lead to red blood cell formation. They are the direct progeny of burst forming erythrocyte (BFU-E) cells. CFU-Ss are colony forming primitive cells of the spleen. Bone marrow preparations can stimulate their formation, and can reconstitute immune systems of irradiated recipients.

colony stimulating factors: CSFs; species specific glycoproteins that regulate survival, differentiation, and some functions of hematopoietic cells, including colony stimulating factor-1 (CSF-1, monocyte colony stimulating factor, M-CSF), colony stimulating factor-2 (granulocyte-macrophage stimulating factor, GM-CSF), granulocyte stimulating factor (G-CSF), and interleukin-3 (multi-CSF). The various types vary widely in amino acid make-up, but perform similar, and overlapping functions. The effects of low concentrations are fairly specific, but high levels of one kind affect the expression and/or functions of others.

colony stimulating factor-1; CSF-1; M-CSF; *see* **macrophage colony stimulating factor**.

colony stimulating factor-1 receptors: *see* **macrophage colony stimulating factor-1 receptors.**

colony stimulating factor-2: GM-CSF: *see* **granulocyte-macrophage colony stimulating factor**.

colostrokinin: a component of colostrum released by the action of kallikreins that promotes contraction of the uterus and intestine, and can lower blood pressure.

colostrum: the yellowish, watery secretion, low in lipid content and devoid of lactose, produced by eutherian mammary glands shortly before and for 1-2 two days after parturition. It contains mononuclear macrophages, granulocytes, lymphocytes, and antibodies that confer infant resistance to bacterial infections, as well as prolactin, much higher levels of epidermal growth factor (EGF) than milk, other hormones, and components that stimulate the infant intestine.

column chromatography: *see* **chromatography**.

colyogenes: DNA segments that direct the synthesis of colyones.

colyones: naturally occurring inhibitors of cell growth and proliferation. The stimulatory effects of estrogens and some other hormones may be accomplished in part by decreasing their production or opposing their actions.

coma: a sustained state of unconsciousness from which arousal cannot be achieved with stimuli that are effective for torpor or sleep.

combinatorial association: association of an immunoglobulin heavy chain with an immunoglobulin light chain.

combined immunodeficiency: dysfunction of systems for both cellular and humoral immunity. Although it involves both T and B lymphocytes, the term is usually applied to defects less serious than *severe* combined immunodeficiency.

commensalism: associations between members of two different species that are beneficial to one of the partners, but neither beneficial nor harmful to the other. *See* also **symbiosis**.

commitment: attainment of a state of differentiation that restricts subsequent development to certain pathways. For example, a hemopoietic stem cell that advances to the promyelocyte stage has the potential for developing into any kind of granulocytic leukocyte, but has lost the ability to become an erythrocyte.

compactin: mevastatin.

compazine: *see* **prochlorperazine**.

compensatory hypertrophy: enlargement in response to some kind of deficiency, for example of the remaining ovary or adrenal gland when one has been removed.

competence: ability to respond to a regulator, usually because of the presence of receptors or other cell components.

competence factors: agents that promote passage of cells from G_1 to M phases of cell cycles, block reversion to G_o, or render cells responsive to progression factors. Platelet derived growth factor (PDGF), fibroblast growth factors (FGFs), and bombesin are competence factors for many cell types.

competence genes: nucleic acid segments that code for competence factors.

competitive binding assays: analytical procedures based on the ability of one ligand to displace another. For example, the amount of radioactively labeled cortisol bound to corticosterone binding globulin that is displaced by unlabeled cortisol in a test sample provides a quantitative measure of the cortisol concentration in that sample.

competitive inhibition: interference with the actions of an enzyme by compounds that bind reversibly to, but are not cleaved by the enzyme; or interference with the actions of a hormone by agents that bind reversibly to its receptors but do not damage them or elicit the responses invoked by the natural ligand. The effects of the first can be attenuated by adding more substrate, and of the second by adding more hormone. *Cf* **noncompetitive** and **uncompetitive inhibition**.

complement: at least 20 heat-labile proteins that collectively account for approximately 10% of total blood globulin, and contribute to nonspecific defenses against infections. Proteins present before activation are distinguished by numbers (C1 through C9), and fragments formed from them (or subtypes) by lower case letters (as in C2a, and C2b). Cascades, initiated by bacterial chemicals or antigen-antibody complexes, lead to assembly of attack complexes that insert into plasma membranes, form ion channels, and cause cell lysis. Some fragments additionally increase vascular permeability, attract granulocytes, monocytes, macrophages and eosinophils to sites of inflammation, facilitate cell adherence and phagocytosis, promote release of histamine and other biogenic amines, activate kinins, and/or contribute to immune system responses. C1 is composed of C1q, C1r, and C1s. The *classical pathway* for complement activation begins with the binding of C1q molecules to a cluster of antigen-antibody complexes that contains immunoglobulins of the IgG or IgM class. Each C1q molecule then activates a C1r, which, in turn, activates a C1s. C1s catalyzes cleavage of C4 to C4a plus C4b, and C4b binds covalently to membranes. This mediates binding of C2 and its cleavage products (made in reactions catalyzed by activated C1 proteins) to C2a and C2b. When a C4b/C2b complex attached to the membrane cleaves C3 to C3a and C3b, the C3b binds to the membrane and facilitates attachment of C5, after which it cleaves the C5. (C4b/C2b is also known as C3 convertase and C5 convertase; and both C3a and C5a are anaphylotoxins). Next, C5b binds C6, and the attack complex that destroys cells is assembled with C6, C7, C8, and C9. An *alternate pathway* can be initiated by bacterial polysaccharides. It involves properdin and other proteins that activate C3 and stabilize the fragments. Some immune system cell types have receptors for complement proteins (*see* **CR-1**, **CR-2**, **CR-3**, and **CR-4**). Naturally occurring inhibitors of activation, the short half-lives of the intermediates, the need for clusters of antigen-antibody complexes to initiate the classical pathway, and some hormones (especially glucocorticoids) usually protect against widespread destruction of host cells. However, small numbers of previously healthy cells are always affected, and some pathological conditions involve extensive damage.

complement cytolysis inhibitor: CLI; *see* **clusterin**.

complement fixation tests: assay systems for specific kinds of antigens or antibodies, based on the abilities of antigen-antibody complexes to initiate classical complement cascades. The specimen is incubated with a solution that contains small quantities of complement, plus the specific kind of antibody (to test for an antigen) or the specific kind of antigen (to test for antibody). After an appropriate time interval, an indicator system is then added to determine if the complement has been used up. Antibody-coated erythrocytes are commonly used, since they are lysed if complement is still present.

complement receptors: *see* **CR-1**, **CR-2**, **CR-3**, and **CR-4**.

complementarity-determining region: CDR; the component of an immunoglobulin variable region that determines its antigen-binding specificity.

complementary base pairs: (1) nitrogenous bases on one strand of a DNA molecule that can hydrogen bond to bases on the other strand. Usually, the combinations are adenine:thymine, and guanine:cytosine; (2) RNA bases that bond to DNA bases (usually uracil to adenine, and guanine to cytosine); (3) components of tRNA triplets (anticodons) that bond to messenger RNA bases.

complementary DNA: *see* **cDNA**.

complementary genes: nonallelic genes that affect a common function. Two or more genes may contribute to expression of a trait; or one type may inhibit activation of the other.

complementary interaction: processes by which two or more genes interact to achieve expression of a trait or realization of a function.

complementary RNAs: cRNAs; DNA transcripts or transcript fragments, synthesized *in vitro*. They can be labeled with radioactive markers and used as probes for locating genes, or used to make DNAs with complementary base sequences.

complete Freund's adjuvant: *see* **Freund's adjuvant**.

complete linkage: associations of genes on the same chromosome that cause them to be passed on as a unit to daughter cells. *See* also **linkage disequlibrium**.

complete medium: a preparation that contains all of the substances required to support the growth and proliferation of cultured cells or microorganisms; *see* also **defined medium**.

compounds A through S: Kendall's nomenclature for steroids; *see* individual types.

compound A: 11-dehydro-corticosterone; *see* **cortisone**.

compound B: corticosterone.

compound C: allopregnane-3α,11β,17α,21-tetral-20-one.

compound D: allopregnane-3β-11β,17α,20β,21-pentol.

compound E: cortisone.

compound F: cortisol.

compound G: adrenosterone.

compound H: allopregane-3β-21-diol-11,20-dione.

compound Q: electrocortin; *see* 11-**deoxycorticosterone**.

compound S: 11-deoxycortisol.

computerized axial tomography: CAT; computer assisted tomography; diagnostic procedures in which computers are used to analyze the patterns obtained, and construct three-dimensional images, when rotating machines direct X-rays through tissues at various angles. One application is determination of the sizes and locations of hormone-secreting tumors.

COMT: catecholamine-*O*-methyltransferase.

conalbumin: ovotransferrin; an estrogen-induced egg white protein that binds and transports iron.

concanavalin A: con A; a 283 amino acid homodimeric lectin obtained from the jackbean, *Canavalia ensiformis*, that binds terminal mannose and glucose moieties of cell surface oligosaccharides (and also Ca^{2+} and some other ions), and promotes agglutination of some cell types. By causing clustering of their membrane-associated receptors, it can mimic the actions of some hormones, promote T lymphocyte proliferation, and "normalize" the growth of some kinds of tumor cells. Con A is used to study cell surface molecule properties and the functions of their carbohydrate groups, and in affinity chromatography.

conception: (1) zygote formation; (2) implantation.

conceptus: a product of conception. The term is variously applied to (1) zygotes; (2) embryos; (3) embryos and their associated membranes; (4) fetuses.

concordance: emergence of a trait in both members of a pair of twins or in siblings; *cf* **discordance**.

conditioned medium: CM; a fluid or other preparation in which cells have been cultured. It contains substances released by the cells, and can be used as a source of growth factors.

conduit vessels: the aorta and the large arteries that rapidly transport blood to smaller vessels. *Cf* **capacitance** and **resistance vessels**.

confluent cultures: cultures in which most cells directly contact other cells, and sufficient numbers have been formed to cover the underlying vessel surface. *See* **contact inhibition** and **contact inhibition of locomotion**.

conformational change: a change in three-dimensional form. Heat, ions, ligands, and substrates are among the factors that affect the spacial arrangements of atoms in protein molecules, and can thereby expose or shield active domains. Ligands and substrates usually change protein and glycoprotein configurations; and translation factors can affect nucleic acids. *See* also **denaturation** and **chaperones**.

congenital: existing at the time of birth. The term can describe defects caused by genetic aberrations or unfavorable prenatal environments.

congenital adrenal hyperplasia: CAH; inherited conditions in which inadequate production of glucocorticoids impairs negative feedback control over adrenocorticotropic hormone (ACTH) secretion. Consequently, the adrenal cortex enlarges, excessive amounts of steroid hormone precursors are made, and the precursors are shunted into pathways for androgen synthesis. Approximately 90% of human disorders are caused by mutations or deletions of a gene on the chromosome that codes for the major histocompatibility complex and also directs formation of 21-hydroxylase (an enzyme that catalyzes conversion of progesterone and 17α-hydroxyprogesterone, respectively to 11-deoxycorticosterone and 11-deoxycortisol). When hydrogenation to cortisol is impaired, much of the 11-deoxycortisol is converted to dehydroepiandrosterone (a testosterone precursor). Conditions that develop very early in life can cause severe masculinization of female fetuses (including development of Wolffian duct derivatives). Depending on the amounts of androgen made and the timing of onset, the appearance of the external genitalia can range from somewhat virilized female, through ambiguous, to totally male. Postnatally, CAH invokes precocious puberty in boys, and virilization in girls. It can be associated with gonadal dysfunction and sterility. In some cases, cortisol deficiency is severe and life-threatening. 11-deoxycorticosterone is also an aldosterone precursor. Although much smaller amounts of aldosterone are needed, some individuals have a "salt-wasting" form of the disease that can be exacerbated by progesterone and 17α-hydroxyprogesterone competition for mineralocorticoid receptors. Salt and water loss may then elevate renin levels and invoke hypertension. Mutations that impair synthesis of 11-β-hydroxylase account for something like 5% of the cases. That enzyme is essential for formation of both glucocorticoids and aldosterone, but 11-deoxycorticosterone and some other mineralocorticoids can be made. Progesterone accumulates, and much of it is converted to androstenedione. Glucocorticoid administration corrects the conditions, since it replaces the missing hormone and inhibits ACTH secretion. Methods for diagnosing CAH in fetuses and instituting early treatment have been developed. *See* also 11-β and 21-**hydroxylases**, **sex determination**, **glucocorticoids**, **mineralocorticoids**, and **adrenal androgens**.

Congo red: direct red; sodium diphenyldiazo-*bis*-α-naphthalamine sulfonate; a dye used to stain amyloid, and to detect its pathological accumulation in tissues. It also stains collagens, spindle fibers, and erythrocytes, and is often used in combination with other dyes. Additionally, it is a probe for nucleotide-binding enzymes, and is used (often in the form of Congo red paper) as an indicator for mineral acid (halide) and thiocyanide determinations.

conjugate pairs: (1) a proton donor and a proton acceptor of a pH buffer system; (2) an electron donor and an electron acceptor of an oxidation/reduction system. *See* also **conjugation**, definition 2.

conjugation: joining; (1) covalent attachment of chemical groups to organic molecules. For example, hepatic enzymes catalyze formation of sulfate and glucuronate conjugates of steroid hormones and related molecules. Most of the derivatives are more hydrophilic than the parent compounds, and therefore more easily transported through body fluids, and more easily excreted to urine. Pharmacological preparations are conjugated with small, hydrophilic groups to increase water solubility, or with more complex chemicals to yield molecules that resist degradation and can be slowly hydrolyzed to release active components over long time periods; (2) temporary union of two single-celled organisms, during which nuclear components are exchanged.

connectin: a 70K protein on the surfaces of some tumor cells that binds laminins and actins.

connecting peptide: C peptide; an amino acid segment within a protein, usually fairly long, and located between two biologically active domains. In most cases, both ends have Arg-Arg, Arg-Lys, or Lys-Lys bonds that can be cleaved by cellular proteolytic enzymes; and the term is also applied to certain peptides that are thereby released. The proinsulin C peptide is needed for correct positioning of disulfide bonds during translation. The prohormone, which has limited biological activity, can be stored until needed, and then rapidly converted (via removal of the C peptide) to active insulin. Measurements of C peptide levels provide a useful estimate of endogenous secretion in individuals receiving insulin therapy (since the injected hormone does not contain the sequence). There have also been suggestions that the C-peptide performs some functions. In contrast, the C-peptides of insulin-like growth factor-I (IGF-I) and some other regulators (named for analogies with proinsulin), are retained by the regulator molecules, and are needed to stabilize the configurations for receptor binding. C peptides released from proopiomelanocortin (POMC) and other hormone precursors are under investigation for possible use as indicators of hormone production rates.

connective tissues: several tissue types derived from embryonic mesoderm, including blood, bone, cartilage, tendon, blood, areolar, adipose, and fibrous forms. They are located internally, between other tissues (not exposed on free surfaces). All contain large quantities of extracellular matter, and all except blood have collagen fibers. Most carry blood vessels (although cartilage vessels are confined to the perichondrium). The functions of the various types include mechanical support, binding and maintaining the locations of body components, cushioning, nutrient, fluid and electrolyte storage, and production of some cell types.

connective tissue diseases: a term applied to several autoimmune diseases associated with connective tissue disorders and inflammation, including rheumatoid arthritis and systemic lupus erythematosus. In most cases, other structures are additionally affected. *See* also **nonsteroidal antinflammatory agents**.

connexon: an assembly of six 32K proteins which forms a membrane hemichannel for passage of hydrophilic molecules. Gap junctions are juxtaposed, communicating connexons of adjacent cells.

Conn's syndrome: primary hyperaldosteronism and the associated effects of mineralocorticoid excess, usually caused by a hormone-secreting adrenocortical adenoma.

conopeptide GV: sleeper conopeptide; Gly-Glu-Gla-Gla-Glu-Gln-Gla-Asn-Glu-Gla-Glu-Ile-Arg-Gla-Lys-Ser-Asn. A peptide in the venom of *Conus Geographicus* that contains carboxyglutamate (Gla) groups, and invokes sleep when injected into mice. It differs in structure from sleep inducing peptides identified in mammalian brains.

conopressin: Lys-conopressin; peptide G; a cyclic peptide, chemically related to lysine vasopressin, in the venom of *Conus geographicus*. It invokes scratching behavior when injected into mice. In the amino acid sequence shown, disulfide bonds connect the two cysteine moieties: Cys-Phe-Ile-Arg-Asn-Cys-Pro-Lys-Gly. *Conus striatus* venom contains peptide S, a noncyclic, neurophysin-binding type in which an arginine moiety replaces the lysine.

conotoxins: several cyclic neurotoxic peptides in the venoms of marine fish-hunting cone snails. An α-conotoxin made by *Conus geographicus* (geographicus toxin I, GI) has the amino acid sequence shown, with disulfide bonds connecting the cysteine moieties at positions 3 → 8 and 3 → 14: H_2N-Glu-Cys-Cys-Asn-Pro-Ala-Cys-Gly-Arg-His-Tyr-Ser-Cys-NH_2. Another α type, with similar bonds (conotoxin M1), from the *Conus magnus* marine snail has the amino acids: Gly-Arg-Cys-Cys-His-Pro-Ala-Cys-Gly-Lys-Asn-Tyr-Ser-Cys-NH_2. Both peptides invoke paralysis by selectively blocking nicotinic type acetylcholine receptors in skeletal muscle and neurons that control Na^+ channels. Conotoxin GIIIA, H_2N-Arg-Asp-Cys-Cys-Thr-Hyp-Hyp-Lys-Lys-Cys-Lys-Asp-Arg-Gln-Cys-Lys-Hyp-Gln-Arg-Cys-Cys-Ala-NH_2, as well as toxins GIIIB, and GIIIC, are similar 22-amino acid peptides that block neurotransmitter release by acting on Na^+ channels. ω-conotoxin promotes persistent inhibition of L and N type Ca^{2+} channels. Disulfide bridges connect the cysteine moieties at positions 1:16, 8:19, and 15:26 in the sequence shown: H_2N-Cys-Lys-Ser-Hyp-Gly-Ser-Ser-Cys-Ser-Hyp-Thr-Ser-Tyr-Asn-Cys-Cys-Arg-Ser-Cys-Asn-Hyp-Tyr-Thr-Lys-Arg-Cys-Tyr-NH_2.

Congo red

CH₃ / CH₂ / N — (chemical structure diagram of Coomassie blue with NaO₃S, SO₃⁻, NH, O—CH₂—CH₃ groups)

CH_3 CH_2 N ... NaO_3S ... SO_3^- ... NH ... $O-CH_2-CH_3$

Coomassie blue

---

consensus sequence: usually, a similar or identical DNA sequence in two or more genes.

conserved sequence: a nucleic acid or protein segment that has undergone little or no change during the course of evolution, and is similar across many species.

conspecific: belonging to the same species.

conspersion: coming together, for example aggregation of melanocyte granules; *cf* **dispersion**.

constant domains: portions of molecules that display little or no variation among individuals of a species, a term usually applied to antibody components that are not directly involved in antigen recognition, or to certain T lymphocyte receptor subunits.

constitutional delay: describes conditions in which maturation (for example of skeletal or reproductive system structures) does not occur at the usual time for the species, but proceeds to completion in a normal manner at a later time.

constitutive: always present, and intrinsic to the system. The term can refer to an enzyme that is always made by a cell type, and displays some activity under basal conditions, or to a reaction product always produced. In most cases, both the synthesis and the activity can be augmented by appropriate stimulants.

contact inhibition of growth: density dependent inhibition; the slowing or cessation of proliferation that occurs when a critical cell mass is attained, so that each cell is in close contact with others. It can result from restricted access to nutrients or growth factors, decreased ability to interact with extracellular matrix components, or the effects of substances made in larger amounts when cell numbers increase. Most normal cells divide only when in contact with extracellular matrix molecules, and they are therefore said to be anchorage dependent. In contrast, many kinds of tumor cells fail to display the inhibition. *Cf* **contact inhibition of locomotion**.

contact inhibition of locomotion: decreased motility of cultured cells caused by close contact with other cells, or restricted access to the substratum. Cells engaged in wound healing cease migration and proliferation when the wound surfaces meet.

contraceptives: usually, agents that block fertilization via mechanisms such as interference with ovulation, spermatogenesis, or sperm:oocyte interactions. *See* **oral contraceptives** and other specific types. Some authors include interceptives and certain abortifacients.

contralateral: on the opposite side; *cf* **ipsilateral**.

Conus: a genus of fish hunting marine snails that includes at least 300 species. Neurotoxins isolated from their venoms are used to study ion channel and receptor functions. Most are 13-30-amino acid peptides; *see* **conotoxins**. Some venoms also contain peptides related to vasopressins (*see* **conopressins**). A nomenclature system that identifies the toxins by the capital letter for the species (for example G for Geographitoxins of *Conus Geographicus*, and S for *Conus striatus*), followed by a Roman number has been proposed, but prefixes (such as α- and γ-) are applied to types that act via specific mechanisms.

convergence: coming together toward a point. The term is used for (1) evolutionary changes in unrelated species that lead to acquisition of similar body components; and (2) eyeball movements that contribute to accommodation for near vision.

Cooley's anemia: Thalassemia.

Coomassie blue: a trade name for anazolene sodium, 4′-anilo-8-hydroxy-1,1′-azonapthalene-3,5′6-trisulfonic acid trisodium salt; a dye used for nonspecific staining of proteins on gels.

Coombs test: procedures for detecting IgG type immunoglobulin antibodies or complement on erythrocytes, or IgM antibodies directed against Rh antigens.

cooperativity: usually, the effects of binding some ligand molecules on the affinity of an enzyme or hormone receptor for additional ligand of the same kind. It can be positive (affinity increased), or negative.

α-COP, β-COP, γ-COP: coat proteins; *see* **coatamers**.

copolymer: a substance composed of repeating units of two or more different chemical subunits.

copper: Cu; an element (atomic number 29, atomic weight 63.45). It is an essential cofactor for dopamine-β-oxidase, lysyl oxidase, cytochrome oxidase, the cholesterol side-chain cleavage system, and some other oxidases. Cu also interacts with heparin, and it affects immune system functions, angiogenesis, blood coagulation, iron transport, and other processes. When incorporated into intrauterine devices, it contributes to contraceptive effectiveness.

coprophagia: ingestion of feces. Rabbits are among the animal types that do this consistently under normal conditions. Similar behavior is displayed occasionally by many other species, and it can be invoked or increased by depriving them of certain nutrients.

coprosterol: 5β-cholestan-3β-ol; a cholesterol degradation product in feces.

copulation: sexual interaction; usually, (1) a term synonymous with coitus in animals that engage in internal fertilization; (2) exchanges of genetic components by microorganisms; *see* **conjugation**.

copulin: a volatile lipid released to monkey vaginal fluids during the periovulatory phases of their menstrual cycles, that arouses sexual interest in conspecific males. Its status as a pheromone is controversial, since, in contrast to related phenomena in insects and some other animal types, the responses of male monkeys are neither stereotyped nor consistently reproducible. A comparable substance has been described for women, but is probably of little functional importance because of the use of deodorants and perfumes, and because human sexual interest and behavior are controlled mostly by very different factors.

copy number: the number of similar base sequences in the genome of a single cell or plasmid.

Co Q: coenzyme Q.

cordycepin: 3′-deoxyadenosine; an antibiotic made by *Cordyceps militaris* that inhibits RNA polyadenylation and prematurely terminates transcription.

cordycepic acid: mannitol.

core protein: *see* **nucleosomes**.

Cori cycle: a metabolic pathway in which glucose released during glycogenolysis in the liver is taken up by skeletal muscle cells and used for glycogenesis. Glycogenolysis in muscle, followed by glycolysis, then yields lactic acid, which travels to the liver, in which it is

cordycepin

converted to glucose and liver glycogen. The reactions are accelerated by amylin.

cornea: the anterior, transparent, convex portion of the outermost tunic of the eye that admits and refracts light. It is composed of surface epithelium, a collagenous stroma, and underlying epithelium. The cornea is said to be an immunologically privileged site, in which low rates of transplant rejection are attributed to the absence of blood and lymphatic vessels. Tissues inserted below the cornea of an experimental animal are easily visualized and can acquire nutrients from the middle tunic.

corona penetrating enzymes: CPE: a general term for enzymes made by spermatozoa that are essential for traversing the corona radiata prior to fertilization. They are said to be inhibited by a decapacitation factor.

corona radiata: the ring of cells that surrounds the oocyte of a preovulatory ovarian follicle, and remains attached to it during and for a short time after ovulation. *See* also **cumulus oophorus**.

coronary: encircling; crown-like; describes blood vessels that supply the heart.

corpus albicans: a white body; usually, the scar-like structure that forms after a corpus luteum deteriorates.

corpus allatum: a retrocerebral insect endocrine organ that synthesizes and secretes juvenile hormone. It contains the axon terminals of neurons that make and release brain (prothoracicotropic) hormone. In the larvae of some species, it is a component of the ring gland.

corpus cardiacum: an insect neurohemal organ. Axons of neurons that synthesize brain (prothoracicotropic) hormone pass through it and terminate in the corpus allatum.

corpus luteum [corpora lutea]: CL: a yellow body; usually, the structure that develops from an emptied ovarian follicle after ovulation. (It is yellow in humans, but not in all mammals.) Corpora lutea secrete progesterone during ovarian cycles and thereby contribute to preparation of the endometrium for implantation. Most additionally secrete estrogens, relaxin, prostaglandins, oxytocin, and other hormones. There are marked species differences in structures and functions. In women, usually just one forms during a cycle, and it deteriorates after 10-12 days if conception does not occur (*see* **luteolysis**). It derives mostly from granulosa cells that undergo extensive morphological and biological changes (luteinization) and secrete mostly progesterone, but the theca interna contributes substantial numbers of smaller luteinized cells; and fibroblasts and macrophages are incorporated. Rabbits are among the animal types that do not incorporate theca. Their corpora lutea do not made estrogens, but depend on steroid made by neighboring ovarian follicles. In females of some species that produce large litters, many corpora lutea form during a single cycle. In some others, corpora lutea that begin maturation during one cycle persist through two or more subsequent ones; and the structures accumulate until conception ensues. (This occurs mostly in rats, mice, and other small mammals with very short estrus cycles, but elephants, with long cycles also accumulate them.) In addition to its roles in ovulation, luteinizing hormone (LH) is required for formation of the CL, and for promoting the early phases of progesterone secretion. The CL rapidly lose dependence on that hormone. Progesterone soon takes over as a stimulant for its own production (and it exerts negative feeback controls over gonadotropin secretion). Prolactin is important contributor to CL formation and maintenance in a few animal types (*see* **luteotropic hormone**). If conception does not occur, the structures involute after a time period characteristic for the species. If it does, they grow, specialize, and form "corpora lutea of pregnancy". In women, chorionic gonadotropin (hCG) made by the trophoblast is the major stimulant. Chorionic gonadotropins perform comparable functions in other mammals, but pituitary hormones are important in some. Corpus luteum steroids support the first two months of human pregnancy, after which the feto-placental unit takes over most of the its functions. In rats and some other species, several corpora lutea are needed for the entire pregnancy, and new ones are formed shortly after parturition.

corpuscles of Stannius: Stannius corpuscles: bilateral endocrine glands on the surfaces of teleost fish kidneys. They have calciferol receptors, and secrete peptides that regulate calcium, monovalent ion, and water metabolism, but were originally believed to secrete steroid hormones.

corpus striatum: the major component of brain basal ganglia, composed of right and left caudate and lenticular nuclei. The lenticular nucleus on each side includes the putamen and the globus pallidus. (The neostriatum includes the caudate nuclei and putamen, whereas the globus pallidus belongs to the paleostriatum). Corpus striatum neurons regulate extrapyramidal functions. The caudate nucleus is also a major site for central control of analgesia, and is affected by acupuncture. Dopamine mediates most of the extrapyramidal functions, but it antagonizes influences on the peripheral release of enkephalins.

correlation coefficient: a statistical measure (usually represented by *r*) of the extent to which two parameters vary in parallel. Values of 0, +1, and -1 indicate, respectively, no correlation, perfect positive, and totally negative correlations.

cortex [cortices]: an outer portion or layer, for example of a kidney or adrenal gland; *cf* **medulla**.

cortexolone: compound S; *see* 11-**deoxycortisol**.

cortexone: compound Q; *see* 11-**deoxycorticosterone**.

cortical granules of oocytes: *see* **cortical reaction**.

cortical nephrons: nephrons whose glomeruli are located close to the renal cortex. Unlike **juxtamedullary** types (*q.v.*), they have short Henle loops.

cortical reaction: a process that occurs in an oocyte soon after fertilization and the zona reaction. It involves sustained changes in the oocyte surface that contribute to protection against entry of additional spermatozoa. In some species, cortical granules are extruded from the plasma membrane.

cortical thymocytes: *see* **thymus gland**.

corticine: a hypothetical factor made by the cortical regions of mammalian embryonic gonads that promotes ovarian differentiation. No factor has been identified; and gonads cultured without exogenous regulators develop into ovary-like structures.

corticoliberin: corticotropin releasing hormone.

corticolipotropes: *see* **corticotropes**.

corticostatins: CSs; 29-31 amino acid peptides of the defensin family. All contain several cysteine moieties and have three disulfide bonds. The group includes CS-1, with the amino acid sequence: Gly-Ile-Cys-Ala-Cys-Arg-Arg-Arg-Phe-Cys-Pro-Asn-Ser-Glu-Arg-Phe-Ser-Gly-Tyr-Cys-Arg-Val-Asn-Gly-Ala-Arg-Tyr-Val-Arg-Cys-Cys-Ser-Arg-Arg. It is present in blood plasma, peritoneal neutrophilic leukocytes, lung, spleen, small intestine, hypothalamus, adrenal medulla, and elsewhere. Some of the peptides are known under two or more names, (for example CS-3 is is identical with the neuropeptide, NP1.) Corticostatins inhibit adrenocorticotropic hormone (ACTH)-stimulated glucocorticoid and aldosterone secretion, probably by competing for receptors, and thereby retard cholesterol conversion to pregnenolone (but do not affect basal or angiotensin-II-stimulated steroidogenesis). CS-1 also dispalys antimicrobial and antiviral activity, and may contribute to inflammatory reactions. Its levels in the hypothalamus rise during responses to infections. In contrast, the peptides in gonadotropes and somatotropes are unaffected by infection, but may be paracrine regulators of adenohypophysial functions.

corticosteroid: (1) any steroid hormone secreted by the adrenal cortex; (2) any steroid made in the adrenal cortex (even if it is not released); (3) a glucocorticoid, mineralocorticoid, or chemically related synthetic compound that exerts similar actions.

corticosteroid binding globulins: CBG; transcortin; plasma proteins secreted by the liver that bind cortisol and corticosterone with high affinity, and also bind some progesterone and related steroids. Usually, approximately 75% of circulating glucocorticoid, and 17% of circulating aldosterone, are associated with CBG. The protein is believed to facilitate steroid transport through body fluids, and to protect the molecules against rapid excretion. According to most observers, the hormones must be released from the proteins before entering target cells.

CBGs may therefore protect against excessive uptake when blood levels of the hormones are too high, and serve as reservoirs that rapidly provide more when it is needed. The high potencies of some synthetic glucocorticoids (such as dexamethasone) are attributed in part to negligible affinity for CBG. However, roles in facilitation of uptake by target cells have also been proposed; and identical or closely related proteins are found in the cytoplasms of some types. CBG synthesis is augmented by estrogens and glucocorticoids in humans. (Triiodothyronine is an additional stimulant in rats.)

corticosteroid receptors: *see* **glucocorticoid** and **mineralocorticoid receptors**.

corticosterone; compound B; 11β-21-dihydroxy-4-ene-3,20-dione; the major glucocorticoid of rats and some other mammals. Humans secrete small quantities, but cortisol is the major glucocorticoid. Dogs are among the species that make approximately equal amounts of the two steroids. Most of the biological actions are similar to those of cortisol, but corticosterone is a stronger mineralocorticoid, and it lacks anti-inflammatory potency.

11-dehydro-**corticosterone**: a steroid secreted in small amounts by adrenal glands. It is biologically inactive, but a hydroxylase in many cell types rapidly catalyzes its conversion to corticosterone. (A dehydrogenase catalyzes the reverse reaction.) *See* also **cortisone**.

11-deoxy-**corticosterone**: *see* 11-**deoxycorticosterone**.

corticotropes: corticotrophs; corticolipotropes; adenohypophysial cells that synthesize and process pro-opiomelanocortin (POMC). The major secretory products are adrenocorticotropic hormone (ACTH), and β-endorphin (derived from the β-lipotropin component), along with some uncleaved β-lipotropin and small amounts of γ-melanocyte stimulating hormone (γ-MSH). Corticotropin releasing hormone (CRH) is the major factor for maintaining cell morphology and functions, for promoting POMC production, and for augmenting hormone secretion in response to stress. The importance of other stimuli varies with the species. In many, arginine vasopressin strongly potentiates CRH influences, but is only moderately effective when presented alone. Larger amounts are released during some forms of stress. Additional stimuli include angiotensin I, epinephrine, oxytocin, and possibly also peptide histidine isoleucine (PHI), vasoactive intestinal peptide (VIP), and cholecystokinins. Glucocorticoids exert negative feedback controls, both directly and via influences on CRH and vasopressin release.

corticotropin: ACTH; *see* **adrenocorticotropin**.

corticotropin-like intermediate peptide: CLIP; a peptide composed of amino acids 18-39 of adrenocorticotropic hormone (ACTH). It is cleaved from pro-opiomelanocortin (POMC) in the pars intermedia of species in which this component of the adenohypophysis persists, and in human fetuses, in which the intermediate lobe degenerates as the gland matures. CLIP is implicated as a regulator of steroidogenesis in fetal adrenal glands (which lack the sensitivity to ACTH displayed postnatally). It may additionally affect other fetal functions such as insulin release. α-melanocyte stimulating hormone (α-MSH) is formed from amino acids 1-13, and some CLIP may be made as a byproduct when that peptide is required.

corticotropin release factor: corticotrophin releasing factor; CRF; a term used for the hypothalamic hormone that stimulates adenohypophysial corticotropes, before the chemical nature of that regulator was known. Some authors continue to use it, but others prefer corticotropin releasing hormone.

corticotropin releasing hormone: corticotrophin releasing hormone; CRH: a peptide initially defined as the major hypothalamic factor that stimulates corticotropes, but now known to be made at many sites, and to perform other functions. Although species specific, it is chemically similar in most mammals. The amino acid sequence for humans and rats is: H-Ser-Glu-Glu-Pro-Pro-Ile-Ser-Leu-Asp-Leu-Thr-Phe-His-Leu-Leu-Arg-Glu-Val-Leu-Glu-Met-Ala-Arg-Ala-Glu-Gln-Leu-Ala-Gln-Gln-Ala-His-Ser-Asn-Arg-Lys-Leu-Met-Glu-Ile-Ile-NH₂. Sauvagine and urotensin I are chemically and biologically related. The hypothalamic paraventricular nuclei contain high levels, and are the major sources of the CRH that acts on corticotropes. CRH co-localizes with peptide histidine isoleucine (PHI) in some neurohypophysial neurons, and with oxytocin in others; and it promotes the release of vasopressin (which potentiates CRH influences on ACTH secretion). In some species, it also stimulates release of α-melanocyte stimulating hormone (α-MSH). CRH secreting neurons with other functions are widely distributed throughout the central nervous system, including the spinal cord as well as the cerebral cortex, limbic system, and brain stem. The central effects include inhibition of gonadotropin releasing hormone (GnRH, LRH) and growth hormone releasing hormone (GRH) secretion, and of GnRH and luteinizing hormone-mediated sexual behavior. CRH also suppresses appetite, and is anxiogenic. The CRH-adrenocortical axis is hyperactive in individuals with anorexia nervosa; and high glucocorticoid levels characterize several forms of psychic depression. It functions subnormally in many with bulimia (although that condition is commonly associated with psychic depression). Additionally, CRH affects memory, promotes arousal and alertness, exerts stimulatory influences on the sympathetic nervous system, and inhibits some parasympathetic functions. At least some effects on the cardiovascular and respiratory systems, adrenal medulla, gonads, lungs, and liver also appear to be centrally mediated. CRH made in Sertoli and Leydig cells of the testis is a negative regulator of steroidogenesis. Its release there (and at some other sites) is

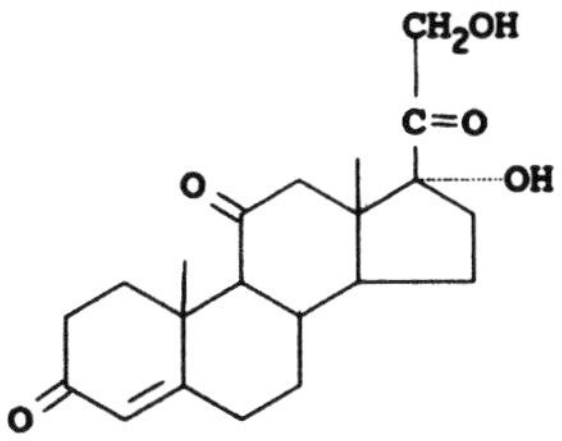

cortisone

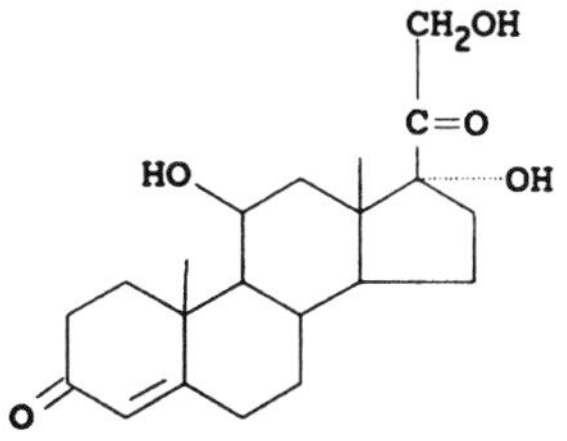

11-dehydrocorticosterone

augmented by serotonin. Pancreatic CRH appears to affect mostly glucagon secretion, but the hormone is also made in the exocrine cells (and is released in large amounts by some pancreatic tumors). In the gastrointestinal tract, CRH decreases gastric acid production, slows gastric emptying, and elevates intestinal bicarbonate levels. Circulating CRH has been observed to depress natural killer (NK) cell cytotoxicity and to be antipyretic, but the effects may be mediated via glucocorticoids. In contrast, CRH released locally from sympathetic and sensory neurons is pro-inflammatory. Its delivery from activated monocytes is inhibited by glucocorticoids. Placental CRH (cCRH), which is chemically identical to the hypothalamic hormone, may regulate both chorionic gonadotropin (hCG) secretion and fetal corticotrope functions. A major clinical use is for differential diagnosis of glucocorticoid deficiency syndromes.

cortisol: hydrocortisone; compound F; 17α-hydroxy-corticosterone; 11β,17α,21-trihydroxy-preg-4-en-3,20-dione; the major **glucocorticoid** (*q.v.*) of humans, guinea pigs and some other species, and one of two glucocorticoids for different animal types. It is made in much larger amounts than aldosterone, and in addition to interacting with type II receptors (specific for glucocorticoids), it binds to and activates type I receptors that mediate aldosterone actions. Cortisol can be made from cortisone (which lacks direct glucocorticoid or mineralocorticoid potency) via a reaction catalyzed by 11-β-hydroxysteroid hydroxylase. An 11-β-hydroxysteroid dehydrogenase catalyzes the reverse reaction. In species whose major glucocorticoid is corticosterone, similar enzymes act on 11-dehydrocorticosterone and corticosterone. Aldosterone is not a substrate for the dehydrogenase, possibly because its alcoholic group is incoporated into a hemiacetal. At some sites, the dehydrogenase protects against excessive amounts of the active hormone. The high activity in placentas and fetuses appears to serve this purpose. In the kidneys, the enzyme is needed to overcome cortisol interference with aldosterone actions on type I receptors. Lower, but substantial levels are also present in the colon. It has been suggested that close regulation of the activity of the enzyme in parotid salivary glands excludes cortisol most of the time, but permits it to act under certain conditions, for example during responses to stress. The hypertension associated with genetic defects and other factors that impair 11-dehydrogenase synthesis or inhibit its activity is attributed to excessive effects of unmetabolized cortisol; *see* also **carbenoxolone**. In contrast to aldosterone target cells, heart and hippocampus are among the structures

that lack the enzyme, and in which cortisol is the primary ligand for type I receptors.

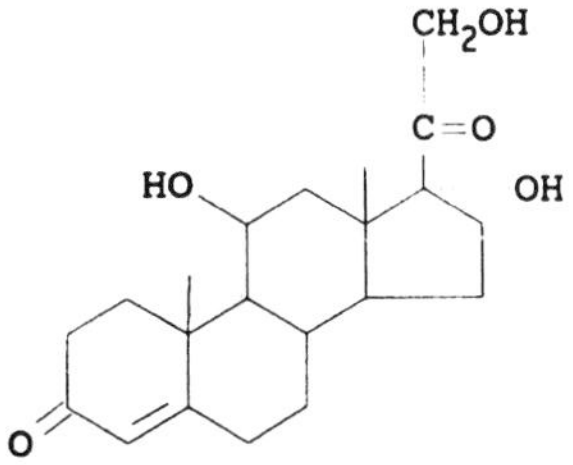

11-dehydro-**cortisol**: cortisone.

11-deoxy-**cortisol**: *see* 11-**deoxycortisol**.

cortisone: 11-dehydro-cortisol; compound E: Cortogen; a steroid secreted directly in small amounts by adrenal cortices of many species, but made in larger quantities from cortisol via a reaction catalyzed by 11β-hydroxysteroid dehydrogenase. It is a component of many preparations used for their anti-inflammatory and anti-allergic effects. Cortisone does not interact directly with type II receptors, which are specific for glucocorticoids, or with type I receptors that also bind aldosterone, but it is rapidly converted to cortisol in many cell types. The same dehydrogenase promotes conversion of corticosterone to 11-dehydrocorticosterone.

cortisol receptors: *see* **glucocorticoid receptors**.

cortolonic acid: 5β-3α,11β,17α,20-tetrahydroxy-21-oic acid; a cortisol metabolite made in the liver and excreted to urine.

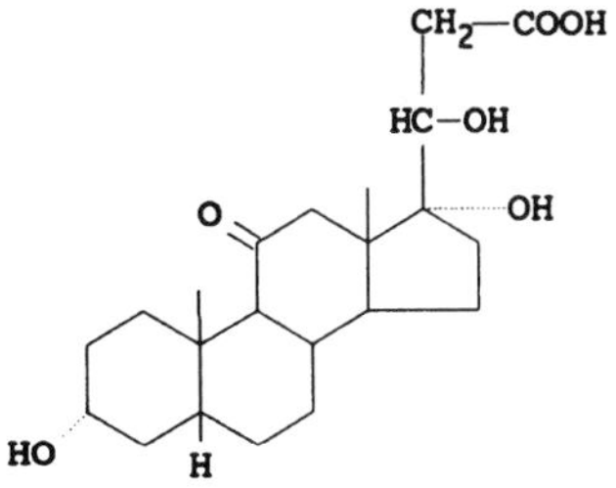

cortol: 5β-pregnane-3α,11β,17,20α,21-pentol; a cortisol metabolite made in the liver and excreted to urine.

cortolone: 3α,17α,20α,21-tetrahydroxypregnan-11-one; a cortisol (and cortisone) metabolite made in the liver and excreted to urine.

155

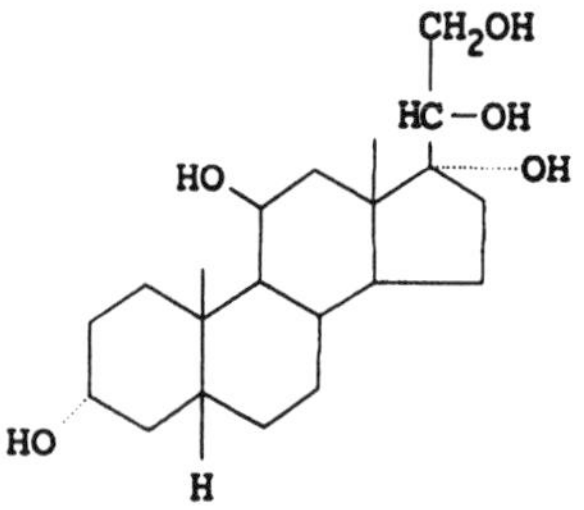

cortol

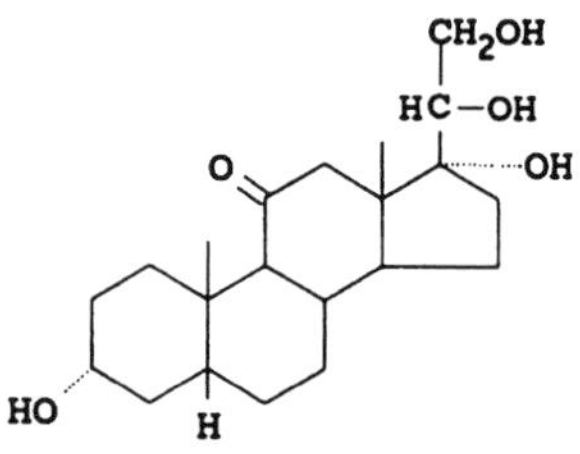

cortolone

COS cells: several cell lines (distinguished by numbers following COS) derived from monkey kidneys, and transformed by integrated SV40 DNA segments that code for T antigen. They support replication of recombinant RNAs that contain an SV40 origin and a foreign gene, but lack origin components for other viral DNAs.

cosmids: plasmid vectors into which lambda phage *cos* sites have been inserted, along with one or more markers, such as antibiotic resistance genes. They are used to clone large eukaryote DNA segments. *See* also **cotransformation**.

cos **sites**: cohesive ends of lambda phage DNA particles. When cosmids are inserted into cells, eukaryote DNA made between two *cos* sites is packaged into particles that are coated by phage proteins.

cosyntropin: $ACTH_{24}$; Synacthen; a synthetic peptide composed of amino acid moieties 1-24 of adrenocorticotropic hormone. It binds to ACTH receptors and displays most of the actions of the native hormone.

cot: in reannealing experiments, the initial concentration of single-strand nucleic acids (in moles per liter) multiplied by the time (in seconds) during which reassociation has been permitted to occur. $C_0t_{1/2}$ is the point at which half the DNA is present as double-stranded fragments.

cothromboplastin: factor VII; *see* **coagulation**.

cotransduction: simultaneous transfer (transduction) of two or more genes to a recipient bacterial cell by the same phage particle. It occurs with greatest frequency when the genes are close to each other, and is therefore useful for gene mapping.

cotransformation: incubation of host cells with two different plasmid types, one of which is selective for a specific phenotype and therefore easily identified, and the other a nonselective transforming factor. It is used to identifify the cells in a culture that have been transformed.

cotransport: symport; simultaneous transport of two different substances across a membrane. For example, active transport of many amino amino acids is associated with simultaneous uptake of sodium ions. *Cf* **counterport**.

coulomb: C: the quantity of electricity transported in one second by a current of one ampere.

Coumadin: warfarin; 3-(α-acetonylbenzyl)-4-hydroxycoumarin; a vitamin K antagonist that blocks hepatic production of prothrombin and other blood coagulation factors, and decreases the γ-carboxyglutamate content of osteocalcin and other vitamin K dependent proteins. The sodium salt is used to protect against formation of intravascular blood clots, and as an insecticide.

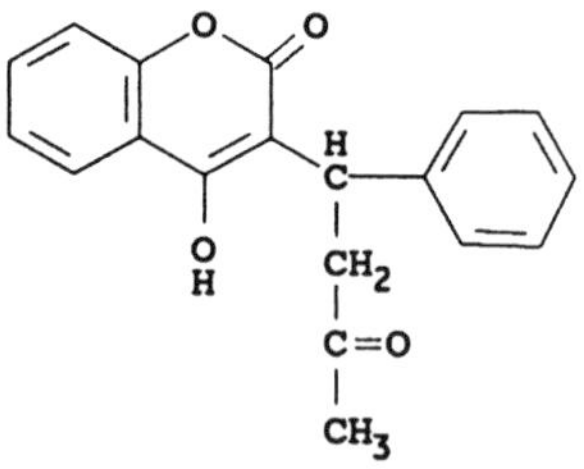

coumarin: cumarin; 2*H*-1-benzopyran-2-one: a component of sweet clover and some other plants. It is used directly as a flavoring agent, and as a component of fluorescent markers and laser dyes. *Cf* **dicoumarol**.

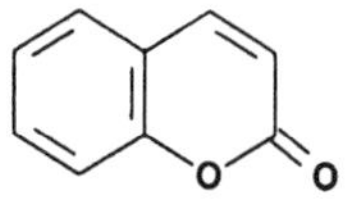

coumermycin A1: an antibiotic that inhibits DNA gryase.

coumestrol: 2-(2,4-dihydroxyphenyl)-6-hydroxy-3-benzofurancarboxylic acid δ lactone; an estrogen in clovers and some other forage crops.

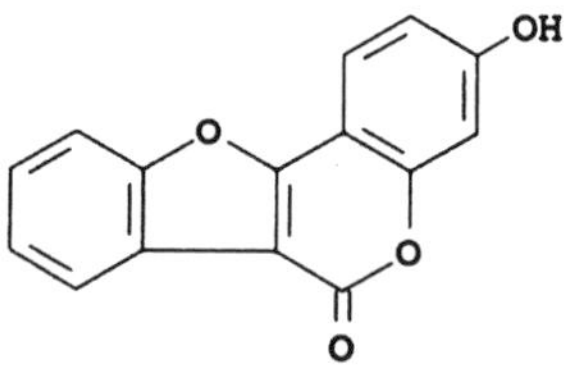

countercurrent exchange: passive exchange of components between two contiguous compartments arranged in parallel, in which flow procedes in opposite directions. It facilitates processes such as heat and water conservation, and the maintenance of osmotic pressure relationships without the need for input of energy from ATP or other sources. For example, during exposure to cold environments, heat is transferred from small blood vessels of the arterial tree that supply the feet, to vessels that return blood to the abdominal cavity. Since the feet are cooled, they lose less heat to cold air than warm ones would; and blood returning to the body requires less re-warming than would otherwise be required. Similarly,

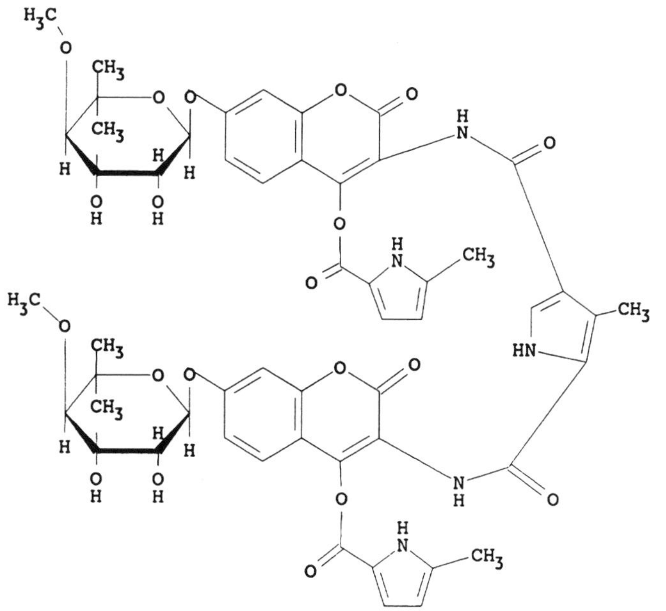

coumermycin A1

water vapor from expired air that traverses respiratory passageways moistens inspired air. *See* also **vasa recta** and *cf* **countercurrent multiplication**.

countercurrent multiplication: exchange of components between two parallel, contiguous channels that are connected at one end, but in which flow proceeds in opposite directions and energy is used to drive the movement of one or more of the substances. It is usually more efficient than countercurrent exchange. *See* **Henle loops**.

countertransport: counterport; antiport; transport of one substance across cell membranes that requires simultaneous movement of another in the opposite direction. For example, Na^+ extrusion can be coupled to Ca^{2+} uptake, and H^+ extrusion to Na^+ uptake. *Cf* **cotransport**.

COUP-TF: chicken ovalbumin upstream promotor transcription factor; a zinc finger protein of the steroid hormone receptor superfamily that binds to upstream promotors of several genes and contributes to transcription initiation. In addition to the one for ovalbumin, it activates genes that code for insulin, proopiomelanocortin (POMC), an apoprotein of very low density lipoprotein particles (VLDLs), and some other proteins. A closely related factor in *Drosophila* activates the *seven up* gene that directs dopamine phosphorylation in the retina. COUP-TF has been called an "orphan receptor", since no ligand has been identified. The possibility that it does not require one is suggested by observations that dopamine acting on its own receptors in some cell types initiates phosphorylations that lead to COUP-TF activation.

coupling factor: a biological agent that links two processes, such as bone resorption with new bone formation, or electron transport with ATP synthesis. Transducers are coupling factors that link hormone-receptor binding to enzyme activation or other responses. Coupling factor-I

(F_1) is a complex of five polypeptide chains on inner mitochondrial membranes that catalyzes ATP synthesis and has ATPase activity. *See* also **uncoupling**.

coupling reactions: reactions that join two chemical groups, for example two iodotyrosyl moieties during thyroid hormone synthesis.

courtship rituals: genetically determined behaviors that precede copulation in many species, and may be important for limiting mating to conspecifics, as well as for arousing sexual interest. The control mechanisms and hormone influences vary widely with the species.

covalent: describes strong bonds between atoms that involve sharing of electrons, for example ones commonly formed between carbon and oxygen atoms. They are stable in aqueous solutions, and are not easily disrupted by high temperatures; *cf* **electrovalent** and **hydrogen bonds**. Covalent modifications, such as phosphorylations, sulfations, and acetylations, affect the surface charges, activities, and other properties of enzymes, hormone receptors, DNA binding factors, and other cell components.

covariance: a statistical measure of concomitant changes in two parameters. For example, if several dosages of an agent are administered to animals that vary in body weights, it can be used to investigate possible influences of body weight on dose-related responses.

cozymase: a heat-stable, dialyzable fraction of yeast extracts that supports glycolysis. The major component is NAD.

CP-96,345: (2*S*,3*S*)-*cis*-2-(diphenylmethyl)-*N*-[(2-methoxyphenyl)-methyl]-1-azabicyclo[2,2,2]-octan-3-mine); a potent, selective NK_1 type substance P receptor antagonist that does not act on NK_2 or NK_3 types. It blocks

157

the ability of substance P to activate the locus ceruleus, invoke salivation, and relax norepinephrine stimulated smooth muscle, but does not interfere with the actions of neurokinins A or B.

CPA: N^6-cyclopentyladenosine; a potent adenosine receptor agonist, selective for A_1 subtypes.

CPD: cis-2,3-piperidine diacarboxylic aid; a GABA$_A$ type γ-aminobutyric acid receptor antagonist.

CPE: corona penetrating enzyme.

C-peptide: the **connecting peptide** (q.v.) of proinsulin, also called the proinsulin C-chain. The human type has the sequence: Arg-Arg-Glu-Ala-Glu-Asp-Leu-Gln-Val-Gly-Gln-Val-Glu-Leu-Gly-Gly-Gly-Pro-Gly-Ala-Gly-Ser-Leu-Gln-Pro-Leu-Ala-Leu-Glu-Gly-Ser-Leu-Gln-Lys-Arg.

cpm: counts per minute.

CPP: 3-(2-carboxypiperazine-4-yl)-propyl-1-phosphonic acid; a highly potent, selective, competitive NMDA receptor antagonist. It displaces glutamate, and is used to localize NMDA receptor sites.

8-CPT-cAMP: 8-(4-chlorophenylthio)-cAMP; a cAMP analog that resists degradation by phosphodiesterases, and does not release butyrate; cf **dibutyryl cAMP**.

CR: complement receptor; see **complement** and specific types (**CR1**, **CR2**, **CR3**, and **CR4**).

CR1: complement receptor 1; 190-290K polymorphic membrane glycoprotein receptors for complement frag-

8-CPT-cAMP

ment C3b on erythrocytes, and C4b on granulocytes, monocytes, macrophages, mast cells and renal epithelial cells; and cofactors for cleaving C3b and C4b. By mediating immune adherence, they contribute to clearance of immune complexes from blood. See also **CD35**.

CR2: 140K membrane B lymphocyte glycoproteins that mediate growth and differentiation. They are receptors for C3 complement fragments, and for the Epstein-Barr virus. See also **CD21**.

CR3: Mac-1 in mice; Mo1 in humans; membrane glycoproteins, and components of granulocyte, mononuclear phagocyte, and natural killer (NK) cell granules, composed of 150-180K α subunits identical to CD11b, and 95K β subunits identical to CD18 (and to the β subunits of LFA-1 and p150,95). They are receptors for complement fragment C3b, contribute to opsonin recognition, and facilitate phagocytosis and leukocyte adhesion to endothelium. Their synthesis is augmented by C5a, f-methionine-leucine-phenylalanine (fMLP), tumor necrosis factor-β (TNFβ), and other mediators of inflammation.

CR4: neutrophil membrane glycoprotein receptors for fragments of complement C3 proteins, and mediators of phagocytosis. One form is identical to p150,95 (CD11b plus CD18).

CRABPs: cytosolic retinoic acid binding proteins; see **retinoic acid**.

CRALBP: cellular retinal binding protein; see **retinoic acid**.

cranin: a 120K integral membrane glycoprotein of neurons that binds laminins and mediates some of its influences on neuroblast proliferation, migration, and differentiation, and on neurite growth. Small amounts are also made by fibroblasts and liver cells, and at other sites.

CRBPs: cytosolic retinol binding proteins.

CRD: carbohydrate recognition domain; usually, the carbohydrate component of a protein that functions as a receptor.

CRE[s]: cAMP regulatory elements: TGACGGTCA base sequences in the promotors of several genes whose activities are regulated by CREBs and some other proteins. In eukaryotes, they directly mediate many of the transcriptional effects of cyclic 3′5′-adenosine monophosphate-activated protein kinase A, and cooperate with other gene segments to increase the activities of some other promoters activated by different translation factors. CREs differ by a single base from AP-1 binding sites (response elements that mediate the effects of some growth promoting protoncogene products, and of phorbol esters and other protein kinase C-dependent factors). cAMP performs different functions in prokaryotes, by complexing with catabolite activator protein (CAP); but the complex associates with CREs closely related to animal types.

C-reactive protein: CRP: an acute phase protein composed of 5 identical 206-amino acid moieties, named for its calcium-dependent binding to the phosphorylcholine component of the C-carbohydrate on the surfaces of *Streptococcus pneumoniae*. It also binds chromatin and the C1q component of complement protein C1. The known effects include complement activation, initiation of agglutination, and stimulatory influences on phagocytosis. Production of the protein increases up to 1000-fold during inflammatory reactions.

creatine: α-methylguanido acetic acid, a compound present in highest concentration in muscle tissue that contributes to energy metabolism; *see* **creatine kinases** and **creatine phosphate**. It is synthesized in two steps: arginine + glycine → guanidoacetate + ornithine, followed by guanidoacetate + *S*-adenosylmethionine → creatine + *S*-adenosylcysteine. *See* also **creatinine**.

$$H_2N-\underset{\underset{H}{\overset{\|}{N}}}{\overset{\overset{CH_3}{|}}{C}}-N-CH_2-COOH$$

creatine kinases: enzymes that catalyzes the reaction: creatine + ATP → creatine-P + ADP, and thereby provide a mechanism for storing high energy phosphate bond energy for later use. (Cells cannot accumulate ATP stores.) Creatine phosphate is synthesized when rates for ATP synthesis exceed those for ATP hydrolysis. During muscle contraction and other processes that consume large quantities of energy, the reaction proceeds in the opposite direction and liberates ATP. Several isozymes with similar amino acid sequences are formed by differential posttranslational processing. The B type was initially called estrogen induced protein, because high estrogen levels stimulate its formation in myometrium. Creatine kinases are also induced by 1,25-dihydroxycholecalciferol in kidneys, and by parathyroid hormone in bone. Arginine undergoes similar phosphorylation and dephosphorylation and performs comparable functions in some invertebrates.

creatine-phosphate: creatine-P; phosphocreatine: *See* **creatine kinase**.

$$^-O-\underset{\underset{O^-}{\overset{\|}{P}}}{\overset{\overset{O}{\|}}{P}}-\overset{H}{N}-\underset{\underset{H}{\overset{\|}{N}}}{\overset{\overset{CH_3}{|}}{C}}-N-CH_2-COOH$$

creatine-phosphate

creatinine: 2-amino-1-methyl-4-imidazolidinone; a creatine degradation product that circulates and is excreted by the kidney. In many species (including humans), it is filtered by glomeruli but neither reabsorbed nor secreted by renal tubules. The urinary levels can therefore be used as indicators of glomerular filtration rates. Since the amounts excreted vary with skeletal muscle mass (which does not change rapidly), and are usually constant from day to day, they are also used to determine the completeness of 24-hour urine collections. (Dogs are among the animal types that actively secrete the molecules.)

$$\underset{O}{\overset{CH_3}{\underset{\|}{C}}}$$

CREBs: cAMP regulated DNA-binding proteins; proteins that form CRE-binding homodimers, and also heterodimers (with other transcription factors) when activated by protein kinase A, calmodulin kinase II, glycogen synthetase III, or some other protein kinases. They mediate transcriptional effects of both cyclic adenosine 3′5′-monophosphate (cAMP) and some factors that elevate cytosolic Ca^{2+}. 38-47K forms have been identified in higher animals, and a related 66K homolog is made by yeasts. In common with AP-1 and other transcription factors, CREBs have multiple sites for posttranslational phosphorylations, and leucine zipper domains that mediate dimerization; and they closely resemble transcription factors that mediate the effects of some viruses.

crenation: usually, the shrinking of erythrocytes, and the associated wrinkling of their plasma membranes, that occurs when the cells are exposed to hypertonic environments.

crepuscular: occurring at dusk or in dim light.

cretinism: a condition caused by thyroid hormone deficiency that begins prenatally or during infancy. The manifestations include dwarfism with infantile body proportions, mental retardation, and failure to undergo puberty. The effects can be averted if replacement therapy is instituted during infancy. However, if treatment is delayed, the skeletal and reproductive systems respond, but the nervous system defects are irreversible. *See* also **critical periods**.

Creutzfeldt-Jakob disease: a progressive, degenerative brain disease believed to be caused by a prion. It is prevalent in cannibals who consume human brains. Since humans respond to growth hormone derived from primates but not from other mammals, GH deficiency was at one time treated with preparations made from human corpses; and some recipients developed the disease. Recombinant growth hormone made by microorganisms is now used.

CRF: corticotropin release factor.

CRH: corticotropin releasing hormone.

CRH-BP: CRH binding protein; a 38K protein that binds corticotropin releasing hormone, and thereby limits its access to target cells. The circulating levels fall during pregnancy.

C ring: the third ring of a **steroid** (*q.v.*), formed by carbons 8, 9, 11, 12, 13 and 14. Carbons 8 and 9 are shared with the B ring, and carbons 13 and 14 with the D. Carbon 18 of steroid hormones is attached to carbon 13.

crinophagy: cell destruction mediated by lysosomal enzymes released within the cell. It proceeds, for example, in lactotropes when termination of lactation reduces the need for large numbers of prolactin-secreting cells.

CRIP: cysteine-rich intestinal protein.

critical periods: limited time periods during which cells can respond in specific ways to certain regulators. For example, central nervous system maturation during infancy is mediated in part by triiodothyronine (T_3); but cells deprived of that regulator cannot respond in the same way at later times (*see* **cretinism**). Similarly, some aspects of reproductive system development are restricted to late embryonic or early fetal stages (*see* **sex determination** and **Müllerian duct inhibitor**). In at least some cases, differences in hormone receptor isoforms parallel the changes in receptivity.

crk: the transforming oncogene of chicken sarcoma CT10 virus. It directs formation of p47^{gagcrk}, a protein that indirectly augments protein kinase A activity by competing with inhibitors, and can invoke continuous activation in some cell types. One domain closely resembles the non-receptor tyrosine kinase regulatory components of some other proteins.

cRNA: complementary RNA.

Cro: *see* **cro protein**.

Crohn's disease: irritable bowel syndrome; a chronic inflammatory disease of the ileum and/or colon. The resulting malnutrition can impair growth and sexual maturation. Abnormally high numbers of substance P receptors in arterioles and venules of intestinal submucosa, muscularis, and serosa contribute to the etiology.

cromokalin: BRL 34915; 6-cyano-3,4-dihydro-2,2-dimethyl-*trans*-4-(2-oxo-1-pyrrolidyl)-2*H*-benzo[*b*]pyran-3-ol; an agent that activates ATP-sensitive K^+ channels in smooth muscle, and, at higher concentrations, in the heart (and can also act on some protein kinase C isozymes). It mimics the effects of hypoxia and ATP deficiency on K^+ extrusion, and thereby relaxes smooth muscle and lowers blood pressure. Glyburide and related agents are antagonists.

cromolyn: 1,3-*bis*(2-carboxychromone-5yloxy)-2-hydroxypropane, an agent that stabilizes mast cell membranes and thereby inhibits histamine release. The sodium salt is used to avert asthma attacks, allergic rhinitis, and some other allergic responses, but is not effective for acute treatment.

Crooke's cells: large, hyalinized, agranular adenohypophysial cells in pituitary glands of some individuals with Cushing's disease. Chronic exposure to high glucocorticoid concentrations is believed to cause the degranulation by inhibiting proopiomelanocortin (POMC) synthesis, and possibly also by promoting microtubule hyalinization.

cro protein: a dimeric protein composed of 7K subunits, made by lambda phage during its lytic phase. It binds DNA and controls viral replication genes, possibly by altering the DNA configuration.

crop sac: a structure that develops from the gullet of some birds. Prolactin stimulates thickening of the walls and formation of "milk" that is regurgitated and fed to the young. A bioassay procedure for prolactin is based on the growth promoting effects in pigeons.

cross: usually, (1) the mating of two individuals of a breeding population to produce offspring with specific kinds of genetic traits derived from one or both parents, or to obtain information on the parental genotype; (2) the offspring of such mating. See also **backcross**.

cross linking: the joining of chemical groups (within the same molecule, or on different ones), usually by formation of covalent bonds.

crossing over: exchange of genetic material between contiguous chromatids of homologous chromosomes during meiosis; *see* **synapsis**. It contributes to genetic variation among gametes made by an individual.

cross-reactivity: usually, binding of an antibody to an antigen different from (but structurally related to) the kind that usually stimulates its formation. The process can create problems when attempts are made to identify specific molecular species with antibodies; and it accounts for some autoimmune attacks against normal cells. See also **monoclonal** and **polyclonal antibodies**.

cross-talk: usually (1) interactions among two or more second messenger types, for example phosphorylation of one type by an enzyme activated by another, or activation by one type when the other elevates cytosol Ca^{2+} levels; (2) the effects of one hormone (or neurotransmitter) on responses by the same target cells to a different regulator.

crotonic acid: *trans*-2-butanoic acid; an intermediate in the pathway for fatty acid degradation.

crotonic acid

croton oil: an oil expressed from *Croton tiglium* seeds that is used as a counterirritant and purgative in veterinary medicine. The components include glycerides of several fatty acids. *See* also **phorbol esters**.

CRP: (1) C-reactive protein; (2) cAMP receptor protein (an alternate term for catabolite activated protein).

Crustacea: a class of mostly aquatic invertebrates of the Arthropod phylum that includes crabs, lobsters, and shrimps. All members have exoskeletons and jointed appendages. The large nerve cells are used in neurophysiology studies.

cryoactivation: activation by freezing and thawing. The process is used, for example, for prorenins. *Cf* **cryopreservation**.

cryoglobulins: globular proteins that precipitate when cooled. In some immune system dysfunctions, blood plasma contains large quantities of IgG and/or IgM immunoglobulins that display the property. *See* also **cryoprecipitates**.

cryoprecipitates: aggregates that form when blood plasma is frozen and then thawed. The components include coagulation factor VIII and fibronectin.

cryopreservation: (1) cooling embryos, gametes, or other organisms, to maintain them in a dormant (but viable) state from which they can be returned to normal functions when rewarmed; (2) preservation of proteins and other substances for later use by freezing and thawing procedures that do not damage the components; *cf* **cryoactivation**.

cryoprotectants: glycerol, DMSO, and other substances used to prevent the formation of ice crystals when organisms, chemicals, or specimens for microscopy are frozen.

cryostats: devices in which specimens for microscopy are hardened by freezing for sectioning. The techniques avert problems associated with the use of chemical fixatives, but some cell types are damaged.

crypt: a deep pit.

cryptic: concealed or camouflaged, a term applied to substances whose functions are unknown, for example amino acid sequences within a prohormone that are released during processing, or nucleic acid components that do not code for messenger RNAs.

cryptic plasmid: a plasmid that does not invoke discernible changes in the host.

cryptic species: sibling species; ones with similar phenotypes that do not breed and produce hybrid progeny.

cryptorchism: cryptorchidism: retention of testes within the abdominal cavities, in humans and other species in which descent to the scrotum normally occurs. The associated loss of fertility is attributed mostly to adverse effects of high abdominal temperatures on the germinal cells; but small decreases in androgen production have been described for some species. Elephants and whales are among the mammalian types in which no scrotum develops (and none is required for sperm maturation).

crystallins: 28K to 8000K, water-soluble proteins whose synthesis is directed by several gene families. The diversities result in part from posttranslational modifications. α, β, and $\delta1$ and γ types account for approximately 90% of the protein content of eye lenses. The gene that directs synthesis of the δ_1 form (used as a lens differentiation marker), also codes for argininosuccinate lyase. It is activated by insulin and insulin-like growth factor I (IGF-I). A more widely distributed αB crystallin that may confer heat tolerance is induced in 3T3 fibroblasts by *v-mos* and *Ha-ras*; and the amounts in several other cell types increase in response to numerous forms of stress. High levels also accumulate in some cell types under pathological conditions. Nonenzymatic glycosylation is one of the mechanisms whereby chronic hyperglycemia causes cataract formation.

Cs: cesium.

CS: (1) calf serum; (2) calsequestrin; (3) cholera toxin.

CSAT: (1) chicken embryo fibroblast cell surface antigen, a 140K complex of three proteins that binds fibronectin and talin, and may be the avian homolog of a mammalian integrin; (2) an antibody directed against that antigen.

CSF: (1) cytostatic factor; (2) cerebrospinal fluid.

CSF-1: colony stimulating factor-1; *see* **macrophage colony stimulating factor**.

CSF-2: colony stimulating factor-2; *see* **granulocyte-macrophage colony stimulating factor**.

CSI: corticostatin.

CSIF: cytokine synthesis inhibitory factor; *see* **interleukin-10**.

CSP: castanospermine.

c-src: *see* **Rous sarcoma virus** and **proto-oncogenes**.

C subunit: usually, the catalytic component of an enzyme that has regulatory subunits.

CT: (1) calcitonin; (2) computerized tomography; (3) cholera toxin.

CTB: cytotactin binding protein.

***C*-terminal**: the end of a peptide or protein that carries the terminal carboxyl (or amide) group. The term can refer to one or many amino acids, or to peptides cleaved from that end. During translation, the amino acid with the free -COOH is the last to be added to the peptide chain. *Cf* **N-terminal**.

CTL: cytotoxic T lymphocytes; T_C cells.

CTP: cytidine triphosphate.

CTR: RG 12851; N^A-propionyl-diAla^{1,7}-desLeu^{19}-sCT; a noncyclic salmon calcitonin analog that exerts the therapeutic effects of calcitonin but invokes fewer side effects, such as anorexia.

cubitus valgus: a deformity of the elbow that causes the forearm to incline away from the midline when the arm is held in the anatomical position. Turner's syndrome is one of the conditions in which the incidence is high.

culture: in biology, (1) to grow *in vitro*; (2) cells or tissues grown *in vitro*.

cumulus oophorus: cells that encircle a preovulatory ovarian follicle oocyte, and are believed to perform functions not shared by other granulosa cells, such as production of factors that regulate meiotic progression. Some authors use the term synonymously with corona radiata; others restrict the corona term to the components closest to the oocyte.

curare: a generic term for high molecular weight alkaloids obtained from the barks of *Strychnos toxifera*, *Chondodendron tomentosum*, and other members of the *Menispermacaeae* family, initially used by South American Indians as arrow poisons and known under names such as woorari and urari. Modifying terms (tube, bamboo, pot, and calabash), refer to the containers in which they were packaged. Low dosages relax, and higher ones paralyze striated muscle, by competing with acetylcholine for postjunctional receptors. Since diaphragm muscle is less sensitive than the kinds that move bones, it is possible to inject animals with dosages that block voluntary activity but preserve vital functions. Hunted animals can be then safely transported long distances while still alive. (Higher doses kill by acting on the heart as well as the muscles used for breathing.) Intocostrin (a standardized extract), **tubocurarine** (*q.v.*), some semi-synthetic derivatives such as metocurarine, and some totally synthesized congeners are used as skeletal muscle relaxants, to control some dysfunctions, and to reduce the amounts of general anesthetics required for surgical procedures. The structure of C-curarine I (from calabash curare) is shown.

curariform: exerting curare-like effects; *see* **tubocurarine**, and *cf* **muscarinic** and **nicotinic**.

curcumin: turmeric yellow; 1,7-*bis*(4-hydroxy-3-methoxyphenyl)-1,6-heptadiene-3,5-dione; the pigment used to color curries and other foods. Its ability to block phorbol ester induced tumorigenesis is attributed to intereference with the influences on *c-jun* gene product activities.

CURL: compartment for uncoupling receptors from ligands; a specialized, acidic "prelysosomal" organelle in which complexes taken up by endocytosis undergo dis-

C-curarine I

sociation. In some cases, receptors are recycled to plasma membranes, but their ligands are taken up by lysosomes. In others, both components are degraded by lysosomal enzymes.

Cushing's disease: disorders in which excessive production of glucocorticoids is stimulated by adrenocorticotropic hormone (ACTH)-secreting pituitary adenomas; *see* also **Cushing's syndrome**.

Cushing's syndrome: disorders caused by excessive production of glucocorticoids. When caused by adrenocortical tumors, the manifestations resemble those for Cushing's disease (although adrenocorticotropic hormone secretion is usually inhibited). They include hypertension, polycythemia, fat redistribution, obesity, impaired immune system functions, mood swings, mild hyperglycemia, and protein depletion that leads to muscle weakness, skin striations, and osteoporosis.

cuticle: (1) an outer rigid or semi-rigid layer, for example on the surfaces of hair follicles, plant leaves, or organisms such as *Paramecia*; (2) the epidermal fold that covers the base of a fingernail; (3) a term applied to some nonmineralized tooth components.

cutin: complexes of long-chain fatty acid esters and other fatty acid derivatives that form cuticles (definition 1) in plants, and are also deposited in the outer walls of epidermal cells.

CV 3988: a synthetic platelet activating factor analog that antagonizes PAF actions.

CV 6209: a selective platelet activating factor (PAF) antagonist that does not affect the actions of histamine, leukotrienes, or acetylcholine.

curcumin

162

C value: a measure of the total amount of DNA in a haploid cell.

cyanide: -C≡N; an anion that binds Fe^{3+} and other metallic cations in their oxidized states. It rapidly arrests cellular oxidation by blocking transfers of electrons from cytochrome a_3 to molecular oxygen, and is used (usually as the potassium salt) to study mitochondrial functions. If accidentally ingested, very prompt treatment with nitrates or thiosulfates can avert lethal consequences, since those compounds oxidize the Fe^{2+} of hemoglobin, and the product (methemoglobin) competes with cytochromes for the ion. (Hemoglobin functions are retained, since only small amounts are affected.) The cyanide is then slowly converted to thiocyanate and excreted. Nitroprusside metabolism yields some cyanide, but therapeutic doses do not produce enough to invoke toxicity. Cyanide also inhibits production of vitamin K-dependent proteins (including blood coagulation factors) by competing with CO_2 for glutamate carboxylase, and similarly affects other carboxylases.

cyano-: a prefix meaning blue.

Cyanobacteria: blue-green algae; prokaryotes that make phycobiliproteins (which impart the characteristic color), and use chlorophyll on intracytoplasmic membranes for photosynthesis. They may be the evolutionary precursors of chloroplasts. Some species fix nitrogen.

cyanocobalamin: extrinsic factor; a form of vitamin B_{12}, and a component of the vitamin B complex. It associates with 5′-deoxyadenosine to form a B_{12}-enzyme required for conversion of methylmalonyl-coenzyme A to succinyl-coenzyme A (a pathway for both carbohydrate and lipid metabolism), and is also needed to make methylcobalamin (required for methyl group transfers affecting, among other things, folic acid use). The vitamin is required in just trace amounts, is easily obtained from foods, and is made by microorganisms that colonize normal colons. However, absorption into the bloodstream requires intrinsic factor (which is made in the stomach), and it is facilitated by gastric HCl. Most vitamin B_{12} deficiencies are caused by inability to provide those factors. Since the coenzymes are essential for cell growth and replication, and for myelin formation, the major effects include pernicious anemia and irreversible neurological damage. *See also* **cobalamin**.

cyanogen bromide: Br-C≡N; a reagent used to split polypeptides at methionine residues, and to brominate organic compounds.

cyanogen chloride: Cl-C≡N; a reagent used to convert alcohols to chlorides, to activate polysaccharide carriers that bind enzymes and other proteins, and in affinity chromatography. It liberates **cyanide** (*q.v.*), and has been used as a military poison gas.

cyanoketone: 2-cyano-4,4,17α-trimethylandrost-5-en-17β-ol; an agent that inhibits 3β-hydroxysteroid dehydrogenase, and thereby the synthesis of most steroid hormones. It is used to study the functions of adrenocortical cells, and to invoke deficiencies in laboratory animals.

cyanoketone

cyanolabe: a pigment in retinal cone cells that absorbs blue light.

cyanosis: bluish discoloration of skin, caused by accumulation of unoxygenated hemoglobin.

cyanuric chloride: 2,4,6-trichloro-1,3,5-triazine; a reagent used for colorimetric determinations of glycine and some other amino acids, and on cellulose columns that immobilize DNAs.

cyclamate: Sucaryl: cyclohexylsulfamic acid sodium salt; an artificial sweetener with no nutritive value that (unlike aspartame) resists degradation by the amounts of heat used in food preparation, and is generally regarded as more palatable than saccharin. It is consumed in Canada (where saccharin is banned), and in some other countries, and is used in studies of taste perception (or to sweeten preparations fed to laboratory animals). Sale for human consumption in the United States has been banned because of purported carcinogenicity.

cyclase associated protein: adenyl cyclase associated protein; CAP; a protein that localizes to the cytoplasmic faces of yeast (*Saccharomyces cerevisiae*) plasma membranes, and is essential for RAS activation of adenylate cyclase and the consequent influences on cell shape, budding, and other effects that involve the cytoskeleton. The *N*-terminal associates directly with the enzyme, and the *C*-terminal participates in a phosphatidylinositol signalling mechanism. Mutants that lack the CAP *N*-terminal domains are unresponsive to RAS. Ones that lack the *C*-terminal enlarge markedly, become rounded, and display budding and nutritional defects. It has been suggested that CAP binds directly to, and affects the polymerization of actin. Different observations implicate profilins in both polymerization control and signalling, via either binding CAP, or acting on another pathway that intersects with the RAS-CAP system. High levels of profilin II can restore morphology in CAP mutants. Although known to block polymerization by complexing with actin monomers, profilins can also promote polymerization by attaching to the rapidly growing ends, and accelerating ATP-ADP exchange. The second effect predominates when ATP levels are high and large quantities of ADP-actin are made (conditions that prevail in activated cells). Tight binding of profilin to phosphoinositides causes the profilins to dissociate from actin; and profilin binding to clusters of inositol 1,4-biphosphate molecules blocks phosphatidylinositol-phosphate (PIP_2) hydrolysis by PI-specific phospholipase Cγ. In other cell types, phospholipase Cγ promotes hydrolysis of prolifin-bound PIP_2, when it is phosphorylated by epidermal or platelet derived growth factor receptor kinases.

cyclazocine: 3-(cyclopropylmethyl)-1,2,3,4,5,6-hexahydro-6,11-dimethyl-2,6-methano-3-benzazocin-8-ol; a benzomorphan type narcotic analgesic with mixed agonist-antagonist properties that binds with highest affinity to μ type receptors, but also acts on other opioid types. It is a less potent analgesic than morphine, but invokes fewer side effects, is not addictive, and is of some use for the treatment of morphine addiction.

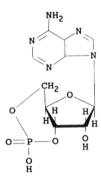

cycle: in biochemistry, a pathway that begins with a compound, and later restores the same kind of compound for a new round of reactions. For example, oxaloacetate combines with acetyl-coenzyme A in the first reaction of the tricarboxylic acid cycle, and a new oxaloacetate molecule is generated by the final reaction.

cyclic adenosine diphosphate ribose: cADP-ribose; cADPR; an NAD^+ metabolite that acts on ryanodine-sensitive channels, and promotes translocation of Ca^{2+} ions from the endoplasmic reticulum to the cytoplasm in pancreatic β cells, cerebellar neurons, sea-urchin oocytes, and some other cell types. It can desensitize cells to ryanodine by depleting Ca^{2+} stores. cADPR synthesis is accelerated by glucose, and it appears to mediate the glucose stimulated elevation of cytoplasmic Ca^{2+} in pancreatic β cells that leads to insulin secretion. Streptozotocin abolishes cADPR effects by depleting NAD^+. The concept that glucose elevates cytosolic Ca^{2+} in pancreatic islets by accelerating phosphatidylinositol hydrolysis is based on observations made with tumor cells. In normal β cells, glucose does not accelerate phosphatidylinositol turnover, and inositol$_{1,4,5}$-triphosphate (IP_3) does not mimic CaDPR actions. Moreover, heparin (which blocks IP_3 binding to its receptors) does not antagonize cADPR-mediated insulin secretion.

cyclic adenosine 3′5′-monophosphate: cyclic AMP; cAMP; a major second messenger for eukaryote hormones and neurotransmitters, formed in the adenylate cyclase catalyzed reaction: ATP → cAMP + P-P. In most cells, the activity of the plasma membrane enzyme is low under basal conditions, but is rapidly augmented in

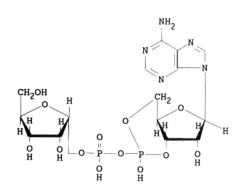

cyclic adenosine diphosphate ribose

eukaryotes when ligands such as glucagon, adrenocorticotropic, follicle stimulating, thyroid stimulating, and parathyroid hormones, epinephrine, and gastrin interact with their receptors (*see* also **G proteins**). In eukaryotes, cAMP exerts most of its effects by activating protein kinase A isozymes. It binds to the regulatory (R) subunits of the enzymes, and releases the catalytic (C) subunits in active form (C*), via the reaction: 4 cAMP + R_2C_2 → 2 cAMP-R_2 + 2 C*. The activated subunits then catalyze phosphorylation of numerous substrates. The major pathway for inactivation is the reaction catalyzed by cyclic nucleotide dependent phosphodiesterases: cAMP → AMP. However, some cAMP is extruded from cells when the levels are high; and kinase A inhibitors contribute to the controls. When the cAMP levels fall, the R subunits reassociate with the catalytic ones. In prokaryotes, cAMP effects are mediated via binding to catabolic activator protein.

cyclic AMP: cAMP; *see* **cyclic adenosine 3′5′-monophosphate**.

cyclic AMP-dependent protein kinases: kinase A; *see* **cyclic adenosine-3′5′-monophosphate** and **protein kinases**.

cyclic AMP-dependent protein kinase inhibitor: H_2N-Thr-Thr-Tyr-Ala-Asp-Phe-Ile-Ala-Ser-Gly-Arg-Thr-Gly-Arg-Arg-Asn-Ala-Ile-His-Asp-OH.

cyclic CMP: cCMP; *see* **cyclic cytosine 3′5′-monophosphate**.

cyclic cytosine 3′5′-monophosphate: cCMP: a cyclic nucleotide made from cytosine triphosphate. Since it is not known to perform functions of the kinds established for cAMP or cGMP, it is used as a control in some second messenger studies.

NH$_2$
N
O
CH$_2$
O
H   H   H
O=P—O   O H
O H

cyclic GMP: cGMP: *see* **cyclic guanosine 3'5'-monophosphate**.

cyclic guanosine 3'5-monophosphate: cyclic GMP; cGMP; a major second messenger for acetylcholine, atrial natriuretic peptides, nitric oxide, and some other endogenous factors, and for some environmental ones. It relaxes smooth muscle, inhibits platelet aggregation, affects macrophage activities, mediates several brain functions, and contributes to vision, olfaction, and fertilization (*see* **resact**). Diverse **guanylate cyclases** (*q.v.*) catalyze its generation from guanosine triphosphate via the reaction: GTP → cGMP + P-P. Some of the enzymes are associated with plasma membranes, whereas others are intracellular. cGMP is degraded by cyclic nucleotide dependent phosphodiesterases, via cGMP → GMP. By binding to regulatory subunits, the nucleotide activates protein kinase G catalytic subunits; but unlike cAMP activation of kinase A, it does not promote subunit dissociation. Since kinase G acts on a few cAMP substrates, and cGMP competes with cAMP for some phosphodiesterases, it can synergize with, or prolong the effects of cAMP at certain sites. However, kinase G also activates some phosphatases that act on compounds phosphorylated by cAMP, and cGMP exerts other forms of antagonism. Some cGMP actions are exerted directly (without kinase G activation), for example on Na$^+$ channels in retinal rod photoreceptors. During darkness, cGMP maintains the channels in partially opened states. Channel closing is initiated by light acting on rhodopsin, and consequent activation of a cGMP phoshodiesterase.

O
HN   N
H$_2$N   N   N
CH$_2$ O
H   H   H
O=P—O   O H
O H

cIMP: cyclic inosine-3'5'-monophosphate.

cyclic inosine-3'5'-monophosphate: cyclic IMP; cIMP; a cyclic nucleotide made from inosine triphosphate. It is not known to function as a second messenger, and is used as a control in studies of cAMP and cGMP functions.

H
O
N   N
N   N
CH$_2$ O
H   H   H
O=P—O   O H
O H

cyclic nucleotides: compounds composed of a nitrogenous base (such as adenine, guanine, or cytidine), covalently linked to a sugar (usually ribose) which is, in turn, linked by two covalent bonds to a phosphate group. Examples include cyclic adenosine 3'5'-monophosphate (cAMP), cGMP, cIMP, and cCMP.

cyclic nucleotide phosphodiesterases: enzymes that catalyze conversion of cyclic nucleotides to their corresponding linear types, via reactions such as cAMP → AMP, and cGMP → GMP. Hormones and other factors affect the synthesis of various types, which differ from each other in substrate affinities and specificities, as well as distribution to specific cell types. *See* also **cyclic adenosine-3'5'-monophosphate** and **cyclic guanosine-3'5'-monophosphate**.

cyclins: thirty or more 60-62K proteins synthesized during various cell cycle phases, and soon afterward inactivated and degraded. They associate with, and activate specific kinds of preexisting cell division cycle kinases (CDKs) to form complexes that undergo dephosphorylations at certain loci. The activated kinases catalyze threonine and/or serine phosphorylation of other proteins, and are components of cascades essential for cell division. C cyclins attain highest levels during early G1 phases of cell cycles, and activate an as yet undetermined CDK type. Cyclins D1, D2, and D3 associate with CDKs 2, 4 and 5, and with proliferating cell nuclear antigen (PCNA) around the time of the restriction point. E cyclins, which associate with CDK2, are implicated as regulators of G$_1$ → S transitions. A types, which also associate with CDK2, reach their highest levels somewhat later, and are believed to control some aspects of DNA synthesis, as well as G$_2$ → M transitions. B types bind CDK1 (cdc2) during late S phases, peak at metaphase, decline at anaphase, and may play roles in both entry into and completion of mitosis. Two subgroups (B1 and B2) are first detectable in perinuclear regions during G2. They persist for some time, enter nuclei during prophase, and associate with spindle caps.

F and G cyclins have been identified, but their functions are not known. Most cyclins must be degraded before cell division is completed. (Protease inhibitors that affect them arrest cells in metaphase). The cyclins contain **PEST sequences** (*q.v.*), flanked by basic amino acids. Consistent with such structures, the degradation is preceded by ubiquitination, and it requires specific ligases. Cyclin functions are affected by phosphorylation; and the proteins are substrates for **cytostatic factor** *(q.v.)*. There is some evidence that dysregulation leads to tumorigenesis. High levels of PRAD1, which is identical with cyclin D1, have been detected in some lymphomas, parathyroid gland adenomas and breast cancers; and the retinoblastoma gene product is a substrate for cyclin activated kinases. Moreover, some of the antitumorigenic effects of transforming growth factor-β (TGFβ) have been linked with inhibition of cyclin E formation. *See* also **MPF**.

1,2-cyclohexanedione: an agent that binds specifically to arginine moieties of peptides and proteins.

2-cyclohexene-1-one: a glutathione (GSH) redox cycle inhibitor that is used to lower glutathione levels in laboratory animals and *in vitro* preparations.

cycloheximide: CHX; cyclohexamide; actidione; 3-[2-(3,5-dimethyl-2-oxocylohexyl)-2-hydroxyethyl]glutarimide; an antibiotic and plant fungicide derived from *Streptomyces griseus*. It binds to the large subunits of eukaryote cytoplasmic (but not prokaryote or mitochondrial) ribosomes, and promotes dissociation of peptidyltransferases from ribosomal RNAs. Consequently, it blocks peptide bond formation, and thereby peptide chain elongation. It also elevates cell messenger RNA content, in part by stabilizing polysomes, but may additionally decrease synthesis of either a direct inhibitor of RNA polymerase II, or of a protein that activates the inhibitor gene.

N^6-**cyclohexyladenosine**: CPA; a selective A$_1$ type adenosine receptor antagonist.

cycloleucine: 1-amino-cyclopentanecarboxylic acid; a leucine analog that is transported across cell membranes but is not incorporated into proteins. It is used to study amino acid transport, and as an immunosuppressant.

2-cyclooctyl-2-hydroxyethylamine: an agent used to inhibit phenylethanolamine-*N*-methyltransferase (PNMT).

cyclooxygenase: prostaglandin synthase; PGH$_2$ synthase; an enzyme system that requires both heme and nonheme cofactors, and catalyzes conversion of arachidonate to prostaglandin G$_2$ (PGG$_2$, an endoperoxide). The product rapidly converts spontaneously to prostaglandin H$_2$ (PGH$_2$), but cyclooxygenase speeds the reaction. The synthase additionally catalyzes its own destruction. PGH$_2$ is a precursor of thromboxanes, prostaglandins, prostacyclin, and other biologically active lipids. The major rate-limiting factor for PGG$_2$ formation is substrate availability. In non-stimulated cells, arachidonate is present mostly as a component of phospholipids (*see* **phospholipases**), with lesser amounts present in cholesterol esters and triacylglycerols. Glucocorticoids act in several ways to decrease arachidonate release, and they oppose many effects of the compounds derived from it. Aspirin irreversibly inhibits the enzyme by promoting its acetylation. Some other nonsteroidal anti-inflammatory agents (NSIFs) are reversible inhibitors. *See* also **lipocortins**.

8-cyclopentyl-1,3-dimethylxanthine: CPT; 8-cylcopentyltheophylline; a selective A$_1$-type adenosine receptor antagonist.

8-cyclopentyl-1, 3-dimethylxanthine

cyclophilins: mammalian proteins that bind to and mediate the immunosuppressive effects of cyclosporins. Since they display peptidyl-prolyl *cis-trans* isomerase (PPI, rotamase) activity, they probably contribute to the control of protein folding, and may affect associations of physiological inhibitors of T cell and mast cell activation with their binding sites. Cyclosporin A (CsA) inhibits the rotamase, but its major immunosuppressant effects are attributed to formation of complexes with cyclophilins that block lymphocyte calcineurin functions; *see also* **immunophilins**. A homologous 26K membrane-bound protein in *Drosophila* eyes exerts posttranscriptional control over rhodopsin levels, possibly by affecting rhodopsin insertion into photoreceptor membranes.

cyclophosphamide: *N,N*-bis(β-chloroethyl)-*N'*,*O*-propyl-enephosphoric acid ester diamide; a compound metabolized to several products, some of which are alkylating agents used to arrest the growth of neoplasms. It can invoke antidiuresis by stimulating vasopressin release.

cyclo(-L-Pro-Gly)₃: a synthetic peptide that binds cations, and is used to study calcium and magnesium binding to endogenous proteins.

cyclopiazonic acid: a potent neurotoxin that diminishes Ca^{2+}-dependent K^+ currents in smooth muscle, and a specific inhibitor of sarcoplamic and endoplasmic reticulum Ca^{2+}-ATPases. It does not affect inositol-1,4,5-triphosphate (IP$_3$) levels, but releases Ca^{2+} from intracellular sequestration sites by augmenting plasma membrane permeability.

cycloserine: seromycine; D-4-amino-3-isoxazolidinone; a serine analog made by *Streptomyces garifalus* that

binds to several cell components, and kills dividing cells. It is used to treat tuberculosis and some other infections, and as a marker for certain kinds of cultured cells. It is also a partial agonist for NMDA receptor glycine sites.

cyclosporines: cyclosporins: several small peptides made by *Tolypocladium inflatum* and related fungi. Cyclosporine A (CsA), is cyclic-(Ala-D-Ala-*N*-methyl-Leu-*N*-methyl-Leu-*N*-methyl-Val-3-hydroxy-N,4-dimethyl-2-amino-6-octenoyl-α-aminobutyryl-*N*-methyl-Gly-*N*-methyl-Leu-Val-*N*-methyl-Leu), an undecapeptide that binds to cyclophilins, inhibits the proliferation and functions of helper type lymphocytes, acts on some B lymphocytes, and blocks mast cell degranulation. It does not interfere with phosphatidylinositol hydrolysis, but appears to inhibit cytoplasmic transport of T cell proteins and mast cell granules, and to block transcription of genes for interleukins-1, 2, and 3, interferon-γ and other regulators by acting on calcineurins; *see also* **immunophilins**. CsA is used as an immunosuppressant to control autoimmune disorders such as myasthenia gravis and some forms of diabetes mellitus, and to block transplant rejection. It also decreases luteinizing hormone (LH) and testosterone secretion, and bone resorption mediated by prostaglandins and other pro-inflammatory factors. It can invoke nephrotoxicity, hepatotoxicity, hypertension, and anemia.

cyclostomes: a class of aquatic, jawless vertebrates with cartilaginous skeletons. The living species are hagfishes (the only vertebrates known to lack true thymus glands, and in which blood osmotic pressure varies with the environment), and the somewhat less primitive lamprey eels.

Cyd: cytidine.

[125]I-**CYP**: iodocyanopindolol-hydrochloride; a radioactive compound made from pindolol (shown), a specific ligand for identifying β-type adrenergic receptors.

CYP genes: genes in the Class III region of the part of human chromosome 6 that codes for complement proteins C4A and C4B. *CYP 21B* directs formation of steroid 21-hydroxylase (an enzyme essential glucocor-

cyclosporine A

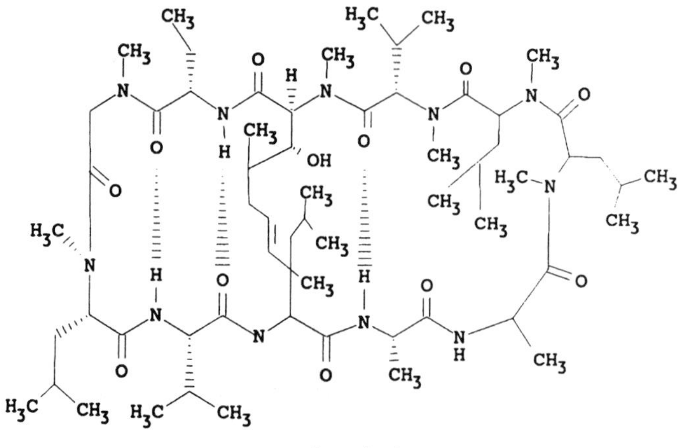

ticoid and mineralocorticoid biosynthesis). *CYP 21A* is a similar, but nonfunctional pseudogene. *See* also **congenital adrenal hyperplasia**.

cyproheptadine: 4-(5*H*-dibenzocyclohepten-5-ylidene) piperidine; an orally effective H_1 type histamine receptor antagonist, used to treat allergies. It also blocks responses to serotonin, and is a cholinergic and central nervous system depressant. Additionally, it affects insulin and growth hormone secretion, and can stimulate appetite.

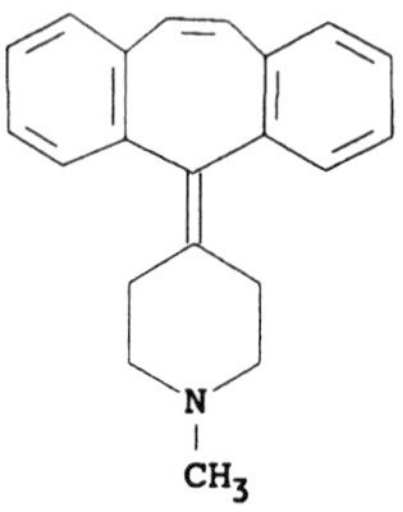

cyproterone: 6-chloro-1,2α-methylenepregnadien-17α-ol-3,20-dione. The acetate (shown below) is an androgen receptor antagonist that also exerts progesterone-like actions and inhibits gonadotropin secretion. It is used to treat prostatic cancer, and to arrest precocious puberty.

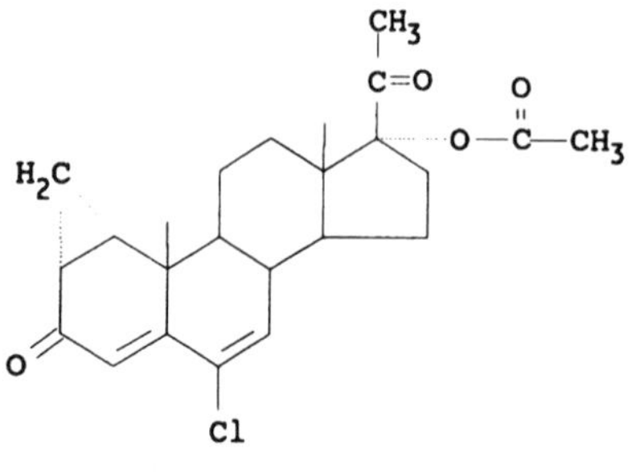

cystathione: an intermediate in the pathway for biosynthesis of cysteine; *see* **cystathioninase.** and **cystathione β-synthetase**.

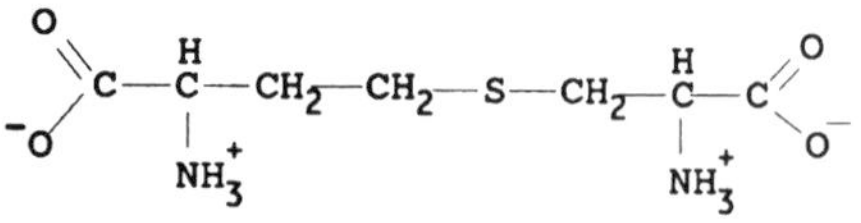

cystathione lyase: an enzyme that degrades excess cysteine by catalyzing its conversion to β-hydroxybutyrate + ammonia.

cystathione β-synthetase: cystathionase; an enzyme that catalyzes the reaction: homocysteine + serine → cystathione + H_2O. Cysteine is then generated via the reaction catalyzed by cystathioninase.

cystathioninase: an enzyme that catalyzes the reaction: cystathione + H_2O → cysteine + α-ketobutyrate.

cystathioninuria: apparently benign conditions in which large amounts of cystathione are excreted to the urine. Excessive amounts of the compound accumulate if cystathione β-synthetase activity is too high, and when a deficiency of a cobalamin enzyme (N^6-methyltetrahydrofolate-homocysteine methyltransferase) channels too much homocysteine into the pathway for biosynthesis. Other causes include vitamin B_6 deficiency, which leads to inadequate production of cystathioninase.

cystatins: naturally occurring protease inhibitors that protect against tissue damage. The group includes 12K cystatins A and B (thiolproteinase inhibitors in human placenta and other tissues), cystatin C (a 13.5K form in blood plasma), and a 12.7K egg white cystatin.

cysteamine: β-mercaptoethanol; 2-aminoethyl mercaptan; an amine made from cysteine that can be converted to taurine. Although a component of coenzyme A, it is not used directly to synthesize that compound, and is not released from it. Cysteamine is a reducing agent that converts disulfide bonds to sulfhydryl types, and protects compounds against oxidation (both *in vivo* and *in vitro*). It is used to treat radiation sickness and chronic leukemias. In the laboratory, it is used to separate protein subunits linked by disulfide bonds, denature proteins for analysis, and remove analytical reagents such as β-hydroxymercuribenzoate.

$$HS-CH_2-\underset{\underset{H}{|}}{\overset{\overset{NH_2}{|}}{C}}-NH_2$$

cysteamine

cysteine: Cys; C; a glucogenic amino acid synthesized via reactions catalyzed by cysteine β-synthetase and cystathioninase. It is a component of many peptides and proteins, of leukotrienes C_4, D_4, E_4, and F_4, and of glutathione. The sulfhydryl groups of two molecules can split out hydrogen atoms and form the disulfide bond of cystine. Bonds of this kind hold protein subunits together, cause many peptides to assume ring structures, and are essential for establishing and maintaining the tertiary and quaternary structures of many proteins (*see* also **zinc fingers**). Cysteine yields pyruvate (via a β-mercaptopyruvate intermediate when transaminated, and via cysteine sulfinate when oxidized). It is also the precursor of taurine, and the major source of urinary sulfate (*see* also **cystinuria**). Since it reacts with cyanide, prompt administration can combat the toxicity.

$$HS-CH_2-\underset{\underset{H}{|}}{\overset{\overset{NH_2}{|}}{C}}-COOH$$

cysteine proteases: thiol proteases; papain and other proteolytic enzymes whose catalytic sites contain a cysteine moiety, and whose activities involve formation of thiol ester intermediates facilitated by adjacent histidine moieties. Some contribute to antigen processing.

cysteine-rich intestinal proteins: 6-9K proteins that mediate zinc transport in the small intestine. A major type is Met-Pro-Lys-Cys-Pro-Lys-Cys-Asp-Lys-Glu-Val-Tyr-Phe-Ala-Glu-Arg-Val-Thr-Ser-Leu-Gly-Lys-Asp-Trp-His-Arg-Pro-Cys-Leu-Lys-Cys-Glu-Lys-Cys-Gly-Lys-Thr-Leu-Thr-Ser-Gly-Gly-His-Ala-Glu-His-Glu-Gly-Lys-Pro-Tyr-Cys-Asn-His-Pro-Cys-Tyr-Ser-Ala-Met-Phe-Gly-Pro-Lys-Gly-Phe-Gly-Arg-Gly-Gly-Arg-Glu-Ser-His-Thr-Phe-Lys.

cyst: a closed cavity.

cystic: (1) a term that refers to the urinary or gall bladder; (2) relating to or characterized by the formation of cysts.

cystic fibrosis: the most common lethal autosomal recessive disease in Caucasians. The incidence is 1 in 2000 live births; and 1 in 20-25 individuals is a carrier. The primary defect is a mutation that impairs chloride transport (*see* **cystic fibrosis gene**). It can secondarily interfere with transport of sodium, bicarbonate, and sulfate ions, and cause fluid and electrolyte loss, and hypovolemia. The most common manifestations are decreased net electrolyte absorption in sweat glands, and accelerated absorption in airway epithelium; but electrolyte transport is also defective in the exocrine pancreas, salivary glands, seminal vesicles, and cervical glands, and in some cases also in the small intestine,

colon and rectum, and possibly at other sites. A major problem is accumulation of viscous mucus in the lungs that impedes gas exchange and predisposes to respiratory infections. The biliary tracts and pancreatic ducts can also become obstructed; and, because of influences on the reproductive tracts, the incidence of infertility is around 85% for afflicted females, and almost 100% for males. The sweat of newborns has a high sodium chloride content, and the small intestines of some are obstructed with meconium. A few have liver disease. Deterioration occurs with advancing age, and secondary pulmonary complications are the most common cause of death. The mean survival time has been increased with treatment from around 29 years to approximately 40.

cystic fibrosis antigen: a protein of the S100 family identified in the blood of individuals with cystic fibrosis, but present in small amounts on the surfaces of normal cells. The levels rise on leukemia cells stimulated to undergo differentiation by retinoic acid or dimethylsulfoxide (DMSO).

cystic fibrosis gene: a DNA segment that directs formation of a 480 amino acid protein (CFTR, cystic fibrosis transport regulator) that displays homology to P-glycoprotein. It integrates into membranes, and is essential for maintaining the normal permeability of exocrine gland chloride ion channels. Although it appears to be a channel component, some observers suggest that it is a regulator of channel proteins, essential for second messenger control. The channels can be activated by kinase A and kinase C catalyzed phosphorylations and inhibited by arachidonic acid. Deletion of a single phenylalanine residue in the CFTR protein has been detected in approximately 75% of individuals with cystic fibrosis, but other point mutations can cause the disease.

cystine: an amino acid composed of two cysteine moieties linked by a disulfide bond. The ring structures and other three-dimensional configurations of many peptides and proteins are created via joining of cysteine moieties within molecules or on adjacent peptide chains. Cystine bridges also provide structural strength for keratins and some other proteins. *See* also **cysteine**.

$$S-CH_2-\underset{\underset{H}{|}}{\overset{\overset{NH_2}{|}}{C}}-COOH$$
$$S-CH_2-\underset{\underset{NH_2}{|}}{\overset{\overset{H}{|}}{C}}-COOH$$

cystinosis: autosomal recessive disorders in which cystine accumulates and deposits in cells, because of defects in amino acid transport and metabolism. In benign forms, no symptoms are associated with the amounts found in cornea, bone marrow, and leukocytes. In more severe types, cystine also accumulates in spleen, lymph nodes, retina, conjunctiva, and elsewhere. Nephrogenic cystinosis, which begins during early infancy, causes growth failure, renal rickets, acidosis, and and progressive renal failure.

cystinuria: conditions in which excessive amount of cystine, lysine, arginine, and ornithine are excreted to the urine. They are caused by impaired transport across renal tubule epithelium, which is usually associated with defective transport in the small intestine.

cyt: cytochrome.

Cyt: C; *see* **cytosine**.

cytarabine: cytosine arabinoside.

cytidine: Cyd: a nucleoside composed of cytosine covalently linked to ribose; *see* **cytidine triphosphate** and **deoxycytidine**.

cytidine 3′-diphosphate: CDP: a nucleotide composed of cytosine, ribose, and two phosphate groups. It reacts with NADPH + H⁺ to yield deoxycytidine (which is used for DNA synthesis). *See* also **cytidine triphosphate**.

cytidine 3′-monophosphate: CMP; cytidylic acid; a nucleotide composed of cytosine, ribose, and a phosphate group; *see* **cytidine triphosphate**.

cytidine 3′-triphosphate: CTP: a nucleotide composed of cytosine, ribose, and three phosphate groups, and made from uridine triphosphate. It is a component of RNAs, and a participant in metabolic pathways for lipid synthesis. CTP reacts with phosphocholine, phosphoserine, phosphoethanolamine, and phosphoinositols to form the corresponding alcohol phosphates (CDP-choline, CDP-serine, CDP-inositol) + P-P. The phosphorylated alcohols then react with 1,2,-diacylglycerols to yield phospholipids (phosphatidylcholine, phosphatidylserine or phosphatidylinositol) + cytidine monophosphate.

cytidylic acid: usually, cytidine-3′-monophosphate; but *see* 2-**cytidilyic acid**.

2′-cytidylic acid: cytidine-2′-monophosphate; 2′-CMP; a cytidine-3′-monophosphate analog that inhibits ribonucleases.

cytoadhesins: β₃ **integrins** (*q.v.*) that mediate platelet aggregation and other cell to cell interactions. The group includes GPIIb/IIIa (unique to platelets and megakaryocytes) and vitronectin receptors.

cytocenter: *see* **microtubule organization center**.

cytochalasins: several mold metabolites (A, B and F types made by *Helminthosporium dermatoideum*, and C and D types by *Metarrhizium anisopliae*). By binding to and blocking actin filament polymerization, and promoting F-actin network disassembly, they alter cell shape, impair cell movement, disrupt cytokinesis, and inhibit glucose transport, phagocytosis, platelet aggregation, and clot retraction (*see* **syneresis**). The ability to inhibit the release of several hormones is attributed to interference with the fusion of secretory granule and plasma membranes. Cytochalasin B is used to study glucose carrier translocation and other microfilament functions.

170

cytochalasin B

cytochemistry: the study of cell components with dyes, specific antibodies, enzymes, or other agents which react with them to form products that can be visualized.

cytochromes: lipophilic, membrane-associated enzymes with heme groups that transport electrons via reversible reduction and oxidation of metallic atoms. The structures of the various types (*q.v.*) are very similar across the species. They are essential for oxidative phosphorylation, for the synthesis of steroid hormones, prostaglandins, and catecholamines and other cell components, and for fatty acid synthesis and oxidation. They also promote degradation or activation of numerous pharmaceutical agents, and oxidation of some procarcinogens to carcinogens; and they can generate superoxides and other toxic metabolites. The numbers included in the names of some types refer to the wavelengths (in nm) for maximum absorption when the cytochrome in its reduced state is associated with carbon monoxide.

cytochromes a_3, b, c, and c_1: enzymes essential for oxidative phosphorylation and some other oxidative processes. The ones described here associate with eukaryote mitochondrial membranes. Related types occur in bacterial plasma membranes. *Ubiquinol-cytochrome c reductase* is a complex that contains several polypeptide chains, a nonheme iron-sulfur protein, two cytochrome b, and two cytochrome c components. Electrons donated by the reduced form of coenzyme Q are passed successively from the iron-sulfur protein to the iron atoms of cytochromes b-566, b-562, c_1, and c. The terminal acceptor is a **cytochrome oxidase complex** (*q.v.*). Some of the energy released by the transfers drives the reaction ADP + P → ATP. The remainder is lost as heat.

cytochrome oxidase complex: an enzyme complex that contains at least eight subunits, including two heme proteins (cytochromes a and a_3) with iron atoms that accept electrons from cytochrome c, and two proteins with copper atoms that accept electrons from cytochrome a and pass them on to molecular oxygen. Each oxygen molecule accepts two electrons and joins with hydrogen ions to form one of water, but incomplete reduction generates superoxide. Some of the energy released is used to synthesize ATP from ADP + Pi.

cytochrome P-450s: cytochrome components of mitochondrial and microsomal mixed function oxidases that contribute to hydroxylation reactions. They accept electrons from iron-sulfur proteins, transfer them to molecular oxygen, and use hydrogen provided by coenzymes. The overall pathway (in which R-H is the substrate) is R-H + NADH (or NADPH) + H^+ + O → R-OH + NAD^+ (or $NADP^+$). Ten families and 15 sub-families have been identified in eukaryotes. Specific substrates for some types are indicated by subscripts (*see*, for example **cytochrome P-450$_{scc}$** and **cytochrome P-450$_{11\beta}$**). Hepatic enzymes participate in pathways for synthesis and degradation of fatty acids, cholesterol, and some other lipids, for drug metabolism, and for conjugation reactions.

cytochrome P-450$_{11\beta}$: a component of the enzyme system that catalyzes oxidation of carbon atoms at position 11 on steroids. It is essential for glucocorticoid and aldosterone biosynthesis.

cytochrome P-450$_{scc}$: a component of the cholesterol side-chain cleavage system; *see* **pregnenolone synthetase**.

cytodifferentiation: progression of cells from primitive to more specialized types.

cytogenesis: cell origin and development.

cytohistogenesis: development of specialized structures within cells.

cytokeratins: intermediate filament proteins of epithelial cells; *see also* **keratins**.

cytokine: a general term for biologically active peptides and proteins that act near their sites of release (*see* **lymphokines** and **monokines**), and for some macrophage peptides that act at longer distances. The group includes nerve growth factor (NGF), as well as immune system regulators such as interleukins 1 and 6, interferons, and tumor necrosis factors.

cytokine receptor superfamily: growth hormone/prolactin superfamily; a group of single chain transmembrane proteins that includes the receptors for growth hormones and prolactins, granulocyte-macrophage colony stimulating factor (GM-CSF), erythropoietin, ciliary neurotropic factor (CTNF), interferons α, β, and γ, interleukins 3, 4, 5, and 7, the interleukin-2 p75 receptor component, and the p130- associated interleukin 6 receptor. All have similar cysteine-rich extracellular domains, but the various types range widely in size (from 54 to more than 600 amino acid moieties), and have quite different transmembrane domains.

cytokinesis: a process that starts with constriction of the cytoplasm in a region between two nuclear components, and leads to formation of two daughter cells. It usually begins during telophase; but karyokinesis can be completed without it.

cytokine synthetase inhibitory factor: CSIF; *see* **interleukin-10**.

cytokinins: kinetin, triacanthin, zeatin, and other *N*-substituted adenine derivatives that regulate plant cell differentiation and proliferation.

cytolipins: glycosphingolipids.

cytological maps: representations of gene loci on chromosomes.

cytolysins: agents that partially or totally destroy cells by inserting into membranes and undergoing calcium-dependent polymerization to form amphipathic pore structures which cause leakage of the cell contents. The term has been applied to specific peptides that accumulate in the granules of natural killer (NK) cells and cytotoxic T lymphocytes, and more broadly to several agents that exert similar overall effects, including not only the functionally related perforins, but also peptides that interact with complement components to invoke the damage.

cytolysis: cell dissolution.

cytomegaloviruses: double-stranded DNA *Herpes* viruses that infect humans and other mammals, and promote cell enlargement. Diseases attributed to various types include infectious mononucleosis, some gastrointestinal disorders, and some forms of hepatitis, retinitis, and pneumonia.

cytometers: devices for counting cell numbers.

cytometry: enumeration of cells in body fluids. In *flow* cytometry, a light or an electrical current is used to monitor the properties of cells as they pass single-file through a narrow aperture.

cytopenia: abnormally low numbers of cells, usually of a specified type.

cytophagy: phagocytosis.

cytophotometry: quantitative measurement of light transmission through various cell parts, used to determine changes in DNA and other substances.

cytoplasm: all of the cell substance outside the nucleus that is enclosed by the plasma membrane.

cytoplasmic inheritance: maternal inheritance: transmission of non-chromosomal cell components to progeny, for example mitochondria (which contain DNA that replicates and directs the synthesis of some mitochondrial proteins), RNAs made by oocytes that function in zygotes, or intracellular parasites.

cytosine: C; 4-amino-2-hydroxypyrimidine; a nitrogenous base of DNA and RNA, and a participant in several metabolic pathways (*see* **cytidine triphosphate**). It undergoes enol-amino:ketol-amino isomerization. Selective inhibition of gene expression, which can be cell type specific, is mediated in part via methylation of the bases at certain DNA loci.

cytosine arabinoside: Cytarabine; ARA-C; β-cytosine arabinoside; a cytidine analog in which arabinose replaces the usual sugar. It incorporates into DNAs, distorts their molecular configurations, and thereby blocks both replication and the actions of reverse transcriptases. Since it kills cells in the S phases of cell cycles, it is used to treat some viral infections and neoplasms. It also suppresses both primary and secondary antibody and cellular immunity responses to new antigens, and can protect against rejection of bone marrow transplants.

cytoskeleton: microfilaments, intermediate filaments, microtubules, and associated cell components that determine cell shape, and affect cell movements and intracellular translocations. The components are indirectly affected by many hormones and other regulators. Interactions with extracellular matrices contribute to differentiation, growth and proliferation.

cytosol: cytoplasm devoid of organelles such as mitochondria, endoplasmic reticulum, lysosomes and secretory granules. It contains microfilaments and other small components that are not enclosed in membranes.

cytosolic inhibiting factor: CIF; a component of estrogen target cells that inhibits steroid receptor binding to DNA.

cytosolic retinoic acid binding proteins: CRABPs: intracellular proteins that bind retinoic acid and related molecules (but not retinol). They may regulate the amounts available for association with nuclear retinoic acid receptors, and in that way contribute to retinoic acid influences on morphogenesis.

cytosolic retinol binding proteins: CRBP: intracellular proteins that bind retinol and related molecules (but not retinoic acid). They may determine the availability of the retinol for binding to nuclear receptors, and/or for conversion to retinoic acid and other metabolites. Roles in morphogenesis have been suggested.

cytostasis: (1) cessation of cell movement, growth, and replication; (2) localized accumulation of cells, for example at sites of inflammation or capillary obstruction.

enol-amino form   keto-amino form

cytosine

cytostatic: characterized by, or promoting cytostasis.

cytostatic factor: CSF: pp39$^{c\text{-}mos}$; p37; a serine/threonine kinase whose synthesis is directed by *c-mos* genes. It arrests secondary oocyte meiosis at metaphase, and can block blastomere cleavage, evidently by inhibiting a protease that degrades **cyclins** (*q.v.*). *See* also **MPF**. CSF must be destroyed before cell division can be completed. It is degraded by calpain, a calcium-activated protease. Fertilization is believed to terminate metaphase arrest via elevation of cytosolic Ca^{2+} in oocytes.

cytotactin: several 190-220K extracellular matrix glycoproteins, similar to or identical with brachionectin and tenascin, whose synthesis is directed by a single gene. They form hexabrachions that surround central cores, and contain domains similar to some that occur in fibronectins and fibrinogen, several epidermal growth factor (EGF)-like repeats, and Arg-Gly-Asp sequences that account for some (but not all) of the attachments to other proteins. The molecules also bind chondroitin sulfate. The distribution is restricted, and changes in the types made during various developmental stages suggest roles in embryogenesis. Cells exposed to cytotaxin round up and stop migrating. The large amounts made by glial cells may mediate neuron:neuroglia interactions.

cytotactin binding protein: CTB: a proteoglycan that binds cytotactin and is believed to modify its functions.

cytotaxins: agents that promotes cytotaxis.

cytotaxis: (1) cell movement in response to agents that promote attraction or repulsion; (2) cell structure reorganization.

Cytotec: a trade name for misoprostol.

cytotoxicity: ability to damage or destroy cells, a term used for noxious agents and some substances generated by immune system components (but not for endogenous factors that promote apoptosis).

cytotoxic lymphocytes: CTLs: usually, T lymphocytes that mediate cellular immunity; *see* **lymphocytes** and **K cells**.

cytotoxic lymphocyte differentiation factor: CDF: an accessory factor (other than interleukins 2 or 4) required for cytotoxic T lymphocyte development. A 24K protein from conditioned media of stimulated mononuclear cells that works in conjunction with IL-2 and dendritic cells (but does not promote cell proliferation) has been identified. It may be produced by helper type T lymphocytes.

cytotrophoblast: Langhans layer; the component of the trophoblast or placenta that contains cells with defined boundaries. It provides cells to the syncytiotrophoblast, produces several kinds of peptide hormones, and is essential for establishing and maintaining pregnancy.

cytotropic: (1) attracted to or moving toward cells; (2) a property of some IgG and IgE type immunoglobulins that involves binding to Fc receptors without prior association with antigens, and sensitizes cells for subsequent anaphylaxis.

D

d: (1) dextrorotary; (2) day; (3) dog, in acronyms, as in dGH (dog growth hormone).

d-: (1) deci-; (2) deoxy-.

D: (1) asparagine; (2) Dalton (also Da); (3) deuterium; (4) right handed configuration (*see* **stereoisomerism**); (5) the human major histocompatibility complex region that codes for class 2 proteins; (6) the mouse H-2 complex that codes for class 1 proteins.

δ: delta; (1) the fourth subunit of a multimeric protein; (2) the third carbon atom to the left of a terminal carboxyl (or amide) group, or the position of a chemical group attached to that carbon atom; (4) the fourth type of a substance that exists in several forms. *See* also **opioid receptors**, δ type.

Δ: when followed by a superscript, the first of two carbons linked by a double bond. *See* also Δ^4 and Δ^5 **pathways**.

D_1, D_2: *see* **dopamine receptors**.

D-600: gallopamil; methoxyverapamil; a calcium channel blocking agent with properties similar to those of **verapamil** (*q.v.*). It acts on L types in both closed and open states, and is used to study channel functions and the effects of Ca^{2+} uptake on responses to other regulators.

2,4-D: 2,4-dichlorophenoxyacetic acid.

dA: deoxyadenosine.

Da: D; *see* **dalton**.

DA: dopamine.

DA, DAB complexes: *see* **transcription**.

DAB: 3′-3′-diaminobenzidine: a chromogen used in immunoperoxidase studies that imparts a brown color when it reacts with catalases.

dabsyl chloride: 4-(dimethylamino)azobenzene-4′sulfonyl chloride; a chromogen that reacts with free α-amino groups of peptides and proteins to form sulfonamide derivatives that are stable during hydrolysis. It is used to study amino acid sequences.

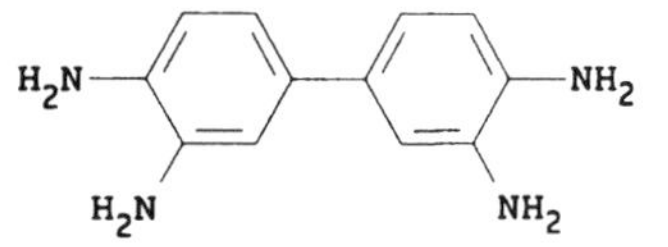

DAB

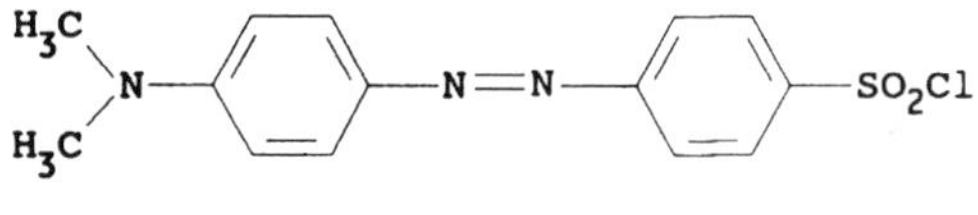

dabsyl chloride

Dactomycin: actinomycin D.

dactyl: a finger or toe.

DADL: DADLE: [D-Ala^2,D-Leu]-enkephalin: a potent δ type opioid receptor agonist, used with radioactive markers to identify those receptors. High concentrations also interact with μ types.

DAF: decay accelerating factor.

DAG: diacylglycerol.

DAGO: [D-Ala^2, *N*-Me-Phe^4,Gly-ol^5]-enkephalin: a μ-type opioid receptor agonist.

Dahl rats: a strain that develops hypertension when fed diets high in NaCl content.

DAKLI: dynorphin A-analog-kappa: [Arg^{11,13}]-dyn(1-13)-Gly-NH(CH$_2$)$_5$-NH$_2$: a dynorphin analog selective for κ type opiate receptors.

dalton: D, Da: a unit equivalent to the mass of a hydrogen atom. Relative molecular weights (Mr) of large molecules are expressed in kilodaltons (Kd, K).

dam: the female parent, a term applied to laboratory, domesticated, and other animal species.

DAMA: D-Ala^2-D-Met-enkephalin; a metenkephalin analog with high affinity for a subtype of δ opioid receptors

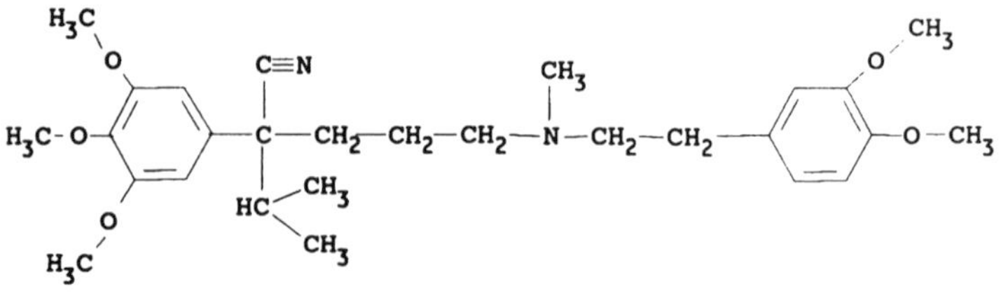

D-600

that mediates immune adherence, cell flattening and elongation, chemokinesis, and chemotaxis.

DAMGO: D-Ala^2-Me-Phe^4-Glycol^5-enkephalin; a metenkephalin analog that is selective for μ type opioid receptors.

dAMP: 2-deoxyadenylic acid; *see* 2-**dexoyadenosine-monophosphate**.

DAMP: *see* **Duolax**.

4-DAMP: 4-diphenylacetoxy-*N*-methylpiperidine methiodide; an M$_2$ type muscarinic acetylcholine receptor antagonist.

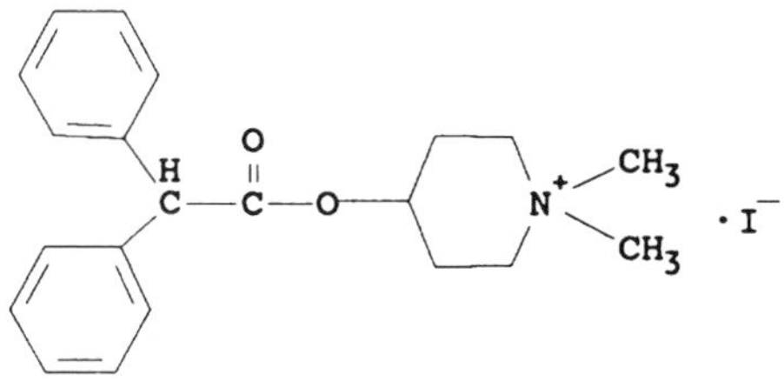

danazol: 17α-pregna-2,4-dien-20-yno[2,3-*d*]isoxazol-17-ol; a weak androgen devoid of estrogenic or progestin potency that reversibly inhibits follicle stimulating and luteinizing hormone (FSH and LH) secretion, the binding of those hormones to gonadotropin receptors in testes and ovaries, and also an esterase that acts on complement factor C1, and elevates C4 levels. When used to treat endometriosis, fibrocystic breast disease, and hereditary angioedema, it invokes virilization and acne; and prolonged use can affect hepatic functions, depress high density (HDL) and elevate low density lipoprotein (LDL) levels, and cause bile duct obstruction.

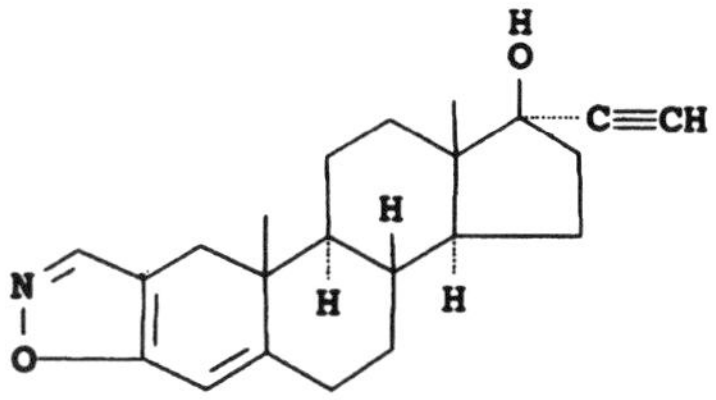

dansyl-: 5-(dimethylamino)naphthalene-1-sulfonyl-; the active group of **dansyl chloride** (*q.v.*) and related compounds.

dansyl amino acids: *see* **dansyl chloride**.

dansylcadaverine: an agent that opposes insulin effects on glycogen metabolism in the liver, and also inhibits transglutaminases, fibrin stabilizing factor, and mechanisms for internalizing epidermal growth factor (EGF). It is used as a fluorescent substrate in transamidation assays. *See* also **dansyl-** and **cadaverine**.

dansyl chloride: DNS: 5-(dimethylamino)naphthalene-1-sulfonyl chloride; a fluorescent reagent used to label amino acids and proteins. It reacts with free α-amino groups to form derivatives that are stable during hydrolysis.

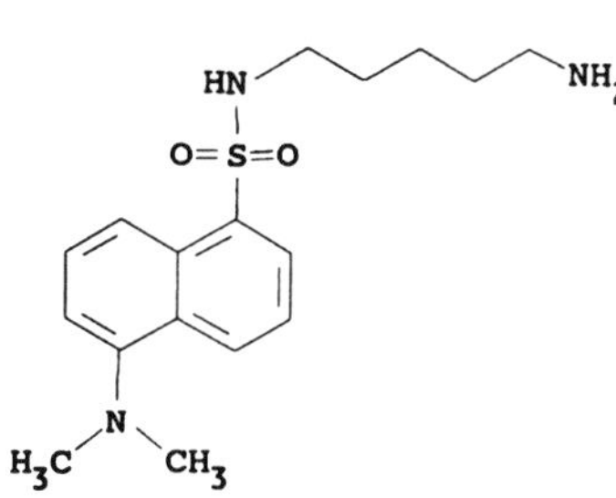

dansylcadaverine

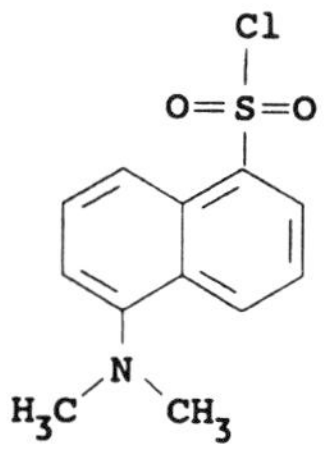

dansyl chloride

dansyl-glutamyl-glycinyl-arginine chloromethylketone: DGGACK: an agent used to inhibit proteases that act on substrates with basic amino acids.

dantrolene: 1-[5-(4-nitrophenyl)-2-furanyl]-methylene-amino-2,4-imidazolidine dione; an agent that inhibits Ca^{2+} ion transport across cell membranes, and thereby slows both uptake from extracellular fluids and intracellular translocation. The sodium salt is used as a muscle relaxant.

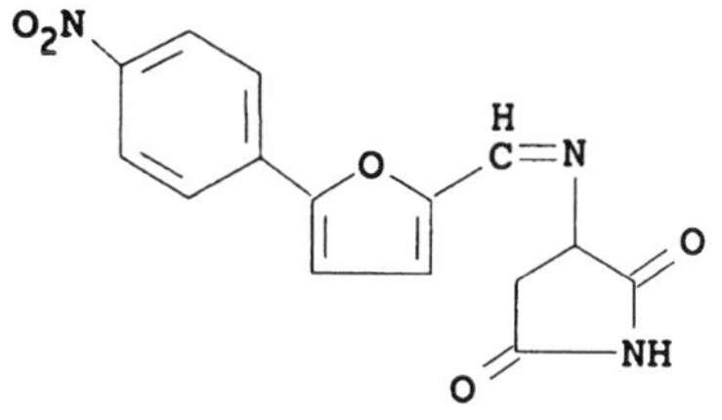

D-AP5: *see* 2-D-**aminoheptanoate**.

D-AP7: *see* 2-D-**aminovaleric acid**.

DAPs: diabetes associated peptides; *see* **amylins**.

DAPT: amphiphenazole; 5-phenyl-2,4-thiazolediamine; a morphine receptor antagonist.

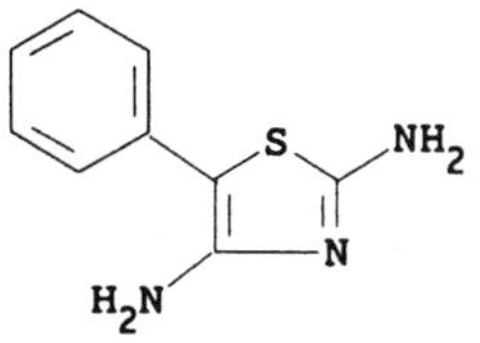

dark current: the flow of electrons in retinal rod cell photoreceptors during darkness, mediated via cyclic guanosine-3'5'-monophosphate (cGMP), which maintains plasma membrane Na$^+$ ion channels in partially open states. Rhodopsin responses to light lead (via transducin) to activation of a phosphodiesterase that degrades cGMP. The current is restored when rhodopsin is inactivated.

dark field microscopy: *see* **microscopy**.

dark reaction: *see* **photosynthesis**.

DARPP: *see* **dopamine and cAMP regulated phosphoprotein**.

Daudi cells: a human lymphoblastoid cell line used for immunological studies. The cells synthesize class 2 proteins, but do not display them on their plasma membrane surfaces because no β_2-microglobulin is made. The exquisite sensitivity of most types to interferon-α (IFNα) is attributed to possesion of large numbers of receptors; but a few subclones that make the receptors do not couple them to responses.

daunomycin: daunorubicin; leukaemomycin C; ribidomycin; (8-*cis*)-8-acetyl-10-[(3-amino-2,3,6-trideoxy-α-L-lyxo-hexopyranosyl)oxy]-7,8,9,10-tetrahydro-6,8,11-trihydroxy-1-methoxy-5,12-naphthacenedione; an antibiotic, made by *Streptomyces peucetius*, that intercalates into DNAs, affects topoisomerase activity, causes double-strand breaks and sister chromatid exchanges, impairs RNA as well as DNA functions, and kills cells in the S phases of their cycles. It also indirectly promotes superoxide radical formation by interacting with cytochrome P_{450} reductase. Daunomycin is highly potent against acute lymphocytic and granulocytic leukemias, and it kills some childhood lymphoma cells (but is not useful for treating most solid tumors). The numerous toxic effects include bone marrow depression, hair loss, gastrointestinal tract dysfunction, skin eruptions, and stomatitis. It is also mutagenic and carcinogenic.

daunorubicin: daunomycin.

dawn phenomenon: early morning hyperglycemia in individuals with diabetes mellitus receiving insulin. It is attributed to excessive growth hormone secretion during the night.

dazoxiben: UK 37248; 15-deoxy-9,11-aza-PGH$_2$: an agent that inhibits thromboxane synthesis and its interactions with receptors.

dB: decibel.

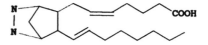

dazoxiben

db mice: a mouse strain that carries a recessive autosomal defect used to study diabetes mellitus. Homozygotes become hyperphagic and obese, and pass through a hyperinsulinemic stage before becoming hormone deficient.

DBH: dopamine β-hydroxylase.

DBI: (1) diazepine binding inhibitor; (2) phenformin.

dbl: a human transforming oncogene that codes for a product related to intermediate filament proteins, but lacks the *N*-terminal segment believed to exert inhibitory controls over the activities of normal types.

DBM paper: diazobenzyloxymethyl paper. The diazo (N=N—) group reacts with single-stranded DNAs and RNAs to form covalent bonds used for Northern blotting procedures and hybridization studies.

DBPs: vitamin D binding proteins.

dC: deoxycytosine.

DCA: 11-deoxycorticosterone acetate; *see* 11-**deoxycorticosterone**.

D-cAMP: dibutyryl cyclic adenosine 3′5′-monophosphate; bucladesine; *see* N^6, 2-dibutyryl-**adenosine-3′5′-cyclic monophosphate.**

DCC: (1) dextran coated charcoal; (2) *N,N*′-dicyclohexylcarbodiimide; (3) deleted in colon cancer; *see* **tumor suppressor genes**.

DCCD, DCCC: *N,N*′-dicyclohexylcarbodiimide.

D, δ cells: (1) A$_1$ delta cells of the pancreas and gastrointestinal tract that secrete somatostatin; (2) a term formerly applied to adenohypophysial gonadotropes identified with special stains under light microscopy.

DCI: dichloroisoproterenol.

DCMB: 2,3-dichloro-α-methylbenzylamine; a reversible inhibitor of phenylethanolamine-*N*-methyltransferase that also acts on α_2 type adrenergic receptors.

DD: continuous darkness; usually, an artificially imposed condition used to study the effects of photoperiods on biological functions.

ddA: 2′3′-dideoxyadenosine.

DDAO: dodecyldimethylene oxide;

DDAVP, dDAVP: Desmopressin.

ddC: 2′3′-dideoxycytidine.

DDC: (1) dopamine decarboxylase; (2) dextran coated charcoal.

o,p′-**DDD**: mitotane; 1,1-dichloro-2-(*o*-chlorophenyl)-2-(*p*-chlorophenyl)ethane; an agent that selectively kills cells of the adrenal cortex by damaging their mitochondria. It is used to treat some neoplasms, and to study steroid hormone deficiency.

DDGACK: dansyl-glutamyl-glycinyl-amine chloromethylketone.

ddI: 2′3′-dideoxyinosine.

ddT: 2′3′-dideoxythymidine.

DDT: dichlorodiphenyl dichlorethane.

deacetylases: enzymes that catalyze removal of acetyl groups. The reactions change the surface charges of the substrates, and their affinities for other molecules. The effects on histones contribute to activation of many genes, probably because of effects on their associations with DNA segments.

DEAE cellulose: diethylaminoethyl cellulose; a trade name for a family of ion exchange resins used in high performance liquid chromatography.

deafferentation: severing of nerves that supply a structure; *cf* **denervation**.

deamidation: removal of a terminal amino group, a process that affects the properties of several hormones.

deamination: removal of a non-terminal amino group. Oxidative deamination replaces the NH_2 with an oxygen atom and thereby forms a ketone. Some reactions convert amino acids to their corresponding glucogenic or ketogenic derivatives.

deamino-: desamino-: a prefix which indicates absence of an amino group that is present on related compounds. It is commonly used with a number that indicates the position of the deletion.

deaminooxytocin: demoxytocin; desaminooxytocin: an analog of **oxytocin** (*q.v.*) in which the amino group of the first cysteine moiety is replaced by a hydrogen atom. It acts like, but is much more potent that the naturally occurring hormone.

5-deaza-adenosine: an analog of **adenosine** (*q.v.*) in which the nitrogen at position 5 is replaced by a hydrogen atom. It is used to inhibit transmethylation reactions.

debouch: to open or empty into another part.

debridement: removal of devitalized tissue, usually from a wound surface.

debt: *oxygen debt* is the amount of oxygen (in excess of the usual requirements during rest), that must be supplied during recovery from a bout of demanding physical activity, to support the oxidative processes that overcome the effects of accelerated anaerobic metabolism. The reactions restore normal levels of circulating oxygen and carbonic acid, and of skeletal muscle creatine-phosphate; and they dispose of the lactic acid that has accumulated. *Lactacid* oxygen debt refers specifically to the oxygen deficit caused by lactic acid accumulation.

deca: ten.

decamethonium: decamethylene-*bis*[trimethylammonium]; the dibromide is used as a skeletal muscle relaxant. In common with succinyl chloride, it invokes prolonged depolarization; but it is more more potent.

decapacitation factors: DF: seminal fluid components said to reverse capacitation of spermatozoa. A 170K glycoprotein that inhibits a corona penetrating enzyme has been reported to perform such a function. *See* also **acrosome stabilizing factor** and **seminalplasmin**.

decapentaplegic gene: *dpp*; a *Drosophila* gene that determines dorso-ventral orientation during development. Its protein product is related to bone morphogenic proteins BMP-2 and BMP-4; and it closely resembles the β subunits of inhibin and transforming growth factor-β (TGFβ).

decarboxylases: enzymes that catalyze liberation of COO from -COOH groups. Various types, which differ in substrate affinities and cofactor requirements, are essential for the biosynthesis of histamine, dopamine, serotonin, and other amine type regulators, and for conversion of pyruvic acid to acetyl coenzyme A.

decay: decomposition, a term applied to (1) deterioration of organic compounds when exposed to oxygen or other environmental factors; (2) degradation catalyzed by enzymes of bacteria and fungi; and (3) the disintegration of radioactive elements.

decay accelerating factor: DAF; plasma membrane glycoproteins on erythrocytes, leukocytes, platelets, epithelial, and other cells that take up protein fragments generated by the complement system. They inhibit amplification of both classical and alternative activation pathways, and protect against complement-mediated damage to host cells. 47K and 70K forms have been identified. Most of the molecules are anchored to plasma membrane phosphatidylinositol moieties, and can be released by phospholipase C isozymes. Others are more permanently fixed by palmitoylation. Paroxysmal nocturnal hematuria is attributed to DAF deficiency; and inability to synthesize sufficient amounts probably contributes to lymphocyte destruction in individuals infected with the AIDS virus.

decay constant: disintegration constant; d; a factor related to the properties of a specific kind of radioactive element that is used to estimate the emission rate at a given time. In the equation $N = N_o e^{-dt}$, N_o = the number of radioactive atoms initially present, e is the natural logarithm, and N = the number still present at time t.

decerebrate rigidity: *see* **spastic paralysis**.

decerebration: destruction of the forebrain. The procedure is performed on anesthetized animals to study the effects of removing influences exerted by upper motor neurons (and other messages that normally descend) on the functions of lower motor neurons, and on spinal reflexes; *see* also **spastic paralysis**.

deci-: one-tenth, as in deciliter.

decibel: dB; a logarithmic unit equivalent to 1 picowatt of sound power. Young human adults with good hearing acuity can detect sound intensities of 1 dB or lower. The intensities for whispers and ordinary conversation are approximately 15 and 45 dB, respectively; and the noise made by a penumatic drill is closer to 90 dB. Intensities above 115 dB invoke pain.

decidua: the endometrial tissue that borders the uterine lumen. When used without modifiers, the term usually refers to the tissue formed during pregnancy that is shed during parturition. It includes all of the endometrium except the deepest layers. However, under the influence of estrogen, progesterone and other regulators secreted during ovarian cycles, the superficial layers of the endometrium specialize for implantation. If fertilization does not occur, the mucous membrane sloughs off, and the term *d. menstrualis* can be applied. If conception does occur, the newly formed cells persist, and new ones are made. The *d. basalis* originates at the site of implantation, is partly penetrated by the cytotrophoblast, and is incorporated into the maternal part of the placenta. It contains cells that secrete placental prolactin, relaxin, and other hormones which subsequently appear in amniotic fluid, and is attached to the myometrium by the *d. spongiosum*, which contains glands and small blood vessels. The *d. parietalis* lines the parts of the cavity of the pregnant uterus that are not incorporated into the placenta. The *d. capsularis* overlies the chorion, and separates it from the d. parietalis. As the chorionic cavity grows, it is stretched and compressed against the parietalis, and it regresses during the 4th month of human pregnancy. The *d. marginalis* is the junction site for the basalis, parietalis and capsularis regions.

decidual proteins: the structural and secreted proteins made by endometrial cells during pregnancy, or following a decidual reaction. In women, they include placental prolactin, relaxin, IGF binding proteins (insulin-like growth factor binding proteins, IG-BPs), and various other types, most of which have molecular weights in the 23-78K range.

decidual reactions: responses of hormone-primed endometrial cells to blastocysts, and to artificial stimuli that lead to deciduoma formation.

deciduoma [deciduomata]: a vascularized cell conglomerate formed by hormone-primed endometrial cells when exposed to artificial stimuli (such as needle pricks and some chemicals). It somewhat resembles the tissue that develops around an implantation site.

deciliter; dl; 100 milliliters.

decondensation: transition of chromatin from a complex, highly ordered coiled state to a more extended form, in which nucleosomes are separated from each other by linear linker DNA segments, and the molecules assume a "beads on a string" appearance. The process exposes DNA segments that can bind to other factors and engage in transcription.

deconditioning: eradication of a conditioned response, a technique used to study factors that affect learning and memory.

decorin: a small, extracellular matrix chondroitin-dermatan sulfate proteoglycan, composed of a core protein with ten identical leucine-rich, 24-amino acid sequences, plus a single glycoprotein chain. It affects cell morphology and growth by binding to transforming growth factor-β (TGFβ). The complexes formed attach to receptors which recognize the decorin component and mediate endocytosis. Decorin appears to be a component of a feedback system in which TGF-β induces decorin, and decorin inhibits TGF-β production and actions. Since TGF-β can cause disease by promoting accumulation of excessive extracellular matrix, and is an autocrine growth factor for some tumor cells, decorin may perform protective as well as growth regulating functions.

decorticate: (1) to remove the outer layer (for example of the cerebral cortex, or of an adrenal gland); (2) describes an individual in which the procedure has been performed on the brain, or the structure that remains when the outer portion has been removed.

decorticate rigidity: skeletal muscle spasms that occur when cerebral cortex damage or other lesions remove the inhibitory influences that normally descend from the premotor areas. *See* also **extrapyramidal system**.

decussation: crossing over.

dedifferentiation: reversion to a more immature cell or tissue type.

defective virus: a virus that lacks intrinsic machinery for replication, but can replicate when co-infected with a "helper" type. Many transforming retroviruses are defective. Some lose essential components when they incorporate into host genomes.

defeminization: the loss of an "inherent" tendency to acquire or display feminine characteristics; *cf* **masculinization**. In female rats, mice an some other rodents, androgen administration during the first few days after birth changes some aspects of central nervous system maturation. After maturity is attained, the animals have male-type patterns for release of gonadotropin stimulating hormone (GnRH), with no luteinizing hormone (LH) surges required to achieve ovulation. Some behavioral responses to hormones are also affected.

defensins: NPs; small (mostly 29-34 amino acid) cationic, arginine and cysteine rich bactericidal peptides, synthesized by neutrophilic leukocytes, and stored in granules. The kinds made by various species share common sequences, but differ in antibiotic potencies and specificities. Letters that precede the neutrophilic protein acronym refer to the species, and numbers that follow to the subtype. HNP-2 (made by humans) is H_2N-Cys-Tyr-Cys-Arg-Ile-Pro-Ala-Cys-Ile-Ala-Gly-Glu-Arg-Arg-Tyr-Gly-Thr-Cys-Ile-Tyr-Gln-Gly-Arg-Leu-Trp-Ala-Phe-Cys-OH. *Cf* **magainins**.

deferoxamine: desferrioxamine B: 1-amino-6,17-dihydroxy-7,10,18,21-tetraoxo-27-(N-acetylhydroxyamino)-6,11,17,22-tetraazaheptaeicosane; a growth factor for microorganisms, obtained by removing iron from a complex made by *Streptomyces pilosus*. It is a potent Fe^{3+} chelator, used to prevent or treat toxicity in individuals with Cooley's anemia, and others who require repeated blood trasnfusions. It impedes intestinal absorption of iron, and inhibits Fe^{3+}-mediated formation of free radicals. Although somewhat effective for removing hemosiderin deposits, it does not gain access to cytochrome enzymes. Derivatives include the mesylate salt (desferol, DFOM), and N-acetyldeferoxamine.

defibrinate: to remove fibrin, usually from blood, and usually to prevent coagulation. Fibrin sticks to a glass rod that is inserted into a liquid and twirled.

defined media: artificial cell culture media, composed of known constituents. They are used to determine which substances are essential for supporting survival, growth, and proliferation of cultured cells, to study their functions, and to eliminate the effects of undefined factors (present, for example, in blood serum) on cell activities.

D genes: DNA components that direct formation of immunoglobulin D segments.

degenerate code: describes messenger RNA triplets that can hydrogen bond to more than one kind of transfer RNA anticodon, and thereby direct insertion of more than one kind of amino acid at a locus.

degrees of freedom: d.f.; the numbers of data items that can vary independently, calculated as the total number of observations minus 1.

dehydratases: enzymes that catalyze removal of water molecules from compounds.

dehydration: removal of water, a term applied to (1) *in vitro* processes used, for example to prepare specimens for electron microscopy, or to protect chemicals against

degradation (2) reactions catalyzed by dehydratases; *see* also **dehydration synthesis**; or (3) loss of more body water than associated solutes, caused, for example by water deprivation or antidiuretic hormone deficiency.

dehydration synthesis: processes of the general type: R_1-OH + R_2H → R_1-R_2 + H_2O (in which an OH from one molecule combines with an H from another, water is released, and a larger compound is formed. Peptide, glycoside, and ester bonds are made in such reactions. *Cf* **digestion**.

dehydroascorbic acid: threo-2,3-hexodiulosonic acid γ-lactone; the oxidized form of **ascorbic acid** (*q.v.*).

5,6-dehydroandrosterone: methandriol.

7-dehydrocholesterol: provitamin D; cholesta-5,7-diene-3-ol; a sterol obtained from food, synthesized in the liver, or made from cholesterol via a reaction catalyzed by intestinal 7-cholesterol dehydrogenase. It accumulates in skin, in which it is converted by ultraviolet light to vitamin D and other secosteroids.

dehydrocholic acid: 3,7,12-triketocholanic acid; a bile acid oxidation product. The sodium salt is used as a choleretic.

11-dehydrocorticosterone: *see* 11-dehydro-**corticosterone**.

dehydroepiandrosterone: DHA; DHEA: prasterone; dehydroisoandrosterone; $Δ^5$-androsten-3β-ol-17-one; a weak androgen made in the adrenal cortex, gonads, and feto-placental unit that can be enzymatically converted to

deferoxamine

testosterone. The sulfate conjugate (DHEAS) is the major adrenal androgen secreted by humans and other species that use Δ^5 pathways, and the major precursor of estrogens in postmenopausal women; but substantial quantities are excreted to the urine. Some virilizing tumors release large amounts. Administration of DHEA to retard atherosclerosis has been advocated, since the steroid can inhibit fibroblast growth and differentiation, antagonize arachidonic acid stimulated platelet aggregation, and lower circulating levels of both total and low density lipoprotein (LDL) cholesterol. Declining DHEA and DHEAS concentrations with advancing age have been attributed in part to the tendencies for insulin levels to rise, since that hormone accelerates clearance of the steroids and inhibits the C17-C20 lyase enzyme required for their synthesis. Rats, mice, and other species whose adrenal glands use Δ^4 pathways for hormone synthesis do not release detectable amounts, but do respond to orally administered DHEA (which exerts profound influences on lipid and carbohydrate metabolism). Moderate amounts markedly reduce body weight and fat content, and accelerate metabolic rate in mutant strains that would otherwise become obese, without affecting food intake. Although some reduction in body fat content (but not body weight), has been observed in men taking DHEA, the effectiveness for treating human obesity has not been demonstrated.

dehydroepiandrosterone

dehydroepiandrosterone-sulfate: DHAS; DHEAS; dehydroisoandrosterone-3-sulfate; a conjugate of **dehydroepiandrosterone** (DHEA, *q.v.*), synthesized by fetoplacental units, and in substantial quantities by adrenocortical cells of species that use Δ^5 pathways. It can be made from sulfate conjugates of cholesterol, (via pregnenolone and 17α-hydroxypregnenolone-3-sulfates), and is interconvertible with DHEA.

dehydrogenases: enzymes that catalyze removal of a pair of hydrogen atoms, usually from parts of molecules with -CHOH groups. The hydrogens are taken up by coenzymes, but are not directly transferred to molecular oxygen. *See* specific types, such as 11β- and 17-**hydroxysteroid dehydrogenases**; and *cf* **oxidases**.

deinduction: return to the basal rate of messenger RNA synthesis, following removal of a stimulatory regulator (or administration of an agent that opposes it).

deiodinases: enzymes that catalyze removal of iodine atoms from thyroxine (T_4), triiodothyronine (T_3), and their metabolites. Type I (in liver, kidney, and other tissues) acts on both inner and outer iodothyronine rings, and is the major isozyme for converting T_4 secreted by thyroid glands to circulating T_3. It also contributes to iodothyronine degradation to inactive products. Thyroid hormone deficiency lowers the activity at most sites, and food deprivation has this effect on the liver. In the thyroid gland, the type I enzyme increases the T_3:T_4 ratio and contributes to iodine conservation. Its activity is increased by thyroid stimulating hormone (TSH), and is therefore higher in iodine and thyroid hormone deficiency states. Propylthiouracil and related agents are inhibitors. Type II, in brain, pituitary gland, placenta, and skin, acts only on the outer ring, is resistant to propylthiouracil, and is important for regulating intracellular T_3 levels. Type III acts on the inner ring, and promotes conversion of T_4 to rT_3 (reverse triiodothyronine). Successive actions of the various types lead to formation of metabolites with lesser numbers of iodine atoms: diiodothyronines (T_2), monoiodothyronines (T_1), and thyronine (T_0).

Delalutin: a trade name for hydroxyprogesterone caproate; *see* **progestins**.

delayed hypersensitivity: delayed type hypersensitivity; DTH; a slowly developing, often destructive allergic reaction in individuals previously sensitized to the stimulating antigens, mediated by activated Td type lymphocytes. The skin is a common site. *Cf* **immediate hypersensitivity**.

deletion: loss or removal of an entity, for example a chromosome segment. Deletion of some DNA base sequences that are not transcribed has little discernible effect, whereas loss of certain others impairs transcriptional controls. When the deletions occur in transcribed regions, the locations and numbers of nucleotides lost determine the effects. In some cases, translation is totally blocked, but in others, abnormal proteins are made. If complete messenger RNA triplets are removed, the proteins lack one or more amino acid moieties. *See* also **frame shifts**.

deletion mapping: use of overlapping deletions to determine the chromosomal locations of specific genes.

deletion methods: techniques for identifying specific messenger RNA segments by hybridizing them with DNA molecules that contain deletions at known sites.

delta: *see* δ and Δ.

delta cells: pancreatic and gastrointestinal tract cells that secrete somatostatin.

delta chains: IgD type immunoglobulin heavy chains.

delta sleep-inducing peptide: DSIP; Trp-Ala-Gly-Asp-Ala-Ser-Gly-Glu.

deltorphins: peptides isolated from the skin of frogs of the *Phyllomedusa* genus with high high affinities and selectivities for δ-type opioid receptors. Each is composed of 7 amino acid moieties, the second of which is in the D-form. The term was initially applied to Tyr-D-Met-

Phe-His-Val-Val-Gly-NH$_2$. Two more potent peptides, [D-Ala^2]-deltorphin-I (Tyr-D-Ala-Phe-Asp-Val-Val-Gly-NH$_2$) and [D-Ala^2]-deltorphin-II (Tyr-D-Ala-Phe-Gly-Val-Val-Gly-NH$_2$) were later identified. *Cf* **dermorphin**.

demeclocycline: 7-chloro-6-demethyltetracyline; an antibiotic that antagonizes the antidiuretic actions of vasopressin.

demecolcine: colcemid.

Demerol:a trade name for meperidine.

denaturation: loss of native three-dimensional configuration, for example after exposure to heat, pH changes, or certain chemicals. It usually involves the rupture of hydrogen (but not covalent) bonds. DNAs undergo melting (separation of the two strands) and shape changes. Proteins and peptide chains often unfold and/or lose associations with other molecules. In addition to effects on physical properties such as solubility, denaturation changes the chemical groups exposed to the microenvironment, and thereby the potential for interactions with other molecules (nucleic acids with proteins or other nucleic acids, enzymes with substrates, and hormones with receptors). Many kinds of analytical procedures are performed on denatured macromolecules.

dendrites: usually, numerous short, slender, branching cytoplasmic projections from a neuron cell body that receive stimuli and convey information to the perikaryon. Some neurons have only one dendrite; and some messages are carried to neurons in other ways. *See* also **retrograde conduction** and **synapses**.

dendritic cells: (1) a leukocyte subset that contributes to T lymphocyte mediated processes such as transplant rejection, allergic reactions, and autoimmune disease, and secondarily affects B cell functions. Other names used for those large mononuclear cells, related to their locations, include Langerhans (in skin), interdigitating (in thymus glands, lymph nodes and spleen), follicular (in spleen germinal follicles and B cell regions), and veiled cells (in circulating lymph). They are not directly related to **dendritic epidermal cells** (*q.v.*). The cytoplasmic extensions range in appearance from blunt pseudopods to indistinct veils. The cells contain little or no acid phosphatase, and are not phagocytic, but appear to be descendants of a macrophage lineage that originates in bone marrow. They express membrane-bound class 2 proteins and CD4 (but no CD3), and have Fc and C3 receptors. Dendritic cells pick up antigens at various sites, process them, present the products (in association with the class 2 proteins) to helper type T cells, bind to those cells, and may contribute in other ways to T cell activation. They also accumulate antigen-antibody complexes in the spleen. The ability of small numbers to mount vigorous

responses is attributed to persistent retention of antigens, rapid stimulation of T lymphocyte conversion to blast cells, and formation of clusters in lymphatic organs and sites of inflammation that attract blast and other T cells responsive to the specific antigen type. The effects on B cell functions may be secondary to helper cell activation and consequent release of lymphokines; (2) branching melanocytes, unrelated to the leukocyte type, that derive from neural crests and migrate to the epidermis.

dendritic epidermal cells: Thy-1-DEC cells; a subpopulation of Thy$^+$ T lymphocytes in mouse skin. The human counterpart has not been clearly identified, but small numbers of similar cells are present in several tissues, and larger ones appear at sites affected by autoimmune processes, such as thyroid glands of individuals with Graves' disease and Hashimoto's thyroiditis, and in synovial fluids of those with rheumatoid arthritis. They have γδ receptors, and are responsive to antigens, but do not express class II proteins on their surfaces, and have been implicated in down-regulation of allergic responses. Natural killer (NK)-like activity has also been observed. There are controversies concerning whether they are immature cells released by thymus glands or, alternatively, mature types that differentiate outside that gland. Their numbers increase in response to γ-interferon, and they produce interleukin-2-like peptides.

denervation: severing or destruction of all afferent nerves entering, and all efferent ones leaving a structure; *cf* **deafferentation**.

denervation hypersensitivity: the heightened responsivity to neurotransmitters that develops after afferent nerves are severed. It is usually associated with increased receptor numbers and/or binding affinities, but can result from (or include) postreceptor changes.

de novo: arising anew; usually describes synthesis of substances from simple precursors (as opposed to modification of more complex compounds).

dense bodies: a general term for small dark-staining entities in electron micrographs. Some resemble the half-desmosomes that associate with thin filaments in vascular smooth muscle cells. Others can be amorphous cell inclusions, or membrane-bound vesicles that contain large quantities of particulate matter.

density: weight per unit volume, often expressed as mg per ml.

density dependent growth inhibition: see **contact inhibition of growth**.

density gradient centrifugation: techniques for separating components of mixtures on the basis of differences in migration rates through layers of solvents that contain various concentrations of inert solutes (such sucrose or cesium chloride). The particles migrate in centrifugal fields until they reach levels at which their densities match those of the surrounding media.

dentin: dentine; the non-cellular, calcified substance that forms most of a tooth. It is harder than bone, but softer than enamel.

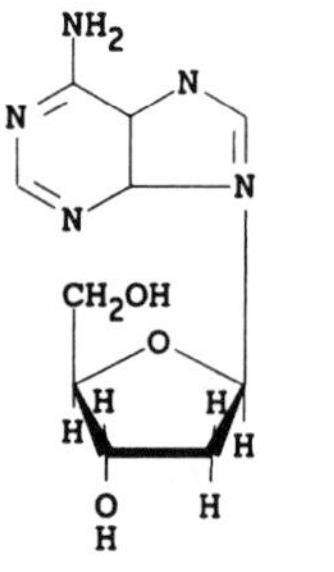

2'-deoxyadenosine

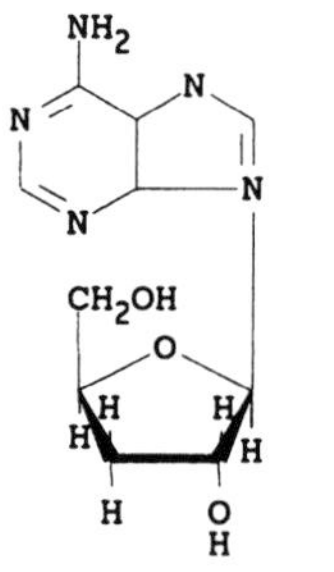

3'-deoxyadenosine

deoxy-: a prefix that indicates an oxygen atom has been deleted. A number can define the position (as in 2-deoxyribose or 11-deoxycorticosterone). Desoxy- is an older term that is still used.

deoxyadenosine: when used without modifiers, dA, 9-(2-deoxy-β-D-ribofuranosyl)adenine; a nucleoside composed of adenine covalently linked to deoxyribose. It is obtained by hydrolyzing DNAs, can be made from adenosine, and is phosphorylated to deoxyadenosine-5'-triphosphate (dATP). Cordycepin is 3'-deoxyadenosine. *See* also 2,5-dideoxy-**adenosine**, and *cf* **adenosine**.

2-deoxyadenosine monophosphate: dAMP; a nucleotide obtained by removing the terminal phosphate group of 2-**deoxyadenosine diphosphate** (*q.v.*).

2-deoxyadenosine diphosphate: dADP, an intermediate in the pathway for biosynthesis of 2-**deoxyadenosine triphosphate** (*q.v.*). It is made from adenosine diphosphate via a reaction catalyzed by ribonucleotide reductase.

2-deoxyadenosine triphosphate: dATP; one of the nucleotides used for DNA synthesis.

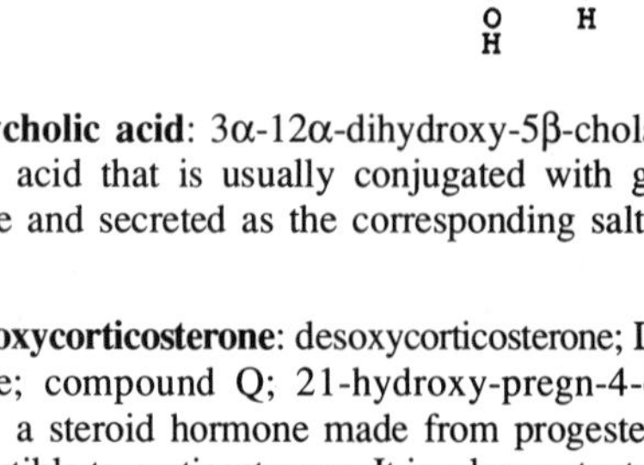

deoxycholic acid: 3α-12α-dihydroxy-5β-cholanic acid; a bile acid that is usually conjugated with glycine or taurine and secreted as the corresponding salt (*see* **bile salts**).

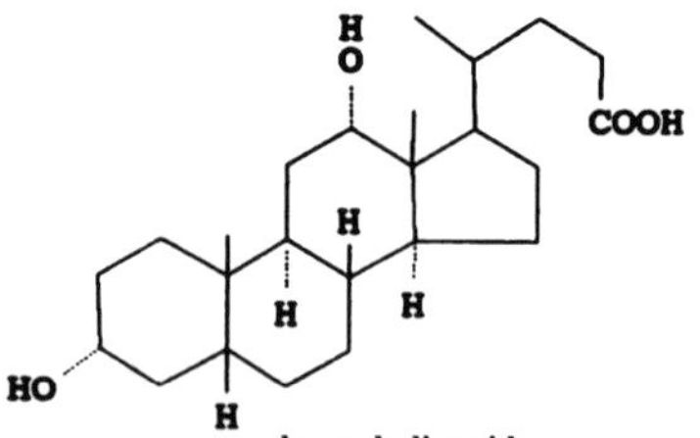

11-**deoxycorticosterone**: desoxycorticosterone; DOC; cortexone; compound Q; 21-hydroxy-pregn-4-ene-3,20-dione; a steroid hormone made from progesterone, and convertible to corticosterone. It is a less potent mineralocorticoid that aldosterone, devoid of glucocorticoid po-

deoxycholic acid

11-deoxycorticosterone

tency at ordinary levels. Small amounts are secreted by the normal adrenal cortex, and transient increases can occur when ACTH levels rise. Under pathological conditions, excessive amounts, and conversion to other steroids such as 19-nor-deoxycorticosterone, can invoke salt and water retention, edema, hypokalemia, and hypertension.

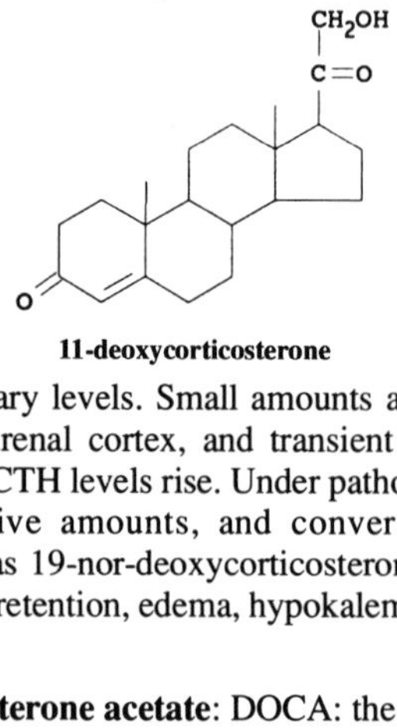

deoxycorticosterone acetate: DOCA: the 21-acetic acid ester of 11-deoxycorticosterone; a compound more polar than the native steroid, and less expensive to prepare than aldosterone. It is used to treat mineralocorticoid deficiency, or to invoke hormone excess in laboratory animals. Large amounts can invoke hypertension and edema.

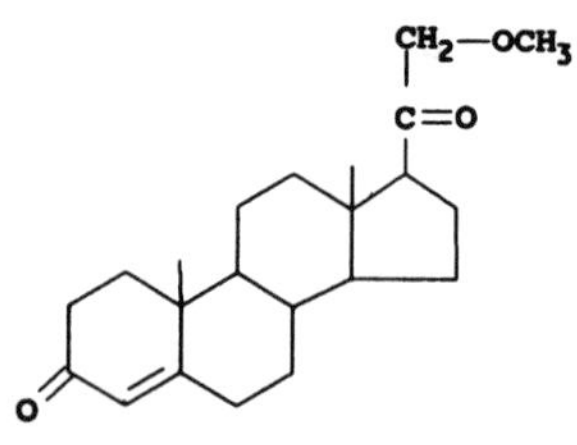

19-nor,11-deoxycorticosterone: a steroid similar to 11-deoxycorticosterone, in which the carbon 19 methyl group is replaced by a hydrogen atom. It is made in large amounts by some individuals with Cushing's syndrome, and is implicated as one cause of hypertension. It circulates mostly as a glycuronate conjugate.

11-**deoxycortisol**: cortexolone; compound S; 11-deoxy, 17-hydroxy-corticosterone: $17\alpha,21$-dihydroxypregn-4-ene-3,20-dione; a steroid synthesized in the adrenal cortex from 17α-hydroxyprogesterone. Usually, most of it is converted to corticosterone and aldosterone; but small amounts are released. 11-β-hydroxylase deficiency leads to accumulation of large amounts (along with 11-deoxycorticosterone). High levels can invoke sodium and water retention, hypokalemia, edema and hypertension.

deoxycytidine: dC; a nucleoside composed of cytosine covalently linked to deoxyribose. It can be obtained from DNAs and RNAs.

2-**deoxyglucose**: 2-DG: a glucose analog that is taken into cells and phosphorylated, but not further metabolized. By competing with glucose for transport carriers and hexokinases, it elevates blood glucose levels and impairs glycolysis. It is used to study glucose transport, differences between hypoglycemia and inability to use the sugar, and the effects of ATP depletion.

deoxymannojiramycin: *see* deoxymanno-**jiramycin**.

deoxynorjiramycin: *see* deoxynor-**jiramycin**.

deoxyribonucleases: DNases; enzymes that degrade DNAs by catalyzing hydrolysis of bonds that link the nucleotides. Intracellular types are used to selectively delete defective DNA segments prior to repair, for recombination, and to destroy foreign nucleic acids, whereas the ones released to pancreatic juice digest foods. Type I DNases are similar to 30K nonspecific endonucleases that bind to minor grooves of the double helices and promote formation of oligonucleotides with 5′-phospho- and 3′-hydroxy-termini. Because of decondensation, regions that are transcriptionally active (and their associated regulatory sites) are the most vulnerable. Pancreas and thymus gland preparations are used to identify such sites, study protein binding, and invoke mutations. They are also administered topically to degrade blood clots and remove exudates. Bacterial **restriction endonucleases** (*q.v.*) are more useful for some purposes, since their actions are restricted to sites with specific base sequences. Type II DNases (made by thymus gland, pancreas, and gastric mucosa) yield fragments with 3′-phospho-termini. In common with type I enzymes, they can release dinucleotides and mononucleotides, and act to a limited extent on single stranded molecules. Some additionally catalyze RNA cleavage and display exonuclease activity. Phosphodiesterases from spleen and snake venoms also degrade DNAs.

deoxyribonucleic acids: DNAs; high molecular weight polymers synthesized from deoxyribonucleoside triphosphates via reactions catalyzed by DNA polymerases. In the most common form, B-DNA, two complementary strands wind around each other to form a right-handed double helix; *see also* **Z-DNA**. The strands are identical in composition but antiparallel (run in opposite directions). Hydrogen bonds between complementary bases (mostly adenine:thymine and guanine:cytosine) hold them together. DNAs carry the genetic codes for all organisms except certain viruses. In eukaryotes, most are components of chromosomes. A typical human haploid cell has 2.9×10^9 base pairs distributed among 23 chromosomes. A diploid cell contains a second set that is similar, but not identical (*see* **alleles** and **sex chromosomes**). Shortly before cell division, the strands separate, and both replicate. During mitosis, one copy of all types is sent to each of the two daughter cells. Limited strand separation also precedes transcription. It was believed until recently that cells transcribe only one ("sense") strand; but some "anti-sense" RNA is made. Artificially constructed anti-sense RNAs can be transfected, and used to block the formation of specific proteins. Some DNA is also made in mitochondria, and in plant chloroplasts. It, too, replicates, and it directs the synthesis of some organelle proteins. *See also* **DNA methylation, DNA replication, DNA polymerases, transcription,** and **reverse transcriptases.**

deoxyribonucleosides: molecules composed of purine or pyrimidine bases linked to deoxyribose. The major purines are adenine and guanine, and the most common pyrimidines are thymine and cytidine. The corresponding nucleosides are, respectively, deoxyadenosine, deoxyguanosine, deoxythymidine, and deoxycytosine. *See also* **deoxyribonucleotides.**

deoxyribonucleotides: phosphorylated **deoxyribonucleosides** (*q.v.*). The triphosphates are used to synthesize DNAs.

2-deoxyribose: the 5-carbon sugar component of DNA, and of the associated nucleosides and nucleotides. It binds to purine and pyrimidine bases, and to phosphate groups.

depactin: an 18K starfish oocyte protein that binds actin, and related proteins made by other species. They shorten actin filaments by promoting release of monomers, one at a time. However, since many short filaments capable of acting as nucleation sites are formed, they can also indirectly accelerate polymerization. When ATP is depleted, myosin blocks depactin binding to actin.

dephosphorylation: removal of one or more phosphate groups, via reactions catalyzed by phosphatase enzymes. Dephosphorylation changes surface charges and associated binding properties. It is a major mechanism for activating some enzymes and inactivating others.

depolarization: dissipation of cell resting potentials. Many neurotransmitters, and some other cell activators accomplish it by opening Na^+ channels. Others directly or indirectly affect channels for different cations. Complete depolarization is the first phase of action potential responses. Partial depolarization does not invoke those changes, but it renders cells more responsive to stimuli. *Cf* **hyperpolarization**.

depolymerization: breakdown of entities composed of repeating subunits to simpler components, a term applied to molecules, filaments, and complex structures such as microtubules.

Depo-provera: a trade name for medroxyprogesterone acetate; *see* **depo-steroids**.

depo-steroids: steroid hormone and synthetic analog conjugates that are slowly hydrolyzed to release the active components. They are used to achieve sustained effects when injected or implanted.

deprenyl: selegiline; R(-)-phenylisopropylmethylpropynylamine; a monoamine oxidase inhibitor with properties similar to those of pargyline. When used to treat Parkinson's disease, it is usually better tolerated than L-DOPA, and can delay the need for L-DOPA (which invokes serious side-effects). The *S*(+) isomer has similar properties but lower activity.

depsipeptides: polypeptides with ester as well as peptide bonds. Examples include actinomycins and some other antibiotics. Valinomycin and some other ionophores are cyclic depsipeptides.

depurination: cleavage of links between purine bases and deoxyribose. When it occurs spontaneously, cell function can be restored by enzymatic repair of the DNA. *In vitro*, low concentrations of acids are more effective for cleaving purine, than pyrimidine nucleosides; and they act more rapidly on DNAs than on RNAs.

derepression: partial or complete antagonism of factors that inhibit the transcription of specific genes. Microorganisms make derepressors when they adapt to changing environmental conditions such as contact with nutrients previously unavailable in adequate amounts. Some mutations also invoke derepression.

dermatan sulfates: 15-40K glycosaminoglycans of skin, blood vessels, heart, and extracellular matrices. They are iduronic acid and galactosamine-4-sulfate heteropolymers.

dermatome: the outermost part of a somite that contains dermal cell progenitors.

dermis: corium; the connective tissue layer of the skin, located between epidermis and subcutaneous tissue. In addition to fibroblasts, large numbers of irregularly arranged collagen fibers, and smaller ones of elastic types, it contains blood and lymph vessels, nerves and sensory structures, and also small numbers of smooth muscle cells, adipocytes, mast cells, and macrophages. Hair follicles, sweat gland ducts, and epithelial components of sebaceous glands extend into it, and provide cells for repair when the epidermis is severely damaged.

dermorphin: Tyr-D-Met-Phe-Gly-Pro-Ser-NH$_2$; a heptapeptide isolated from the skin of frogs of the genus *Phylomedusa* that displays strong affinity and selectivity for μ-type opioid receptors; *cf* **deltorphins**.

DES: diethylstilbestrol.

desensitization: (1) diminished responsivity (usually rapidly developing and reversible) to a hormone, neurotransmitter, or other regulator that is continuously presented. *Homologous d.* requires receptor occupancy, and affects only responses to agents that act on the same receptor types. It usually involves translocation and sequestration, and/or phosphorylation of the receptors, and consequent loss of ability to couple to transducers; *cf* **down regulation**. *Heterologous d.* is mediated by different enzymes. It additionally affects responses to other regulators that use the same transducers, and can affect the functions of unoccupied receptors; (2) reduction or eradication of a hypersensitivity response to an antigen. In most cases, the hypersensitivity is caused by excessive amounts of IgE type antibodies. Repeated exposure to gradually increasing doses of the antigen can desensitize by stimulating production of specific kinds of IgGs that inhibit IgE formation and/or IgE binding to target cells; (3) the transient loss of responsivity to an antigen that follows an anaphylactic reaction to that antigen.

desferrioxime diamide, desferrioxime mesylate: deferoxamine conjugates. They chelate Fe^{3+}, and are used to treat iron poisoning.

desipramine: noripramine: 10,11-dihydro-*N*-methyl-5*H*-dibenzapine-5-propanamine; a tricyclic antidepressant that inhibits neuronal uptake of amine neurotransmitters (especially norepinephrine). It additionally counteracts malaria parasite resistance to chloroquine. Although effective for relieving some forms of psychic depression, it can invoke sedation or anxiety in healthy individuals.

desmin: a 51K intermediate filament protein, similar to vimentin and to the glial fibrillary acidic protein (GFAP) of astrocytes and Schwann cells, but most abundant in skeletal muscle, in which it links Z disks to each other and to the sarcolemma and provides sites for attachment of other proteins. Desmin is also made in smooth muscle, and it is a desmosome component in some cell types.

desmocollins: two or more closely related plasma membrane glycoproteins that contribute to cell adhesion, and are components of desmosomes.

desmogleins: 110-120K transmembrane linker glycoproteins of desmosomes. They insert into epithelial cell cytoplasmic plaques that contain desmoplakins, extend across plasma membranes, and project to extracellular spaces where they associate with desmogleins of adjacent cells.

desmolase: usually (1) the cholesterol side-chain cleavage system; *see* **pregnenolone synthetase**; (2) any enzyme system that catalyzes oxidative cleavage of side chains.

desmoplakins: 83-250K desmosome glycoproteins that form cytoplasmic plaques and thereby provide attachment sites for intermediate filament proteins and desmogleins.

Desmopressin: DDAVP: 1-deamino-8-D-Arg-vasopressin; an arginine vasopressin analog that acts on V_2-type vasopressin receptors, and is used to treat diabetes insipidus. It is a weak agonist for V_1 receptors; *cf* **DVAP**.

desmosine: complexes, each assembled by oxidative cross-linking of four lysine molecules that hold four polypeptide chains in radial array. They account for much of the ability of elastin to stretch in two directions.

desmosome: macula adherens; a specialized kind of adhesion site between adjacent cells that strengthens tissue, increases rigidity, and provides attachment sites for intracellular fibers and extracellular molecules. Desmosomes are cytoplasmic plaques that contain desmoplakins, vinculin, and transmembrane **desmogleins** (*q.v.*). The kinds of intermediate filament proteins inserted into them vary with the cell types. Keratins predominate in skin (which contains large numbers of junctions), desmin in cardiac muscle, and vimentin in the brain.

desmosterol: cholesta-5,24-dien-3-ol; a sterol made by both vertebrates and invertebrates that accumulates in skin and can be converted to a vitamin-D like secosteroid when exposed to ultraviolet light.

desogestrel: 17α-ethynyl-18-methyl-11-methylene-Δ⁴-estren-17β-ol; a progestin component of combination type oral contraceptive pills that appears to be more effective and less toxic than steroids previously introduced.

Desonide: 16α-hydroxyprednisolone-16α,17-acetonide; a synthetic glucocorticoid analog used for its anti-inflammatory properties.

desoxy-: a prefix now largely replaced by deoxy-.

Desoxin: a trade name for methamphetamine.

desynapsis: (1) the separation of paired homologous chromosomes that normally occurs during the diplotene stage of meiosis prophase I; (2) failure of chromosomes associated during the pachynema stage to remain together during diplonema.

detergents: surface-active molecules with both hydrophilic and hydrophobic domains that break up lipid molecule aggregates by increasing the water solubilities of the components. Naturally occurring types include bile salts (which contribute to lipid digestion and are essential for absorption) and phospholipids (which, among other functions, maintain membrane structures). Tritons are used in low concentrations to augment plasma membrane permeabilities, and thereby facilitate inward diffusion of substances in extracellular fluids and/or release cytoplasmic components, and in higher ones to disrupt surface and intracellular membranes. SDS (sodium dodecylsulfate) is used to denature proteins and separate them from lipids for electrophoresis studies.

determinant: usually, the component of an antigen (the epitope) that is recognized by and binds to an antibody paratope.

determination: establishment of properties that specify the directions along which embryonic or stem cells can differentiate.

detirelix: a potent gonadotropin releasing hormone (GnRH) analog, in which five of the ten amino acid moieties have D configurations. It is used to inhibit gonadotropin secretion.

detoxification: (1) conversion of poisons to substances that are biologically less active or totally ineffective. The liver is the major site for chemical mechanisms, such as oxidation, reduction, or conjugation; but the kidneys contribute, and some reactions are accomplished by other cell types. The abilities of some toxins to interact with receptors, or directly damage cells is diminished or abolished; and accumulation of damaging levels is averted by changing the substances to kinds that are more rapidly transported and excreted; (2) a term more generally applied to chemical reactions of the kinds that modify foreign substances. Some liver enzymes generate products that are more toxic than the parent types.

deuterium: D; ^{2}H; heavy hydrogen; a stable isotope (atomic number 1, atomic weight 2.016). Since the chemical properties resemble those of the more common form of hydrogen, deuterium can be used to label relatively large molecules that are followed through metabolic pathways (sometimes in conjunction with radioactive markers at other sites). However, although the presence of extra neutrons has little effect on the physical properties of most atoms, the weight of deuterium is twice that of ^{1}H; *see* **deuterium oxide**.

deuterium oxide: D₂O; heavy water; water in which deuterium (^{2}H) replaces the common hydrogen isotope, [1]H. It inhibits microtubule polymerization.

development: acquisition of the specializations and characteristics of more mature forms. The term is applied to tissues, organs, systems, and whole organisms, often in conjunction with descriptive adjectives such as embryonic, postnatal, or abnormal, whereas *differentiation* is more commonly used for cells.

dexamethasone: 9α-fluoro-16α-methylprednisolone; a long-acting, orally and topically effective synthetic glucocorticoid with virtually no mineralocorticoid activity in the doses usually administered. Its high potency is related to very low affinity for corticosteroid binding globulin, as well as resistance to degradation by hepatic enzymes. Dexamethasone is used to study glucocorticoid receptors, and clinically for its anti-inflammatory properties. It also arrests the growth of some neoplasms and is highly effective against some forms of leukemia.

dexamphetamine: dextroamphetamine.

Dexedrine: a trade name for dextroamphetamine.

dextran[s]: high molecular weight polysaccharides composed of glucose units, mostly with 1 → 6 linkages, initially obtained from beets (in which they are produced by microorganisms). They can be hydrolyzed to smaller forms of desired sizes. 70-75K, 40K, and other derivatives are used to expand blood volume. When infused, they are retained for many hours in the bloodstream, where they attract water molecules from extracellular spaces. The do not enter cells, and can protect against the blood sludging that often otherwise occurs during shock. Although antigenic, large doses more commonly invoke transient immunological paralysis than anaphylaxis. Since they reversibly bind many substances, polymers of various sizes can be linked to pharmaceutical agents to achieve slow, steady release of the active components. *See* also **dextran sulfates**, **dextran coated charcoal**, and **Sephadex**.

dextran coated charcoal: DCC; an adsorbent that takes up unbound steroid hormone receptors, and is used for hormone-receptor binding studies and receptor assays.

dextran sulfates: sulfuric acid esters of dextrans. They are charged polymers that bind many substances, used for their anticoagulant and cholesterol lowering properties. They also bind several kinds of envelope coated viruses (including HIV-I and *Herpes* types), inhibit viral replication, and can protect T lymphocytes against infection.

dextrins: oligosaccharides formed by partial digestion of starches. They can be further degraded to maltose and glucose.

dextroamphetamine: dexamphetamine; the *d* isomer of **amphetamine** (*q.v.*). It is a more potent central nervous system than the *l* form. Many of its effects are attributed to catecholamine release from sequestration sites, but it also lowers monoamine oxidase activity. Interactions with special binding sites in the brain have been described, some of which may receptors for phenylethylamine. Although still used to treat narcolepsy, dextroamphetamine has been largely replaced by other agents for Parkinson's disease and attention deficits in children. Because of undesirable side-effects (that can include anxiety, insomnia, cardiovascular disturbances, habituation, and severe psychic manifestations) it is no longer prescribed for appetite suppression; but it is taken illegally for this purpose, and for the effects on mood. The stimulation is usually followed by psychic depression and fatigue.

dextromethorphan: the *d* isomer of racemethorphan (3-methoxy-17-methylmorphinan); a morphine derivative with codeine-like properties, used mostly to suppress coughing. It is also an allosteric antagonist for NMDA controlled ion channels, and an antagonist for voltage controlled types.

dextrose: glucose.

dextrorotary: *d*; +; describes substances that, when dissolved in aqueous media, rotate the plane of polarized light to the right; *cf* **levorotary** and **D configuration**.

d.f.: degrees of freedom.

DFMO: difluoromethylornithine.

DFO: *see* **deferoxamine**.

DFP: diisopropylfluorophosphate.

2-DG: 2-deoxyglucose.

D genes: DNA segments located between ones that code for immunoglobulin V and J components, and for T lymphocyte receptor α and β chains. They direct the synthesis of 2-10 amino acid peptides that link the V and J segments of immunoglobulin heavy chains.

DG: diacylglycerol.

2-DG: 2-deoxyglucose.

DGG: α-D-glutamyl-glycine.

DGGE: denaturing gradient gel electrophoresis.

DGLA: dihomogammalinoleic acid.

DHA: (1) DHEA; *see* **dehydroepiandrosterone**; (2) docosahexenoic acid.

DHAS: DHEAS; *see* **dehydroepiandrosterone-sulfate**.

DHEA: DHA; *see* **dehydroepiandrosterone**.

DHEAS: DHEAS; *see* **dehydroepiandrosterone-sulfate**.

DHETEs: dihdydroxyeicosatetraenoic acids; *see* **hydroxyeicosatetraenoic acids**.

DHFR: dihydrofolate reductase.

DHP: dihydropyridine.

DHPG: dihydroxyphenylethylglycol.

DHT: (1) 5α-dihydrotestosterone; (2) dihydrotachysterol.

DI: diabetes insipidus.

DIA: *see* **differentiation inhibiting activity**.

Diabenal: a trade name for chlorpropamide.

diabetes: increased urine flow; polyuria. *See* **diabetes insipidus**, **diabetes mellitus**, and **renal diabetes**.

diabetes associated peptides: DAPs; *see* **amylins**.

diabetes insipidus: DI: a disorder in which very large volumes of hypotonic, glucose-free urine are excreted. Hemconcentration occurs in severe cases, despite the associated compelling thirst and polydipsia. The major cause is vasopressin deficiency. More rarely, the hormone is made, but the receptors are defective. *See* also **Brattleboro rats**, and *cf* **diabetes mellitus** and **renal diabetes**.

diabetes mellitus: DM; several diseases in which insulin deficiency or defects that affect its use lead to the development of hyperglycemia, glycosuria, thirst, polydipsia, and hunger (usually with hyperphagia), other metabolic problems, and tendencies to develop microangiopathy, nephropathy, neuropathy, retinopathy, and arteriosclerosis. *Type I* DM is also called *insulin dependent* DM (IDDM), because little or no hormone is secreted, and replacement therapy is absolutely required. Since in most cases the symptoms are first manifested early in life (sometimes before the end of the second year), it has also been called juvenile onset diabetes (JOD), or juvenile onset in the young (JODY). However, it does begin later in some individuals; and other forms of diabetes mellitus can affect children. The most common cause of IDDM is autoimmune destruction of pancreatic β cells that leads to absolute hormone deficiency. Some viruses can directly attack the cells (at least in laboratory animals); but more often, viral infections and/or other environmental factors initiate the destruction in individuals with genetically defective immune systems. Certain histocompatibility complex patterns have been associated with susceptibility, and some others with conferring protection, but the patterns vary with geographical locales, and with other genetic factors; and IDDM can develop in just one member of a pair of identical twins. If insulin replacement therapy is not provided, the consequences include impaired growth, fat depletion, ketoacidosis, coma, emaciation, and death. *Type II* DM has been called *maturity onset diabetes mellitus* (MOD), since it typically develops in adults, often during the fourth decade or later. It is less severe than IDDM, and is associated with different histocompatibility antigen patterns. Many individuals are hyperinsulinemic, but resistant to the hormone during the early stages, and most are at least moderately obese at the time of onset. Since hyperphagia stimulates the pancreatic β cells, it contributes to the etiology in many cases. (Possible factors related to the disease that predispose to hyperphagia have not been adequately explored.) Chronically elevated insulin levels can promote down regulation of insulin receptors and invoke postreceptor defects, both of which lead to insulin resistance. In some cases, an obese twin displays the symptoms, whereas a lean one remains healthy. (However, many obese individuals with hyperinsulinemia and mild forms of resistance do not develop DM; and there are examples of onset in both members of a twin pair at almost the same time, even when the individuals live far apart and have different life styles.) Ketoacidosis is rare in type II disorders. Many individuals are effectively treated (at least in the early stages) by dietary restrictions alone (or with diet control in combination with oral hypoglycemic agents). Since long-term overactivity of the islet cells sometimes leads to exhaustion, deterioration and true insulin deficiency, insulin is administered to some patients. Most individuals with type II DM have some insulin resistance that is not directly related to low receptor numbers. Rarer forms of type II DM develop in lean individuals; and the term maturity onset diabetes mellitus in the young (MODY) has been applied when the symptoms begin during childhood or adolescence. Abnormal insulin receptors and postreceptor defects have been identified in many individuals. One form has been linked with mutations of the gene that codes for glucokinase (an enzyme required for normal insulin release, as well as for glucose phosphorylation in the liver), and others with genetic defects that impair different aspects of carbohydrate and lipid metabolism. Glucagon, glucocorticoids, growth hormone, and epinephrine oppose many insulin actions, and excessive secretion can invoke DM-like symptoms. Diabetes of pregnancy is a rare kind of metabolic dysfunction that usually resolves after parturition, and has been attributed to secretion of placental lactogen (chorionic somatomammotropin). Latent, *"chemical"* DM, in which overt symptoms are not manifested, but responses to glucose tolerance and other tests are abnormal, has been detected in some close family members of individuals with DM, substantial numbers of which later develop overt disease.

diabetogenic factor: a component of pituitary gland extracts enriched in growth hormone that invokes diabetes mellitus-like symptoms. There are controversies concerning how much of the activity results from direct effects of growth hormone (or of a fragment derived from it), indirect influences that involve release of secondary mediators, or actions of contaminants extracted with the hormone.

Diabinese: a trade name for chlorpropamide.

diacetyl morphine: heroin.

diacylglycerols: DGs: molecules composed of two fatty acid moieties (R_1 and R_2 in the structure shown), covalently linked to glycerol. Phospholipase C isozymes catalyze their release from phospholipids. DGs activate some kinase C isozymes by binding to them and lowering their requirements for Ca^{2+} to levels usually present in the cytoplasm, and may additionally exert other regulatory influences. Some phorbol esters (which are DG analogs) acutely mimic the effects, but prolonged presentation eventually diminishes, and can totally abolish the activity. DGs can be hydrolyzed to release arachidonic and other fatty acids, and can be phosphorylated to phosphatidic acid.

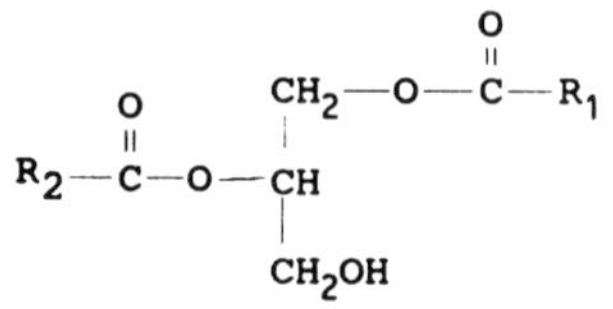

diacylglycerol kinases: enzymes that catalyze formation of phosphatidic acids from diacylglycerols + ATP. The products are key intermediates for phospholipid biosynthesis.

diacylglycerol kinase inhibitors: organic molecules synthesized for use in studies of diacylglcerol functions. One type, diacylglycerol kinase inibitor II, 3-[2]-4[*bis*(4-fluoro-phenyl)methylene]-1-piperidinyl]ethyl]-2,3-dihydro-2-thioxo-4(1*H*)-quinazolinone, is shown.

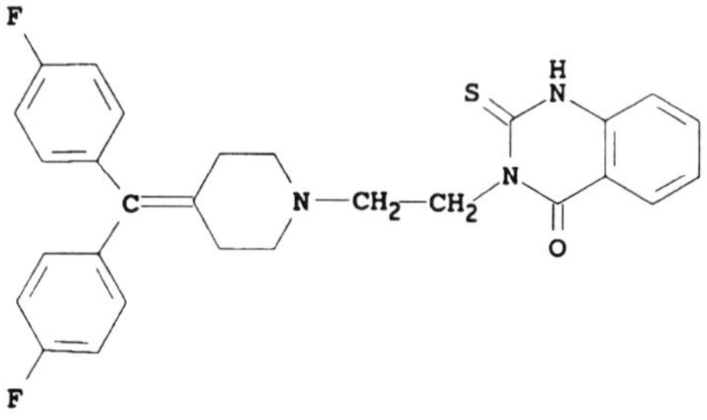

diacylglycerol-3-phosphates: phosphatidic acids.

diakinesis: the final stage of the first prophase of meiosis, during which chromosomes complete condensation and attach to spindle microtubules, the nucleolus disappears, and nuclear membrane fragments disperse.

diallelic: having two different alleles at a given locus.

dialysis: procedures in which a liquid (which can contain particulate matter), enclosed in a semi-permeable membrane, exchanges substances (via passive diffusion that can proceed in both directions) with a surrounding solvent. The nature of the membrane can be varied to selectively affect the kinds of molecules and/or ions that traverse it; and the concentrations of solutes in the surrounding solvent can be adjusted to determine the directions in which there is net movement. *Hemodialysis* is used to correct electrolyte and other extracellular fluid imbalances caused by renal dysfunction or other diseases. As blood passes through the compartment, urea and other nitrogenous wastes, along with excessive quantities of some electrolytes, travel down their concentration gradients to the solvent, but plasma proteins and formed elements are retained. Nutrients and other desired substances can be added to the solvent for diffusion into the blood. Dialysis is used *in vitro* to remove impurities from proteins and other large molecules. In *equilibrium dialysis*, antibodies are enclosed within the membrane compartments, and associated antigens are permitted to diffuse inward until no additional net changes occur. The binding affinities and valences of the antibodies can then be assessed by determining differences between the amounts of antigen bound (inside) vs the amounts retained in the solvents.

diamide: 1′,1′bis(*N,N*-dimethylformamide); a thiol oxidizing agent that acts on glutathione. It also interacts with enzyme disulfide groups, and is used to inhibit the activities of some phosphorylases.

diamines: compounds with two amino groups.

diamine oxidases: copper containing flavoprotein enzymes that catalyze oxidative deaminations. Most require ascorbic acid as a cofactor. In addition to substrates such as spermine and spermidine, they act on histamine, dopamine, norepinephrine, and some other monoamines, and on tryptophan and a few other amino acids. They are major factors for adjusting the levels of some of the substrates, but also contribute to some metabolic pathways, and to the cross-linking of collagen and elastin fibers.

2,4-diaminobutyrate: an agent used to prolong the effects of gamma aminobutyric acid (GABA) by inhibiting its uptake into nerve terminals.

cis-**diaminodichloroplatinum**: Cisplatin.

2,6-diaminopurine: a purine analog that blocks the actions of adenylate pyrophosphorylase and adenine phosphoryltransferase, and is used as a mutagen. Its inhibitory effects on bacterial growth can be reversed with adenine or folic acid.

diamorphine: diacetyl morphine; heroin.

Diamox: a trade name for acetazolamide.

2,6-diaminopurine

Dianabol: a trade name for methandrostenolone.

diapause: usually (1) delayed implantation. In seasonal breeders, it assures that young will be born at a time of the year favorable for survival, and is regulated by neuroendocrine mechanisms that respond to photoperiod changes by affecting the secretion of gonadal steroids and/or adenohypophysial hormones; *see* also **melatonin**. In rats, mice, and some other animals, *lactational* diapause is important when large litters are delivered, because the mothers cannot simultaneously nourish fetuses and provide sufficient milk for the young. It is initiated by stimuli associated with suckling four or more pups (and can be terminated if two or more are removed). In kangaroos and some other marsupials, implantation is delayed until a joey becomes sufficiently mature to detach from the teat and nurse intermittently. Diapause regulated in different ways occurs during times of severe drought and/or food shortages; (2) any pause in embryonic development; (3) a period of delay in the life cycle of an insect.

diapedesis: usually, leukocyte migration across blood vessel walls.

diaphorase: a general term for enzymes that catalyze reactions in which pyridine nucleotides are oxidized. Some are specific for NADH, and others for NADPH. *See* also **nitric oxide synthase**.

diaphoresis: sweating.

diaphysis: the shaft of a long bone.

diastereoisomerism: *see* **stereoisomerism**.

diastase: an obsolete term for α-amylase.

diastole: the relaxation phase of the cardiac cycle; *cf* **systole**.

diazepam: Valium; 7-chloro-1-methyl-5-phenyl-3*H*-1,4-benzodiazepin-2-one; an orally effective benzodiazepine type tranquilizer, muscle relaxant, and anti-convulsant. It mimics some gamma aminobutyric acid (GABA) actions, depresses spinal cord polysynaptic activity, and inhibits some mesencephalic reticular neurons.

diazepam binding inhibitor: DBI; anxiety peptide; species specific peptides that block the binding of diazepam and related agents to GABA$_A$ type γ-aminobutyric acid receptors. The human form is H_2N-Gln-Ala-Thr-Val-Gly-Asp-Ile-Asn-Thr-Glu-Arg-Pro-Gly-Met-Leu-Aso-Phe-Thr-Gly-Lys-OH.

diazo: the chemical group -N=N-.

diazoxide: 3-methyl-7-chloro-1,2,4-benzothiadiazine; an agent used to lower blood pressure. Unlike chlorothiazide, it does not promote sodium depletion, but may exert its effects by directly lowering the sodium content of arterioles. It also raises blood glucose levels.

Dibenamine: a trade name for the hydrochloride of *N*-(2-chloroethyl)-dibenzylamine, a haloalkylamine chemically related to nitrogen mustards. It is a potent but non-specific, noncompetitive adrenergic receptor antagonist, used to study adrenergic functions, in the diagnosis of pheochromocytoma, and to treat some forms of hypertension and cardiac dysrhythmias.

dibenzoxazepines: a class of neuroleptics that includes chlorpromazine, perphenazine, and other phenothiazines.

dibenzyline: phenoxybenzamine hydrochloride; an α-type adrenergic receptor antagonist, used to treat some forms of hypertension. It is pharmacologically similar to dibenzamine, but much more selective for α_1 type receptors. It additionally exerts anti-histamine effects, and can invoke sedation and local irritation.

dibucaine hydrochloride: Nupercaine; 2-butoxy-*N*-[2-(diethylamino)ethyl]-4-quinoline-carboxamide monochloride; a long-acting, but toxic local anesthetic. It also acts on acidic vesicles and inhibits receptor recycling.

dibutyryl cyclic adenosine 3′5′-monophosphate: bucladesine; DBcAMP; N^6,2'-*O*-dibutyryl adenosine; a hydrophobic cAMP analog that penetrates plasma mem-

branes, mimics most actions of cAMP, and resists hydrolysis by cyclic nucleotide phosphodiesterases. It is used to study cAMP functions; but slow release of butyrate is a disadvantage for some. *See N^6,2'-O-*dibutyryl-**cAMP** for the structure.

dibutyryl cAMP: dibutyryl cyclic adenosine-3′5′-monophosphate.

dicentric: describes chromosomes or chromatids with two centromeres.

o,p′-**dichlorodiphenyl dichloroethane**: DDD; mitotane: *see o′*, p′-**DDD**.

dichlorodiphenyltrichloroethane: DDT: an insecticide widely used before 1972, but discontinued because of its toxicities in humans and other animals. It prolongs action potentials and invokes repetitive firing after a single stimulus, by blocking both inactivation of axon Na^+ channels, and activation of K^+ channels. It accumulates in adipose tissue, and can therefore exert delayed effects. Although this limits the amounts presented to neurons, high doses deliver enough to invoke convulsions and ventricular fibrillation in vertebrates. Hepatic enzymes degrade DDT, and high doses induce mixed function oxidases.

dichloroisoproterenol: DCI; dichloroisoprenaline; 3,4-dichloro-α(isopropylaminomethyl)benzyl alcohol; a nonspecific adrenergic receptor antagonist that affects both β_1 and β_2 subtypes. It is used mostly as a laboratory tool.

5,-7-dichlorokynurenic acid: a potent excitatory amino acid agonist that binds to strychnine-insentive glycine sites of NMDA receptors.

2,3-dichloro-α-methylbenzylamine: an agent used to inhibit phenylethanolamine-*N*-methyltransferase (PNMT).

2,4-dichlorophenoxyacetic acid: 2,4-D; Hedonal; a phytohormone used to stimulate latex production, and to kill weeds. Small amounts can cause contact dermatitis, eye irritations, and gastrointestinal upsets in humans. Al-

2,3-dichloro-α-methylbenzylamine

2,4-dichlorophenoxyacetic acid

though rapidly excreted to urine, large amounts impair neuromuscular function in laboratory animals, and massive ones invoke coma and ventricular fibrillation.

dichorionic: describes twins with separate chorions.

dichroism: circular dichroism; the property of absorbing light polarized to the right to a different extent than light polarized to the left, and assuming different colors when viewed under transmitted, as compared with reflected light. It is useful for studying the orientations of some macromolecules and supramolecular complexes.

dictyate: dictyotene; a prolonged diplotene stage of meiosis I prophase in which primary oocytes of many mammalian species are arrested before undergoing further maturation. In human females, oocytes enter this stage during the third trimester of the gestation period. After puberty, a few complete meiosis I during each ovarian cycle; and one or more prepare for meiosis II (which occurs after fertiliazation). Some are arrested for five decades or longer.

dicumarol: Dicoumarol; Dicoumarin; 3,3″-methylene[4-hydroxydroxycoumarin]; a compound initially identified as the component of spoiled clover that causes hemorrhagic disease in cattle. It impairs the synthesis of several vitamin K-dependent proteins (including coagulation factors), and is used to protect against formation of intravascular blood clots.

N,N′-**dicyclohexylcarbodiimide**: DCC; DCCD; an agent that activates carboxyl groups and facilitates formation of peptide bonds. It is used for the chemical synthesis of peptides and proteins. It also inhibits ATP-dependent proton pumps of secretory granules, clathrin-coated vesicles, Golgi vesicles, and lysosomes, and exerts oligomycin-like effects on mitochondria.

Dictyostelium discoideum: a slime mold used to study cell:cell interactions during development. The life cycle includes a motile, unicellular stage, and another in which 10^5 cells aggregate to form a spore-producing fruiting body. cAMP is a major mediator of the effects of nutrient deprivation, and adenosine is an important inhibitor. The simple genome is useful for mutation studies. The cells can synthesize receptors and other molecules not easily made by bacteria because they require glycosylation.

2′,3′-dideoxyadenosine: a deoxyadenosine analog that crosses plasma membranes, and is converted by cells to a triphosphate that incorporates into DNAs and terminates chain elongation. It is a potent inhibitor of reverse transcriptases that blocks the replication of several viruses (including HIV-I). It also inhibits eukaryote DNA β and γ (but not α) polymerases. Because it is less toxic to bone marrow than zidovudine, it is under investigation for use (alone, especially in individuals who cannot tolerate zidovudine side effects, or along with low doses of zidovudine) for treating acquired immunodeficiency syndrome (AIDS). The triphosphate is used directly in DNA base sequence studies. Cells make an adenosine kinase, but the first phosphorylation is catalyzed mostly by deoxycytidine kinase. The ddA-monophosphate formed is then believed to be acted upon by a purine nucleoside monophosphate kinase, and the product of that reaction by a purine nucleoside diphosphate kinase. ddA is also deaminated to 2′3′-dideoxyinosine. The degradation products are hypoxanthine and dideoxyribose-phosphate.

2′,3′-dideoxycytidine: a deoxycytidine analog with properties similar to those described for 2′,3′-dideoxyadenosine.

2′3′-dideoxyinosine: a deoxycytidine analog derivable from, and with properties similar to those of 2′3′-dideoxyadenosine.

2′3′-dideoxythymidine: a deoxythymidine analog with properties similar to those described for 2′3′-dideoxyadenosine.

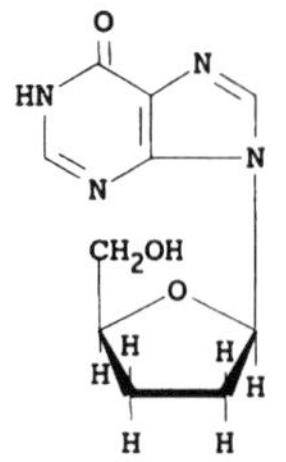

2′3′-dideoxyinosine

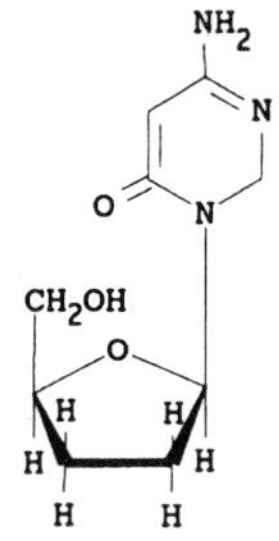

2′3′-dideoxythymidine

Didronel: a trade name for disodium etidronate.

DIDS: 4,4-diisothiocyanato-2,2′-stilbenedisulfonic acid; an agent that binds covalently to cell membranes, blocks anion channels, cross-links anion sites, and can inhibit adenylate cyclases.

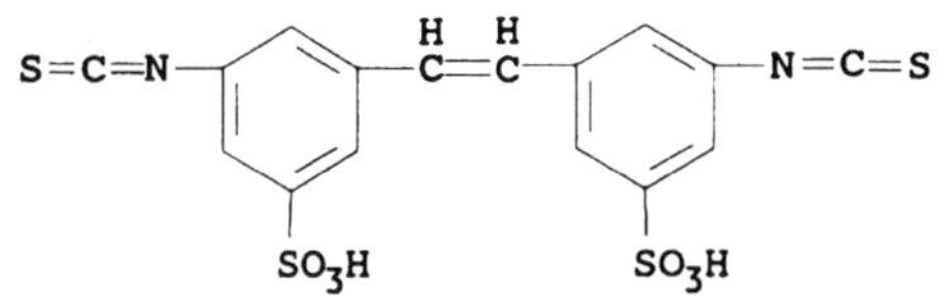

diecious: dioecius.

dielectric: an insulating medium between two plates of a capacitor.

diencephalon: the brain region that includes the thalamus, hypothalamus, and epithalamus.

dietary fiber: cellulose, lignins, pectins, and other high molecular weight polymer components of fruits, grains, and vegetables that cannot be digested by vertebrate gastrointestinal enzymes. *Soluble* types in fruits, vegetables, and grains absorb water, and form gel-like conglomerates that soften stools, aid evacuation, and appear to protect against development of diverticulosis. They contribute to satiety (a property especially useful to obese individuals attempting to lose weight) by creating a sense of fullness. In addition, by binding bile salts, they decrease the absorption of cholesterol and other lipids, and can lower blood cholesterol levels. Some slow carbohydrate absorption and thereby protect against prandial hyperglycemia. However, they can also impair absorption of essential fatty acids and fat-soluble vitamins; and large quantities of phytates interfere with calcium and zinc absorption. *Insoluble* fibers, in rinds and seed coats, do not absorb water, but do add bulk to the intestinal contents. They mechanically stimulate the lower intestine and, by accelerating evacuation of wastes (including products made by bacteria), they protect against constipation, and are believed to remove substances that increase the risks for developing colon cancers.

diesterases: enzymes that catalyze hydrolytic degradation of compounds with two ester linkages, for example phospholipases and cyclic nucleotide phosphodiesterases.

diestrus: the quiescent (and usually longest) phase of the estrous cycle. It follows metestrus and precedes the next proestrus. The blood levels of ovarian hormones are low, and vaginal smears contain mostly small, nucleated epithelial cells and a few leukocytes, along with some mucus and cell debris.

diethylcarbamoyl-4-aza-5-α-androstan-3-one: DMAA; 4-MA; an androgen analog used to inhibit the 5α-reductase that converts testosterone to 5α-dihydrotestosterone.

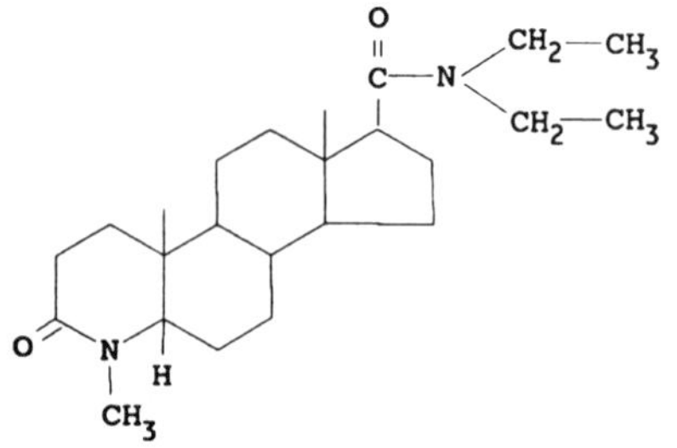

1,3-diethyl-8-phenylxanthine: DPX; an A_1-type adenosine receptor antagonist.

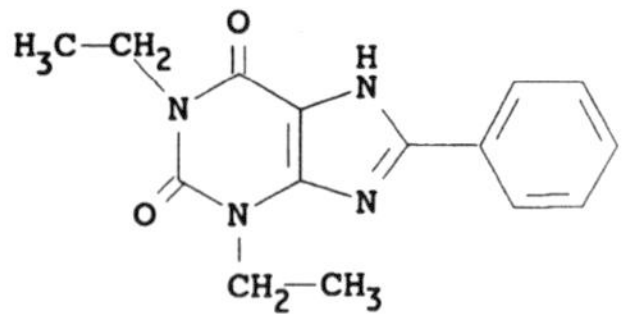

diethylpropion hydrochloride: a sympathomimetic agent that depresses appetite.

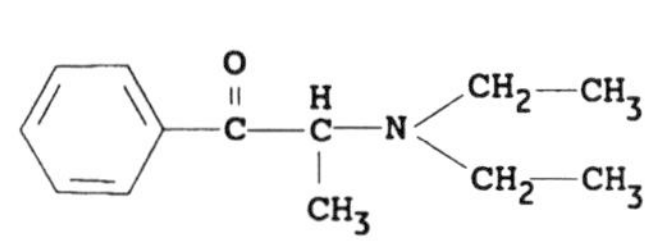

diethylstilbestrol: DES; stilbestrol; 3,4-bis-(*p*-hydroxyphenyl)-3-hexene; a potent, orally effective nonsteroidal estrogen receptor agonist. It was once used to prevent spontaneous abortions; but estrogens are no longer regarded as suitable agents for such purposes. Some adverse effects of DES on fetuses do not become apparent for many years. They include impaired vaginal maturation, and in some cases reproductive system cancers. The incidences of prostate gland abnormalities, and impaired development of the external genitalia in males is somewhat lower. Because of the potential toxicity, DES has been replaced by other estrogens for alleviating menopausal symptoms and slowing the development of postmenopausal osteoporosis. It is still used to a limited extent to treat some breast and prostate gland cancers.

diethylstilbestrol

DIF: *see* **differentiation inhibitory activity**.

differential centrifugation: techniques for separating subcellular components on the basis of sedimentation velocities. Nuclei (the heaviest particles of cell homogenates) form pellets when the mixture is subjected to moderately high gravitational fields. Progressively stronger fields successively promote sedimentation of mitochondria, and then ribosome fractions. At each stage, the supernatant can be removed, and the pellet resuspended for further purification.

differentiation: the changes associated with maturation and specialization, a term commonly reserved for cells (*cf* **development**), but also used for tissues. Cell differentiation is usually accompanied by a decline in (or total loss of) the potential for proliferation. *See* also **commitment**, and **sex differentiation**.

differentiation antigens: entities that appear on cell surfaces during specific stages of cell differentiation (or are present in large amounts at such times, but barely detectable at later stages); (2) substances expressed on only certain kinds of cell types that are used as markers of specialization (*see* **cluster of differentiation antigens**). The amounts of some types increase when the cells are exposed to certain stimulants, or when they are transformed. Most of the compounds are glycoproteins. They are called antigens, because they have been identified with monoclonal antibodies.

differentiation inhibitory activity: DIA; leukemia inhibitory factor; LIF; differentiation retarding factor; DRF; human interleukin stimulant for DA cells; HILDA; a 45-56K multifunctional glycoprotein, initially identified as the factor secreted by fibroblast-like feeder cells that is essential for growing embryonic stem cells from blastocyst inner cell mass. It supports proliferation, but inhibits differentiation in that system, and exerts similar influences on myeloid hematopoietic cell lines, some kinds of leukemia cells, and cultured testicular teratomas. DIF is believed to play roles in implantation and blastocyst growth, and also in cells of mature individuals that proliferate rapidly and then undergo specializations. Estrogens stimulate endometrial glands to produce large amounts shortly before the time of implantation (even in the absence of viable blastocysts); and trophectoderm has DIF receptors. The levels in endometrium fall rapidly shortly after implantation is completed, but small amounts are consistently found in postimplantation embryos and fetuses. Fairly large amounts are made in neonatal skin, and in adult small intestine (both of which contain populations of rapidly proliferating cells). DIF also stimulates bone growth and accelerates remodeling. Additionally, it augments acute phase responses in hepatocyte cultures, and it promotes establishment of cholinergic phenotypes in sympathetic system neurons. Large doses invoke cachexia in mice. Although the acronym LIF is used by some investigators, DIF is distinguishable from a different protein that inhibits leukocyte migration.

diffusion: passive movement of molecules or ions down a concentration gradient, driven by intrinsic kinetic activity. The rates for *simple* diffusion vary directly with the temperature, and inversely with the viscosity of the medium; and are also related to particle size and shape. At some sites, they are affected by the sizes of the pores through which the substances pass. The concentration gradients are major determinants of the net effects. *Carrier mediated* (facilitated) diffusion requires a factor (carrier) that travels to the cell surface, attaches to the diffusing substance, transports it to the cell interior, and returns without it to the membrane. Although subject to all of the factors described for simple diffusion, carrier mediated diffusion rates are additionally affected by the quantities of carrier available in active form, and by the presence of substances that compete for it. (For example, high levels of deoxyglucose interfere with glucose uptake). In some cell types, carrier availability is regulated by hormones. (Insulin promotes transport of carriers from intracellular sequestration sites to plasma membranes in skeletal muscle and adipose tissue). *Cf* **active transport**.

diffusion coefficient; diffusion constant: a factor calculated for a specific kind of molecule or ion, determined from the rate of net passive transfer per unit of concentration gradient under defined conditions (*see* **diffusion**). Its value is related to the molecular size and shape of the transported substance, and to the nature of the solvent.

DIFP: DFP: diisopropylfluorophosphate.

2-**difluoromethylornithine**: α–difluormethylornithine; eflornithine; DFMO: an ornithine analog used to irreversibly inhibit ornithine decarboxylase, to kill Trypanosomes, and to arrest the growth of some cancers.

digametic: describes organisms that produce two kinds

of gametes with different sex chromosomes, for example X and Y type spermatozoa.

DiGeorge syndrome: human disorders caused by failure of the third and fourth embryonic branchial pouches to undergo normal development. Since neither thymus nor parathyroid glands differentiate, T lymphocyte functions are not acquired, and hypocalcemia can be a major problem. Other manifestations can include heart and blood vessel deformities.

digestion: hydrolytic cleavage; reactions of the general type: R_1-R_2 + HOH → R_1-OH + R_2-H, catalyzed by proteases, lipases, and other enzymes; *cf* **dehydration synthesis**. Some reactions proceed extracellularly, for example in the gastrointestinal tract, and when enzymes are taken up by blood or formed there; and some intracellular enzymes are enclosed in lysosomes. Several kinds with potential for damaging the cells that make them are synthesized in inactive forms; *see*, for example **trypsinogen**.

digitalin: digitoxin: a steroid glycoside component of digitalis that inhibits Na^+/K^+-ATPases, and is used to treat myocardial insufficiency. By causing Na^+ ions to accumulate within the cells, it accelerates Na^+/Ca^{2+} exchange, and thereby elevates intracellular Ca^{2+}. The toxic effects can include vomiting, diarrhea, delirium, and convulsions, as well as cardiac arrhythmias.

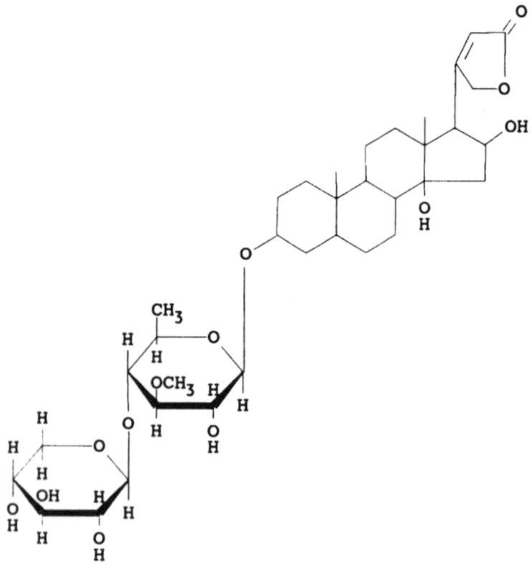

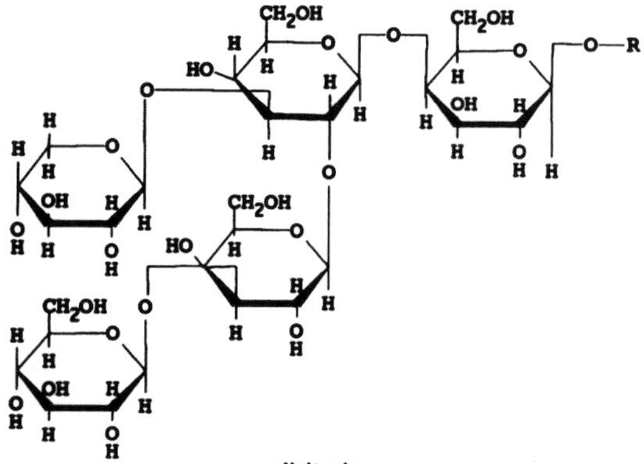

digitonin

digitoxigenin

digitalis: a mixture of substances obtained from the leaves of *Digitalis purpurea* (purple foxglove) and related plant species, and used to stimulate the myocardium. The components include digitalin and digitonin.

digitogenin: (25R)-5α-spirostan-2α,3β,15β-triol; the alycone of digitonin.

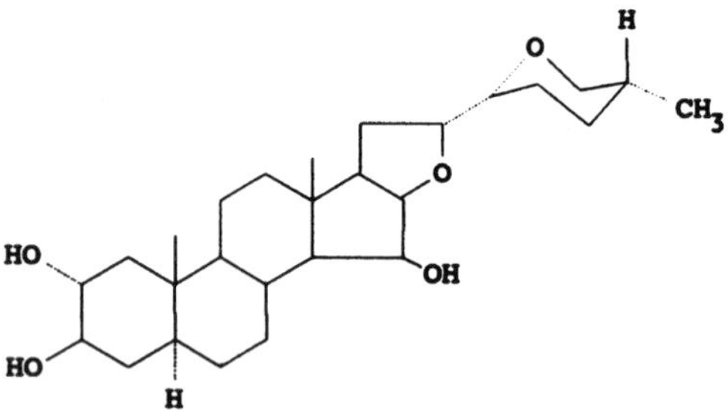

digitonin: digitin; a detergent extracted from the leaves of *Digitalis purpurea*. It is used in procedures for measuring cholesterol and bile in blood and body tissues. The R in the structure shown is digitogenin.

digitoxigenin: 3,4-dihydroxycard-20(22)-enolide; an aglycone of digitoxin and related plant derivatives, released from digitalis by hydrolysis. Its actions closely resemble those of **digitalin** *(q.v.)*.

digitoxin: digitalin.

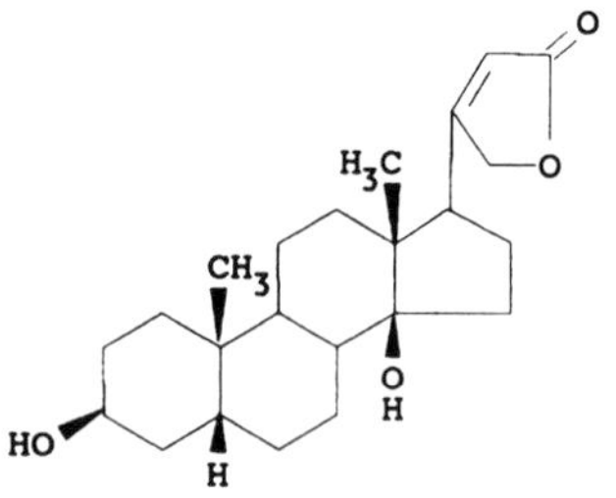

dihaploid: describes a diploid cell with two identical sets of chromosomes, acquired by replication of a haploid genome.

dihomogammalinoleic acid: DGLA; Δ 8,11,14-eicosanoic acid; an essential fatty acid, obtained from foods and used to synthesize prostaglandins and related lipids. Liver cells can make it from linoleic acid, and can convert it to arachidonic acid.

dihybrid: an individual that is heterozygous at two loci.

dihydrobiopterin: oxidized tetrahydrobiopterin coenzyme, formed in reactions catalyzed by tyrosine hydroxylase and some other enzymes. It is reduced in the reaction: dihydrobiopterin + NADPH + H^+ → tetrahydrobiopterin + NADP.

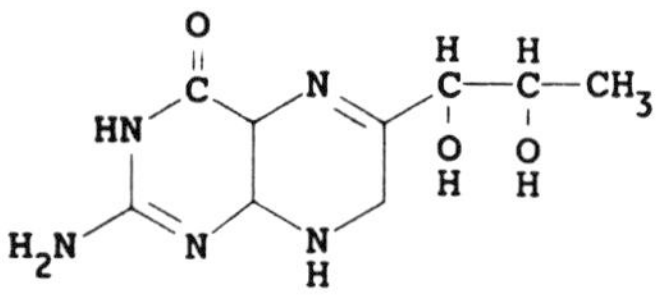

dihydrocortisol: an intermediate in the pathway for hepatic degradation of cortisol. It is converted to tetrahydrocortisol and other metabolites, which are excreted mostly as glucuronic acid conjugates.

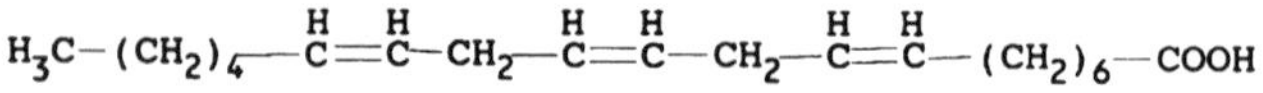

dihomogammalinoleic acid

194

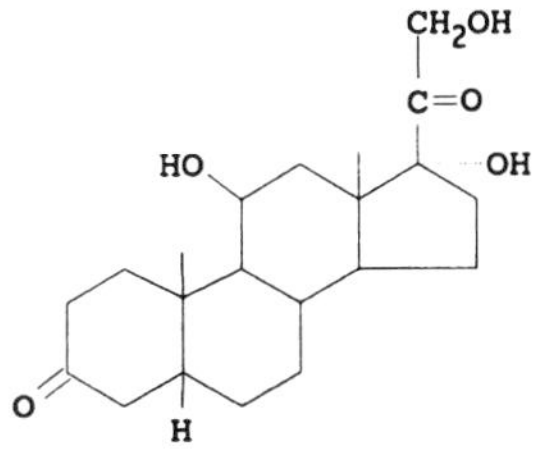

dihydrocortisol

dihydrocortisone: an intermediate in the pathway for degradation of cortisol and cortisone. It is converted to tetrahydro derivatives and other metabolites which are excreted mostly as glucuronic acid conjugates.

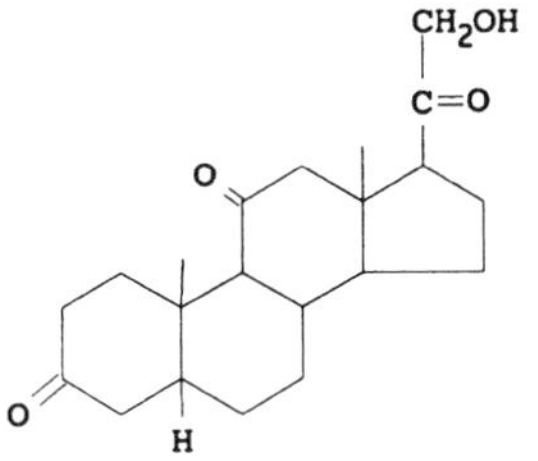

dihydroergotamine: 9,10-dihydro-12′-hydroxy-2′-methyl-5′5-(phenylmethyl)-ergotaman-3′,6′18-trione; a hydrogenated derivative of ergotamine. The mesylate is used to treat migraine headaches. The usual dosages do not stimulate uterine muscle, and have minimal effects on systemic blood pressure.

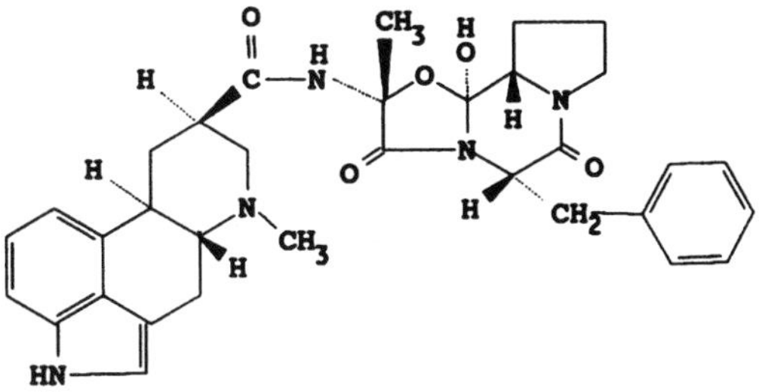

dihydrofolate: *see* **folic acid** and **dihydrofolate reductase**.

dihydrofolate reductase: DHFR; an enzyme that catalyzes the reaction: 7,8-dihydrofolate + NADPH → 5,6,7,8-tetrahydrofolate + NADP. Tetrahydrofolate reacts with serine to form N^5,N^{10}-methylene tetrafolate, a coenzyme for thymidylate kinase. The enzyme catalyzes conversion of deoxyuridine-monophosphate (dUMP) to deoxythymidine-monophosphate (dTMP), and is therefore essential for DNA synthesis. Methotrexate and aminopterin are dihydrofolate analogs that competitively inhibit DHFR, and are used to treat leukemias, choriocarcinomas, and other malignancies with rapidly dividing cells. Trimethoprim is an inhibitor in prokaryotes. *See* also **folic acid**.

dihydrolipoic acid: 6,8-dimpercaptoocanoic acid; the reduced form of lipoic acid; *see* **pyruvate dehydrogenase**.

$$H_3C - CH_2 - CH_2 - CH_2 - CH_2 - CH_2 - CH_2 - COOH$$

dihydromorphine: 4,5α-epoxy-17-methylmorphinan-3, 6α-diol; a highly addictive morphine derivative that invokes euphoria. It is a potent analgesic.

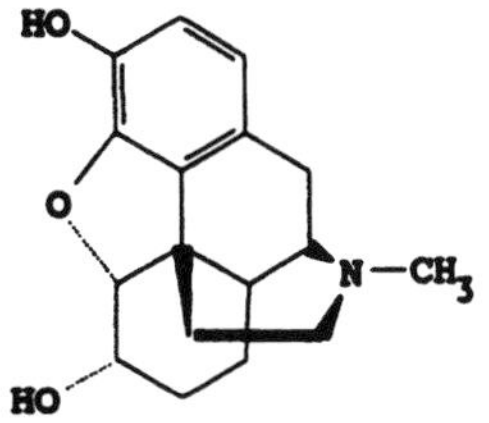

dihydroorotase: an enzyme that catalyzes the reaction: carbamoylaspartate → dihydroorotate + H_2O. It is a component of the CAD complex, which includes carbamoyl phosphate synthetase.

dihydroorotate: an intermediate in the pathway for uridylate biosynthesis, made from carbamoylaspartate via a reaction catalyzed by dihydroorotase. Dihydroorotate dehydrogenase then catalyzes dihydroorotate + NAD^+ → orotate + NADH + H^+. Orotate phosphoribosyl transferase acts on the product: orotate + PRPP → orotidylate + P-P. Carboxylation of orotidylate yields uridylate (UMP).

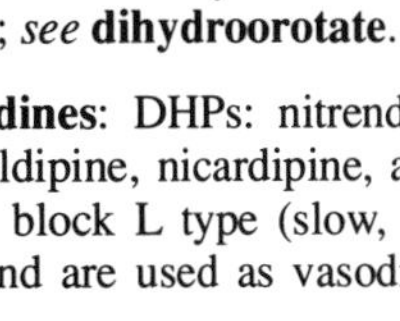

dihydroorotate dehydrogenase: an enzyme essential for DNA synthesis that catalyzes conversion of dihydroorotate to orotate; *see* **dihydroorotate**.

1,4-**dihydropyridines**: DHPs: nitrendipine, nifedipine, nimodipine, nisoldipine, nicardipine, and related agents that bind to and block L type (slow, voltage-sensitive) Ca^{2+} channels, and are used as vasodilators, as well as

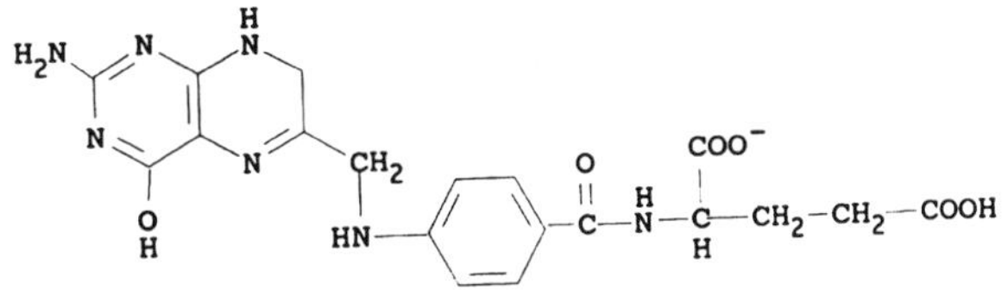

dihydrofolate

Bay K 8644 and a few other compounds that are Ca^{2+} channel agonists.

dihydropyridine receptors: large transmembrane complexes, composed of α_1, α_2, β, γ, and δ subunits, that mediate excitation-contraction coupling and Ca^{2+} entry into muscle cells via L type ion channels. The α_1 component, which contains only small amounts of carbohydrate, is the major functional site for the coupling, ion entry, and binding of dihydropyridine agonists and antagonists. The α_2, γ, and δ subunits are heavily glycosylated, whereas the β component appears to totally lack sugar groups. Endothelin, a vasoconstrictor, binds to the receptors.

dihydrosphingosine: an intermediate in the pathway for sphingosine biosynthesis. Its precursor, dehydrosphinganine, is formed in a condensation reaction with palmitoyl-coenzyme A and serine, in which one of the carbons is eliminated. An NADPH-catalzyed reaction then converts the precursor to dihydrosphingosine. Oxidation of the product by an FAD enzyme yields sphingosine.

dihydrotachysterol: DHT: AT10: 9,10-secoergosta-5,7,22-trien-3B-ol; an orally effective vitamin D_2 analog, used to treat hypoparathyroidism and osteodystrophy. It is activated by hepatic 25-cholecalciferol hydroxylase, but does not require 1-hydroxylation to bind to and activate 1,25-dihydroxyvitamin D receptors.

5α-dihydrotestosterone: DHT; the major testosterone metabolite that acts on androgen receptors in most target cells. It is formed in a reaction catalyzed by 5α-reductase, an enzyme induced by testosterone. DHT is essential for differentiation, maturation, and functions of the male external genitalia, for spermatogenesis, and for the maturation and functions of male accessory reproductive organs. It also mediates most androgen effects on skeletal muscle, skin, bone, liver, kidney, brain, and other structures. However, testosterone can act directly on skeletal muscle receptors, affects some brain functions, and is the promoter of Wolffian duct differentiation. Unlike testosterone and some other androgens, DHT cannot be aromatized to estrogens.

5β-dihydrotestosterone: a testosterone metabolite that acts on receptors in bone marrow, and stimulates erythropoiesis. It does not exert the effects described for 5α-dihydrotestosterone.

dihydrouridine: a nucleoside derived from uridine. It is present in transfer, but not in most other RNAs.

dihydroxyacetone-phosphate: an intermediate in the glycolysis pathway, formed along with 3-phosphoglyceraldehyde when aldolase catalyzes cleavage of fructose-1-6-biphosphate. It is the major precursor of glycerol-3-phosphate in the adipose tissue of most species, an intermediate for ether lipid biosynthesis, and a component of the glycerol phosphate shuttle. In one pathway for gluconeogenesis, dihydroxyacetone-phosphate is

dehydrosphingosine   dihydrosphingosine   sphingosine formed from glycerol-3-phosphate. It then combines with 3-phosphoglyceraldehyde to yield fructose-biphosphate.

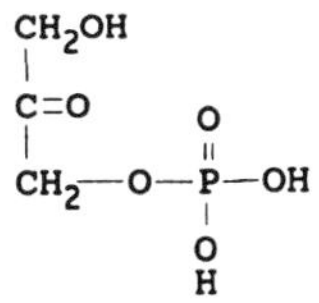

dihydroxyphenylacetic acid: *see* **DOPAC**.

L-dihydroxyphenylalanine: DOPA; 3-hydroxytyrosine; L-DOPA; levodopa: an intermediate in the pathway for catecholamine and melanin biosynthesis. Its formation from phenylalanine is catalyzed by tyrosine hydroxylase (the rate-limiting enzyme for dopamine and norepinephrine synthesis). Systemically administered DOPA crosses blood-brain barriers, and is converted to dopamine in the central nervous system. It is used to study catecholamine effects on the brain, and to treat Parkinson's disease (but *see* also **selegiline**). Most influences on the adenohypophysis (including inhibition of prolactin secretion) are attributed to its conversion to dopamine; but direct inhibition of growth hormone release has been suggested.

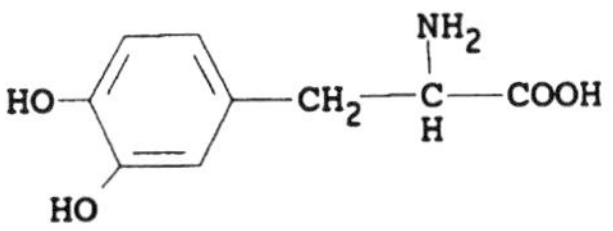

dihydroxyphenylethylglycol: DHPG; DOPEG; a biologically inactive epinephrine and norepinephrine metabolite formed in the brain. Monoamine oxidases catalyze conversion of those catecholamines to dihydroxyglycoaldehye, and aldehyde reductase acts on the product to yield DOPEG. Catecholamine-*O*-methyltransferase (COMT) converts most of the DOPEG to 3-methoxy,4-hydroxyphenylethylglycol (MOPEG, MHPG). The major end-product excreted to the urine is MOPEG-sulfate. (Most of the dihdyroxyglocylaldehyde made outside the central nervous system is oxidized to dihydroxymandelic acid.)

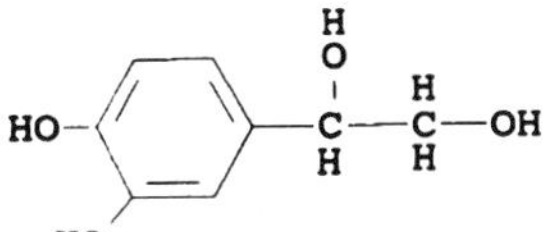

dihydroxyphenylserine: DOPS; an agent used to study noradrenergic functions in the central nervous system. When administered systemically, it crosses the blood-brain barrier, and is converted in the brain to norepinephrine.

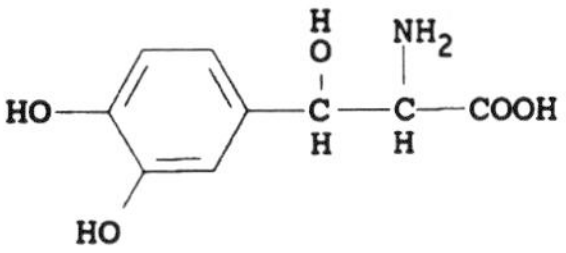

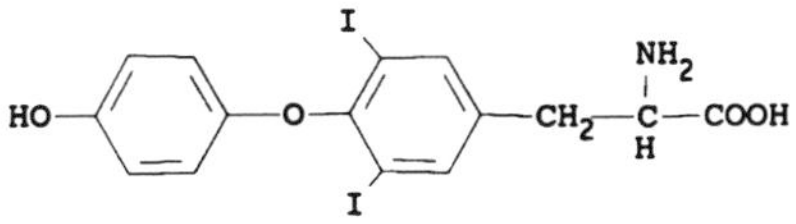

3'5'-T$_2$

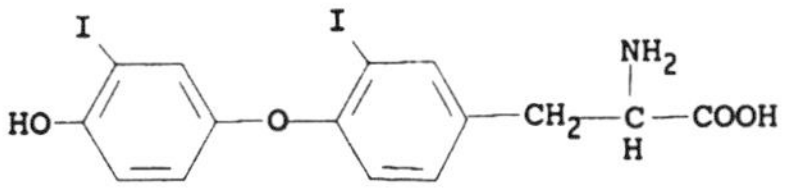

5,5'-T$_2$

diiodothyronines

dihydroxyphenylserine

dihydroxytetraeneoic acid: *see* **hydroxyeicosatetraenoic acids**.

1,25-**dihydroxyvitamin D**: *see* 1,25-dihydroxy-**cholecalciferol**.

24,25-**dihydroxyvitamin D**: *see* 24,,25-dihydroxy-**cholecalciferol**.

diiodothyronines: T$_2$; biologically inactive metabolites formed when deiodinases act on thyroxine, triiodothyronine, and reverse triiodothyronine. The most common types are 3'5'-T$_2$ and 5,5'-T$_2$, but other forms can be made. T$_2$s can be further degraded to monoiodothyronines, thyronine, and sulfated derivatives.

3,5-**diiodotyrosine**: DIT: a biologically inactive compound released when iodinated thyroglobulin undergoes proteolysis to yield thyroxine and triiodothyronine. It can be deiodinated within the thyroid gland to monoiodotyrosine and tyrosine; and both the free amino acid and the iodine can be recycled for thyroid hormone synthesis. (Iodotyrosines are not directly incorporated into thyroglobulin.)

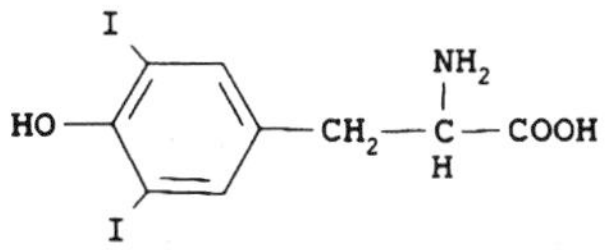

diisopropylfluorophosphate: DFP; DIFP; isofluorophosphate; an irreversible inhibitor of acetylcholinesterase, chymotrypsin, and other serine proteases, once used as a military nerve gas. By prolonging the effects of acetylcholine, it can invoke severe gastrointestinal tract disturbances, hypotension, and respiratory arrest. Low concentrations are administered topically (to a limited extent) to treat glaucoma. Higher ones are used for studies of acetylcholine functions, and as insecticides.

Dilantin: a trade name for phenytoin.

Dilaudid: a trade name for hydromorphine hydrochloride.

diltiazem: 3-(acetyloxy)-5-[2-(dimethylamino)-ethyl]-2,3-dihydro-2-(4-methyoxyphenyl)-1,5-benzothiazepin-4-(5*H*)-one; a benzodiazepine that blocks L-type Ca^{2+} channels and inhibits Na$^+$-dependent calcium efflux from

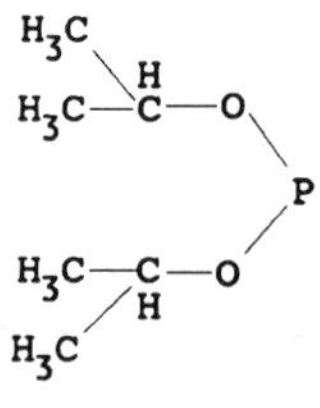

diisopropylfluorophosphate

dimestrol

mitochondria by binding to a site different from the dihy-dropyridine receptor. It is used as a coronary vasodilator.

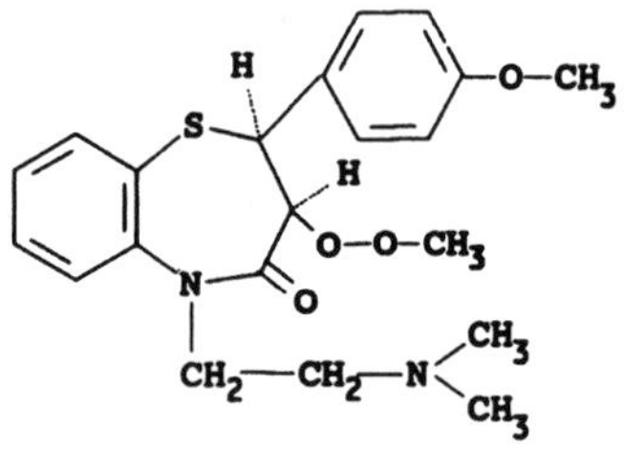

dimethisterone

dimaprit: (3-imino, 3-amino)-thio,1-dimethylamino-propane; an H_2 type histamine receptor agonist.

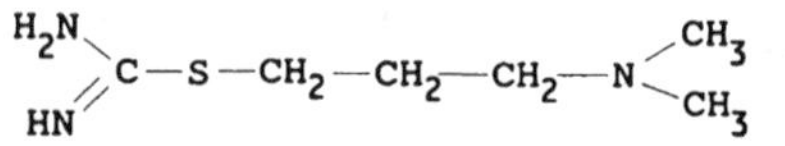

dimethylbenzylamines: several β-type adrenergic receptor agonists with similar properties. R_1, R_2, and R_3 in the structure shown mark the sites where they differ.

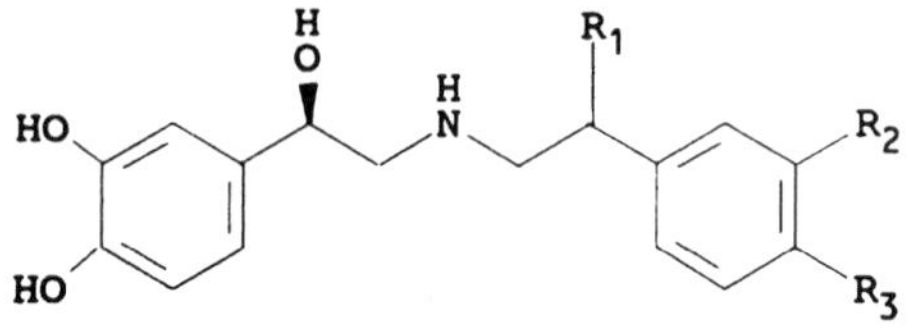

dimenhydrinate: Dramamine; a preparation composed of equal parts of 8-chloro-3,7-dihdyro-1,3-dimethyl-1*H*-purine-2,6-dione (structure A) and 2-(diphenylmethoxy)-*N*,*N*′-dimethylethanamine (structure B). It is an H_1-type histamine receptor antagonist, used mostly to prevent motion sickness, but to a lesser extent to control vomiting during pregnancy.

N^2-**dimethylguanosine**: a nitrogenous base component of transfer, but not of other RNAs.

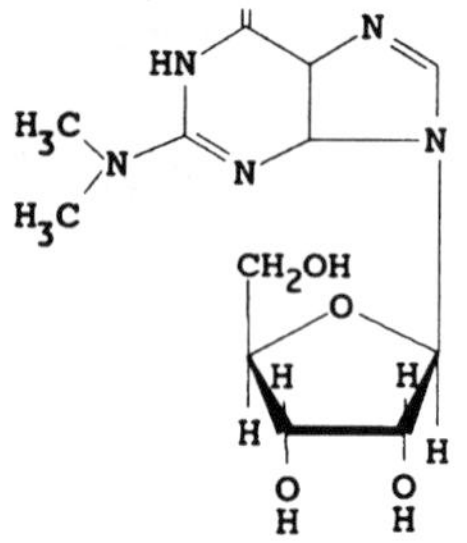

dimer: usually, a peptide composed of two subunits (which are identical in homodimers, and different in heterodimers).

dimercaprol: *see* **BAL**.

dimestrol: diethylstilbestrol dimethyl ether; a non-steroidal estrogen receptor agonist, used in depot preparations for prolonged effects. Its biological properties are similar to those of diethylstilbestrol.

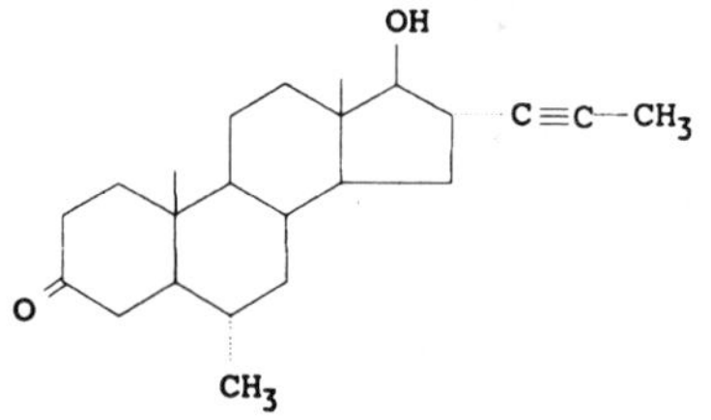

dimethisterone: 17α-hydroxy-6-methyl-17-(1-proponyl) androst-4-en-3-one; an orally effective progestin, used to treat some ovarian dysfunctions, and as an oral contraceptive component.

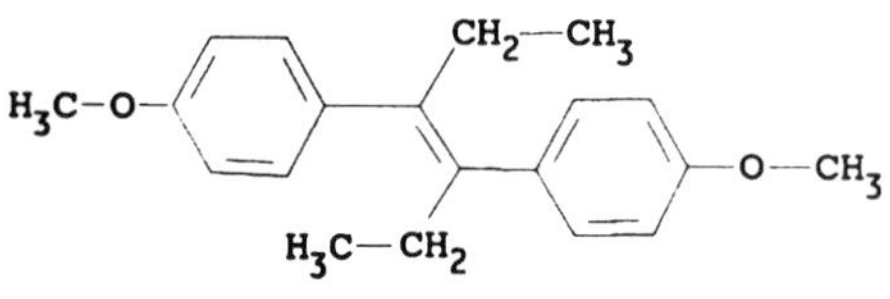

dimethylmaleate: an agent used to inhibit the glutathione oxidation-reduction cycle.

dimethylmorphine: thebaine.

dimethylsulfate: an agent used to methylate DNA; *see* **DNase protection**.

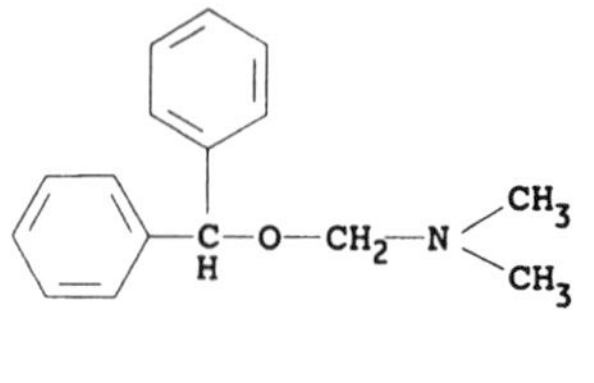

A

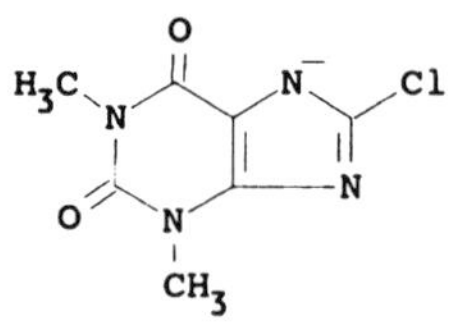

B

dimenhydrinate

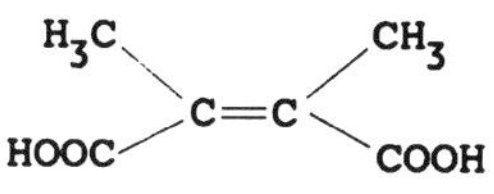

dimethylmaleate

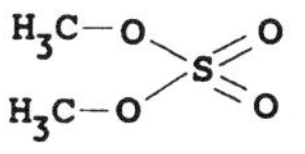

dimethylmorphine

dimethylsulfoxide: DMSO: an analgesic that also affects DNA methylation, promotes differerentiation of some leukemia cells, exerts anti-inflammatory effects, and activates epidemermal growth factor (EGF) receptors. It is used as a solvent that penetrates tissues, to deliver topically applied therapeutic agents and promote uptake of substances that affect microtubules and other organelles, and to preserve tissues prior to freezing.

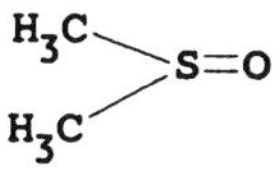

dimethyltryptamine: a tryptophan metabolite believed to invoke hallucinations and other brain dysfunctions when made in large amounts.

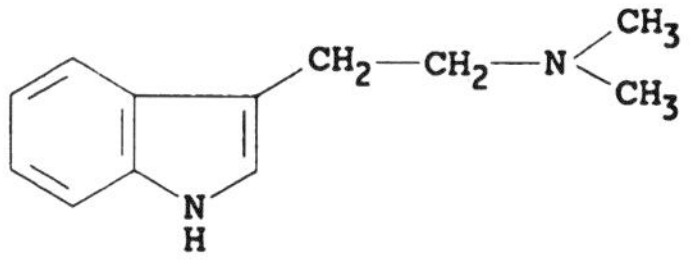

dimethylurea: a scavenger for hydroxyl radicals. It protects against some kinds of oxidative damage, for example in the pancreas (where it blocks development of diabetes mellitus in streptozotocin treated animals).

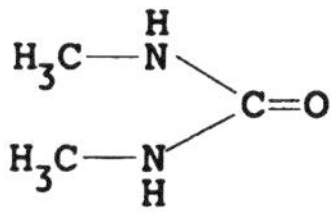

dimorphism: existing in two different forms; usually, phenotypic differences in females, as compared with males of the same species; *see* **sexual dimorphism**.

3,5-**dinitrocatechol**: an orally effective inhibitor of catechol-*O*-methyltranferase (COMT) that enters cells and penetrates blood-brain barriers.

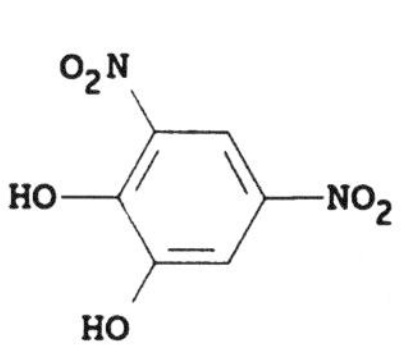

2,4-**dinitrophenol**, DNP: a laboratory tool for studying mitochondrial functions. It uncouples oxidative phosphorylation by blocking inorganic phosphate uptake. It also binds to many proteins, and is used as a hapten in immunology studies, and as a chemical reagent. Since it elevates metabolic rates, it was once believed that DNP could be a useful adjunct for treating obesity. However, it invokes cataract formation, agranulocytosis, and hyperthermia that can be fatal.

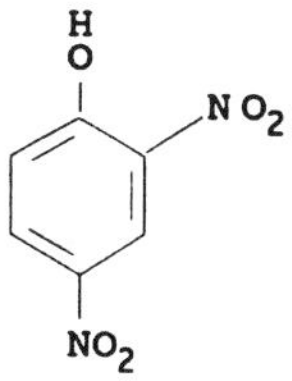

dinoflagellates: minute, aquatic organisms with both animal and plant-like characteristics that retain nuclear envelopes during mitosis, and have permanently condensed chromosomes with DNA that is not associated with histones. They are used to study some aspects of cell division, and as a source of several toxins; *see*, for example **saxitoxin**.

dinoprost: prostaglandin PGF_2.

dinor: 2,3-dinor-6-keto-PGF1; a prostacyclin metabolite. The amount excreted to urine varies directly with the amount of prostacyclin synthesized.

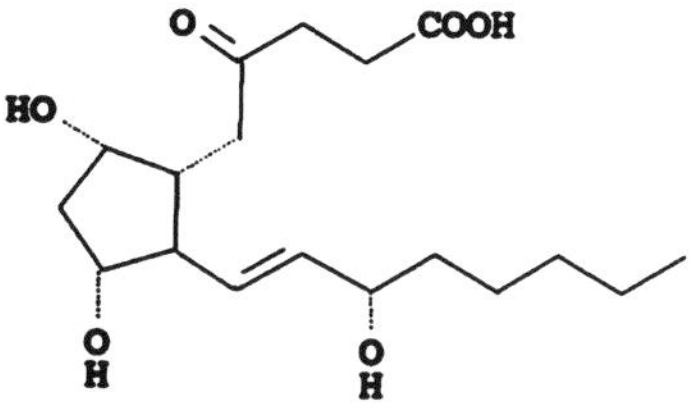

Diodrast: a trade name for iodopyracet.

dioecious: diecious; describes species in which individuals have either male or female type reproductive organs, but not both; *cf* **monoecious**.

dioxygenases: enzymes that catalyze reactions in which both oxygen atoms of O_2 are incorporated into the products; *cf* **mixed function oxidases**.

dipeptidases: enzymes that catalyze hydrolytic cleavage of dipeptides to yield their constituent amino acids.

diphenylhydantoin: *see* **phenytoin**.

diphenhydramine: an H_1 type histamine receptor antagonist used to suppress allergic reactions and decrease motion sickness.

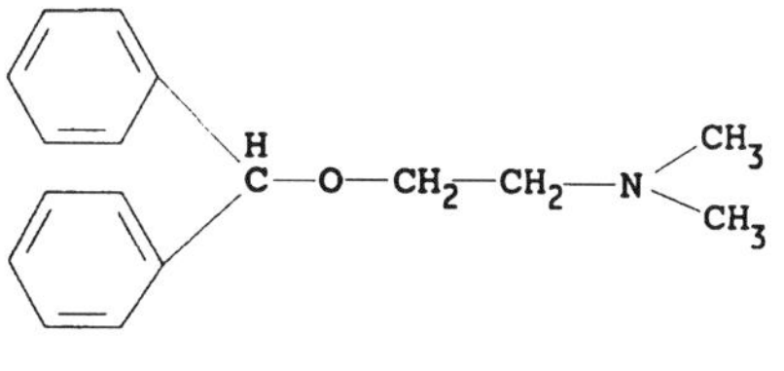

diphosphatidyl glycerols: cardiolipins.

2,3-**diphosphoglycerate**; 2,3-biphosphoglycerate. a glycolysis pathway intermediate, formed from 1,3-diphosphoglycerate via a reaction catalyzed by biphosphoglycerate mutase, and converted to 3-phospho-glycerate via a reaction catalyzed by 2,3-biphos-phoglycerate kinase that is coupled to ATP synthesis from ADP + Pi. Phosphoglyceromutase then catalyzes forma-tion of 2-phosphoglycerate. 2,3-diphosphoglycerate is a physiological competitive inhibitor of its own formation. In erythrocytes, which contain high levels, it binds tightly to, and stabilizes the deoxygenated form of hemoglobin, markedly lowers hemoglobin affinity for oxygen, and thereby accelerates oxygen delivery to tissue cells.

diphosphopyridine nucleotide: DPN: an old term for nicotine amide dinucleotide.

diphthamide: 2-[3-carboxyamido-3-(trimethylammo-nio)propyl]-histidine: a component of elongation factor EF-2. The site at which diphtheria toxin inactivates it by catalyzing ADP ribosylation is indicated by X.

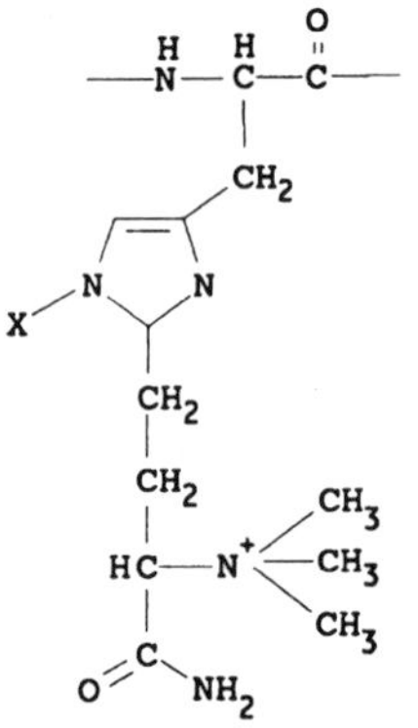

diphtheria toxin: diphtherotoxin; a 62K exotoxin made by lysogenic strains of *Corynebacterium diphtheriae*. The B domain facilitates entry into the cell by binding to a plasma membrane receptor. The A domain inhibits protein synthesis by catalyzing ADP-ribosylation of the diphthamide component of elongation factor EF-2. Since peptide chain elongation is arrested, a single A fragment can kill a cell. Mucous membranes are the major sites affected.

diploblastic: containing, or formed from two embryonic germ layers.

diploid: possessing two complete sets of homologous chromosomes; *cf* **haploid**. Most eukaryote somatic cells are diploid.

diplotene: the fourth and final stage of the meiosis I prophase, during which all four tetrad chromatids are

visible, and paired homologous chromosomes begin to separate (but remain attached at chiasmata).

1,3-dipropyl-8-(2-amino-4-chlorphenyl)-xanthine: PACPX; a potent adenosine receptor antagonist, selective for A_1 subtypes.

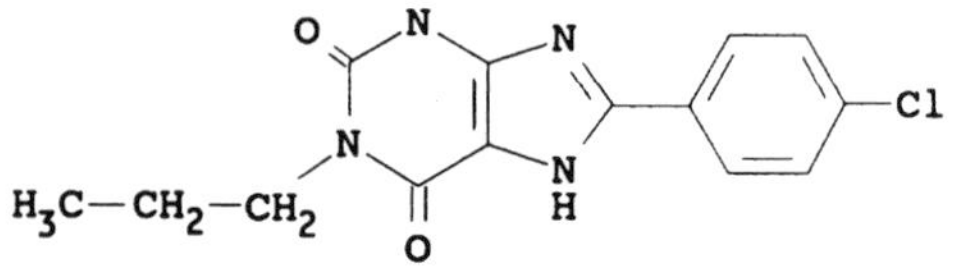

N.N-**dipropyl-5-carboxamidotryptamine maleate**: a potent serotonin receptor antagonist, selective for 5-HT$_{1A}$ subtypes.

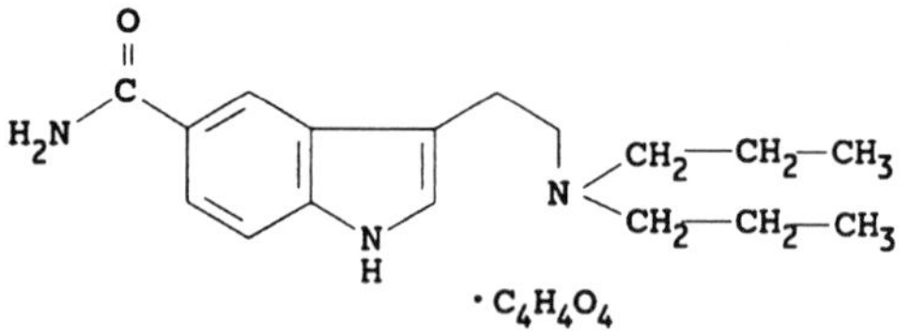

dipsogens: agents that invoke thirst and promote drinking.

dipyridamole: DPM: 2,6-*bis*-(diethylamino)-4,8-dipiper-idinopyrimido-(5,4-*d*)-pyrimidine; an orally effective agent used to dilate coronary vessels and suppress platelet aggregation. The effects on platelets are attrib-uted to inhibition of cyclic nucleotide phosphodiesterase activity and/or potentiation of prostacyclin actions. DPM also inhibits carrier mediated transport of adenosine and other nucleosides across plasma membranes, and it potentiates the therapeutic (but not toxic) effects of zidovudine and dideoxycytidine in patients with acquired immune deficiency syndrome (AIDS). It is under inves-tigation for possible use (in conjunction with nucleotide synthesis inhibitors) for arresting the growth of some neoplasms.

discoidins: galactose binding lectins that accumulate in some differentiating cell types, and mediate cell:cell ad-hesion. They are used as differentiation markers, and in studies of development. *Dictostelium discoidin* (slime mold) discoidins 1 and II closely resemble lectins made by myoblasts and other embryonic and fetal cells.

discordance: expression of different phenotypes in in-dividuals that are genetically identical or closely related. The term usually refers to expression of a trait in one

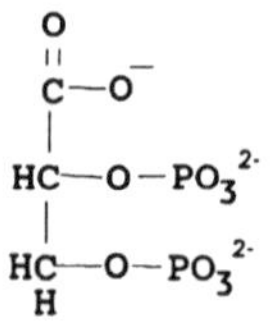

2,3-biphosphoglycerate

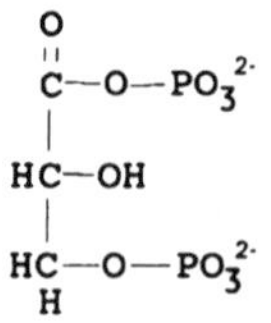

1,3-biphosphoglycerate

dipyridamole

monozygotic twin but not in the other, but is also used for siblings and other pairs. *Cf* **concordance.**

disequilibrium: *see* **linkage disequilibrium.**

disintegration constant: decay constant; a factor calculated for a specific kind of atom that is related to its rate of conversion to other types. In the equation: $N = N_o e^{-dt}$, d is the disintegration constant. N is the number of radioactive atoms present at time t, N_o = the number initially present, and e is the natural logarithm.

disintegrins: components of viper venoms that bind integrins with high affinity and block their associations with ligands. Most have Arg-Gly-Asp (RGD) domains that bind integrin types $\alpha_v \beta_1$, $\alpha_v \beta_3$, $\alpha_v \beta_5$, and $\alpha_5 \beta_1$. Barbourin contains a KGD (Lys-Gly-Asp) sequence specific for GPIIb/IIIa.

disjunction: separation of paired chromosomes during anaphase; *cf* **nondisjunction.**

dismutases: mutases; enzymes, such as phosphoglyceromutase, that catalyze **dismutation** (*q.v.*).

dismutation: reactions catalyzed by dismutases, in which electrons and/or atoms are rearranged within a molecule to yield a new product, for example conversion of 3-phosphoglycerate to 2-phosphoglycerate.

disodium etidronate: sodium etidronate; Didronel; a pyrophosphate derivative that slows both formation and dissolution of hydroxyapatite crystals. It is used to treat Paget's disease, in which it can lower alkaline phosphatase activity and decrease urinary excretion of hydroxyproline. It also protects against soft tissue calcification caused by toxic levels of calciferols, but can invoke focal osteomalacia. Intermittent use in conjunction with other agents is reported to slow bone resorption and facilitate bone mass augmentation in women with postmenopausal osteoporosis.

dispermy: fertilization of one oocyte by two spermatozoa.

dissociation constant: K_D: pK; the reciprocal of the equilibrium constant, a measure of the separation rate for

molecules that associate reversibly, and therefore (inversely) of binding affinity. (The higher the value, the greater the tendency to dissociate). The K_D is used to calculate receptor occupation at given ligand concentrations, but does not provide information on biological activity. For simple, direct association of a hormone, H with its receptor R, in the relationship $H + R \rightleftarrows H\text{-}R$, K_D = [H]•[R]/[H-R]. The constant is also used in studies of enzyme-substrate interactions and for preparation of buffers. For dissociation of a weak acid, $HA \rightleftarrows H^+ + A^-$, K_D = $[H^+]•[A^-]/[HA]$, and pH = pK + log $[A^-]/[HA]$.

distal: farthest removed from the attachment site, or from the midline of the body.

distal convoluted tubule the nephron component that connects the ascending Henle loop with the collecting tubule or collecting duct. The cells contribute to the control of electrolyte balance, and participate in urinary excretion of many pharmacological agents.

disulfide bond: S-S bond. Cysteinyl S-S bonds determine the secondary structures of many peptides and proteins, and they link subunits of dimers and more complex molecules.

disulfiram: disulfuram: tetraethylthioperoxydicarbonic diamide; an agent that inhibits dopamine-β-hydroxylase, and promotes accumulation of acetaldehyde after ethanol ingestion by competing with hepatic aldehyde dehydrogenase for NAD^+. It has little effect alone, but ingestion of ethanol following disulfiram leads to intense vasodilation, tachycardia, hypotension, nausea, and vomiting (and in some cases unconsciousness and death). Small amounts are used to increase the motivation to abstain from ethyl alcohol ingestion.

DIT: diiodothyronine.

1,4-dithiothreitol: DTT; Cleland's reagent; *threo*-1,4-dimercapto-2,3-butanediol; an agent that reduces peptide and protein disulfide bonds and blocks sulfhydryl oxidation. It is used to protect the sulfhydryl moieties of hormones and other molecules during analytical procedures. Comparisons of electrophoresis patterns of treated vs untreated compounds provide information on the locations of disulfide bonds.

diuresis: increased urine flow.

diuretics: agents that augment urine flow.

diurnal: (1) occurring during daytime; (2) describes species that are normally most active during the light phases of light-dark cycles; *cf* **nocturnal.**

diurnal rhythms: cyclical changes with approximately 24 hour periodicities. Most have free-running lengths of 23.5-26 hours, but are entrained by light/dark cycles and/or other signals, such as feeding times.

divalent: having two combining sites. The term can describe cations such as Ca^{2+} or Mg^{2+}, anions (e.g. SO_4^{2-} or HPO_4^{2-}), or antibodies.

divergence: moving apart; a term applied to evolutionary changes in structures and/or functions of molecular species that derive from a common ancestral type and lead to acquisition of different phenotypes, as well as to changes in whole organisms.

diversity segment: D segment; a small region of an immunoglobulin heavy chain, located between the V_H and J_H segments.

dividin: a nuclear phosphoprotein synthesized by cells that are committed to divide.

dizygotic twins: genetically dissimilar twins that develop from two different oocytes during the same pregnancy; *cf* **monozygotic twins**.

Djungarian hamsters: *see* **hamsters** and **pineal gland**.

DLAs: dog histocompatibility antigens.

DM: diabetes mellitus.

DMAA: diethylcarbamoyl-4-methyl-4-aza-5-α-androstan-3-one; a testosterone analog that inhibits 5α-reductase; *see* 4-**MA**.

6-DMAP: 5-dimethylaminopurine; an inhibitor of some protein kinases that can invoke premature meiosis in oocytes.

DMD: Duchenne muscular dystrophy.

DMPP: 1,1-dimethyl-4-phenylpiperazinium; a nicotinic type acetylcholine receptor agonist. The iodide salt is used as a autonomic ganglion stimulant.

DMSO: dimethylsulfoxide.

DNA: *see* **deoxyribonucleic acid**.

cDNAs: complementary DNAs; single-stranded deoxyribonucleic acid molecules, synthesized via reactions catalyzed by reverse transcriptases, with base sequences complementary to those of the chosen RNA.

DNA gyrase: an *Escherichia coli* type II topoisomerase essential for DNA replication. It catalyzes cleavage (nicking) and subsequent resealing of circular DNA phosphodiester bonds, and can promote or relax supercoiling.

DNA glycosidases: DNA glycosylases; at least 20 enzymes that catalyze cleavage of covalent bonds between deoxyribose and nitrogenous bases. Endogenous types are used for DNA repair.

DNA helicases: enzymes that promote DNA unwinding prior to DNA replication.

DNA hybridization: techniques for determining the degrees of similarity between DNA segments (derived from different individuals of the same or different species), or the locations of specific base sequences within a genome. A radioactively labeled DNA segment is used as a probe. The complementary components of the test material pair with the probe, and can be visualized in autoradiographs; (2) formation of diploid cells with DNAs from two different sources.

DNA inversion: a change that occurs when a DNA molecule is cleaved at two internal sites, and the fragment released flips before re-inserting between the cleavage sites. It alters the kinds of RNAs subsequently transcribed. Spontaneously occurring inversions are known to cause several kinds of diseases. When the process is accomplished *in vitro*, the altered DNA can be used to direct the formation of special kinds of proteins.

DNA library: genomic library; gene bank: a collection of cloned DNA fragments that includes all of the base sequences of an organism.

DNA ligases: enzymes used for DNA replication and repair. They catalyze joining of the 3'-OH end of one DNA molecule to the 5-'phosphate of another.

DNA methylation: replacement of hydrogens on DNA bases with methyl groups. Under natural conditions, the loci affected are both species and cell type specific. Methylation can inactivate some genes, and confer resistance to DNase degradation.

DNA polymerases: enzymes used for DNA replication, repair, and recombination that catalyze stepwise 5' to 3' elongation of DNA strands via addition of nucleotide phosphates. The 3' ends interact with nucleotide triphosphates, form diester bonds, and release P-P. The first reaction releases some of the energy that drives the reactions, and P-P hydrolysis facilitates its completion. Bacterial DNA polymerase I (Pol I) is a 103-109K zinc-containing monomer that requires a DNA primer and a DNA template. It binds to all four nucleotide types, and can function only when all are present. It is also an exonuclease, essential for removing RNA primers, filling in gaps at primer release sites, and repairing DNA. Pol II is a 120K monomer with similar synthethesizing, but no exonuclease activity. Pol III, the major bacterial enzyme for DNA replication, is a zinc-containing 180K trimer that requires Mg^{2+}, and has exonuclease activity. Its functions are initiated by formation of 400K holoenzyme complexes (replicons) and RNA primers with free 3'OH groups. In eukaryote cells, the most abundant enzyme is DNA polymerase α, a 300K multimer that attaches to lagging strands, and is essential for chromosome duplica-

dobutamine

tion. Its activity is augmented by androgens and some other hormones. However, pol δ attaches to the leading strand and is a major enzyme for DNA replication in the nucleus. Pol β appears to be most important for DNA repair, whereas polymerase γ catalyzes most of the replication in mitochondria. Some viral DNA polymerases are reverse transcriptases. *See* also **DNA replication**.

DNA probe: a labelled DNA segment used to determine the loci of other DNA segments with complementary base sequences.

DNA puff: see **chromosome puff**.

DNA replication: formation of new DNA molecules identical to the parent types; *see* also **DNA polymerases**. In eukaryote cells, the process is preceded by chromosome decondensation and nucleosome unfolding. It begins with formation of a replicon composed of at least 20 enzymes and other factors. A DNA helicase catalyzes use of energy derived from ATP hydrolysis to unwind segments of the DNA duplex, separate the two strands, and form replication forks. Proteins then attach to the separated strands and prevent their reassociation. A short RNA primer with bases complementary to those of the parent leading ($5' \rightarrow 3'$) strand is synthesized, after which a DNA polymerase (pol III in prokaryotes and pol δ in eukaryotes) begins continuous synthesis of a new DNA molecule by catalyzing successive additions to the $3'$ end of the primer, of nucleotides with bases complementary to those of the leading strand. DNA polymerases I and α (in prokaryotes and eukaryotes, respectively) catalyze cleavage of parent DNA lagging strands to Okazaki fragments. Primases direct synthesis of very short RNA primers with bases complementary to those of Okazaki fragments, and polymerases I and α catalyze additions to short primers, of DNA nucleotides with bases complementary to those of the Okazaki fragments. They, too work in the $5' \rightarrow 3'$ direction. DNA ligases then join the segments. Polymerases I and α additionally remove RNA primers when they are no longer needed. *See* also **reverse transcriptases**.

DNases: *see* **deoxyribonucleases**.

DNase protection: resistance to degradation by endonucleases, conferred by proteins that bind to specific DNA segments. The size, location, and nature of the affected segment can be determined by degrading adjacent, unprotected regions with endonucleases. Protein binding also protects adenine and guanine bases within the bound region against methylation by dimethyl sulfate.

DNA topoisomerases: enzymes that mediate DNA relaxation and supercoiling by catalyzing cleavage and re-establishment of covalent linkages. They contribute to chromosome condensation and decondensation, and to strand separation and rejoining during replication and transcription. Mutations, and agents that impair their functions, can cause abnormal gene recombinations, possibly via influences on the three-dimensional structures of the DNA molecules. Type I enzymes act on one strand at a time, and form enzyme-DNA intermediates. Type II enzymes use energy derived from ATP hydrolysis to promote double strand breaks. Bacterial and eukaryote enzymes perform comparable functions, but are not homologous proteins.

DNA virus: a virus with a single or double-stranded DNA genome. Adenoviruses, Epstein Barr virus, and some others invoke tumor formation in animals. *Cf* **RNA virus**.

DNFB: *see* **Sanger's reagent**.

DNP: dinitrophenol.

DNQX: 6,7-dinotroquinoxaline-2,3-dione; an NMDA-type excitatory amino acid receptor antagonist.

DNS: dansyl chloride.

dobutamine: 3,4-dihydroxy-*N*-[3-(4-hydroxyphenyl)-1-methylpropyl]-β5D-phenylethylamine; a β-type adrenergic receptor agonist, used as a cardiac stimulant.

DOC: *see* 11-**deoxycorticosterone**.

DOCA: 11-deoxycorticosterone acetate.

docking protein: an endoplasmic reticulum protein that binds to, and serves as the receptor for **signal recognition particles** (*q.v.*).

docosa: twenty-two, as in docosahexenoic acid.

docosahexenoic acid: DHA; (C22:6 ω-3); a 22 carbon polyunsaturated fatty acid with six double bonds. It is a component of some brain lipids.

dodeca: twelve, as in dodecapeptide (a peptide with 12 amino acid moieties).

dodecyldimethylamine oxide: DDAO; a nonionic detergent used in protein exchange chromatography.

dodecyl sulfate sodium: SDS; an anionic detergent that disrupts intramolecular noncolvalent bonds. It is used in polyacrylamide gel electrophoresis methods for determining molecular weights, and in some chromatography procedures. Its ability to disrupt protein-protein and protein-lipid interactions is employed in studies of membrane components.

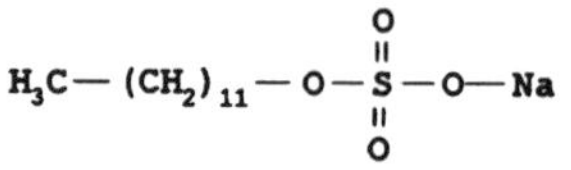

$$H_3C-(CH_2)_{11}-O-\overset{\overset{O}{\|}}{\underset{\underset{O}{\|}}{S}}-O-Na$$

dodecyltrimethylammonium bromide: DTAB; a detergent used in exchange chromatography to separate proteins from other compounds.

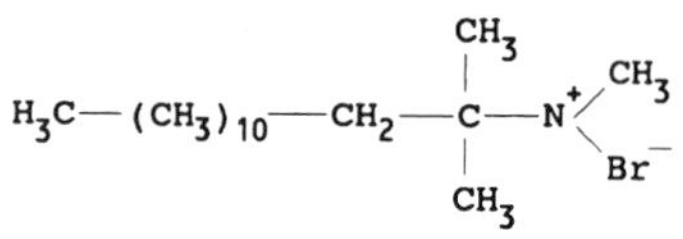

$$H_3C-(CH_3)_{10}-CH_2-\overset{\overset{CH_3}{|}}{\underset{\underset{CH_3}{|}}{C}}-\overset{+}{N}\overset{CH_3}{\diagdown}\,\, Br^-$$

R(-)-**DOI**: 2, 5-dimethoxy-4-iodo-amphetamine; a potent serotonin receptor agonist, selective for 5-HT$_2$-5HT$_{1C}$ subtypes, that crosses blood-brain barriers. The *S*(+) isomer is less active.

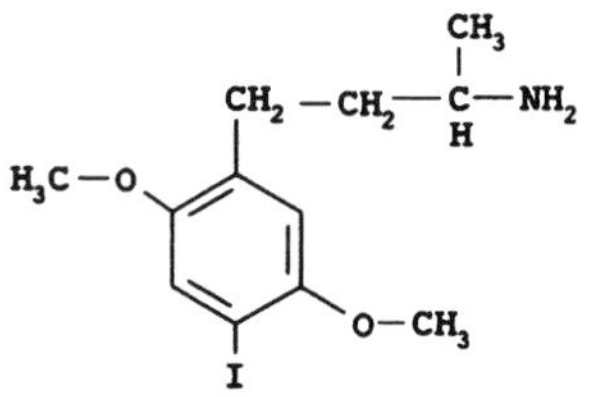

dolicho-: a prefix meaning elongated. It can describe linear stretches of compound components, and also anatomical structures, as in dolichocephalic (having an elongated head).

dolichol phosphate: an endoplasmic reticulum membrane terpenoid used for glycoprotein biosynthesis, composed of 13-24 isoprene units and a terminal phosphate that faces the cytoplasm. It successively acquires two *N*-acetylglucosamine and five mannose moieties from cytoplasmic intermediates, and then four mannose and three glucose types from another dolichol phosphate. The oligosaccharide blocks are then transferred to growing polypeptide chains. In the structure shown, n can be any number from 13 to 24.

domain: a segment of a large molecule (usually a protein) with a special chemical structure, physical property, or function.

dominance: *see* **dominant gene**.

dominant gene: in diploid organisms, an allele that determines a phenotype trait in a heterozygote; *cf* **recessive gene** and **incomplete dominance**.

domino effect: a complex response in which each stage promotes the one that follows; *cf* **sustained action effect** and **cascades**.

domoic acid: 2-carboxy-3-carboxymethyl-4-isohexenoic-pyrrolidine acetic acid; a kainate type excitatory amino acid receptor agonist in crab viscera. It can invoke blood vessel injury and memory loss in vertebrates.

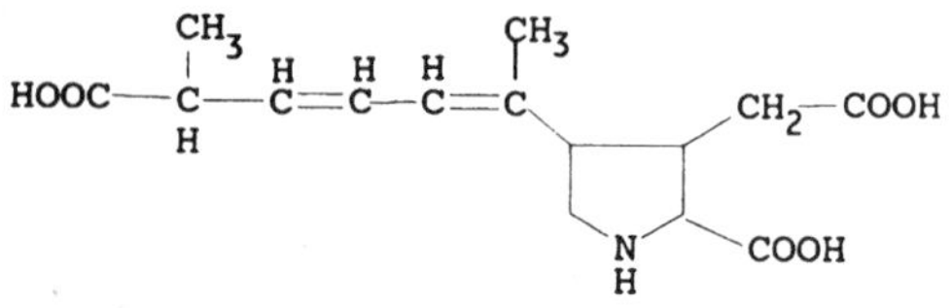

domperidone: 5-[chloro-1-[1-[3-(2,3-oxo-1-benzimida-zolinyl)propyl]-4-piperidyl]-2-benzimidazolinone]; a D$_2$-type dopamine receptor antagonist that affects Na$^+$ ion excretion and other processes. It is used mostly to control vomiting.

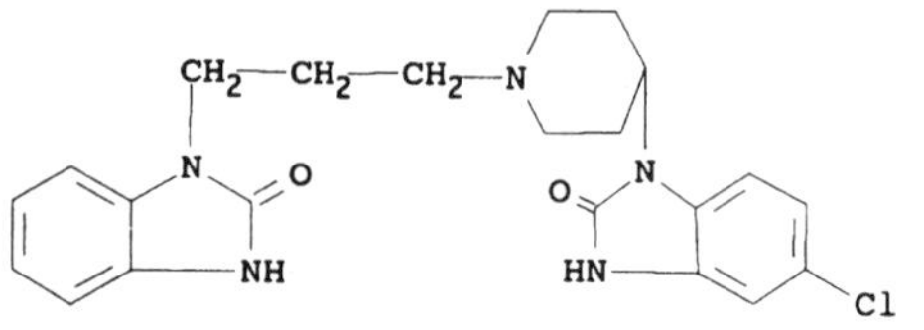

Donnan equilibrium: the state attained at equilibrium when small ions diffuse freely across a plasma membrane that blocks the egress of large, charged macromolecules. Intracellular anions that cannot cross the membranes attract small cations inward. Since the movements of small ions are also affected by concentration gradients (which usually promote egress of the kinds attracted inward by the macromolecules), the net effect is unequal charge distributions and ion concentrations on the two sides of the membrane. Donnan equilibria contribute to the establishment of resting potentials.

DOPA: *see* **dihydroxyphenylalanine**. L-Dopa is the naturally occurring isomer.

6-hydroxy-**DOPA**: 6-OH-DOPA: a dihydroxyphenylalanine analog best known as a neurotoxin that penetrates the blood-brain barrier, promotes acute degeneration of noradrenergic nerve terminals and depletes norepinephrine, but does not destroy adrenomedullary cells. Low concentrations are physiological cofactors for amine oxidases.

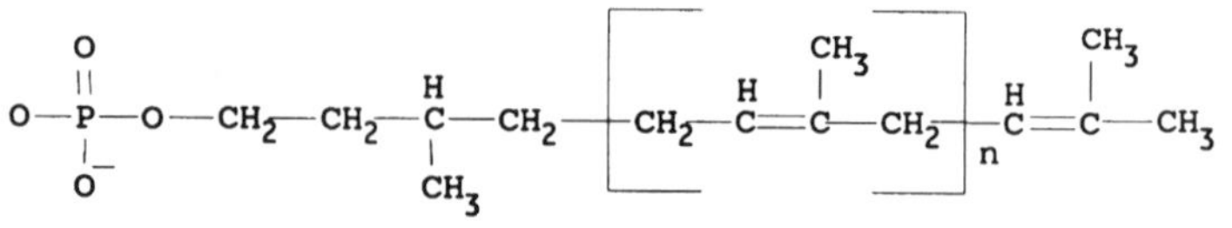

dolichol phosphate

6-OH-DOPA

DOPAC: dihydroxyphenylacetic acid; a dopamine metabolite formed in a reaction catalyzed by mitochondrial monoamine oxidase. Catecholamine-*O*-methyltransferase (COMT) converts most of it to homovanillic acid.

dopachrome: 2-carboxyindole-5,6-quinone; an intermediate in the pathway for biosynthesis of melanins from dihydroxyphenylalanine; *see* **dopaquinone**.

DOPA decarboxylase: DDC; an enzyme that catalyzes conversion of dihydroxyphenylalanine (DOPA) to dopamine, and is essential for catecholamine biosynthesis. It is similar to or identical with the enzyme that catalyzes conversion of 5-hydroxytryptophan to serotonin.

dopamine: DA; 3,4-dihydroxyphenylalanine: 3-hydroxytyramine; a hormone and neurotransmitter. It is the major mediator for extrapyramidal system neurons in the brain, and the primary precursor of norepinephrine and epinephrine. The rate-limiting step for its biosynthesis is usually tyrosine conversion to dihydroxyphenylalanine (DOPA) via the reaction catalyzed by tyrosine hydroxylase. (However, when severe protein deficiency depletes the tyrosine supply, substrate availability assumes importance.) The dopa decarboxylase that converts DOPA to dopamine is present in relatively large amounts. DA is taken up by, and stored in synaptic vesicles and secretory granules. Some contain dopamine hydroxylase (which hydroxylates DA to norepinephrine). Others release it directly in response to acetylcholine and other neurotransmitters. Most actions are rapidly terminated, because dopamine is taken back into the nerve terminals that release it. High levels in the vinicity of dopaminergic neurons exert negative feedback controls over DA synthesis by inhibiting the tyrosine hydroxylase. Additionally, DA is degraded by enzymes that act on other catecholamines (*see* **monoamine oxidases** and **catecholamine-*O*-methyltransferase**). Blood plasma contains more dopamine than norepinephrine and epinephrine combined, but most of it is in the form of sulfate conjugates which may not be directly active. Most circulating DA originates in the nerve endings of various organs; but some comes form adrenomedullary cells, and small amounts of the amine are made in kidneys and other organs. Peripherally, DA stimulates the heart, dilates renal, mesenteric, and coronary blood vessels, directly accelerates Na^+ excretion and inhibits aldosterone secretion, and indirectly increases water loss. The functions of the dopaminergic neurons and DA receptors that are concentrated in the corpus striatum and in related basal ganglion regions that control them are regulated, in part by acetylcholine. Parkinson's disease is attributed to degeneration of those DA neurons, and (at least in some cases) the symptoms appear to be exacerbated by loss of inhibitory controls over cholinergic types. Since the numbers of DA receptors increase as neurons die, considerable damage can occur before the symptoms become apparent. The effectiveness of treatments with L-DOPA and monoamine oxidase inhibitors is evidently directly related to elevation of brain DA levels (and the gradually diminishing responsivity to continued neuron deterioration). Acetylcholine inhibitors are beneficial in some cases. Unilateral lesions of the associated regions cause laboratory animals to rotate in the direction away from the lesions; and DA injections in the same regions cause rotation in the opposite direction. Dopamine is also made in parts of the cerebral cortex; and the limbic system is richly supplied with dopaminergic neurons and DA receptors. The neurotransmitter contributes to the initiation of voluntary locomotor activity; and large doses invoke hyperactivity and stereotyped behavior in laboratory animals. Brain DA is also a component of visual and olfactory systems. It additionally contributes to the control of food and fluid intake, influences mood and memory, and may mediate some forms of addiction. Excessive production of DA and/or DA receptor dysfunctions have been implicated as participants in the etiology of schizophrenia, manic depression, and other forms of mental illness. (Common side-effect of DOPA in Parkinson patients include psychic depression and loss of appetite). Many of the agents used to treat mental illness are dopamine receptor inhibitors. Most stimulate the appetite; and prolonged use of some invokes tardive dyskinesia (which in many ways resembles Parkinsonism). DA is metabolically converted to least thirty other substances. Many are biologically active, and a few are hallucinogenic. It also interacts with numerous other regulators. Influences on cAMP generation, and on induction of Fos, Fra, and related transcription factors, have been linked with elevated levels of messenger RNAs for substance P, dynorphin, and enkephalin precursors. A negative feedback loop, in which neuropeptide Y promotes DA release, and DA inhibits NPY synthesis has been described, and some effects of cocaine and amphetamines (both of which inhibit neuronal uptake of DA) are associated with NPY depletion. DA colocalizes at various sites with cholecystokinin (CCK), neurotensin, and other neuropeptides and affects their release. DA neurons also regulate the functions of substance P, dynorphin, enkephalin, serotonin, acetylcholine, ATP, and other neurotransmitters, and those regulators, in turn, affect both dopaminergic neurons and dopamine receptors. Additionally, DA exerts some histamine-like actions that cannot be blocked by the usual kinds of histamine receptor antagonists. Many tuberoinfundibular neurons are dopaminergic, and DA made in hypothalamic neurons tonically inhibits prolactin release. Regulators that augment release of that hormone act in part by lowering DA levels. DA also promotes thyrotropin and gonadotropin secretion, and stimulates normal somatotropes (but inhibits growth hormone release in some adenohypophysial tumor cells and, is useful for treating some cases of acromegaly). In species that possess a pars intermedia, DA lowers POMC levels and diminishes α-melanocyte stimulating hormone (α-MSH) secretion by decreasing messenger RNA stability. Some effects may be related to dopamine conversion to norepinephrine. Discrete, but overlapping distributions of various kinds of **dopamine receptors** *(q.v.)* have been mapped with ligands and other tools, and shown to exist on many cell types. A single cell can have more than one type, each of which can generate more than one kind of second messenger. Discrepancies between mRNA levels, as compared with binding affinities, support the belief that receptors made at some sites are translocated to others, and that a single kind can assume multiple forms.

dopamine β-hydroxylase: DBC; *see* **dopamine β-monooxygenase.**

dopamine β-monooxygenase: an enzyme that catalyzes conversion of dopamine to norepinephrine via a reaction that uses molecular oxygen and requires ascorbic acid as a cofactor. Older terms still in use include dopamine β-oxidase, and dopamine β-hydroxylase.

dopamine receptors: several kinds of cell components that bind dopamine and mediate its actions. Two major types were initially described: D_1 (D_e, excitatory), which interact with G protein α_s subunits to activate adenylate cyclases, and D_2 (D_i, inhibitory) that act via α_i subunits to decrease the enzyme activity. It is now recognized that each class includes numerous subtypes, at least some of which are convertible to truncated forms with different properties, and that there are other kinds with different structures, distributions, second messengers, and functions. A single cell can have two or more interacting types; and D1/D2 combinations occur in many brain neurons. The synergistic stimulation of neuron firing at some sites, but antagonistic influences at others, may be related to observations that binding to a single kind of receptor type can lead to generation of two or more second messengers, and that presynaptic members of a sub-type differ from ones located postsynaptically. Some receptors copurify with α subunits of G_o proteins (with no effects on adenylate cyclases), and many dopamine effects depend on (or are modified by) either cosecretion with other mediators, or influences on neurons that make them (*see* **dopamine**). The effects of ligand binding can include phospholipase C activation, phosphatidylinositol hydrolysis, and stimulatory or inhibitory influences on arachidonic acid release. D_{1A} subtypes are widely distributed, and are implicated as mediators of olfaction, cardiac stimulation, blood flow through mesenteric and renal vessels, the natriuretic and diuretic influences on nephron proximal convoluted tubules, and the release of some hormones. D_{1B} receptors differ from them in ligand binding affinities, and are restricted to special central nervous system regions including the hippocampus. They mediate visual and limbic system effects. A third D_1 subtype inhibits neurite outgrowth in embryos. A type in thick ascending Henle loops of the kidney also has D_1-like properties. D_{2A} subtype composed of 444 amino acid moieties (D_{2L}, $D_{2[444]}$) predominates in the corpus striatum and cerebral cortex, and appears to be a major regulator of extrapyramidal system functions; but some is also present in the hypothalamus. A smaller, D_{2B} form (D_{2S}, $D_{2[415]}$), with 415 amino acids and different properties, is cleaved from the same mRNA. D_{2K}, identified in inner medullary collecting ducts, shares some properties with the other D_2 receptors, but is the product of a different gene (and differs from a renal D_1 type). D_3 receptors do not activate adenylate cyclases, but they, and D_4 types otherwise resemble D_1 receptors. They seem to be the mediators of behavioral effects. The D_4s have been most closely linked with mental diseases, and the existence of special alleles in afflicted individuals has been suggested. They are especially sensitive to clozapine, which (unlike most other antagonists) has minimal (if any) influences on extrapyramidal functions. D_5 receptors, which resemble D_1 types, mediate adenylate cyclase activation at low concentrations, but inhibit it at higher ones, possibly by interacting with different enzyme isoforms.

6-OH-dopamine: 6-hydroxydopamine; 3,4,6-trihydroxyphenylethylamine; an agent that selectively promotes acute degeneration of noradrenergic nerve terminals and causes almost total depletion of norepinephrine in sympathetically innervated structures, but has little effect on the adrenal medulla. Unlike 6-OH-DOPA, it does not cross the blood-brain barrier.

dopamine regulated phosphoprotein: DARPP; DARP-32; a 32K protein in neurons and thick ascending Henle loop cells that undergoes phosphorylation when D_1 type dopamine receptor activation leads to generation of cAMP and activation of kinase A. The reaction may also be regulated high Ca^{2+} levels. The phosphorylated form inhibits protein phosphatase-1 (a major intracellular regulatory enzyme). In thick ascending loop cells, it promotes diuresis by blocking dephosphorylation of the Na^+/K^+-ATPase.

dopaminergic: describes (1) neurons that synthesize and release dopamine; (2) nerve tracts composed of axons that release dopamine; (3) effects exerted by dopamine.

dopaquinone: 4-(2-amino-carboxyethyl)benzo-1,2-quinone; phenylalanine-3,4-quinone; an intermediate in the pathway for melanin biosynthesis, formed from dihydroxyphenylalanine via an oxidation reaction catalyzed by tyrosinase. It spontaneously rearranges to dopachrome, and a dopachrome conversion factor promotes formation of 5,6-dihydroxyindole. A different conversion factor then facilitates formation of indole-5,6-quinone, which polymerizes to melanins. Dopaquinone can also

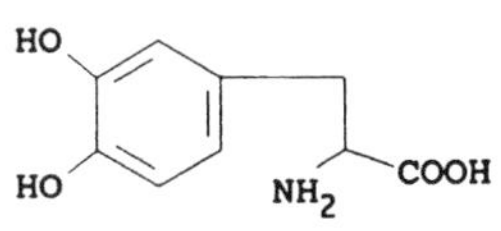

DOPA

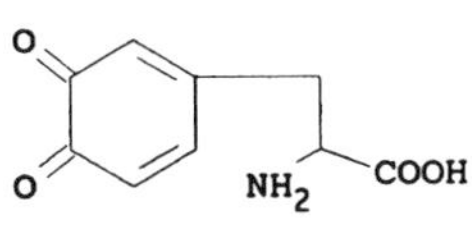

dopaquinone

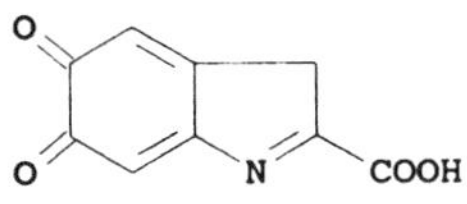

dopachrome

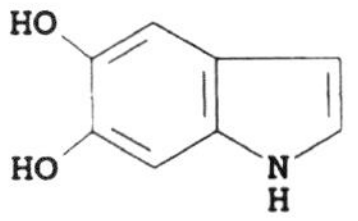

5,6-dihdyroxyindole

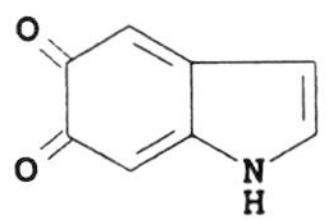

indole-5,6-quinone

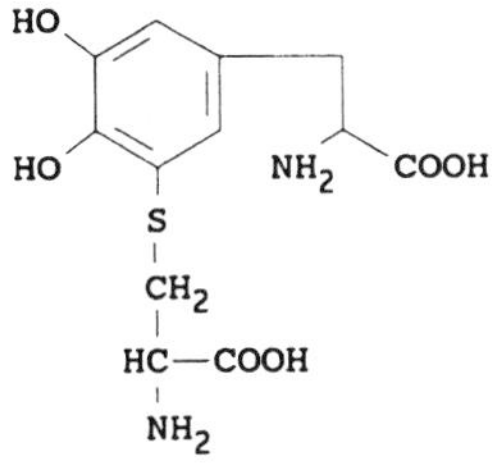

cysteinyl-DOPA

react with cysteine to form cysteinyl-DOPA, an intermediate in the pathway for pheomelanin biosynthesis.

DOPEG: dihydroxyphenylethylglycol.

dopexamine: 4-[2-[[6-(phenylethylamino)hexyl]amino] ethylpyrocatechol; a selective dopamine and β_2-adrenergic receptor agonist, used as a cardiac stimulant.

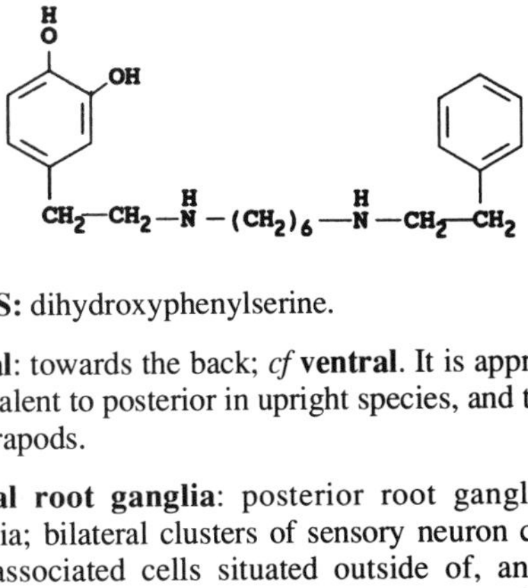

DOPS: dihydroxyphenylserine.

dorsal: towards the back; *cf* **ventral**. It is approximately equivalent to posterior in upright species, and to superior in tetrapods.

dorsal root ganglia: posterior root ganglia; spinal ganglia; bilateral clusters of sensory neuron cell bodies and associated cells situated outside of, and running parallel to the spinal cord. Peripherally located dendrites, activated by receptors for touch, temperature, pressure, pain, and other stimuli, send information to perikarya in the ganglia, from which it is transmitted via the nearest spinal nerve dorsal roots to the posterior regions of the cord.

dorsomedial hypothalamic nuclei: bilateral neuron clusters functionally associated with ones in the anterior hypothalamic area, and with some preganglionic autonomic neurons.

dosage compensation: usually (1) random inactivation of much of the second of two X chromosomes of normal females (with XX patterns), and of supernumerary X chromosomes in individuals with XXY, XXX, and other

abnormal numbers; (2) a term sometimes used to describe other forms of gene activation and/or inactivation.

double-blind study: procedures in which neither the observer nor the subject is provided with information that could affect the results of an investigation. For example, if various dosages of an agent are given to several groups, prepartion differences are disguised, and control subjects are given a placebo that externally resembles the active compounds. Investigators who examine subjects (or materials derived from them) do not know which form of treatment was administered.

double cross: matings that produce progeny heterozygous for two traits, but otherwise genetically similar. For example, individuals of a species homozygous for allele A are mated with others homozygous for allele a to obtain Aa offspring. Similarly, C and c homozygotes are mated to yield Cc type progeny. The double cross is accomplished by then mating Aa with Cc individuals. The procedures are used to study gene functions and inheritance patterns, and to produce hybrid plants or animals with special characteristics.

double negative: describes an individual or a cell type in which neither of two traits that can occur in normal representatives of the population is expressed. For example, T lymphocytes that express neither CD4 nor CD8 surface antigens are said to be double negative (T4⁻8⁻). *Cf* **double positive**.

double positive: describes individuals or cell types that express two specific genes, although other members of the population can express just one or neither. For example, T lymphocytes that express both CD4 and CD8 surface antigens are said to be double positive (T4⁺8⁺). Different T lymphocytes can be T4⁺8⁻, T4⁻8⁺ or T4⁻8⁻.

double sieve mechanisms: physiological processes that minimize or correct translation errors. Amino acids are usually inserted in the right places because each transfer RNA type bears both a binding site for a specific kind, and an anticodon complementary to a specific kind of messenger RNA anticodon. However, substitutions can occur. RNA synthetases reject amino acids too large to fit the allotted spaces, and they catalyze hydrolysis of bonds when ones too small attach.

double stranded: having two closely associated linear components. The term describes (1) the most common forms of eukaryote DNA when it is not involved in replication or transcription, in which hydrogen bonds link the complementary bases of the two polynucleotide strands. (2) RNAs formed by some replicating viruses, or ones that are artificially made. Double stranded RNAs (dsRNAs) are major stimulants for host production of interferons.

doubling time: the time required to complete one cell cycle (produce two daughter cells from each parent cell).

Dowex: a trade name for a group of ion exchange resins; *see* **cholestyramine**.

down regulation of receptors: reduction of the numbers of functional hormone or neurotransmitter receptors, usually via lysosomal degradation of endocytosed ligand-receptor complexes. It can diminish cell responsivity to the regulators, and protect against overstimulation. Chronic elevation of the levels of many circulating hormones leads to accelerated endocytosis, and accounts in part for hormone resistance. *Cf* **desensitization**.

Down's syndrome: trisomy 21 syndrome; a congenital disorder in humans attributed to the presence of an extra chromosome # 21 (or to duplication of the distal long arm of that chromosome). The condition arises most commonly via non-disjunction during meiosis, and the incidence rises in parallel with gonad age. More rarely, the problem is a translocation that leads to fusion of chromosomes 14 and 21. The altered DNA directs synthesis of excessive amounts of S100 and some other proteins. The manifestations include moderate to severe mental retardation, impaired growth, poor muscle tone, enlarged tongue, characteristic facial deformities, defective immune system responses, and often also heart disease and intestinal stenosis. High levels of β−amyloid protein accumulate in the brains of young individuals, and Alzheimer's disease develops in most who survive four or more decades.

downstream: usually describes (1) the position of a compound component located closer to the site at which synthesis terminates than a reference component of the same molecule, for example a DNA or RNA base sequence closer to the 3′ end, or an amino acid sequence closer to the *C*-terminal of a protein. Promoter regions of genes are commonly located downstream with respect to modifying elements; (2) the nucleotide sequences of a chromosome located 3′ with respect to the last exon; (3) the direction of transcription (5′ to 3′), or of translation (amino to carboxyl); (4) an event that occurs at a later stage of a sequence, such as a post-receptor reaction, as compared with binding of the hormone to its receptor. *Cf* **upstream**.

doxantrazole: an agent used to stabilize mast cells.

doxazosin: 1-(4-amino-6,7-dimethoxy-2-quinazolinyl)-4-[(2,3-dihydro-1,4-benzodioxin-2-yl)carbonyl]-piperazine; a selective α₁ type adrenergic receptor blocking agent, chemically and pharmacologically related to prazosin, but longer-acting.

doxepin: 3-dibenz[*b,e*]oxepin-11(6*H*)-ylidene-*N,N*-dimethyl-1-propanamine; a **tricyclic antidepressant** (*q.v.*), with some anti-histamine properties.

doxorubicin: adriamycin.

doxyl: 4,4-dimethyl-3-oxazolinyloxy)4,4-dimethyloxzolidine-*N*-oxyl: a free radical that is attached to compounds for use in electron spin spectroscopy.

doxylamine: 2-dimethylaminoethoxyphenylmethyl-2-picoline; a histamine receptor antagonist, used in combination with other agents to alleviate nausea associated with pregnancy. High doses are hypnotic.

DPA: dual photon absorptiometry, a technique used for measuring bone mass.

8-OH-DPAT: 8-hydroxy-2-(di-*N*-propylamino)-tetralin; a 5-HT₁ₐ-type serotonin receptor agonist.

Δ⁴ pathway: the major pathway for androgen biosynthesis in rats and some other species. Pregnenolone is converted to progesterone (which has a Δ⁴ double bond). Oxygen is then introduced at the 17 position, and the side chain of 17α-hydroxyprogesterone is cleaved to yield Δ⁴-androstenedione. *Cf* Δ⁵ **pathway**.

Δ^5 **pathway:** the major pathway for androgen biosynthesis in humans and some other species. Pregnenolone is converted to 17α-hydroxypregnenolone, and the side-chain attached to carbon-17 is cleaved to yield dehydroepiandrosterone (DHEA). *Cf* Δ**4 pathway.**

DPCX: 1,3-dipropyl-8-cyclopentylxanthine; a highly selective A_1 type adenosine receptor antagonist.

DPD; deoxypyridinolone; *see* **hydroxylysine.**

DPDPE: a D-penicillamine enkephalin analog that binds specifically to δ-type opioid receptors.

dpm: disintegrations per minute, a measure of the rate of radioactive decay.

DPM: dipyridamole.

DPMA: N^6-[2-(3,5-dimethoxyphenyl)-2-(2-methylphenyl)-ethyl]adenosine; an adenosine receptor agonist, selective for A_2 subtypes.

DPN: diphosphopyridine nucleotide; an obsolete term for nicotine adenine dinucleotide.

dpp: decapentaplegic gene.

DPP-C: decapentaplegic gene complex.

DPPD: *N,N′*-diphenyl-*p*-phenylenediamine; 1,2-dianilomethane; an anti-oxidant used to protect against the formation of free radicals, and as a preservative for animal foods. In industry, it is used to protect rubber and petroleum oils against oxidation, and to inhibit polymerization of some compounds.

DR: VDR; *see* **vitamin D receptors.**

DRE: vitamin D response elements; VDRE; *see* **vitamin D receptors** and **vitamin D response elements.**

δ **receptors:** *see* **opioid receptors.**

D ring: the five-membered, fourth ring of a **steroid** (*q.v.*), formed by carbons 13 through 17. C13 and C14 are shared with the C ring.

dromic: describes nerve impulses that travel in the most common direction, for example from dendrite to perikaryon to axon; *cf* **antidromic.**

dromotropic: affecting conductivity; *cf* **chronotropic** and **inotropic.**

Drosophila melanogaster: the common fruit fly, a widely used subject for studies of development and inheritance. Many mutant forms with specific defects are available.

drug resistance: ability to tolerate agents toxic to other members of the species; *see* also *mdr* (multiple drug resistant genes) and **P glycoprotein.**

drumstick: a small, stalked, knob-like extension from the nucleus of some neutrophilic leukocytes in individuals with more than one X chromosome per cell. The DNA at those sites is highly condensed and transcriptionally inactive. Two or more can be present in some cells, if larger numbers of X chromosomes are present. *Cf* **Barr bodies.**

ds: double-stranded, as in dsDNA or dsRNA.

D segment: *see* **diversity segment** and **immunoglobulins.**

DSP-4-hydrochloride: *N*-(2-chloroethyl)-*N*-ethyl-2-bromobenzylamine hydrochloride; a neurotoxin that selectively destroys noradrenergic nerve terminals.

DTH: delayed type hypersensitivity.

dTMP: deoxythymidine monophosphate; *see* **dihydrofolate reductase.**

DTT: dithiothreitol.

dual recognition hypothesis: an outmoded concept that a T lymphocyte possesses one kind of receptor for foreign antigens, and a separate, different kind for histocompatibility antigens.

Duchenne muscular dystrophy: a severe, progressive X-linked hereditary disorder caused by inability to synthesize **dystrophin** (*q.v.*), in which skeletal muscle fibers undergo degeneration and necrosis, and are replaced by fibrous and fatty connective tissue. It occurs mostly in males, but also in females with Turner's syndrome. Afflicted individuals usually lose the ability to walk before the end of the second decade, and rarely survive beyond the third. Becker's muscular dystrophy is a related, milder form in which an abnormal dystrophin is made.

dulcitol: galactitol.

Dulcolax: a trade name for the cathartic, (4,4′-diacetoxydiphenylmethyl)pyridine. It is also known under several other trade names, and as DAMP, but is different from 4-**DAMP** (*q.v.*).

$$CH_3COO - \text{---} - \underset{H}{\overset{C}{-}} - \text{---} - OOCH_3$$

dUMP: deoxyuridine monophosphate; *see* **dihydrofolate reductase**.

duodenum: the short, uppermost, widest part of the small intestine. It receives chyme, pancreatic juice, and bile, and contains cells that secrete gastrin, glucose-dependent insulinotropic peptide (GIP), and other regulators. Considerable amounts of calcium can be absorbed, but most nutrients are taken up in the jejunum and ileum. It is a common site for ulcer formation.

DVAP: D-amino[Val⁴, D-Arg⁸]VP; a vasopressin analog that mimics the antidiuretic (but not pressor) effects of arginine vasopressin; *cf* **DDAVP**.

dwarf: a very short individual who, if surviving to adulthood, never attains a stature within the normal range for others of the same species and sex; *see* **dwarfism**. (2) to cause to become (or to appear) very small.

dwarfism: any condition in which growth is severely impaired, and untreated individuals have subnormal statures when they attain adulthood. In humans, the most common cause of *pituitary* dwarfism is "simple" growth hormone deficiency (not accompanied by inability to make other adenohypophysial hormones). Growth retardation becomes apparent during infancy or early childhood and puberty is delayed, but intelligence is not affected. The individuals are otherwise normal in appearance, and fertile as adults. Growth hormone replacement therapy instituted during childhood is usually effective. *Laron* type dwarfs make growth hormone, but lack the ability to synthesize insulin-like growth factor I (IGF-I), and are unresponsive to the growth-promoting effects of exogenous GH. In at least some cases, the problem is directly linked to absence of normal growth hormone receptors. Malnourished, but otherwise normal children usually secrete large amounts of growth hormone, but make very little IGF-I. If the deficiency is of limited duration, they respond to feeding. Renal dysfunctions in which nutrients are lost to the urine can have similar effects; but nitrogen retention impairs growth, and some kidney disorders lead to the development of renal rickets. Insulin is an essential regulator of protein and lipid, as well as carbohydrate metabolism, and children with untreated diabetes mellitus display growth retardation. Severe thyroid hormone deficiency that begins early in life causes *cretinism*, in which mental retardation is

severe, infantile body proportions are retained, and reproductive system organs fail to undergo maturation. The problems can be averted by thyroid hormone administration that begins during infancy, but the central nervous system defects cannot be corrected when treatment is delayed. *Achondroplasia* is caused by mutations that impair cartilage growth. Affected individuals have short limbs and other skeletal system defects, but can be fertile and acquire normal intelligence.

dynamin: a 100K protein with GTPase activity that induces microtubule bundling in the brain, and budding of endocytic vesicles from plasma membranes. It is homologous to different proteins that participate in spindle pole separation during cell division and contribute to sorting of molecules to vesicles.

dynein: 1500 to 2000K proteins composed of 9-12 polypeptide chains that form the arms of microtubule, cilium and flagellum tubulin A subfibers, and mediate sliding of outer axoneme doublets. They have two or three globular heads linked by slender, flexible stalks to a common multimer base. Three-headed molecules are attached by their bases to microtubule A rods, and their head ATPase activity is augmented by the association. Cycles of ATP binding, ATP hydrolysis, and ATD/ADP exchange cause conformational changes in the heads and stalks that promote attachments to B rods of adjacent filaments, filament sliding, and disengagement from the B rods. In conjunction with other factors, dynein contributes to organelle transport.

dynorphins: dynorphin A[1-17], dynorphin A[1-8], dynorphin B, and several other, closely related neuropeptides cleaved from prodynorphin, all of which contain an *N*-terminal leu-enkephalin sequence that can interact with κ type opioid receptors. Porcine dynorphin A has the amino acid sequence: H_2N-Tyr-Gly-Gly-Phe-Leu-Arg-Arg-Ile-Arg-Pro-Lys-Leu-Lys-Trp-Asp-Asn-Gln-OH. Dynorphin B (rimorphin) is H_2N-Tyr-Gly-Gly-Phe-Leu-Arg-Arg-Ile-Arg-Pro-Lys-Leu-Lys-OH. Dynorphin A [1-8] additionally binds to δ and μ receptors. Age-associated elevation of the levels in the hippocampus has been linked with memory loss. Dynorphins also affect smooth muscle contraction (for example in vas deferens), autonomic, and other functions. Their synthesis (in basal ganglia, nucleus tractus solitarius, hypothalamic magnocellular neurons, adrenal medulla and at some other sites) is regulated by neuronal activity.

dys-: a prefix meaning defective or abnormal; *cf* **eu-**.

dyscrasias: abnormal conditions. The term usually refers to hematological disorders.

dysgammaglobulinemia: immune system defects caused by deficiency of one or more (but not all) classes of immunoglobulins that increase susceptibility to infection; *see* also **agammaglobulinemia**.

dysgenesis: (1) abnormal development; (2) genetic selection of traits that are deleterious or disadvantageous to a population.

dysgerminomas: malignant gonadal tumors. Some occur in testes, but ovaries are the most common sites.

dysgeusia: abnormal taste perception.

dyslipidosis: any lipid metabolism disorder.

dysmenorrhea: painful menstruation.

dysostosis: defective bone formation, caused by impaired ossification of fetal cartilage.

dyspareunia: persistent genital pain in women, during and following coitus.

dyspepsia: indigestion; (1) short term discomfort that follows ingestion of certain kinds of foods; (2) chronic conditions in which discomfort after eating is caused by gastrointestinal system defects.

dysphagia: difficulty with swallowing. The causes include pressure exerted on the esophagus by other organs, defects that impair normal contraction and relaxation of esophageal muscles, and tumors.

dysphoria: restlessness, anxiety, malaise, feelings of discomfort, or other mood disturbances. The term has also been applied to some forms of abnormal perception such as hyperalgesia, and to abnormal psychological responses to environmental stimuli.

dysplasia: incomplete or abnormal development.

dyspnea: labored breathing.

dystroglycans: 43K and 156K glycoproteins in skeletal muscle and at some other sites that mediate associations of cell components with extracellular matrices. *See* **dystrophin**.

dystrophin: a 3685 amino acid rod-shaped, homodimeric cytoskeletal protein chemically related to α-actinin and spectrin, on the inner surfaces of skeletal muscle sarcolemma and T tubules. It attaches to the membranes via an ankyrin or protein 4.1-like molecule, and is believed to interact with the myofibril actin filaments. Proposed functions include coupling of triads to the myofibril system, membrane stabilization, influences on Ca^{2+} transport, and roles in T tubule morphogenesis. It forms complexes with dystrophin associated glycoproteins that link the sarcolemma with the extracellular matrix. The complexes contain one molecule each of 59K cytoskeletal, 43K, 35K, and 25K transmembrane, and 156K laminin-binding glycoproteins. (The 43K and 156K types are also made at other sites, including heart, liver, stomach, and kidney). Individuals with Duchenne muscular dystrophy cannot synthesize dystrophin and have very low levels of the glycoproteins. Loss of muscle associations with extracellular matrices appears to contribute to necrosis in this disease by increasing osmotic fragility and disrupting calcium-regulating mechanisms.

dystrophin associated glycoproteins: *see* **dystrophin**.

dystrophy: any disorder that involves degeneration of structure and/or function.

E

E: (1) glutamic acid; (2) epinephrine; (3) vitamin E.

e: equine, as in eFSH.

E$_1$: estrone.

E1A genes: adenovirus early region genes; *see* **E1A proteins**.

EIA proteins: 243 and 289 amino acid peptides expressed in host cells soon after adenovirus infection. They bind to and affect the functions of several proteins that contribute to the control of cell division, including a 60K cyclin, the retinoblastoma gene product, CRE-BP, and transcription factor IID (TFIID) which binds to TATA boxes. After binding, they display kinase activity, and can catalyze phosphorylations of viral gene products, as well as histone H1 and several other host cell proteins. Although better known for their abilities to invoke transformation, they exert some anti-oncogenic effects.

E$_2$: estradiol.

E$_3$: estriol.

E$_4$: estetrol.

EA: antibody-coated erythrocytes; *see* **EA-rosettes**.

EAA: excitatory amino acids; *see* **glutamate**.

EAC-rosettes: clusters of erythrocytes coated with anti-erythrocyte antibodies and complement that form around B lymphocytes. The antigen-antibody complexes promote release of complement component C3 and its incorporation into a complex that binds to lymphocyte C3 receptors. *Cf* **E-rosettes** and **EA-rosettes**.

Eadie-Hofstee plot: a graph in which V (the velocity of a reaction) is plotted along the ordinate, and V/S (where S is the initial substrate concentration) along the abscissa.

EAE: experimental autoimmune encephalitis.

ear: *erbA*-related genes. They code for proteins closely related to thyroid hormone (triiodothyronine, T$_3$) receptors. However, since no specific ligands have been identified, they are called "**orphan receptors**" (*q.v.*). The messenger RNA for Erb-1 (Rev-erbA) is transcribed from the anti-sense strand of the DNA that codes for c-erbAα. It binds to the thyroid hormone response element (TRE), but has little affinity for T$_3$. The *ear-7* gene is on the sense strand of the same DNA, and it contains an exon that overlaps with two of *ear-1*. The protein product is processed to yield erb-71 (with very high affinity for T$_3$) and ear-72 (which binds to the TRE but not to the hormone). An *ear-2* has also been identified. *Ear-3* codes for COUP transcription factor (which has also been called an orphan receptor; but observations that it is indirectly activated by a dopamine regulated protein kinase have raised the possibility that it functions without a ligand). Other potential activators of *ear* genes include nutrients, environmental factors, and kinase cascade components. The corresponding human genes are named *hear*. *See* also *erb*.

Eagles's medium: blood serum supplemented with amino acids, vitamins, salts, and glucose. It is used to support the growth of cultured cells.

early antigens: cell surface antigens whose synthesis is directed by viral genes very soon after the viruses infect cells (before viral nucleic acid synthesis begins). *See* also **immediate early genes**.

early genes: *see* **immediate early genes**.

early pregnancy factor: EPF; several glycoproteins detected in maternal blood plasma soon after conception. They are believed to be made by syncytiotrophoblast, and to be components of mechanisms for protecting conceptuses against immunological rejection by maternal immune systems.

EA-rosettes: clusters of erythrocytes coated with anti-erythrocyte IgG type immunoglobulin that form around B lymphocytes by binding to their Fc receptors. The numbers made provide a measure of B populations in test aliquots. *Cf* **E-rosettes** and **EAC-rosettes**.

EBPS: estrogen binding proteins.

EBV: Epstein-Barr virus.

EC$_{50}$: the dosage that invokes a half-maximal effect.

E-cadherin: *see* E-**cadherin**.

E-CAM: epithelial cell adhesion molecule; *see* E-**cadherin**.

EC cells: (1) endothelial cells; (2) enterochromaffin cells that secrete serotonin and peptide regulators.

ecchymosis: skin discoloration caused by extravasation of blood.

eccrine: secretion (such as watery sweat) that does not involve loss of cell structural components; *cf* **apocrine** and **merocrine**.

ecdysis: shedding of the outer layer of skin, or of a shell.

ecdysones: ecdysteroids; usually (1) molting hormones; Y hormone; polyhydroxylated steroid hormones synthesized from cholesterol that promote maturation, metamorphosis, and ecdysis, and protect against apoptosis of some cell types. Chromosomal puffs form at the transcription sites. In arthropods, they are made in prothoracic or in ventral (ring) glands. Stimulation of their production by brain hormones may be mediated via cAMP. In

α-ecdysone

β-ecdysone

immature insects, juvenile hormones antagonize the effects on morphogenesis (but not on molting). In many species, α-ecdysone (1,2,14,22,25- pentahydroxycholest-7-en-6-one) is secreted and converted peripherally to β-ecdysone (20-OH-ecdysone), the biologically active form. The term *zooecdysones* is applied to hormones made by animals; (2) *phytoecdysones* made by some plants that kill insects by invoking premature molting.

ECFs: ECF-A; eosinophil chemotactic factors.

ECGFs: endothelial cell growth factors.

Echinodermata: an invertebrate phylum that includes sea urchins and sea-stars. All have calcareous external skeletons and water vascular systems, and undergo developmental stages consistent with links to vertebrate evolution.

echistatin: H$_2$N-Glu-Cys-Glu-Ser-Gly-Pro-Cys-Cys-Arg-Asn-Cys-Lys-Phe-Leu-Lys-Glu-Gly-Thr-Ile-Cys-Lys-Arg-Ala-Arg-Gly-Asp-Asp-Met-Asp-Asp-Tyr-Cys-Asn-Gly-Lys-Thr-Cys-Asp-Cys-Pro-Arg-Asn-Pro-His-Lys-Gly-Pro-Ala-Thr-OH; a single-chain peptide with four cysteine bridges isolated from the venom of the saw-scaled viper, *Echis carinatus*. It is chemically and biologically similar to trigramin; and both peptides contain an Arg-Gly-Asp (RGD) sequence that binds fibrinogen. Echistatin inhibits platelet aggregation stimulated by ADP, thrombin, collagen, epinephrine, and platelet activating factor (PAF). It also attaches to vitronectin receptors, and promotes osteoclast detachment from bone surfaces; but its ability to inhibit bone resorption may additionally involve inhibitory influences on recruitment and differentiation of osteoclast precursors.

echocardiograms: diagnostic procedures that use images generated by ultrasound waves which are directed at the heart and reflected from tissue interfaces.

echoviruses: several viruses that inhabit human intestines. Most appear to be harmless, but some invade other tissues and cause disease.

ECL cells: enterochromaffin-like cells of the stomach that secrete histamine.

eclipsed antigen: a parasite antigen that does not invoke antibody production because it resembles, and is treated like a tolerated host type.

eclipse period: the time interval between virus entry and the first appearance of virions.

eclosion hormones: 62-amino acid, species specific hormones produced in the brain and accumulated in the

corpus cardiacum of some insects. They promote emersion of adults from pupal cases by acting on epidermis and muscle, and by triggering behavioral responses.

ECM: ecm; extracellular matrix.

ECM RIII: type III extracellular matrix receptor; *see* **CD44** and **heterotypic adhesion receptors**.

E. coli: *Escherichia coli*; bacterial strains that ferment lactose. They are used to study metabolic processes, and for production of specific kinds of proteins. Some strains colonize normal human intestines, and are ingested with drinking water and foods. When present in limited numbers, they protect against the growth of pathogens in the gut, and make some vitamins. Different strains release endotoxins, cause diarrhea, and invade urinary tracts and other parts of the body.

ecological niche: the position occupied by an organism within its community, and its interactions with other organisms and with the environment.

EcoRI: a type II restriction endonuclease derived from *E. coli* that generates sticky ends. It cleaves DNAs between G and A nucleotides of GAATC sequences.

ECP: eosinophilic cationic proteins.

E-CSF: eosinophil colony stimulating factor; *see* **eosinophil differentiation factor**.

ecosystem: the organisms within a locale, and their interactions with each other and with the environment.

ecotropic virus: a virus that integrates into the genome of, or replicates only within the cells of a specific host species; *cf* **xenotropic virus**.

ecstacy: (1) overwhelming emotion, especially of the joyful kind, or religious fervor; (2) MDMA, an illegal drug that invokes euphoria; *see* 3,4-**methylene dioxymethamphetamine**.

ectoderm: a surface layer, usually the outermost of the three embryonic primary germ layers. Structures derived from it include nervous system components and epidermis. *Cf* **endoderm** and **mesoderm**.

ectoenzymes: exoenzymes; enzymes whose catalytic sites face interstitial fluids or other external environments.

ectohormones: pheromones and other regulators released externally that act on other organisms.

ectolecithal: describes ova or oocytes with mostly cortical distribution of yolk; *cf* **telolecithal**.

ectomorphy: the body type of tall, lean, long-limbed individuals. It is often associated with asthenia. *Cf* **endomorphy** and **mesomorphy**.

ectopic: out of place; describes tissues, cell types, or cell products outside locations in which they normally reside; *see* also **ectopic hormone production** and **ectopic pregnancy.**

ectopic hormone production: hormone synthesis at sites within the body where detectable amounts are not usually made. Many kinds of tumors cells secrete large quantities of regulators normally made within typical endocrine glands, or substances with closely similar biological properties. Normal cell types are now known to make small amounts of regulators previously believed to be restricted to just one or a few sites.

ectopic pregnancy: pregnancy in which implantation occurs at a site other than the uterus (most commonly the Fallopian tubes, and more rarely the ovary or abdominal cavity).

ectotherms: animals whose body temperatures vary with environmental factors such as temperature and the amounts of ultraviolet radiation. The term "cold-blooded" has been applied, since the body temperatures are usually lower than those of mammals and birds. Related terms include poikilotherms and exotherms; *cf* **endotherms.**

eczema: usually, an inflammatory skin reaction.

ED$_{50}$: the dose that affects 50% of organisms, cells, or other responding entities.

EDCF$_2$: *see* **endothelium-derived contracting factor**.

edema: excessive accumulation of interstitial fluids. The causes include liver diseases and malnutrition that impair the synthesis of plasma proteins and thereby lower blood oncotic pressure, kidney damage that leads to protein loss to the urine, augmented capillary permeability, blood vessel injury, pressure that interferes with fluid reabsorption and/or promotes excessive filtration across capillary vessel walls, lymph channel obstruction, and excessive production of mineralocorticoids or vasopressin.

edentate: toothless.

edetate calcium disodium: calcium disodium versenate; ethylenediamine tetraacetic acid; calcium disodium che-

late; a chelating agent used to treat heavy metal poisoning. (It does not recruit tissue-bound mercury.) Since the affinity for lead, zinc, iron, manganese and other metals is greater than for calcium, it does not invoke hypocalcemia. *cf*. **edetate sodium**.

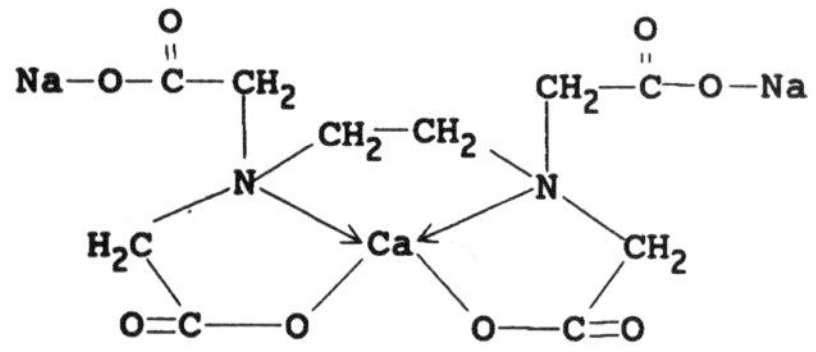

edetate sodium: salts of ethylenediamine tetraacetic acid that contain one, two, three, or four sodium atoms. They bind metals, and are used as chelating agents. However, when used to treat metal poisoning, they also bind calcium; and large amounts can invoke hypocalcemia. The trisodium salt is shown.

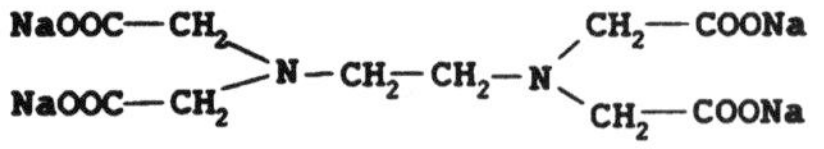

Edetin: ethylenediamine tetraacetic acid.

EDF: eosinophil differentiation factor.

Edman degradation: a technique for determining amino acid sequences of small peptides. Phenylisothiocyanate attaches to the free amino groups of *N*-terminal amino acid moieties. Acid hydrolysis then cleaves the terminal peptide bond, shortens the chain by just one residue, and releases the affected amino acid as a phenylthiohydantoin (PTH) derivative that can be isolated and identified by chromatography. The process is then repeated for the next, and succeeding terminal amino acids.

EDRF: endothelium-derived relaxation factor.

edrophonium bromide: *N*-ethyl-3-hydroxy-*N,N*-dimethyl-benzaminium bromide; an acetylcholinesterase inhibitor, used to counteract the effects of curare and related agents, and in the diagnosis of myasthenia gravis.

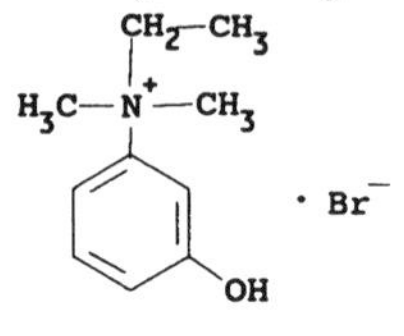

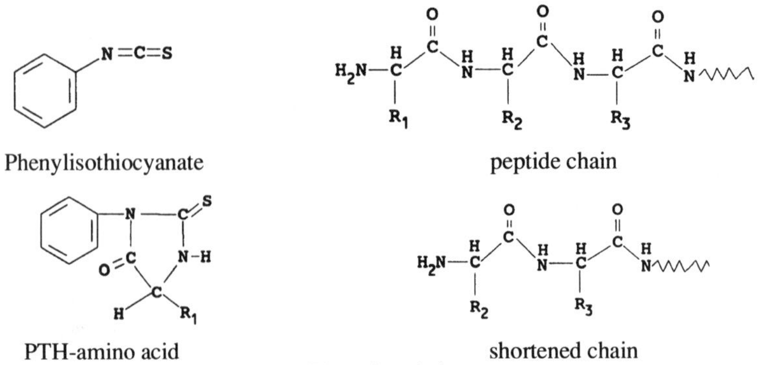

Phenylisothiocyanate

peptide chain

PTH-amino acid

shortened chain

Edman degradation

EDS: ethylene dimethanesulfonate.

EDTA: ethylenediamine tetraacetate.

EEG: electroencephalogram.

E_1E_2-ATPases: membrane-associated enzymes that use energy released by ATP hydrolysis to catalyze ion movements against concentration gradients; *see*, for example **Na^+-K^+-ATPases**. The activity involves interconversion of E_1 and E_2 conformational states. Inhibitors include ouabain, oligomycin, and orthovanadate.

EETS: epoxyeicosatetraenoic acids.

EFs: EF-1, EF-2, EF-Tu, EF-Ts, and EF-G: *see* **elongation factors**.

E face: the inner surface of the outer layer of a plasma membrane lipid bilayer, obtained by freeze fracture techniques; *cf* **P face**.

effector: a cell or organ that responds to a stimulus.

efferent: conveying outward or away from the center; describes, for example axons or nerve impulses that travel from the central nervous system to peripheral targets, or vessels that carry blood away from structures.

effluvium: fluids, hair, or other substances shed from a surface.

effusion: a fluid discharge.

EF hand: a configuration common to troponin C, parvalbumin, calmodulins, and some other calcium binding proteins, in which two helices (E and F) are positioned, respectively, as the index finger and thumb of the right hand, with the calcium binding site in a loop that connects the helices. Most of those proteins contain two such units.

EF-G: *see* **elongation factors**.

Efudex: a trade name for a topical preparation of 5-fluorouracil.

Eg-1: the protein product of a maternally derived messenger RNA in oocyte animal poles that plays roles in differentiation.

EG cells: gastrointestinal tract cells that secrete enteroglucagon.

egestion: elimination of unassimilated material from the digestive tract.

EGF: epidermal growth factor.

EGFRc: epidermal growth factor receptor.

egg: although the term means ovum, it is also used for mature secondary oocytes, and for structures that contain them and can have overlying yolk, other proteins, and shells.

egg laying hormone: ELH: a peptide isolated from *Aplysia californica* that invokes egg laying behavior. It is cleaved from a prohormone that yields other regulators involved in the responses. *See* **bag cell peptides**.

egg peptides: cysteine-rich, 77K species-specific extracellular matrix glycoproteins that surround the mature oocytes of many aquatic species. They are chemoattractants for sperm and stimulants of sperm motility and metabolism. The actions involve elevation of cytosolic Ca^{2+}, H^+ efflux, and cAMP generation. cGMP levels are also elevated, possibly via interaction of a closely related peptide with an oocyte guanylate cyclase.

EGR proteins: at least three serum-inducible zinc-finger nucleoproteins (EGR-1, 2, and 3), that function as transcription regulators. EGR-1 (also known as Knox 24, *zif*268, TIS-8, and NGF1-A) is believed to contribute to cell repair after injury. Its levels rise rapidly in response to ionizing radiation and some other factors that damage cells.

EGTA: ethyleneglycol *bis-N,N′*-tetraacetate; ethylene glycol bis(β-aminoethyl ether)-*N,N,N′N′*-tetracetate; a cation chelator that avidly binds calcium, but has much lower affinity for magnesium and other metals bound by ethylene diamine tetraacetate (EDTA).

EHDT: etidronate.

Ehlers-Danlos syndrome: several autosomal or X-linked connective tissue disorders, in which inability to synthesize a procollagen peptidase leads to short stature, hypermobile joints, weakened dermis with excessively stretchable skin, and impaired wound healing. A rare, severe form can cause death from blood vessel rupture or intestinal perforation. Dermatosparaxis is a related autosomal recessive disease of cattle.

eicosa: icosa; twenty, as in eicosapentaenoic acid.

eicosanoids: icosanoids; prostaglandins, prostacyclins, thromboxanes, leukotrienes, and other metabolites of arachidonic and related 20-carbon polyunsaturated fatty acids.

5,8,11,14,17-eicosapentaenoic acid: a 20-carbon polyunsaturated fatty acid precursor of prostaglandin E_3 (PGE_3) and other eicosanoids with three double bonds. It is classified as essential, since most animals cannot synthesize it from acetyl-coenzyme A; but it can be made from other polyunsaturated fatty acids. The form assumed in solution is shown.

5,8,11,14-eicosatetraenoic acid: arachidonic acid.

5,8,11,14-eicosatetraynoic acid: ETYA; an arachidonic acid analog that competes with AA as a substrate, and thereby blocks formation of metabolites made in cyclooxygenase, lipoxygenase, and epoxygenase pathways.

eIF-1, **EIF-2**: eukaryote **initiation factors** (q.v.).

EIPs: estrogen induced proteins.

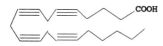

5,8,11,14-eicosatetraynoic acid

ejaculation: rapid discharge, usually of semen.

ELAM-1: endothelial-leukocyte cell adhesion molecule-1.

Elasmobranchs: a class of cartilaginous fishes that includes sharks, rays, and dogfish.

elastases: serine proteases that degrade elastin and closely related proteins. A basic 25K glycoprotein made by neutrophils acts mostly on bonds formed by small aliphatic amino acids, and is implicated as a mediator of tissue damage during inflammatory responses, and a major contributor to the development of emphysema when inadequately opposed by naturally occurring inhibitors. It displays 43% homology with a pancreatic juice elastase that digests food proteins.

elastic tissue: a highly distensible connective tissue type. The extracllular matrix contains large quantities of elastins, along with some collagens and elastonectin.

elastins: the major components of elastic connective tissues, assembled from tropoelastin subunits. They are approximately 70K extracellular matrix scleroproteins, with numerous glycine, alanine, proline and valine moieties (but very little hydroxyproline and no hydroxylysine or carbohydrate). Lungs, vertebral ligaments, and large arteries contain substantial amounts. The ability to stretch in two directions and rapidly recoil is attributed to **desmosine** cross-links (*q.v.*), and the yellow color to the polymeric structure and coiling as well as the positioning of cross-linkages. Long, interwoven, inelastic collagen fibrils limit the stretch and protect against tearing.

elastonectin: a 120K extracellular matrix protein made by fibroblasts that binds elastins.

Elavil: a trade name for amitriptyline hydrochloride.

Eldepryl: a trade name for deprenyl.

electrical coupling: cell-to-cell communication via exchanges of ions across gap junctions or electrical synapses. Hepatocytes, cardiac myocytes, some neurons, lens epithelial, and intestinal smooth muscle cells, are among the types that communicate in this way.

electrical gradient: the electrical charge difference measured at two points (usually on opposite sides of a cell membrane). For physiology studies, it is expressed in millivolts.

electrical synapse: a functional coupling between adjacent excitable cells that permits rapid communication, mediated by ion exchanges across gap junctions. Most vertebrate neurons use chemical synapses.

electric eel: *see Electrophorus electricus*.

electric organ: *see* **electrocytes**.

electrochemical gradient: in biological systems, chemical and electrical differences measured at two points on opposite surfaces of a membrane that result from the combined effects of differences in solute concentrations and electric charges. Net movements of ions into (or out of) a cell, mediated by a high concentration gradient that drives passive diffususion, can be accelerated by electrical attraction or opposed by repulsion.

electrochemical potential: a quantity, usually expressed in joules/mole, that defines (1) the amount of energy released by ions that move passively down an electrochemical gradient, or (2) the work required to move them in the opposite direction. *See* **Nernst equation**.

electrocortin: an obsolete term for aldosterone.

electrocytes: specialized muscle fibers of *Electrophorus electricus*, *Torpedo californicus*, and some other fishes, organized into non-contracting electrical organs. They contain large amounts of Na^+/K^+-ATPases, and generate high voltages when stimulated by acetylcholine.

electrodialysis: dialysis (*q.v.*) in which electrical fields accelerate the movements of charged molecules.

electroencephalographs: EEG; instruments that amplify and record the electrical activities of brain regions. They are used in the diagnosis of epilepsy and some other brain disorders. Usually, electrodes attached to the scalp transmit the messages to devices with pens that write on moving drums covered with paper calibrated in time and voltage units.

electrofocusing: techniques that employ electrical fields to concentrate specific chemical species.

electroimmunodiffusion: diffusion of antigens and antibodies assisted by electric fields.

electrokymographs: instruments used to record changes in densities, or motions of anatomical structures, by sensing passage of narrow radiation beams and transmitting signals to fluorescent screens or photographic plates.

electrolysis: in chemistry, use of electric currents to decompose molecules.

electrolytes: compounds that ionize when dissolved in water. The solutions conduct electrical currents.

electromyography: recording of electrical changes associated with muscle activity.

electron carrier: a coenzyme or other compound that undergoes reversible reduction and oxidation by taking up electrons from one substance and transferring them to another.

electron dense: describes regions on electron micrographs that appear dark because the passage of electrons is blocked by high concentrations of macromolecules, or by substances that have bound heavy metals.

electron microscopy: *see* **microscopy**.

electron-spin resonance: ESR; spectroscopic methods for locating electrons within paramagnetic substances, based on energy differences between two possible alignment states of unpaired electrons in magnetic fields. They provide information on molecular structure, and are used, for example to study free radicals, and cholesterol binding to cytochrome P450$_{scc}$.

electron transferring protein: ETF; a flavoprotein that participates in fatty acid oxidation. It accepts electrons from reducd flavine adenine dinucleotide (FADH$_2$), donates them to an iron-sulfur protein, ETF:ubiquinone reductase, and thereby promotes ubiquinone conversion to ubiquinol.

electron transport chain: a series of enzymes and associated factors used for orderly transfer of electrons from donor molecules to a final acceptor. The ones on eukaryote cell inner mitochondrial membranes accept electrons and hydrogen ions from coenzymes and transport them, via a series of oxidation-reduction reactions, to molecular oxygen. Much of the energy released is used to actively transport protons and drive oxidative phosphorylation (mitochondrial synthesis of ATP from ADP + Pi). The remainder is lost as heat. When NADH + H$^+$ (produced by tricarboxylic acid cycle and other reactions) is the primary donor, NADH-Q reductase catalyzes transfer of the hydrogen atoms and electrons to flavine mononucleotide (FMN), formation of FMNH$_2$, and release of energy sufficient to form one ATP from ADP + Pi for each NADH + H$^+$ oxidized. FADH$_2$ can also serve as the primary donor. The reduced form of ubiquinone transports electrons from either of the reduced flavoproteins to cytochrome reductase (a complex which includes heme b-562, b-566, and c$_1$). Reduction of two molecules of cytochrome c$_1$ releases energy for the synthesis of a second ATP. Cytochrome oxidase (a complex that includes cytochromes a and a$_3$) then promotes transfer to molecular oxygen, and a third ATP can be made. Oxygen in its reduced from (O^{2-}) simultaneously accepts hydrogen ions to from water, A maximum of three ATP can be therefore be synthesized when NADH + H$^+$ is the initial donor, and a maximum of two from a reduced flavoprotein. Somewhat different electron transport chains are used in photosynthesis light reactions.

electron volt: eV; 1.6 x 10^{19} joule; the amount of electrical energy acquired by an electron that passes through a vacuum at a potential difference of one volt.

electrophoresis: movement of solute particles in an electrical field. Mixture components can be separated on the basis of differences in surface charges and other properties (such as size and configuration) that affect mobility rates. Filter paper, cellulose, gels (composed of starch, agar, or polyacrylamide, with specified pore sizes that block passage of large molecules), or other supports, are used to generate bands of solute components that can be identified by staining or radiological methods and isolated. When used for molecular weight determinations, proteins are pretreated with sodium dodecylsulfate (an anionic detergent that disrupts noncovalent interactions), and mercaptoethanol (which cleaves disulfide bonds) to permit assumption of random coil configurations. Small molecules can be separated from larger ones with *pulsed field gel electrophoresis*, since they reorient and migrate

more rapidly when the direction of the electrical field is changed at specified time intervals.

Electrophorus electricus: the Amazon electric eel. Its electrical organs are used to study nicotinic type acetylcholine receptors, Na$^+$/K$^+$-ATPases, and sodium channels, and as a source of acetylcholinesterase.

electroplax: a stack of specialized muscle fibers (electrocytes) arranged in series and organized into an acetylcholine-sensitive electrical organ. *See* also ***Electrophorus electricus***.

electroporation: techniques in which brief electrical pulses are used to reversibly increase the permeabilities of membranes, and thereby facilitate the entry of nucleic acids and other large and/or hydrophilic molecules.

electrotaxis: movement of cells or organisms in response to electric currents. It can be positive (toward the current source) or negative.

electrotonus: (1) a state produced in a cell, tissue, organ, or organism subjected to a steady, depolarizing current; (2) changes in excitability and conductance imposed by steady, depolarizing currents.

electrovalent bond: the kind of chemical bond formed when a cation combines with an anion. Compounds formed this way dissociate (ionize) when dissolved in water. *Cf* **covalent** and **hydrogen** bonds.

eledoisin: pyr-Gln-Pro-Ser-Lys-Asp-Ala-Phe-Ile-Gly-Leu-Met-NH$_2$; a hormone secreted by the salivary glands of *Eledone* (a small octopus), and a precursor of several other biologically active peptides. It is a tachykinin, biologically related to substance P and physalaemin that relaxes vascular, but stimulates extravascular smooth muscle. In some species, it stimulates salivary and lacrimal gland cells.

elephantiasis: chronic, severe tissue swelling with fluid retention. The most common cause is lymphatic vessel obstruction by parasites.

ELH: egg laying hormone.

ELISA: enzyme-linked immunosorbent assay; very sensitive immunological assay systems that do not require radioactive markers. An antibody directed against the substance investigated is linked to an enzyme (for example, horseradish peroxidase or a phosphatase) that catalyzes a color-generating reaction when the antibody binds to the antigen. The color intensity varies directly with the amount of test substance (antigen) that binds.

Elk-1: a protein of the ets family, similar to or identical with p62^{TCF} (ternary response factor). It binds to DNA sequences immediately upstream from *fos* promoter response elements, as a component of a ternary complex that activates that gene, and may function as a cell type specific regulator of *fos* and other immediately early genes.

elongation factors: EFs; peptides required for amino acid chain elongation during translation. Bacterial EF-Tu elongation factor bound to GDP is inactive, with little affinity for amino-acyl-tRNAs. When it associates with

EF-Ts, GTP exchanges for GDP. EF-Tu-GTP then tightly binds an amino-acyl-tRNA that holds the first amino acid of the chain, and positions it at the ribosome A site. (It does not recognize the *f*-met-tRNA that enters into formation of the initiation complex.) GTP is then hydrolyzed to GDP + Pi, and EF-Tu-GDP leave the ribosome. After the peptide bond is formed, EF-G (translocase, a different GTPase with high affinity for GTP) promotes transfer of the dipeptidyl-tRNA to the ribosome P site, and the A site becomes available for attachment of the next amino acid. In eukaryotes, EF-1α (which delivers amino-acyl-tRNAs to ribosomes), EF-1$\beta\gamma$ (a guanine nucleotide exchange factor), and EF-2 are the functional equivalents, respectively, of prokaryote EF-Tu, EF-Ts, and EF-G. Diphtheria toxin blocks protein synthesis by promoting ADP-ribosylation of EF-2.

elution: separation of one or more components from a mixture or complex. Solvents specific for certain solutes are used to dissolve and remove those molecules from chromatography columns.

Embden-Meyerhof pathway: *see* **glycolysis**.

embolus: usually, something that clogs a blood vessel, for example a thrombus or air bubble.

embryo: an organism in the early stages of development, during which the major organs or organ precursors are formed. In mammals, the term is variously applied to conceptuses during the time interval that begins with fertilization, the first blastomere cleavage, implantation, or the establishment of the primary germ layers, and terminates when structures characteristic of the species can be identified. From then to the end of the gestation period, the organism is called a fetus. (In humans, the fetal stage extends from eight weeks post-conception to the time of birth.). In some animal species, the embryo is enclosed in egg membranes. Although the organism that hatches is usually called a larva, some authors prefer the term embryo. Plants in early stages of development are also called embryos.

embryoblast: inner cell mass; the part of a blastocyst that gives rise to the new individual, and to some extra-embryonic tissues; *cf* **trophoblast**.

embryo culture: *in vitro* growth of embryos.

embryogenesis: usually, development of an embryo. The term is sometimes applied to all stages of prenatal development.

embryonal: (1) embryonic; (2) poorly differentiated, a term applied to some malignant cells or tissues.

embryonal carcinomas: malignant epithelial tumors, composed of poorly differentiated (embryonal) cells or tissues, usually derived from germ cells, and more common in testes than in ovaries.

embryonic: (1) immature, with potential for development; (2) derived from or characteristic of an embryo or its components.

embryonic germ layers: the primary tissues of a young vertebrate embryo; *see* **ectoderm**, **mesoderm**, and **endoderm**.

embryonic inducers: hormone-like substances released by some cells of an embryo that affect the development of other (usually neighboring) cells.

embryo transfer: artificial insertion of one or more young embryos into the oviduct or uterus, a procedure used in women to overcome some causes of infertility such as Fallopian tube obstructions, or to accomplish development in surrogate mothers when the woman is incapable of sustaining a pregnancy. Surrogate animal mothers are used to nurture endangered species when natural mothers are scarce, or to breed animals regarded as especially valuable (for example disease-resistant cattle, or race horses) in less expensive hosts. They are also used to nurture fertilized oocytes and/or embryos into which DNA from other species has been injected, and to investigate some aspects of reproduction in laboratory animals.

EMD 21388: 3-methyl-4′6-dihydroxy-3′-dibromoflavone; a thyroxine analog that displaces T$_4$ and T$_3$ from transthyretin binding sites. It is a potent *in vitro* inhibitor of hepatic 5′-deiodinase. In rats (in which transthyretin is a major transport protein for iodinated thyroid hormones), it transiently affects plasma levels of total and free T$_4$ and T$_3$ and secondarily lowers TSH levels.

EMD-23488: 3-[4-(4-phenyl-1,2,3-6-tetrahydropyridyl-1)-butyl]-indole; a selective dopamine autoreceptor agonist.

emeiocytosis: exocytosis.

emerogens: anti-oncogenes; DNA segments that code for proteins which suppress transformation.

emesis: vomiting.

emetic: an agent that invokes vomiting.

emetine: 6′,7′10,11-tetramethoxymetan; an alkaloid derived from ipecac, that inhibits protein synthesis in eukar-

EMD-23488

yotes by blocking translocation of peptidyl-tRNAs from acceptor to donor sites of ribosomes. The compound and some preparations made from it (usually the hydrochloride or camphosulfonate), are used to treat resistant amebic and lungworm infections.

enalapril

EMF: (1) erythrocyte maturation factor; (2) electromotive force.

Eminase: *see* **streptokinase**.

eminence: a protrusion or bulging structure.

emollients: softening agents.

emphysema: usually, (1) pulmonary emphysema; (2) any collection of air in connective tissues.

empty sellar syndrome: conditions in which the sella turcica is filled with cerebrospinal fluid, and the pituitary fossa appears empty when examined radiologically (although the pituitary gland is present in flattened form). They can be associated with inadequate, normal, or excessive secretion of pituitary gland hormones.

emulsification: dispersion of the lipid droplets of an emulsion, usually by addition of a substance with detergent properties. (Mechanical agitation can break large droplets into smaller ones, but large ones usually reform afterward.)

emulsion: a stable dispersion of lipid droplets in an immiscible liquid.

EMS: (1) ethyl methane sulfonate; (2) eosinophilia myalgia syndrome; *see* **tryptophan**.

en-2: the mammalian homolog of a *Drosophila* engrailed protein (which directs anterior/posterior pattern formation in insects). It is induced by anterior mesoderm, and is an early marker for neural differentiation. Its expression in specific muscle groups indicates roles in establishing muscle identity and neuronal recognition targets.

enalapril: MK-421; 1-[*N*-[1-ethoxycarbonyl)-3-phenylpropyl]-L-proline; a rapidly absorbed, long-acting agent used to treat some forms of hypertension. It is converted to a dicarboxyl derivative that inhibits **angiotensin converting enzyme** (*q.v.*).

enameloblasts: ameloblasts.

enanthic acid: heptanoic acid.

enantiomers: mirror image pairs of chemical compounds; *see* **stereoisomerism**.

encephalization: (1) formation of the brain; (2) concentration of sensory, coordinating, and other structures in the head region.

encephalon: brain.

enclomiphene: zuclomiphene; the *cis* isomer of **clomiphene citrate** (*q.v.*). It is a non-steroidal mixed agonist-antagonist for estrogen receptors.

endemic: characteristic of a specific geographical locale.

endemic goiters: thyroid gland enlargements prevalent in certain geographic locales. The most common cause is iodine deficiency, in regions where the soil and foods are low in iodine content, and where iodized table salt or other supplements are not used. Thyroxine synthesis is impaired (or shut down), and loss of its negative feedback control leads to excessive secretion of thyroid stimulating hormone (TSH). *See* also **goiters**, **colloid goiters**, and **goitrogens**.

endergonic reactions: reactions that take up free energy; *cf* **endothermic reactions**. They are usually coupled to exergonic types that provide the energy.

endochondral: occurring or formed within cartilage.

endochondral ossification: replacement of cartilage with bone, a process that contributes to the development and maturation of most parts of the vertebrate skeleton; *cf* **intramembranous ossification**. Formation of a long bone in a young fetus begins with a cartilaginous template enclosed in perichondrium. A periosteal collar then surrounds the perichondrium of the mid-diaphyseal region, sets up a primary ossification center by replacing chondrocytes with osteoblasts, and sends blood vessels and cells to the interior that carve out a marrow cavity. Secondary ossification centers then form within the **epiphyses** (*q.v.*), and these become the sites for bone elongation. *See* also **bone remodeling**.

endocortin: *see* **lipomodulin**.

endocrine: describes (1) hormones secreted by one kind of cell that travel through body fluids to act on other cell types. Some authors restrict the term to regulators that are transported via the bloodstream, but others include paracrine types; (2) cells or organs (glands) that secrete hormones to surrounding fluids, for transport by blood (or other fluids) to their target sites. *See* also **endocrine glands**, and *cf* **autocrine**, **intracrine**, and **exocrine**.

endocrine glands: organs that synthesize substantial quantities of specific hormones types, and release them to extracellular spaces for uptake by the circulating blood and delivery to target organs. This "classical" definition is not as useful now as when it was formulated. Many hormones are made by cells that are not organized into glands (for example in the hypothalamus and gastrointestinal tract); and angiotensin II is one of several synthesized extracellularly. Moreover, many regulators now classified as hormones do not travel through the bloodstream. Insulin and some others exert both endocrine and paracrine actions; and some types released by glands function at other sites as neurotransmitters and/or neuromodulators.

endocrine pancreas: organized, innervated cell clumps (islets of Langerhans) embedded within exocrine pancreatic tissue. All contain insulin-secreting β, glucagon-secreting α, and additional cell types (mostly somatostatin-secreting δ in some, and mostly pancreatic polypeptide-secreting F in others). Some islets also contain gastrin-secreting G and other kinds.

endocrinomas: tumors that contain hormone-secreting endocrine cells. Most types make large quantities of the regulators, and are insensitive to the feedback controls exerted over their normal counterparts.

endocytic vesicles: *see* **endosomes**.

endocytosis: a physiological mechanism for taking up substances that do not enter directly via diffusion or active transport. The plasma membrane extends projections that encircle the substances, and then join to form vesicles, which are internalized; *see* also **pinocytosis** and **phagocytosis**. *Receptor-mediated* endocytosis requires expression of specific kinds of surfaces components, with outwardly directed ligand binding sites. Some are enclosed in clathrin coated pits. When low density lipoproteins (LDLs) are taken up in this way, the nutrients are retained, and the receptors are recycled to the plasma membranes. Some hormone-receptor complexes are sent to lysosomes, in which both components are degraded (*see* also **down regulation**), whereas receptors for some others return to the membranes. In thyroid glands, endocytosis contributes to hormone synthesis. Follicular cells take up thyroglobulin from the lumens via endocytosis, and they form phagolysosomes in which selective proteolysis releases free T_4 and some T_3.

endoderm: entoderm; the innermost of the three embryonic germ layers. Structures derived from it include the epithelia of the digestive, respiratory, and urinary tracts, much of the lung, liver, and pancreatic tissue, and the major components of the parathyroid, thyroid, and thymus glands. *Cf* **mesoderm** and **ectoderm**.

endoenzymes: enzymes that act (1) within cells; *cf* **ecto-enzymes**; (2) on internal components of molecules (*see*, for example **endopeptidases** and *cf* **exopeptidases**).

endogamy: inbreeding; the mating of individuals descended from a recent common ancestor; *cf* **exogamy**.

endogenous: developing or originating within a cell or organism; *cf* **exogenous**.

endogenous pyrogen: (1) interleukin-1; (2) any regulator produced within an organism that elevates body temperature; *see*, for example **tumor necrosis factor-α** (TNFα), interleukin-6, and **prostaglandin E$_2$** (PGE$_2$).

endoglycosidases: enzymes that catalyze hydrolysis of bonds between sugar (or sugar derivative) moieties of glycoprotein and glycopeptide oligosaccharides. Several types obtained from microorganisms are used in analyses, or to obtain specific kinds of products. Endoglycosidase D (Endo-D) from *Diplococcus pneumoniae* is a 280K protein with an optimum pH of 6.5 assayed with (mannose)$_5$(N-acetylglucosamine)$_2$-acetyl-Asn. Endoglycosidase F (endo-F), a 32K protein from *Flavobacterium meningosepticum* acts optimally in the pH range 5.0-7, and is assayed with dansyl-Asn(N-acetylglucosamine)$_2$ (mannose)$_5$. Endoglycosidase H, a 29K enzyme with an optimum pH range of 5.5-6.0, is assayed with the same substrate. It is made by *Streptomyces griseus* and *S. plicatus*, and is available as a recombinant obtained from *S. lividans*. Endo-β-galactosidase from *Bacteroides fragilis* is a 30K protein with a 5.8 pH optimum that releases galactose from bovine corneal keratin. Endo-α-N-acetylgalactosaminidase from *Diplococcus pneumoniae* has a pH optimum of 6.0-7.3, and is assayed with asialofetuin.

endolymph: the fluid within the membranous labyrinth (tunica media) of the inner ear. When sound waves initiate tympanic membrane (eardrum) vibrations, auditory ossicles amplify the signals and transmit them to the perilymph which, in turn, sets up vibrations in the endolymph. Auditory perception is mediated via hair cells in the endolymph compartment, which are activated when deformed by the vibrations.

endometrial cycles: regularly recurring changes in the cell layers that border the uterine lumen, in response to hormones released during ovarian cycles; *see* **endometrium**.

endometriosis: conditions caused by the presence of ectopic, hormone-responsive endometrial tissue (usually in the pelvic cavity or ovary). The manifestations include pelvic pain and dysmenorrhea.

endometritis: inflammation of the endometrium.

endometrium: the uterine lining, composed of epithelial cells directed toward the lumen, and underlying, vascularized stroma composed mostly of spindle shaped cells. In primates, it is functionally divisible into a stratum basale, and a stratum functionale (which includes stratum spongiosum and stratum compactum). Estrogen secreted during follicular phases of ovarian cycles initiates its preparation for implantation by stimulating cell proliferation and the lengthening of tubular gland-like structures, and by inducing progesterone receptors, and augmenting blood flow. Progesterone secreted during luteal phases promotes specializations that include gland coiling, and glycogen accumulation in the epithelial cells. It further augments stromal vascularity, promotes water retention, lowers estrogen receptor numbers, and suppresses mitotic activity. If conception does not occur, progesterone levels decline during late luteal phases, and prostaglandins mediate necrotic changes in the superficial cells and blood vessels; *see* **menstruation**. *See also* **implantation** and **parturition**.

endomitosis: endopolyploidy; chromosome replication that is not followed by formation of a mitotic apparatus and nuclear division. The process, which leads to aneuploidy, occurs under normal conditions in the salivary glands of some insects, and in many plant species.

endomixis: self-fertilization; union of sperm and ovum nuclei derived from the same individual.

endomorphy: the somewhat round body type of humans in which soft tissues and viscera predominate. It is commonly associated with moderately short stature; *cf* **ectomorphy** and **mesomorphy**.

endoneurium: (1) the thin layer of connective tissue that surrounds the axon of a myelinated nerve; *cf* **axolemma** and **perineurium**; (2) the Schwann cell layer that surrounds an unmyelinated axon.

endonexin: a fibroblast endoplasmic reticulum membrane protein that engages in calcium-dependent binding to some phospholipids (but not to cholesterol or sphingomyelin). It is related to a 36K brush border membrane protein that is phosphorylated by a *src* encoded tyrosine kinase, and to synexin with which it is co-distributes.

endonucleases: phosphodiesterases that catalyze cleavages of DNA and RNA internal bonds to yield polynucleotides and oligonucleotides. Endogenous enzymes are used for DNA repair, and during meiosis. *See* **restriction endonucleases**, and *cf* **exonucleases**.

endopeptidases: enzymes that catalyze cleavage of peptide and protein internal bonds, and thereby generate smaller proteins and peptides. Examples include pepsin and trypsin. *Cf* **exopeptidases**.

endoperoxides: highly reactive organic compounds that contain internal peroxide (O-O) groups, for example prostaglandins G_2 and H_2 (PGG_2 and PGH_2), and other precursors of thromboxanes, prostaglandins, and related eicosanoids.

endoperoxide isomerases: enzymes that act on the endoperoxide groups of prostaglandin G_2 (PGG_2) and related molecules, generate hydroxy and ketone derivatives, and are essential for the biosynthesis of prostacyclin, E type prostaglandins, thromboxanes, and other eicosanoids.

endoplasmic reticulum: ER; a network of interconnected membranes and vesicles that communicates with the Golgi apparatus and plasma membrane, and mediates intracellular trafficking of ions and molecules. *Rough* endoplasmic reticulum (RER), which is studded with ribosomes, provides sites for translocation of nascent proteins that are to be inserted into plasma membranes or incorporated into secretory granules (*see* **signal sequences**). *Smooth* ER holds enzymes for fatty acid, phospholipid, and steroid biosynthesis. In hepatocytes, it contains enzymes that catalyze conjugation and detoxification reactions.

endoplasmin: GRP; a 100K stress glycoprotein present in highest concentrations in endoplasmic reticulum. *See also* **glucose regulated proteins**.

endopolygeny: a type of asexual reproduction used by some parasites, that leads to formation of more than two individuals within the parent organism.

endopolyploidy: endomitosis.

endorphins: "endogenous morphines". The term was initially used for α-, β-, and γ-endorphins, and other peptides cleaved from the β-lipotropin component of proopiomelanocortin (POMC), that have common *N*-terminal metenkephalin pentapeptide sequences, and act on opioid receptors. It has been extended to include to peptides such as α- and β-neoendorphins made from prodynorphins and other precursors, and to the minute amounts of morphine, codeine and related compounds made in the brain. Various members of the group affect (among other things) mood and motivation; feeding, sexual, social, and other behaviors; memory; pain perception; immune system functions; smooth muscle contraction; and the secretion of adrenocorticotropic hormone (ACTH), growth hormone (GH), corticotropin releasing hormone (CRH) and other regulators. The major circulating peptide is β-endorphin that originates in adenohypophysial corticotropes. In the central nervous system, the highest endorphin levels are in the arcuate nuclei (with lesser amounts in the limbic system, midbrain, nucleus tractus solitarius and spinal cord). Endorphins are also made in the adrenal medulla, pancreatic islets, gastrointestinal tract, reproductive system, liver, kidney, some immune system cells, and elsewhere. The levels at some sites rise in response to several forms of stress. Production of POMC-derived types is inhibited indirectly by glucocorticoids.

α-endorphins: peptides identical to the first 15-17 amino acids of β-endorphins, and cleaved from those peptides. No specific target cells or receptors are known, but there are indications that they antagonize some effects of the parent peptide. The human type [β-lipotropin (1-16)], has the sequence H₂N-Tyr-Gly-Gly-Phe-Met-Thr-Ser-Glu-Lys-Ser-Gln-Thr-Pro-Leu-Val-Thr-OH.

β-endorphins: the most abundant endorphins derived from proopiomelanocortin (POMC). All vertebrate species make similar molecules. The human type [β-lipotropin (61-91), has the sequence:H₂N-Tyr-Gly-Gly-Phe-Met-Thr-Ser-Glu-Lys-Ser-Gln-Thr-Pro-Leu-Val-Thr-Leu-Phe-Lys-Asn-Ala-Ile-Ile-Lys-Asn-Ala-Tyr-Lys-Lys-Gly-Glu-OH. The circulating peptides originate primarily in corticolipotropes. They interact mostly with μ-type opioid receptors and invoke morphine-like effects; but high levels also activate δ and κ types. The processes affected include locomotor activity, food intake, body temperature control, immune system functions, responses to stress, the secretion of growth hormone, prolactin, gonadotropins, glucagon, insulin, and other hormones, and the release of some neurotransmitters. Roles in normal delay of puberty onset in juveniles, and in suppression of reproductive system functions in individuals who engage in very strenuous exercise, or with eating disorders, have been proposed. Many effects are linked with inhibition of adenylate cyclase activity (and compensatory synthesis of additional enzyme leads to hyperactivity when the peptide is withdrawn). In species possessing pars intermedia melanotropes, the peptides can be cleaved to β-endorphin 1-26 (a β-endorphin antagonist). They also undergo acetylation, which abolishes analgesic potency.

γ-endorphin: β-lipotropin(61-77); H$_2$N-Tyr-Gly-Gly-Phe-Met-Thr-Ser-Glu-Lys-Ser-Gln-Thr-Pro-Leu-Val-Thr-Leu-OH; a peptide cleaved from β-endorphin, with properties similar to those of α-endorphin.

endosmosis: **osmosis** (*q.v.*) in which water moves into the cell interior, or toward an internal cavity.

endosomes: uncoated (clathrin-free) vesicles formed during endocytosis. They fuse with CURL vesicles (which are acidic), and thereby provide an environment that facilitates uncoupling of ligands from receptors.

endosteum: the membrane that lines bone marrow cavities and Haversian canals. It contains osteoclasts, osteoblasts, and blood vessels, and is essential for bone remodeling.

endothelial cells: epithelial cells derived from mesoderm. They form a continuous lining layer for the blood vascular system (the heart, and all blood vessels) and for the lymphatic system, and are the major components of blood and lymph capillaries. In addition to providing smooth surfaces that protect erythrocytes and thrombocytes, and separate the platelets from collagens and other components of blood vessel walls, the cells perform numerous functions that vary with their locations and associations with other cell types, and with regional differences in cell sizes. Capillary endothelium is the site for passive diffusion of respiratory gases in the lungs, for delivery of nutrients to body tissue cells, and for removal of wastes from extracellular fluids. The cells play active roles in hemostasis by affecting platelet aggregation, exerting both stimulatory and inhibitory influences over blood coagulation, and promoting fibrinolysis. They contribute to leukocyte recruitment and inflammation, angiogenesis, blood pressure control, immune system responses, and acid-base balance; and they sequester natriuretic peptides and some other circulating hormones. Activators at various sites include histamine, thrombin, interleukins 1, 4, 6, and 8, tumor necrosis factor-α (TNF-α), and lipopolysaccharides. Regulators induced in activated cells include ELAM-1 (endothelial-leukocyte adhesion molecule-1), platelet activating factor (PAF), prostaglandins, prostacyclins, nitric oxide, urokinase type plasminogen activator, plasminogen activator inhibitor-1, some growth factors, and a factor that augments eosinophil toxicity. *See* also **endothelins**.

endothelial cell adhesion factor-1: *see* **endothelial cell-leukocyte adhesion molecule-1**.

endothelial cell growth factors: ECGFs; (1) hormones similar to or identical with α-fibroblast growth factors, that promote endothelial cell proliferation and migration, and contribute to wound repair. They are also potent mitogens for bone cells, but are less effective on smooth muscle, and appear to be inactive on fibroblasts and chondrocytes. (2) a term sometimes applied to any growth factor made by epithelial cells.

endothelial cell leukocyte adhesion molecule-1: ELAM-1; LECAM-2; E-selectin; glycoproteins expressed on the surfaces of endothelial cells activated by interleukin-1β, tumor necrosis factor-α (TNFα), lipopolysaccharides, and some other stimulants, that mediate adhesion to myeloid lineage leukocytes (neutrophils and eosinophils), to monocytes, to homing receptors for dermal T lymphocytes, and to some tumor cells (including human colon carcinoma types). They contribute to leukocyte margination, migration, and extravasation at sites of injury, and are implicated as major mediators of cutaneous inflammation and delayed hypersensitivity responses. In common with other selectins, they contain lectin domains that bind ligands described for CD62, as well as epidermal growth factor (EGF)-like domains, and amino acid sequences for binding fucosylated, sialylated ceramides. The major form is 115K, but small amounts of a 97K type (which may be a precursor) are also made. Dimers composed of 115K and 110K chains have also been identified.

endothelins: ETs; 21-amino-acid peptides made by epithelial cells that share sequence homologies and biological properties with sarafotoxins. Various isoforms (all with disulfide bonds that link cysteine moieties at positions 1→15 and 3→11) have been identified in the lungs, spleen, heart, kidneys, brain, eyes, bone, and gonads, as well as in the heart and intimal layers of large and small arteries and arterioles. They are cleaved from precursors via reactions catalyzed by endothelin converting enzyme (which acts on Trp-Val bonds). Expression of the subtypes (ET-1, ET-2, ET-3, and VIC, each controlled by its own gene) is tissue-specific and developmentally regulated. Endothelins are the most potent smooth muscle stimulants known. The greater potencies on resistance vessels of older individuals (as compared with young adults) are attributed to diminished opposition by relaxation factors, and may account for some of the hypertension that develops late in life. ETs also act on intestinal and respiratory tract smooth muscle. Most effects appear to be exerted locally. The peptides are continuously made in the aorta and large arteries, and their formation at those sites can be augmented by thrombin and oxidized low density lipoproteins (LDLs). Although there have been reports that substantial amounts are released to the bloodstream in some forms of hypertension, and that some ischemic damage is caused by toxic levels, the amounts that circulate in unstimulated healthy individuals appear to be very small. In smaller arteries and arterioles, stimulants for ET production include hypoxia and transforming growth factor-β (TGFβ). Prostaglandins exert some negative feedback control (but cyclooxygenase inhibitors do not exacerbate ET effects). Only minute amounts are required to elevate arterial blood pressure, in part because the peptides release renin, aldosterone, and catecholamines, exert both chronotropic and inotropic effects on the myocardium, and augment the effects of norepinephrine, serotonin, and other vasoconstrictors. Blood pressure can rise substantially if the amounts remain constant while inhibitors of nitric oxide generation are administered. Under physiological conditions, the duration of action is limited, because ETs release **endothelium derived relaxation factors** (*q.v.*), accelerate dissociation of natriuretic peptides from their binding sites, and inhibit Na^+/K^+-ATPases. However, stimuli that release large amounts can overcome the effects of antagonists. The vasoconstriction is preceded by a brief interval during which vasodilation occurs. High mean arterial blood pressure can then be sustained in most vascular beds, as renal plasma flow and glomerular filtration rates fall substantially. ETs contribute to the control of blood flow to the gastrointestinal tract, promote contraction of hepatic vessels, and also accelerate gluconeogenesis. They additionally stimulate mitogenesis in smooth muscle, fibroblasts, and glomerular mesangial cells (processes associated with induction of *c-fos* and *c-myc*), and may augment the effects of some transforming factors. Other effects include modulation of synaptic transmission, and contributions to hypothalamic control over growth hormone, gonadotropins, and possibly other pituitary gland hormones. In the ovaries, they are reported to protect against premature luteinization, and in bone ET-2 can stimulate osteoblasts. Endothelin receptors are widely distributed throughout the central nervous system, and are also found in the heart, lungs, kidney, adrenal gland, and pituitary gland. An ET_A type displays highest affinity for ET-1, but binds some ET-2, whereas an ET_B type binds all three peptides with approximately equal affinities. Both types have structures consistent with coupling to G proteins. Some effects are mediated via phospholipase C and induction of phosphoinositide cascades. Others involve activation of phospholipase A_2 and production of eicosanoids.

endothelin-1: ET-1; H_2N-Cys-Ser-Cys-Ser-Ser-Leu-Met-Asp-Lys-Glu-Cys-Val-Tyr-Phe-Cys-His-Leu-Asp-Ile-Ile-Trp-COOH; an **endothelin** (*q.v.*) that exerts potent, long-lasting effects on vascular smooth muscle and is also present in the dorsal root ganglia, spinal cord, and hypothalamus.

endothelin-2: ET-2: H_2N-Cys-Ser-Cys-Ser-Ser-Trp-Leu-Asp-Lys-Glu-Cys-Val-Tyr-Phe-Cys-His-Leu-Asp-Ile-Ile-Trp-COOH; an **endothelin** (*q.v.*) believed to exert mostly paracrine effects, and observed to promote bone formation.

endothelin-3: ET-3; H_2N-Cys-Thr-Cys-Phe-Thr-Tyr-Lys-Asp-Lys-Glu-Cys-Val-Tyr-Tyr-Cys-His-Leu-Asp-Ile-Ile-Trp-COOH; an endothelin made in neural and other tissues. It is less potent that endothelin-1 for stimulating vascular smooth muscle, and the hypertension invoked is preceded by greater vasodilation.

endothelin converting enzyme: *see* **endothelins**.

endotheliochorial: the placenta type in dogs, cats, ferrets, and some other mammals. The trophoblast interacts with maternal endothelium, but blood vessel walls are not disrupted during parturition; *cf* **hemochorial**.

endothelium: a tissue type that shares major properties with surface epithelium, but derives from mesoderm. The term is often used synonymously with vascular endothelium. *See* **endothelial cells**.

endothelium derived contraction factor: ECF_2; cyclooxygenase dependent endothelium derived contraction factor; one or more regulators released by endothelial cells that blunt the effects of acetylcholine, ADP, serotonin, and other mediators of vasodilation. The major component appears to be prostaglandin H_2.

endothelium-derived relaxation factor: EDRF; incompletely defined regulators made by endothelial cells that promote vasodilation, increase blood vessel permeability, and inhibit platelet aggregation. Small amounts are released by unstimulated cells, and larger ones in response to hypoxia, acetylcholine, histamine, bradykinin, and other vasoactive agents. They are essential for realization of the effects of those agents, and also of substance P, arachidonic acid, ATP and ADP on vascular smooth muscle, and for opposing excessive effects of endothelins and some other vasoconstrictors. However, they do not seem to interact with catecholamines, adenosine, or vasoactive intestinal peptide (VIP). Although **nitric oxide** (NO), *q.v.*, appears to be the major component at many sites, and inhibitors of NO synthesis elevate the levels at some, nitrosamines, nitrosothiols, and other nitric oxidation products may contribute; and prostacyclin and other as yet unidentified arachidonic acid metabolites derived via the epoxygenase pathway may also be involved.

endotherms: homeotherms; animals that maintain fairly constant body temperatures despite substantial variations in environmental temperatures and/or exposure to sunlight. The term "warm blooded" has been applied, since, in most locales, the body temperatures are higher than those of the environment. *Cf* **ectotherms**.

endothermic: describes chemical reactions that take up heat from the environment; *cf* **endergonic** and **exothermic**.

endotoxins: (1) poisons released by microorganisms when their membranes are disrupted; *cf* **exotoxins**; (2) specifically, LPS (bacterial pyrogen), a lipopolysaccharide released from the cell walls of gram-positive bacteria. The lipid A component, composed of six fatty acid chains linked to two glucosamine moieties, promotes release of tumor necrosis factor-α (TNF-α), interleukin-1, and other mediators; and most manifestations of serious infections (including fever, leukopenia, thrombocytopenia, and circulatory shock) are attributed to those peptides. LPS molecules additionally contain a core oligosaccharide and a polysaccharide.

endozepine: diazepine binding inhibitor; DBI; an 8.2K somewhat acidic brain protein that modulates chloride channel activity by inhibiting diazepam binding to $GABA_A$ type γ-aminobutyric acid receptors. It also acts peripherally on mitochondrial membranes of many cell types and accelerates cholesterol side-chain cleavage; *see* **steroidogenesis**.

end-product inhibition: inhibition of a metabolic pathway by a final product that acts on one or more of the enzyme components. Usually, a single, rate-limiting step is affected.

end-product repression: inhibition of a metabolic pathway by high levels of a final product that acts on the operon, and thereby controls the synthesis of one or more key enzymes.

energy: the capacity to do work. One form (chemical, electrical, mechanical, or photic) can be converted to another; *see* also **kinetic**, **potential**, **activational**, and **free** energy, **thermodynamics**, and **transducers**.

energy-rich bonds: chemical bonds (such as the ones between the α and β, or β and γ phosphate groups of ATP and GTP) that require large amounts of energy to form, and release substantial amounts when the molecules are hydrolyzed. Although some of the energy released is lost as heat, much of it is used to drive endergonic reactions.

Engrailed: a *Drosophila* gene that determines segment polarity.

engrams: sets of neuronal changes associated with memory.

enhancers: *cis*-acting eukaryotic DNA base sequences, located mostly upstream from promoters, that accelerate RNA polymerase II-directed gene transcription. A single enhancer can act on many promoters, but it usually exerts its major effects on the nearest one. Enhancers retain their ability to stimulate when relocated to other gene regions, and when re-inserted after deletion and inversion. *See* also **enhancer proteins**.

enhancer proteins: proteins that augment gene transcription by binding to enhancers. Examples include ligand bound receptors for steroid, thyroid, and other some hormones, and many oncogene and proto-oncogene products that form DNA-binding dimers.

enkephalins: opioid pentapeptides made in the brain, pituitary gland, adrenal medulla, reproductive tract, and other parts of the body. They interact with δ type opioid receptors to affect behavior, the release of several neurotransmitters and hormones, and other functions. *See* **leu-enkephalin**, **metenkephalin**, **prodynorphin**, and **proenkephalin**.

enkephalin convertase: a carboxypeptidase E that catalyzes cleavage of precursor proteins to yield enkephalins. It also degrades atrial natriuretic peptides and acts on some other substrates. *See* also **prohormone converting enzymes** and **furin**.

enkephalinases: metalloproteinases that catalyze rapid degradation of enkephalins and related peptides.

enolases: (1) enzymes that catalyzes reversible reactions of the general type shown; (2) the enzyme of the glycolysis pathway that catalyzes conversion of 2-phosphoglycerate to phosphoenolpyruvate. A specific isoform (neuron specific enolase) is used as a marker for neuroendocrine cells.

Enovid: a trade name for several oral contraceptive preparations that contain mestranol (a synthetic estrogen), and norethynodrel (a synthetic progestin). Enovid E contains 100 μg of mestranol and 2.5 mg. of norethynodrel per pill. Enovid 5 has 75 ug mestranol plus 5.0 mg

$$\underset{\text{enolases}}{\overset{\displaystyle \begin{array}{l} | \\ \text{HC}-\text{O}-\text{X} \\ | \\ \text{CH}_2-\text{OH} \end{array} \rightleftharpoons \begin{array}{l} | \\ \text{HC}-\text{O}-\text{X} \\ \| \\ \text{CH}_2 \end{array} + \text{HOH}}{}}$$

norethynodrel, and Enovid 10 has 150 μg mestranol and 9.85 mg norethynodrel.

entactin: nidogen; a basement membrane glycoprotein that mediates cell adhesion.

enteramine: an undefined intestinal smooth muscle stimulant; it may be identical to serotonin.

enteric: related to the intestine.

enterochromaffin cells: EC cells: gastrointestinal tract cells that secrete serotonin and other amines, named for their staining with chromium and silver dyes. Some secrete catecholamines, and small numbers in the ileum make substance P.

enterocrinin: an undefined hormonal stimulant of intestinal motility. The candidates include glucose-dependent insulinotropic peptide (GIP), and vasoactive intestinal peptide (VIP).

enterocytes: intestinal epithelial cells.

enterogastrone: an undefined hormone released from the duodenum following fat ingestion that inhibits gut motility, gastric emptying, and gastric gland secretion, and functions as a satiety factor. Glucose-dependent insulinotropic peptide (GIP, formerly called gastric inhibitory peptide) may exert much of the activity.

enteroglucagons: gut hormones that cross-react with antibodies directed against pancreatic glucagon, and exert similar (but less potent) effects on carbohydrate metabolism. They also affect stomach and intestine motility, gastric gland functions, and sugar absorption. Pancreatectomy augments the secretory responses to meal ingestion. The major forms are **oxyntomodulin** and **glicentin** (*q.v.*). They are made from precursors that yield glucagon at other sites, but have *C*-terminal extensions.

enterohepatic circulation: recycling of body chemicals via biliary secretion followed by intestinal absorption. It permits recovery of useful molecules. For example, bile salts are made in the liver and released (directly or after storage in the gall bladder) to the small intestine. After performing their roles in digestion and absorption of dietary lipids, they are returned to the liver. Some of the thyroxine that enters the bile is lost to the feces; but substantial amounts can be reabsorbed into the bloodstream.

enteroinsular axis: control systems that involve interactions between pancreatic islet and intestinal cells. For example, food-related stimuli in the gut relay hormonal and parasympathetic system messages to the endocrine pancreas that promote insulin secretion and inhibit glucagon release, and thereby protect against development of prandial hyperglycemia. Insulin promotes rapid disposal of absorbed sugars (by promoting its uptake into muscle, adipose tissue and others cells, and more slowly affecting its metabolism); but it also accelerates the absorption of glucose and some other sugars. If the blood sugar levels rise too steeply, both the gut and the islet cells release somatostatin (which slows food absorption and adds to the inhibition of glucagon release). If food high in protein and low in carbohydate content is ingested, insulin facilitates amino acid use; but it can at such times invoke hypoglycemia. The problem is averted by then releasing glucagon. Enteroglucagon can contribute, since it promotes glycogenolysis and exerts several kinds of inhibitory influences on digestion; but it can also promote more insulin release. *See* also **gut-islet-gut axis** and **anticipatory controls**.

enterokinase: an endopeptidase released by cells of the small intestine following meal ingestion, that initiates trypsinogen conversion to trypsin. When sufficient amounts are formed, trypsin then becomes the major activator of the remaining trypsinogen.

enteron: the gut.

enterooxyntin: EO; a putative regulator of gastric acidity, different from gastrin, that acts indirectly by promoting histamine or acetylcholine release.

enterotoxins: exotoxins released by *Vibrio cholera, Clostridium birefringens, Staphylococci,* some *Escherichia coli* strains, and some other microorganisms that infect the intestines. Several types cause diarrhea by disrupting normal controls over water and electrolyte transport in the intestines. They augment guanylate cyclase activity, increase chloride excretion, and decrease water and sodium ion reabsorption; see also **guanylin**. Other diseases initiated by enterotoxins involve disruption of immune system functions that lead to overproduction of interleukin-2 and other cytokines (see **superantigens**). The consequences can include toxic shock syndrome, auto-immune attacks against previously normal cells, and possibly also, deterioration of T cell functions in individuals with acquired immune deficiency syndrome (AIDS).

enterovirus: any microorganism of the genus *Picornaviridae*. Most types preferentially replicate in the intestines, but some enter other structures. The group includes *polioviruses, echoviruses,* and *Coxsackie viruses*.

enthalpy: a measure of the heat content of a system, usually represented by the symbol H. *See* also **endother-**

mic and **exothermic reactions, free energy** and **entropy**.

entoderm: endoderm.

entropy: (1) a measure of the amount of energy in a system that is not available for useful work, usually represented by the symbol S; (2) a measure of the randomness or disorder of a system. Entropy increases, for example when spontaneous processes such as diffusion down concentration gradients, or reversible chemical reactions are permitted to proceed to equilibrium, and when macromolecules are converted to smaller products. It is related to enthalpy and free energy by the equation: $\Delta G = \Delta H - T\Delta S$, where ΔG = the change in free energy at constant temperature and pressure, ΔH is the change in enthalpy, and ΔS the change in entropy. Reactions can proceed spontaneously (i.e. without energy input from external sources) if the value of ΔG is negative, and if the sum of the change in entropy of the system plus the change in entropy of the environment has a positive value.

ENU: *N*-ethyl-nitrosourea.

env: structural retrovirus genes that code for envelope glycoproteins. The products are essential for virus replication, and they contribute to the associated pathogenesis.

enzyme[s]: organic molecules that bind to and catalyze cleavage of specific substrates. They accelerate reaction rates in both directions by lowering activation energies, but do not directly affect equilibrium points. Most enzymes are proteins, but *see* **ribozymes**.

enzyme-linked assays: sensitive methods for identifying specific metabolites or cell types that employ enzyme markers linked to specific antibodies. *See* **ELISA**.

enzyme-linked immunosorbent assays: *see* **ELISA**.

EO: enterooxyntin.

EO-CSF: eosinophil colony stimulating factor; *see* **interleukin-5**.

eosins: acidic dyes that bind proteins, and are used as histological stains (directly, or as counterstains with hematoxylin or methylene blue). Secretory granules of eosinophilic leukocytes, somatotropes, lactotropes, and parathyroid hormone secreting cells avidly take up the dyes. Eosin yellowish (YS) (2′,4′,5′,7-tetrabromofluore-

eosin yellowish

eosin I bluish

scein) imparts a bright red color, and is also used in cosmetics. Eosin I bluish is 4′,5′-dibromo-dinitro-fluorescein sodium salt.

eosinophil: (1) any cell that stains with eosin; (2) *see* **eosinophilic leukocytes**.

eosinophilia: excessive numbers of circulating eosinophilic leukocytes. The condition is most often invoked by environmental or food allergens, or parasitic infections.

eosinophilia myalgia syndrome: EMS; blood dyscrasias, skeletal muscle pain and paralysis, and other symptoms attributed to ingestion of contaminants in tryptophan preparations used as food supplements or to treat insomnia. *See* **tryptophan**.

eosinophil cationic proteins: ECP: at least 7 proteins released from the granules of activated eosinophilic leukocytes that act most effectively at alkaline pHs and mediate toxicity. Some adhere directly to parasites and promote formation of plasma membrane pores. The term is also applied to a specific 21K form that kills helminths.

eosinophil chemotactic factors: ECF; peptides that stimulate directed migration of eosinophilic leukocytes. The ones produced by activated T lymphocytes and mast cells contribute to inflammatory reactions. Estradiol stimulates ECF production in uterine stroma, where eosinophils are implicated as mediators of water imbibition, augmented blood flow, and other early (nongenomic) responses to that hormone. Progesterone and glucocorticoids antagonize the estrogen effects.

eosinophilic chemotactic peptides: a term applied to certain chemotactic factors released during allergic responses, including some made by eosinophilic leukocytes, but also to tetrapeptides Val-Gly-Ser-Glu and Ala-Gly-Ser-Glu, which are released by mast cells.

eosinophil-derived neurotoxin: a heavily glycosylated 53-amino acid peptide made by eosinophilic leukocytes that contributes to trypanosome killing. It has ribonuclease activity and is identical with a ribonuclease found in human urine, but does not appear to be cytotoxic when presented alone. Its entry into cells may depend on the simultaneous presence of eosinophil cationic proteins that act on plasma membrane channels.

eosinophil differentiation factor: EDF; (1) **interleukin-6** (*q.v.*); (2) any peptide that promotes maturation of eosinophilic leukocyte precursor cells. Interleukin-3 (also known as eosinophil stimulating factor, ESF) acts on hemopoietic stem cells. Granulocyte-macrophage colony stimulating factor (GM-CSF) affects more mature cells types. Neither peptide is specific for eosinophilic lineages.

eosinophilic leukocytes: eosinophils; white blood cells with granules that stain bright red with acidic dyes. They differentiate from bone marrow myeloid precursors, and normally account for 2-6% of the total circulating blood leukocytes. They are activated by IgE type immunoglobulins, and their numbers increase during allergic and some inflammatory reactions, and following parasitic infestation. Eosinophils contribute to inflammation, are directly cytotoxic to some protozoa and helminths, and

can (under some conditions) injure healthy body cells. Many of the effects are mediated via eosinophil cationic proteins, major basic protein, leukotrienes C_4 and D_4, eosinophil peroxidase, and other factors they release from secretory granules; but they also stimulate other cells to secrete tumor necrosis factors and other cytokines.

eosinophil peroxidase: EPO; an enzyme released from the granules of activated eosinophilic leukocytes that generates free radicals, contributes to parasite killing, and can damage normal cells. It is implicated as one of the factors that mediates respiratory tract damage in individuals with asthma.

eosinophil stimulating factor: ESF; *see* **eosinophil differentiating factor**.

eosinophilopoietin: a small peptide that regulates eosinophilic leukocyte maturation. It may be identical with interleukin-5.

epalrestat: 3-carboxymethyl-5-(2-methylcinnamylodine)rhodanine; an inhibitor of **aldose reductase** (*q.v.*). It is used to protect against the development of cataracts and neuropathies in individuals with diabetes mellitus.

ependyma: usually, (1) the central nervous system layer

formed by ependymal cells; (2) the inner cell layer of the embryonic neural tube.

ependymal cells: tanycytes; neuroglial cells that line cerebral ventricles. They regulate transfers of substances between blood and cerebrospinal fluid. Some make vasopressin and/or other regulators, and have hormone receptors.

ependymins: acidic glycoproteins identified in goldfish brain ependyma, and implicated as mediators of learning and memory.

EPF: early pregnancy factor.

ephedrine: 1-phenyl-2-methylaminopropanol; a long-acting, orally effective, nonspecific agonist for both α and β type adrenergic receptors that also displaces catecholamines from synaptic vesicles. It relaxes respiratory tract smooth muscle, but promotes vasoconstriction and mydriasis, and stimulates the myocardium and central nervous system neurons. Although initially extracted from *Ephedra* species, it is now synthesized. Various preparations (including nasal sprays) are used to treat asthma, relieve congestion, and counteract the hypotension associated with anesthesia.

226

epi-: a prefix (1) that means up, above, over, outside, or next to; (2) used to name isomers; *see* **epimers**.

epiandrosterone: isoandrosterone; 3β-hydroxy-17-androstan-17-one; a 17-ketosteroid excreted to urine in small amounts. It is a weak androgen.

epiblast: the outer part of the embryonic ectoderm that gives rise to the skin and its derivatives.

epicanthus: a vertical skin fold that extends upward from the lower eyelid along the side of the nose.

epidermal chalone: *see* **epidermal mitosis inhibitor**.

epidermal derivatives: structures that derive from epidermis, such as hair, fur, feathers, fingernails, claws, and also sweat, mammary, and sebaceous glands.

epidermal growth factor: EGF; Asn-Ser-Tyr-Pro-Gly-Cys-Pro-Ser-Ser-Tyr-Asp-Gly-Tyr-Cys-Leu-Asn-Gly-Gly-Val-Cys-Met-His-Ile-Glu-Ser-Leu-Asp-Ser-Tyr-Thr-Cys-Asn-Cys-Val-Ile-Gly-Tyr-Ser-Gly-Asp-Arg-Cys-Gln-Thr-Arg-Asp-Leu-Arg-Trp-Trp-Glu-Leu-Arg; a 53-amino acid, 6K peptide hormone with disulfide bonds that link the cysteine moieties at positions 6:20, 14:31, and 32:42. In addition to two EGF sequences, the 72K precursor from which it is cleaved also contains two 29K arginine esteropeptidase domains similar to ones in nerve growth factor (NGF) precursors, that liberate the 6K peptides. Urogastrone is a urinary protein with 70% amino acid homology that exerts similar actions. In humans, most circulating EGF originates in the kidneys. Other sources include blood platelets and some tumor cell types. Lactating mammary glands secrete it to milk; and local production for mostly paracrine (and possibly also autocrine) functions has been described for adenohypophysis, placenta and other organs. EGF shares substantial sequence homology with transforming growth factor-α (TGFα) and amphiregulin, and is more distantly related to the growth factors of vaccinia, Shope fibroma, and myxoma viruses. Other proteins that contain EGF-like domains include tissue plasminogen activator, clotting factors VII, IX, X, and XI, proteins C and S, several basement membrane and extracellular matrix proteins (including laminin, entactin, proteoglycan core particles, and fibronectins), some *Drosophila* types (for example the Notch protein that directs sensory organ differentiation), and proteins identified in nematodes, sea urchins, and malaria parasites. EGF exerts numerous influences on growth, proliferation, and differentiation, and on the activities of several epithelial and mesoderm-derived cell types; and it is a major contributor to fetal development and wound healing. Some effects involve induction of c-*fos* and c-*myc* products, and activation of ornithine decarboxylase, phospholipase C-II isozymes, numerous protein kinases (including mitogen activated [MAP]

types, as well as casein kinase II, S-6 kinase and thymidine kinase). It also binds to and modulates the activity of inositol-3-phosphate kinase, promotes phosphorylation of several plasma membrane components, accelerates nutrient uptake, exerts influences on Na^+/K^+-ATPases, and causes cytoplasmic alkalinization by increasing Na^+/H^+ counterport. Since it additionally modulates growth hormone release, stimulates the secretion of prolactin, of corticotropin releasing, adrenocorticotropic, and luteinizing hormones (CRH, ACTH, and LH), and of chorionic gonadotropin, placental prolactin, and cortisol, some effects in whole organisms are indirect. EGF additionally promotes eicosanoid synthesis, but inhibits testosterone, estrogen, progesterone, and thyroxine secretion. It stimulates proliferation and keratinization of skin epithelium, proliferation of glial cells, mammary gland growth, and lung maturation, and can promote growth of cartilage, and of the liver, kidneys, and adrenal glands. In the stomach, it inhibits acid secretion, but exerts trophic effects on gastric mucosa and facilitates the healing of peptic ulcers. Its ability to inhibit adipocyte differentiation may be physiologically important, since *ob/ob* rodents are among the obese animal strains that are deficient in either the hormone or its receptors. EGF additionally reduces thymus gland weights, inhibits collagen synthesis in osteoblasts, promotes bone resorption, and antagonizes the antidiuretic effects of vasopressin. In infant rodents, exogenous EGF accelerates eye opening, tooth-eruption, and hair growth, and is implicated in neuron maturation. Large amounts of the hormone are made in the submaxillary glands of adult males, in which the production is controlled by androgens, and from which norepinephrine-regulated release appears to promote aggression. EGF also stimulates salivary gland growth factor secretion. In female rodents, the salivary gland levels rise during pregnancy, the placenta acquires large numbers of receptors, and roles in fetal development and survival have been described. Dysregulation can invoke or contribute to transformation and tumorigenesis. Gene amplification has been observed in human glioblastomas, squamous cell carcinomas, and some other tumor types. Excessive numbers of EGF receptors, and/or abnormal forms occur in several other kinds of carcinoma cells; but coexistence of neu and possibly other proteins may be needed to elicit transformation in some (*see* also **epidermal growth factor receptors**). In breast cancers, the numbers of EGF receptors correlate negatively with the numbers for steroid hormones. Mechanisms that protect normal cells include negative controls over EGF production by triiodothyronine (T_3), estrogen, and other regulators, decreased sensitivities that accompany maturation in some cell types, and EGF down-regulation of its own receptors, as well as influences on the numbers for receptors for T_3 and other hormones. Some defects associated with diabetes mellitus (including oligospermia) have been linked with EGF deficiency.

epidermal growth factor receptors: EGFRcs. The major type identified in rodents that binds EGF with high affinity and mediates most of its actions is a ERBB1, a 1186-amino acid, 170K transmembrane glycoprotein with many *N*-linked oligosaccharide groups whose synthesis is directed by the *c-erbB-1* proto-oncogene. The very similar human counterpart is HER-1. The extracellular (ligand recognition) domains also bind transforming growth factor-α (TGF-α), amphiregulin, and a vaccinia virus growth factor. (However, although some actions are mediated via the EGF receptor, TGFα additionally acts on its own receptors, and is a more potent stimulant for angiogenesis, bone decalcification, and some other effects). Several hormones exert localized controls over ERBB1 expression. For example, the receptor numbers are increased by follicle stimulating hormone (FSH) in granulosa cells of the ovary, by thyroid hormones in the liver, skin, and mammary glands, by retinoic acid in the kidneys, by growth hormone in the liver, and by 1,25-dihydroxyvitamin D in bone. EGF binding activates a cytoplasmic tyrosine kinase domain, and promotes autophosphorylation. The activated receptor acts on phospholipase CII, phosphatidylinositol-3-kinase, Raf-1, progesterone receptors, gastrins, growth hormone, myosin light chains, glycolytic enzymes, and calpactins. Topoisomerase activity co-purifies with the receptor, but may be a contaminant. Some of the substrates are kinase components of cascades that catalyze serine-threonine phosphorylations. Transmodulation of the receptor, with consequent diminution of affinity for EGF, by phorbol esters, bombesin, arginine vasopressin, and platelet derived growth factor has been linked with activation of kinase C isozymes. A truncated (95K) protein that lacks the transmembrane domain derives from the *erbB1* gene. It is secreted, and is believed to be a ligand for some membrane-bound growth factor receptors. The possibility that it limits the activities of the larger EGF receptor by competing for the ligand has also been suggested. A *c-erbB2* protooncogene on the same chromosome codes for a very similar product (ERBB2; neu, p185, in rodents and HER-2 in humans). The *neu* gene was initially identified in neuroblastomas. Its product does not bind directly to EGF receptors, but is phosphorylated by the ligand bound EGF receptor. Overexpression has been described for some mammary gland and ovarian tumors, and is linked with poor prognosis. It also occurs in some other tumor types. A mutant form of the receptor is made by an avian erythroblastosis virus, and is directly implicated in the etiology of erythroid leukemia in chickens, and of some angiosarcomas. A related *c-erbB3* gene resides on a different chromosome. Some cell types (such as keratinocytes) express all three kinds of receptors, whereas others have one or two. *V-erbB* is a related, but mutated gene that codes for a truncated intracellular protein that lacks the ligand-binding domain and is constitutively active.

epidermal Langerhans cell *see* **Langerhans cells**.

epidermal mitosis inhibiting peptide: pGlu-Glu-Asp-Ser-Gly-OH; a tetrapeptide implicated as a chalone that protects against excessive cell proliferation in the epidermis.

epidermis: the outer epithelium of a plant or animal. In skin, mitosis proceeds only in the germinal layer closest to the underlying dermis. As the cells are pushed outward by ones newly formed, they undergo terminal differentiation (*see* also **keratinocytes** and **melanocytes**). Those closest to the free surface (farthest from the blood supply) then deteriorate, die, and are eventually sloughed. In addition to providing protection against mechanical injury, entry of many chemicals and microorganisms, and dehydration, skin epidermis produces parathyroid hormone-like peptide and other regulators, and contributes to immune system functions. In many species, cells exposed to ultraviolet radiation accumulate 7-dehydrocholesterol, which is converted by ultraviolet radiation to cholecalciferol (vitamin D_3) and related secosteroids. The epidermis of some ectothermic vertebrates contains poison glands, and is a major source of thyrotropin releasing hormone.

epididymal fluid: the aqueous fluid secreted to the lumen of the epididymis. It contains glycoproteins that are deposited on sperm surfaces, some of which may inhibit premature capacitation, glycerophosphorylcholine (which stabilizes the membranes, acts in conjunction with potassium ions to maintain a high osmotic pressure, and is hydrolyzed by an esterase in the female tract), and substances essential for sperm survival, maturation, storage, and transport. Carnitine is a component taken up by sperm and released in small amounts with semen. Additional factors act on the seminal vesicles and prostate gland.

epididymis [**epididymides**]: paired male accessory reproductive organs, located within the scrotum in most species, that receive spermatozoa from the efferent ductules of the testes, and later deliver them to the vas deferens. The organs are essential for sperm maturation, storage, and transport, and for phagocytosis of abnormal and deteriorating gametes. As sperm travel successively through caput, corpus, and cauda regions, they gradually acquire the ability to swim. (However, they are not yet capable of fertilization; *see* **capacitation**). Testosterone directly promotes differentiation of the epididymides from the Wolffian ducts, but dihydrotestosterone is the major regulator of pubertal growth and maturation, and is essential for maintaining the functions. The levels required are much higher than those of the blood plasma. They are achieved by taking up testosterone from the testes via countercurrent exchange mechanisms, and by the high 5α-reductase activity of epididymal cells. A contraceptive method under investigation employs androgen doses sufficient to maintain adequate levels in the bloodstream. By exerting negative feedback control over LH secretion, the steroids inhibit testosterone secretion in the testis and thereby deprive the epididymis of the amounts required for sperm maturation. Progestins administered along with the androgens augment the effects.

epidural: overlying the dura mater; *cf* **subdural**. The epidural space, which is filled with fatty connective tissue and contains blood vessels, separates the dura mater from the vertebral canal wall. Spinal anesthetics and other agents are injected into the space.

epiestriols: 16-epiestriol(16β,17β), 17-epiestriol(16α, 17α), 16,17-estriol(16β,17α), and certain other estriol isomers. Some are synthesized in fetoplacental units, and taken up by the maternal bloodstream. Small amounts are directly excreted to maternal urine, but most are first conjugated with sulfate or glucuronate in the liver.

epigamic: attractive or stimulatory to the opposite sex during courtship.

epigamous: occurring after fertilization.

epigastrium: the abdominal wall above the navel.

epigenesis: the concept that development is initiated in undifferentiated, pluripotential cells, and proceeds via a series of orderly changes. **Preformation** (*q.v.*) is an older idea that has been rejected.

epigenetics: the study of mechanisms by which genes invoke gradually developing changes that culminate in attainment of adult phenotypes.

epiglycans: high molecular weight cell surface sialo-glycoproteins that mask histocompatibility antigens and thereby block immune system attacks. They have been identified on some mouse carcinoma cells.

epilepsy: several neurological disorders in which spontaneous episodic electrical discharges spread across wide regions of the brain, and cause convulsions and loss of consciousness. The kindling is attributed to abnormal NMDA type excitatory amino acid receptor activity. It can be opposed by bicuculline (a $GABA_A$ agonist).

epiligrin: a glycoprotein in most epithelial cell basement membranes that binds integrin $\alpha_3\beta_1$, and co-localizes with integrin $\alpha_6\beta_4$ in hemidesome-like anchoring contacts. It is a major cell adhesion molecule for skin epidermis; *see* also **very late antigens**.

epimers: diastereoisomer pairs (for example D-glucose and D-mannose, or D-glucose and D-galactose), whose members differs from each other only in the the positions of chemical groups attached to a one asymmetric carbon atom. *See* **epimerases**, and *cf* **enantiomers**.

epimerases: enzymes that catalyze translocations of chemical groups form one position to another around a single asymmetric carbon atom. For example, one type catalyzes conversion of uridine-diphosphate-α-D-gluco-pyranose (UDPG) to UDP-galactose.

epimere: the dorsal part of a somite that gives rise to muscles innervated by a nearby spinal nerve dorsal ramus.

epimestrol: 3-methoxy-17-epiestriol; an estriol derivative that stimulates gonadotropin release and ovulation.

epimorphin: a 150K protein made by fibroblasts, and identified on the surfaces of embryonic mouse mesen-

epimestrol

chymal cells. It induces epithelial cell differentiation, and is essential for normal organization of epithelium, possibly via influences on cytoskeletons. Its expression appears to be regulated posttranscriptionally (since it is made in cells organized into mesenchymal tissues, but not in monolayers of cells derived from them).

epimorphosis: (1) regeneration of organized tissue in which cell proliferation precedes specialization; (2) regeneration that begins with cell proliferation at a cut surface.

epimutation: DNA changes that do not involve base substitutions, for example translocations or insertions that affect gene activation.

epinephrine: E; adrenalin; 1-(3,5-dihydroxyphenyl)-2-(methylamino)ethanol; a hormone and neurotransmitter synthesized from norepinephrine (N) in some adrenal medulla cells, and in limited numbers of brain neurons, via a reaction catalyzed by phenylethanolamine-*N*-methyl-transferase (PNMT). Glucocorticoids released by the adrenal cortex into blood vessels that travel directly to the adrenal medulla directly induce the enzyme. In common with N, it acts via β_1 receptors to exert potent inotropic and chronotropic effects on the myocardium, and via α_1 types to promote vasoconstriction in skin and mucous membranes of the respiratory and gastrointestinal tracts, and to inhibit gastrointestinal tract motility. However, unlike N, which exerts only vasoconstrictor effects on blood vessels, elevates both systolic and diastolic pressures, and invokes reflex bradycardia, E additionally acts on β_2 type receptors. Since it dilates blood vessels that supply liver and skeletal muscle, it does not usually raise the diastolic blood pressure. Rather, it tends to elevate only systolic pressure, accelerate the heart rate, and increase cardiac output. Another β_2-mediated response, relaxation of respiratory tract smooth muscle, makes it useful for emergency treatment of asthma. It also indirectly raises blood glucose levels by stimulating glycogenolysis in skeletal muscle. The glucose-phosphate released enters the glycolysis pathway (and

16-epiestriol

17-epiestriol sulfate

16,17-epiestriol

provides energy for contraction). Much of the lactic acid formed travels to the liver, in which it is converted to glucose. Some is taken up by cardiac muscle and used directly as fuel; and circulating lactic acid provides a stimulus for the respiratory center in the medulla oblongata. E stimulates lipolysis in white adipose tissue, and acts on β_3 type adrenergic receptors in brown adipose tissue to augment oxygen consumption and metabolic rate. In the brain, it increases alertness and can invoke sensations of anxiety. Most β receptor effects are mediated via cAMP, whereas most α types involve elevation of cytosolic Ca^{2+} levels. The stimuli for increased E release include hypoglycemia and stress. The effects are short-lived, if the hormone is not continuously released, because (in common with other catecholamines), E is rapidly taken up by synaptic vesicles, and by secretory granules of the adrenal medulla. It is also slowly degraded by monoamine oxidases and catecholamine-*O*-methyltransferase (COMT).

epinine: *N*-methyldopamine; an amine synthesized in small amounts by catecholamine-secreting cells under normal conditions, and in larger ones when the metabolism is altered, for example with monoamine oxidase (MAO) inhibitors. Although classified as a **false transmitter** (*q.v.*), it exerts mostly dopamine-like effects, and can be converted to epinephrine.

epiphysial line: *see* **epiphysis**.

epiphysis: (1) the part of a long bone between the metaphysis and the articular cartilage that develops from a secondary ossification center. In juveniles, an *epiphyseal plate* separates the diaphysis from the epiphysis. One component, a quiescent "zone of reserve cartilage", composed of small chondrocytes in extracellular matrix, anchors the plate to epiphysial bone. Directly beneath it, a "zone of proliferating cartilage" supplies new cells, and contributes to growth of the plate. The older cells of the proliferating region enter the "zone of hypertrophic cartilage", in which further elongation is accomplished by cell growth. The enlarged cells then enter the "zone of calcified cartilage", in which minerals are deposited into the matrix, and chondrocytes die. New bone is added to the diaphysis when phagocytes take up the calcified matrix, and the region is invaded by osteoblasts and blood vessels. During adolescence, the epiphysial plate is gradually replaced by a narrow, calcified epiphysial line; (2) the epiphysis cerebri; *see* **pineal gland**.

epiphysis cerebri: the pineal gland.

episome: a genetic element that can function as an autonomous replicating unit, or integrate into and replicate within chromosomes.

epistatic: describes nonreciprocal interactions between nonallelic genes. For example, gene A suppresses expression of gene B, but gene B does not control gene A.

epitectin: CA antigen.

17α-epitestosterone: a testosterone epimer and metabolite made in skeletal muscle that lacks androgenic potency.

epithelial: characteristic of, or derived from **epithelium** (*q.v.*).

epithelial cell adhesion molecule: E-CAM: *see* E-**cadherin**.

epithelial thymic-activating factor: an undefined component of epithelial cell cultures that stimulates thymocyte growth. It may be interleukin-1.

epitheliochorial: the type of placenta formed by pigs, horses, lemurs, whales, and some other mammals, in which endometrial structures undergo only minor changes, and very little blood is lost during parturition; *cf* **endotheliochorial** and **hemochorial**.

epithelioid: resembling epithelium, a term applied for example to the flattened macrophages in granulomas.

epithelium: the tissue type that lines internal, and covers external surfaces, and is a major component of endocrine and exocrine glands. It is composed mostly of cells supported by a basal lamina (with very little extracellular matrix). Since it is avascular, the cells depend on neighboring or underlying connective tissue for nourishment. *Simple* types are single-layered. *Stratified e.* has several cell layers, only one of which rests on the basal lamina. *Pseudostratified* describes tissues in which all cells contact the basal lamina, but differences in heights and locations of nuclei impart a stratified appearance. Epithelial cell sizes and shapes vary from *squamous* (flattened, scalelike), through *cuboidal*, to *columnar*. Specializations at various sites include brush borders which increase surfaces for absorption, desmosomes that link one cell to another, and cilia. A few types (for example in the kidney and small intestine) are polarized (have specific components in the plasma membranes at one surface that differ from those on the opposite side). In some regions, the cells communicate via gap junctions, whereas in others passage of substances between cells is blocked by tight junctions. *See* also **desmosomes**, **endothelium**, **mesothelium**, and **epidermis**.

epitope: an antigen determinant; the part of an antigen that binds to an immunoglobulin paratope.

epizoic: living on the surface of an animal, a term applied, for example to ectoparasites.

epo: EPO; *See* **erythropoietin**.

EPO: (1) erythropoietin; (2) eosinophil peroxidase.

Epogen: a trade name for a recombinant human erythropoietin preparation.

epoprostenol: prostacyclin.

epostane: 4, 5-epoxy-3, 17-dihydroxy-4, 17-dimethyl-Δ_2-androstane-2-carbonitrile; a synthetic steroid that inhibits 3ß-hydroxysteroid dehydrogenase (and thereby the synthesis of progesterone and other steroid hormones). It can terminate early pregnancy in women and laboratory animals, and inhibit ovulation in rats.

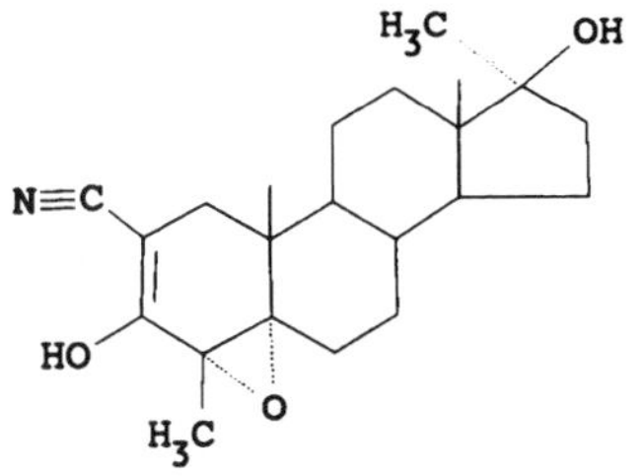

epoxide: an organic compound that contains a reactive bridge formed by the union of an oxygen atom with two other (usually carbon) atoms; *see*, for example **leukotriene A$_4$** (LTA$_4$) and **thromboxane A$_2$** (TXA$_2$).

epoxyeicosatetraenoic acids: EETs; several epoxides synthesized from arachidonic acid. 14,15-epoxyeicosatetraenoic acid (14,15-EET, shown below) affects *c-fos* expression, and potentiates vasopressin stimulation of DNA synthesis in mesangial cells.

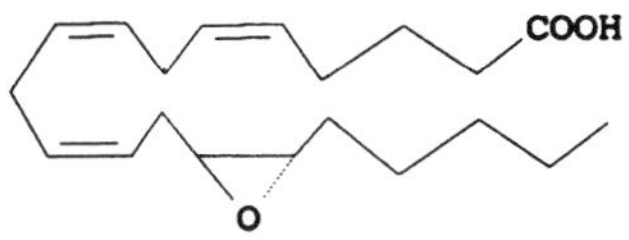

EPS: exophthalmos producing substance.

epsilon cells of hypophysis: a subset of acidophilic adenohypophysial cells, believed to be lactotropes.

EPSP: excitatory postsynaptic potential.

Epstein-Barr virus: EBV; a DNA virus of the *Herpes* family that attaches to C3b receptors on B lymphocytes, and to some helper type T cells. It is the major cause of acute infectious mononucleosis, and can also invoke nasopharyngeomas. The virus carried by mosquitoes is believed to initiate most cases of Burkitt's lymphoma. Relationships to "chronic fatigue syndrome" have been suggested. EBV can transform B cells by establishing autocrine loops, in which host cells are stimulated to secrete factors that support their proliferation. Interleukin-6, CD23, and to a lesser extent interleukin-1, may contribute to the growth, but lactic acid appears to be the most important host factor. BCRF1, an EBV gene prod-

uct, exerts interleukin-10-like inhibition of cytokine synthesis, but lacks mast-cell stimulating and other IL-10 properties. The virus is used as a vector in transfection studies.

equilenin: 3-hydroxyestra-1,3,5,7,9-pentaen-17-one; an estrogen made by stallions and mares, and excreted to urine in both free and conjugated forms. Sodium salts of conjugates extracted from the urine are components of some preparations used to treat estrogen deficiency states.

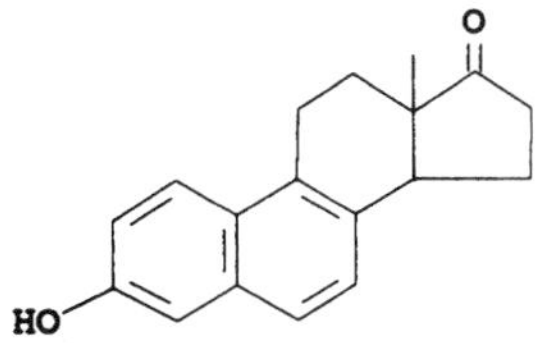

equilibrium: stable conditions, in which factors that tend to drive the components of a reversible system in one direction are exactly balanced by opposing forces. In chemistry, the state in which a reversible reaction proceeds in both directions at the same rate (*see* **equilibrium constant**). True chemical equilibrium is seldom attained in biological systems, mostly because of different rates for substrate presentation and product removal. See also **Donnan equilibrium**.

equilibrium constant: K; a value obtained under standardized conditions that defines the relative concentrations of specific kinds of reactants when chemical equilibrium is attained (but provides no information on reaction rates). In a system of the general type $A + B \rightleftarrows AB$, it is equivalent to the dissociation constant, and the reciprocal of the association constant, calculated as $K = \dfrac{[AB]}{[A] \cdot [B]}$ where [AB], [A] and [B] are respectively, the molar concentrations of AB, A, and B. For reactions of type $A + B \rightleftarrows C + D$, $K = \dfrac{[C] \cdot [D]}{[A] \cdot [B]}$. A high value indicates that the reaction tends to go to the right (when no complicating factors affect substrate availability or product removal).

equilibrium dialysis: techniques for measuring interactions between ligands (such as substrates or haptens) that can diffuse across membranes, and macromolecules (enzymes or antibodies) that cannot. The macromolecule is placed in a membrane-bound compartment surrounded by a second one. The ligand (in both compartments) is then permitted to diffuse in both directions, and to combine with the macromolecule. The concentrations of free and bound ligand are determined when the ligand concentrations on the two sides stabilize.

equilin: 1,3,5,7-estratetraene-3-ol-17-one; an estrogen made by stallions and mares and excreted to urine in both free and conjugated forms.

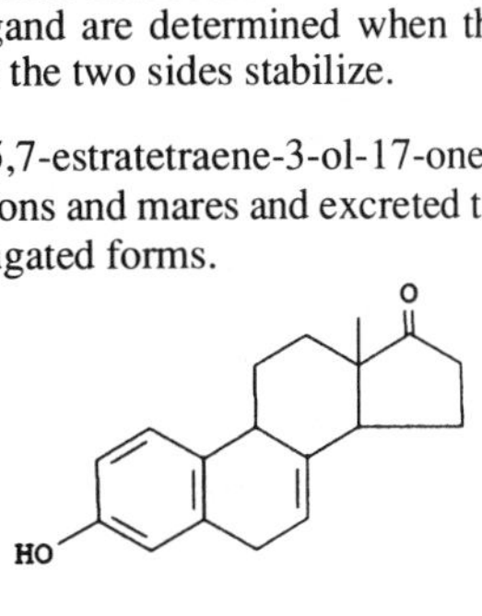

equine: characteristic of or derived from horses and related species.

er: endoplasmic reticulum.

ER: (1) endoplasmic reticulum; (2) estrogen receptor.

erabutoxins: neurotoxins isolated from the venom of the sea-snake *Laticauda semifasciata*, that block neurotransmission by acting on postsynaptic membranes, and on autonomic ganglia. The two major types (A and B) are very similar 61-amino acid peptides with four disulfide bonds.

c-erbA: proto-oncogenes that direct formation of zinc finger, DNA-binding proteins of the thyroid hormone, steroid hormone, calciferol, retinoid receptor superfamily, some of which function as triiodothyronine (T_3) receptors. The *c-erbA*α gene codes for erbA$α_1$, a 410 amino acid protein expressed at high levels in skeletal muscle and brown fat, and in lower ones in most other tissues. A second product of the same gene is erbA$α_2$, a 492 amino acid protein of similar structure except for an extended *C*-terminal region, is expressed at high levels in Sertoli cells, and in lower ones in brain and elsewhere. Since the messenger RNA levels in some cell types are high (compared with those of the protein), truncated forms that do not recognize antibodies directed against erbA$α_1$ may be made. A *c-erbA*β gene on a different chromosome directs formation of at least two related proteins. The ones identified are erbA$β_1$, with a more restricted distribution than erbAα types, but expressed in the placenta, and in spermatids, spermatocytes, and some other cell types, and erbA$β_2$, which may be restricted to the adenohypophysis and some hypothalamic nuclei. Most cell types express more than one kind, but some investigators find no erbA proteins in thymus glands or spleen. All erbA proteins form dimers that bind to thyroid response element (TRE) DNA sequences. However, only erbA$α_1$ (thyroid hormone receptor α-1, TR$α_1$) and the erbAβ forms (TR$β_1$ and TR$β_2$) bind T_3 with high affinity and mediate thyroid hormone actions. Their effects are enhanced by TRAP (T_3 receptor auxiliary protein) and possibly some other factors. There are indications that the non-T_3 binding erbA$α_2$ is a negative regulator of gene transcription. It may either compete with hormone binding forms for TREs, or directly repress the activities of TREs not bound to hormone-receptor complexes. However, a 44K glycoprotein ligand that activates the gene has been described. *V-erbA* is an avian erythroblastosis oncogene that codes for v-erbA, a 435 amino acid protein that, in cooperation with a *v-erbB* gene product, stimulates erythroblast proliferation in some animal types, possibly by interfering with the differentiation promoting effects of erbA$α_1$. The antisense DNA strand of the *c-erbA*α gene codes for ear-1, which may also be a repressor.

c-erbB: proto-oncogenes that code for several transmembrane proteins with tyrosine kinase domains and common DNA binding sites. The component of the *erbB1* product, ERBB1 (HER-1) that faces the cell exterior binds epidermal growth factor (EGF), transforming growth factor-α (TGF-α), amphiregulin, and some related proteins, and is believed to be the major EGF receptor (but *see* also **epidermal growth factor receptors**).

The avian and mammalian forms are chemically and functionally similar, but the avian type displays preferential affinity for TGF-α. Avian leukosis virus inserts at the c-erbB locus, and promotes formation of a truncated protein (v-erbB) that lacks the ligand binding domain and displays constitutively active tyrosine kinase activity. The *c-erbB-2* (*neu*) gene codes for ERBB2 (HER-2, neu, MAC 117, p185), a protein homologous to the EGF receptor. It does not bind EGF, but is a substrate for the EGF receptor tyrosine kinase, and is activated by the hormone. Roles in normal development have been proposed, but excessive production of p185 (with or without gene amplification) has been detected in mammary gland, ovarian, pancreatic, and some other glandular carcinomas; and this seems to be associated with poor prognosis and metastasis. In the presence of EGF receptor, p185 can invoke transformation and tumorigenesis. A third gene, *ERBB3* (*HER-3*) has also been identified in normal cells.

ERCC genes: excision repair cross-complementing genes; a gene cluster that codes for proteins required for DNA repair. Defective ERRC2 products are implicated in the etiology of xeroderma pigmentosa, a rare autosomal recessive disease characterized by photosensitivity and the tendency to develop skin cancers in regions exposed to sunlight. The product of a related *RAD3* gene in *Saccharomyces cerevisiae* (Rad3), has helicase and ATPase activities.

ERE: estrogen response element.

erg: a unit of work, equal to one dyne-centimeter.

erg: a proto-oncogene of the *ets* family (*q.v.*) that codes for 40K and 52K transcription factors.

ergocalciferol: activated ergosterol; vitamin D_2; viosterol; 9,10-secoergosta-5,7,10(19),22-tetraen-3-ol; a secosteroid present in small amounts in some fish oils, and obtained commercially by subjecting ergosterol to ultraviolet radiation. It is an inexpensive, orally effective substitute for cholecalciferol (vitamin D_3) in humans, but is too rapidly degraded for use in chickens and some other species.

ergocornine: 12'-hydroxy-2',5'α-*bis*(1-methylethyl)ergotaman-3',6',18-trione; an ergot alkaloid derived from lysergic acid. It is a dopamine receptor agonist, used to inhibit prolactin secretion.

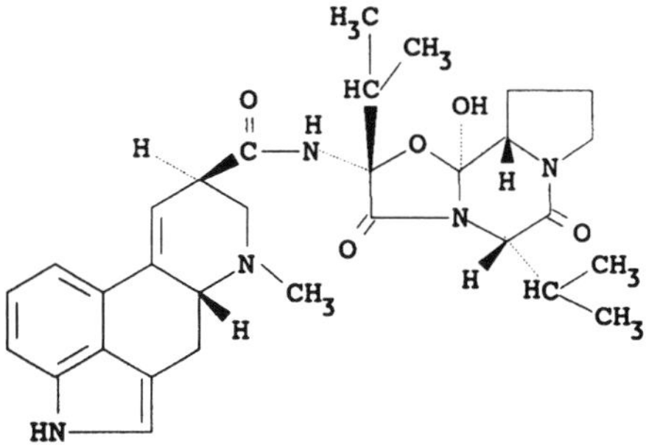

ergocornine

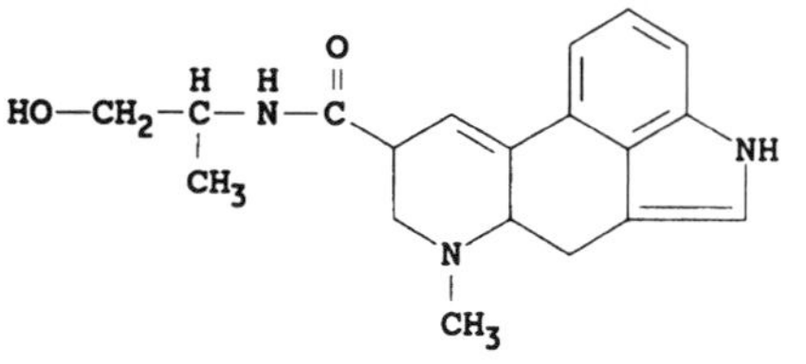

ergonovine

ergosterol

ergocristine: 12-hydroxy-2'-(1-methylethyl)-8α-ergota-man-3'6',18-trione; a naturally occurring alkaloid derived from lysergic acid. It is a dopamine receptor agonist, used to inhibit prolactin secretion.

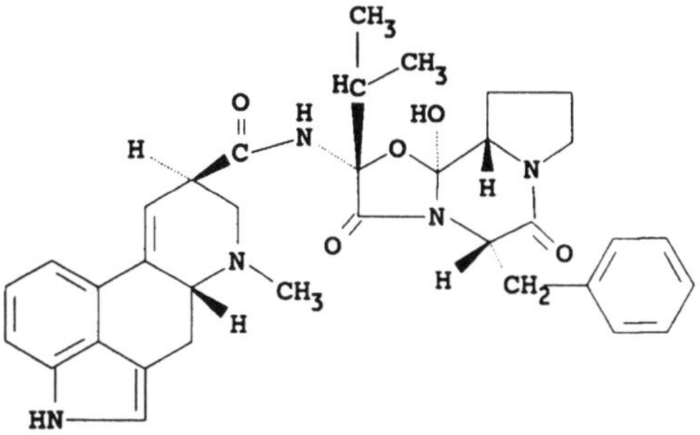

ergocryptine: two chemically related alkaloids derived from ergot. α-ergocryptine is 12'-hydroxy-2'(1-methyl-ethyl)-5'α-(2-methylpropyl)ergotaman-3'6',18-trione. The β form has a slightly different side-chain. Both are dopamine receptor agonists, used to inhibit prolactin secretion.

ergonovine: 9,10-didehydro-*N*-(2-hydroxy-1-methyl-ethyl)-6-methylergoline-8-carboxamide; an alkaloid derived from ergot. It, and methylergonovine are highly potent uterine muscle stimulants. They are less toxic than other ergot derivatives, and are used to protect against postpartum hemorrhage.

ergosterol: ergosta-5,7-22-trien-3β-ol; a plant sterol that can be converted to ergocalciferol when subjected to ultraviolet radiation.

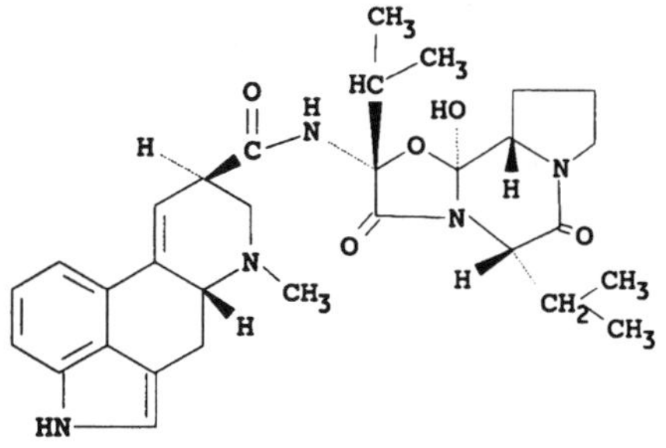

ergot: *Claviceps purpurea*, a parasitic fungus on spoiled rye and other grains. Its components and their derivatives include lysergic acid, lysergic acid amides, ergotamine, ergocornine, ergocristine, ergocryptine, ergonovine, tri-methylamine, histamine, and acetylcholine. Nausea, vomiting, diarrhea, tachycardia, abdominal pain, and coma are the most common early effects of ingesting the grains. Prolonged vasoconstriction can lead to develop-ment of gangrene. *See* also **ergotoxins**.

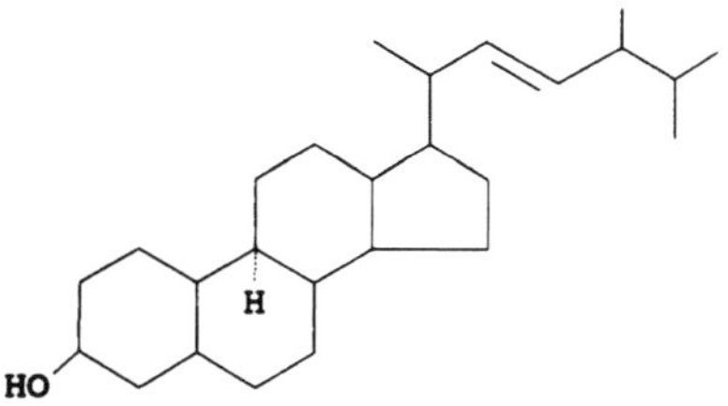

ergotamine: 12'-hydroxy-2'-methyl-5'α-(phenylmethyl) ergotaman-3',6',18-trione; an ergot alkaloid. The dihydro derivative is used to treat migraine headache, and the tartrate to stimulate uterine muscle contraction.

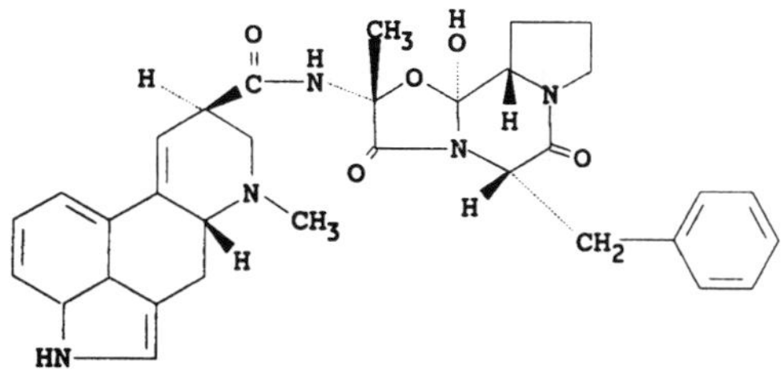

ergotoxins: several ergot alkaloids. Most stimulate smooth muscle, but depress the vasomotor center. The early signs of toxicity include vomiting, diarrhea, and

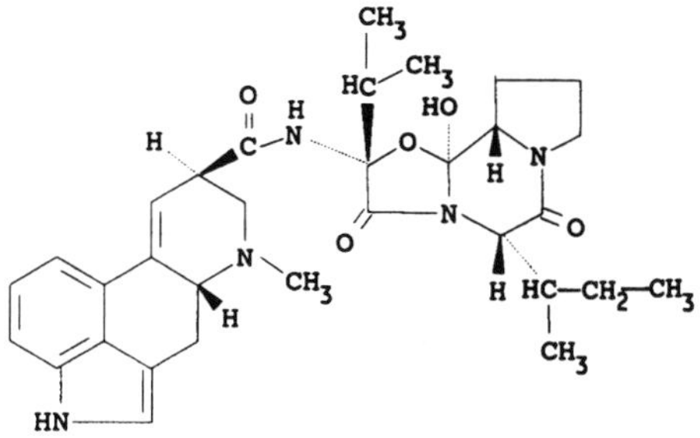

α-ergocryptine

β-ergocryptine

thirst, and cardiovascular collapse; and loss of consciousness can follow. The strong stimulation of uterine muscle can cause abortion, and the prolonged vasoconstriction leads to development of gangrene. Most of the stimulation is mediated via α-adrenergic receptors, with possible participation of serotonin types. However, inhibition of prolactin secretion results from the dopamine agonist activity. Some purified components are used in controlled dosages for therapeutic purposes; *see*, for example **ergocryptine** and **ergonovine**. Ergotoxine (ecboline) is a 1:1:1 mixture of ergocornine, ergocristine, and ergocryptine.

eriochromes: several dyes used in chemical analyses. Eriochrome black T, 3-hydroxy-4-[(1-hydroxy-2-naphthalenyl)azo]-7-nitro-1-naphthalenesulfonic acid monosodium salt (shown below), is used for calcium and magnesium determinations.

ERKs: extracellular signal regulated kinases; kinases with extracellular domains that are activated when they bind ligands. *See* **mitogen activated kinases**.

erk: proto-oncogenes that direct formation of ERK-1 and ERK-2, proteins with ligand activated kinases that catalyze phosphorylations of serine, threonine, and tyrosine residues. The substrates include microtubule-associated protein-1 and myelin basic protein. The forms made by bacteria into which the gene has been inserted also catalyze ERK autophosphorylation.

E-rosettes: *see* **T-rosettes**.

ERPF: effective renal plasma flow.

ERPp99: *see* **glucose regulated proteins**.

erucic acid: 13-docosenoic acid; a major component of rapeseeds, and of mustard, nasturtium, and some other plant seeds. Purported beneficial effects of rapeseed triglycerides in children with adrenoleukodystrophy have been publicized; but no consistent changes have been found; and the toxic effects include thrombocytopenia caused by disruption of blood platelet plasma membranes.

erythema: reddening, usually of the skin, and usually caused by capillary dilation.

erythritol: 1,2,3,4-butanetetrol; an alcohol made by *Aspergillus niger* and *Penicillium herquei*, by algae,

lichens and grasses, and derived commercially from starches. It is used to dilate coronary blood vessels.

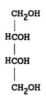

erythroblast: a generalized term applied to nucleated erythrocyte precursor cells, including normoblasts and more primitive types.

erythroblastomas: soft tissue masses composed mostly of erythroblasts.

erythroblastosis: usually, conditions in which erythrocyte precursors proliferate excessively, and the nucleated cells enter the circulating blood; but *see* **erythroblastosis fetalis**.

erythroblastosis fetalis: a hemolytic disease of Rh^+ infants born to Rh^- mothers, caused by maternal anti-Rh antibodies that cross the placenta; *see* **Rh factor**. Although fetal antigens enter the maternal circulation, the antibody titers during a first pregnancy usually inflict only mild fetal injury. In untreated mothers, exposure to the antigens during parturition markedly stimulates antibody production, and the amounts formed during subsequent pregnancies can invoke serious damage by destroying fetal erythrocytes and causing accumulation of bilirubin.

erythrocruorins: high molecular weight oxygen transporting proteins, carried in extracellular fluids of some annelid worms and molluscs with open circulatory systems.

erythrocyte[s]: mature red blood cells, the smallest and most numerous of the circulating formed elements. Healthy adult men have 5-5.4 million or more per cubic milliliter of blood, and healthy, non-pregnant women 4.5-5.0 million. Some of the difference is related to stimulatory influences of androgens, and inhibitory ones of estrogens, on erythropoiesis. The major functions are respiratory gas transport and participation in blood pH control (*see* **chloride shift**); but they also sequester excessive amounts of some regulators and perform other functions. Unique features that facilitate the roles in gas exchange include the biconcave disk shape (which provides a large surface for diffusion), and the high hemoglobin content. The cells lack mitochondria, and do not use molecular oxygen for metabolic reactions. The major energy source is glycolysis, supported by circulating glucose. The sugar is also used in the hexose monophosphate pathway to convert $NADP^+$ to NADPH (a process that seems to be essential for protection against excessive fragility). However, since mammalian red cells also lack nuclei and ribosomes (used by other cell types for repair), and are subjected to mechanical insults when ejected from the heart and squeezed through narrow capillaries, the survival time averages only around 120 days; *see* also **Kupffer cells** and **bilirubin**. The immediate precursors are reticulocytes; *see* also **erythropoietin, interleukin-3**, and **activins**. Erythrocytes are used to investigate membrane transport and other processes that do not depend on RNA and protein synthesis. "Ghosts" prepared by subjecting them to hypotonic solutions which cause hemolysis, are used in cytoskeleton and plasma membrane protein studies.

erythrocyte differentiation factor: erythrocyte maturation factor; EMF: *see* **activins**.

erythrocyte stimulating factor: *see* **erythropoietin**.

erythrocyte transketolase: a thiamine-dependent erythrocyte enzyme used in the hexose monophosphate pathway. The activity levels are measured in some thiamine deficiency studies.

erythrogenin: an enzyme proposed to be released by kidneys, that cleaves an erythropoietinogen secreted by the liver to yield erythropoietin.

erythroid: red, a term usually applied to hematopoietic cells capable of developing into erythrocytes and their precursors.

erythroid differentiation factor: activin A.

erythroleukemias: conditions in which malignant proliferation of bone marrow erythrocyte precursor cells leads to the formation of abnormal cells, release of erythroblasts to the bloodstream, and anemia.

erythroleukemic cells: transformed erythrocyte precursor cells. Some types transformed by viruses and grown in culture undergo differentiation when treated with dimethylsulfoxide (DMSO).

erythromycin: erythromycin A (shown below) is an orally effective, broad-spectrum antibiotic isolated from a *Streptomyces erythreus* strain, that inhibits protein synthesis in some microorganisms by binding to 50S ribosomal subunits. Erythromycins B and C are fermentation products. The major untoward effects are exerted on the gastrointestinal tract, but several kinds of allergic reactions have been described.

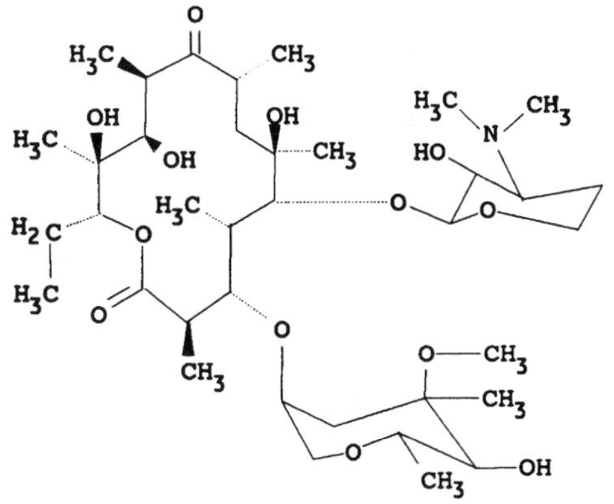

erythrophores: chromatophores that contain red pigments.

erythropoiesis: formation of red blood cells. Since the cells are short-lived, a healthy human adult must replace at least 2.5 million per second (around 0.25 trillion per day), to maintain normal blood levels. The processes require proteins, iron, vitamin B_{12}, other nutrients, and several humoral regulators. *See* **erythrocytes, erythropoietin, interleukin-3**, and **activins**.

erythropoietin: epo; EPO; erythrocyte stimulating factor: a heavily glycosylated, species-specific 34K (166 amino acid) protein made in fetal livers. After birth, the kidneys are the major source. The sites implicated include proximal tubule, peritubular, glomerular, and juxtaglomerular (especially mesangial) cells. Small amounts may also be made in the livers of healthy adults. Epo promotes commitment of pluripotential stem cells in bone marrow to erythroid type differentiation, and synergizes with interleukin-3 (IL-3) and granulocyte-macrophage colony stimulating factor (GM-CSF) to stimulate proliferation of erythroblast precursor cells and newly formed erythroblasts. It additionally promotes erythroblast maturation and synthesis of hemoglobin, spectrin, and other proteins. Epo is therefore a major regulator of circulating erythrocytes numbers. Discharge of reticulocytes to the bloodstream accelerates when the levels are high. Actions on some spleen and other cell types have also been suggested. Growth hormone and factors that invoke hypoxia (such as chronic blood loss, high altitudes, or high metabolic rates) augment Epo synthesis; and substantial amounts can be made in the livers of anemic individuals. The effectiveness is regulated by the amount of Epo receptor translocated to the plasma membranes. Epogen is a preparation used to stimulate erythrocyte production in some forms of anemia (for example in individuals with chronic renal failure or acquired immune deficiency syndrome [AIDS]). It can ameliorate sickle cell anemia symptoms by promoting the synthesis of fetal type hemoglobin.

D-**erythrose**: (*R*)-2,3,4-trihydroxybutanol.

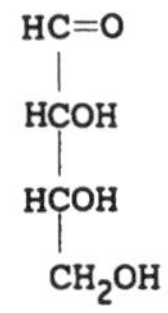

escape: (1) development of resistance to the effects of a regulator that is presented continuously, or administered repeatedly at short time intervals. Animals chronically overdosed with deoxycorticosterone initially retain excessive quantities of sodium and water, but accelerate their rates of sodium and water excretion after a few days. The escape involves increased secretion of antagonistic regulators (*see* **natriuretic hormones**), as well as the effects of augmented extracellular fluid volume on glomerular filtration. Escape mechanisms displayed by target cells for calcitonin and some other hormones can include accelerated hormone inactivation, covalent modification, translocation, and/or down-regulation of hormone receptors, and post-receptor changes. *See* also **desensitization**; (2) assumption of control by a secondary pacemaker in the heart, for example when the sinoatrial node is damaged, or when other cardiac tissue becomes hyperexcitable.

ES cells: embryonic stem cells.

Escherichia coli: rod-shaped gram-negative bacilli, used as models for prokaryote functions, and for synthesizing specific kinds of molecules. A few strains are directly pathogenic when they infect the intestines. Other, harmless types normally inhabit human intestines, but can cause disease if they gain access to the urinary tract or other structures. *See* **E.Coli.**

eserine: physostigmine,

ESF: eosinophil stimulating factor; *see* **eosinophil differentiating factor**.

esmolol: methyl-*p*[2-hydroxy-3-(isopropylamine)propyl hydrocinnamate; a selective, short-acting β_1-type adrenergic receptor antagonist, used for acute treatment of some cardiac dysrhythmias. Brevibloc is a trade name for the hydrochloride.

ESNs: estrogen-stimulated neurophysins.

ESP: extrasensory perception.

ESR: electron spin resonance.

essential amino acids: amino acids that must be supplied from external sources (food) because they cannot be made *de novo* by organisms who require them for protein synthesis and other functions. In most mammals, they include histidine, methionine, tryptophan, threonine, isoleucine, leucine, lysine, valine, and phenylalanine. Arginine may also be required during growth.

essential fatty acids: fatty acids with at least two conjugated double bonds (such as linoleic and linolenic), that are needed in small amounts, but cannot be synthesized by the organism, and must therefore be supplied by the diet. Hepatic enzymes can convert some types to others. A few act directly on target cells, but most are used as precursors for eicosanoids and other regulators. Most phospholipids and diacylglycerols contain one or more unsaturated fatty acid moieties that can be liberated by A type phospholipases. The middle carbon of the glycerol component is the major attachment site.

essential hypertension: high blood pressure of unknown etiology.

essential oils: oils that (1) contain essential fatty acids; (2) are volatile and aromatic.

esters: compounds of the general type R_1-CO—O—R_2, in which at least one of the R groups is organic. They do not ionize in water. Examples include ethyl acetate, and cholesterol covalently linked to a fatty acid. Phospholipids, triacylglycerols, and nucleic acids contain such ester bonds.

esterases: enzymes (for example lipases, cholesterol esterases, and acetylcholinesterases) that catalyze hydrolysis of ester bonds. *See* also **phosphodiesterases**.

estetrol: E_4: estra-1,3,6(10)-triene, 3,15,16,17-tetraol; an estrogen metabolite made in the placenta that circulates in the blood of pregnant women.

esthesia: ability to perceive sensory stimuli.

estivation: aestivation; a reversible state of lowered metabolic activity and torpor, or one that resembles hibernation, that occurs during the summer months (usually in locales that have seasonal droughts). Lungfishes, some snails, some reptiles, some insects, and some small mammals avert otherwise fatal dehydration in that way.

estradiol: E_2: *see* **estradiol-17β**.

estradiol-17α: estra-1,3,5(10)triene-3,17α-diol; a naturally occurring estradiol-17β isomer and metabolite with little or no known biological activity. It is used as a control in studies of estrogen actions.

estradiol-17β: estradiol; E_2: estra-1,3,5(10)triene-3,17-diol; the most potent, and most abundant of the naturally occurring **estrogens** (*q.v.*), secreted in largest amounts by ovaries, and in smaller ones by testes. Luteinizing hormone (LH) promotes synthesis of its major precursor, testosterone. Aromatases that catalyze conversion of androgens to estradiol are made, not only in gonads, but also in placenta, adipose tissue, skin, some neurons, and elsewhere. Estradiol dehydrogenase catalyzes a reversible reaction that converts E_2 to estrone; *see* also **estriol**. The hormone is administered in free form (which must be injected), and also as a component of long-acting conjugates (for example with benzoate, cypionate, enanthate, or valerate) to correct estrogen deficiencies, and in laboratory studies. Synthetic analogs that resist degradation by hepatic and other enzymes are components of oral contraceptive preparations.

esmolol

236

estradiol-17β

estradiol dehydrogenase: an enzyme that catalyzes conversion of estradiol-17β to estrone. Progesterone augments its synthesis.

estrane: 18-methyl cyclopentanoperhydrophenanthrene. A structure used for the nomenclature of estrogens and related steroids.

estriol: E₃; a steroid hormone synthesized in large amounts by fetoplacental units, and a metabolite of estrone and estradiol-17β. Its short-term effects are similar to those of estradiol-17β, but it must be administered repeatedly or continuously to invoke the long-range actions. Suggestions that it performs special functions during pregnancy, and that it protects against the development of breast cancer have not been substantiated.

estrocolyones: it has been proposed that mitosis is a constitutive property of estrogen target cells that can divide, and that estrocolyones arrest the cells in the G₀ phases of the cycles, and thereby provide physiological protection against hyperplasia and tumorigenesis when the hormone is not present (and, also, that estrogens accelerate proliferation by lifting the inhibition). Several possible mechanisms have been suggested. Estrogens could directly inactivate the colyones by binding to them, displace the peptides from their binding sites, or interfere with the coupling to transducers. Transforming growth factor-β (TGFβ) may exert such activity in mammary glands and at some other sites.

estrogens: naturally occurring 18-carbon steroid hormones with aromatic A rings (for example, estradiol-17β and estrone), and synthetic agents (including non-steroidal types such as diethylstilbestrol) that invoke similar responses. The hormones are made from androgen precursors via reactions catalyzed by aromatase enzymes. In gonads, luteinizing hormone (LH) is the major stimulant for androgen synthesis, and follicle stimulating hormone (FSH) for aromatase induction. Substantial quantities of estrogens are also made from dehydroepiandrosterone (DHA, DHEA) and its sulfate (DHAS, DHEAS), secreted by adrenal glands and aromatized in adipose tissue, skin, brain, and elsewhere. The hormones travel to some sites via the bloodstream, and use paracrine and/or autocrine mechanisms at others. The target organs include not only ovary, endometrium, myometrium, uterine cervix, vagina, and mammary gland, but also testis, thymus and pituitary glands, skin, liver, bone, brain and other structures. Estrogens are essential for oogenesis, for the maturation and functions of female accessory reproductive organs, and for the emergence of adult female phenotypes. The influences on pituitary glands and on some hypothalamic regions contribute to ovulation, and the ones on endometrium to implantation and pregnancy maintenance. They promote myometrial growth and contraction, initiate mammary gland maturation, contribute to parturition, participate in cyclical changes in Fallopian tubes, vagina, and uterine cervix glands, and affect mood in humans and reproductive behavior in laboratory animals. They also facilitate bone maturation and contribute to the maintenance of normal bone mass in adults, modulate immune and hemopoietic system functions, influence skin texture, adipose tissue distribution, and hepatic enzyme synthesis, and exert many other effects. Functions in birds include stimulation of egg white production. In addition to direct actions, they can, at various sites, promote the synthesis and/or release of prolactin, dopamine, and other regulators, induce progesterone receptors, affect the numbers of receptors for estrogen and other hormones, and serve as precursors for catechol derivatives. Although all long-range responses appear to be mediated via estrogen receptors that interact with the genome (*see* **estrogen response elements**), some rapidly invoked types are accomplished via direct effects on plasma membranes and other cell components. Estrogens can, for example, promote histamine release and water retention in the uterus within minutes after it is presented to the target cells.

estrogen binding proteins: blood plasma and intracellular proteins that bind estrogens with high affinities. *See* also **testosterone-estrogen binding proteins** and **estrogen receptors**.

estrogen induced proteins: EIPs; proteins whose synthesis is substantially accelerated by estrogens. The creatine kinase isozyme in the uterus was formerly called estrogen induced protein, but it is just one of many affected by the hormones.

estrogen receptors: ERs; ERcs; the term usually refers to 65-70K species-specific phosphoproteins made in estrogen target cells that mediate the effects of the hormone on messenger RNA synthesis, cell growth and cell proliferation. They are members of a superfamily that includes receptors for progesterone, glucocorticoids, mineralocorticoids, thyroid hormones, retinoids, calciferols, and peroxisome proliferators. The ligand binding domain, which is hormone-specific, binds estradiol-17β with highest affinity. Estrone and estriol bind with lower affinities, and some agonists, including nonsteroidal types such as diethylstilbestrol, attach to the same sites. (However, some estrogen antagonists interact with different amino acid sequences.) In unstimulated cells, most of the receptors reside in nuclei. Estrogen binding leads to "activation", which includes release from other proteins. A zinc finger domain contains the component that binds to estrogen response elements, and additional functional sites (including ones for dimerization) contribute to transcription *trans*-activation properties. Proteins with functions analogous to those described for thyroid receptor auxiliary protein (TRAP) have also been identified. Different kinds of receptors on plasma membranes mediate nongenomic actions. It has been suggested that estrogens exert some of their influences by binding to non-histone proteins of the nuclear matrix.

estrogen response elements: EREs; DNA base sequences that interact with activated estrogen-receptor complexes and contribute to the genomic actions of estrogens. Most are enhancer components of specific genes that resemble the response elements for several other hormone-receptor complexes (*see* also **estrogen receptors**). Some may be functionally associated with RNA polymerase I.

estromedins: estrogen-induced proteins that mediate estrogen actions on target cells.

estrone: E_1; 3-hydroxyestra-1,3,5(10)trien-17-one; a steroid hormone that interacts weakly with estrogen receptors, and is interconvertible with estradiol-17β.

16α-hydroxy-**estrone**: a naturally occurring estrogen metabolite that may have oncogenic potency.

estrophilins: intracellular estrogen binding proteins; estrogen receptors.

estrous cycles: ovarian cycles of subprimates. Unlike menstrual cycles, they are associated with behavioral changes (*see* **estrus**), require gonadotropin releasing hormone (LRH) surges for ovulation, and usually involve only limited preparation of the endometrium for implantation (with no obvious sloughing or blood loss when conception does not occur).

Estrovis: a trade name for quinestrol.

estrus: the phase of the estrous cycle, preceded by proestrus and followed by metestrus, during which estrogen levels are high, and females display receptivity, lordosis when stimulated, and associated behavioral changes

(which can include increased motor activity, ear-wiggling, and decreased food intake). It is the only phase during which females accept sexual advances of males. The timing contributes to the probability that sperm will arrive in the female reproductive tract when oocytes have been freshly prepared for fertilization.

ET[s]: *see* **elongation factors**.

ETA (η) cells: adenohypophysial acidophils believed to secrete prolactin. The numbers increase during pregnancy and lactation.

etafedrine: 2-methylamino-1-phenyl-propanol; a $β_2$-type adrenergic receptor agonist, used as a bronchodilator.

ETF: electron transferring protein.

ethacrynic acid: 2,3-dichloro-4-(2-methylene-1-oxobutyl) phenoxy]acetic acid; a potent "high-ceiling" type diuretic that inhibits chloride transport across Henle loops (*see* also **loop diuretics**). Na^+ excretion is secondarily increased, in part because effects on blood flow to the proximal tubules retard salt absorption. The agent is used to treat edema of cardiac, hepatic, or renal origin. Ca^{2+}, K^+, and Mg^{2+} are also lost to the urine, and excessive excretion of hydrogen and ammonium ions by distal segments of the nephron can invoke metabolic alkalosis. Ethacrynic acid can additionally augment renin secretion and affect transmembrane electrolyte transport by other cell types. The toxic effects include hearing impairment secondary to changes in endolymph composition.

ethamoxytriphetol: MER-25; α-[4-[2-(dimethylamino) ethoxy]phenyl]-4-methoxy-α-phenylbenzene ethanol; a non-steroid estrogen receptor antagonist that augments gonadotropin secretion by impairing negative feedback control.

ethane dimethyl sulfonate: busulfan; 1,4-butanediol dimethanesulfonate; Myleran; Mitosan; an alkylating agent used to treat chronic granulocytic leukemia, as an insecticide, and as a laboratory tool to destroy Leydig cells. It is carcinogenic.

ethanol: ethyl alcohol; the major pharmacological component of alcholic beverages. It is a central nervous system depressant that in small doses gives the illusion of

$$H_3C-\overset{\overset{\displaystyle O}{\|}}{\underset{\underset{\displaystyle O}{\|}}{S}}-O-(CH_2)_4-O-\overset{\overset{\displaystyle O}{\|}}{\underset{\underset{\displaystyle O}{\|}}{S}}-CH_3$$

ethane dimethyl sulfonate

$$Cl-CH_2-CH_2-\overset{\overset{\displaystyle O}{\|}}{\underset{\underset{\displaystyle H}{\underset{\displaystyle |}{O}}}{P}}-OH$$

ethephon

stimulation by inhibiting the activities of some cerebral cortex neurons. Small amounts are widely used to invoke relaxation and elevate mood (and sometimes to impart a sense of warmth). Amounts sufficient to raise pain thresholds adversely affect mental and circulatory system functions. The tendency for some individuals to become addicted has been attributed to the presence of D_2 subtype dopamine receptor alleles that are not made by other persons. Some of the toxic effects of large doses are attributed to direct influences on plasma and mito-chondrial membrane components, augmentation of γ-aminobutyric acid (GABA)-mediated synaptic inhibition, and conversion to acetaldehyde. Chronic ingestion of large amounts can damage the liver, kidneys, and brain, depress gonadotropin secretion, accelerate bone resorp-tion, and lower 1,25-dihydroxyvitamin D levels. The withdrawal effects can include tremors, as well as hal-lucinations and other manifestions of "alcohol psycho-sis", which subside after some time. Exceedingly high levels invoke coma and can be lethal. Teratogenic effects in embryos and fetuses of mothers who take substantial amounts during early pregnancy, and lesser damage (for example to bone formation) when the exposure comes later, may involve direct ethanol and/or acetaldehyde in-hibition of cell proliferation, as well as influences on the placenta that impair nutrition delivery. Yeasts and some other microorganisms synthesize large amounts of ethanol under anaerobic conditions that accelerate glycolysis. Pyruvate decarboxylase catalyzes the reac-tion: pyruvate + H^+ → acetaldehyde + CO_2. An alcohol dehydrogenase then promotes the second reaction of the pathway, acetaldehyde + NADH → ethanol + NAD^+. Ethanol is used as a solvent for many agents, in graded concentrations to fix tissues for microscopy, and in 70% solutions as a local antiseptic.

$$H_3C-CH_2-OH$$

ethanolamine: an amine formed by decarboxylation of serine. It is a component of phosphatidylethanolamine and some other essential compounds, and an intermediate in pathways for biosynthesis of others, including choline and its derivatives.

$$H_2N-CH_2-CH_2-OH$$

ethanolamine-O-sulfate: an agent that prolongs γ-aminobutyric acid actions by inhibiting GABA trans-aminase.

$$H_2N-CH_2-CH_2-O-\overset{\overset{\displaystyle O}{\|}}{\underset{\underset{\displaystyle O}{\|}}{S}}-OH$$

ethephon: Florel; 2-chloroethylphosphonic acid; an agent used to release ethylene from plants (for controlling the growth and ripening of fruit crops), and to study ethylene functions.

ether: (1) any compound that contains an R—O—R' group, in which both Rs are organic moieties; (2) diethyl ether, a volatile general anesthetic that is used for some surgical procedures, but is inflammable and explosive. Since it irritates mucous membranes and increases mucus secretion, has a disagreeable odor, and requires a long induction period, other agents are usually given before it is administered. The after-effects include gastrointestinal distress. Vinyl ether is more potent, and requires a shorter induction period, but otherwise shares most of the draw-backs. Diethyl ether is also used as a lipid solvent in extraction, chromatography and other laboratory proce-dures.

$$H_3C-CH_2-O-CH_2-CH_3$$

diethyl ether

$$H_2C{=}\overset{\overset{\displaystyle H}{|}}{C}-O-\overset{\overset{\displaystyle H}{|}}{C}{=}CH_2$$

vinyl ether

ethidium bromide: homidium bromide; the bromide salt of 3,8-diamino-5-ethyl-6-phenanthridinium; an inter-calating agent that can decrease DNA supercoiling, re-versibly slow transcription by inhibiting the actions of RNA polymerases, and invoke frame-shift mutations. Complexes with DNAs fluoresce under ultraviolet light, and can be used to detect double-stranded nucleic acid molecules in agarose gels. Since ethidium bromide dis-plays greater affinity for linear duplexes than for covalent DNA circles, it is used in conjunction with differential centrifugation to separate the two kinds of molecules.

ethinyl estradiol: 17α-ethynyl-1,3,5(10)-estratriene-3, 17β-diol; the most potent of the synthetic estrogens used in oral contraceptive preparations, most commonly in combination with norethindrone, norgestrel, or ethyn-odiol diacetate. It is also used alone to treat estrogen deficiency, postmenopausal symptoms, some uterine dis-orders, and some forms of cancer.

ethinylestrenol: lynestrenol; 19-*nor*pregn-4-en-20-yn-17-ol; a potent synthetic progestin that does not exert androgenic or anabolic effects. It is used in combination with mestranol for oral contraception.

Ethiodol: a trade name for an iodine-poppyseed oil fatty acid ester preparation, used as a contrast medium in roentgenography.

ethion: ethyl methylene phosphorodithioate; an acetylcholinesterase inhibitor, used as an ascaricide.

ethionamide: 2-ethyl-4-thiocarbamoylpyridine; an agent that impairs nucleic acid synthesis and blocks some acetylation reactions. It used in conjunction with other agents to inhibit the growth of tuberculosis-causing bacteria, but is hepatotoxic, and can invoke sensory disturbances, nausea, vomiting, drowsiness, psychological depression, tremors, and convulsions.

ethionine: *S*-ethyl-homocysteine; an amino acid analog that deranges protein and nucleic acid synthesis, and inhibits some acetylation reactions. It is used in laboratory studies to invoke mutagenesis.

ethisterone: 17α-ethynyltestosterone; Proluton C; one of the first synthetic progestins used in oral contraceptive preparations. It is mildly androgenic, and has been replaced by other steroids.

ethnology: the study of human races.

ethology: the study of behavior.

ethoxyacetazolamide: an acetazolamide derivative used to inhibit carbonic anhydrases.

ethyl chloride: a highly volatile liquid that cools surfaces as it evaporates, and is used as a local anesthetic.

ethylene: ethene; a volatile phytohormone that diffuses rapidly from its site of production. It terminates dormancy in plants, acts in conjunction with auxins to promote growth of short, thick lateral roots, strengthens cell walls, and accelerates fruit ripening and senescence. By opposing the effects of gibberellic acid on microtubule orientation, it limits longitudinal, but facilitates lateral expansion. **Ethephon** (*q.v.*) is used to release it for commercial purposes, and to study its effects. Ethylene also participates in plant **systemic acquired resistance** responses (*q.v.*) that induce pathogen resistance proteins, and contributes to the production of chitinase, β1,3-glucanase, and other enzymes that attack parasites. Its synthesis increases following plant injury, and is induced by jasmonic acid. In animals, ethylene is a hypnotic, used as an inhalation anesthetic in veterinary medicine. Toxic doses can cause narcosis and asphyxia in humans.

1,1-ethylene *bis*-tryptophan: a contaminant of some tryptophan preparations taken orally as dietary supplements, and implicated as one of the factors that contributes to development of eosinophilia-myalgia syndrome; *see* **tryptophan**.

ethylenediamine tetracetic acid: Edetin; EDTA; (ethylene dinitrilo)tetraacetic acid; a divalent cation chelator that avidly binds calcium and has lower affinity for magnesium and some other metals; *cf* **ethyleneglycol bis-*N,N'*-tetraacetate (EGTA).**

ethylene dimethylsulfate: EDS; an alkylating agent used as a laboratory tool to damage Leydig cells.

ethylene glycol: a compound widely used as anti-freeze for automobiles. If inhaled in large amounts, it directly causes central nervous system depression that can lead to narcosis, coma, and death. Other toxic effects, the most common of which is renal failure, are attributed to its metabolism. Alcohol dehydrogenase catalyzes conversion of ethylene glycol to glycoaldehyde, and aldehyde dehydrogenase converts the product to glycolic acid. Both reactions alter redox potentials by converting NAD^+ to NADH, and invoke metabolic acidosis by facilitating lactose formation from pyruvate. Glycolic acid is further metabolized to other products that include oxalic acid, which chelates Ca^{2+}, causes muscle spasms (*see* **tetany**), and precipitates in renal tubules.

ethyleneglycol bis-*N,N'*-tetraacetate: EGTA; ethylene glycol bis(β-aminoethyl-ether)-*N,N,N'N'*-tetraacetate; a divalent cation chelator that avidly binds calcium. Its affinity for other metals is much lower than that of ethylenediamine tetraacetate.

ethylestrenol: 19α-*nor*-preg-4-ene-17-ol; Orabolen; Dura-bolen; Maxibolin; an **anabolic steroid** (*q.v.*).

ethyl ether: *see* **ether**.

ethylketocyclazocine: a benzorphan derivative with very high affinity for *k*-type opioid receptors, used to identify those receptors, and as an agonist. It also interacts with μ- and δ- type receptors, and has analgesic potency, but is not addictive, does not affect morphine withdrawal symptoms, and is not antagonized by concentrations of naloxone that block the effects of morphine and β-endorphin. Large doses invoke dysphoria, hallucinations, aversive reactions, and sensory disturbances, and can delay extinction of conditioned responses.

N-**ethylmaleimide**: NEM: *see* *N*-**ethylmaleimide**.

ethylmethanesulfonate: EMS; methylsulfonic acid ethyl ester; ethyl mesylate; an alkylating agent used as a mutagen. When it donates ethyl groups to DNA guanine bases, those bases pair with thymine during replication.

N-**ethyl-nitrosourea**: ENU; EtNU: an extremely potent carcinogen that invokes multiple mutations in spermatozoa and is used to accomplish germ-line mutations.

ethylnorepinephrine: a $β_2$-type adrenergic receptor agonist that relaxes bronchiolar muscle. Therapeutic doses exert only minimal effects on the myocardium.

α-**ethyltryptamine**: a highly potent monoamine oxidase inhibitor.

ethynodiol: ethinylestranol: 19-nor-pregnen-4-en-20-yne-3,17-diol; a synthetic progestin. The diacetate is used for oral contraception (for example with ethinyl estradiol in Demulen, and with mestranol in Ovulen and Metrulen).

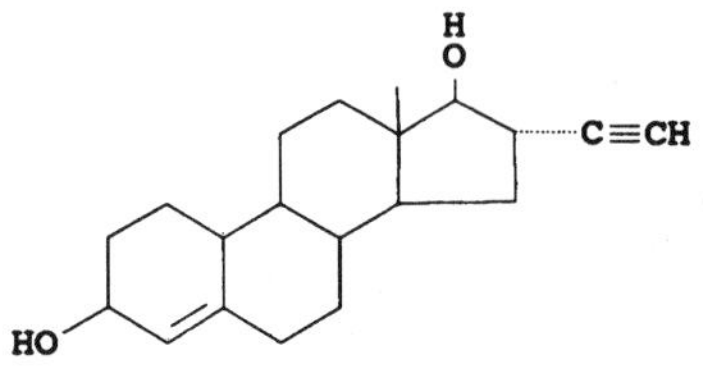

ethynodiol

etidronate: etidronic acid; Etidron; EHDP; (1-hydroxy-ethylidene)biphosphonate. The disodium salt (Didronel, shown below) slows bone resorption and hydroxyapatite crystal deposition. It is used to treat Paget's disease, to protect against soft tissue calcification, and in bone scanning.

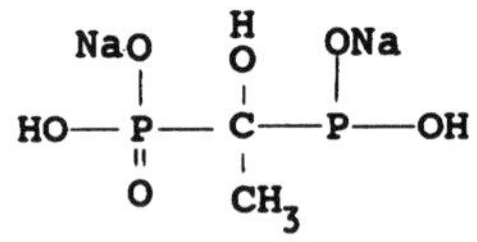

etiocholanolone: 3α-hydroxy-5β-androstan-17-one; a steroid hormone metabolite (one of the 17-ketosteroids excreted to urine). It exerts actions on bone marrow similar to those of 5β-dihydrotestosterone, and is reported to provide some protection against the development of atherosclerosis. High blood concentrations invoke fever.

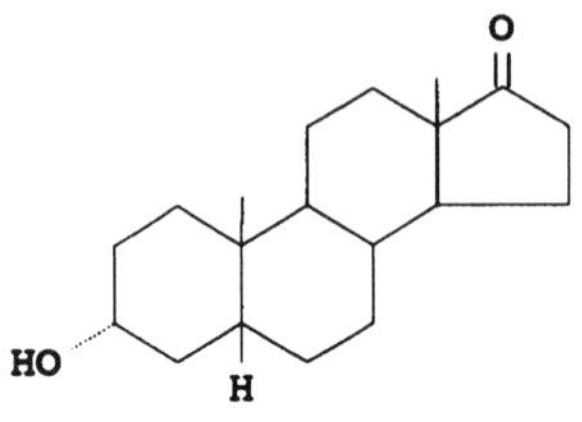

$S(-)$-**etioclopride hydrochloride**: a potent, selective D_2 type dopamine receptor antagonist. The $R(-)$ isomer is inactive.

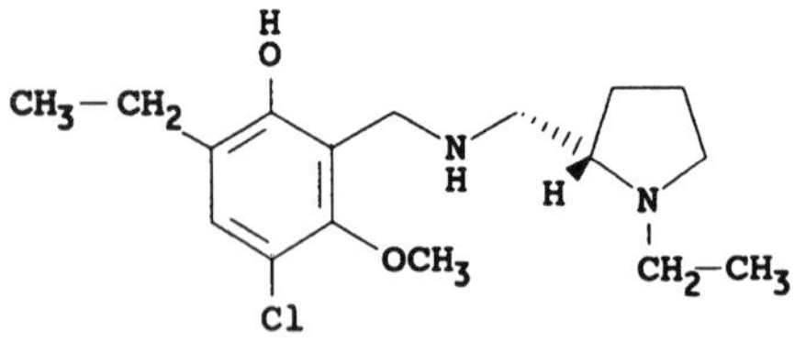

etiolation: lightening; usually, (1) a process in light-deprived plants, in which chlorophyll synthesis and leaf growth are inhibited, but shoots elongate; (2) skin pallor in light-deprived individuals.

etiology: the study of causes, usually of diseases.

EtNU: *N*-ethyl-nitrosourea.

c-ets: a large family of proto-oncogenes related to *v-ets* (one of two E26 avian leukemia virus oncogenes), and to some other viral oncogenes. The group includes cellular types *ets-1*, *ets-2*, *elk-1*, *elk-2*, and *erg* (usually represented in humans in upper case letters, as in *ETS-1* and *ETS-2*). The genes have been identified in chickens, sea-

urchins, *Drosophila*, and other animal types, as well as in mammals. All code for phosphoproteins with very similar, approximately 85 amino-acid domains that bind to specific sites on DNAs and affect transcription. Some of the complexes formed with other proteins interact with AP-1 sites, and others with serum response elements; and many effects are additive with those of *myb* products. *ETS-1* is expressed at high levels in quiescent CD4+CD8- thymocytes and T cells, in which it is believed to contribute to maintenance of the inactive state. The levels fall when the antigens bind to the T cell receptors, and the train of events that follows (augmentation of phospholipase C and tyrosine kinase activities, and then of kinase C, and elevation of Ca^{2+} levels) leads rapidly to expression of *ETS-2*. *ETS-2* then directs synthesis of a 52K protein that appears to be essential for completing activation and accomplishing replication (and can be detected before DNA synthesis begins). The ETS-2 product is also made by fibroblasts, hepatocytes during liver regeneration, and brain astrocytes, and is believed to play roles in proliferation and differentiation of many cell types. Very high levels can transform cells and abolish the requirements for serum. The gene is present in all three copies of chromosome #21 in individuals with Down's syndrome trisomy; and translocation to chromosome 8 occurs in individuals with acute myelogenous leukemia. Different members of the gene family code for TCF1-αT and other proteins that affect the synthesis of T lymphocyte receptor subunits. Since the effects of the gene products vary with the levels of other regulators, it has been proposed that they mediate gene switching in response to second messengers and environmental factors.

ETYA: 5,8,11,14-eicosatetraynoic acid.

eu-: a prefix meaning (1) good or normal, as in euglycemia; (2) true or typical, as in euchromatin.

Eubacteria: a major prokaryote subdivision that includes most gram positive bacteria, cyanobacteria, mycoplasms, pseudomonads, and enterobacteria. The plasma membranes contain ester-linked lipids, and the chromosomes appear to lack introns.

eucaryote: eukaryote.

euchromatin: chromatin that uncoils during interphase and condenses during mitosis, and stains strongly in polytene chromosomes (but less densely in most others). It contains smaller amoutns of repetitive DNA than heterochromatin, associates with more nonhistone proteins, and contains base sequences that are transcribed.

eugenics: the study or practice of altering phenotype traits through selective breeding. It can be positive (selection for "good" traits) or negative (discouraging or preventing breeding of individuals with "bad" traits).

Euglena: a genus of unicellular flagellated protoctists used in genetics studies. The organisms are classified as protozoa, but they make chlorophyll and display other plant-like characteristics when exposed to light.

euglobulins: globulins that are insoluble in water, soluble in dilute salt solutions, and precipitated with half-saturated ammonium sulfate; *cf* **pseudoglobulins**.

euglycemia: blood or serum glucose concentrations within the normal range.

eukaryotes: eucaryotes: animals and plants whose cells have membrane-enclosed nuclei, multiple chromosomes, and mitotic cycles.

eumelanins: dark brown and black pigments synthesized from dopamine; *see* **melanins** and *cf* **phaeomelanins**.

eunuchoidism: usually (1) conditions in males caused by androgen deficiency, in which secondary sex characteristic are incompletely developed, and delayed epiphysial closure leads to excessive growth of the long bones. *Hypogonadotropic* types can be caused by pituitary gland defects that impair the ability to secrete sufficient luteinizing hormone (LH). When the problem is gonadotropin releasing hormone (GnRH, LRH) deficiency, it is often accompanied by anosmia or hyposmia (*see* **Kallmann's syndrome**). In *hypergonadotropic* types, LH levels are high, but Leydig cell responses are subnormal (*see* also **Klinefelter's syndrome**); (2) *female eunuchoidism*, analogous disorders in females, usually caused by ovarian defects that impair estrogen secretion.

euphenics: treatment of phenotypic disorders. (Most are caused by genetic defects.)

euphoria: an abnormally exaggerated sense of well-being. It is usually followed by (or alternates with bouts of) psychic depression. Excessively high glucocorticoid levels, some brain disorders, and many pharmacological agents (including anabolic androgens, heroin, cocaine, and amphetamines) are among the factors that can invoke euphoria/depression cycles.

euploidy: describes cells with chromosome numbers characteristic of the species; *cf* **aneuploidy**, **triploidy** and **tetraploidy**.

eupnea: normal breathing during times of rest or low activity; *cf* **hyperpnea** and **dyspnea**.

euryhaline: capable of adapting to wide ranges of environmental saline concentrations, a term usually applied to fish species that can survive in fresh, brackish, and salt water. Hormones related to prolactin are essential for adaptations to fresh water in most species.

eurythermal: capable of maintaining growth over a wide temperature range.

eutectic: usually, having the lowest possible melting point, a term applied to mixtures with melting points lower than those of any of the constituents.

eutelolecithal: describes ova with very large quantities of yolk and other components that do not directly contribute to formation of embryonic cells.

euthanasia: mercy killing; deliberate, painless killing, or failure to employ special measures to prolong life. The term is applied to the killing of anesthetized laboratory animals when studies are terminated, and sometimes to the administration of lethal agents to (or withdrawal of life-sustaining support from) humans with intractable pain and incurable, debilitating illnesses who request it.

euthenics: the science of improving human welfare by modifying environments.

Eutheria: a vertebrate subclass that includes all placental mammals; *cf* **Metatheria** and **Monotremes**.

eutopic: entopic; occurring in the normal location; *cf* **ectopic**.

eutrophic: characterized by, or conducive to good nutrition.

eutrophication: excessive growth of one type of organism within an ecosystem to the disadvantage of others in the same system, usually because of increased nutrient supply to the former.

eV: electron-volt.

ev-1: a Moloney virus oncogene that integrates into host genomes, and causes myeloid leukemia in mice.

evagination: outpocketing, usually of a tissue layer, for example during gastrulation.

Evans blue: T-1824; 4,4′-bis[7-(1-amino-8-hydroxy-2,4-disulfo)naphthylazo]-3,3′bitolyl tetrasodium salt; a dye soluble in blood plasma that does not cross capillary membranes. It is used to measure blood volume.

eversion: turning outward or inside-out; *cf* **inversion**.

Evipal: a trade name for hexobarbital.

evocator: an embryonic inducer; a morphogen released by an organizer.

evolution: gradual, irreversible changes in hereditary components, caused by successive mutations (or other DNA changes) that are transmitted to, and affect the characteristics of successive generations. *Convergent* evolution is acquisition of similar characteristics by two or more phylogenetic lineages, a term sometimes restricted to changes in which the descendants resemble each other more than the progenitors did. The term *parallel* evolution is used when the descendants are as similar to each other as the ancestors were.

evolutionary clock: the rate at which a gene accumulates mutations.

exchange pairing: the association of homologous chromosomes that leads to crossing over.

Evans blue

exchange transfusion: replacement of the blood of one individual with blood from others, a procedure used, for example, to treat infants with severe erythroblastosis fetalis.

excipient: a pharmacologically inactive substance that is combined with a drug to facilitate its administration or distribution.

excision repair: physiological mechanisms for replacing damaged DNA strands with normal types, in which endonucleases recognize and remove defective base sequences, complementary DNA strands serve as templates for DNA polymerase-mediated synthesis of the correct sequences, and DNA ligases promote insertion of the new sequences.

excitable cells: cells with plasma membrane voltage-gated ion channels that develop action potentials when stimulated.

excitation-contraction coupling: the linking of events initiated by stimuli acting on plasma membranes to mechanical mechanisms for muscle cell shortening. In skeletal muscle, depolarization in response to acetylcholine acting on postjunctional receptors leads to release of Ca^{2+} from the sarcoplasmic reticulum. Calcium then combines with a **troponin** (*q.v.*), and thereby initiates changes in the actin-myosin system.

excitation-secretion coupling: the linking of cell stimulation to exocytosis, and consequent release of hormones, neurotransmitters, enzymes, or other substances. The intermediate steps usually include depolarization in response to a regulator, and elevation of cytoplasmic Ca^{2+} levels (and/or release of other messengers). High Ca^{2+} levels affect cytoskeletons and promote fusion of secretory granule membranes with plasma membranes.

excitatory amino acids: EAA: glutamic acid, aspartic acid, and related regulators that act on plasma membrane receptors and mediate cell excitation. The term is usually restricted to amino acids that act on voltage-gated ion channels within the central nervous system. Excessive amounts are excitotoxins. *See* also **NMDA, kainate**, and **quisqualate receptors**, and **nitric oxide**.

excitatory postsynaptic potentials: EPSP; partial depolarizations of postsynaptic neuron membranes invoked by subthreshold level stimuli. They do not generate action potentials, but do augment sensitivities to subsequent stimulation. *See* also **summation**, and *cf* **inhibitory postsynaptic potentials**.

excitotoxins: excitatory amino acids or other agents that stimulate neurons excessively, and thereby damage the cells. Some promote generation of oxidants and free radicals that cause much of the injury.

exclusion principle: the concept that two species cannot coexist in the same locale if they have identical ecological requirements.

excrescence: projection of abnormal tissue from the surface of skin, a mucous membrane, a heart valve, or other structure.

exergonic: describes processes that release free energy to the surrounding environment; *cf* **endergonic**. Exergonic reactions tend to proceed spontaneously. They can be endothermic or exothermic.

exfetation: ectopic pregnancy.

exochorion: the part of the chorion that develops from embryonic ectoderm.

exocoelom: primitive yolk sac; a temporary cavity that develops in very young conceptuses (around 12 days after fertilization in humans). It is lined by a thin layer of endoderm, and is surrounded by extra-embryonic mesoderm. *Cf* **extra-embryonic coelom**.

exocrine: secreting in the direction of a free (internal or external) surface, a term applied, for example to salivary, sweat, and acinar pancreatic glands. *Cf* **endocrine, paracrine**, and **intracrine**.

exocrine pancreas: the part of the pancreas composed mostly of acinar (exocrine) cells that secrete proenzymes and other pancreatic juice components. *Cf* **endocrine pancreas**.

exocytosis: the major process for releasing cell products stored in granules to extracellular spaces. It is calcium dependent, and involves migration of secretory granules to the plasma membrane, fusion of granule and plasma membranes, and release of granular components. *Cf* **endocytosis**.

exoenzyme: ectoenzyme.

exogamy: outbreeding; (1) reproductive union of gametes from individuals that are not descended from a common ancestor; (2) mating of members of different tribes, communities, or other social groups.

exogenic heredity: transmission of nongenetic information (such as knowledge or customs) from one generation to the next.

exogenous: from the outside, a term that can refer, for example, to nutrients, injected agents, or the effects of light and other environmental factors.

exogenous virus: a virus that replicates vegetatively, and is not transmitted via the genome.

exohormone: a pheromone or other regulator that is released externally, and acts on other individuals.

exons: gene components that can be transcribed, and their RNA counterparts. In most genes of complex species, some exons are separated from each other by introns; and formation of mature messenger RNAs from direct transcripts requires removal of introns, followed by joining of exons. Since RNA processing can involve union of only some of the exons, a single kind of transcript can generate more than one mRNA. *See*, for example, **calcitonin gene related peptides**.

exonucleases: enzymes that cleave terminal nucleotides from nucleic acids. They are important for maintaining DNA replication fidelity, and for DNA repair. *Cf* **endonucleases**.

exopeptidases: carboxypeptidases and aminopeptidases; enzymes that cleave single amino acids (and in some cases dipeptides) from peptide and protein *N*- or *C*-terminals; *cf* **endopeptidases**.

exophthalmic goiter: thyroid gland enlargement that is associated with exophthalmos. *See* also **Graves' disease** and **exophthalmos producing substance**.

exophthalmos: protrusion of the eyeball, usually caused by glycosaminoglycan and fluid accumulation in and/or hyperplasia of retro-orbital tissues. The condition occurs in individuals with Graves' disease and Hashimoto's thyroiditis, and is now believed to be an organ-specific autoimmune disorder. *See* also **exophthalmos producing substance**.

exophthalmos producing substance: EPS; one or more factors that contributes to the development of exophthalmos. An old concept that human EPS is either thyroid stimulating hormone, or a pituitary gland factor secreted along with TSH has been discarded (although thyroid hormone levels affect the condition, and massive amounts of TSH promote eye protrusion in amphibians). The factors appear to be substances generated by defective immune systems that act on fibroblasts.

exoskeletons: the rigid or semi-rigid supporting substances on the external surfaces of arthropods and some other invertebrates. Chitin is the major component for many species.

exotherm[s]: "cold-blooded animals"; animals whose body temperatures vary with environmental factors such as temperature and ultraviolet radiation; *cf* **endotherms**.

exothermic: giving off heat; *cf* **endothermic**. Exothermic reactions are not necessarily exergonic.

exotoxins: poisons secreted by microorganisms. Some are used as laboratory tools to inhibit specific kinds of enzymes; *see*, for example **botulinum**, **cholera**, and **diphtheria toxins**, and *cf* **endotoxins**.

experiment: a procedure performed to test a hypothesis.

experimental: describes conditions deliberately imposed by an investigator.

experimental allergic autoimmune encephalitis: EAE: an autoimmune disease invoked by injecting brain or spinal cord homogenates along with adjuvant, or of myelin. The effects include focal infiltration of lymphocytes and macrophages into some brain regions, demyelination, disruption of blood brain barriers, and skeletal muscle paralysis. There are controversies concerning whether the conditions provide suitable models for the study of multiple sclerosis and other demyelinating diseases.

experimental autoimmune thyroiditis: autoimmune diseases invoked by injecting thyroid gland extracts along with an adjuvant. They are used as models for studying some thyroid gland disorders. Similar conditions arise spontaneously in a few species, including Buffalo rats and a strain of obese chickens.

explants: tissues, organs, or organ fragments removed from the body and grown in culture. The cultures can provide large numbers of cells of the desired types, and can be used to investigate the effects of hormones, inhibitors, and other factors on growth and/or differentiation. Some interactions between the various cell types are retained, but not all *in vivo* conditions are preserved. Many cells soon display abnormal responses, or give rise to ones that do.

expression: in molecular biology, gene transcription, or the appearance of proteins whose synthesis is directed by the messenger RNAs formed.

expression vector: a construct designed to promote expression of a specific gene in a different (prokaryotic or eukaryotic) cell type. It is usually a plasmid that contains a recombinant DNA (cDNA) derived from the messenger RNA transcript, attached to a suitable promotor. The cDNA does not contain introns. Expression vectors are used to synthesize large quantities of host type proteins (such as human insulin and human growth hormone) by bacterial cells (which lack enzymes for intron excision).

extant: living today.

extended haplotypes: sets of major histocompatibility complex genes that display positive linkage disequilibrium.

extendin-3: His-Ser-Asp-Gly-Thr-Phe-Thr-Ser-Asp-Leu-Ser-Lys-Gln-Met-Glu-Glu-Glu-Ala-Val-Arg-Leu-Phe-Ile-Glu-Trp-Leu-Lys-Asn-Gly-Gly-Pro-Ser-Ser-Gly-Ala-Pro-Pro-Pro-Ser; a peptide in the venom of the gila monster, *Hiloderma horridum*, that promotes insulin release. It is chemically related to members of the glucagon family.

external genitalia: externally visible reproductive organs, for example penis, scrotum, clitoris, labia, and vagina, and their embryonic and fetal precursors.

exteroceptor: a structure specialized for reception of environmental stimuli; *cf* **interoceptor**.

extinction: (1) progressive weakening of a conditioned response. It is used to study the effects of hormones and other factors on learning and memory; (2) disappearance or annihilation of a species; (3) loss of an allele from a population.

extra-: a prefix meaning outside of, or in addition to.

extracellular fluid: ECF. The term usually refers to the bulk extracellular fluid that surrounds most cells, and is stored in loose connective tissue (but is also applied to smaller amounts of specialized types such as cerebrospinal and bone extracellular fluids, aqueous humor, endolymph, and perilymph, which are confined to certain compartments). The major ions are Na^+ and Cl^-, but the fluid also contains other inorganic ions, solutes such as glucose and amino acids, and small quantities of protein. The volume usually varies directly with the total ECF sodium content. When hydration and electrolyte balance are maintained, it is approximately three times that of blood plasma. Under normal conditions, it increases when sodium is retained, and decreases when the diet provides inadequate amounts of the mineral, or when large amounts of Na$^+$ are excreted. However, water deprivation, salt loading, and changes in vasopressin levels can upset the balance. Bulk ECF freely diffuses across capillary walls in both directions. The composition and volume of fluids in specialized compartments are regulated by the cells that make them.

extracellular matrix: ECM: the nonliving matter secreted by cells that accumulates along cell surfaces and fills intercellular spaces. It is especially abundant in connective tissues. Epithelial tissue contains very little intercellular matter, but the cells rests on basal laminae. The matrix made by each cell type has unique features that are related to special combinations of fibrous components (collagens, elastin, and reticulin), linking proteins (such as fibronectin, vitronectin, laminins, thrombodspondin, and osteopontin), and space-filling molecules (proteoglycans, hyaluronic acid, and glycoproteins). It can vary from semi-fluid (in loose connective tissues) to rigid (in bone). The functions, which vary with the types, include support and protection. In soft tissues, matrix components play essential roles in cell adhesion and contact inhibition, provide traction for cell motility (regulated in part by protein gradients that draw cells to higher concentrations), and contribute to growth and morphogenesis. Many contain domains recognized by cell surface receptors. For example, RGD (Arg-Gly-Asp) amino acid sequences are recognized by integrins. Metastasis is usually preceded by detectable changes in the ECM components and their receptors.

extracellular signal-related kinases: ERKs: ERK-1, ERK-2, ERK-3, and related serine-threonine protein kinases activated by insulin, nerve growth factor, and other growth stimulants, that link growth factor receptor mediated tyrosine phosphorylation to covalent modification of target proteins. *See* **MAP kinases**.

extrachromosomal inheritance: extranuclear inheritance; transmission of hereditary material via elements other than chromosomes, for example mitochondria, chloroplasts, or plasmids.

extraembryonic coelom: a cavity formed by coalescence of smaller ones which develops in the mesoderm that surrounds young mammalian embryos. Extra-embryonic splanchnopleuric mesoderm covers the **exocoelomic cavity** (*q.v.*), whereas extra-embryonic somatopleuric mesoderm lines the amnion and cytotrophoblast.

extranuclear inheritance: extrachromosomal inheritance.

extrapyramidal: outside the pyramidal tract, a term that refers to the structures and activities of the basal ganglia, red nucleus, vestibular nucleus, reticular formation, and descending nerve tracts that mediate involuntary control of skeletal muscle functions.

extrinsic: exogenous; *cf* **intrinsic**.

extrinsic factor: **vitamin B$_{12}$** (*q.v.*); *see* also **intrinsic factor**.

extrinsic pathway: *see* **blood coagulation** and **complement**.

exudates: discharges, usually of fluid from blood vessels into extracellular spaces. They can contain fibrin and other proteins, cells, and cell debris. Their formation accelerates when excessive pressure is exerted on blood vessels, and when capillary permeability increases during inflammatory reactions.

eye derived growth factors: growth-promoting peptides initially isolated from the eyes. *Eye-derived growth factor-1* is identical with a β-fibroblast growth factor, and *eye-derived growth factor-2* is an α-fibroblast growth factor.

F

F: (1) phenylalanine; (2) fluorine; (3) Fahrenheit; (4) factor; (5) F factor; (6) farad; (7) variance ratio; (8) the fibrous form of a protein, as in F-actin.

F: Faraday's constant.

f: feline.

f: (1) formyl, as in *f*-**Met**; (2) femto; (3) frequency.

F_o: a transmembrane mitochondrial protein with four kinds of polypeptide chains. The hydrophobic domain forms the $F_o F_1$-ATPase proton channel.

F_1: (1) the first generation of a mating; (2) coupling factor 1; a multimeric 380K protein component of F_o-F_1-ATPase proton channels, composed of five kinds of polypeptide chains ($\alpha_3\beta_3\gamma\delta\epsilon$), that catalyzes ATP synthesis in the presence of a proton gradient, but promotes the reverse reaction when solubilized. *See* also F_1 **inhibitor.**

F_2: the progeny of an F_1 generation, produced by mating two F_1 individuals (or by self-fertilization of one F_1 parent).

FA: (1) fluorescent antibody; (2) fluorescin labelled antibody; (3) fluorescent assay; (4) Fanconi's anemia.

Fab fragment: one of the two 45K proteins cleaved by papain from an immunoglobulin molecule, composed of one light, and a portion of one heavy chain. It has a single antigen-binding site. Fab fragments can bind to and prevent agglutination or precipitation of bivalent antibodies, but cannot cross-link antigens.

Fab′ fragment: one of the two pieces of an immunoglobulin molecule obtained by reducing the disulfide bonds between the heavy chain components of an $F(ab')_2$ fragment. It has a single antigen binding site. FAB′ fragments cannot promote agglutination or precipitation.

$F(ab')_2$ fragment: the 95K protein cleaved by pepsin from an immunoglobulin molecule. It has two antigen-binding sites, two light chains, and portions of two heavy chains. The fragments can cross-link antigens, and cause agglutination or precipitation.

Fabc fragment: a protein obtained by limited papain digestion of an immunoglobulin molecule, composed of one Fab and one Fc fragment. It has one antigen-binding site. The fragments cannot cause agglutination or precipitation.

FABP: fatty acid binding protein.

Fabricius, bursa of: *See* **Bursa of Fabricius.**

Fabry's disease: an inherited, X-linked disease in which a defective α-galactosidase gene leads to glycosphin-golipid accumulation in endothelial cell lysosomes. The resulting blood vessel damage can cause corneal lesions and adversely affect the cardiovascular and renal systems.

Facb fragment: a protein obtained by plasmin digestion of an acid-denatured IgG type immunoglobulin molecule. It has two antigen-binding sites, and retains the complement-fixation properties of the parent molecule. The fragments can cause agglutination or precipitation.

facilitated diffusion: carrier-mediated passive transport; *see* **diffusion**, and *cf* **active transport.**

facilitation: (1) processes whereby one hormone (or other regulator) increases the effectiveness of, lowers the requirements for, or shortens the latent period for another; (2) the enhanced synaptic efficiency that follows presynaptic stimulation; *see*, e.g. **excitatory postsynaptic potential**.

FACS: fluorescence activated cell sorter; *see* **flow cytometry.**

facteur serum thymique: FST; see **thymulin.**

F-actin: *see* **actin**.

factor: F; (1) a component of a body fluid, cell fraction, cell, tissue extract, conditioned medium, or other biological material that reproducibly displays a special kind of activity. Numbers and/or letters distinguish members of a group involved in a common function; *see*, for example **coagulation**, **complement fixation**, **initiation**, and **elongation factors**; (2) a term applied to many regulators that affect cell growth and/or differentiation; *see* **growth factors** and specific types, such as epidermal, fibroblast, and platelet derived (EGF, FGF, and PDGF); (3) a hormone whose activity is known, but whose chemical nature has not as yet been defined. For example, the hypothalamic extract component that stimulates the secretion of thyroid stimulating hormone (TSH, thyrotropin) was initially called thyrotropin release factor (TRF). The structure is now known, and most authors use the term thyrotropin releasing hormone (TRH), although some still prefer older designation; (4) a hormone-like regulator that acts via paracrine, autocrine, or intracrine mechanisms.

Factrel: a commercial preparation of porcine or ovine gonadotropin releasing hormone (GnRH).

facultative: describes organisms that preferentially use a metabolic pathway under some conditions, but can substitute alternate (often less efficient) ones when the environment changes. For example, some yeasts are called facultative anaerobes, because they obtain most of their energy for ATP synthesis from oxidative phosphorylation when oxygen is plentiful, but can switch to glycolysis as the primary source when oxygen deprived.

facultative heterochromatin: (1) heterochromatin that is condensed under some conditions; (2) heterochromatin that is condensed in some cells but not in others. Much of the chromatin of the second X chromosome of a normal (XX) female is condensed (inactivated) in somatic cells; but it is decondensed in ovarian cells when they are engaged in oogenesis.

FAD, FADH$_2$: the oxidized and reduced forms, respectively, of flavin adenine dinucleotide.

fa/fa obese rats: Zucker rats; homozygous members of a rat strain used in obesity studies. They are hyperphagic, hyperinsulinemic, hyperlipidemic, hypothyroid, and hypothermic, and have hypersensitive glucocorticoid receptors. They also display augmented parasympathetic, and low sympathetic nervous system tone, and have abnormal hypothalamic neurons. Morning blood corticosteroid levels are high in both sexes. Males also have high evening levels and exaggerated adrenocorticotropic hormone (ACTH) and corticosterone responses to stress.

Fahrenheit: F: a system for defining temperature, in which the freezing point of water at atmospheric pressure is 32°, and the boiling point 212°; *cf* **Celsius** and **Kelvin**. One degree Fahrenheit = 5/9 degree Celsius. °F = 32 + 9/5 x °C.

falces: plural of falx.

Fallopian tubes: mammalian oviducts; paired female reproductive organs that receive and transport oocytes and spermatozoa, provide sites for capacitation and fertilization, support blastocyst development, and deliver blastocysts to the uterine cavity. Moveable, finger-like projections (fimbriae) lie close to the ovaries around the time of ovulation and direct the oocytes towards the openings (ostia). Cilia and smooth muscle contractions then aid in gamete propulsion to the fertilization site. Regulators of Fallopian tube structure and function include estrogens, progesterone, and catecholamines.

false negative: failure to detect something sought, although it is present; *cf* **false positive**.

false positive: describes a test result in which something appears to exist but is not, in fact present; *cf* **false negative**.

false transmitter: a substance chemically similar to a neurotransmitter that acts as a weak agonist when presented alone, but interferes with the effects of the more potent physiological ligand by competing with it for receptor binding. False transmitters are made in small amounts under normal conditions, and in larger ones when enzyme defects or pharmacological agents impair neurotransmitter synthesis and/or degradation. For example, administration of monoamine oxidase inhibitors accelerates formation of octopamine and synephrine.

falx: a sickle-shaped structure. The *falx cerebri* is a dura mater fold that separates the right and left cerebral hemispheres and encloses the superior and inferior sagittal

sinuses. The *falx cerebelli* partially separates the right and left cerebellar hemispheres.

familial: occurring in a family, or affecting more members of a family than would be predicted on the basis of chance.

familial hypercholesterolemia: *see* **low density lipoproteins**.

familial multiple endocrine neoplasia: *see* **multiple endocrine neoplasia**.

family: (1) a social group, such as parents, children, and other close relatives; (2) a set of entities (for example proteins or genes) with similar chemical compositions, three-dimensional structures and/ or biological properties; *cf* **superfamily**.

famotidine: Pepcid: 3-[[[2-[(aminoiminomethyl)amino]-4-thiazolyl]-methyl-thio]-*N*-(aminosul-fonyl)-propanimidamine; an H$_2$ type histamine receptor antagonist used to treat peptic ulcers.

Fanconi's anemia: FA: an inherited disease in which chromosome fragility caused by impaired transport from cytoplasm to nucleus, of enzymes required for DNA repair leads to lowering of the numbers of all formed elements of the blood, and increases the risk for developing leukemia.

Fanconi syndrome: congenital or acquired proximal tubule defects that cause excessive loss of phosphate, amino and imino acids, sodium, potassium, bicarbonate, and in some cases also glucose and proteins to the urine, and thereby metabolic acidosis and rickets or osteomalacia.

farad: F; a capacitance unit, equal to 1 coulomb/volt.

Faraday's constant: *F*; a unit equivalent to 96493.5 coulombs per mole (the electron charge on one mole of a univalent ion).

farnesenes: several chemically related terpenes made by animals and plants; *see* α and β types and **farnesyl pyrophosphate**. Laminin, active transducin, and ras proteins are among the molecular species that anchor to plasma membranes via covalently linked farnesyl groups. The linkages seem to be essential for guanine nucleotide binding and other functions. *See* also **isoprenylation**.

α-**farnesene**: 3,7,11-trimethyl-1,3,6-10-dodecatetraene; a fire ant trail, and aphid alarm pheromone. It is also made by plants, and released to the skins of apples and other types, where it contributes to defenses against insects.

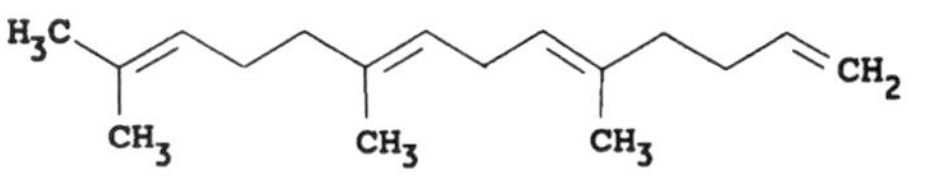

α-farnesene

β-farnesene: 7,11,dimethyl-3-methylene-1,6,10-dodecatriene; an aphid pheromone, and a component of many essential (aromatic) oils.

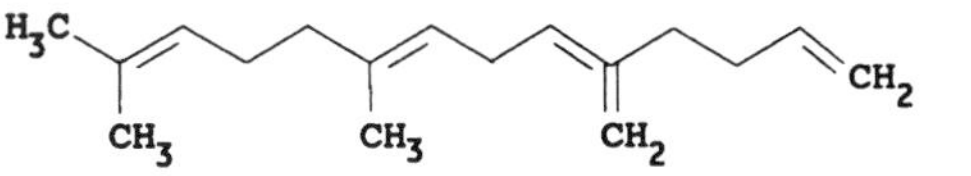

farnesol: several isomers of 3,7,11-trimethyl-2,6-10-dodecatrien-1-ol. They are components of essential oils used in the perfume industry.

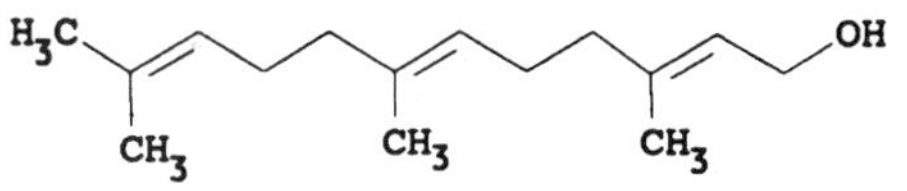

farnesyl pyrophosphate: FPP; 3,7-dimethyl-2-6-octadien-1-ol; an intermediate in the pathway for biosynthesis of cholesterol and some other lipids, made in the reaction: geranyl-PP + isopentyl-PP → FPP + P-P. It, and several derivatives, are components of essential oils used in the perfume industry and as insect attractants.

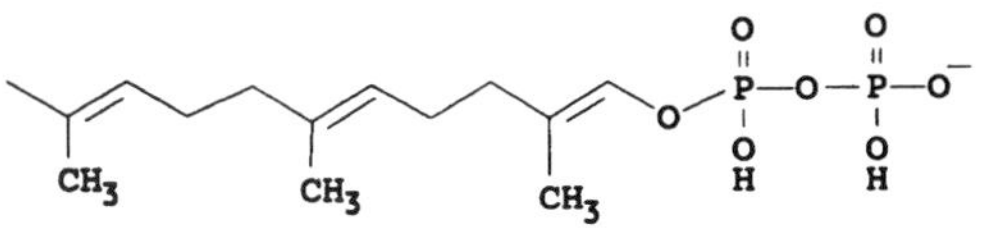

farrow: to give birth to swine.

Fas: a cysteine-rich, 36K protein that resembles CD40 and the receptors for tumor necrosis and nerve growth factors (TNFs and NGFs). It inhibits apoptosis, and is believed to play roles in embryogenesis and clonal deletion of T lymphocytes. Overexpression invokes transformation in some cell types.

fascia: a layer of fibrous connective tissue.

fascicle: fasciculus; a small bundle or cluster, a term usually applied to fibrous connective tissue that surrounds small groups of nerve, muscle, or tendon fibers.

fasciculation: (1) formation of functional units composed of small numbers of nerve fibers held together by connective tissue; *see also* **fascicle**; (2) repeated contractions of small numbers of muscle fibers following discharge of impulses from a single nerve fiber.

fasciculin II: a 6.7K protein made by *Dendroaspis angusticeps* snakes that inhibits acetylcholinesterases and butyrylcholinesterases.

fasciculus [fasciculi]: plural of fascicle.

fascin: a 58K actin bundling protein in intestinal microvilli, and in sea-urchin eggs.

fast green: *N*-ethyl-*N*-[4-[[4-[ethyl[3sulfonphenyl)-methyl]amino]phenyl])-4-hydroxy-2-sulfophenyl)methylene]-2,5-cyclohexadien-1-ylidene]-3-sulfobenzene-methanaminium hydroxide disodium salt; a biological stain for muscle, cornified epithelial cells, and collagen. It is also used to identify proteins separated by electrophoresis.

fat: *see* **triacylglycerols**.

fate map: a diagram of the cell types, tissues, or regions of a young embryo and the structures into which they develop.

F-ATPase: *see* **F₁F₂-ATPase** (under FF).

fatty acids: compounds of the general type R—COOH. Most R groups of phospholipids, cholesterol esters, and animal triacylglycerols are long hydrocarbon chains; *see*, for example **palmitic**, **oleic**, and **arachidonic acids**. Dairy products are among the foods with butyric and other short-chain types. *See* also **essential fatty acids**, **fatty acid oxidation** and **fatty acid synthetase**.

fatty acid oxidation: oxidative degradation of fatty acids. Most cell types use short-chain fatty acid fuels, but cannot degrade the long-chain types released by lipolysis or obtained from food. The liver takes up the long ones, shortens the chains, mostly via β-oxidation, and sends the products it does not use to the bloodstream. The fatty acid is first activated on the outer mitochondrial membrane via a reaction catalyzed by **acyl-CoA synthetase** (*q.v.*). Delivery to the mitochondrial matrix requires coupling of the activated acid to a carnityl carrier via a reaction catalyzed by carnityl transferase I, and a translocase that mediates the transport. The carnityl moiety is cleaved within the mitochondrial compartment by carnityl transferase II. Oxidation of saturated fatty acids then proceeds directly in the matrix, but epimerases are needed for unsaturated types. Acyl-CoA dehydrogenases with varying chain length specificities catalyze the first reaction of the fatty acid oxidation cycle: acyl-CoA + E-FAD → *trans*-Δ^2-enol-CoA + E-FADH₂ (where acyl-CoA is the activated fatty acid, and E is the enzyme). Enoyl-CoA hydratase (crotonase) then catalyzes *trans*-Δ^2-enol-CoA

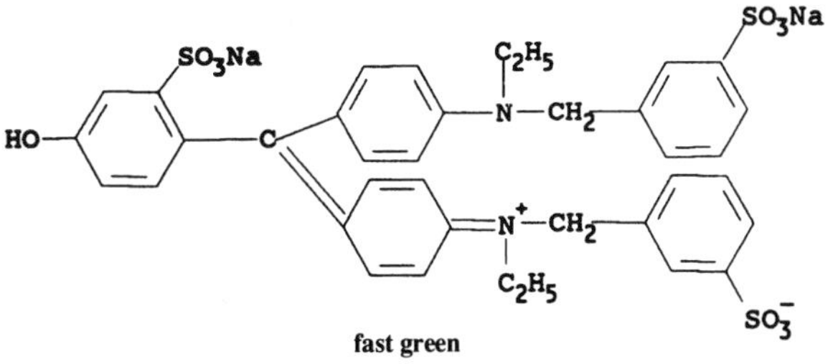

fast green

249

$$R—CH_2—CH_2—CH_2—\overset{O}{\overset{\|}{C}}—S—CoA$$

acyl-CoA

$$R—CH_2—\overset{H}{\underset{}{C}}=\overset{H}{\underset{}{C}}—\overset{O}{\overset{\|}{C}}—S—CoA$$

enoyl-CoA

$$R—CH_2—\overset{H}{\underset{H}{\overset{O}{\underset{}{C}}}}—CH_2—\overset{O}{\overset{\|}{C}}—S—CoA$$

L-hydroxyacyl-CoA

$$R—CH_2—\overset{O}{\overset{\|}{C}}—CH_2—\overset{O}{\overset{\|}{C}}—S—CoA$$

ketoacyl-CoA

$+ H_2O \rightarrow$ L-3-hydroxyacyl-CoA. Next, L-3-hydroxyacyl-CoA dehydrogenase catalyzes L-hydroxyacyl-CoA + NAD$^+$ $\rightarrow$ 3-ketoacyl-CoA + NADH + H$^+$. Finally, β-ketothiolase catalyzes shortening of the 3-ketoacyl-CoA to a fatty acyl-CoA with 2 fewer carbons than the initial metabolite, and the release of a molecule of acetyl-CoA. Each time the fatty acid cycle is repeated, another acetyl-CoA is released, and the substrate chain is shortened by two carbons. The end products are usually acetyl-CoA and either acetoacetyl-CoA (for fatty acids with even numbered carbons) or propionyl-CoA (for the less common odd-numbered ones). The overall pathway for oxidation of palmityl-Co A can be summarized as: palmityl-CoA + 7 FAD + 7 NAD$^+$ + 7 CoA + 7 H$_2$O $\rightarrow$ 8 acetyl-CoA + 7 FADH$_2$ + 7 NADH + 7 H$^+$. Coenzyme oxidation in electron transport chains releases sufficient energy for synthesis of 35 ATP from 35 ADP + 35 Pi, and oxidation of the 8 acetyl-CoA molecules liberated for 96 additional ATP. Since formation of palmityl-Co A from palmitic acid requires ATP degradation to AMP + P-P, the net yield for complete oxidation of each palmitic acid is 129 ATP. *See also* **ketones**.

fatty acid synthetase: fatty acid synthase: a cytosolic enzyme complex used to make fatty acids from acetyl CoA, and to lengthen fatty acid chains. When acetyl-Co A is the initial substrate, the first step is formation of malonyl-CoA (*see* **acetyl-CoA carboxylase**). Acetyl transacylase and malonyl transacylase convert acetyl-CoA and malonyl-CoA, respectively to acetyl-ACP and malonyl-ACP (*see* **acyl carrier proteins**). The first round of chain elongation begins with a reaction catalyzed by acyl malonyl-ACP condensing enzyme: acetyl-ACP + malonyl-ACP $\rightarrow$ acetoacetyl-ACP + ACP + CO$_2$. The next step, catalyzed by β-ketoacyl-ACP reductase is acetoacetyl-ACP + NADPH + H$^+$ $\rightarrow$ D-3-hydroxybutyryl-ACP + NADP$^+$. 3-hydroxyacyl-ACP dehydratase then catalyzes D-3-hydroxybutyryl-ACP $\rightarrow$ crotonyl-ACP. In the final step of the elongation cycle, enoyl-ACP reductase catalyzes crotonyl-ACP + NADPH

$+ H^+ \rightarrow$ butyryl-ACP + NADP$^+$. Butyryl-ACP enters a second round of chain elongation by condensing with malonyl-ACP, and the process continues until the appropriate length is attained. Finally the ACP is removed by hydrolysis. The overall pathway for palmitic acid synthesis can be summarized as: acetyl-CoA + 7 malonyl-CoA + 14 NADPH + 14 H$^+$ $\rightarrow$ palmitic + 7 CO$_2$ + 14 NADP$^+$ + 8 CoA + 6 H$_2$O. (Formation of 7-malonyl-CoA also requires 7 ATP$\rightarrow$ 7 ADP + 7 Pi.)

fatty streak: a region just below the endothelium of an artery that contains large numbers of foam cells. It is the earliest morphologically recognizable lesion in the wall of a vessel undergoing atherosclerosis.

fauna: the animal life present in a habitat, area, or time period.

favism: hemolysis and other defects that develop following consumption of *Vicia fava* beans by individuals deficient in glucose-6-phosphate dehydrogenase. It is attributed to enzymatic hydrolysis of bean components to quinones that generate oxygen radicals.

Fb fragment: a peptide generated by subtilisin digestion of an immunoglobulin molecule, composed of the constant domains of Fab fragments.

FBJ murine osteogenic sarcoma virus: FBJMSV; a retrovirus that invokes osteogenic tumors in mice, in part by directing production of p55^{fos}.

FBS: fetal bovine serum; *see* **fetal calf serum**.

Fc: an immunoglobulin domain that binds to an Fc receptor. The immunoglobulin class is usually specified, as in Fcε for IgE, and Fcγ for IgG. *See also* **Fc fragments**.

FCA: Freund's complete adjuvant.

FCCP: carbonyl cyanide trifluormethoxy phenyl-hydrazine.

F cells: pancreatic and gastrointestinal cells that secrete pancreatic polypeptide.

$$H_3C—\overset{O}{\overset{\|}{C}}—S—ACP$$

acetyl-ACP

$$^-OOC—CH_2—\overset{O}{\overset{\|}{C}}—S—ACP$$

malonyl-ACP

$$H_3C—\overset{O}{\overset{\|}{C}}—CH_2—\overset{O}{\overset{\|}{C}}—S—ACP$$

acetoacetyl-ACP

$$H_3C—\overset{H}{\underset{\underset{H}{O}}{\overset{}{C}}}—CH_2—\overset{O}{\overset{\|}{C}}—S—ACP$$

D-3-hydroxybutyryl-ACP

$$H_3C—\overset{H}{\underset{}{C}}=\overset{H}{\underset{}{C}}—\overset{O}{\overset{\|}{C}}—S—ACP$$

crotonyl-ACP

$$H_3C—CH_2—\overset{O}{\overset{\|}{C}}—S—ACP$$

butyryl-ACP

F⁺ cells: "male" bacterial cells, with plasmids that contain F (fertility) factor and can donate it to F⁻ types during conjugation; *see also* **Hfr**.

F⁻ cells: "female" bacterial cells that lack F (fertility) factor, but receive it from F⁺ cells during conjugation.

Fc receptors: glycoproteins on the surfaces of several cell types that interact with Fc regions of immunoglobulins. Greek letters indicate the immunoglobulin classes, and numbers and/or letters the subtypes (isoforms). *See* **Fcε** and **Fcγ receptors**.

Fc region: the component of an immunoglobulin molecule that contains the site for interaction with Fc receptors; *see also* **Fc fragment** and **Fc receptors**.

Fcε receptors: FcεR; cell surface glycoproteins that interact with Fc regions of IgE class immunoglobulins. When IgE binds to FcεRI (a high affinity type on mast cells and basophilic leukocytes), it promotes release of histamine (and also of serotonin in some species), and thereby promotes the vasodilation and increased capillary permeability associated with allergic reactions such as hay fever and hives, and contributes to asthmatic attacks (but *see* **leukotrienes**). The rat type has a 35K alpha chain, a 27K beta chain, and two 7K gamma chains. FcεRII (CD23) is a monomeric, low affinity receptor on several cell types that enhances phagocytosis by monocytes, eosinophil cytotoxicity, lymphocyte immunological functions, and the release of inflammatory mediators by blood platelets.

Fc fragments: 50K, crystallizable portions of immunoglobulin molecules, generated by papain digestion of IgGs, or trypsin digestion of IgMs. Each molecule is composed of the *C*-terminal halves of both heavy chains plus part of the hinge region. Since they do not contain variable regions, all Fc fragments from the same Ig class are identical. The fragments do not bind antigens, but contain immunoglobulin components that interact with Fc receptors.

FcγR: Fcγ receptors.

Fcγ receptors: glycoproteins on the surfaces of neutrophils, monocytes, B and T lymphocytes, blood platelets, natural killer cells, and syncytiotrophoblast. Human FcγRI is a monomeric 72K high affinity receptor that binds IgG1 and IgG3 immunoglobulins, and enhances phagocytosis by monocytes. The 40-60K FcγRII isoforms include FcγRII-B1 (CD32), which is expressed on B lymphocytes, is phosphorylated in unstimulated cells, and is a substrate for kinase C, and a modulator of B cell functions. FcγRII-A and FcγRII-B2 on macrophages mediate endocytosis of antigen-antibody complexes and promote the release of inflammatory reaction cytotoxic agents. FcγRIIIs are also expressed on neutrophils, eosinophils, and platelets. FcIIIs are the most abundant of the receptors. Human FcγRIIIs (CD16) are 50K proteins expressed on neutrophils, eosinophils, natural killer cells, and macrophages (but not on monocytes). Paroxysmal nocturnal hemoglobinuria is attributed to insufficient numbers on neutrophils.

FcR: Fc receptor.

FCS: fetal calf serum.

Fd piece: the heavy chain segment of an Fab fragment.

fd phage: a bacteriophage that attacks F (fertility) factor-directed surface components of *E. coli*.

F-duction: sexduction; transfer of a genetic fragment along with F (fertility) factor from one bacterium to another.

FDIM: fluorescence digital imaging microscopy.

FDNB: DNFB; 2,4-dinitro-1-fluorobenzene; *see* **Sanger's reagent**.

Fe: Iron.

FEBs: fetal or feto-neonatal proteins that bind estrogens; *see* α-**fetoproteins**.

fecundation: to make fertile. Artificial fecundation is artificial insemination.

fecundity: reproductive potential; ability to conceive, a term that usually refers to the numbers (and sometimes the quality) of gametes produced. *Cf* **fertility**.

feedback control: regulation of one component of a reaction system by another of the same system, for example regulation of the synthesis and/or activity of a rate-limiting enzyme by an intermediate or end-product of a biochemical pathway, or of the numbers of hormone receptors by the hormone that acts on those receptors. *See* also **negative** and **positive feedback controls**.

feedback loops: pathways that mediate feedback controls. In endocrine system *long* loops, hormones travel via the systemic bloodstream to distantly located target organs. In *short* loops, they are transported to nearby targets via hypothalamo-hypophysial portal blood vessels. *Ultrashort* loops are used for paracrine effects on neighboring cells.

feeder cells: cells of one type added to culture media to support growth of another, for example by releasing growth factors and/or providing suitable substrates (definition 2). They are usually irradiated or pretreated in other ways to block their abilities to proliferate.

feed-forward: the effect (negative or positive) of one intermediate in a pathway on another that follows, or on an end-product of the same system.

feeding "centers": brain regions said to stimulate food intake; *cf* **satiety "centers"**. The concept that any one set of neurons can exert such controls is no longer accepted.

Feldine: a trade name for piroxicam.

feline: *f*: derived from, or characteristic of members of the cat family.

feline leukemia viruses: oncogenic RNA viruses that cause leukemia in cats. The major oncogenes of McDonough and Gardner-Rasheed types are, respectively, p180$^{gag\text{-}fms}$ and p70$^{gag\text{-}fgr}$.

Felis catus: the domesticated cat.

female: ♀; describes members of an animal population that (1) produce, can acquire the ability to produce, or resemble those that produce ova; (2) possess the genetic components associated with the development of ovaries (for example XX chromosome patterns in mammals or WZ types in birds), or (3) display characteristics such as phenotype, behavior patterns, neuron organization, levels of specific enzymes, or numbers and types of hormone receptors associated with those chromosomes. *Cf* **male**. The term is also applied to (1) plants that produce (or can develop the ability to produce) female type gametes, or possess the characteristics of members of the species that do; and (2) microorganisms, such as F$^-$ bacteria, that are recipients of genetic components made by F$^+$ individuals (males), and other small organisms that receive analogous substances.

feminine: displaying female characteristics.

feminizing testis: a form of pseudohermaphroditism caused by androgen insensitivity, in which individuals with male karyotypes acquire predominantly female phenotypes. When no functional androgen receptors are made, testes form and secrete testosterone, but are usually retained in the abdominal cavity. Müllerian ducts undergo atrophy, but Wolffian ducts do not develop, and the external genitalia look like those of normal females at the time of birth. When the hypothalamus matures, and increased production of luteinizing hormone (LH) more strongly stimulates the testes, larger amounts of testosterone are secreted. They are aromatized to estrogens that promote maturation of female-type secondary sex characteristics. The individuals then externally resemble normal adult females. The first overt indication of abnormality may be failure to initiate menstrual cycles. The conditions differ from forms of pseudohermaphroditism in which some functional androgen receptors are made, but 5α-reductase defects impair testoterone conversion to dihydrotestosterone (DHT). Then, Wolffian ducts differentiate (since they respond directly to testosterone), and the high testosterone levels made after puberty affect the development of skeletal muscle, mammary glands, and some other targets; but the external genitalia (which require DHT for masculinization) appear female.

feminotropin: feminizing factor; FF; an uncharacterized regulator, said to be secreted by pituitary glands, that directs acquisition of female type hepatic enzyme patterns. Most observers attribute the effects to sex-related differences in growth hormone secretion patterns.

femoxetine: (+)-*trans*-1-methyl-3-(*p*-(methoxy)phenoxymethyl)-4-phenylpiperidine; an agent that inhibits serotonin uptake by synaptic vesicles. Unlike some other inhibitors, it is ineffective for alleviating psychic depression.

femto: *f*: 10^{-15}, as in femtomole or femtogram.

fenamates: *N*-phenylanthranilic acid derivatives that exert aspirin-like effects, and are used as anti-inflammatory agents. *See*, for example **flufenamic, mefenamic, and meclofenamic acids**.

fenfluramine: *S*(+)-2-ethylamino-1-(3-trifluoromethylphenyl)propane; an orally effective agent with sympathomimetic properties, that blocks serotonin uptake by secretory granules and synaptic vesicles, and accelerates glucose oxidation. The hydrochloride (Pondimin) is used as an anorectic to treat some forms of obesity. The side effects can include sedation and psychic depression in some individuals, and mood elevation, insomnia, and/ or anxiety in others, as well as dizziness, and either diarrhea or constipation. The *R*(-) enantiomer is less active.

fenofibrate: 2-[4-(4-chlorobenzoyl)phenoxy]-2-methylpropanoic acid 1-methylethyl ester; an agent used to prevent the progression of coronary artery disease by lowering plasma triglyceride, total cholesterol, LDL-cholesterol and very low density lipoprotein (VLDL) levels, and elevating HDL-cholesterol. It augments lipoprotein lipase activity, and may additionally accelerate hepatic clearance of VLDLs, but can invoke allergic responses and flu-like symptoms, and increase the risk for developing cholelithiasis or cholecystitis.

fenoldopam: 6-chloro-2,3,4,5-tetrahydro-1-(4-hydroxyphenyl)-1*H*-3-benzazepine-7,9-diol; a selective D$_1$-type dopamine receptor agonist that is used to lower blood pressure.

fenoprofen: Nalfon; Progesic; α-methyl-3-phenoxybenzeneacetic acid; an analgesic and anti-inflammatory agent with properties similar to those of ibuprofen. It is used to treat rheumatoid and osteoarthritis.

fenoterol: 1-(3,5-dihydroxyphenyl)-1-hydroxy-2-[(4-hydroxyphenyl)isopropylamino]ethane; a β$_2$ type adrenergic receptor agonist, used as a bronchodilator, and to arrest premature labor.

fenoprofen

fenoterol

fentanyl: *N*-phenyl-*N*-[1-(2-phenylethyl)-4-piperidinyl] propanamide. The citrate is a short-acting analgesic with morphine-like effects. Chronic use can lead to addiction.

feral: wild; not domesticated, cultured, or maintained under laboratory conditions. The term usually describes animals living in their natural habitats.

fermentation: energy yielding, anaerobic degradation of organic substances by microorganisms, a term often specifically applied to glucose metabolism by yeasts that leads to formation of ethyl alcohol and CO_2.

ferning: formation of leaf-like patterns in uterine cervix mucus collected during the estrogen-dominated perifollicular phase of a menstrual cycle, dried on a glass slide or coverslip, and viewed under a light microscope. It is used as an indicator of the timing of ovarian cycle phases.

ferredoxins: several 6-24K electron transporting proteins made by microorganisms, plants, and animals that contain iron and sulfur (as Fe_2S_2, Fe_4S_4, or $[Fe_4S_4]_2$) and participate in respiration, nitrogen fixation, and photosynthesis. Adrenodoxin is a specific kind of mitochondrial protein, required for synthesis of adrenocortical steroid hormones, that donates electrons to cytochrome P450s; *see* also **cholesterol side-chain cleavage system.**

ferri, ferric: indicates the presence of iron in its trivalent state (Fe^{3+}).

ferritin: the major iron storage protein, in most (possibly all) animal and plant cell types, and especially abundant in liver, spleen, and intestinal mucosa. Each molecule is composed of an apoferritin shell that surrounds a hydrated iron oxide/iron phosphate core capable of holding up to 4500 Fe atoms. Ferritin conserves iron for cell use, is essential for cell growth and proliferation, and protects against toxic effects of excess Fe^{3+}, such as free radical and peroxide formation. The amounts made are directly related to extracellular iron levels (*see* **ferritin inducer, ferritin repressor protein** and **iron response elements**), and are regulated by several hormones. Ferritin also binds zinc and provides some protection against excessive amounts. Since the iron atoms scatter electrons, ferritin conjugated to immunoglobulins and other proteins is used to determine the locations of specific compounds in electron micrographs.

ferritin inducer: a cell component that accelerates formation of the messenger RNA that directs ferritin synthesis. Hemin is a primary candidate, since changes in its levels are inversely related to those of iron, and hemin can inactivate ferritin repressor protein.

ferritin repressor protein, FRP: a 90K protein that binds to iron response elements and inhibits production of ferritin messenger RNA when iron levels are low. Hemin can accelerate ferritin synthesis by inactivating FRP.

ferro, ferrous: indicates the presence of iron in its divalent state (Fe^{2+}).

fertility: ability to produce (or production of) offspring; *cf* **fecundity**.

fertility factor F: F; *see* **F factor**.

fertilization: syngamy; union of two gametes to form a zygote. *See* also **zona pellucida proteins**.

fertilization cone: a somewhat pointed projection from an oocyte surface that forms at the site of entry of a spermatozoan. It is covered by an extension of the plasma membrane, and contains clear cytoplasm continuous with that of the oocyte.

fertilization membrane: fertilization envelope: the specialized, hardened surface membrane elaborated by an oocyte soon after fertilization. It confers some protection against polyspermy; but *see* **fertilization potential**. *See* also **fetuins**.

fertilization potential: the change in the electrical properties of an oocyte plasma membrane that occurs almost immediately after fertilization. It rapidly confers protection against polyspermy (before fertilization membrane formation is completed).

fertilization site: the place where the sperm and oocyte unite. In most mammals, it is at or near the Fallopian tube ampullary-isthmic junction.

fertilizins: species-specific glycoproteins on the surfaces of jellies that coat extruded oocytes of species that use external fertilization. They attract spermatozoa and bind to sperm surface antifertilizins.

fertilysin: *N,N'*-octamethylene-*bis*(2,2-dichloroacetamide); an orally effective agent used to inhibit spermatogenesis in laboratory animals without inhibiting gonadotropin synthesis.

ferulic acid: 3-methoxy-4-hydroxy-cinnamic acid; caffeic acid methyl ether; a compound made in small amounts by many plants, and used as a food preservative. *See* also **caffeic acid**.

$$HC=\overset{\overset{\displaystyle H}{|}}{C}-COOH$$

fes: a Fujinami sarcoma virus oncogene of chickens that codes for a 92K non-receptor tyrosine kinase. The cat homolog is *fps*.

fetal: pertaining to, derived from, or characteristic of a fetus.

fetal bovine serum: FBS; *see* **fetal calf serum**.

fetal calf serum: FCS; fetal bovine serum; serum obtained from calf fetuses, used in diluted form to support the culture of many cell types when defined media are not required. It contains nutrients, and a wide variety of growth factors. *See* also **fetuin** and α-**fetoprotein**.

fetal hemoglobin: hemoglobin F; *see* **hemoglobin**.

fetal membranes: *see* **amnion**, **chorion**, **allantois**, and **placenta**.

fetation: intrauterine fetal growth and development.

feticide: (1) killing or destruction of a fetus (usually by artificial means); (2) a substance that kills fetuses.

fetoplacental unit: a complex formed from placental and fetal components, across which nutrients, respiratory gases, metabolites, and regulators are exchanged. In primates, it is essential for estrogen synthesis. The fetus converts pregnenolone to dehydroepiandrosterone and its sulfate (DHEA and DHEAS), which are taken up and aromatized by the maternal component. The size in laboratory animals varies with the magnitude of genetic difference between the mother and the fetus.

α-**fetoprotein**: AFP; alpha fetoprotein: 65-70K species specific glycoproteins related to albumin, produced in the yolk sac, fetal liver, and fetal gastrointestinal tract. They accumulate in amniotic fluid and fetal blood plasma, and are components of umbilical cord blood and fetal calf serum. Although not directly mitogenic, their abilities to enhance the effects of epidermal growth factor (EGF), transforming growth factor-α (TGFα), and some other growth stimulants suggest roles in fetal growth and development. Amniotic fluid levels are elevated in human fetuses with neural tube defects, and subnormal in those with Down's syndrome. Other proposed functions include maintenance of oncotic pressure in fetuses. Human type AFP is also present in maternal blood and on T lymphocytes during early pregnancy, and is believed to contribute to protection against immunological rejection of fetuses. Small amounts of AFPs are made postnatally by normal liver cells, and are released to the bloodstream in infants. Much larger ones are made by individuals with hepatic cirrhosis and viral hepatitis, and by hepatocellular and embryonal carcinoma cells. Rodent (but not primate) types share homology with a vitamin D binding protein,

avidly bind estrogens, and are believed to protect the female hypothalamus against defeminization. They may also facilitate estrogen transport to some target cells. Additionally, they bind other lipids (including different steroids and arachidonic acid), bilirubin, and cations.

fetuins: the major anionic, low molecular weight α-globulins obtained from the sera of fetal and newborn calves and other ungulates. They possess growth promoting and trypsin-inhibiting properties. Roles in blocking premature hardening of oocyte membranes (*see* **fertilization membrane**) by inhibiting conversion of ZP2 to ZP2f have been proposed.

fetus: a conceptus that has acquired the morphological features characteristic of its species. The human embryo becomes a fetus at 8 weeks post conception.

Feulgen method: a procedure for staining DNA in cells, in which aldehyde groups released by mild acid hydrolysis react with periodic acid Schiff (PAS) stain to form a purple colored derivative.

fever: elevated body temperature in which thermoregulatory mechanisms are retained, but the set-point is above the normal range. The most common causes are bacterial toxins and cytokines released in response to them. *See* **pyrogens**, and *cf* **hyperthermia**.

FF: (1) feminizing factor; *see* **feminotropin**; (2) follicular fluid factor.

F factor: F; fertility factor F; sex factor F; F plasmid: a 94.5 kilobase genetic component of F$^+$ bacteria that can be donated to an F$^-$ type. *See* also **F$^+$ cells** and **Hfr**.

F$_1$F$_2$-ATPase: H-ATPase; the mitochondrial protein complex that catalyzes synthesis of ATP from ADP + Pi. See also **F$_1$** (definition 2), **F$_1$ inhibitor**, **F$_2$**, and **oxidative phosphorylation**.

FGFs: *see* **fibroblast growth factors**, and individual types.

fgr: a Gardner-Rasheed feline sarcoma oncogene that directs formation of a 55-60K protein of the *src* tyrosine kinase family.

fiber: (1) an elongated threadlike or rope-like structure; *cf* **filaments**; (2) a term that assumes special meanings when preceded by others, as in muscle, nerve, collagen, or dietary fiber.

fibric acids: several chemically related agents used to lower circulating triacylglycerol and cholesterol levels; *see*, for example **clofibrate**, **fenfibrate**, and **gemfibrozil**.

fibril: a fine, thread-like structure; *see*, for example **myofibrils**. Fibrils are smaller than fibers, and can contain microfilaments.

fibrillar center: a pale-staining region of a nucleolus, surrounded by dense fibrillar components, that contains DNA which is not actively transcribed.

fibrillin: a 350K connective tissue glycoprotein. It is the major component of microfibrils. Marfan's syndrome is attributed to an autosomal dominant gene mutation that impairs formation of normal fibrillin.

fibrin: usually, fibrin-i, an insoluble multimeric protein. *Fibrin-s* is soluble monomeric 323K protein cleaved directly from fibrinogen via a reaction catalyzed by thrombin when blood clots (*see* **coagulation**), fibrinogen leaks from damaged blood vessels, or inflammatory reaction mediators increase capillary permeability. After soft clots composed of fibrin-s networks organize, thrombin activates fibrin stabilizing factor, which catalyzes polymerization to form the fibrin-i of firm clots. Blood clots (which trap formed elements) arrest hemorrhaging by plugging small blood vessels. Fibrin clots in extracellular spaces provide temporary barriers (later fortified by fibers) that slow the spread of toxins and infectious agents during inflammatory reactions.

fibrin stabilizing factor: FSF; a proenzyme in blood plasma, activated by a thrombin catalyzed reaction. *See* **fibrin**.

fibrinogen: a soluble 340K globular protein composed of 6 peptide chains, synthesized in the liver and secreted to the bloodstream. In addition to serving as the fibrin precursor, it binds to gp IIb/IIIa on activated platelets and enhances aggregation.

fibrinolysin: an enzyme that catalyzes fibrin degradation, and destroys clots that are no longer needed; *see* **plasmin**.

fibrinopeptides: peptides cleaved from fibrin, via reactions catalyzed by thrombin. Human fibrinopeptide A is Ala-Asp-Ser-Gly-Glu-Gly-Asp-Phe-Leu-Al-Glu-Gly-Gly-Gly-Val-Arg, and human fibrinopeptide B is pGlu-Gly-Val-Asn-Asp-Asn-Glu-Gly-Phe-Phe-Ser-Arg-Ala-Arg.

fibrinoid layer: an acellular film on the outer surface of the trophoblast, implicated as one of the factors that protects fetuses against rejection by maternal immune systems.

fibroblast[s]: widely distributed spindle-shaped connective tissue cells derived from mesoderm. They synthesize collagen, form connective tissue fibers, and can differentiate into chondroblasts, osteoblasts, adipocytes, and muscle cells. Fibroblasts proliferate at sites of inflammation and wound healing, and in mixed cell cultures (in which they can interfere with the growth of other cell types). They are also sources of interferon-β and some other cytokines. Several cell lines (some of which resemble mesodermal stem cells) have been developed for studies of platelet derived growth factor (PDGF) and other stimulants of cell growth, differentiation, proliferation, and transformation. *See* also 3**T3 cells**.

fibroblast derived growth factor: *see* **platelet derived** and **fibroblast growth factors**.

fibroblast growth factors: FGFs; a family of regulators, also known as heparin binding growth factors, with primary structures that resemble those of interleukins 1α and 1β. Seven types (along with some subtypes), have been identified (*see* items that follow). Several genes (including ones located on human chromosomes 4, 5, 11, and 12) code for various types, all of which may derive from a common ancestral DNA segment. The terminology is confusing, since not all of the peptides act on or originate in fibroblasts. Moreover, interleukin-3, macrophage colony stimulating factor (M-CSF), and many other regulators that are not structurally or biologically related also interact with heparin (and with heparan sulfates). Before the identities were established, at least thirty different names, related to the sites of action, were introduced. (Examples include ovarian, seminiferous, chondrocyte, kidney, hypothalamic, pituitary, hepatic, retinal, and melanocyte growth factors.) At least twenty are FGF-1 or FGF-2 subtypes. The kinds and amounts expressed vary with the cell types, and with developmental stages. The range of functions includes support of survival, growth, proliferation, and differentiation of cell types derived from all three embryonic germ layers, influences on cell motility, cytoskeletal organization, extracellular matrix composition, the activities of some proteases, the secretion of other regulators, and contributions to angiogenesis, vasodilation, wound healing and tissue repair. However, some FGFs act on only certain kinds of cells, not all are mitogenic, and ones that are mitogenic additionally act in other ways. Their effects are mediated by a variety of high-affinity receptors, some of which display ligand-activated tyrosine kinase activity. Different, low-affinity receptors include proteoglycan components. In some cell types, two or more peptides bind to the same kind of high-affinity receptor, and display overlapping biological properties; but in others the actions are mutually antagonistic. One member of the FGF family can also bind to its own receptor but augment the activity of another. When overexpressed or continuously presented, some FGFs invoke transformation that is reversed after withdrawal. Others have stronger, persistent transforming potential; and high levels of some types (made in small amounts by normal cells) are present in specific kinds of cancers. FGFs anchored to plasma membranes affect mostly neighboring cells, but truncated forms that lack *N*-terminal amino acids are secreted; and intracrine effects that include induction of FGF receptors are also known.

fibroblast growth factor-1: *see* acidic **fibroblast growth factor**.

fibroblast growth factor-2: *see* basic **fibroblast growth factor**.

fibroblast growth factor 3: *see* **int-2**.

fibroblast growth factor 4: K-FGF; *see* **Kaposi sarcoma fibroblast growth factor** and **hst** (human stomach tumor growth factor; heparin binding secretory transforming factor).

fibroblast growth factor-5: FGF-5; heparin binding growth factor-5; HBGF-5; a member of the fibroblast growth factor family identified in many parts of the brain and spinal cord, and in embryonic cells that differentiate into neurons and neuroglia. It is implicated as a trophic factor for those cells.

fibroblast growth factor-6: FGF-6; heparin binding growth factor-6; HBGF-6; hst-2; *see* **hst**.

fibroblast growth factor-7: KGF; *see* **keratinocyte growth factor**.

acidic fibroblast growth factor: aFGF; α-fibroblast growth factor; αFGF; heparin binding growth factor-1; HBG-1; closely related members of the fibroblast growth factor family with acidic (5.6) isoelectric points. The subtypes appear to be identical with all of the following: astroglial growth factor 1, embryonic kidney-derived angiogenesis factor, endothelial cell growth factor (ECGF), endothelial growth factor, eye-derived growth factor II, heparin-binding growth factor class I, and prostatotropin. The major form has 140 amino acids; another (des 1-6 aFGF) lacks the first 6 *N*-terminal amino acids. The mitogenic potency is weak (compared with that of β-FGF), but is potentiated by heparin binding (which increases the affinity for receptors, and causes endothelial cells to respond). The actions include inhibition of myoblast differentiation (which is stimulated by basic FGFs). Although encoded by genes on different chromosomes, and displaying different distributions, they are structurally related to basic FGFs, and can act on the same receptors. Both types share amino acid sequences with interleukin-1β, and with some neuropeptides, and both bind to fibronectin RGD (Arg-Gly-Asp) sequences.

basic fibroblast growth factor: beta fibroblast growth factor; bFGF; β-FGF; fibroblast growth factor-2; heparin binding growth factor-2; HBGF-2: several widely distributed peptides with basic (9.6) isoelectric points that participate in the regulation of growth, differentiation, and proliferation of many cell types, affect the secretion of several hormones, and contribute to bone remodeling. One form has 146 amino acids, some others have a few more moieties, and des 1-15 bFGF lacks the first 15 *N*-terminal amino acids. They appear to be identical with all of the following: astroglial growth factor-2, cartilage-derived growth factor 1, chondrosarcoma growth factor, embryonic kidney-derived angiogenesis factor 2, eye-derived growth factor I, heparin binding growth factors class II, human placenta purified factor, hepatoma growth factor, leukemia growth factor, macrophage growth factor, myogenic growth factor, prostatic growth factor, and uterine-derived growth factor. Many cell types derived from mesenchyme and neuroectoderm (including ones in brain, retina, bone, placenta, kidney, ovary, pituitary, adrenal, and thymus) make and respond to them. Monocytes, macrophages, vascular endothelial cells, and eye lens epithelial cells are additional targets; and tumor types affected include melanoma, hepatoma, and chondrosarcoma. Hypothalamic bFGF stimulates of the growth of neurons that make gonadotropin releasing hormone (GnRH). β-FGF made in folliculostellate cells plays roles in maintaining hypothalamo-hypophysial blood vessels, promotes lactotrope and thyrotrope proliferation, and augments thyroid stimulating hormone (TSH), and thyrotropin releasing hormone (TRH)-stimulated prolactin secretion. Pituitary bFGF released to the bloodstream is mitogenic for cells of the adrenal cortex, and locally released peptide suppresses follicle stimulating hormone (FSH)-stimulated estrogen secretion, luteinizing hormone (LH)-stimulated testosterone pro-

duction, and the formation of LH receptors in gonads. Heparin binding does not augment the potency, but does protect it against degradation.

fibroblast pneumocyte factor: a regulator believed to be made by fibroblasts, that affects surfactant production in the lungs.

fibrocytes: mature, fiber-forming fibroblasts.

fibroid tumors: fibromyomas: *see* **leiomyomas**.

fibroin: the major protein of silk, made in large amounts by the silkworm, *Bombyx mori*, and in smaller ones by some other arthropods. It has a rigid, filamentous, antiparallel beta-pleat type structure with many Gly-Ser-Gly-Ala-Gly-Ala sequences.

fibrolipomas: adipocyte tumors that contain considerable amounts of fibrous connective tissue.

fibromatosis: formation of large numbers of tumor-like connective tissue lesions that contain fibers and actively proliferating cells.

fibromyositis: inflammation of muscle and associated connective tissue.

fibronectins: FNs: α$_2$SB glycoproteins; α$_2$-opsonins; several chemically related high molecular weight glycoproteins, composed of disulfide linked 210-250K peptide chains, present on cell surfaces, in blood plasma, amniotic and other fluids, in soft connective tissue matrices, and in most basement membranes. Similar molecules are made by insects, yeasts, and bacteria. Multiple forms within a species arise from differential, cell regulated splicing of messenger RNAs, and from posttranslational modifications that include phosphorylation, glycosylation, acylation, tyrosyl sulfation, and self-association. They contain domains that bind to numerous cell surface, intracellular, and extracellular components, including all collagen types, glycosaminoglycans, proteoglycans, prothrombin, fibrinogen, fibrin, IgG type immunoglobulins, C3 complement component, thrombospondin, plasminogen activator, plasminogen, heparin, some seminal plasma proteins, and DNA. The binding affinities are affected by the structures, and by associations with other proteins, such as tenascin. Arg-Gly-Asp (RGD), Arg-Gly-Asp-Ser (RGDS) and other FN sequences are recognized by many cell adhesion factors and growth promoting peptides, and at least five kinds of receptors are present on cell surfaces (*see* also **integrins** and **very late antigens**). Some mediate interactions with cytoskeletal proteins. FNs regulate cell adhesion (including platelet aggregation), cell shape, cell migration, morphogenesis and wound healing, and are used as attachment factors for cell and tissue cultures. The processes affected in embryos include gastrulation and the migration of neural crest cells. FNs are also involved in immunoglobulin switching by B lymphocytes, and in some other functions of specialized mature cells. Circulating forms, made mostly in the liver, function as opsonins, contribute to blood coagulation and phagocytosis of cell debris, and can be incorporated into extracellular matrices. Abnormal changes in FN and FN receptor expression are believed to contribute to metastasis.

fibronectin inhibitors: several synthetic peptides (for example Arg-Gly-Asp-Ser and Arg-Gly-Asp-Ser-Pro), that bind to fibronectin and block the abilities of FN (and also of vitronectin, Von Willebrand factor, and some other proteins) to bind to other molecules.

fibroneuromas: benign peripheral nerve neoplasms that contains fibrous as well as neuronal components.

fibronexus: a plasma membrane region in which the cytoskeletal components link to the extracellular matrix. In most cases, the connection is established by cytoplasmic vinculin binding to both intracellular actin filaments and a transmembrane protein (that, in turn, binds extracellular fibronectin).

fibroplasia: usually, excessive formation of fibrous tissue. Substantial amounts of the tissue can be made during normal wound healing. When not adequately regulated, it can severely affect blood vessels.

fibrosarcomas: malignant tumors composed mostly of cells derived from collagen-secreting fibroblasts.

fibrosis: usually, replacement of normal tissues by fibrous connective tissue; scar formation. When preceded by other terms (as in cystic fibrosis), it describes specific kinds of degenerative lesions.

ficin: a proteolytic enzyme (or the whole latex) extracted from fig trees of the *Ficus* genus. It is used to digest proteins, and for Rh factor determinations.

Ficoll: a nonionic sucrose polymer used for density gradient centrifugation, and to isolate lymphocytes from whole blood.

"fight or flight": a set of coordinated, catecholamine-mediated responses to stress that includes cardiac stimulation, vasoconstriction in the skin, mucous membranes and most viscera, bronchodilation, mydriasis, inhibition of visceral smooth muscle contraction, increased blood flow to skeletal muscle, improved neuromuscular transmission, arousal, and often anxiety (*see* also **norepinephrine** and **epinephrine**). The responses support the ability to engage in sustained skeletal muscle activity, and to cope in other ways with emergency situations and stress. They usually subside soon after the stimulus is removed. Excessive or prolonged responses deplete metabolic reserves and can adversely affect the cardiovascular, immune, and other systems.

filaggrin: a protein made by keratinocytes; *see* **profilaggrin**.

filaments: thread-like structures; *see*, for example **micro-**, **intermediate**, **myo-**, and **neurofilaments**.

filamin: the most abundant cytoskeletal cross-linking and bundling protein, composed of two identical, head-to-head linked 260K subunits. The tails bind F-actin, and block the binding of tropomyosin to α-actinin. Filamin monomers are used as gel electrophoresis standards, and dimers as antigens for immunological studies.

filial: describes any generation that follows the parental one; *see* F_1 and F_2.

filigree cells: gonadotropes believed to secrete luteinizing hormone.

filiform: thread-like.

filipin: a polyene antibiotic complex made by *Streptomyces filipenensis*. 4,6,8,10,12,14,16,27-octahydroxy-3-(1-hydroxyhexyl)-17,28-di-methyloxacyclooctacosa-17,19,21,23,25-pentaen-2-one, the filipin-III component shown, is an antifungal agent that augments plasma membrane permeability by interacting with cholesterol. Low concentrations are used in laboratory studies to enhance cell uptake of some substances, to mimic rapidly developing effects of 1,25-dihydroxy-cholecalciferol actions on intestinal mucosa and of some other hormones on plasma membranes, and to invoke an experimental form of arthritis. Very high concentrations destroy membranes.

filly: a young female horse, usually less than 4 years old.

fimbria [fimbriae]: a fringe-like structure; a component of a fringed border or edge. See also **Fallopian tube**.

fimbrin: a 68K cytoskeleton protein of microvilli that binds actin filaments and contributes to the formation of tight bundles.

fingers: *see* **zinc fingers**.

fingerprinting: in molecular biology, techniques for detecting small differences in the primary structures of proteins and nucleic acids, used, for example to identify abnormal hemoglobins, search for common gene characteristics in the relatives of individuals with familial diseases, or compare DNAs of parents and offspring for legal or other purposes. The test materials are cleaved by enzymes that act at specific sites, and the fragments are separated by electrophoresis and chromatography. After staining, the patterns are compared with those obtained from closely related control substances treated in the same way.

finger swap: techniques for studying the properties of hormone-receptor complexes that bind to specific DNA base sequences; *see* **zinc fingers**.

finickiness: describes eating behaviors of the kinds observed in animals with lesions of the ventromedial nuclei and other hypothalamic regions. The animals eat voraciously and become grossly obese when given free access to palatable food, but reject unappetizing diets accepted by hungry intact animals, and refuse to "work" for their food (for example by lifting heavy lids or repeatedly pressing bars).

F$_1$ inhibitor: an oligomycin-sensitive protein within the stalk that joins F$_o$ and F$_1$ proteins of eukaryote ATP synthase complexes. It regulates proton flow and ATP synthesis.

firefly luciferin: 4,5-dihydro-2-(6-hydroxy-2-benzothiazolyl)-4-thiazolcarboxylic acid; a compound obtained from *Photinus pyralis*, used to study photochemical reactions, and for ATP determinations.

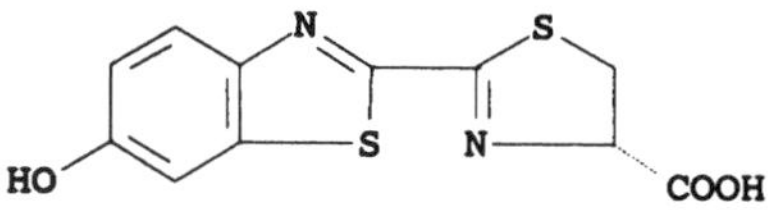

first law of thermodynamics: (1) energy cannot be created or destroyed, but can be changed in form; (2) the energy lost (or gained) by a system is exactly equivalent to the energy gained (or lost) from its surroundings. *See* also **second** and **third law of thermodynamics**.

first order reactions: chemical reactions in which enzymes are present in larger amounts than required, and the rates of product formation vary directly with the substrate concentrations; *cf* **zero order reactions**.

first polar body: *see* **polar bodies**.

FISH: fluorescence *in situ* hybridization; techniques in which fluorescent probes are used to identify specific kinds of compounds or other cell components. When two different dyes are employed, duplication of interphase chromosome genes can be visualized.

fission: splitting. The term is applied to (1) a form of asexual reproduction in microorganisms (binary fission), in which one cell gives rise to two daughters; (2) disintegration of heavy atom nuclei.

fissure: a groove or tear.

fistula [fistulae]: an abnormal communication between two cavities, caused by tissue destruction, or made surgically for therapeutic or investigational purposes.

FIT: FITC: fluorescein isothiocyanate.

fitness: ability of an organism to survive and reproduce, relative to that of others (usually of the same species).

fixation: (1) physical and/or chemical preparation of biological material for histology that binds it to slides or coverslips, or facilitates embedding. It usually involves protein denaturation and precipitation that protects the specimens against degradation by cell enzymes or microorganisms; but it can distort some structures; (2) removal of complement components from serum, for example with immune complexes, antibody-coated cells, or bacteria; (3) immobilization.

fixatives: agents used for fixation (definition 1), such as ethyl alcohol, formalin, Bouin's fluid, or glutaraldehyde.

FK 366: an agent used to inhibit **aldose reductase** (*q.v.*).

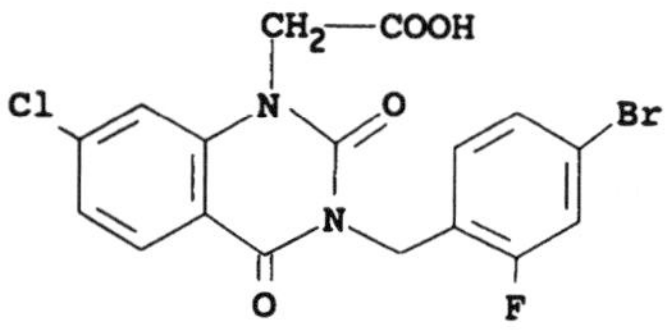

FK 506: 17-allyl,1,14-dihydroxy-12-[2-(4-hydroxy-3-methoxycyclohexyl)-1-methylvinyl]-23,25-dimethoxy-

FK 366

13,19,21,27-tetrmethyl-11,28-dioxa-4-azatricyclo[22.3. 10^{4,9}]octacos-18-ene-2,3,10,16-tetraone; a potent immunosuppressant structurally related to rapamycin, isolated from *Streptomyces tsukubaensis*, and used to block transplant rejection. It inhibits T cell activation and transcription of T cell early activation genes (for interleukins 2, 3, and 4, granulocyte-macrophage colony stimulating factor [GM-CSF], and interferon γ), in part by modifying the synthesis of NF-AT. In common with rapamycin, it binds to and inhibits the activities of FKBPs (immunophilins that bind it with high affinity), but does not affect the rotamase inhibited by cyclosporin A. FK506 also inhibits exocytosis of mast cell granules that is mediated via IgE type immunoglobulin receptors, and a pathway in common with the one that affects T lymphocytes has been suggested. 506BD and rapamycin reverse the FK506 inhibition, but do not affect cyclosporin A effects. *See* also **immunophilins**.

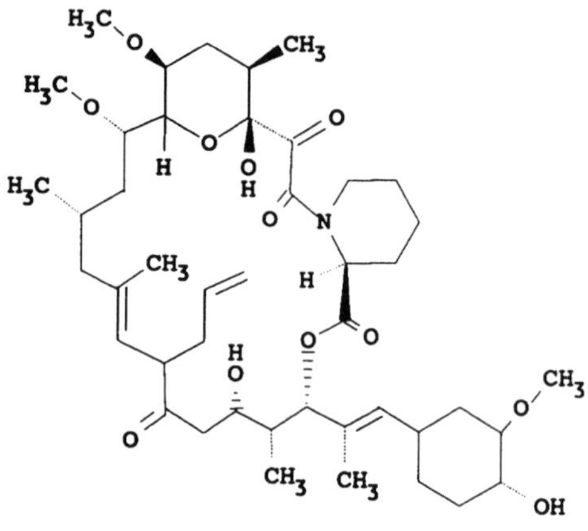

FK 506

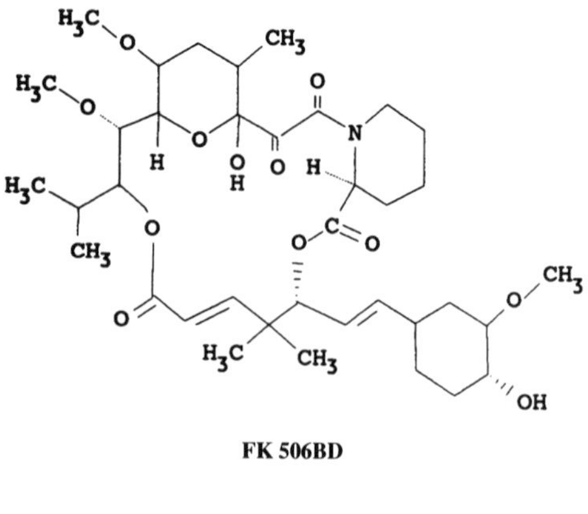

FK 506BD

FK 33-824: an enkephalin analog used to study receptor functions.

FKBPs: FK 506 binding proteins; **immunophilins** (*q.v.*) that form complexes with, and mediate the immunosuppressant effects of FK 506 and rapamycin. Various types display rotamase activity that is inhibited by the ligands, are chemotactic for leukocytes, attach to heat shock proteins, are components of unoccupied steroid hormone receptor complexes, and/or are implicated in other functions.

FLA-63: *bis*-(1-methyl-4-homopiperazinyl-thiocarbonyl)disulfide; an agent used to inhibit dopamine β-hydroxylase.

flaccid: weak, lax, or soft; describes the condition of skeletal muscles deprived of tonic stimulation by their motor neurons.

flagella: plural of flagellum.

flagellins: the major proteins of flagella. Eukaryotes types have 53K subunits. Bacterial types, with 20K subunits, are antigenic in mammals.

flagellum [flagella]: a long, thread-like structure that extends from a cell surface, and is used for locomotion. Bacterial types are simple helical, filamentous tubes composed of flagellin attached by flexible hooks to protein disks embedded in the plasma membranes. The disks function as motors that derive energy from proton gradients. Eukaryote flagella extend from bases similar to those of cilia, but are longer and usually occur singly or in pairs. Dynein arms attached to the microtubules are mechano-ATPases that promote microtubule sliding.

flanking sequence: a short DNA segment adjacent to one that can be transcribed.

flatus: gas generation (usually in the stomach or intestine) or gas expulsion (usually from the anus).

flatworm: any worm of the phylum **Platyhelminthes** (*q.v.*).

flavins: riboflavin and related isoalloxazines. They are yellow, and the oxidized forms fluoresce. *See also* **flavin adenine dinucleotide** and **flavin mononucleotide**.

flavin adenine dinucleotide: FAD; isoalloxazine flavine dinucleotide; a coenzyme for succinic dehydrogenase, xanthine oxidase, D-amino acid oxidases, acyl-CoA dehydrogenase, and some other enzymes, synthesized from flavin mononucleotide via the reaction FMN + ATP → FAD + P-P. In electron transport chains, the oxidized form (FAD) accepts H^+ and electrons from NADH + H^+. The reduced form ($FADH_2$) passes electrons to ubiquinones. $FADH_2$ is also a hydrogen and electron donor

for reactions catalyzed by pyruvate dehydrogenase and several other reactions.

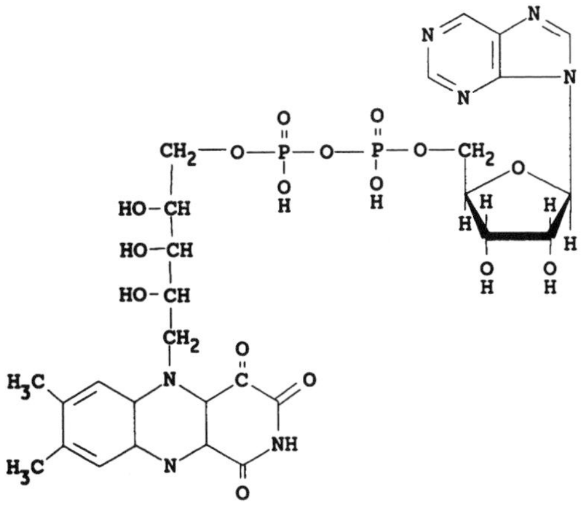

flavin mononucleotide: FMN; isoalloxazine-ribityl-phosphate; riboflavin-5′-phosphate; a coenzyme for L-amino acid oxidases and some other enzymes, and the direct precursor of flavin adenine mononucleotide. The oxidized form (FMN) accepts electrons and H^+ to yield $FMNH_2$.

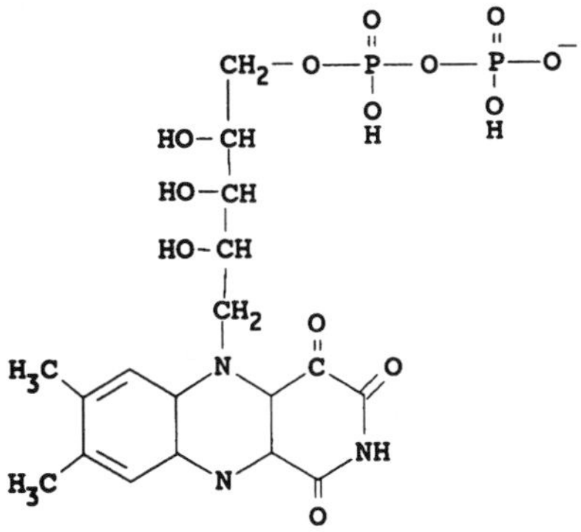

flavin nucleotides: *see* **flavin adenine dinucleotide** and **flavin adenine mononucleotide**. The oxidized forms of the flavin components take up two hydrogen ions and two electrons when they are converted to the reduced forms.

flavo-: a prefix meaning yellow.

flavone: 2-phenyl-4*H*-1-benzopyran-5-one; a colorless compound made by *Primula malacoides* and other plants that forms crystals and can decrease capillary permeability.

flavonoids: anthocyanins, citrin, rutin, and other compounds chemically related to flavone.

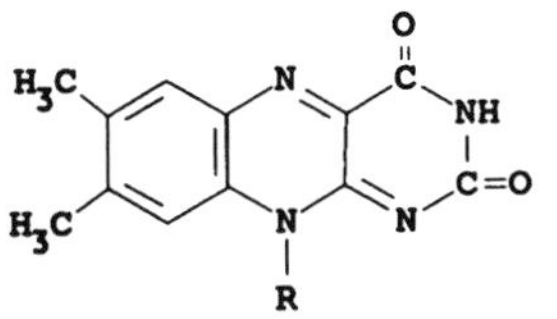

oxidized form

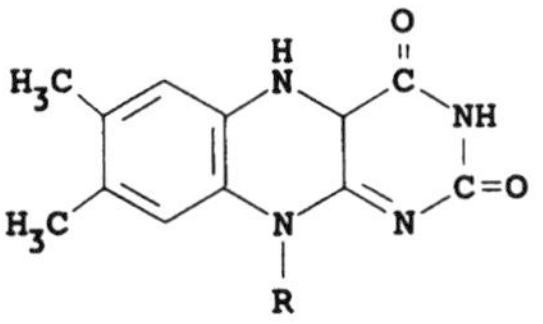

reduced form

flavin nucleotides

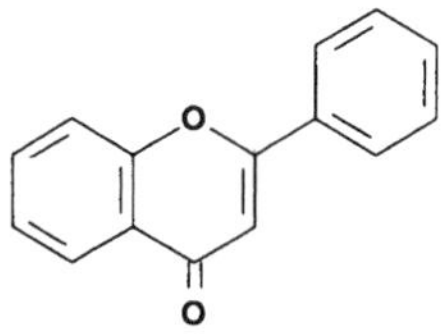

flavone

flavoprotein: any yellow protein that contains a flavin group; *see*, e.g. **flavin adenine mononucleotide**.

Flaxedil: a trade name for gallamine triethiodide.

Fletcher factor: a plasma prekallikrein.

flip flop: (1) a change in the orientation of a pair of phospholipid molecules within a membrane, in which the polar head of one goes from the intracellular to the extracellular surface, and the polar head of the other goes in the opposite direction. Unlike the very rapid lateral diffusion of membrane lipids, flip flop is believed to occur only once in several hours. (Similar movements of membrane proteins have not been observed.); (2) alternation in the expression of two genes via recombinase directed changes in the locations of promoters and repressors.

flocculation: formation of fluffy, "woolly", or lumpy precipitates, for example when particulate antigens in colloidal suspension combine with antibodies over a narrow concentration range. Antibodies on *Salmonella* bacteria, and on lymphocytes of individuals with thyroiditis are among the preparations used for diagnostic purposes.

flora: (1) the plants of a geographical locale or era; (2) microorganisms that reside in the intestine, mouth, vagina, or other organs.

florigens: plant factors that promote flowering. *See* **phytohormones**.

Florinef: a trade name for fludrocortisone.

flow cytometry: *see* **fluorescence activated cell sorting**.

floxuridine: FUdR; fluorodeoxyuridine; 2′-deoxy-5-fluoruridine; an agent metabolized via several enzymatic pathways to derivatives that disrupt nucleic acid synthesis. It is used mostly to arrest the growth of colon metastatic carcinomas, but is also effective against some viruses and fungi. However, it is toxic to bone marrow and to oral and gastrointestinal epithelium. FUdR can be directly phosphorylated by thymidine and uridine kinases to fluordeoxyuridylate (F-dUMP), a dUMP analog converted by thymidylate synthase to F-dTMP (fluro-deoxythymidylate). The product, in conjunction with the folate co-factor, N^5,N^{10}-methylentetrahydrofolate, attaches to, and becomes a suicide inhibitor of the thymidylate synthase (and thereby blocks its ability to convert dUMP to dTMP). FuDR can also be made from, and converted to **5-fluorouracil** (*q.v.*).

fludarabine: 2-fluoro-9-β-D-arabinofuranosyl-adenine; a purine nucleoside antimetabolite that resists degradation by adenosine deaminase. It inhibits DNA synthesis, and is used to treat some leukemias.

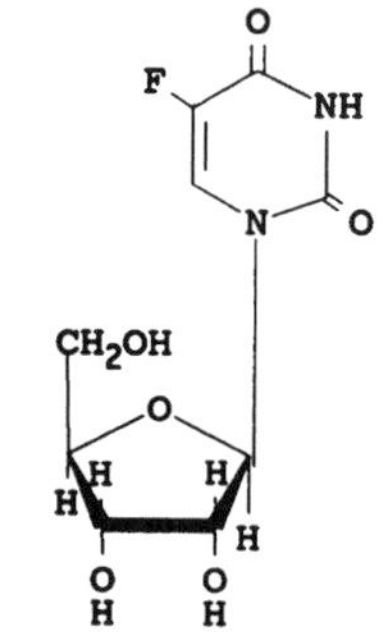

floxuridine

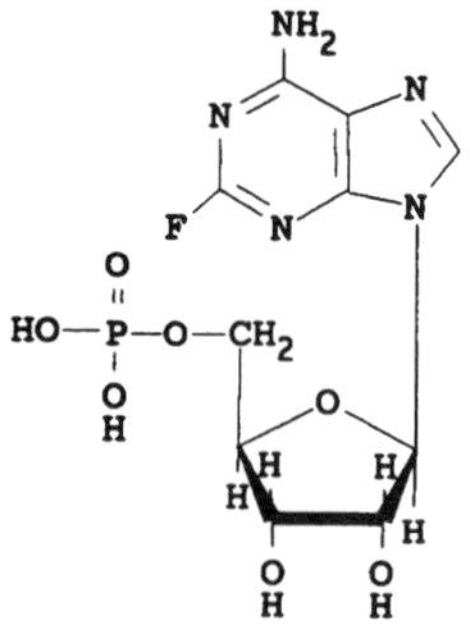

fludarabine

fludrocortisone: Florinef acetate; Astromin-H; 9α-fluoro-11β,17,21-trihydroxy-pregn-4-ene-3,20-dione; a potent synthetic steroid that exerts strong mineralocorticoid, and some glucocorticoid effects. It is used to treat Addison's disease and salt-losing forms of congenital adrenal hyperplasia.

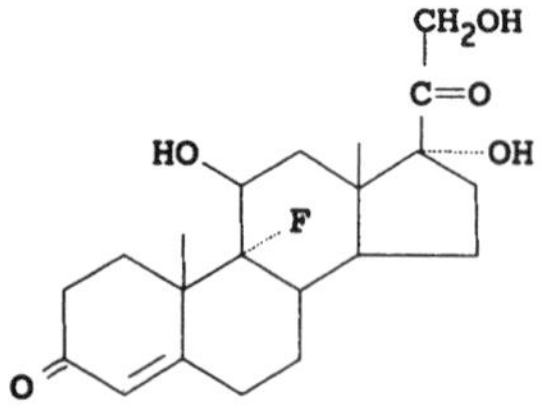

flufenamic acid: 2-[[3-(trifluormethyl)phenyl]amino] benzoic acid; a nonsteroidal anti-inflammatory agent and analgesic that inhibits prostaglandin synthesis.

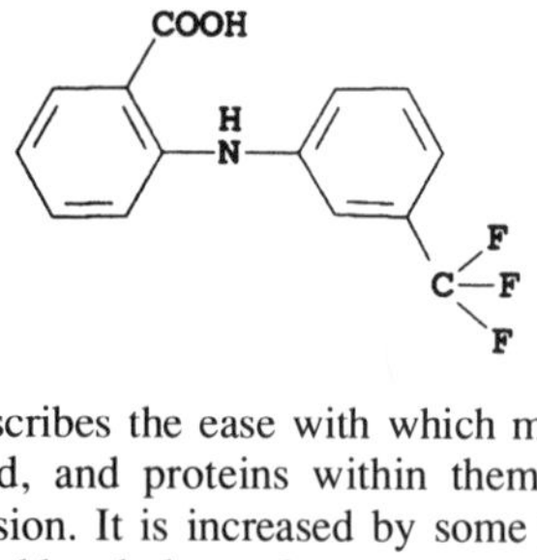

fluidity: describes the ease with which membranes can be deformed, and proteins within them can undergo lateral diffusion. It is increased by some phospholipids and decreased by cholesterol.

fluid mosaic model: the concept that plasma membranes are composed predominantly of phospholipid bilayers with polar heads facing extracellular and cytoplasmic faces, cholesterol and other lipids that affect fluidity interspersed among them, integral proteins that can move laterally trapped within the layers, and peripheral proteins that project from inner and outer surfaces anchored to the layers. *See* **phospholipid bilayers**. The model has undergone modifications to accommodate more recent findings, since it is now known that the mobility of some proteins is restricted by factors such as linkages to cytoskeletal components, that some glycans are attached to phospholipids, and that several kinds of compounds are anchored to membranes via covalent prenylation or myristoylation.

fluke: any flatworm of the class Trematoda. Some species are parasites that infect vertebrate livers and lungs.

Flumadine: a trade name for rimantadine.

flumazenil: Ro 15-1788: 8-fluoro-5,6-dihydro-5-methyl-6-oxo-4*H*-imidazo[1,5-a][1,4]benzo-diazepine-3-carboxylic acid ethyl ester; a competitive benzodiazepine receptor agonist, used to counteract excessive sedation, and reported to facilitate learning and memory.

flumethasone: 6α-fluoro-dexamethasone; a potent synthetic glucocorticoid, used as a topical anti-inflammatory agent to treat some skin conditions.

flunarizine: 1-cinnamyl-4-(di-*p*-fluorobenzhydryl)piperazine; a dihydropyridine type calcium channel blocker, used to dilate blood vessels. It also affects neurotransmission in the brain, and has anticonvulsant potency.

flunitrazepam: 5-(2-fluorophenyl)-1,3-dihydro-1-methyl-7-nitro-2*H*-1,4-benzodiazepin-2(1*H*)-one; an anxio-

lytic that acts on γ-aminobutyric acid (GABA) receptors; *see* **benzodiazepines**.

fluocinolone acetonide: 6,9-difluoro-11,21-dihydroxy-16,17-[(1-methylethilidene)bis(oxy)]-pregna-1,4-diene-3,20-dione; a synthetic glucocorticoid used as a topical anti-inflammatory agent to treat some skin disorders.

fluorapatite: apatite in which some hydroxide groups are replaced by fluorine atoms. Small amounts form during tooth enamel development and maturation, and they increase the resistance to caries. Minute amounts also accumulate in, and can harden bone.

fluorescein: 9-(*o*-carboxyphenyl)-6-hydroxy-isoxanthen-one; resorcinol phthalein; a compound that emits green fluorescence in alkaline solutions. It is used to detect ophthalmic lesions, and (in combination with other agents), to localize brain tumors. The diacetate is a pH sensitive vital stain, used to monitor of changes in cell acidity. *See* also **fluorescein isothiocyanate**.

fluorescein isothiocyanate: FITC; a fluorescent chromogen that binds to proteins. It is used with antibodies to locate intracellular molecules such as hormone receptors, and to follow intracellular transport (for example of substances taken up by endocytosis). *See* also **ATPases** and **fluorescence activated cell sorting**.

fluorescence: emission of photons, a property of some naturally occurring substances that can be induced in many others with ultraviolet light, X-rays, or laser beams.

fluorescein isothiocyanate

fluorescence activated cell sorting: FACS; flow cytometry; techniques for identifying, analyzing, and separating specific cell types without incurring injury. (Up to 18 million per hour can be studied.) Suspended cells are pretreated with fluorescein isothiocyanate labeled antibody, exposed to laser beams, and sent through very narrow nozzles, in some cases one at a time. The staining intensities of the emerging droplets are determined with photocells. Cell sizes can also be estimated from light scattering patterns. When sent between charged plates, cells with positively charged, negatively charged, and uncharged surfaces can be collected separately. The techniques are especially useful for sorting cells with similar characteristics, for example CD^{4+} from CD^{8+} lymphocytes, and can also provide information on receptor numbers.

fluorescence enhancement: techniques based on increases in photon emission displayed by some compounds when their hydrophobic sites are blocked. They are used, for example to study molecular associations such as antigen-antibody binding.

fluorescence quenching: techniques used to determine association constants, based on decreases in fluorescence that result from ligand binding.

fluorescence recovery after photobleaching: FRAP; techniques based on recovery of the ability to emit photons that has been abolished by radiation. They are used to study rhodopsin functions, and lateral diffusion of proteins in membranes exposed to laser beams.

fluorescent: emitting photons (displaying fluorescence).

fluorexon: *see* **calcein**.

fluorine, F: an element (atomic number 9, atomic weight 18.998). Under normal conditions, minute amounts of fluorides are ingested with plant foods and water, and they enter all cell types. Limited quantities are added to drinking water, and to toothpastes and other dentrifices, to protect against dental caries. The ions are filtered by renal glomeruli. Although also reabsorbed by proximal tubules, they are excreted in urine. Substantial amounts can be lost with sweat, and smaller ones leave with the feces; and they also enter milk. Since fluorides are absorbed via the skin and lungs, as well as the gastrointestinal tract, coal burning and other industrial processes that elevate environmental levels can cause accumulation of excessive amounts, which tend to concentrate in thyroid glands, and aorta (and to a lesser extent in kidneys), as well as in hard tissues. They can mottle and discolor tooth enamel, increase bone fragility, and damage pulmonary tissue. Acute poisoning by toxic doses invokes nausea,

vomiting, diarrhea, hypocalcemia, and hypoglycemia, and it can directly damage the heart. Fluoride ions react with many organic and inorganic compounds, and are potent inhibitors of enolase, ATPases, and other enzymes. By attaching to G proteins, they maintain adenylate cyclases in persistently active states, and by chelating calcium, can cause hypocalcemia and tetany. They also indirectly activate some proteolytic enzymes, accelerate phosphatidylinositol hydrolysis, and promote cell acidification via influences on Na^+/H^+ exchange. The effects on bone cells are used to treat Paget's disease. When given alone, they can somewhat increase bone mass in individuals with osteoporosis, but may not protect against fractures, since the new bone is brittle. However, intermittent administration with other agents that stimulate bone formation is reported to confer beneficial effects. Since calcium chelation stops coagulation, and enzyme effects block glycolysis, fluoride salts are added to blood drawn for glucose determinations. However, aluminum fluoride (AlF_4) can be a troublesome laboratory glassware contaminant.

fluorodeoxyuridine: FUdR; *see* **floxuridine**.

5-fluorouracil, 5-FU: 5-fluoro-2,4(1*H*, 3*H*-pyrimidine-dione; a pyrimidine analog that is metabolized via several endogenous enzymes to fluorouridine monophosphate (F-UMP) and to its deoxy derivative, F-dUMP. The latter incorporates into RNAs and inhibits of protein synthesis by impairing RNA processing and functions. (It also incorporates into DNA, but this does not seem to be a major mechanism of action). 5-FU undergoes other metabolic reactions, and can also be made from floxuridine via reactions catalyzed by thymidine and deoxyuridine phosphorylases. A dihydrouracil dehydrogenase inactivates it by reducing the pyrimidine ring. 5-FU is used to treat gastrointestinal tract, oropharyngeal, breast, pancreatic, ovarian, prostatic, urinary bladder, liver, and malignant skin carcinomas, but is toxic to all rapidly proliferating cell types; and amounts that are therapeutically effective can cause stomatitis, diarrhea, mucosal ulceration, and bone marrow depression.

fluorosulfonylbenzoyl adenosine: FSBA; an agent that inhibits protein kinases by forming covalent bonds with the Mg-ATPase binding sites.

fluoxetine: Prozac; *N*-methyl-γ-[4-(trifluoromethyl)phenoxy]benzenepropanamine; an agent that inhibits serotonin uptake by synaptic vesicles and secretory granules. It is used to treat individuals with compulsions, obsessions, depression, and other psychological problems not related to schizophrenias, and is reported to influence personality. Its ability to depress appetite in moderately obese persons may be secondary to effects on mood and self-esteem. Although a few suicides have occurred, the agent is generally regarded as less toxic and

fluorosulfonylbenzoyl adenosine

less likely to invoke undesired side effects than tricyclic type anti-depressants and monoamine oxidase inhibitors.

fluoxymesterone: 9-fluoro-11β,17β-dihydroxy-17-methylandrost-4-ene-3-one; an orally effective synthetic androgen, used to treat male hypogonadism and some forms of breast cancer.

cis-**flupentixol**: flupenthixol: 2-trifluoromethyl-9-[3-[4-(β-hydroxyethyl)-1-piperazinyl]propyl-idine]thioxanthene; a non-selective D_1 and D_2 type dopamine receptor antagonist, used for its antipsychotic effects.

fluphenazine: 4-[3-[2-(trifluormethyl)-10H-phenothiazin-10-yl]propyl]-1-piperazine ethanol; a D_1 type dopamine receptor antagonist. The hydrochloride, enanthate, and decanoate are used as antipsychotic agents.

flurazepam: 7-chloro-1-[2-9-diethylamino)ethyl]-5-(2-fluorophenyl)-1,3-dihydroxy-2H-1,4-bendodiazepin-2-one; a benzodiazepine type antipsychotic agent.

flutamide: 2-methyl-N-[4-nitro-3-(trifluoromethyl)propanamide; an agent metabolized to the androgen receptor antagonist, hydroxyflutamide. It is used to investigate hormone functions, and to treat prostate gland cancer.

fluvoxamine: 5-methoxy-1-[4-(trifluoromethyl)phenyl]-1-pentanone; an agent that inhibits serotonin uptake by synaptic vesicles. It is used to treat some forms of psychic depression.

FMBs: forward mobility proteins.

f-**Met**: formylmethionine; the amino acid that enters into the formation of initiation complexes for translation in bacteria; *see* also *f*-**met-tRNA**. Methionine is used by eukaryote ribosomes.

f-**Met-Leu-Phe**: FMLP; *formyl*-methionyl-leucyl-phenylalanine; a peptide made by *E. coli* that acts in low concentrations on specific neutrophilic leukocyte and macrophage cell surface receptors and stimulates chemotaxis. Higher levels promote respiratory burst activity, leukotriene production, release of lysosomal enzymes, formation of complement receptor CR3, and actin polymerization. The consequences are potentially damaging to normal body cells, but usually subside within minutes because of both homologous and heterologous desensitization (which also affects the functions of other chemotaxins, including platelet activating factor and a C_5 complement fragment). Most of the effects are mediated via a G_i-like, pertussis sensitive G protein transducer that activates kinase C isozymes and promotes phosphatidylinositol hydrolysis. FMLP also acts on different kinds of receptors as a chemoattractant for spermatozoa. Related peptides are released by some bacteria and some epithelial cells, and have been identified in extracts of disrupted mitochondria. Several different small, formylated peptides with chemoattractant potencies contain isoleucyl or lysyl moieties. The actions can be antagonized with *f*-Met-Leu-Phe-Phe, *boc*-Phe-Leu-Phe-Leu-Phe, and related compounds.

f-Met-tRNA: formylmethionine-transfer RNA; a component of bacterial translation initiation complexes, formed in the reaction catalyzed by a transformylase: methionyl-tRNA + *N*-formyltetrahydrofolate → *f*-Met-tRNA + tetrahydrofolate.

FMLP: *see f*-**Met-Leu-Phe**.

FMN, FMNH$_2$: oxidized and reduced forms, respectively, of flavin mononucleotide.

FMRFa, FMRF amide: Phe-Met-Arg-Phe-NH$_2$; a neuropeptide made by some invertebrates that exerts calcium-dependent presynaptic inhibition of acetylcholine release by slowing Ca^{2+} influx and decreasing the sensitivity to intracellular Ca^{2+}.

fms: *c-fms*; *CSFR1* in humans; proto-oncogenes expressed by monocytic macrophages and their precursors, that direct the synthesis of species specific receptors for mast cell stimulating factor (M-CSF, CSF-1). The products are 180K homodimeric, transmembrane glycoproteins that reside in clathrin coated pits. Ligand binding activates their tyrosine kinase domains, promotes receptor phosphorylation, and (in time) receptor down regulation. The genes are essential for growth factor stimulation of the proliferation and differentiation of myeloid lineage cells, and for maintaining the differentiated phenotypes. The ligands are also chemotactic; and one function is recruitment of phagocytes to sites of inflammation and tissue injury. Influences on osteoclast differentiation have also been described. The receptor made by trophoblast cells is believed to contribute to trophoblast development. The genes are located close to the ones for platelet derived growth factor (PDGF), code for similar products, and may have originated from common ancestral DNA sequences. The *c-fms* product is also similar to, and uses mechanisms in common with the protein whose synthesis is directed by *c-kit*. The McDonough feline sarcoma retrovirus oncogene, *v-fms*, directs the synthesis of a related glycoprotein, p180$^{gag-fms}$, which differs somewhat in amino acid composition glycosylation, and conformation. Its transforming potential appears to be directly linked to persistent, ligand-independent tyrosine kinase activity. Related oncogenes have been found in some humans with acute myelogenous leukemia (and in some leukemic cats). Different kinds of mutations lead to formation of nonfunctional receptors, and severe disturbances in monocytic functions.

FNs: fibronectins.

foam cells: pathological cell types, laden with cholesterol esters, that accumulate in fatty streaks of arteries undergoing atherosclerosis. Most are derived from circulating monocytes or tissue macrophages that take up modified low density lipoproteins via scavenger receptors; but some come from the smooth muscle of blood vessel tunica medial layers. *See* also **apolipoprotein (a)**.

focal contacts: *see* **adhesion plaques**.

fodrin: a spectrin-like tetrameric cytoskeletal protein with 240K α, and 235K β subunits, identified in intestinal and some other epithelial cells, and in the brain and adrenal medulla. It binds actin, links adjacent actin bundles to each other and to plasma membranes, and plays essential roles in exocytosis. It is degraded by calpains.

folic acid: folacin; pteroylglutamic acid; vitamin M; 5-formyl-5,6,7,8-tetrahydropteroyl-L-glutamic acid, a component of the B-vitamin complex. (Vitamin B$_c$ is a polyglutamate derivative.) It is converted to tetrahydrofolate, a coenzyme for reactions that transfer one-carbon groups, and is needed for DNA synthesis, RNA methylation, and the formation of choline and creatine. It also contributes to amino acid metabolism and other metabolic functions. Deficiency causes a form of megaloblastic anemia. Folic acid is not included in non-prescription multivitamin supplements, because most diets contain sufficient amounts, and excessive ones mask the effects of cyanocobalamin deficiency on hematopoiesis but do not ameliorate the associated nervous system defects. However, there is some evidence that ingestion by pregnant women lowers the incidence of neural tube defects in fetuses.

folinic acid: *see* **citrovorum factor**.

follicles: sac-like structures. They can be hollow, or composed mostly of cells. *See*, for example **ovarian, thyroid, lymph node**, and **hair follicles**.

follicle regulatory protein: FRP; a peptide made by ovarian granulosa cells and released to follicular fluid, that attenuates several responses to follicle stimulating hormone (FSH), including adenylate cyclase activation, and induction of numerous proteins (aromatase, 3β-hydroxysteroid dehydrogenase, luteinizing hormone receptors, and others). The consequences of excessive amounts include delayed follicle maturation associated with impaired estrogen secretion, and delayed ovulation (attributed in part to progesterone deficiency). A component of testicular extracts exerts similar effects on ovaries. Exogenous FRF delays sperm maturation, but augments Sertoli cell production of androgen binding protein and transferrin.

follicle stimulating hormone: FSH; follitropin; an approximately 36K, species specific glycoprotein hormone secreted by gonadotropes, composed of an α subunit (with 92 amino acid moieties in humans), similar to or identical with the α subunits of thyroid stimulating hormone (TSH), luteinizing hormone (LH), and human chorionic gonadotropins (hCG), noncovalently linked to a β subunit (118 amino acids in humans) that is unique for the hormone type. Gonadotropin releasing hormone (GnRH, LRH) is the major stimulant for maintaining the morphology and functions of gonadotropes that synthesize it; but activins also promote FSH secretion. Some evidence for the existence of a hypothalamic FSH-RH that does not also promote luteinizing hormone secretion has been presented. Small amounts of FSH are constitutively released; and androgens are implicated as additional direct stimulants (although they inhibit GnRH release). Inhibin and some other gonadal products decrease the secretion. Androgens and estrogens regulate the glycosylation; and the resulting microheterogeneities affect the biological half lives. FSH promotes growth and maturation of ovarian granulosa and testicular Sertoli cells, induces aromatase, androgen binding protein, inhibin, testibumin, and several other factors that affect reproduction. It also stimulates the formation of receptors for estrogens and LH.

follicle stimulating hormone binding inhibitor: FSH-BI; an ovarian peptide that attenuates follicle stimulating hormone (FSH) actions on the ovary by decreasing hormone-receptor binding. It may be identical with or related to follicle regulatory protein.

follicle stimulating hormone release factor: FRF; FSH-RF; *see* **follicle stimulating hormone releasing hormone**.

follicle stimulating hormone releasing hormone; FSH-RH; an uncharacterized regulator (different from gonadotropin releasing hormone, GnRH), believed by some investigators to be secreted by hypothalamic neurons, and to specifically stimulate FSH, but not luteinizing hormone (LH) release. However, although there are phases of ovarian cycles during which the two gonadotropins are not released in parallel, other explanations have been offered. *See* also **gonadotropes**.

follicle stimulating hormone releasing peptide: FRP; ovarian peptides that promote the release of follicle stimulating hormone; *see* **activins**.

follicular cells: (1) cell components of follicles; (2) granulosa or pregranulosa ovarian cells; (3) thyroid gland cells that make iodinated thyroid hormones; (4) adenohypophysial folliculo-stellate cells. *See* also **follicular dendritic cells**.

follicular dendritic cells: lymph node or spleen cells, with receptors for immunoglobulin Fc, and C1 and C3 complement components, that extend slender cytoplasmic processes between B lymphocytes, and are believed to contribute to germinal center formation. They do not express class II histocompatibility proteins on their surfaces.

follicular fluid factor: FF; ovarian follicular fluid components that inhibit the secretion of follicle stimulating hormone (FSH). *See* **inhibins** and **folliculostatin**.

follicular phase: the part of an ovarian cycle during which substantial amounts of estrogen are secreted, and

one or more follicles matures and prepares for ovulation; *cf* **luteal phase**.

folliculostatin: follistatin; FSH suppressing protein, FSP; activin binding protein: 32-38K monomeric proteins (some of which are glycosylated) that inhibit follicle stimulating hormone (FSH) secretion, at least in part by binding activins. They differ chemically from inhibins (which are dimers), and are less potent for acute effects, but can sustain more persistent responses. Low affinity binding to inhibins may affect the ability of those peptides to interact with their receptors. Ovarian granulosa FSPs directly augment progesterone and 20α-hydroxyprogesterone formation in theca types, and indirectly increase the amounts of Δ^4-androstenedione. The relative amounts of activins and FSPs are believed to determine whether partially matured follicles progress to preovulatory types or undergo atresia. The ones in Sertoli cells may modulate activin stimulation of spermatogenesis. In pituitary glands, activins are reported to promote FSP synthesis. FSPs have additionally been identified in the kidneys, brain and blood, and also in the uterus and placenta during early stages of gestation.

folliculo-stellate cells: stellate cells; marginal cells; neuroglia-like adenohypophysial cells that form follicles, predominantly in the vicinity of the hypothalamic cleft. Most are ciliated. They express glial acidic fibrillary protein (GFAP), S-100, and other proteins that distinguish them from other adenohypophysial cell types. Although they lack secretory granules (and were once classified as chromophobes), they secrete basic fibroblast growth factor (bFGF), interleukin-6, a vascular endothelium growth factor, and other regulators, and are believed to perform several localized functions that include contributions to the maintenance of the hypothalamo-hypophysial portal vessels, regulation of the growth and functions of lactotropes and thyrotropes, and removal of debris. Peptides released peripherally also affect adrenocortical cell proliferation and other endocrine functions.

follicle-stellate growth factor: *see* **glioma derived growth factor**.

folliculotropes: folliculotrophs: adenohypophysial cells that secrete follicle stimulating hormone (FSH); but *see* **gonadotropes**.

follistatin: folliculostatin.

follitropin: follicle stimulating hormone.

footprinting: techniques for identifying DNA segments that bind specific proteins such as RNA polymerases and transcription activators, based on the ability of the proteins to protect the nucleic acid regions to which they bind against degradation by endonucleases. The DNA is labeled (usually with ^{32}P), and one aliquot is treated with the protein. Both aliquots are then subjected to endonuclease digestion, and the fragments are separated (according to length) by polyacrylamide gel electrophoresis. The bands obtained from the DNA control samples that are missing from the protein treated ones contain the binding sites.

foramen [foramina]: a hole, opening, or perforation.

forebrain: prosencephalon; the most anterior portion of the embryonic brain. It gives rise to the telencephalon and diencephalon.

formaldehyde: a gas that irritates mucous membranes. It is generated when methanol is ingested, and accounts for most of the toxicity. *See also* **formalin**.

$$\underset{\text{H}}{\text{H}}C=O$$

formalin: an aqueous solution of formaldehyde. It cross-links proteins and is used as a fixative for biological specimens.

formamide: an agent used to denature double-stranded DNA. It combines with the free NH_2 groups of adenine and thereby blocks pairing with thymine.

$$\underset{\;}{\overset{O}{\text{HC}}}-\text{NH}_2$$

formed elements: usually, the membrane enclosed components of blood: erythrocytes, leukocytes, and platelets.

formic acid: the smallest and most water-soluble of the fatty acids. It is a toxic, irritating metabolite of methanol that can invoke metabolic acidosis, albuminuria and hematuria. Large amounts are made by some ants. It has limited use as an astringent and counterirritant, and is employed as a reducing and decalcifying agent.

$$\text{H}-\text{COOH}$$

formins: two or more (69K and 164K) DNA-binding proteins with proline-rich cores that play essential roles in limb and kidney development.

formylmethionine, formylmethionine-tRNA: *see f*-**Met** and *f*-**Met-tRNA**.

formylmethionyl-leucyl-phenylalanine: *see f*-**Met-Leu-Phe**.

fornix: a major myelinated nerve tract component of the limbic system. It originates in the hippocampus, and sends projections to the thalamus, mammillary bodies and habenular nuclei.

forskolin: 7β-acetoxy-8,13-epoxy-1α-,6β,9α-trihyoxyl-*abd*-14-en-11-one; a terpene from the roots of *Coleus forskohli*, that acts directly on adenylate cyclase catalytic subunits, and thereby activates the enzymes via mechanisms that bypass ligand-receptor binding and the need for G proteins. Although used to study cAMP functions, it additionally interacts directly with G proteins, and exerts several effects unrelated to cAMP generation. The inotropic influences of low doses on the heart are attributed to cAMP-dependent augmentation of Na^+ permeability that leads to increased Na^+/Ca^{2+} exchange and elevation of intracellular Ca^{2+} in myocytes. Higher doses act indirectly via cAMP to relax vascular and other smooth muscle. However, its ability to elevate cytosolic Ca^{2+} levels in some other cell types, inhibit GABAᴀ receptor functions, modify acetylcholine and voltage

regulated K^+ channels, and inhibit glucose transport in adipocytes and muscle cells, have been linked with anesthetic-like perturbations of plasma membrane lipid bilayers. Forskolin also exerts cAMP-independent inhibition of cholecalciferol 24-hydroxylase, and is more potent than parathyroid hormone (which acts via cAMP). *See* also 1,9-dideoxy-**forskolin**.

1,9-dideoxy-forskolin: a forskolin analog that inhibits adenylate cyclase and mimics some forskolin effects that are not directly linked with activation of that enzyme. It is a more potent inhibitor of cholecalciferol 24-hydroxylase than forskolin when tested on isolated renal tubules.

Forssman antigen: a glycolipid chemically related to the A type blood group antigen, expressed on the surfaces of erythrocytes and some other cells of several species. When injected into rabbits, it stimulates production of antibodies that mediate complement-dependent sheep red cell lysis. It is a tumor-associated antigen in humans, but is also present on normal gastrointestinal cells.

forward mobility protein: FMB: a component of epididymal fluid, implicated as a promoter of sperm maturation and acquisition of the ability to swim in a forward direction.

fos: FOS, the product of the *c-fos* proto-oncogene, is a leucine zipper nuclear protein that forms heterodimers with *jun* products and other transcription factors. The dimers bind to specific TGACTCA DNA base sequences, interact with serum response elements, and regulate the expression of several other genes; *see* also **AP-1**. (Although FOS:FOS monomers form, they are unstable and do not bind effectively.) FOS is required for quiescent cell entry into G_1 phases of cell cycles, and it plays essential roles in embryogenesis, hematopoiesis, bone development, spermatogenesis, and other functions in which cells proliferate and then differentiate. It is very rapidly induced by platelet-derived (PDGF), epidermal (EGF) and several other growth factors, and by phorbol esters, other protein kinase C activators, some ionophores, and some factors that elevate inositol 1,4,5-triphosphte (IP_3) levels. In the suprachiasmatic nuclei

(SCN), it contributes to the control of body rhythms, and is induced there by light. In addition to directly fostering cell proliferation, it suppresses the expression of *Rb* and some other genes that exert opposing influences; and deregulation of the mechanisms that control its expression leads to transformation. Under normal conditions, high FOS levels exert negative feedback control over the gene. *C-fos B* is a related gene. *V-fos* is a transforming oncogene identified in tumors of mice infected with FBJ osteosarcoma virus.

foscarnet sodium: Foscavir; phosphonoformic acid; dihydroxyphosphinecarboxylic acid trisodium salt; an agent that inhibits viral DNA polymerases and reverse transcriptases by interacting with phosphate binding sites. It is effective against cytomegalovirus, human immune deficiency viruses (HIVs), and some strains of *Herpes simplex* resistant to acyclovir and ganciclovir, but is not available for use in the United States. It can impair renal function, and cause malaise, nausea, vomiting, anemia, tremors, and seizures.

fosphomycin: fosfomycin; *See* **phosphomycin**.

fossa: a depression or hollow region.

founder cell: a cell that proliferates and gives rise to a tissue. In complex animals, several kinds adhere to extracellular matrix components at specific regions and initiate histogenesis in embryos.

fourth polar body: *see* **polar bodies**.

foxglove: any plant of the *Digitalis* genus.

α-FP: α-fetoprotein.

F particle: a mitochondrial particle involved in coupling ATP synthesis to electron transport. F_1 has ATPase activity.

FPF: fibroblast pneumocyte factor.

fps: a Fujinami sarcoma virus oncogene identified in domestic cats that is homologous to the Fujinami chicken sarcoma *fes* gene. It directs formation of p98^{fps}, a protein with non-receptor tyrosine kinase activity.

fra-1: a proto-oncogene related to *fos* that codes for a 38K nuclear protein. The product forms DNA-binding heterodimers with *jun* gene products.

fragile X: a defective X chromosome that can undergo breakage or deletion. A form of mental retardation in humans (often associated with large ears), in which bands 27 and 28 of the long arm of are affected, occurs mostly in males (who have just one X). It is transmitted by symptom free females.

fragmin: a 42K cytoskeletal protein chemically related to gelsolin, villin and severin, initially identified in *Physarum polycephalum*. Its ability to bind to the ends of, and to sever actin filaments is affected by Ca^{2+} levels.

frame-shift mutations: DNA changes caused by insertions or deletions of one or two base pairs (or of larger numbers that are not multiples of 3). They alter the coding functions of all base pairs downstream from the mutation sites.

FRAP: fluorescence recovery after bleaching.

fraternal twins: dizygotic twins; two non-identical siblings that develop during the same pregnancy, but are products of different zygotes. *Cf* **monozygotic twins**.

FRc: ferritin receptor.

FRE-BP: *see* **iron response elements**.

free energy: G; energy available for work. The change in the free energy in Calories per mole (ΔG), for a system undergoing transformation at constant temperature and pressure, is related to the change in enthalpy (ΔH) and the change in entropy (ΔS) by the equation: $\Delta G = \Delta H - T\Delta S$, where T is the absolute temperature. The process can proceed spontaneously if the value is negative (and is associated with a gain in entropy). The *standard* free energy change for a chemical reaction (ΔG_o) is the amount lost or gained when all of the reactants are present in 1 molar concentrations under standardized conditions. It is related to the molecular structures of the reactants, but is independent of the chemical pathway. The free energy released (or taken up) by a chemical reaction that proceeds at constant temperature and a pressure of 1 atmosphere is related to the equilibrium constant (K) by the equation: $\Delta G = \Delta G_o + RT\ln K$, where R is the gas constant (1.987 Cal per mole per degrees Kelvin) ln the natural logarithm, and T the absolute temperature. For many reactions, it is convenient to calculate $\Delta G_o'$, the standard free energy at pH 7.0. A negative value of ΔG indicates that the reaction is exergonic (free energy is released). A positive one indicates that it is endergonic, and must be coupled to another that is negative. At equilibrium, $\Delta G = 0$. The ΔG does not provide information on heat gain or loss. (An exergonic reaction is not necessarily exothermic.) There is also no direct relationship to the reaction rate; *see* **free energy of activation**.

free energy of activation: a measure of the amount of energy required to initiate a chemical reaction. The value is inversely related to the reaction rate, but is not related to the free energy change. Enzymes accelerate reversible reactions in both directions by lowering activation energies.

free fatty acids: FFAs; the term usually refers to fatty acids in blood plasma or serum that are not covalently linked to other compounds (i.e. are not components of triacylglycerols, phospholipids, or other lipids), and are not contained within lipoprotein particles or chylomicrons.

freemartin: a virilized or hermaphroditic calf with female type (XX) chromosomes, whose abnormal development is attributed to Müllerian duct inhibitor, testis determining antigen, and/or other factors released prenatally by a normal male twin fetus that shares the same placental circulation. In most freemartins, the gonads are ovotestes, but in some, one or both can resemble a true testis. Similar conditions occur in pigs and other species in which fetuses share placentas.

free radicals: superoxide (O^{2-}), semiquinone intermediates (QH•) and other highly reactive, short-lived, charged substances with unpaired electrons. Small quantities are formed on a regular basis. The much larger ones generated during inflammatory reactions, and under some pathological conditions, contribute to destruction of microorganisms, but can damage normal body cells. Some of the metabolic derangements they invoke are attributed to activation of cytoplasmic guanylate cyclases.

free living: (1) not metabolically dependent on other organisms; not symbiotic or parasitic; (2) motile; not permanently attached to a substratum.

free running rhythms: intrinsic biological rhythms that persist and establish their own periodicities when not restrained by synchronizing signals. Most circadian types have cycle lengths in the general range of 22.5 to 26.5 hours, with individual differences among members of the same species. They are usually entrained to 24 hour periodicities by diurnal changes in environmental lighting (or by other cues, such as food presentation at regular times). Members of a population exposed to the same entraining factors have rhythms that are in phase.

freeze drying: lyophilization; techniques for preserving hormones, vaccines, antibiotics, and other biological materials in stable form without refrigeration. The substances are rapidly frozen in an environment that contains an inert gas (such as liquid nitrogen), dried under a vacuum, and placed in sealed containers. Most proteins retain their native forms. *See* also **freeze etching** and **freeze fracture**.

freeze etching: techniques for preparing biological specimens for electron microscopy that avert the distortions caused by chemical fixation, and preserve three-dimensional organization. The specimens are usually freeze dried in liquid helium (which protects against formation of large ice crystals), sectioned under vacuums, and fractured with knives. Water sublimation then etches surfaces that are not covered by lipid bilayers. Replicas of the resulting contours (which reflect the types and distributions of cell components) are made by shadowing with platinum vapor, and are protected by carbon films. The organic matter is then dissolved away. Finally, the replicas are stripped off and placed on grids for viewing.

freeze fracture: techniques used to prepare biological specimens for electron microscopy studies of membrane and cellular proteins. The procedures are similar to those described for freeze etching, but a cryoprotectant is added before freezing to minimize water sublimation. Fractures that pass between the two parts of the plasma membrane lipid bilayer permit visualization of a P face (the inner component as viewed from outside the cell), and an E face (the outer component as viewed from the inside). Fractures that separate the plasma membrane from the cytoplasm provide information on intracellular components. The techniques can also be applied to endoplasmic reticula.

"freeze" response: immobilization, a catecholamine-invoked component of "fight or flight" responses to perception of danger in some species. It can render animals less visible or less attractive to predators.

freeze-squeeze: techniques for recovering DNA from agarose gels. The segment that contains the desired DNA is frozen, and is then squeezed between two sheets of parafilm to eject the DNA.

freeze-thaw: techniques used to disrupt cell membranes without chemicals, and for cryoactivation of some enzymes (*see*, for example **renin**), accomplished by freezing and then rewarming.

Freund's adjuvants: water-oil emulsions used to enhance immune system responses. The *incomplete* type contains weak antigens. Since it invokes granuloma formation at the injection site, it is not used in humans. Freund's *complete* adjuvant (FCA), which contains killed *Mycobacteria*, is a more potent (but more toxic) stimulant.

FRF: (1) follicle regulatory protein; (2) follicle stimulating hormone release factor.

Friedman (rabbit) test for pregnancy: a test based on the ability of human chorionic gonadotropin (hCG) in pregnancy urine to promote ovulation when injected into immature rabbits (*see* **reflex ovulators**). It is no longer used because it is expensive, requires considerable skill, can yield false positive results, is time-consuming, and involves killing of the test animals. Moreover, since hCG deteriorates in urine, the test cannot be later repeated on the same urine specimen.

frictional coefficient: a measure of the resistance of molecules to movement in an electrical field or ultracentrifuge. Its magnitude is related to the shapes and masses of the particles.

Friend leukemia virus: a complex of two viruses that slowly invokes erythroleukemia in mice. One is a replication defective spleen focus forming virus that codes for an env-like protein, promotes replication, and induces a preleukemic condition. The second, which is replication competent, can also serve as a helper virus for other replication defective types.

"frog" (Galli-Mainini) test for pregnancy: a test, usually performed on the African toad, *Xenopus levis*, based on the ability of human chorionic gonadotropin (hCG) in pregnancy urine to promote spermiation in amphibians. Since little skill is required to identify spermatozoa released to surrounding fluids, amphibians are cheaper to purchase and maintain than rabbits, the animals are not killed for the test, and results can be obtained within a few hours, it is preferable to the Friedman test. However, since the responses of the toads vary with the season of the year, and with several other factors, both false negative and false positives results are often obtained. The test has largely been superseded by immunological methods.

frontal organ: a component of the pineal gland complex of some amphibians.

FRP: (1) ferritin repressor protein; (2) follicle regulatory protein; (3) follicle stimulating hormone releasing peptide.

fructokinase: an enzyme that catalyzes the reaction: fructose + ATP → fructose-1-phosphate + ADP; *cf* **phosphofructokinase**.

fructose: levulose; fruit sugar; a ketohexose sugar, usually present in furanose form. It is a component of honey and many fruits, of inulin and some other polysaccharides, of some glycoproteins, and a product of sucrose digestion. It is rapidly absorbed by intestinal cells via insulin-independent transport. Fructokinase and phosphohexoisomerase catalyze its conversion, respectively, to fructose-1-phosphate, and glucose. Fructose is a major direct energy source for spermatozoa, and a component of human and bull seminal fluid. When excessive amounts are taken up by some cell types, much of it is reduced to **sorbitol** (*q.v.*). *See* also **fructose-1-phosphate**.

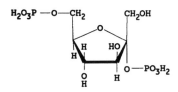
fructose 2,6-biphosphate

α-D-fructofuranose

fructose 1,6-biphosphatase: a gluconeogenesis pathway enzyme that catalyzes the reaction: fructose-1,6-biphosphate + H_2O → fructose-6-phosphate + Pi. Its activity is augmented by glucagon and ADP, and is inhibited by insulin and ATP.

fructose 1,6-biphosphate: a metabolite formed from fructose-6-phosphate in the irreversible reaction of the glycolysis pathway, catalyzed by phosphofructokinase-1: fructose-6-P + ADP $\rightleftarrows$ fructose 1,6-biphosphate + ADP. The reaction is rate-limiting for the steps of that pathway that lead to phosphoenolpyruvate.

fructose 2,6-biphosphate: a metabolite made in small amounts from fructose-6-phosphate via a reaction catalyzed by phosphofructokinase-2. It is a major regulator of phosphofructokinase-1 activity, and therefore of glycolysis.

fructose 1-phosphate: a ketohexose phosphate formed from fructose via the reaction catalyzed by fructokinase: fructose + ATP → fructose-1-P + ADP. Since fructose-1-P aldolase catalyzes its cleavage to **dihydroxyacetone phosphate + glyceraldehyde** (*q.v.*), it can be used for glycolysis, and for the synthesis of triacylglycerols and other lipids.

fructose-6-phosphate: a ketohexose phosphate, formed mostly in the reversible reaction catalyzed by phosphohexoisomerase (an enzyme used for both glycolysis and gluconeogenesis): glucose-6-P 6 $\rightleftarrows$ fructose-6-P. Phosphofructokinase-1 catalyzes its conversion to fructose-1,6-biphosphate (an intermediate in the glycolysis pathway), and phosphofructokinase-2 to fructose-2,6-biphosphate.

fructosuria: an autosomal recessive disorder, attributed to hepatic fructokinase deficiency, in which dietary fructose is excreted to urine. Other than nutrient loss, no harmful effects are known.

fruit fly: *see* **Drosophila**.

fruiting body: *see* **slime molds**.

frusemide: furosemide.

FSH: follicle stimulating hormone.

FSH-BI: follicle stimulating hormone binding inhibitor.

FSH-RF: follicle stimulating hormone release factor; *see* **follicle stimulating hormone releasing hormone**.

FSH-RH: follicle stimulating hormone releasing hormone.

FSH-RP: (1) follicle stimulating hormone regulatory protein; (2) follicle stimulating hormone releasing peptide.

FST: facteur serum thymique; *see* **thymulin**.

FSV: Fujinami sarcoma virus.

F test: a statistical measure used in analysis of variance, obtained by dividing the mean square of data values for one group by the mean square for another. Tables based on the degrees of freedom are then consulted to determine the probability that an F as high (or higher) can occur by chance (i.e. when the two groups are samples of the same population). If the first mean square derives from a treated group and the second is a measure of random variation (error), a large F value is consistent with a statistically significant effect of the treatment.

FTS: facteur thymique serique; *see* **thymulin**.

FTX: funnel web spider toxin.

fuchsins: several dyes that impart pinkish, red, or purple coloration to biological materials. Acid fuchsin, 2-amino-5-[(4-amino-sulfophenyl)(4-imino-3-sulfo-2,5-cyclohexadien-1-ylidene)methyl]-3-methylbenzenesulfonic acid disodium salt (shown below) is a component of some connective tissues stains. Since it changes from red to pink to colorless over the pH range 10-12, it is also used as an indicator. Basic fuchsin (a dye mixture), is the major component of Schiff stains.

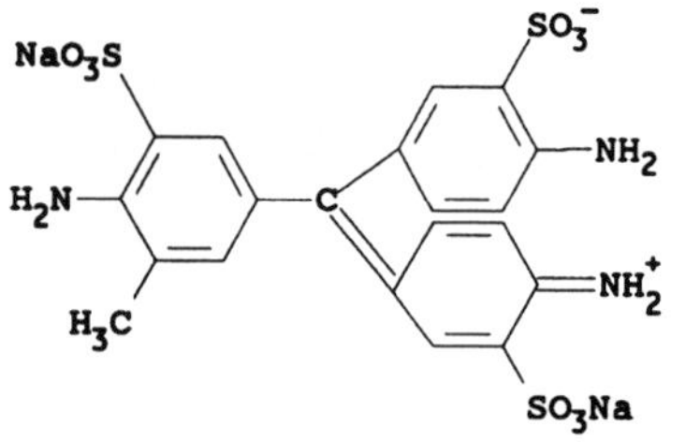

fucose: L-fucose (6-deoxy-L-galactose) is a component of many animal glycoproteins with *N*-linked oligosaccharides. It is made from galactose. D-fucose (6-deoxy-D-galactose) is a component of several plant glycosides.

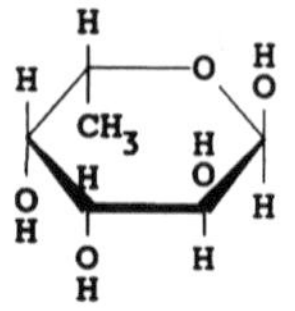

L-fucose 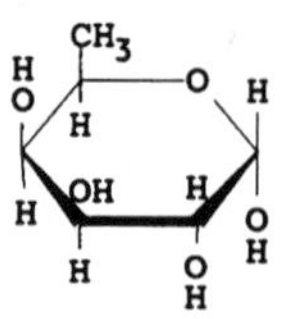   D-fucose

FUDR: fluorodeoxyuridine; *see* **floxuridine**.

Fujinami sarcoma virus: *see fes*.

Fuller's earth: an aluminum magnesium silicate kaolin, used as a filtering agent that adsorbs impurities.

fumarate {**fumaric acid ion**}: an intermediate of the tricarboxylic acid cycle, formed in the reaction catalyzed by succinic dehydrogenase: succinate + FAD → fumarate + $FADH_2$. Fumarase then catalyzes: fumarate + H_2O → malate. Fumarate is also formed from arginosuccinate in the urea cycle, and can additionally be derived from aspartic acid, phenylalanine, and tyrosine.

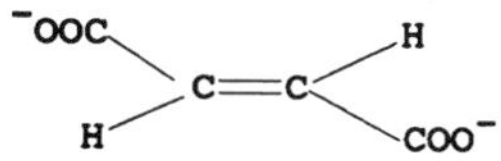

fundus: usually, the deepest part of an organ, such as the stomach or uterus.

Fundulus heraclitus: the killifish. Since the animals are small, have short life cycles, engage in courtship rituals, display pituitary-dependent ability to survive in environments that vary markedly in saline content, and express gene-related variations in coloration, they are used for studies of genetics, evolution, hormone functions, and behavior.

fungus [fungi]: any of at least 100,000 species of the Fungi kingdom, which includes mushrooms, molds, and yeasts. All form spores at some stage of the life cycle, lack flagella, and display some plant-like characteristics (but do not make chlorophylls). Most are saprophytic; and several types grow on human tissues. Some are sources of antibiotics, and of laboratory tools used to inhibit specific processes.

funnel web spider toxin, FTX: 200-400K components extracted from the venoms of the American funnel web spiders, *Agelenopsis aperta*, *Hololina curta*, and *Calilena*. They block P type Ca^{2+} channels of Purkinje cells and of squid optic lobes that are insensitive to dihydropyridines and ω-conotoxin.

fur: a mammalian gene (named for its location in the *fes/fps* upstream region) that codes for furins.

Fura-2: 1-[2-(5-carboxyoxazol-2-yl)-6-aminobenzofuran-5-2(2′amino-5′methylphenoxy)eth-ane-*N,N,N′,N′*-tetracetic acid; a dye that penetrates cells and fluoresces when it binds calcium. Fura-2/AM penetrates cell more rapidly, and is one of the most useful agents for monitoring intracellular Ca^{2+} changes. In the structure shown, R = —Na for fura-2, and —CH_2—O—CO—CH_3 for fura-2/AM.

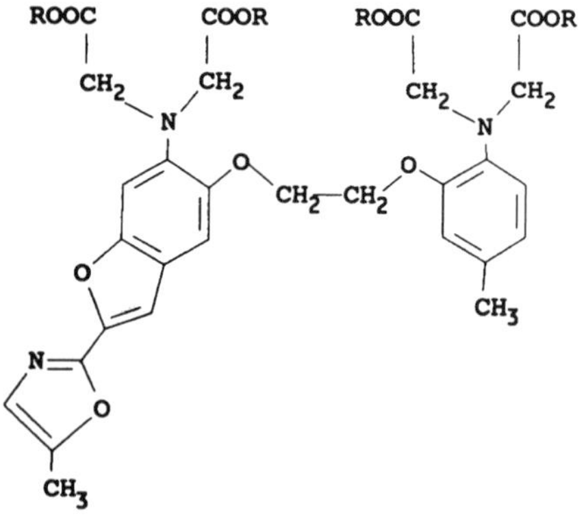

furanose: a sugar with a ring structure composed of one oxygen and four carbon atoms. *See* **fructose** and *cf* **pyranose**.

furins: Golgi-associated endoproteases whose synthesis is directed by *fur* genes. The enzymes, which are closely related to yeast *kex2* gene products, catalyze cleavage of precursor molecules that move through the Golgi apparatus, and thereby promote formation of the corresponding mature proteins. Although they act at specific sites on many substrates, they differ from PC1, PC2, and PC3 proteases of neuroendocrine cell granules which act mostly on prohormones. Furins can, however, potentiate the effects of PCs in some cell types.

furosemide: frusemide: Lasix; 4-chloro-*N*-furfuryl-5-sulfamoylanthranilic acid; a high ceiling loop diuretic used to treat some forms of hypertension. Its major effect is inhibition of ion transport across ascending Henle loops, but acceleration of renal blood flow with consequent slowing of reabsorption by proximal tubules contributes to the diuresis. Prolonged use can cause hemoconcentration, hyponatremia, hypokalemia, alkalosis (because of H^+ loss), and calciuria. Large doses also invoke hypoglycemia in laboratory animals. Furosemide also inhibits carbonic anhydrases, but this action is too weak to affect the responses.

fusaric acid: 5-butyl-2-pyridinecarboxylic acid; an antibiotic made by the fungus, *Fusarium heterosporium*. Its ability to lower blood pressure is attributed to inhibition of dopamine β-hydroxylase (an enzyme essential for norepinephrine synthesis).

fushi tarazu: *ftz*; a mutant form of a *Drosophila* homeobox gene essential for establishing paired body components. The defect causes loss of odd-numbered segments.

fusidic acid: ramycin; 3α,11α,16β-trihydroxy-4α,8,14-trimethyl-18-nor-5α,8α-9β,13α,14β-cholesta-17(20),24-dien-21-oic acid 16-acetate; a steroid antibiotic obtained from the fermentation broth of *Fusidium coccineum* that blocks translation by interfering with translocation of nascent peptides from A to P sites on ribosomes, possibly by inhibiting GTPase.

fusidic acid

fusion gene: a hybrid gene composed of parts from two different sources. Naturally occurring types usually form during unequal crossing over, or when a segment between two linked genes is deleted. Fusion genes are created artificially to put the expression of one under the control of a stronger promoter from the other, or to create fusion proteins.

fusion protein: a hybrid molecule composed of joined amino acid sequences from two different proteins. It can be made by transfecting a fusion gene to direct synthesis of the messenger RNA, or by displacing a stop codon (which otherwise terminates transcription) with a transfected DNA segment inserted into a plasmid. Fusion proteins are usually more easily identified than their native counterparts, and can be used to study the functions of specific amino acid sequences.

fusogenic protein: a protein that mediates membrane fusion. Viral envelope proteins activated by the acidic environments of endosomes fuse with endosome membranes, and this facilitates movement of viral nucleic acids to the cytoplasm. Related proteins that contribute to translocations have been described for eukaryote cells.

futile cycles: metabolic pathways in which the substrates are regenerated from the products of the reactions, for example phosphorylation of fructose-6-phosphate to fructose-1,6-biphosphate (catalyzed by phosphofructokinase-1), followed by dephosphorylation (catalyzed by a phosphatase) to yield fructose-6-phosphate, or hydrolysis of a triacylglycerol to fatty acids plus glycerol, followed by regeneration of the triacylglycerol from activated fatty acids plus glyceraldehyde-3-phosphate. Although some are regarded as metabolic imperfections, other futile cycles perform regulatory functions. Since ATP hydrolysis liberates heat, the fatty acid cycle is used for nonshivering thermogenesis in response to cold environments. It consumes large quantities of ATP (because activation of each of the fatty acids requires conversion of an ATP to AMP + P-P, and more ATP is required to make glyceraldehyde-3-P from glucose). Futile cycles can also amplify metabolic signals. For example, if conversion of substrate A to product B proceeds more rapidly than regeneration of A, the cycle can increase the effectiveness of a hormone on B production if the hormone accelerates A uptake or A → B conversion.

Fv fragment: an immunoglobulin component with a single antigen binding site, obtained by pepsin digestion. It contains one V_H and one V_L domain.

fyn: a proto-oncogene that codes for a 56K protein of the *src* tyrosine kinase family, whose activity is augmented by dephosphorylation. In T lymphocytes, the enzyme is a substrate for CD45 phosphatase.

G

G: (1) glycine; (2) guanine; (3) guanosine; (4) free energy; (5) giga.

g: (1) gram; (2) gravity.

γ: gamma; usually (1) the third member of a group, for example the third (terminal) phosphate of ATP or GTP, the third carbon atom from the carboxyl end of a fatty acid, the third subunit of a polypeptide or protein, or the third most rapidly moving molecular species in an electrical field; (2) microgram, 10^{-9} gram.

G_o: (1) standard free energy; *see* **free energy**; (2) the "resting" (nonproliferating) phase of a cell cycle; (3) *see* **G proteins**.

G_o': standard free energy at pH 7.0.

G_1, G_2: *see* **cell cycles**.

G-14, G-17, G-34: *see* **gastrins**.

G-37: oxyntomodulin; *see* **glicentin**.

G-69: glicentin.

Ga: gallium.

GA: gibberellin.

GABA: gamma aminobutyric acid.

GABA-cuculline: a more potent GABA$_A$ receptor antagonist than **bicuculline** (*q.v.*).

gabaculline: 3-amino-2,3-dihydrobenzoic acid hydrochloride; a potent, irreversible inhibitor of GABA α-oxoglutarate transaminase.

GABA-ergic: gabergic; describes neurons that release, or target cells that respond to gamma aminobutyric acid.

GABA-glutamate transaminase: GABA α-oxoglutarate transaminase.

gabamodulin: an endogenous protein inhibitor of high affinity GABA receptors; *see* also **GABArins**.

GABA α-oxoglutarate transaminase: GABA transaminase; GABA-T; GABA-glutamate transaminase; the major enzyme for GABA degradation. It catalyzes the reaction: GABA + α-oxoglutarate → succinate semialdehyde + glutamate. Pyridoxal-5-phosphate is an essential cofactor.

GABArins: uncharacterized endogenous inhibitors of GABA interactions with GABA receptors. Gabamodulin may be a member of the group.

GABA T: GABA-α-oxoglutarate transaminase.

γ-vinyl-GABA: gamma-vinyl GABA; GVG; Sabril; vigabatrin; 4-amino-5-hexanoic acid; an irreversible inhibitor of gamma aminobutyric acid transaminase. It prolongs the effectiveness of GABA-generating regulators, and is used as an anti-convulsant.

gabexate: *p*-hydroxybenzoic acid ethyl ester 6-guanidinocaproate: a selective inhibitor of proteolytic enzymes that acts on thrombin, plasmin, and kallikreins (but not chymotrypsin).

GABOB: Gabomade; gamibetal; 4-amino-3-hydroxybutanoic acid; a GABA$_A$ receptor agonist, used as an anticonvulsant.

gaboxadol: THIP; 4,5,6,7-tetrahydroisoxazolo[5,4-*c*-pyridin-3-ol; a GABA$_A$ receptor agonist, used to study the receptors.

G-actin: *see* **actin**.

GAD: (1) glutamic acid decarboxylase; (2) generalized anxiety disorder.

GADPH: glyceraldehyde phosphate dehydrogenase.

GAG: glycosaminoglycan.

gag: a viral gene essential for virion synthesis and production of infectious particles. In retroviruses, it acts in conjunction with an adjacent *pol* gene to direct formation of gag-pol messenger RNAs.

galactagogues: agents that promote the flow of breast milk; *see* also **oxytocin**.

galactaric acid: mucic acid; a galactose oxidation product. It is a component of some glycosaminoglycans, and of wood and other high molecular weight plant products.

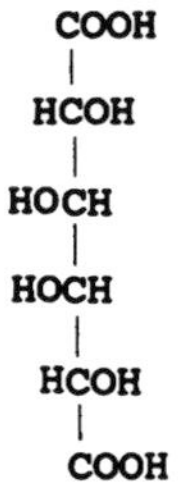

COOH
|
HCOH
|
HOCH
|
HOCH
|
HCOH
|
COOH

galactitol: dulcitol; a sugar alcohol component of the Madagascar manna, *Melampyrum nemorosum*, and of some other plants. It can be made in animals by reducing the aldehyde group of galactose. Very little accumulates under normal conditions, since **galactose-1-phosphate uridyl transferase** (*q.v.*) converts most ingested galactose to glucose. Genetic defects that impair synthesis of the enzyme cause galactitol accumulation when the alcohol (or a precursor) is ingested; *see* also **galactosemia**. Since it does not diffuse across plasma membranes, galactitol formed in cells osmotically draws in water, and can cause cataract formation. *See* also **aldose reductase**.

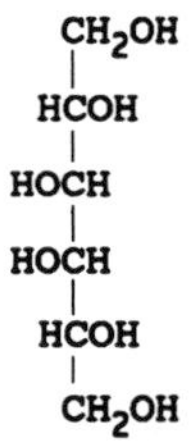

CH₂OH
|
HCOH
|
HOCH
|
HOCH
|
HCOH
|
CH₂OH

galactocerebrosides: **cerebrosides** (*q.v.*), in which the hexose component is galactose. Substantial amounts are made in nervous tissues.

galactoflavin: 6,7-dimethyl-9-(1-deoxy-D-galactitol) iso-alloxazine; a riboflavine antagonist used in nutrition studies. It invokes congenital malformations when fed to pregnant mothers.

galactokinase: an enzyme that catalyzes the reaction: galactose + ATP → galactose-1-phosphate + ADP. The product can be converted to glucose-phosphates; *see* **galactose-1-phosphate uridyl transferase**.

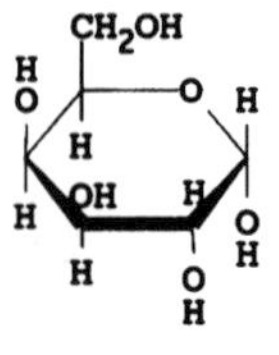

galactose

galactose-1-phosphate

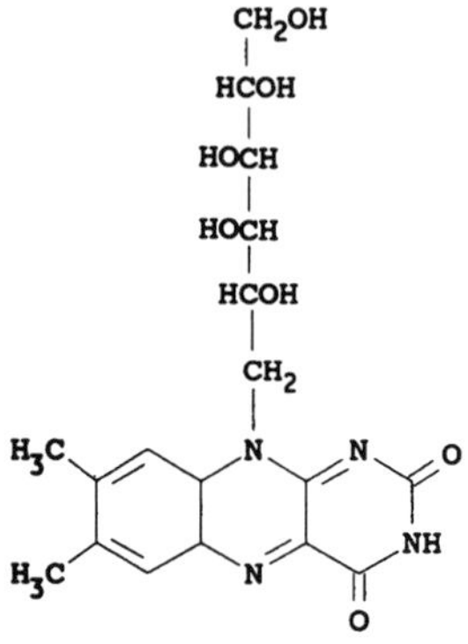

galactoflavin

galactolipids: lipids that contain covalently linked galactose or galactose derivative moieties.

galactopoiesis: lactogenesis; maintenance of established lactation.

galactopoietic: (1) stimulating milk production; (2) an agent that stimulates milk production.

galactorrhea: inappropriate milk secretion (for example in males, or in females that have not recently been pregnant and are not nursing an infant), usually caused by excessive prolactin secretion.

galactosamine: chondrosamine; 2-amino-2-deoxy-D-galactose; a component (often *N*-acetylated) of chondroitin sulfate, keratan sulfate, and some other glycosaminoglycans. High concentrations inhibit hepatic RNA synthesis, and are used to invoke an experimental form of hepatitis. *See* also **galactose**.

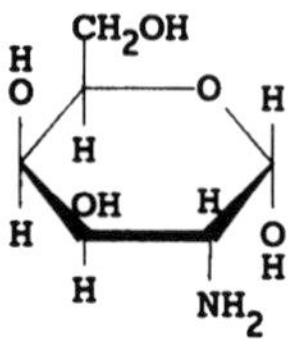

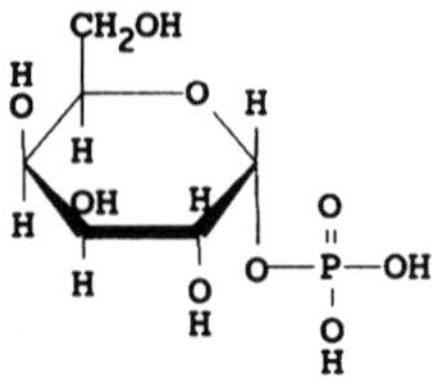

galactose: α-D-galactose; an aldohexose component of lactose, cerebrosides, some glycoproteins, and other body constituents. It is absorbed by intestinal cells via insulin-regulated active transport that uses a carrier shared with glucose. Conversion to glucose in the liver requires phosphorylation (*see* **galactokinase**), reaction of the product with uridine diphosphate glucose (UDPG) to yield UDPG-galactose + glucose-1-P, and, finally, dephosphorylaton of glucose-1-P. Since the reactions are reversible, galactose can also be made from glucose. UDP-galactose can combine with glucose to yield lactose and some other glycosides; and it can enter other metabolic pathways. Galactose can be oxdized to **galactitol** (*q.v.*) and galactaric acid, and it is used to synthesize some glycosaminoglycans and other large molecules.

galactosemia: excessively high blood galactose levels. The consequences can include liver enlargement, jaundice, mental retardation, and cataract formation. Most dietary galactose is obtained from lactose (which yields one molecule of galactose plus one of glucose when digested); but small amounts are released from glycosaminoglycans and other compounds. When healthy individuals ingest large amounts of galactose or its precursors, substantial quantities of the sugar are excreted in the urine, and smaller amounts are used in various metabolic pathways (*see* **galactose**). Autosomal recessive defects that impair production of galactokinase and/or galactose-1-phosphate uridyl transferase cause galactose accumulation, and galactose conversion to toxic metabolites (*see* also **galactitol**). The problems can be averted with low-galactose diets.

galactose-1-phosphate: *see* **galactose** and **galactokinase**.

galactose-1-phosphate uridyl transferase: an enzyme that catalyzes the reaction: galactose-1-phosphate + UDPG → UDP-galactose + glucose-1-phosphate. *See* also **galactose**.

galactosidases: enzymes that catalyze hydrolysis of glycoside bonds formed by galactose moieties. Fabry's disease is attributed to impaired production of a lysosomal α-galactosidase. β-galactosidase is a bacterial enzyme whose synthesis in *E.coli* is controlled by the lac operon.

galactosides: compounds formed by reactions in which galactose aldehyde groups combine with alcoholic groups of other compounds, and water is released.

galactosyl transferases: enzymes that catalyzes transfers of galactose moieties from uridine-diphosphate galactose (UDP-galactose) to acceptor molecules such as *N*-acetylglucosamine. They are needed for the synthesis of galactose containing compounds, such as some glycosaminoglycans, and are used as markers for Golgi membranes in cell homogenates. In nonlactating mammary glands, the *A protein* of the lactose synthase system promotes formation of *N*-acetyllactosamine from galactose + *N*-acetylglucosamine. Prolactin induces *B protein*, which decreases the affinity for *N*-acetylglucosamine, increases it for glucose, and thereby promotes lactose synthesis.

galacturonic acid {**galacturonate**}: the product obtained when the —CH$_2$OH group of galactose is oxidized to —COOH. It is a component of pectins and some other polysaccharides, and of some glycosaminoglycans, and is used by hepatic cells for conjugating a wide variety of compounds.

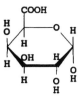

galanin: Gly-Trp-Thr-Leu-Asn-Ser-Ala-Gly-Tyr-Leu-Leu-Gly-Pro-His-Ala-Ile-Asp-Asn-His-Arg-Ser-Phe-His-Asp-Lys-Tyr-Gly-Leu-Ala-NH$_2$; a peptide in sensory and some sympathetic system neurons, in supraoptic, paraventricular and arcuate nuclei, and in pancreatic islets, adrenal and thyroid glands, several kinds of adenohypophysial cells, the small intestine, and elsewhere. Co-localization with acetylcholine, catecholamines, gamma aminobutyric acid (GABA), serotonin, vasopressin and other regulators occurs at various sites. It acts via diverse mechanisms as a neurotransmitter, neuromodulator, or hormone. Influences on exocytosis in many cell types inhibit the release of insulin, somatostatin, pancreatic polypeptide, and dopamine, but the secretion of several pituitary hormones is stimulated. Galanin also directly promotes contraction of intestinal smooth muscle, but antagonizes acetylcholine stimulation. In the central nervous system, it antagonizes acetylcholine effects on memory, suppresses appetite (possibly via release of cholecystokinin), and exerts anti-nociceptive effects by antagonizing the facilitatory influences of substance P and calcitonin gene related peptide (CGRP), and by potentiating the spinal analgesic effects of morphine. Galanin synthesis is regulated in a cell type-specific manner. Estrogen is a potent stimulant in the adenohypophysis, but not in most neurons.

gallamine triethiodide: Flaxedil; 1,2,3-tris(2-triethylammonium ethoxy)benzene-triiodide; a curare-like agent used to relax skeletal muscle during surgery.

gall bladder: an organ specialized for receiving, concentrating, and storing bile, and delivering it to the small intestine. *See* also **cholecystokinin** and **cholelithiasis**. Rats and some other mammals do not have gall bladders.

Galli-Mainini test: *see* "**frog**" **test for pregnancy**.

gallinaceous: resembling domesticated fowl.

gallium: Ga; an element of the rare metal group (atomic number 31, atomic weight 69.74). Gallium salts decrease

gallamine triethiodide

the solubility of bone crystals and inhibit tartrate resistant acid phosphatase in osteoclats. The nitrate is used to slow calcium release in hypercalcemia of malignancy.

Gallus domesticus: the domesticated chicken.

GAL14 protein: a yeast protein that binds specific DNA base sequences, and activates transcription of genes essential for converting galactose to glucose.

GALT: gut-associated lymphatic tissue.

galvanometers: instruments for measuring the amounts of electric current that flow through wires or coils moving in magnetic fields.

gametes: sex cells; *see* **spermatozoa** and **ova**.

gamete intrafallopian tube transfer: *see* **GIFT**.

gameticides: gametocides: agents that kill gametes.

gametogenesis: gamete formation; spermatogenesis or oogenesis.

gamma: *see* γ.

gamma aminobutyric acid; γ-aminobutyric acid; GABA: a neurotransmitter made in largest amounts in the cerebellum, basal ganglia, hypothalamus, olfactory bulbs, and other parts of the central nervous system, and in the retina, and adrenal medulla. Small amounts are present in sympathetic ganglia and some peripheral nerves, and in the heart, liver, and spleen. GABA is also made in the nervous systems of arthropods and some other invertebrates. It exerts mostly inhibitory influences on the central nervous system; and agonists that act on specific brain regions are used as anti-convulsants. The major effects may be exerted on interneurons, or via presynaptic inhibition, but some involve influences on neurons that release other neurotransmitters. Co-release with acetylcholine and other regulators from some neuron types complicates interpretation of the actions. GABA also inhibits the secretion of corticotropin releasing hormone (CRH), gonadotropins, and insulin, but augments prolactin, growth hormone, and somatostatin release. It is implicated in the timing of ovulation, modulation of photoreceptor and olfactory receptor responses, and many other processes. Neurons synthesize it from glutamic acid, and also take it up from extracellular fluids via ATP-dependent mechanisms. GAT-1 may be the major transporter, but other carriers have been identified. They differ from proteins that mediate ATP-dependent, proton driven uptake into synaptic vesicles. Release is accomplished at various sites by both calcium-dependent exocytosis and calcium-independent carrier mechanisms. The major degradation pathway is catalyzed by GABA α-oxoglutarate transaminase. *See* also **gamma aminobutyric acid receptors**.

$$H_2N-CH_2-CH_2-CH_2-COO$$

gamma aminobutyric acid receptors; GABA receptors; several transmembrane glycoproteins that mediate GABA effects. GABA$_A$ types promote opening of chloride channels and consequent cell hyperpolarization.

At least six α-, three β-, and two γ-subunit types, each coded for by a separate gene, contribute to the diversity; and posttranslational processing accounts for additional variations. The receptors do not display protein kinase activity, but some of the subunits are substrates for kinase C and/or kinase A. BZ-1 and BZ-2 subtypes bind benzodiazepines, and a third subtype interacts with the ethyl alcohol antagonist, Ro15-453a. Anxiolytic agents (benzodiazepines), and anti-convulsants (barbiturates) bind to sites different from the ones that bind GABA. Taurine also binds to α subunits. Muscimol is an agonist. Antagonists include convulsants such as picrotoxin, bicuculline, and anxiogenic agents such as β-carbolines. GABA$_B$ types promote opening of K$^+$ channels and exert inhibitory influences on L type calcium channels. At least some effects involve interactions with G proteins. Baclofen is an agonist.

gamma cells: adenohypophysial cells identified under light microscopy that are believed to secrete adrenocorticotropic hormone (ACTH) or and/or α-melanocyte stimulating hormone (α-MSH).

gamma globulins: γ-globulins; the most positively charged of the serum globulins. Most are immunoglobulins.

gamma rays: electromagnetic radiation released by some radioactive atoms. They resemble X-rays, but have shorter wave-lengths and travel faster. The rays rapidly penetrate, and can damage living cells. Isotopes that release them are used as markers in metabolic studies.

gamone: (1) a chemical inducer of reproductive system development; (2) a chemotaxin or other substance produced by gametes that contributes to fertilization.

GAMS: γ-D-glutamylamino-methylsulfonic acid; a broad spectrum excitatory amino acid antagonist that is most effective against kainate subtypes.

ganciclovir: 2′-nor-2-deoxyguanosine; DHPG; a cytosine nucleoside analog effective against all *Herpes* viruses, including cytomegalovirus and Epstein-Barr types. It is used to control secondary infections in patients with acquired immunodeficiency syndrome (AIDS). Phosphorylation catalyzed by viral thymidine kinases converts it to a product that competes with deoxyguanosine triphosphate (dGTP) for incorporation into viral DNA, and terminates DNA synthesis by inhibiting DNA polymerases.

ganglion: an aggregation of neuron cell bodies and their associated processes. The term usually refers to peripheral nervous system components (sympathetic, parasympathetic, and dorsal root ganglia), whereas *nucleus* is used for most central nervous system clusters; but *see* **basal ganglia**.

ganglioneuroblastomas: malignant tumors that contain neurofibrils, partially differentiated neuroblasts, and mature ganglion cells, all of which derive from neural crest cells.

ganglioneuromas: benign tumors derived from sympathetic ganglion cells.

ganglionic blocking agents: usually, compounds that disrupt message transmission from preganglionic to postganglionic neurons. Some types, such as nicotine, stimulate first, and then desensitize via persistent depolarization of postsynaptic membranes. Others, such as hexamethonium, inhibit directly by competing with neurotransmitters for postsynaptic receptors. Since acetylcholine is the major presynaptic transmitter for all autonomic ganglia, most inhibitors affect both sympathetic and parasympathetic target cell functions. Some authors include agents that block transmission to skeletal muscle. However, the since the target cell receptors are different, others prefer terms such as *curariform* or *curare-like* blocking agents for those types.

gangliosides: 15 or more classes of complex glycosphingolipids, all of which contain at least one *N*-acetyl-neuraminic acid (NAN) moiety. They are present in all plasma membranes, but are most abundant in the grey matter of the brain, with substantial amounts at nerve endings and in the vicinities of some hormone receptors. The types differ mostly in carbohydrate content, and are distinguished by letters M, D, and T which denote the presence of one (mono), two (di), or three (tri) NAN moieties, respectively. Subscripts are used for the subtypes, as in GM_1, GM_2 (shown below) and GD_{1a}. All have negatively charged polar heads and nonpolar tails, and are implicated in several functions, including interactions with fibronectin and other extracellular matrix components, modulation of hormone-receptor binding, and signal transduction. GM_1 inhibits the activities of some protein kinase C isozymes by blocking their translocation to plasma membranes, and it protects against glutamate neurotoxicity. Ganglioside biosynthesis from glucosylceramide is continuous in the Golgi apparatus, and accomplished via sequential additions of galactose, *N*-acetylgalactosamine, and NAN moieties. The molecules are continuously degraded by sequential removal of terminal sugar moieties, via reactions catalyzed by substrate-specific lysosomal enzymes (*see* also **gangliosidoses**).

gangliosidoses: several inherited disorders in which lysosomal enzyme defects impair ganglioside metabolism. The lipids accumulate in the central nervous system and invoke pathological changes. *See* also **Tay-Sach's disease**.

Ganite: a trade name for gallium nitrate; *see* **gallium**.

gap: a space; in molecular biology, a missing segment on one strand of double-stranded DNA. (The DNA is single stranded at that site.)

GAP: (1) gonadotropin releasing hormone associated protein; (2) GTPase activating protein.

GAP-43: a 43K protein in growth cone membranes of developing neurons, and at sites of axonal elongation and regeneration. It is implicated as a regulator of nerve terminal remodeling, and may contribute to plasticity, learning, and memory. Roles in signal transduction are suggested by its ability to bind calmodulin and regulate production of phosphatidylinositol-4,5-biphosphate (IP_3). Changes in phosphorylation are associated with long term potentiation. When transfected into non-neuronal cells, it stimulates formation of cytoplasmic processes.

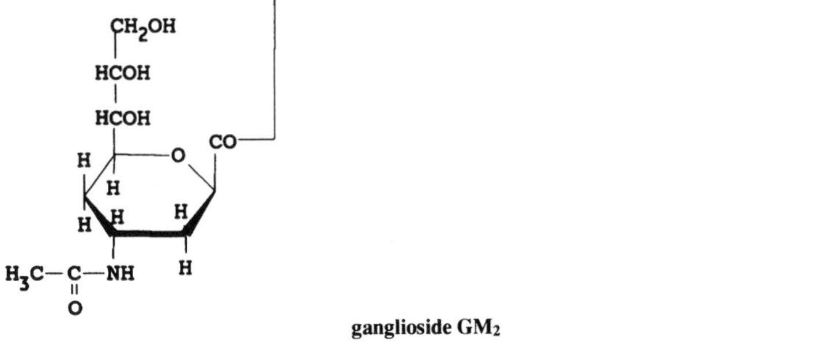

ganglioside GM_2

gap junctions: channels formed by plasma membranes of adjacent cells that permit exchanges of ions and small molecules. The pores are hexagonal arrays of transmembrane proteins (connexons) that resemble synaptophysins, with subunit weights in the 27-43K range for vertebrates. (Lighter ones are made by other animal types). Loops that project from the extracellular face of one cell interact with those of the adjacent cell. Pore sizes are regulated by phosphorylation, calmodulin binding, cytoplasmic acidity, voltage changes, and hormones. The junctions play roles in oocyte development, ovulation, implantation, parturition, morphogenesis, paracrine actions of some regulators, contraction synchronization in the heart, and other functions.

gargoyle cells: fibroblasts that have accumulated excessive amounts of glycosaminoglycans, present in individuals with inherited defects that impair the synthesis of degrading enzymes. *See* also **Hurler's disease** and **Huntington syndrome**.

gastero-: gastro-: a prefix meaning stomach.

gastric: affecting, relating to, or originating in the stomach.

gastricsin: a pepsin isomer in gastric juice.

gastric juice: the watery secretion made by stomach cells. Its components include hydrochloric acid, pepsin (and some pepsinogen), mucin, and intrinsic factor, as well as small quantities of gastrin and other regulators.

gastrins: species specific, chemically and biologically related peptides, including G-14s (*minigastrins* with 14 amino acid moieties), G-17s (*little gastrins*), and G-34s (*big gastrins*). Type II hormones have sulfated tyrosyl moieties, whereas type I peptides do not; but sulfation does not affect biological potency. Human minigastrin I is Trp-Leu-Glu-Glu-Glu-Glu-Glu-Ala-Tyr-Gly-Trp-Met-Asp-Phe-NH$_2$. Little gastrin II is pGlu-Gly-Pro-Trp-Leu-Glu-Glu-Glu-Glu-Glu-Ala-Tyr-Gly-Trp-(SO$_3$H)-Met-Asp-Phe-NH$_2$. Big gastrin has an additional *N*-terminal sequence, pGlu-Leu-Gly-Pro-Gln-Gly-His-Pro-Ser-Leu-Val-Ala-Asp-Pro-Ser-Lys-Lys-Gln-Gly-Pro-, which includes a Lys-Lys bond that can be cleaved by pepsin. Stomach gastrin (G) cells are the major sites for synthesis, but small amounts of the hormone are made in the duodenum, and in fetal and neonatal pancreatic islets. Adults have G cells scattered among other types in both exocrine and endocrine pancreas that make minute amounts of gastrin which may perform paracrine roles. Large amounts of stomach G-17 are rapidly released in response to meal ingestion, vagal stimulation, and hypoglycemia. It is the major stimulant for hydrochloric acid production by stomach parietal cells; and high acidity in the stomach lumen exerts negative feedback control. G-17 also directly stimulates stomach motility, but its ability to augment pepsinogen release may be secondary to the effects on pH. G-14s (and G-13s) are equipotent, and may be true hormones or degradation products. During fasting, the levels of G-34 (which has a long half-life) exceed those of G-17s; and duodenal gastrin is mostly G-34. It is a less potent stimulant of HCl production, but exerts trophic effects on gastric and duodenal mucosa,

and on the exocrine pancreas. The terminal tetrapeptide, -Trp-(SO$_3$H)-Met-Asp-Phe-NH$_2$, is identical with that of cholecystokinins, and this probably accounts for common effects of the two regulators at some sites (for example on stimulation of pancreatic enzyme production and bile formation). Competition for binding sites may explain the antagonistic influences on stomach motility. Some gastrin is additionally made in the brain, in which it may serve as a neurotransmitter. *See* also **pentagastrin** and **gastrinoma**.

gastrin cells: G cells; cells that synthesize gastrins. Under normal conditions, the largest numbers are in the stomach. *See* also **gastrins** and **gastrinoma**.

gastrin inhibitory peptide: GIP: an old name for glucose-dependent insulinotropic peptide.

gastrinomas: tumors derived from gastrin cells that secrete large quantities of the hormone. Most originate in the pancreas. *See* also **Zollinger-Ellison syndrome**.

gastrin releasing peptides: GRPs; tachykinins chemically related to alytesin and ranatensin that share a common *C*-terminal peptide with them, act on the same bombesin receptors, and are believed to be the mammalian counterparts of those amphibian regulators. The major human GRP (GRP-27) is Ala-Pro-Val-Ser-Val-Gly-Gly-Gly-Thr-Val-Leu-Ala-Lys-Met-Tyr-Pro-Arg-Gly-Asn-His-Trp-Ala-Val-Gly-His-Leu-Met-NH$_2$, but a GRP-10 composed of the last ten amino acid moieties has been identified in human prostate glands, Leydig cells, semen, and female genital tracts; and the hypothalamus contains more GRP-10 than GRP-27. At least 2 genes direct formation of premessenger RNAs that undergo differential splicing. The peptides are made in neuroendocrine cells of the gastrointestinal and pulmonary tracts, brain and spinal cord neurons, and pituitary glands; and some are secreted to milk. Large amounts are made by fetal lungs, and by small cell lung and thyroid medullary carcinomas. GRPs act at some sites as neurotransmitters that depress appetite and grooming, affect other forms of behavior, lower body temperature, augment sympathetic system activity, promote smooth muscle contraction (in some cases indirectly), and stimulate the release of gastrin, somatostatin, vasoactive intestinal peptide (VIP), glucose-dependent insulinotropic peptide (GIP), and glucagon, but inhibit insulin secretion. At other sites they are growth promoting paracrine and/or autocrine hormones which act in part via activation of kinase C isozymes. They stimulate proliferation of fibroblasts and some tumor cells; and excessive amounts can invoke gastric hyperplasia. They also promote gall bladder contraction, enhance gastrointestinal motility, and augment DNA synthesis and proenzyme secretion in the pancreas, but inhibit acid production. Stimulatory effects on adrenocorticotropic hormone (ACTH) secretion are attributed to corticotropin releasing hormone-like potency, whereas inhibitory influences on growth hormone and prolactin are probably secondary to somatostatin and dopamine release.

gastroentero-: a prefix meaning gastrointestinal.

gastroliths: (1) concretions composed mostly of calcium carbonate, along with some calcium phosphate, formed by some crustaceans when they absorb their exoskeletons during molt cycles. They are storage forms of minerals used for formation of the new shells; (2) similar concretions formed in vertebrate stomachs under pathological conditions.

Gastropod: a class of mollusks that includes snails, slugs, whelks, and abalones. Some are primary or intermediate hosts for organisms that infect humans and other animals.

gastrotropin: an uncharacterized component of canine and porcine ileal mucosa extracts that mobilizes intracellular Ca^{2+}, stimulates growth and proliferation of some cell types, and augments hydrochloric acid and pepsinogen secretion.

gastrula: an early embryonic stage in the development of most complex organisms (*see* **gastrulation**). In vertebrates and many other animal types, it is a bilaterally symmetrical, centrally located primitive gut (archenteron) that opens into a blastopore at the posterior end, and is surrounded by endoderm. External to the endoderm are layers of mesoderm and ectoderm.

gastrulation: the process by which a blastula develops into a gastrula. In most higher animals, it begins with mesoderm cell migration along the inner wall of the blastocoele to form a solid, cylinder-like cell conglomeration. The archenteron is then molded by invagination of endoderm.

GATs: proteins that mediate cell uptake of GABA. Of the several identified, GAT-1 is believed to be the most important.

gated ion channels: pores formed by transmembrane proteins that permit passage of specific kinds of ions. The openings and closings are differentially regulated; *see* **voltage gated** and **ligand gated channels**.

gating: the opening and closing of gated ion channels.

Gaucher's disease: several autosomal recessive disorders in which glycosphingolipid metabolism is impaired. The most common defect is glucocerebrosidase (β-glucosidase) deficiency. The manifestations, which depend upon the sites at which excessive cerebrosides accumulate, can include liver enlargement, neurological defects, anemia, and reduced bone mass.

Gaussian distribution: normal distribution; the values for a parameter in a total population, in which all variations are random. It is represented by a bell-shaped curve, in which the parameter values are plotted along the X axis, and their frequencies along the Y. *See* also **standard deviation**.

G banding: the patterns obtained when chromosomes are treated first with trypsin, and then with Giemsa stain. Most heterochromatin stains darker than most euchromatin.

GC boxes: DNA sequences that contain mostly guanine and cytosine bases, and serve as promoters for constitutively transcribed eukaryote genes.

G cells: cells that secrete **gastrin** (*q.v.*). Most are in the stomach, but smaller numbers occur in the duodenum, fetal pancreas, and elsewhere. Fetal types also make thyrotropin releasing hormone (TRH).

GC/MC: computerized gas chromatography/mass spectrophotometry.

GCN4: a 281-amino acid yeast transcription factor. It contains a leucine zipper domain, and associates with DNA regions that bind AP-1 proteins.

G-CSF: granulocyte colony stimulating factor.

GDEE: glutamate diethyl ester.

GDP: guanosine diphosphate.

GDPβS: a nonhydrolyzable GDP analog, used as a laboratory tool to inhibit the activation of G proteins.

GD-VEGF: glioma-derived vascular endothelial cell growth factor.

GEF: (1) guanine nucleotide exchange factor; *see* **GTPases**; (2) glycosylation enhancing factor.

GE: glycyrrhetinic acid; *see* **carbenoxalone**.

gelding: a castrated horse.

gel: (1) a semi-liquid phase; in many gels, resistance to flow is attributed to the cross-linking of molecular chains; (2) an inert matrix used for separating molecules or other particles, for example, agarose for nucleic acids, or polyacrylamide for RNAs and proteins; (3) to set or solidify.

gelatin: denatured collagen.

gel electrophoresis: *see* **electrophoresis**.

gel filtration chromatography: methods for separating molecules or other particles on the basis of size, by percolating liquids that contain them through suspensions of chemically inert, solvent-permeable beads with pore sizes similar to those of the smallest types. Particles that can enter the beads take a longer path, and therefore pass through more slowly.

gelsolins: widely distributed cytoskeletal proteins that contribute to phagocytosis, and to cell motility and changes in cell shapes. When present in substantial amounts and activated by Ca^{2+}, they bind to actin monomers, retard actin filament polymerization, and sever noncovalent actin:actin bonds. At low Ca^{2+} concentrations, they are nucleation sites for actin assembly. The cytoplasmic and circulating forms have apparent molecular weights of 90K and 93K, respectively.

Gelusil: Gelusil II; Gelusil M; trade names for aluminum and magnesium hydroxide preparations used to decrease gastric acidity.

gemfibrozil: 5-(2,5-dimethylphenoxy)-2,2-dimethylpentanoic acid; one of several fibric acid derivatives used to treat some lipid metabolism disorders. It lowers circulating very low density lipoprotein (VLDL), VLDL cholesterol, and triacylglycerol levels, has lesser effects on low density lipoproteins (LDLs), and elevates high density lipoprotein (HDL) cholesterol. *See also* **clofibrate**.

gender: a category (male or female) to which an individual of a species is assigned, usually on the basis of phenotypic sex. *See also* **gender identity**.

gender identity: the subjective sense of belonging to the male or female gender; *cf* **gender preference** and **gender role**. Some individuals with phenotypes associated with one gender identify with the other.

gender preference: the gender of the species to which an individual is sexually attracted; *cf* **gender identity** and **gender role**.

gender role: the behavior patterns displayed by or expected of members of a species of a given gender. Since it is determined to a great extent by external factors such as social setting and education, it can vary with the locale, and with the time period.

gene: a hereditary unit or nucleic acid segment (DNA for most organisms, but RNA for some viruses) that performs a specific function. *Structural* genes code for messenger RNAs that direct translation. *Regulatory* genes (which are not transcribed) serve as recognition sites for promoters, enhancers, operators, and other proteins that regulate DNA replication, transcription, recombination, and/or repair. Different genes direct formation of ribosomal and transfer RNAs (which are not translated).

gene activation: a change in a gene that leads to initiation or acceleration of transcription. Some genes function only in specific cell types, or only when certain proteins, such as hormone-receptor complexes or transcription factors, interact (directly or indirectly) with promoter and/or enhancer regions. Others are active under basal conditions, but can be affected by such factors. Demethylation at specific sites, and detachment from histones and other nuclear proteins, are among the mechanisms that can lead to activation.

gene amplification: formation of additional copies of a gene. Multiple copies of genes that code for ribosomal

RNAs are made during oogenesis in many species; and development of resistance to some drugs is associated with amplification of specific structural types. Amplification can occur when fragments of broken DNA strands join, and transcribing segments come under the control of efficient promoters, when certain viral nucleic acid segments incorporate into host genomes, and following unequal crossing over during meiosis. The rapid growth of some kinds of cancer cells is attributed to amplification of genes that direct formation of growth factors, or permit use of alternate substrates, and metastasis with ones that alter interactions with extracellular matrices. Artificial amplification accomplished by DNA manipulation is used to study some functions. When the duplicated nucleic acid sequences are joined head-to-tail, they are said to be tandemly repeated. *See also* **gene conversion** and **genetic recombination**.

gene bank: *see* **gene library**.

gene cloning: generation of many copies of the same DNA segment. It can be accomplished by inserting the segments into vectors that propagate in host cells. *See also* **polymerase chain reaction**.

gene cluster: a set of contiguous genes on the same chromosome. The components often derive from a common ancestral type that has undergone duplication and mutation.

gene conversion: replacement of a DNA segment from one gene with a segment from another, for example by template switching during chromosome replication. Transcription can be accelerated (or blocked) if the positions of promoters and other regulatory elements are altered. The kinds of messenger RNAs made change if the conversion shifts open reading frames. In some cases, the consequences are trivial. In others, they seriously disrupt functions, or invoke effects compatible with survival that lead to diversity and speed evolution.

gene dosage: the number of copies of a given gene in a cell nucleus.

gene duplication: formation of an additional DNA segment adjacent to, and identical with or very similar to one previously present, in a manner that does not change the open reading frame of the original gene. It can result from unequal crossing over during meiosis, or from defective replication. In some cases, segments that code for "stop" RNA triplets are affected, and longer proteins are made. If the new segment is not identical with the original one, it can become a nonfunctioning pseudogene, or can code for variant products with new properties. Some aspects of evolution are attributed to selective transmission of altered genes.

gene expression: usually (1) gene transcription; (2) the phenotypic manifestations of a genome that result from transcription and processes affected by it. *See also* **gene activation**.

gene extinction: gene repression.

gene family: *see* **gene cluster** and **multigene family**.

gene flow: gene exchanges between different populations of the same species.

gene frequency: the percentages of the various allele types at a given locus expressed by members of a population.

gene insertion: addition of one or more genes (usually from an outside source) to the genome. It can occur during viral infections, and can be accomplished artificially by transduction or cell fusion.

gene interactions: the mechanisms whereby two or more genes affect the expression of the same trait. In some cases, one gene codes for a product that is regulated by another, nonallelic gene. In others, simultaneous expression of two (or more) alleles affects the phenotype; **see** also **codominance**. One gene can also inhibit or augment expression of another.

gene library: gene bank: a collection of cloned DNA fragments from a single individual that contains all of the base sequences characteristic of the genome.

gene locus: the position of the gene on a chromosome.

gene mapping: determination of the chromosomal loci for specific gene types.

gene pair: a set of two alleles at analogous loci on homologous chromosomes.

gene pool: the total genetic information possessed by a reproductively competent population of a single species.

generation time: the time required for a cell population to double in number. In actively proliferating cells, it is roughly equivalent to the time required to complete one cell cycle.

gene regulatory protein: a protein that affects transcription by interacting (directly or indirectly) with a specific genome component.

gene repression: inhibition of gene expression. It is usually accomplished via proteins that bind directly to regulatory components (or affect other proteins that bind those regions), and is usually reversible.

generic: (1) of or relating to a genus; (2) describes a preparation that is not protected by a trade name, but is pharmacologically identical (or nearly so) to one that is.

gene splicing: *in vitro* manipulation of genetic material, usually to achieve deletions, insertions, or rearrangements that affect transcription.

genetic: heritable; pertaining to or controlled by genes.

genetic block: disruption of a biochemical reaction or pathway because a a gene is defective, or unable to function in a normal manner.

genetic burden: *see* **genetic load**.

genetic code: information contained in nucleic acid triplets that directs the synthesis of specific kinds of messenger RNAs; *see* also **codons**.

genetic distance: a measure of the heritable differences (numbers of allelic changes) between two popula-

tions of a species that have accrued during the course of evolution.

genetic drift: random fluctuations of gene frequencies observed when the samples selected for testing do not accurately reflect the characteristics of the entire population. It occurs most commonly when small numbers of individuals are examined.

genetic engineering: artificial manipulation of genes, for example to produce large quantities of specific kinds of proteins (*see* also **gene cloning**), to make probes for investigation, to breed species with new characteristics useful for understanding gene functions or for commercial purposes, or to treat inherited disorders caused by gene defects.

genetic fitness: the ability of individuals of a specific genotype to transmit traits to the next generation, compared with the contributions of individuals of the same population with different genotypes.

genetic linkage: the tendency for two or more genes to be inherited together; *see* also **linkage disequilibrium**.

genetic load: genetic burden; in a population, the (1) difference between the observed mean fitness and the value that would be expected if all individuals possessed the genotype most compatible with survival and reproduction; (2) decrease in fitness caused by deleterious mutations; (3) average number of lethal equivalents per individual.

genetic markers: genes whose expression can be used to identify the cells, or the individuals in which they occur. Specific DNA segments can be used as probes to determine the chromosomal loci, or to detect the presence of mutated forms.

genetic mosaic: an individual with some cells that differ in DNA composition from other cells. Zygotes can acquire abnormal chromosome patterns if more than one spermatozoan fertilizes an oocyte, if a polar body adheres to an oocyte and is incorporated, or if nondisjunction, chromosome lag, or chromosome duplication occurs during gametogenesis. Cells with extra chromosomes often undergo uneven cleavages that lead to formation of daughter cells with different make-ups. Loss, duplication, or translocation of chromosomes in some cells can also occur during later stages of embryonic development. *See* also **chimeras**.

genetic obesity: conditions in which inherited defects lead to the accumulation of excessive amounts of body fat. Several animal models have been developed. In most cases, the obesity is associated with other metabolic problems. *See*, for example *fa/fa* **rats** and *ob/ob* **mice**.

genetic polymorphism: occurrence of two or more genotypes in a population in frequencies not accounted for by recurrent mutation, for example when one genotype provides special advantages under the imposed living conditions.

genetic recombination: formation of sets of alleles in offspring that differ from those of the parents; *see* **crossing over** and **gene conversion**.

genetics: the study of heredity.

genetic sex: chromosomal sex; the numbers and kinds of sex chromosomes in the genome of an individual. In most mammalian species, normal females have two X chromosomes, whereas normal males have one X and a smaller Y. Abnormal patterns include XO, XXY, XXYY, XYY, and XXX. (Survival is not possible without an X). Usually, individuals with at least one complete Y chromosome are phenotypic males (although more than one X type can impair development). Those lacking a Y are usually phenotypic females. However, since male-determining components of the Y chromosome can be deleted, or translocated to an X or autosome type, discrepancies between chromosome morphology and phenotype can occur; *see* **sex determination**. Reproductive system development also requires contributions from autosomes; *see* **sex differentiation**. In birds and some other vertebrates, normal females have one W and one Z, whereas males have two of the Z type.

gene transduction: *see* **transduction**.

genic balance: the X:A ratio (numbers of X chromosomes compared with numbers of autosomes). In some animal types, for example many insect species, individuals with X:A ratios of 0.5 or less are males, and ones with ratios of 1 or greater are females.

geniculate: knee-shaped, a term used, for example to describe some formations in the brain such as the thalamic medial and lateral geniculate nuclei.

genistein: 4,5,7-trihydroxyisoflavone; an isoflavone isolated from the fermentation broth of *Pseudomonas* species. It is a potent inhibitor of tyrosine kinases, and of epidermal growth factor (EGF)-mediated phosphorylations.

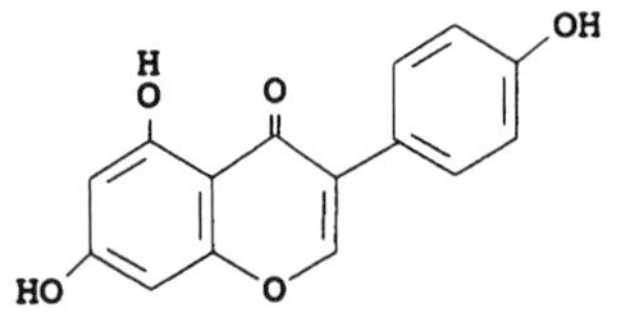

genital: relating to the reproductive system organs.

genitalia: genitals; usually, the externally visible reproductive organs.

genital folds: urogenital folds.

genital ridges: urogenital ridges; bilateral protuberances in young embryos that contain cells which give rise to gonads and associated structures.

genital swellings: the embryonic precursors of the scrotum in males, and the labia majora in females.

genital tubercle: the embryonic precursor of the glans penis and corpora cavernosa in males, and the clitoris in females.

genome: usually (1) the complete set of DNA segments present in a diploid nucleus. The human genome contains approximately 100,000 genes; (2) a term also applied to the DNA in haploid nuclei of gametes, to heritable components of chloroplasts and mitochondria, and to the nucleic acids of viruses.

genotype: the genetic make-up (chromosome pattern) of an individual; *cf* **phenotype** and *see* also **gene expression**.

gentamycin: gentamicin; several antibiotics, including gentamicin C_1 (shown below), gentamycins C_{1a} and C_2, tobramycin, netilmicin, and amikacin (produced by *Micromonosperma purpurea* and related organisms). All contain two or more special amino sugars (garosamine and purpurosamine) linked to two hexoses (deoxystreptamines). They inhibit initiation of protein synthesis in bacteria by attaching to 23S core proteins of 30S ribosomal subunits that bind messenger RNAs, and are effective against both gram positive and gram negative bacteria, but can cause irreversible ear damage.

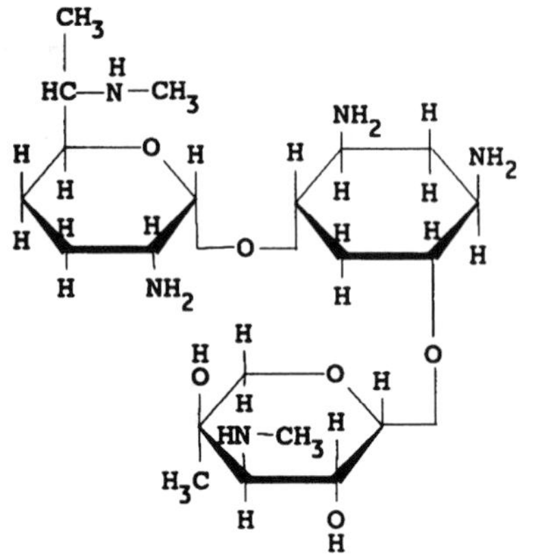

gentian violet: crystal violet; hexamethyl-pararosanaline chloride; N-[4-[*bis*[4-(dimethylamino)-phenyl]methylene]-2,5-cyclohexadien-1-ylidene]-N-methyl-methanaminium chloride; a biological stain used to identify gram positive bacteria, and as an indicator. It is is applied topically to treat mucosal yeast infections, and to protect individuals with severe burns against infections; and it also kills some parasitic helminths. Systemic use can cause nausea, vomiting and diarrhea.

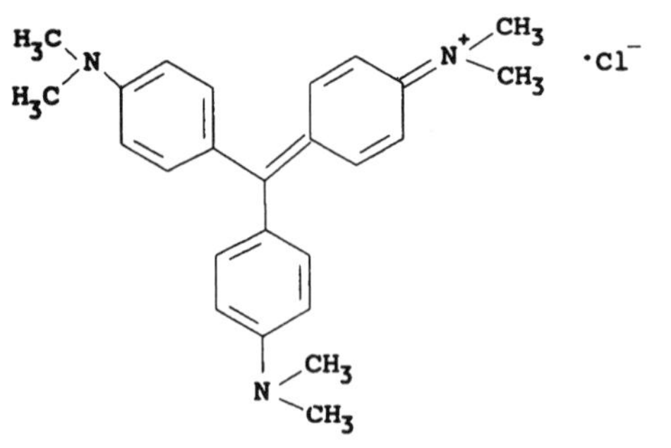

gentianose: a naturally occurring, nonreducing trisaccharide, composed of two glucose and one fructose moiety joined by glycosidic bonds.

gentiobiose: amygdalose; 6-O-β-D-glucopyranosyl-D-glucose; a naturally occurring disaccharide.

gentianose

gentiobiose

gentisic acid: 2,5-dihydroxybenzoic acid; a compound made by *Penicillium patulatum*, a component of gentian dye, and a salicylate metabolite excreted to the urine.

COOH
OH
HO

genus: a taxonomic group that includes one or more species. In most classification systems, it is a subdivision of a family.

gepirone: 4,4-dimethyl-1-[4-[4-(2-pyrimidinal)-1-piper-azinyl]butyl]-2,6-piperidinedione; a tranquilizer with properties similar to those of buspirone.

H₃C
H₃C
O
N — (CH₂)₄ — N   N — N
O
N

geraniol: 3,7-dimethyl-2,6-octadien-1-ol; a pheromone used by some bee species to signal the location of food. It is also a component of rose and palmarosa oils, citronella, lemon grass, and other plant derivatives used in the perfume industry and as insect attractants.

CH₃   CH₃
H₃C   OH

geranyl-geranyl pyrophosphate: *see* **geranyl pyrophosphate**.

geranyl pyrophosphate: geraniol diphosphoric acid ester, an intermediate in the pathway for biosynthesis of cholesterol and some other lipids, formed in the reaction: dimethylallyl-pyrophosphate + isopentenyl pyrophosphate → geranyl pyrophosphate + P-P, catalyzed by geranyl pyrophosphate synthetase. It condenses with another molecule of isopentenyl pyrophosphate to yield farnesyl pyrophosphate. Some proteins are anchored to plasma membrane lipids via geranyl and related terpene moieties. Geranyl-geranyl pyrophosphate is a 20 carbon terpene made by condensation of geranyl pyrophosphate units. The chain is elongated by successive additions of 5-carbon units to form phytoene and other intermediates of the pathway for biosynthesis of carotene and related plant pigments. *See* also **isoprenylation**.

CH₃   CH₃   O   O   O
H₃C   O—P—O—P—O—P—O⁻
                   O   O   O
                   H

GERL: Golgi-endoplasmic reticulum-lysosomal system; a term that has fallen into disuse because of recently acquired insights into the mechanisms for molecular trafficking through cell membrane systems.

germ cells: gametes (spermatozoa and ova). Some authors additionally apply the term to their immediate precursors (spermatocytes and oocytes), to reproductive system cells that divide by mitosis to form the precursors (spermatogonia and oogonia), and to gonocytes. Others prefer the term *germinal cells* for the immature types.

germ free animals: animals raised under sterile (axenic, gnotobiotic) conditions to avoid the effects of contact with foreign antigens, or to support survival of animals with impaired immune systems. Diet restrction may also be necessary, because sterilized foods often contain the antigens of dead microorganisms. Under natural conditions, healthy animals are exposed to many kinds of antigens. Deprivation of the stimuli they provide can impair immune system maturation and production of normal quantities of immunoglobulins.

germinal cells: *see* **germ cells**.

germinal centers: clusters of rapidly proliferating cells in the spleen and lymph nodes, in which large numbers of new lymphocytes are produced.

germinal epithelium: the epithelium that forms the outer surface of gonads. It does not contain germ (germinal) cells.

germinal vesicle: the enlarged nucleus of a primary oocyte that has grown during the follicular phase of an ovarian cycle and is arrested in prophase of meiosis I.

germinal vesicle breakdown: GVBD: disintegration of the germinal vesicle membrane that occurs when an oocyte arrested at meiosis I prophase resumes division. It can be invoked by progesterone in amphibian oocytes, or by removal from the surrounding follicular cells. *See* also **oocyte maturation inhibitor**.

germinomas: rare malignant neoplasms derived from germ cells that can arise in pineal glands, mediastinum, or retroperitoneal regions. *See* also **testicular seminoma** and **ovarian dysgerminoma**.

germ layers: the primary cell layers formed during early embryonic development, usually just before or during gastrulation. In higher animals, which are triploblastic, they are ectoderm, mesoderm, and endoderm. Diploblastic organisms have only ectoderm and endoderm.

283

germ line: describes (1) cells that give rise to gametes; *cf* **somatic cells**; (2) mutations transmitted to progeny by those cells.

gerontology: the study of aging.

gestagens: progestins.

gestation: prenatal development in viviparous species.

gestation period: the time normally required to complete prenatal development. Its duration varies widely with the species, and is related to the size, complexity, and maturity of the young at the time of birth.

gestodene: 17α-ethynyl-17β-hydroxy-18-methyl-4,15-estradien-3-one: a recently developed progestin component of oral contraceptive preparations that appears to be more effective and less toxic than types formerly used.

gestrinone: ethynylnorgestrien-one; RU 2323; a synthetic steroid with anti-estrogen and anti-progesterone properties, used to treat fibrocystic breast disease, and under investigation for use as an oral contraceptive component.

GEW: gram equivalent weight.

GFAP: glial fibrillary acidic protein.

GFR: glomerular filtration rate.

GGF: glial cell growth factor.

GH: growth hormone.

GHBPs: growth hormone binding proteins.

GH cells: several tumor cell lines, distinguished by subscripts (as in GH_1, GH_3, and GH_4C_1) that secrete growth hormone, prolactin, or both.

GHF-1: *see* **pit-1**.

GHIH: growth hormone inhibiting hormone; *see* **somatostatin**.

ghosts: erythrocyte ghosts; the colorless structures obtained when erythrocytes are exposed to hypotonic solutions, or to other agents that leach out hemoglobin. Since they retain many of the features of untreated cells, ghosts are used to study some transport processes, and also the structures, arrangements, and other properties of membrane and cytoskeletal components.

GHRH: growth hormone releasing hormone.

GHRP-6: His-DTrp-Ala-Trp-DPhe-Lys-NH$_2$; growth hormone releasing peptide-6; a synthetic hexapeptide more potent that growth hormone releasing hormone (GRH) for promoting growth hormone release. It synergizes with the natural hormone; and its effects are augmented by pyridostigmine (which inhibits somatostatin release). At least some of its effects appear to be mediated via binding to receptors different from the ones that bind GRH.

GI: gastrointestinal.

G$_i$: *see* **G proteins**.

giant axons: very large unmyelinated axons of squid, crayfish, and some other invertebrates, used to study neurotransmission and adaptation, because of their size, electrical synapses, and abilities to display plasticity.

giant cells: usually, large, multinucleate phagocytes.

gibberellic acid: 2,4a,7-trihydroxy-1-methyl-8-methylenegibb-3-ene-1,10-dicarboxylic acid-1,4α-lactone; *see* **gibberellins**.

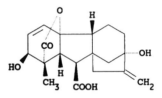

gibberellins: GAs: 60 or more growth factors chemically related to gibberellic acid, made by plants, and especially abundant in embryonic cell types. They promote the release of starch degrading enzymes when seed coats are sensitized by dehydration, and later promote formation of cortical arrays of microtubules that are perpendicular to the long axes of cells (*cf* ethylene), cause rapid shoot and (in conjunction with auxins) stem elongation.

Giemsa method: *see* **G banding**.

Giemsa stain: an aqueous mixture of azure II eosin (an acidic dye), azure II (a basic dye), and glycerin. It is used to stain blood films, bone marrow preparations, chromosomes, and parasites.

GIF: glycosylation inhibiting factor.

GIFT: gamete intrafallopian tube transfer; a procedure used to accomplish conception for couples with fertility problems. Follicle stimulating hormone (FSH), or a preparation that contains it, is used first to stimulate maturation of several ovarian follicles. Luteinizing hormone (LH) or human chorionic gonadotropin (hCG) is then administered to promote ovulation, after which secondary oocytes are aspirated with a laparoscope fitted with a suction device. The oocytes, mixed with freshly ejaculated spermatozoa, are then inserted into the Fallopian tubes. The success rate is limited, especially when only two or three oocytes are inserted. Some of the difficulties may be related to abnormal endometrial preparation for implantation caused by the hormone treatments, or premature ovulation of incompletely prepared oocytes. In common with other *in vitro* procedures, insertion of large numbers of oocytes increases the risk for formation of more zygotes than can be nurtured in the uterus at any one time. *See also* **ZIFT**.

giga: G; billion; 10^9.

gigantism: excessive body growth especially of the long bones. Body size is determined by heredity, nutrition, and other factors, but is most obviously affected by growth hormone (GH). In mammals, secretion of very large amounts during the juvenile period causes rapid elongation of long bones, and enlargement of visceral and other organs. (One man with a pituitary gland tumor attained the height of 8 feet 10 inches.) Giant laboratory animals have been produced by transfecting growth hormone genes. GH also exerts several effects on intermediary metabolism and other processes. Some derangements invoked by excessive amounts (including a form of diabetes mellitus) are more apparent when the hormone acts after skeletal system growth has been completed. *See* **acromegaly**.

gilt: a young female swine, especially one that has not produced a litter.

gill[s]: surface evaginations, richly supplied with capillaries, used by marine animals for gas exchange, waste elimination, and maintenance of electrolyte balance. Rapid movements of the materials are facilitated by countercurrent exchange mechanisms (achieved by the anatomical arrangements), and by active transport. The gills of various fish species respond to hypocalcin (which affects Ca^{2+} transport), paralactin (which affects Na^+/K^+-ATPases), and steroids that act on chloride-secreting cells. Gill retraction reflexes in *Aplysia* are used to study neuronal functions.

gill pouches: pharyngeal pouches; lateral expansions of the pharyngeal region of the digestive tract that form in all chordate embryos. They are temporary structures in most vertebrates, but give rise to gill slits in cephalochordates and urochordates.

gill slits: surface structures derived from gill pouches in cephalochordates. They are used for respiratory gas exchange, and to maintain electrolyte balance. In *Amphioxus* and some others, water enters the mouth, passes through the gill slits into an atrium, and exits via an atriopore.

ginger: the dried rhizomes of *Zingiber officinale*. The preparations are used as flavoring agents, carminatives, stimulants, and anti-emetics, and to protect against motion sickness. The structure of 6-gingerol, (*S*)-5-hydroxy-1-(4-hydroxy-3-methyoxyphenyl)-3-decanone is shown. It is the major biologically active component of ginger oil.

gingiva: the gums of the mouth.

ginseng: energofit; *Panax ginseng* root; a preparation composed mostly of saponin glycosides, variously

6-gingerol

known as ginsenosides, panaxosides, and panaquilins. It is used in Chinese medicine as a tonic.

GIP: (1) an acronym initially used for gastric inhibitory peptide; *see* **glucose-dependent insulinotropic peptide**; (2) granulocyte inhibiting protein.

Girard's reagent T: (carboxymethyl)trimethyl ammonium chloride hydrazide; a reagent used to isolate 17-ketosteroids and some other carbonyl compounds.

GIS: gonadotropin inhibitory substance.

gitalin: gitalignin; an extract of *Digitalis purpura* used to treat myocardial insufficiency. It contains digitoxin, gitoxin, and some other glycosides.

gitogenin: dignin; spirostan-2-3-diol; an aglycone obtained from *Digitalis purpura* that does not exert digitalis-like effects on the myocardium.

F-**gitonin**: gitogenin β-lycotetraoside; a saponin made by *Digitalis purpurea*.

gitoxin: 3-[*O*-2-dideoxy-β-D-ribohexopyranosyl-(1→4)-2,6-dideoxy-β-D-ribohexopyranosyl)oxy]-14,16-dihydroxycard-20(22)-enolide; a glycoside obtained from *Digitalis purpura*, used as a myocardial stimulant.

gla: GLA; carboxyglutamate; a chemical group made from glutamic acid via addition of bicarbonate followed by dehydration. It is the calcium-binding component of osteocalcin, of some coagulation factors, and of other vitamin K-dependent proteins.

glabrous: smooth; bare; describes skin that lacks terminal hair.

gland: glandula [glandulae]; an organ specialized for secretion. Although mucous-secreting types are single

285

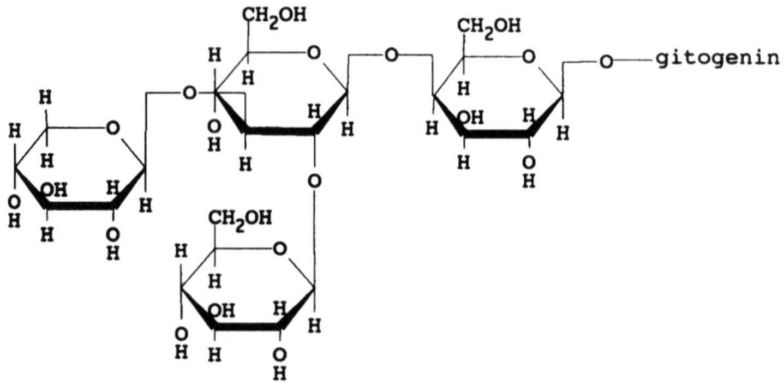

F-gitonin

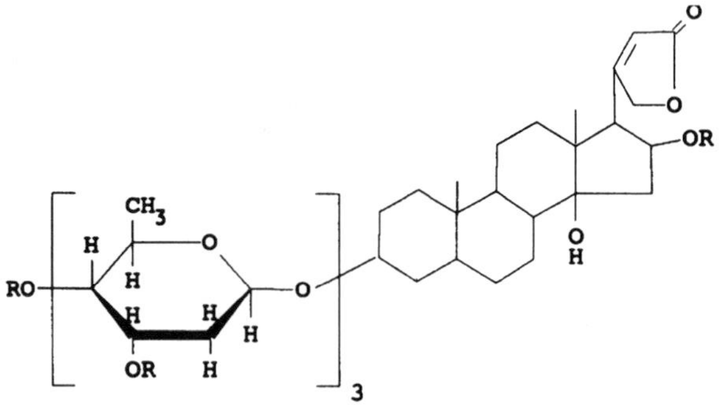

gitoxin

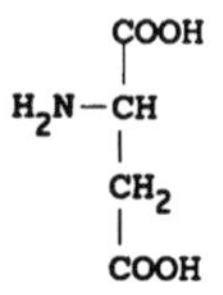

glutamic acid

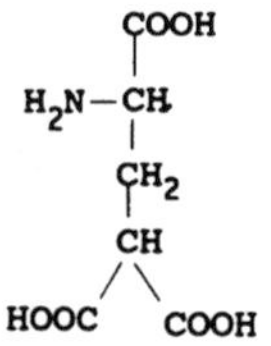

γ-carboxyglutamic
acid

goblet cells, most are multicellular. *Exocrine* types release their secretions to free internal or external surfaces, and usually have ducts. The components that make and store the products can be *acinar* (sac-like) or *tubular* (elongated), and can be coiled or branched. In *simple* types, one or more branches empties into a single duct, whereas *compound* glands have branching ducts. *See* also **apocrine, holocrine**, and **merocrine**. *Endocrine* glands release their products to surrounding extracellular fluids (*see* also **endocrine, paracrine**, and **intracrine**). They can contain two or more different kinds of secretory cells.

glans: (1) a small rounded or acorn-shaped structure; (2) the glans penis.

glans clitoridis: the rounded, free end of the body of the clitoris. It is the female counterpart of the glans penis.

glans penis: the expanded region of the corpus spongiosum at the distal extremity of the penis that derives from the embryonic genital tubercle.

Glanzmann's disease: thrombasthenia; an autosomal recessive disorder in which blood platelet numbers are within the normal range (or only slightly decreasedl), but the functions (and/or morphology) are defective. The consequences include prolonged coagulation time associated with internal hemorrhages and excessive bleeding from external injury sites.

glassy membrane: the basal lamina of the stratum granulosum of a vesicular follicle.

glaucoma: conditions in which intraocular pressure is elevated. A major cause is narrowing of the Canal of Schlemm, and consequent accumulation of aqueous humor. Acetylcholine and other agents that stimulate circular and ciliary muscle facilitate drainage by enlarging the opening, but have limited effects when the canal is obstructed. Epinephrine opposes the effects by activating β-type adrenergic receptors that mediate contraction of radial muscle.

GLC: gas-liquid chromatography.

GlcNAc: *N*-acetyl-glucosamine.

GLI: glucagon-like immunoreactivity; *see* **glicentin**.

glia: glial cells; neuroglia; non-neural central nervous system cells (astrocytes, oligodendrocytes, ependymal cells, and microglia). Some authors include peripheral nervous system Schwann cells. All derive from the neural crests and associated embryonic structures. *See* specific types.

glia derived neurite promoting factor: *see* **protease nexins**.

glibenclamide

glial cell growth factor: GGF; a partially characterized 31K peptide in brain and pituitary gland extracts, that somewhat resembles platelet derived growth factor (PDGF). It stimulates the growth of cultured Schwann cells, astrocytes, and fibroblasts.

glial fibrillary acidic protein: GFAP; a 50K intermediate filament protein made by, and used as a specific marker for astrocytes, but also made by some Schwann cells. Transforming growth factor-β (TGFβ) stimulates its production during development, and in response to injury. Castration and glucocorticoids decrease GFAP synthesis in male animals. Estrogens accelerate formation of the messenger RNAs for both GFAP and clusterin (which colocalizes with GFAP) in deafferented hippocampus.

glibenclamide: Glyburide; N-[4-(β-(2-methoxy-5-chlorobenzamido)ethyl)benzo-sulfonyl]-N^2-cyclohexylurea; a "second generation" sulfonyl-urea type oral hypoglycemic agent, used to treat some forms of type II diabetes mellitus, and as a laboratory tool that inhibits ATP-sensitive K^+ channels.

glicentin: G-69; an 8.1K peptide made in intestinal L, and pancreatic islet α cells, initially believed to contain 100 amino acid moieties, but now known to have 69. It comprises the 30-amino acid glicentin-related peptide, followed by a C-terminal extension composed of -Lys-Arg- plus the entire 29-amino acid sequence of glucagon, followed, in turn, by -Lys-Arg-Asn-Lys-Asn-Asn-Ile-Ala-COOH. G-69 is released in response to meal ingestion, and it exerts some glucagon-like actions. It also undergoes tissue-specific processing that varies with the species. Human enteroglucagon is approximately 80% G-69 and 20% oxyntomodulin. (Oxyntomodulin is also known as G-37, and glicentin 33-69). In pancreatic α cells, G-69 is cleaved to "true" glucagon (moieties 33-61) plus glicentin-related pancreatic polypeptide.

glicentin-related peptide: glycentin-related polypeptide: GRPP; glycentin 1-30; NH$_2$-Arg-Ser-Leu-Gln-Asn-Thr-Glu-Glu-Lys-Ser-Arg-Ser-Phe-Pro-Ala-Pro-Gln-Thr-Asp-Pro-Leu-Asp-Asp-Pro-Asp-Gln-Met-Thr-Glu-Asp-COOH. It is made by glicentin secreting intestinal and pancreatic cells, and in small amounts in the brain and adrenal medulla.

glioblast: spongioblast.

glioblastomas: highly malignant brain tumors, usually in the cerebral cortex, that contain poorly differentiated neuroglia type cells and regions of endothelial cell proliferation and necrosis.

gliomas: neoplasms derived from non-neuronal components of the brain, neurohypophysis, pineal gland or retina. All contain neuroglial cells and/or their precursors, and are named for the specific types (for example astrocytomas or oligodendriomas), or for the locations (e.g. pinealomas or retinoblastomas). Most are malignant, but metastasis outside the central nervous system is uncommon.

glioma derived growth factor: a peptide identical to platelet derived growth factor (PDGF), secreted by glial cell tumors.

glioma derived vascular endothelial cell growth factor: GD-VEGF; human vascular permeability factor; folliculostellate growth factor; a 46K protein secreted by glial and folliculo-stellate cells that promotes endothelial cell proliferation and augments vascular permeability. It is structurally similar to platelet derived growth factor (PDGF), but the amino acid sequences of the two equal-sized subunits differ.

glioma mesenchymal extracellular matrix antigen: tenascin.

gliosis: excessive proliferation of astrocytes, with scar formation. It can occur in response to injury in previously healthy individuals. Interleukin-1 (IL-1) made by microglia is a potent stimulant for the synthesis of glial fibrillary acidic protein and brain type S-100, and is believed to contribute the gliosis commonly found in Alzheimer's disease and Down's syndrome. Gliosis also occurs in some individuals infected with the acquired immunodeficiency syndrome (AIDS) virus.

glipizide: Glucotrol; 1-cyclohexyl[[p[2-(5-methylpyrazinecarboxamido)ethyl]phenyl]sulfonyl]urea; a "second generation" sulfonylurea type oral hypoglycemic agent, used to treat type II diabetes mellitus.

Gln: glutamine.

glipizide

globins: species specific protein components of hemo-globins, myoglobins and related proteins that share common amino acid sequences, tertiary structures, and abilities to associate with prosthetic groups that mediate oxygen transport. Hemoglobulins have two α and two β chains, whereas myoglobins and leghemoglobins are monomeric.

globular proteins: globins, globulins, and other proteins (including many enzymes) with polypeptide chains that fold to complex spherical configurations.

globulins: several related globular proteins, abundant in blood plasma, milk, eggs, and plant seeds. Most are *euglobulins* (insoluble in water, but soluble in saline solutions). *Pseudoglobulins*, which are soluble in water, more closely resemble albumins. Globulins can be fractionated into $α_1$, $α_2$, β, and γ subgroups on the basis of differences in solubility, surface charge, and other properties. Plasma types that contribute to protein, lipid and metallic element transport include thyronine binding globulin (TBG), corticosteroid binding globulin (CBG), and testosterone-estrogen binding protein (TeBG). Prothrombin and fibrinogen are among the kinds that play essential roles in hemostasis, coagulation, and immune system functions. Most γ globulins are antibodies.

glomerular filtrate: an ultrafiltrate of blood plasma, formed when blood traverses the the renal glomerular capillaries. It enters **Bowman's capsules** (*q.v.*), from which it is passed to proximal convoluted tubules. Under normal conditions, it contains water, small molecules (including sugars, amino acids, vitamins, and some peptides), inorganic ions, and minute amounts of several proteins. Excessively high glomerular filtration pressure augments the protein content. Glomerulonephritis is one of the conditions in which formed elements as well as large amounts of protein enter the filtrate.

glomerular filtration pressure: the net pressure in the capillaries of the renal glomeruli. It is roughly equivalent to the sum of the hydrostatic pressure within the blood vessels, the negative hydrostatic pressure of the surrounding structures, and the tissue oncotic pressure (all of which facilitate filtration) minus the blood oncotic pressure (which opposes).

glomerular filtration rate: GFR; ml of glomerular filtrate formed per minute. The major determinants include renal blood flow, glomerular filtration pressure, glomerular capillary permeability, and the numbers of functioning glomeruli. An average sized healthy human adult produces 120-125 ml of filtrate per minute when ingesting the usual quantities of food and water.

glomerulitis: inflammation of renal glomeruli. It can affect limited numbers of glomeruli, or be more generalized, and is almost always associated with endothelial cell proliferation and/or leukocyte infiltration. The causes include infections and auto-immune disorders.

glomerulonephritis: a term usually applied to inflammatory conditions more severe than glomerulitis, or to certain non-inflammatory conditions that affect renal glomeruli and tubules. Transforming growth factor-β (TGFβ) is a suspected contributor to the cellular damage. Antibodies directed against it (and against the Thy-1 antigen expressed on mesangial cells) suppress the associated cell proliferation.

glomerulus [glomeruli]: (1) a ball-like knot of capillaries or nerve fibers; (2) a renal glomerulus; a capillary tuft composed of fenestrated endothelium that rests on a basement membrane, receives blood under high pressure from an afferent arteriole, and delivers it to an efferent arteriole with a smaller diameter. The resulting high capillary pressure, and the endothelial pores (which permit passage of water and small solutes, but not of formed elements or most proteins) facilitate formation of the glomerular filtrate. The fluid then enters a **Bowman's capsule** (*q.v.*). *See* also **podocytes**.

GLP-1 and **GLP-2**: *see* **glucagon-like peptides**.

GLT: *see* **glucose transport carriers**.

Glu: glutamic acid; E.

glucagon: a 29-amino acid hormone cleaved from a proglucagon (*see* **glicentin**), and secreted in largest amounts by pancreatic islet α cells. It is chemically related to secretin, vasoactive intestinal peptide (VIP), and glucose-dependent insulinotropic peptide (GIP). The type made by humans and most other mammals is H_2N-His-Ser-Gln-Gly-Thr-Phe-Thr-Ser-Asp-Tyr-Ser-Lys-Tyr-Leu-Asp-Ser-Arg-Arg-Ala-Gln-Asp-Phe-Val-Gln-Trp-Leu-Met-Asn-Thr-OH. Low levels of glucagon provide short-term protection against hypoglycemia, mostly by promoting glycogenolysis in the liver. Somewhat higher concentrations additionally stimulate gluconeogenesis, and yet higher ones ureagenesis, lipolysis, and ketogenesis. Glucagon also acts both systemically and within the islets to inhibit insulin secretion. High circulating levels exert inotropic effects on the heart. In rodents, glucagon can elevate metabolic rates, mostly by accelerating lipolysis in brown adipose tissue. Most of the actions are mediated via cAMP generation and kinase A catalyzed phosphorylation of numerous proteins. The substrates include hepatic glycogen phosphorylase kinase, and L-type cardiac calcium channels. A few effects may additionally involve inhibition of cyclic nucleotide phosphodiesterases. Target organ responsivity requires the "permissive" presence of glucocorticoids. Glucagon release from pancreatic islets is inhibited by high glucose levels, and by insulin and somatostatin. The stimulants include glucogenic amino acids and catecholamines. Excessive amounts, or usual ones insufficiently opposed by insulin are believed to contribute to the symptoms of diabetes mellitus in some individuals. Small amounts of glucagon are also made in the brain, where one function may be inhibition of appetite and food intake. However, the hormone is not useful for treating obesity related to hyperphagia because the levels required also stimulate insulin release and exert unfavorable effects on the myocardium. Similarly, although pharmacological levels can exert anti-inflammatory effects, they are not used for this purpose.

glucagon-like immunoreactivity: GLI; describes substances that bind antibodies directed against glucagon with high affinity. **Glicentin** (*q.v.*) accounts for most of the activity.

glucagon-like peptides: peptides derived from the *C*-terminal region of proglucagon, most of which are amidated. GLP-I (1-37) is composed of proglucagon amino acid moieties 72-108. In the intact precursor, it is adjacent to the glucagon sequence, but separated from it by an intervening peptide. It undergoes processing to yield a hexapeptide, His-Asp-Glu-Phe-Glu-Arg, plus GLP-I(7-37): Ala-Glu-Gly-Thr-Phe-Thr-Ser-Asp-Val-Ser-Ser-Tyr-Leu-Glu-Gly-Gln-Ala-Ala-Lys-Glu-Phe-Ile-Ala-Trp-Leu-Val-Lys-Gly-Arg. GLP-I(7-37) appears to be the most abundant of the *C*-terminal peptides, but some GLP-I(7-36) is also made. GLP-II is composed of proglucagon moieties 126-159, and has the sequence: H$_2$N-His-Ala-Asp-Gly-Arg-Phe-Ser-Asp-Glu-Met-Asn-Thr-Ile-Leu-Asp-Asn-Leu-Ala-Ala-Arg-Asp-Phe-Ile-Asn-Trp-Leu-Ile-Gln-Thr-Lys-Ile-Thr-Asp-Arg. Additional smaller peptides have been identified, but they may be degradation products.

glucagonomas: tumors, usually derived from pancreatic islet α cells, that secrete large quantities of glucagon. The associated symptoms include a mild form of diabetes mellitus, stomatitis, and often also anemia.

glucans: starch, glycogen, cellulose, and other polysaccharides composed of glucose moieties.

glucocorticoids: 21-carbon steroid hormones synthesized by the adrenal cortex that act on virtually all cell types. The major type in humans, monkeys, guinea pigs, and some other species is cortisol. Rats, mice, and some others make mostly corticosterone, whereas dogs are among the animal types that secrete approximately equal amounts of the two kinds. The steroids maintain blood glucose levels during times of fasting, by inducing hepatic enzymes that indirectly accelerate gluconeogenesis (*see* **tyrosine aminotransferase** and **tryptophan oxidase**), inhibiting glucose uptake and oxidation in insulin-sensitive cell types that can use alternate fuels, supporting glucagon actions, and accelerating lipolysis in catecholamine-innervated tissues; but they also promote glycogen synthesis in the liver, lipogenesis at other sites, and insulin secretion. High levels deplete the fat stores of appendicular structures, but increase them on the face, back of the neck, and abdomen. The effects on gluconeogenesis and glucose uptake account in part for glucocorticoid invoked protein depletion in skeletal muscle, skin dermis, and at some other sites. Excessive secretion causes osteoporosis, and weakening of soft connective tissues. Small amounts are needed to maintain immune system functions, but high levels promote thymus gland atrophy, lower lymphocyte numbers, and depresss the functions in other ways; and pharmacological amounts are administered to treat autoimmune diseases and protect against transplant rejection. In contrast, erythropoiesis is stimulated. Glucocorticoids contribute to the control of blood pressure levels by acting directly on the heart, maintaining the tone of vascular smooth muscle, promoting albumin synthesis in the liver, and normalizing water and electrolyte transport across plasma membranes. They are used to treat some forms of edema; but high levels can invoke hypertension. Glucocorticoids also stimulate the appetite, maintain the tone of digestive tract smooth muscle, accelerate production of hydrochloric acid and some other digestive system secretions, and facilitate food absorption. In fetuses, they promote maturation of the intestine, and also of the liver and lungs (and are major stimulants for surfactant production); and roles in initiation of parturition have been established for some species. Moderate amounts act on the brain to promote a sense of well-being. Individuals with **Addison's disease** (*q.v.*) suffer apathy and psychic depression; ones with **Cushing's disease** have cycles of euphoria and depression. Both beneficial and deleterious influences are exerted on the hippocampus. Although the actions of corticosterone and cortisol are similar at many sites, the former exerts stronger mineralocorticoid activity, but lacks anti-inflammatory potency. Suppression of inflammatory responses involves stabilization of lysosomal membranes, and of leukocyte and mast cell degranulation, as well as inhibition of eicosanoid production (*see* also **lipocortins**). Although most actions are exerted on the genome, and are manifested after latent periods of one or more hours (*see* **glucocorticoid receptors** and **glucocorticoid response elements**), a few directly affect plasma membranes; and some involve permissive actions and/or influences on the secretion of other hormones. Glucocorticoid binding to synaptosomes that do not have "classical" type receptors, rapid influences on the firing of some neuron types, influences of glucocorticoid metabolites on GABA$_A$ type receptors, and on behavior (including inhibition of sexual activity in the males of some species), have all been demonstrated. Glucocorticoid receptor binding to mitochondria has also been observed. The major stimulus for glucocorticoid secretion is adrenocorticotropic hormone (ACTH). Secretion of that hormone is, in turn stimulated by corticotropin releasing hormone (CRH). Vasopressin exerts only limited direct effects on the pituitary gland (along with some on the adrenal cortex), but is a potent synergist for CRH. Circadian rhythms raise glucocorticoid levels during mornings in many mammals (but in evenings for nocturnal species). Diurnal variations in adrenocortical cell sensitivity to ACTH contribute. Moreover, and many factors affect CRH release. Large amounts are secreted in response to stressing stimuli; and high glucocorticoid levels contribute in major ways to the abilities to respond to stress, and to sustain demanding physical activity. They also induce phenylethanolamine-*N*-methyltransferase (PNMT), an enzyme essential for converting norepinephrine to epinephrine. Glucocorticoids exert negative feedback control over CRH release, and over the synthesis of proopiomelanocortin (POMC, the precursor of ACTH, β-endorphin, and melanotropins) in corticotropes, and also act on the neurohypophysis to inhibit vasopressin release. Excess hormone is degraded mostly in the liver. Some of the products are weak androgens.

glucocorticoid receptors: GRc; GR; molecules that bind glucocorticoids with high affinity and mediate most of the hormone actions on target cells. The best known types are intracellular 94K zinc-finger phosphoproteins that closely resemble receptors for other steroid hormones, calciferols, triiodothyronine, retinoids, the products of some proto-oncogenes, factors involved in peroxisome proliferation, some orphan receptors, some molecules that bind nonhormonal ligands, and some *Drosophila* proteins. A type I receptor that binds mineralocorticoids is present in some target cell types, and enzymes that promote oxidation of steroid alcoholic groups at carbon 11 facilitate the glucocorticoid binding. A different, type II receptor is specific for glucocorticoids; and a third type that binds molecules with 6α substitutions and promotes Na^+ retention has also been detected. Receptors on nuclear envelopes may be a fourth. The most widely occurring glucocorticoid receptors contain ligand binding domains (which also display some affinity for progesterone and related progestins), dimerization sites, amino acid sequences that can attach to glucocorticoid response elements, and "immunogenic" sites (named for their ability to bind antibodies) that are essential for realization of the influences on gene transcription. It has been accepted until recently that (in contrast to observations for estrogen and progesterone types), most glucocorticoid receptors not bound to their ligands, reside in the cytoplasm; but there is evidence for predominant nuclear localization. The unbound forms exist in complexes with several proteins, and cannot, in that state, attach with high affinity to genomic hormone response elements. One function of the other proteins is protection of the receptors against degradation by endogenous enzymes. Heat shock protein 90 (hsp90) binds as a dimer. Although it masks the hormone binding site, it appears to play roles in hormone attachment. Heat shock protein 70 (hsp70) facilitates hsp90 binding, and may be involved in receptor translocation. Other components of the complex may contribute to receptor maturation. When glucocorticoids bind, the receptors dissociate from the other proteins, and undergo time and temperature dependent activation processes that facilitate dimerization and confer high DNA binding affinity. The resulting changes probably include phosphorylations at specific sites. The activated receptors then associate with specific DNA sequences, and (depending on the cell type and other factors) either accelerate or inhibit the transcription of specific genes. Since some other steroid hormone-receptor complexes can attach to the same response elements, control of glucocorticoid influences on genomes probably involves interactions with translation factors. Some rapid effects of glucocorticoids on neurons may be mediated via direct interactions with yet different kinds of plasma and synaptic membrane receptors; *see* also **glucocorticoids**. Others appear to involve influences on gangliosides and other membrane components, on GABA$_A$ type gamma aminobutyric acid receptors, and/or on the release of different mediators.

glucocorticoid response elements: GREs; DNA sequences that bind glucocorticoid-receptor complex dimers and mediate the effects of the hormones on the transcription of specific genes. Some are enhancers, but others contribute to repression. The response elements closely resemble the ones for other regulators (*see* **glucocorticoid receptors**), and can interact with some of them; and similar DNA sequences are found in certain viral genomes. The functions are affected by nonhormonal proteins that interact with glucocorticoid-receptor complexes, or exert influences at other DNA loci.

glucogenic amino acids: alanine, serine, glutamine, and other amino acids that can serve as glucose precursors. The conversions (which are accelerated by glucocorticoids and glucagon) maintain blood sugar levels during times of fasting, and when the diet contains very little carbohydrate. In contrast, leucine and lysine are examples of amino acids that are degraded to acetyl-coenzyme A, and are therefore said to be ketogenic. Isoleucine, phenylalanine, tryptophan, and tyrosine can be converted to both glucose and ketones.

glucogenic: promoting glucose formation.

glucokinase: type IV hexokinase; a hexokinase isozyme made in liver and pancreatic islet β cells that functions at high glucose concentrations, and is resistant to inhibition by glucose-6-phosphate. It catalyzes the reaction: glucose + ATP $\rightarrow$ glucose-6-phosphate + ADP, and is induced by glucose and insulin. *Cf* **hexokinases I**, **II**, and **III**.

gluconeogenesis: glucose formation from amino acids, lactate, pyruvate, glycerol, and other non-sugars. Reactions in the liver, which are accelerated by glucagon, glucocorticoids, and other hormones, protect against hypoglycemia. Those in the kidneys contribute to euglycemia during times of food deprivation, but are used primarily for production of NH_4+ to maintain acid-base balance. Insulin inhibits most of the reactions, and thereby protects against amino acid depletion and hyperglycemia. *See* also **glucose-alanine cycles**.

gluconic acid {**gluconate**}: the product obtained when the aldehyde group of a glucose molecule is oxidized; *see* also **hexose monophosphate shunt** and *cf* **glucuronic acid**.

COOH
|
HCOH
|
HOCH
|
HCOH
|
HCOH
|
CH$_2$OH

glucosamine: GlcN; 2-amino,2-deoxyglucose; a glucose metabolite used directly, and after conversion to *N*-acetylglucosamine, for the biosynthesis of chondroitin sulfate, heparan sulfate, chitin, bacterial wall components, other complex polysaccharides, some glycolipids, and some glycoproteins. It can also be phosphorylated, and serve as a precursor for galactosamine, mannoseamine, and other metabolites. A major pathway for biosynthesis is fructose + glutamine $\rightarrow$ glucosamine + glutamate.

glucose: usually, the aldohexose, D-glucose (dextrose). It is present in free form in fruits and some other foods, and is derived when sucrose, lactose, maltose, starches, and glycogens are digested. Glucose is the major circulating sugar, and the major anaerobic source of energy for ATP synthesis (*see* **glycolysis**). It is essential for the survival of erythrocytes (which lack the mitochondria required for oxidation of alternate fuels), and also for normal functions of neurons, and for supporting the activities of vigorously contracting skeletal muscle. Limited amounts are stored as glycogen (*see* **glycogenesis** and **glycogenolysis**). Oxidation via the **hexose monophosphate pathway** (*q.v.*) provides cells with NADPH and pentoses. Glucose is also a component of glycoproteins, glycolipids and many other large molecules, and a precursor of galactose, fructose, mannose, lactose, other sugars, glucuronic acid, and glucosamine. It can be made from fructose, mannose, and other hexoses, and from some amino acids. In aqueous solutions, glucose assumes the pyranose form. The α anomer (shown below) is recognized by most enzymes of higher animals, but can be reversibly converted to the β form. *See* also **glucose transport**, **glucose oxidation**, and **gluconeogenesis**, and glucose metabolites. Some compounds made by microorganisms, and some pharmaceutical preparations contain L-glucose.

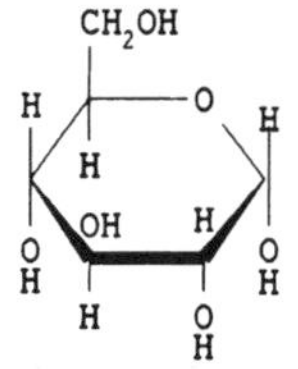

CH$_2$OH structure (α-D-glucose pyranose ring)

2-deoxy-**glucose**: *see* 2-**deoxyglucose**.

3-O-methyl-**glucose**: a glucose analog that enters cells by associating with glucose carriers, but is not oxidized. It is used to study glucose transport.

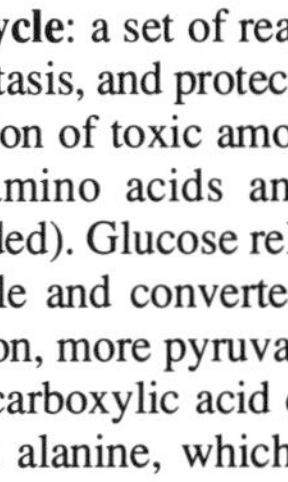

HC=O
|
HCOH
|
H$_3$C—O—CH
|
HCOH
|
HCOH
|
CH$_2$OH

glucose-alanine cycle: a set of reactions that contributes to glucose homeostasis, and protects skeletal muscle cells against accumulation of toxic amounts of NH$_3$ (which is produced when amino acids and adenosine monophoshate are degaded). Glucose released from the liver is taken up by muscle and converted to pyruvate. During vigorous contraction, more pyruvate is made than can be oxidized in the tricarboxylic acid cycle. Some combines with NH$_3$ to form alanine, which leaves the cells, and travels to the liver, in which it is used to make glucose. The cycle delays fatigue by diverting some pyruvate from the lactic acid pathway. Some NH$_3$ is removed in other ways. It forms NH$_4^+$ ions for the reaction: N$_4^+$ + α-ketoglutarate + NADPH + H$^+$ → glutamate + NADP$^+$ + H$_2$O. The α-ketoglutarate is restored via a reaction catalyzed by alanine transferase: glutamate + pyruvate → alanine + α-ketoglutarate.

glucose 1,6-biphosphate: an intermediate in the pathway for interconversion of glucose-6-P and **glucose-1-P** (*q.v.*). It is not released from the enzyme.

glucose-dependent insulinotropic peptide: GIP; a peptide chemically related to glucagon and secretin, made by intestinal cells, and released in response to glucose in the gut lumen. Low levels promote insulin release, and are believed to confer hormonal protection against development of hyperglycemia when dietary sugar is absorbed. The human type is H$_2$N-Tyr-Ala-Glu-Gly-Thr-Phe-Ile-Ser-Asp-Tyr-Ser-Ile-Ala-Met-Asp-Lys-Ile-His-Gln-Gln-Asp-Phe-Val-Asn-Trp-Leu-Leu-Ala-Gln-Lys-Gly-Lys-Lys-Asn-Asp-Trp-Lys-His-Asn-Ile-Thr-Gln-COOH. The peptide was initially believed to be a major regulator of gastrointestinal functions, and was then called gastrin inhibitory peptide. However, it is a weak inhibitor of hydrochloric acid and pepsin secretion, and a weak stimulant of intestinal motility. Pharmacological levels are required to inhibit gastric motility.

glucose oxidase: a flavoprotein made by *Aspergilli*, *Penicillia* and other fungi that catalyzes the reaction: β-D-glucose + O$_2$ → D-glucono-1,5-lactone + H$_2$O$_2$. It is used, in conjunction with a dye whose color is affected by the H$_2$O$_2$, to determine glucose concentrations in blood and urine, with catalase to remove glucose and oxygen from foods and other products, and to retard spoilage.

glucose paradox: when glucose is abundant (for example during absorption of dietary sources), only some is used directly for glycogen synthesis. Substantial amounts are degraded to triose sugars, which are then used to form new glucose molecules.

glucose-6-phosphatases: enzymes that catalyze: glucose-6-P + H$_2$O → glucose + HPO$_4^{2-}$. The hepatic enzyme is required for release of free glucose to the bloodstream when glucose-phosphate is formed during glycogenolysis. It is induced by glucocorticoids and triiodothyronine (T$_3$); and its activity is augmented by glucagon and inhibited by insulin. Type I glycogen storage disease (von Gierke disease) is an autosomal recessive disorder attributed to impaired production of the enzyme. Different isozymes are made in the small intestine, brain, and other organs. In cell fractionation studies, they are used as markers for endoplasmic reticulum. Skeletal muscle cells do not make the enzymes, and are thereby protected against loss of essential fuel (since glucose-phosphate does not diffuse across the plasma membranes). Muscle glucose-6-phosphate enters glycolytic or hexose monophosphate shunt pathways.

glucose-1-phosphate: a metabolite formed when glycogen phosphorylase catalyzes glycogenolysis (and also made from galactose-phosphate). Phosphoglucomutase catalyzes its reversible conversion to glucose-6-phosphate in a reaction whose rate is controlled mostly by substrate levels. Glucose-1,6-biphosphate is an intermediate in the pathway that does not dissociate from the enzyme.

glucose-1-P   glucose-1,6-biphosphate   glucose-6-P

glucose-6-phosphate: the first intermediate formed in all major metabolic pathways for glucose use. Unlike the free sugar, it does not diffuse across plasma membranes. Hexokinases catalyze its formation via the irreversible reaction: glucose + ATP → glucose-6-phosphate + ADP. Usually, the reaction is rate-limiting for glycolysis and other pathways; but **glucose-1-phosphate** (*q.v.*) is an additional source. When hyperglycemia leads to intracellular accumulation of glucose at a rate that exceeds it phosphorylation, the sugar can be shunted to alternate pathways; *see* **aldose reductase**.

glucose-6-phosphate dehydrogenase: G6PD: several variant forms of the first enzyme of the hexose monophosphate shunt. Synthesis of the erythrocyte type is directed by genes on X chromosomes that are closely linked to ones that code for hypoxanthine-guanine phosphoribosyl transferase (HPRT). The cells need that enzyme to make NADPH, which is used to reduce the oxidized form of glutathione. Reduced glutathione plays essential roles in maintaining normal erythrocyte membrane structure, conserving the ferrous state of hemoglobin iron, and destroying hydrogen peroxide and organic oxides. Individuals unable to make sufficient glucose-6-phosphate dehydrogenase develop a form of hemolytic anemia when certain pharmacological agents (such as pamaquin) are administered. However, mild deficiency appears to confer resistance to malaria infection.

glucose-regulated proteins: GRPs: proteins whose synthesis is substantially induced or inhibited by glucose, including endoplasmin and some other heat shock (stress) proteins, gp96 (a 96K glycoprotein implicated as a stimulant of immune system responses to methylcholanthrene and infectious agents), glucokinase, and some glucose transport carriers. *See* also **glucospondins**.

glucose tolerance: ability to restore euglycemia after glucose loading, tested by measuring blood glucose levels at several time intervals following administration of a large quantity of the sugar. It is affected most obviously by insulin (which promotes glucose uptake by several cell types), and by glucocorticoids, glucagon, growth hormone, epinephrine, triiodothyronine (T_3), and other hormones that antagonize insulin actions. Impaired tolerance has been detected in substantial numbers of close relatives of individuals with diabetes mellitus, some of whom subsequently develop overt symptoms of the disease.

glucose transport proteins: at least five structurally related proteins, each encoded by a separate gene, that mediate stereospecific glucose uptake. *GLUT-1* (HepG2, brain glucose transporter, erythrocyte transporter), a high-affinity, low K_m type that facilitates glucose uptake when sugar concentrations are low, is made by all animal cell types, and is especially abundant in ones with high glucose demand, and in cells that transport glucose across barriers. It mediates insulin-independent, facilitated diffusion that is not associated with Na^+ counterport or energy use, and is present in intracellular vesicles (different from the ones that hold GLUT-4) as well as in plasma membranes. A 55K transmembrane glycoprotein, initially identified in HepG2 hepatoma cells, is similar to or identical with a type made by insulinoma cells, and it (or a closely related protein) is made in erythrocytes, fibroblasts, cardiac muscle, adipocytes, and kidneys, in blood vessels that supply the retina, iris, and optic nerves, and in brain regions associated with the blood brain barriers (but not in choroid plexus). Substantial levels are also found in fetal tissues, and in the placenta. The protein varies little across vertebrate species. It is negatively regulated by glucose, and is induced, in parallel with structurally unrelated stress proteins GRP-78 and GRP-94, and by starvation (but not by heat shock). Other inducers include epidermal growth factor (EGF), some fibroblast growth factors, insulin-like growth factor-I (IGF-I), and platelet derived growth factor (PDGF). Its synthesis is also augmented by *src*, *fps*, and some other oncogenes, by phorbol esters, and by serum in cultured cells. Vanadate elevates the levels, in part by stabilizing the messenger RNA. Since GLUT-1 is a protein kinase A substrate, some influences of vanadate may be related to its ability to inhibit phosphatases. Glucocorticoids decrease GLUT-1 levels, evidently by accelerating degradation and/or promoting cellular redistribution. *GLUT-2* (liver type glucose transporter) is a 522-amino acid protein, 55% homologous with Glut-1. It appears to be essential for regulating pancreatic β cell responses to glucose, but is also made in intestines and kidneys (but not in brain, heart or fibroblasts). It has a high Km, and appears to be restricted to cell types that regulate glucose homeostasis. The levels are affected by hyperinsulinemia, certain immunoglobulins, and other factors, and are subnormal in some forms of diabetes mellitus. Variations in its make-up are attributed mostly to differences in glycosylation. *GLUT-3* (the brain isoform) is more like GLUT-1 than GLUT-2, but displays greater variation in composition, and also in cell distribution across the species. It has the lowest Km, and is important for neuronal uptake of glucose, but is also made in kidney and placenta. *GLUT-4* (the muscle-fat isoform, GT-2, IRGT) is abundant in skeletal and cardiac muscle, and in adipocytes of both brown and white fat tissue. It predominates in cells in which insulin accelerates glucose uptake. Insulin induces GLUT-4, and also promotes its translocation from intracellular vesicles to plasma membranes. The molecules are constitutionally phosphorylated. However, although epinephrine, glucagon, adrenocorticotropic hormone, and other regulators that augment adenylate cyclase activity promote addition of more phosphate groups, their influences on glucose transport appear to involve other mechanisms. Food deprivation lowers GLUT-4 levels, at least in part via influences on insulin release. The levels are also low in individuals with insulin-resistant diabetes mellitus. Small amounts of GLUT-4 are also made in the kidneys, but none has been found in brain tissue. *GLUT-5* (the small intestine isoform) is expressed predominantly in the jejunum (a major site for active glucose absorption), but small amounts are made in kidney, adipose tissue and skeletal muscle cells. *GLUT-6* is the name given to what would be the product of a pseudogene related to other GLUT genes, but there is no evidence that a functional protein is made. The term *SGLUT* has been applied to a carrier that mediates active, Na^+-dependent glucose uptake in the kidneys and small intestine.

Glucotrol: a trade name for glipizide.

glucuronic acid {**glucuronate**}: the product obtained when the —CH_2OH group on carbon 6 of glucose is oxidized. It is a component of many glycosaminoglycans, proteoglycans, and other compounds. Hepatic enzymes use it to conjugate steroids, indoles, other endogenous substances, and many pharmaceutical and toxic agents. Since the glucuronates formed are more polar than the parent compounds, they are more easily transported through the bloodstream, and more easily excreted by the kidneys. In olfactory epithelium, odors perceived by the receptors cause enhanced glucuronic acid conjugation of several proteins, and this leads to lowering of adenylate cyclase activity.

glucuronidases: lysosomal enzymes that catalyze hydrolysis of glucuronic acid conjugates. β-*glucuronidases* are made in liver and spleen, and in endocrine, reproductive system, and other tissues, and are released by activated mast cells. Androgens induce them in the kidneys of rats and some other species. Enzymes extracted from the tissues, and from microorganisms are used in chemical analyses.

GLUT-1—GLUT-6: *see* **glucose transport proteins**.

glutamate: *see* **glutamic acid**.

glutamic acid

glutamate diethyl ester: GDEE; a weak, but selective quisqualate type excitatory amino acid receptor antagonist.

glutamate oxaloacetate transaminase: GOT; an enzyme that catalyzes the reaction: glutamate + oxaloacetate → α-ketoglutarate + aspartate. Its activity is augmented by glucocorticoids. Since the enzyme escapes from injured cells, the blood levels are used to assess the extent of myocardial injury after heart attacks. *See also* **glutamic acid**.

glutamic acid: Glu; E; {glutamate}: an acidic, glucogenic amino acid. It functions directly as the major excitatory neurotransmitter in the central nervous system, in which it is involved in rapid transmission, long term potentiation, learning, memory, neuron-glia interactions, astrocyte differentiation, and the control of hypothalamic endocrine functions such as inhibition of gonadotropin releasing hormone (LRH) release. It also contributes to the formation of growth hormone, and to photoreceptor functions in at least some species. At various sites, it is co-released with substance P, or converted to γ-aminobutyric acid (GABA, *see* **glutamic dehydrogenase**), and in the cerebellum, it activates a nitric oxide synthetase by elevating Ca^{2+} levels. Excessive amounts are released in response to hypoxia and ischemia; and toxic levels can invoke epileptic seizures and neuronal degeneration. Impaired glutamate metabolism is implicated as a contributor to amyotrophic lateral sclerosis and Parkinson's disease, and to some forms of obesity, hypoglycemia, and memory loss. Limited protection is provided by associated increases in cell acidity that attenuate the effects on neurons, and by glutamate uptake into glial cells. Glutamate is also a precursor of ornithine, arginine, and proline, a component of glutathione and other biologically important molecules, and a metabolite formed in several pathways. It undergoes oxidative deamination in the liver and kidneys via the reaction: glutamate + NAD^+ + H_2O → α-ketoglutarate + NH_4^+ + NADH + H^+. The α-ketoglutarate can enter the tricarboxylic acid cycle, and renal tubules use the ammonium ions to conserve Na^+. Transaminases catalyze reversible reactions of the general type: α-ketoglutarate + amino acid ⇄ glutamate + α-keto acid. For substrates alanine, aspartic acid, leucine, and tyrosine, the keto acids are, respectively, pyruvate, oxaloacetate, α-ketoisocaproate, and *p*-hydroxyphenylpyruvate. Glutamine synthetase catalyzes several reactions of the general type: glutamate + NH_4^+ + ATP → glutamine + ADP + Pi, in which glutamyl-5-phosphate serves as an intermediate. They provide glutamine for

glutamine

urea synthesis. *See* also **glutamic acid receptors** and **nitric oxide**.

glutamic acid decarboxylase: glutamate decarboxylase; GAD; several isozymes that catalyze the reaction: glutamate $\rightarrow$ γ-aminobutyric acid + CO_2. They are used as markers for GABAergic neurons. *See* also **gamma-aminobutyrate**.

glutamic acid receptors: receptors on neurons and glial cells that mediate glutamate effects. On the basis of responses to agonists and antagonists, they have been grouped into **NMDA, kainate,** and **quisqualate** types *(q.v.)*. Functionally, the ones that directly affect Na^+ and Ca^{2+} uptake are classified as inotropic. Metabotropic types associate with G proteins, activate phospholipase C isozymes, promote diacylglycerol and inositol phosphate generation, activate kinase C isozymes, affect *c-fos* expression, accelerate glial cell differentiation, and inhibit the proliferation of some cell types.

glutaminase: a mitochondrial enzyme in kidneys that catalyzes the reaction: glutamine $\rightarrow$ glutamate + NH_3, and thereby provides ammonium ions for excretion to the urine. Its activity increases when metabolic acidosis or sodium depletion requires Na^+ conservation.

glutamine: Gln; Q; a glucogenic amino acid. In animals in which ammonia is the major nitrogenous waste product, its synthesis from **glutamic acid** *(q.v.)* provides a mechanism for converting NH_4^+ ions to a nontoxic form for transport across gill membranes. *See* also **glutaminase**. Additionally, glutamine is an intermediate in pathways for purine and pyrimidine biosynthesis, and it forms peptide bonds that cross-link fibrin and other proteins. By inhibiting arginosuccinate synthetase, it blocks citrulline conversion to arginine, and thereby diminishes production and release of nitric oxide. Glutamine is also a substrate for glutamine:fructose-6-P amidotransferase, which generates hexosamines that contribute to desensitization of glucose transport system responses to insulin.

γ-D-glutamylaminomethylsulfonate: a γ-aminobutyric acid (GABA) receptor antagonist.

glutamyl-cysteinyl-glycine: glutathione.

γ-glutamyl-glycine: γDGG: a kainic acid type glutamate receptor antagonist.

γ-D-glutamyltaurine: a weak glutamate receptor antagonist.

glutamyl transpeptidase: a membrane bound enzyme that facilitates amino acid transport by catalyzing the

γ-D-**glutamyltaurine**

reaction: glutathione + amino acid $\rightarrow$ glutamyl-amino acid + cysteinyl-glycine. The glutamyl-amino acid undergoes intracellular cyclization to 5-oxoproline, and glutamate is released. Glutathione synthetase then catalyzes a reaction that restores the glutathione.

glutaraldehyde: 1,5-pentanedial; a fixative for light and electron microscopy that preserves fine detail and permits enzyme localization. Since it reacts with norepinephrine but not epinephrine, it is used to distinguish the two kinds of catecholamine-secreting cells in the adrenal medulla.

α-keto-**glutarate**: *see* α-**ketoglutarate**.

glutaredoxin: an enzyme that acts in conjunction with ribonucleotide reductase to convert nucleotide ribosyl moieties to their deoxyribosyl derivatives.

glutaryl-Co A reductase: an enzyme that catalyzes the reaction: glutamate + acetyl-coenzyme A + ATP $\rightarrow$ glutaryl-CoA + ADP + Pi. Glutaryl-Co A can then be converted to acetoacetyl-CoA, which is used to make cholesterol.

glutathione: glutamyl-cysteinyl-glycine; a major physiological anti-oxidant that is essential for mitochondrial and other cell functions. It protects against the formation of methemoglobin and other undesirable compounds, and against cell damage that would otherwise be caused by radiation and by some products released during inflammatory reactions; and it reduces dihydroascorbic to ascorbic acid. Large amounts accumulate in, and protect eye lenses. Glutathione peroxidase catalyzes reactions in which the reduced form (GSH) removes excess hydrogen peroxide and other peroxides, as it is converted to the oxidized form: 2GSH + R-O-OH $\rightarrow$ GS—SG + ROH + HOH. Buthionine sulfoximine depletes glutathione, and thereby exacerbates the deleterious effects of radiation and some drugs, and causes mitochondrial damage and structural changes in cells of skeletal muscle, lung, and eye lens, as well as severe degeneration of the gastrointestinal mucosa. However, glutathione is also a cofactor for prostaglandin isomerases, and an intermediate in the pathway for leukotriene C_4 biosynthesis; and high peroxidase activity impairs the peroxidase-dependent steps required for

reduced form, GSH   oxidized form, GS-SG
glutathione

thyroid hormone synthesis. High levels of glutathione also block dopamine conversion to norepinephrine. Other glutathione functions include contributions to the degradation of excessive amounts of insulin and several other compounds that contain disulfide bonds, and provision of the cysteine groups required for phaeo-melanin synthesis. In Tc type lymphocytes, it regulates interleukin-2 binding and internalization, and is required for cell proliferation. Glutathione synthesis is accomplished in two steps (with glutamyl-cysteine as an intermediate) via reactions catalyzed by the cytoplasmic enzymes, γ-glutamyl cysteine synthetase and glutathione synthetase. *See* also **glutamyl transpeptidase.**

glutathione peroxidase: an enzyme that catalyzes oxidation of **glutathione** (*q.v.*), and reduces peroxides. Its active site contains a selenium analog of cysteine.

glutathione reductase: a flavoprotein enzyme that catalyzes the reaction: $GS—SG + NADPH + H^+ \rightarrow 2\ GSH + NADP^+$, and thereby restores the reduced from of **glutathione** (*q.v.*). The reduced form deters oxidation of the ferrous groups of hemoglobin and other compounds, is needed to maintain normal erythrocyte membrane structure, and performs other protective functions.

glutathione synthetase: *see* **glutathione.**

glutethimide: 3-ethyl-3-phenyl-2,6-piperidinedione; Doriden; an agent seldom used for its sedative and hypnotic effects, because it is addictive and invokes unpleasant after-effects. It induces some heptic enzymes.

Glx: a symbol used when it is not known if a peptide or protein moiety is glutamate or glutamine, or when either of the amino acids can occur at that position.

Gly: G; glycine.

Glyburide: a trade name for glibenclamide.

glycan: any sugar polymer.

glyceraldehyde-3-phosphate: 3-phosphoglyceralde-hyde; glyceraldehyde-3-P; an aldose phosphate formed during glycolysis via a reaction catalyzed by aldolase: fructose-1,6-biphosphate → glyceraldehyde-3-P + dihydroxyacetone-P. The next step is catalyzed by **glyceraldehyde-3-phosphate dehydrogenase** (*q.v.*). Since triose phosphate isomerase catalyzes reversible interconversion with dihydroxyacetone-P, both products of the aldolase reaction are used to make pyruvate. Dihydroxyacetone phosphate is also the direct precursor of **glycerol-3-phosphate** (*q.v.*). Glyceraldehyde-3-phosphate is made form ribulose-1,5-biphosphate in the hexose monophosphate pathway, and during photosynthesis.

glyceraldehyde-3-phosphate dehydrogenase: GAPDH; an enzyme of the glycolysis pathway, induced by insulin,

glyceraldehyde-3-phosphate

that catalyzes the reaction: glyceraldehyde-3-phosphate + NAD^+ + Pi → 1,3-bisphosphoglycerate + NADH + H^+. The product then reacts with ADP to form 3-phosphoglycerate + ATP.

α-phospho-**glycerate**: 3-phosphoglycerate.

β-phospho-**glycerate**: 2-phosphoglycerate.

2-phospho-**glycerate**: β-glycerophosphate; a metabolic intermediate of the glycolysis pathway, formed from 3-**phosphoglycerate** (*q.v.*), and converted to phosphoenol pyruvate via a reaction catalyzed by enolase. It inhibits some phosphatases, facilitates phosphorylation of some pancreatic islet proteins, and promotes insulin release.

3-phospho-**glycerate**: α-phosphoglycerate; a metabolic intermediate, formed in a substrate-linked phosphorylation step of the glycolysis pathway catalyzed by phosphoglycerate kinase: 1,3 bisphosphoglycerate + ADP → 3-phosphoglycerate + ATP. It is then converted by a phosphoglyceromutase catalyzed reaction to 2-phosphoglycerate. In common with 2-phosphoglycerate, it facilitates phosphorylation of pancreatic islet proteins, and thereby stimulates insulin secretion.

1,3-biphospho-**glycerate**: an intermediate in the glycolysis pathway, formed from 3-phosphoglyceraldehyde + Pi via a reaction catalyzed by **glyceraldehyde phosphate dehydrogenase** (*q.v.*).

glycerol: glycerin: trihydroxypropane; a metabolite formed during hydrolysis of triacylglycerols, phospholipids, and some other lipids. It augments glucagon release, and is implicated as a physiological appetite suppressant. A hepatic enzyme, glycerol kinase, catalyzes the reaction: glycerol + ATP → glycerol-3-phosphate + ADP, and the product is used for the synthesis of triacylglycerols and other lipids. It can also be converted to dihydroxyacetone-phosphate for use in glycolysis. A similar enzyme is made in adipose tissues of some species. It is not detectable in humans and some others under normal conditions, but genetic defects that lead to its formation may account for some forms of genetic obesity. Since glycerol takes up water, forms viscous solutions, and interacts with membrane lipids, it is used to treat glaucoma, and also as an emulcent, a vehicle for drug administration, a cryoprotectant, and an agent for permeabilizing plasma membranes (to facilitate cell uptake or extrusion of substances that do not otherwise readily diffuse across the membranes). *See* also **diacylglycerols**.

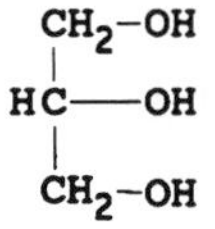

$$CH_2-OH$$
$$HC\!\!-\!\!-OH$$
$$CH_2-OH$$

glycerol kinase: an enzyme that catalyzes the reaction: glycerol + ATP → glycerol-3-phosphate + ADP. *See* **glycerol**.

glycerol-3-phosphate: a metabolite generated from dihydroxyacetone phosphate in a reaction catalyzed by **glycerol-3-phosphate dehydrogenase** (*q.v.*), and from glycerol via a reaction catalyzed by glycerol kinase. It is an intermediate in pathways for the biosynthesis of several kinds of lipids, including triacylglycerols and phospholipids, and is used by microorganisms for pyridoxal synthesis. It promotes glucagon secretion and is implicated as a physiological regulator of food intake. *See* also **glycerol phosphate shuttle**.

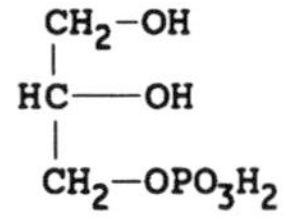

$$CH_2-OH$$
$$HC\!\!-\!\!-OH$$
$$CH_2-OPO_3H_2$$

glycerol-3-phosphate dehydrogenase: an enzyme that catalyzes the reaction: dihydroxyacetone-phosphate + NADH + H$^+$ → NAD$^+$ + **glycerol-3-phosphate** (*q.v.*). Its synthesis is accelerated by triiodothyronine (T$_3$). The enzyme also protects hemoglobin by reducing the Fe^{3+} of methemoglobin to Fe^{2+}.

1-oleoyl-2-acetyl-glycerol: a diacylglycerol analog used to activate kinase C isozymes.

glycerol phosphate shuttle: a set of reactions that facilitates transfers of hydrogen ions and electrons from cytoplasmic NADH + H$^+$ to mitochondria, for oxidative phosphorylation. It is needed because NADH (generated during fuel oxidation in the cytoplasm) does not diffuse across mitochondrial membranes. Glycerol-3-phosphate enters the mitochondrion, and a flavoprotein enzyme on the mitochondrial membrane catalyzes the reaction: glycerol-3-phosphate + FAD → dihydroxyacetone-phosphate + FADH$_2$. The FADH$_2$ is sent to an electron transport chain, and the dihydroxyacetone phosphate diffuses to the cytoplasm, in which glycerol-3-phosphate dehydrogenase promotes its conversion to glycerol-3-phosphate. The overall effect is NADH + H$^+$ + FAD → NAD$^+$ + FADH$_2$. (Therefore, only two ATP can be synthesized when NADH and H$^+$ are made in the cytoplasm, whereas three can be made from mitochondrial NADH.) The shuttle pathway is impaired in some forms of obesity.

glycine: Gly; G; the simplest and most soluble of the common amino acids, present in substantial amounts in body fluids and cell proteins, and a major component of collagens. It is used to conjugate bile acids and other compounds in the liver, and is a participant of pathways that generate porphyrins, nucleic acids, glucose, and other biologically important compounds. Glycine is also a neuromodulator that potentiates glutamate actions on brain NMDA receptors by binding to sites different from the ones that associate with glutamate, decreasing desensitization, and enabling channel opening. In the spinal cord, it acts on different receptors which appear to be confined to inhibitory interneurons, and increases chloride conductance. The effects on the cord are antagonized by strychnine. Although readily obtained from dietary proteins, a major source is the reaction catalyzed by serine hydroxymethyltransferase: serine + tetrahydrofolate → N^5,N^{10}-methylene tetrafolate + glycine + H$_2$O (a reaction important for transfer of one-carbon moieties). Since it switches reversibly from protonated (NH$_3$+) to nonprotonated (NH$_2$) forms, it is a useful buffer.

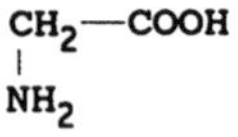

$$CH_2\!\!-\!\!COOH$$
$$NH_2$$

glycine amidinotransferase: an enzyme that catalyzes the reaction: glycine + arginine → guanidoacetate (glycocyamine, shown below) + ornithine. Ornithine is a component of the urea cycle, and is used for polyamine synthesis. Guanidoacetate reacts with *S*-adenosylmethionine to yield creatine + *S*-adenosylhomocysteine.

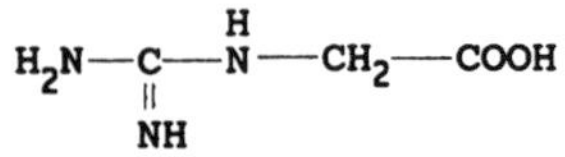

$$H_2N\!\!-\!\!\overset{H}{\underset{\parallel}{C}}\!\!-\!\!\overset{}{N}\!\!-\!\!CH_2\!\!-\!\!COOH$$
$$NH$$

glycinuria: excessive loss of glycine to the urine, a condition that occurs when any of several autosomal dominant disorders impairs renal tubule reabsorption of the amino acid.

glycocalyx: the "fuzzy coat" on the surfaces of many cell types, composed mostly of glycoproteins and glycos-

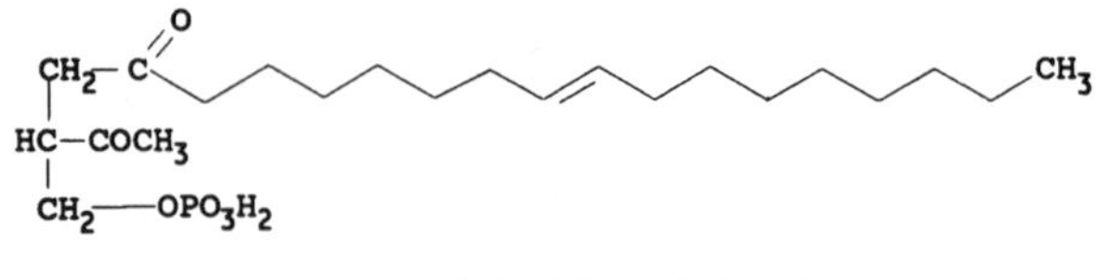

$$CH_2\!\!-\!\!C\overset{O}{\diagup}\ \diagdown\!\!/\!\!\diagdown\!\!/\!\!\diagdown\!\!/\!\!\diagdown\!\!/\!\!\diagdown CH_3$$
$$HC\!\!-\!\!COCH_3$$
$$CH_2\!\!-\!\!-OPO_3H_2$$

1-oleoyl-2-acetyl-glycerol

aminoglycans. It slows cell uptake of nonpolar substances, restricts some forms of cell adhesion, and contains surface antigens.

glycocholic acid: N-[3α,7α,12α-trihydroxy-24-oxocholan-24-glycine; a bile acid.

glycocyamine: guanidoacetic acid; *see* **glycine amidotransferase**.

glycogen: a branched glucose polymer with 1→4 and some 1→6 glycosidic linkages. It is the major carbohydrate storage form in animals. The liver makes the largest amounts, mostly for use by other cell types. Insulin accelerates its synthesis when the glucose supply is abundant. Glucagon stimulates glycogenolysis and release of free glucose to the bloodstream when blood sugar levels fall; *see* **glycogen phosphorylases**. In contrast, although skeletal muscle stores more than most other tissues outside the liver, its glycogen is not used directly to replenish blood glucose; but *see* **epinephrine**. Many other cell types make small amounts for local use. The major rate-limiting reaction for glycogenesis, catalyzed by glycogen synthase, is uridine diphosphate glucose (UDPG) + glycogen$_{(n\ glucose\ moieties)}$ → UDP + glycogen$_{(n+1\ glucose\ moieties)}$. Dietary glycogen is digested to dextrins, maltose, and glucose.

glycogenin: a protein with glucose oligosaccharides in 1 → 4 linkages, attached to a tyrosyl residue. It functions as an essential primer for initiating glycogen synthesis. Glycogen synthetase catalyzes addition of glucose moieties to the glycogenin oligosaccharide, or to the ends of preexisting glycogen chains, but cannot initiate glycogenesis if no oligosaccharide is present.

glycogenesis: glycogen synthesis; *see* **glycogen synthetase**.

glycogenolysis: glycogen conversion to glucose-1-phosphate; *see* **glycogen phosphorylases**.

glycogen phosphorylases: two or more closely related enzymes, most abundant in liver and skeletal muscle but present in many cell types, that catalyze the reaction: glycogen$_{n\ glucose}$ + Pi → glycogen$_{n-1\ glucose}$ + glucose-1-phosphate. In the liver, the product is rapidly converted, via reactions catalyzed by phosphoglucomutase and glucose-6-phosphatase, to free glucose, which enters the bloodstream. In skeletal muscle and other tissues, which contain the mutase but not the phosphatase, glucose-6-phosphate enters glycolytic or hexose monophosphate pathways. When glucose supplies are abundant, the liver enzyme is present as glycogen phosphorylase *b*, which has little activity; and phosphorylase *b* kinase, the enzyme that activates glycogen phosphorylase *b*, is also inactive. When falling blood sugar levels accelerate glucagon release, glucagon initiates a cascade that leads to rapid formation of large quantities of free glucose. It acts via cAMP and protein kinase A to catalyze the reaction: glycogen phosphorylase *b* kinase (inactive, dephosphorylated) + ATP → glycogen phosphorylase *b* kinase (active, phosphorylated) + ADP. The active kinase then catalyzes: glycogen phosphorylase *b* (inactive, dephosphorylated) + ATP → glycogen phosphorylase *a* (active, phosphorylated) + ADP. When blood sugar levels rise, insulin opposes the glucagon effects by activating protein phosphatases that dephosphorylate the enzymes (and by promoting glycogen synthesis). In skeletal muscle, epinephrine binds to β_2 type adrenergic receptors, and acts via cAMP and protein kinase A on the muscle system for degrading glycogen. Enzyme phosphorylation augments the sensitivity to Ca^{2+}. Since muscle glycogen phosphorylase contains a calmodulin subunit, high Ca^{2+} levels can directly activate glycogen phosphorylase *b* (without phosphorylase *b* kinase). Motor nerve stimulation leads to elevation of cytosolic Ca^{2+} in skeletal muscle, and norepinephrine released during exercise augments the effects by acting on α_1 type receptors. Very high norepinephrine levels, and high levels of other regulators (for example vasopressin) that elevate cytosol Ca^{2+} can activate the liver enzyme; but ordinary amounts usually have little effect. Other factors that affect glycogen phosphorylase activity in the liver include high

glycogen

glucose levels (which inhibit), and some phosphatase inhibitors.

glycogen phosphorylase kinase: a calcium-dependent enzyme that promotes phosphorylation (and thereby activation) of **glycogen phosphorylase** *(q.v.). See also* **glycogen phosphorylase phosphatase**.

glycogen phosphorylase phosphatase: an enzyme, activated by insulin, that catalyzes the reaction: glycogen phosphorylase *a* → glycogen phosphorylase *b* + Pi; *see* also **glycogen phosphorylases**.

glycogen synthase: glycogen synthetase.

glycogen synthetase: glycogen synthase; the rate-limiting enzyme for glycogen synthesis, induced and activated by insulin. It catalyzes transfers of glucose moieties from uridine-diphosphate glucose (UDPG) to the ends of pre-existing glycogen chains. Glucocorticoids also promote synthesis of the liver enzyme, but are most important in fetuses. Insulin converts glycogen synthetase D, active only in the presence of high glucose-6-phosphate levels (and named for *d*ependence on that metabolite), to glycogen synthetase I ("independent"), by enhancing the activity of a phosphatase that catalyzes the reaction: glycogen synthetase D (phosphorylated, low activity) + HOH → glycogen synthetase I (dephosphorylated, high activity) + Pi. Glucagon opposes its effects by activating kinase A and promoting phosphorylation of **glycogen synthetase kinase** *(q.v.)*, and by initiating the glycogenolysis cascade.

glycogen synthetase kinase: glycogen synthase kinase; an enzyme that catalyzes phosphorylation (and thereby inactivation) of **glycogen synthetase** *(q.v.)*, via the reaction: glycogen synthetase I + ATP → glycogen synthetase kinase D + ADP. The synthetase kinase is activated by kinase A (which is, in turn, activated by cAMP generated by glucagon). It is inactivated by insulin, which increases the activity of a phosphatase.

glycolipids: lipids that contain covalently linked carbohydrate groups; *see*, for example sphingolipids, cerebrosides and gangliosides.

glycolysis: Embden-Meyerhof pathway; the biochemical pathway that converts glucose-6-phosphate to pyruvate, and thereby provides the major anaerobic source of energy for ATP synthesis. Glucose is prepared for entry into the pathway via reactions catalyzed by hexokinase isozymes that are irreversible under biological conditions: glucose + ATP → glucose-6-P + ADP. Hexoseisomerase converts glucose-6-P to fructose-6-P in a reversible reaction whose direction is controlled by substrate concentrations. The major rate-limiting step that "pushes" the sugar phosphate into glycolysis is catalyzed by phosphofructokinase, an allosteric enzyme induced by insulin, whose activity is augmented by that hormone, and also by adenosine monophosphate (AMP), and fructose 2,6-biphosphate, and is suppressed by glucagon and ATP: fructose-6-P + ATP → fructose 1,6-biphosphate. Thus, two molecules of ATP must be hydrolyzed before energy can be derived from glucose. Aldolase then promotes cleavage of fructose 1,6-biphosphate to glyceraldehyde-3-phosphate + dihydroxyacetone phos-

phate. The products are interconvertible, and can enter other pathways. The next reaction, catalyzed by **glycerol phosphate dehydrogenase** *(q.v.)*, provides useful energy by reducing NAD$^+$, and by yielding 1,3-bisphosphoglycerate, which enters the reaction catalyzed by phosphoglycerate kinase: 1,3-bisphosphoglycerate + ADP → 3-phosphoglycerate + ATP. (Since each glucose molecule provides two glyceraldehyde-3-phosphates, two substrate-linked phosphorylations are accomplished.) Phosphoglyceromutase then converts each 3-phosphoglycerate to its 2-isomer, and enolase catalyzes 2-phosphoglycerate → phosphoenolpyruvate (PEP) + H$_2$O. The rate-limiting reaction that "pulls" glycolysis to completion and involves a second substrate linked phosphorylation that yields two ATP per initial glucose, is catalyzed by pyruvate kinase: PEP + ADP → pyruvate + ATP. It is accelerated by insulin and inhibited by glucagon. The overall effects can be summarized as: glucose + 2 ADP + 2 Pi + 2 NAD$^+$ → 2 pyruvate + 2 ATP + 2 NADH + 2 H$^+$. Glycolysis is the primary source of energy for erythrocytes (which lack mitochondria). It is also essential for normal neuron functions, and a major source of energy for white skeletal muscle fibers and some other cell types. In cells with large numbers of mitochondria, pyruvate is converted to acetyl coenzyme A for entry into the tricarboxylic acid cycle. When pyruvate accumulates in skeletal muscle, much of it is reduced to **lactic acid** *(q.v.,* and *see* also **glucose alanine cycles**). Brewer's and baker's yeasts maintained under anaerobic conditions convert pyruvate to ethanol and CO$_2$. Glycolysis also provides dihydroxyacetone-phosphate and other metabolites that can enter different pathways. The reactions are summarized below, with associated enzymes enclosed in parentheses.

glucose-6-P $\rightleftarrows$ fructose-6-P (hexoseisomerase)

fructose-6-P + ATP → fructose-1,6-biphosphate + ADP (phosphofructokinase)

fructose-1,6-biphosphate $\rightleftarrows$ glyceraldehyde-3-P + dihydroxyacetone-P (aldolase)

dihydroxyacetone-P $\rightleftarrows$ glyceraldehyde-3-P (triose isomerase)

glyceraldehyde-3-P + NAD$^+$ + Pi → 1,3-biphosphoglycerate + NADH + H$^+$ (glyceraldehyde-phosphate dehydrogenase)

1,3-biphosphoglycerate + ADP → 3-phosphoglycerate + ATP (phosphoglycerate kinase)

3-phosphoglycerate $\rightleftarrows$ 2 phosphoglycerate (phosphoglyceromutase)

2-phosphoglycerate → phosphoenolpyruvate + HOH (enolase)

phosphoenolpyruvate + ADP → pyruvate + ATP (pyruvate kinase)

glycopeptides: peptides covalently linked to carbohydrate, including some hormones. Several types made by fishes protect against otherwise deleterious effects of very cold environments by lowering the freezing points of intracellular and extracellular fluids.

glycophorins: sialic acid-rich glycosylated integral membrane proteins of erythrocytes. Glycophorin A is a 131-amino acid monomer that contains MN blood group antigens and holds approximately 100 sugar moieties arranged in 16 units. It binds to extracellular matrix oligosaccharides, and to cytoskeletal actin and spectrin. Gp60 is a closely related glycoprotein on endothelium that interacts with albumin and contributes to the control of permeability to specific extracellular components. Glycophorins restrict erythrocyte adherence to endothelium and uptake by the spleen, and they protect against nonspecific hemagglutination. However, they also bind some bacteria and viruses.

glycoprotein[s]: proteins with covalently linked carbohydrate groups. Some are identified as gp, followed by a cardinal number that relates to the molecular weight of the whole molecule (as in gp90), or the weights of its subunits (as in gp150/225). Roman numbers, often used with upper case letters, can designate the orders in which they were identified, as in GPIV. Others are referred to by the term *glycoprotein*, followed by a qualifier, as in glycoprotein G. Follicle stimulating hormone (FSH), luteinizing hormone (LH), thyroid stimulating hormone (TSH), and human chorionic gonadotropin (hCG) are examples of hormones that require the carbohydrate groups to function (and are inactivated by deglycosylation). Many others regulators exist in both glycosylated and carbohydrate-free isoforms, but do not require sugar groups to interact with their receptors. Different kinds of glycoproteins are cell adhesion molecules. *See* specific types.

glycoprotein IIb/IIIa: *see* **platelets** and **integrins**.

glycoprotein III: a protein that displays 72% identity with human SP-40 and 67% with rat clusterin. It is stored in chromaffin granules of the adrenal medulla, and is released when acetylcholine stimulates exocytosis.

glycoprotein IV: a glycoprotein on malaria-infected erythrocytes.

glycoprotein G: *see* **thrombospondin**.

glycoprotein hormones: hormones that contain covalently linked carbohydrate groups essential for biological activity. Follicle stimulating hormone (FSH), luteinizing hormone (LH), thyroid stimulating hormone (TSH), and human chorionic gonadotropin (hCG) have similar or identical α-subunits, but unique β-subunits related to their functions. Prolactin, adrenocorticotropic hormone (ACTH), and many others exist in both glycosylated and carbohydrate-free isoforms. Although their deglycosylated forms are biologically active, the carbohydrate groups affect clearance rates, water solubility, and other properties.

glycosaminoglycans: GAGs; polysaccharides initially called mucopolysaccharides, composed mostly or exclusively of polymers of amino-sugars linked to other sugar derivatives. Some are components of proteoglycans. *See*, for example **hyaluronic acid**, **heparin**, **chondroitin sulfate**, **keratan sulfate**, and **dermatan sulfate**.

glycosidases: enzymes that catalyze hydrolysis of covalent bonds between two sugar moieties, or between a sugar and other kind of chemical group. Most are selective for α or β type linkages, but many act on a variety of substrates.

glycosides: compounds formed by dehydration reactions in which reducing groups (aldehydes or ketones) of sugars combine with alcohol groups of other compounds to form larger molecules. Examples include disaccharides, oligosaccharides, 3-O-methyl-glucose, and carbohydrate-containing plant derivatives such as digitalis. The sugars can be released by glycosidases. The hydrolytic products of complex glycosides are aglycones.

glycostatic: maintaining carbohydrate levels, a term applied, for example to growth hormone mediated preservation of muscle glycogen stores.

glycosuria: loss of sugar to the urine. Although also applied to fructose, galactose, and other sugars, the term usually refers to glucose loss. The causes include renal defects that impair proximal tubule reabsorption, and hyperglycemia (in which the rate of sugar delivery to the glomerular filtrate exceeds the maximum reabsorption capacity). Severe glycosuria leads to dehydration.

glycosylation: covalent attachment of sugar groups. Many enzyme controlled glycosylation reactions occur in the Golgi apparatus, where specific kinds provide signals for intracellular sorting. Protein glycosylation usually increases the water solubility. It can also affect the conformation, biological activity, and metabolic clearance rate. *See* also **nonenzymatic glycosylation**.

glycosylation enhancing factor: GEF; a substance released by activated spleen cells that augments IgE type immunoglobulin-mediated responses, by promoting formation of a glycosylated IgE binding factor.

glycosylation inhibiting factor: GIF; a 15K fragment of phosphorylated lipomodulin that promotes spleen cell interactions with unprimed T lymphocytes, and T cell production of an IgE suppressor factor.

glycotropic hormones: glucagon, epinephrine, growth hormone, glucocorticoids, and other hormones that contribute to the control of glucose concentrations and glucose metabolism.

glycyrrhetinic acid: the steroid component of glycyrrhizic acid; *see* **glycyrrhiza** and **carbenoxolone**.

glycyrrhiza: licorice; the dried roots of *Glycyrrhiza glabra*. It is used as a flavoring agent, demulcent, and expectorant. Glycyrrhizic acid is a biologically active component that affects mineral metabolism; *see* **carbenoxolone**.

glycyrrhizic acid: glycyrrhizin; glycyrrhetinic acid glycoside; *see* **carbenoxolone**.

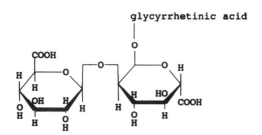

glycyrrhetinic acid

Gly-His-Lys: glycyl-histidyl-lysine); *see* **angiogenic factors**.

glyoxylate: *see* **glyoxylate cycle**.

$$HC=O$$
$$|$$
$$COOH$$

glyoxylate cycle: a biochemical pathway in plants and some microorganisms that permits synthesis of tricarboxylic acid cycle intermediates (and glucose) from acetyl coenzyme A, summarized as: 2 acetyl-CoA + $NAD^+ + H_2O \rightarrow$ succinate + NADH + H^+ + 2 CoA. In reactions identical to those of the tricarboxylic acid cycle, acetyl-CoA combines with oxaloacetate to form citrate, which isomerizes to isocitrate. Isocitrate lyase then catalyzes cleavage of the product to glyoxylate + succinate; and malate synthase catalyzes the reaction: glyoxylate + acetyl-CoA $\rightarrow$ malate + coenzyme A. Malate proceeds through the cycle to regenerate a new molecule of oxaloacetate.

glyoxysomes: organelles of germinating oil-forming seeds (for example those of cotton, corn, peanuts, and castor beans) that contain glyoxylate cycle enzymes.

glypiation: covalent addition of phosphatidylinositol moieties, usually to proteins. In most cases, phosphoryl ethanolamine attaches to the *C*-terminal amino acid and provides the linkage. The additions anchor integral membrane proteins to phospholipid bilayers.

gm: gram; g is now more commonly used.

GM_1, GM_2: *see* **gangliosides**.

Gm allotype: any human IgG type immunoglobulin marker.

GM-CSF: granulocyte-macrophage colony stimulating factor.

GMP: guanosine monophosphate.

cGMP: guanosine 3′5′ cyclic monophosphate; *see* **cyclic GMP**.

GMP-140: protein-140; PADGEM protein; a membrane glycoprotein of platelet and endothelial cell secretory granules that enhances calcium-mediated leukocyte adhesion to endothelium, and appears to be essential for integrin functions. It is a member of the lectin-binding

selectin family, is related to ELAM-1 (endothelial-leucocyte adehesion molecule-1) and MEL-1, and contains domains similar to those of epidermal growth factor (EGF) and some complement binding proteins.

GMW: gram molecular weight.

G/N: *see* **G proteins**.

gnath-: a prefix meaning jaw.

gnoto-: a prefix meaning germ-free.

GNRF: bacterial guanine nucleotide replacing factor; *see* **GTPases**.

GnRH: gonadotropin releasing hormone.

GNRPs: guanine nucleotide releasing proteins; *see* **GTP binding proteins**.

goblet cells: dilated, specialized epithelial cells that function as unicellular exocrine glands. The ones that face the external surfaces of the respiratory, digestive, and genitourinary tracts secrete mucus. Avian oviduct types make avidin, and are regulated by estrogen and progesterone.

goiter: any thyroid gland enlargement; *see* **endemic** and **iodine deficiency goiters**, **Graves'** and **Hashimoto's diseases**, and **goitrogens**. The major cause is excessive stimulation by either thyroid stimulating hormone (TSH), or antibodies that mimic its actions. TSH secretion increases when negative feedback controls exerted by thyroid hormones are impaired, for example in iodine deficiency states. Other dietary causes include ingestion of large quantities of goitrogens, or of walnuts and other foods that accelerate thyroxine loss to the feces.

goitrin: 5-vinyl-2-thiooxazolidone; a component of cabbage, kale, onions, and some other vegetables that, when ingested in large amounts, blocks thyroid hormone synthesis, and thereby invokes goiters. *See* also **goitrogens**.

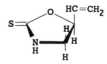

goitrogen: any agent that causes excessive thyroid gland growth. The term is most commonly applied to goitrin, and to thiouracils, thionamides and other synthetic agents that exert similar effects but are more potent. They impair thyroid hormone synthesis by inhibiting iodine incorporation into thyroglobulin and the subsequent coupling reaction. Thiocyanate and some other anions block iodide concentration in thyroid gland follicular cells.

gold, Au: an element (atomic number 79, atomic weight 199.97). Since the free metal is virtually inert at physiological pH, it is used in dentistry. Monovalent gold linked to sulfur atoms transfers to nitrogen, sulfur, and carbon (but not oxygen) groups of organic compounds. Colloidal preparations, which are taken up by phagocytic cells and concentrated in lysosomes, are administered to arrest the progress of rheumatoid arthritis that does not respond to salicylates, and to treat lupus erythematosus. However, they are toxic to skin and mucous membranes, and can impair hematopoiesis and cause kidney damage. The compounds most commonly used are auranofin, aurothioglucose (**gold thioglucose**, *q.v.*), and gold sodium thiomalate (mercaptobutanedioic acid monogold sodium salt, shown below). Radioactive isotopes (especially [198]Au) can slow the growth of some neoplasms. Several gold preparations are used in light and electron microscopy, and in blotting techniques. *See* also **aurintricarboxylic acid**.

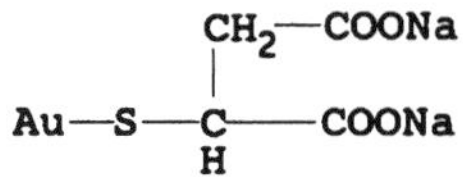

$$Au-S-\underset{\underset{H}{|}}{\overset{\overset{CH_2-COONa}{|}}{C}}-COONa$$

Goldberg-Hogness box: *see* **TATA box**.

golden hamster: an animal species used for studies of hibernation, reproduction, and pineal gland functions; *see* **hamsters** and **pineal gland**.

gold thioglucose: GTG; aurothioglucose; a gold preparation that forms colloidal solutions and binds to glucose carriers. It is used to treat some diseases (*see* **gold**), and to destroy brain cells at specific sites in laboratory animals. Insulin accelerates its accumulation in cells that avidly take up and metabolize glucose.

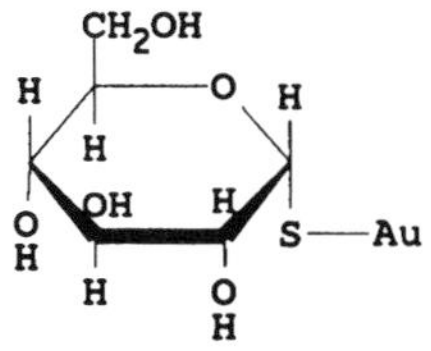

Golgi apparatus: Golgi complex; a set of intracellular stacks of flat and rounded membrane-bound vesicles, usually located close to the nucleus. It is continuous with the endoplasmic reticulum (ER), from which it receives newly synthesized lipids and proteins, processes some of them, retains a few, and distributes others to lysosomes, secretory vesicles, and plasma membranes. Some proteins that are not released directly to the cytoplasm undergo *N*-linked glycosylation before entering the Golgi. A branched chain oligosaccharide with two *N*-acetyl-glucosamine and five mannose moieties is assembled at the cytoplasmic face of the ER, on a dolichol phosphate molecule embedded in the ER membrane. After translocation to the ER lumen, four mannose and three glucose moieties are added, and the assembled oligosaccharide is linked to the amino group of an asparagine residue on the protein. The carbohydrate is believed to confer the appropriate configuration for subsequent processing. Before transfer to the *cis* face of the Golgi, the glucose components are removed one at a time. Proteins destined for incorporation into lysosomes retain high-mannose oligosaccharides and undergo phosphorylation. They are recognized by mannose-6-phosphate receptors on the luminal faces of the Golgi membranes, and are subsequently transported through the medial compartment to the *trans* component, where they are enclosed in clathrin coated vesicles that bud from the *trans* Golgi membrane (the major site for molecule sorting). The molecules are then dephosphorylated, and directed to lysosomes. Soon afterward, the vesicle membranes fuse with those of the lysosomes. The synthesis of many proteins that will be secreted or inserted into the plasma membrane begins with the formation of **signal sequences** (*q.v.*). After small numbers of amino acids are added, those sequences facilitate transfer of the nascent chains (attached to ribosomes) to the endoplasmic reticulum lumen, in which translation is completed. Some then acquire carbohydrate groups, and undergo processing that includes removal of mannose moieties and addition of glucosamines and fucose in the medial compartment of the Golgi, (and, in some cases, addition of sialic acid groups in the *trans* region). A few additionally undergo *O*-linked glycosylation (on serine, threonine, and/or tyrosine moieties); and sulfate groups may be added. The molecules are then incorporated into vesicles different from the ones for lysosomal enzymes. Those vesicles can contain proteolytic enzymes, for processes such as conversion of prohormones to hormones. The Golgi additionally contains enzymes that catalyze *selective* deletion and/or addition of carbohydrate moieties to molecules (and galactosyl transferase is used as a marker in cell and tissue homogenate studies). It also has permeases for taking up nucleotide-linked sugars such as UDP-galactose, and mechanisms for hydrolyzing them and ejecting free nucleotides.

Golgi's method: a histological technique for studying nervous tissue. The specimens are treated with potassium dichromate, and then impregnated with silver nitrate.

gomitoli: networks of specialized capillaries that surround the terminal arteriolar branches of hypothalamo-hypophysial portal system arteries (superior hypophysial in humans and other upright species, and anterior in quadrupeds.)

Gomori methods: (1) cytochemical techniques for localizing acid phosphatases, in which substrates such as 2-glycerophosphate liberate phosphate ions that precipitate with lead in the stain. Addition of yellow ammonium sulfide then generates a brown sulfide; (2) aldehyde fuchsin techniques for staining elastic fibers; (3) silver impregnation methods for staining reticular fibers.

gonad: any organ specialized for the production of gametes. The term is applied to ovaries, testes, and ovotestes, and also to embryonic or fetal structures that give rise to them.

gonadal sex: the kinds of gonads present within an individual (testes in normal male animals, and ovaries in normal females). *See* also **ovotestes**, **hermaphrodites**, **pseudohermaphrodites** and **phenotypic sex**; and *cf* **chromosomal sex**.

gonadal steroids: androgens, estrogens, progestins, and related steroids made by gonads.

gonadectomy: usually, surgical removal of the gonads; orchidectomy (orchiectomy) or ovariectomy. It is performed in laboratory animals to study feedback controls over gonadotropin and gonadotropin releasing hormone (GnRH) secretion, and the roles of gonadal hormones in reproduction and behavior. Controlled amounts of individual regulators can be administered to gonadectomized animals, to study mechanisms that control ovulation and gametogenesis, effects of the hormones on nongonadal functions, and other processes. In humans, the surgery is performed to remove diseased organs, or to eliminate stimulatory effects of the hormones on tumor growth. *See* also **chemical castration**.

gonadocrinins: peptides in gonads, follicular and seminal fluids, and chorionic villi that act within reproductive system organs and on gonadotropes by binding to receptors responsive to gonadotropin releasing hormone (GnRH). Although messenger RNAs for hypothalamic type GnRHs have been identified at those sites in some species, most gonadal gonadocrinins have different amino acid compositions. (They do not cross-react with specific antisera, and, unlike GnRH, are heat-labile.) Two peptides, approximately 2.6K and 5K, have been isolated but not characterized. They may function as paracrine regulators. Exogenous GnRH can inhibit steroidogenesis, decrease gonadotropin receptor numbers and gonadal weights, and inhibit spermatogenesis, follicle maturation and ovulation.

gonadoliberin: GnRH; LRH; *see* **gonadotropin releasing hormone**.

gonadostat: hypothalamic components that regulate reproductive system functions, including neurons that secrete gonadotropin releasing hormone (GnRH), and factors that affect their activities. GnRH synthesis and release are controlled by several neurotransmitters, and are under negative feedback control by gonadal steroids. They also respond to inhibins, activins, and other regulators. It is widely believed that pubertal maturation involves lowering of hypothalamic sensitivity to negative feedback controls, and to decreased release of opioid peptides and other inhibitors.

gonadotropes: gonadotrophs; adenohypophysial cells that make and release gonadotropins. At least some secrete both follicle stimulating hormone (FSH) and luteinizing hormone (LH). Folliculotropes that secrete only FSH, and interstitiotropes that secrete only LH have been described, but there are controversies concerning whether these are distinct cell types (or transitional forms capable of making both regulators, whose activities are modified by their microenvironments). Pulsatile release of gonadotropin releasing hormone (GnRH) is essential for maintaining gonadotrope functions. (The cells undergo atrophy when deprived of that regulator, and become desensitized if it is continuously presented.) Some FSH secretion appears to be constitutive, and androgens can increase its release (although androgens inhibit GnRH and LH secretion). Other factors that differentially affect FSH include activins, inhibins, follistatins, and possibly also a specific FSH-LH. High progesterone levels usually inhibit; but progesterone release close to the time of ovulation stimulates. Steroids affect not only the amounts of gonadotropins made, but also the secretory patterns, the numbers of gonadotropin receptors, and, to some extent, the chemical nature of the hormones. The prefixes *gyno-*, *andro-*, and *neuter-* have been applied to types secreted, respectively, by normal adult females, normal adult males, and castrated animals. The forms differ in glycosylation that affects their half-lives. Gonadotropes also make other regulators (*see*, for example gonadotropin associated peptide, GAP); and they interact with other adenohypophysial cell types via paracrine mechanisms.

gonadotropin[s]: hormones that maintain the structures and functions of the gonads. The term is usually applied specifically to **follicle stimulating hormone** (FSH) and **luteinizing hormone** (LH, *q.v.*). *See* **gonadotropes**, and *see* also **gonadotropin releasing hormone** (GnRH), and **glycoprotein hormones**.

gonadotropin inhibitory substance: GIS; a peptide identified in human urine that is believed to originate in the pineal gland. It suppresses gonadotropin secretion and may be similar to or identical with a substance called *pineal antigonadotropin*.

gonadotropin releasing hormone: GnRH; gonadoliberin; a term often used synonymously with luteinizing hormone releasing hormone (LH-RH, LRH), a peptide, cleaved from a precursor that also yields gonadotropin associated peptide. It is secreted by hypothalamic neurons, and is essential for maintaining gonadotrope morphology and functions. Under physiological conditions, GnRH is released in pulses (one or more hours apart, with timing dependent on the species), and this stimulates formation of GnRH receptors. Continuous administration of the natural hormone (or its agonists) leads to down-regulation of GnRH receptor numbers, and can totally suppress gonadotropin secretion; *see* **chemical castration**. The human type is pGlu-His-Trp-Ser-Tyr-Gly-Leu-Arg-Pro-Gly-NH$_2$. In mammals with estrus cycles, a rapid, massive release (GnRH surge) is required for accomplishing ovulation; but in primates the major controls involve changes in sensitivities to the hypothalamic hormone. Catecholamines stimulate GnRH neurons by acting on α_1 type receptors. Opioid peptides inhibit, in part by diminishing catecholamine release. The negative feedback controls by estrogens and progesterone are mediated in part via interactions with the opioid system. Progesterone can facilitate gonadotropin release by acting on different neurons.

gonadotropin releasing hormone associated peptide: GAP; a 56-amino acid hypothalamic hormone that is cleaved from the prohormone for gonadotropin releasing hormone (GnRH). It inhibits prolactin secretion, and exerts some influences on the release of follicle stimulating hormone (FSH) and luteinizing hormone (LH).

gonaducts: structures specialized for gamete transport. In males, the seminal ducts convey semen (spermatozoa and seminal fluid). In female mammals, oviducts (Fallopian tubes) transport sperm and support capacitation; and in most species, they are the sites for fertilization. They also support early embryonic development, and then send blastocysts to the uterus. In birds and some other vertebrates, oviducts make the proteins and shells that surround oocytes, and are the organs for egg laying.

gonane: sterane; dimethylcyclopentanoperhydrophenanthrene; a structure used for the nomenclature of steroid hormones and their metabolites. The letters for each of the rings, and the numbers for each of the carbon positions are shown.

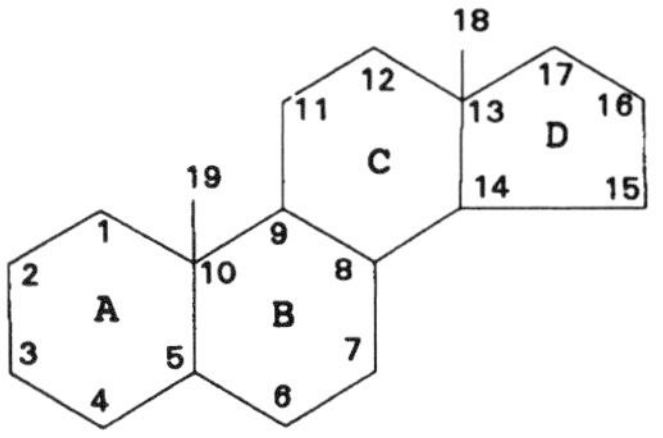

gonarche: initiation of spermatogenesis, or of ovarian cycles at puberty.

gonochorism: describes dioecious sexual systems, in which each individual is either a male or a female. *Cf* **monoecious** and **hermaphroditism.**

gonocytes: primordial germ cells that originate in embryonic yolk sacs, and serve as the direct precursors of spermatogonia and oogonia. They are large diploid cells that divide rapidly by mitosis before and after migrating to the urogenital sinuses and colonizing the developing gonads.

Goodpasture's syndrome: an autoimmune disease in which antibodies directed against renal glomeruli and pulmonary alveoli invoke severe glomerulonephritis and hemorrhagic pneumonia.

gossyplure: 7,11-hexadecadien-1-ol-acetate; a sex attractant made by the pink bollworm.

gossypol: 2,2′bis[8-formyl-1,6,7-trihydroxy-5-isopropyl-3-methylnapthalene]); a component of some cotton seed oils that reversibly inhibits reproductive system functions, and is believed to account for the low fertility in some parts of China. It is under investigation for possible use as a contraceptive in males. It can invoke hypokalemia, but co-administration of potassium salts corrects the condition without diminishing the effects on spermatogenesis.

GOT: glutamate-oxaloacetate transaminase.

gout: several inherited disorders in which monosodium urate crystals accumulate, most commonly in the joints of the big toes. The causes include metabolic derangements that lead to production of excessive quantities of uric acid, or renal defects that impair its excretion. The crystals initiate inflammatory reactions that attract neutrophilic leukocytes. After ingesting the crystals, the cells release lysosomal enzymes, which cause most of the tissue damage. Agents used to treat the condition include allopurinol, colchicine, and probenecid.

gp: GP; glycoprotein. The acronym is usually followed by a cardinal number that designates the molecular weight of the entire molecule (as in gp120), two or more numbers that relate to the subunit weights (as in gp150/225), or a Roman numeral that refers to the order of discovery. The latter can be followed by a lower case letter or asterisk if subtypes are then detected, as in gpIIa or gpIc*. Many of the glycoproteins referred to in these ways are known under different names.

gpIa/IIa: VLA-2; a β_1-type **integrin** (*q.v.*) of blood platelets, monocytes, and some T lymphocytes that binds collagens and laminins. **CD49b** and **CD31** (*q.v.*) are identical, respectively to the gpIa and gpIIa.

gpIb: a β_1-type integrin of platelets that binds von Willebrand factor.

gpIc/IIa: VLA-6; a β_1-type integrin glycoprotein complex that binds laminins. GpIc and gpIIa are identical, respectively to **CD49f** and **CD31** (*q.v.*).

gpIc*/IIa: VLA-5; a β_1-type integrin glycoprotein complex that binds fibronectin. GPIc* is identical to **CD49e** (*q.v.*).

gpIIb/IIIa: a β_3-type integrin glycoprotein complex composed of equal amounts of glycoprotein IIb (a 136K dimer identical with **CD42** (*q.v.*), and glycoprotein IIIa (a 95K monomer identical with **CD61** (*q.v.*). The dimer is also known as CD41. It is the fibrinogen receptor that is essential for platelet aggregation, and accounts for 18% of the mass of activated platelet membranes. Aggregation occurs when dimeric fibrinogen simultaneously binds to two platelets. In inactive platelets, the complex resides within the cytoplasm. Factors that promote its translocation to the cell surface include thrombin, adenosine diphosphate (ADP), epinephrine and thromboxane A$_2$ (TXA$_2$). gpIIb/IIIa is also expressed on the surfaces of macrophages; and it additionally binds fibronectin, von Willebrand factor, vitronectin, and possibly also thrombospondin.

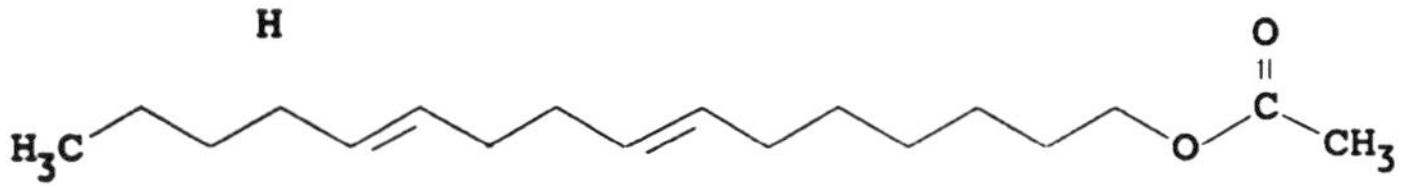

gossyplure

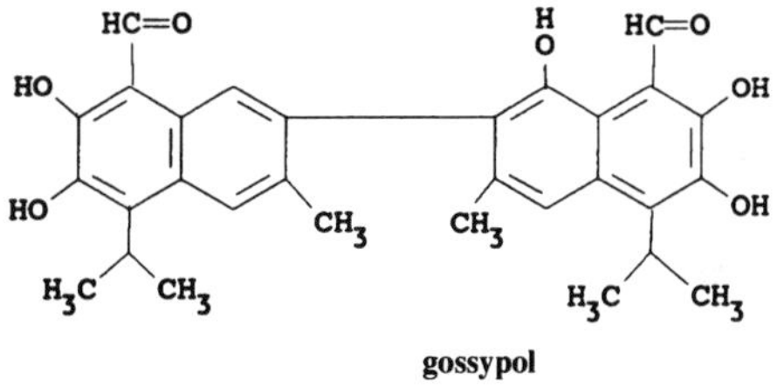

gossypol

gpIV: an integrin that binds thrombospondin and collagen.

gp40: a protein of the acquired immune deficiency syndrome (AIDS) virus envelope that associates noncovalently with gp120.

gp60: a sialoglycoprotein chemically and biologically related to glycophorins.

gp90: gp100: *see* **MEL-14**.

gp120: the major acquired immunodeficiency syndrome (AIDS) virus envelope glycoprotein.

gp130: a signal transducing component of the receptors for interleukin-6, ciliary neurotropic factor, leukemia inhibitory factor, and some related regulators.

gp 150/225: a complex composed of two glycosylated polypeptides isolated from human fetal brain that contains domains homologous to ones in epidermal growth factor (EGF) and fibronectin.

gp44/55/65: CD24.

G6PD: glucose-6-phosphate dehydrogenase.

gp L115: a membrane glycoprotein on the surfaces of lymphocytes that enhances responses to microorganisms. It is identical to **CD43** (*q.v.*).

GPLA: guinea pig histocompatibility antigens.

G phase: *see* **cell cycles**.

Gpp(CH$_2$)p: 5'-guanylylmethyldiphosphate; a nonhydrolyzable GTP analog. It is used to study the actions of G proteins and other molecules that bind guanosine nucleotides.

$$\text{guanosine} - \overset{\overset{O}{\parallel}}{\underset{\underset{H}{O}}{P}} - O - \overset{\overset{O}{\parallel}}{\underset{\underset{H}{O}}{P}} - CH_2 - \overset{\overset{O}{\parallel}}{\underset{\underset{H}{O}}{P}} - OH$$

Gpp(NH)p: 5'guanylimidodiphosphate; a GTP analog that resists hydrolysis, and is used to study the actions of G proteins and other molecules that bind guanosine nucleotides.

$$\text{guanosine} - \overset{\overset{O}{\parallel}}{\underset{\underset{H}{O}}{P}} - O - \overset{\overset{O}{\parallel}}{\underset{\underset{H}{O}}{P}} - \overset{H}{N} - \overset{\overset{O}{\parallel}}{\underset{\underset{H}{O}}{P}} - OH$$

G proteins: a term usually restricted to trimeric proteins that bind guanine nucleotides, possess GTPase activity, and serve as transducers that couple perturbation of the plasma membrane (by arrival of a hormone, neurotransmitter, or other stimulus) with cell responses. Some authors additionally include smaller (nontrimeric) types that also bind and promote hydrolysis of GTP, but function in different ways. However, the term *small GTP-binding proteins* is generally preferred for the monomers; *see* **GTP binding proteins**. The roles of trimeric types, formerly known as *N* (for nucleotide) and *G/N* proteins, in mediation of responses to hormones are described

here. In "resting" cells, the α-subunit of the $\alpha\beta\gamma$ trimer binds GDP, and displays high affinity for the hormone-receptor complex. When it binds the complex, GTP exchanges for GDP, and the α-GTP dissociates from the $\beta\gamma$ components (which remain togther as a dimer). Since the affinity for the ligand diminishes, the hormone-receptor complex is freed to interact with a new G protein. (The hormone continues to function until it is destroyed or otherwise removed from the system). In GTP-depleted cells, the ligand is ineffective, because it binds tightly to G$\alpha\beta\gamma$-GDP, and the G protein subunits do not dissociate. Many kinds of cell responses are initiated by G$_\alpha$-GTP interactions with enzymes, ion channels, or other cell components (and can be inhibited by very high $\beta\gamma$ dimer concentrations). They are terminated when the enzyme component of the α subunit catalyzes hydrolysis of GTP $\rightarrow$ GDP and releases Pi. The trimers then reform and can bind more of the stimulant. Cholera, pertussis and some other toxins invoke persistent effects by inhibiting the GTPase. Less commonly, the $\beta\gamma$ dimers that dissociate from G$_\alpha$-GTP trimers directly mediate the responses. There are at least nine different α, four β, and three γ subunit types. G$_s$ proteins contain α_s subunits that bind to and activate adenylate cyclases in species as diverse as humans and yeasts. α_{olf} is a special subtype in olfactory epithelium. G$_i$ proteins have α_{i1}, α_{i2}, or α_{i3} subunits that bind to and inactivate those enzymes. The α_{Tr} and α_{Tc} kinds in rods and cones, respectively, are components of transducins (G$_T$) that activate a cyclic guanosine monophosphate (cGMP) phosphodiesterase in the retina. The functions of G$_o$ proteins, which are abundant in the nervous system, have not been fully defined. Some evidently act on ion channels; and both G$_T$ and G$_o$ types can activate phospholipase A$_2$ in some cell types. The nomenclature for yet different types has not been standardized. Terms such as G$_k$ and G$_p$ are used by some authors for G proteins that act, respectively, on potassium channels and phospholipase C isoforms. G$_\epsilon$ appears to be a unique type that mediates exocytosis, but may act in conjunction with another G protein that activates phospholipase C and causes secondary activation of kinase C isozymes (but does not affect phosphatidylinositol hydrolysis). The name G$_q$ has been given to a 42K pertussis toxin insensitive brain type similar to α_{i1} that appears to be specific for phosphatidylinositol hydrolysis; and G$_z$ may be yet another form specific for different phospholipases. A G protein that directly activates voltage-gated cardiac calcium channels resembles G$_s$ but does not act via cAMP. In some cases, activation of one kind of G protein affects the functions of another.

GPT: glutamine-alanine aminotransferase.

GR: GRc; glucocorticoid receptor.

GR-64349: a peptide that selectively activates NK-2 type tachykinin receptors.

GR-73632: a peptide that selectively activates NK-1 type tachykinin receptors.

Graafian follicle: *see* **preovulatory follicle**.

gradients: usually, the differences in concentration, electrical charge, pressure, or other parameters on one side of a membrane or other special region, as compared with those on the other side.

gradualism: the concept that evolution proceeds via a series of small, cumulative steps.

graft[s]: implanted organs or tissues. Qualifying prefixes can indicate the donor sources, as in *auto-* (a different part of the same individual), *iso-* (another individual with the same genetic make-up, such as an identical twin or a member of the same highly inbred animal strain), *homo-* (another individual of the same species that resembles, but is not genetically identical with the host), *allo-* (a genetically different member of the same species), or *hetero-* (also *xeno-*, a member of a different species). Autografts implanted into the same tissue type (for example from one part of skin to another) are usually rapidly integrated into the host tissue, and can be used to repair large wounds or severely burned regions. In laboratory studies, grafts can be placed in easily visualized (or accessible) sites, to study wound healing, factors that affect growth and differentiation of grafted structures, the kinds of microenvironments required, the effects of hormones and other regulators, or the importance of the natural location. Autografts are also used to deliver secretions to specific sites within the body, for example ones from which the molecules can be circulated to other organs before encountering the degrading enzymes in the liver. Since isografts behave like autografts, several can be implanted to study the effects of hormone excess. Neither type initiates immunological rejection responses if no normally sequestered antigens are exposed. Homografts selected for their genetic similarity to the host are often also accepted, but it may be necessary to administer immunosuppressants to avoid rejection. When they survive, they can replace factors missing in a host unable to make them, or take over the functions of a damaged or defective host organ. Homografts that are rejected can be used to study immune system responses to foreign antigens and the effects of immunosuppressants. Allografts are usually rejected, but can be accepted by recipients with severe immune system defects (*see*, **nude** and **SCID** mice).

graft rejection: immune system responses to foreign cells or tissues, usually mediated by T lymphocytes, that lead to destruction of allografts and heterografts (*see* **grafts** and **cellular immunity**).

graft versus host reactions: GVH reactions; deleterious conditions caused by allografts or heterografts that contain immunocompetent cells, in hosts unable to reject the grafts. They occur, for example in recipients that have immature or defective immune systems (because of genetic defects or neonatal thymectomy), and in ones that have been subjected to procedures such as radiation or the injection of anti-lymphocytic sera. The effects, which are caused mostly by cytokines, can be fatal. Acute forms commonly begin with skin rashes. Liver and lung damage, cardiac dysrhythmia, diarrhea, and increased susceptibility to infections soon follow. Chronic responses can take days or weeks to develop, and can include severely stunted growth and cachexia.

gram: g: a unit of weight approximately equivalent to 1/28 ounce.

gram atomic weight: a mass in grams numerically equivalent to the atomic weight of an element.

gram equivalent weight: GEW; the gram molecular weight of an element or compound divided by the valence number of the multivalent component. For example, the magnesium ion has a valence of 2, and one **gram molecular weight** (*q.v.*) of $MgCl_2 = 95.211$ grams. One GEW of $MgCl_2 = 95.211/2 = 47.606$ grams. A 1 Normal (1N) solution contains 1 GEW dissolved in 1 liter of water.

gramicidins: several peptide antibiotics made by *Bacillus brevis* that contain D-amino acid moieties, and are used topically to control infections by gram positive bacteria. Some have formyl and ethanolamine side chains. Gramicidin A, HCO-Val-Gly-Ala-D-Leu-Ala-D-Val-Val-D-Val-Trp-D-Leu-Trp-D-Leu-Trp-D-Leu-Trp-NHCH$_2$-CH$_2$OH is a linear type that forms dimers which insert into membranes and establish channels for monovalent ions. Some other types inhibit enzymes of the glycolysis pathway. The amino acid backbone of Gramicidin S, a cyclic type with numerous side-chains, is shown.

gram molecular weight: GMW; mole; a mass equivalent to the sum of the gram atomic weights of a compound. For example, the gram molecular weight of $MgCl_2 =$ 24.305 (for Mg) + 2 x (35.453) (for two Cl) = 95.211 grams. A 1 molar (1M) solution contains 1 GMW dissolved in 1 liter of water. *Cf* **gram equivalent weight**.

Gram negative, Gram positive: *see* **Gram stain**.

Gram stain: a technique for distinguishing two types of bacteria on the basis of cell wall composition. Heat-fixed smears are stained with crystal violet, treated with 3% iodine/ potassium iodide, and then counterstained with a red dye. Gram positive bacteria, with thick walls that contain teichoic and lipoteichoic acids complexed to peptidoglycans, retain the crystal violet, and appear purple. Gram negative bacteria, with thin peptidoglycan walls bounded by liposaccharide rich membranes, release the crystal violet when treated with the iodine solution, but retain the counterstain and appear pink.

grana [singular, granum]: chlorophyll-laden stacks of chloroplast disks.

granulocytes: circulating leukocytes with prominent cytoplasmic granules. The term can refer to neutrophils, basophils, and eosinophils, but often designates just neutrophils. *See* specific types.

granulocyte colony stimulating factor: G-CSF; granulocyte cell stimulating factor; granulocyte CSF; pluripoietin: one of several cytokines essential for normal hematopoiesis, made by macrophages, monocytes, endothelium, placental cells, and probably also by bone marrow stroma. It acts on bone marrow precursor cells committed to myeloid type differentiation, and stimulates proliferation, colony formation, and terminal maturation of granular leukocytes (especially neutrophils). It also promotes differentiation of myeloid leukemia cells. High concentrations can initiate (but not sustain) proliferation of erythroid and megakaryocyte and precursor cells, and pluripotential progenitor cells. G-CSF additionally prolongs the survival and enhances the functions of mature neutrophils; but, unlike granulocyte-macrophage colony stimulating factor (GM-CSF), does not inhibit their migration. The human hormone, which is synthesized from a 207 amino-acid precursor that contains a 30 amino acid leader sequence, is active in other species. Very small amounts enter the bloodstream. Exogenous G-CSF can increase the numbers of circulating neutrophils and decrease susceptibility to infections in individuals with some forms of neutropenia (including ones invoked by cancer chemotherapy), but is beneficial only in the presence of precursor cells.

granulocyte inhibitory protein: GIP; a 28K acidic protein in the serum of uremic individuals that is implicated as a cause of leukocyte dysfunction. It inhibits glucose uptake, chemotaxis, oxidative metabolism, and bactericidal actions.

granulocyte-macrophage colony stimulating factor: GM-CSF; granulocyte-macrophage stimulating factor; colony stimulating factor-2; CSF-2; a cytokine essential for normal hematopoiesis, secreted by activated T cells, macrophages, endothelial cells, fibroblasts, some tumor cells, and possibly also by bone marrow stromal cells. It promotes proliferation of bone marrow pluripotential stem cells, and maturation as well as proliferation of cells committed to differentiation to neutrophils, eosinophils, and monocytes. It also sustains the viability and augments the functions of mature eosinophils, neutrophils, and macrophages, enhances neutrophil chemotaxis, phagocytosis and oxidative metabolism, and facilitates neutrophil retention at sites of inflammation by inhibiting migration. Addtionally, it potentiates the tumoricidal activities of monocytes and macrophages, and exacerbates antibody-dependent cellular toxicity. In the presence of erythropoietin, it promotes megakaryocyte differentiation; and high levels stimulate erythropoiesis *in vitro*. In patients with acquired immune deficiency syndrome (AIDS), it can increase the numbers of circulating neutrophils and eosinophils. Human GM-CSF is synthesized from a 144 amino acid precursor with a 17 amino acid leader sequence. The murine type has 118 amino acids. GM-CSF production by T cells is augmented by antigens, interleukin-1, and some lectins.

granulocytopenia: abnormally low numbers of circulating granular leukocytes. It can be caused by genetic defects that impair hematopoietic system maturation, autoimmune processes that affect the bone marrow, and many pharmacological agents.

granulocytosis: excessive numbers of circulating granular leukocytes. The term usually refers to neutrophils, but can be applied to eosinophils and basophils. Responses to many kinds of bacterial infections include marked increases in the numbers of mature neutrophilic types; and

allergies and worm infestations are stimulants for the eosinophils. In granulocytic leukemias, most of the circulating cells are immature and/or abnormal.

granuloliberin: Phe-Gly-Phe-Leu-Pro-Ile-Tyr-Arg-Arg-Pro-Ala-Ser-NH$_2$; a peptide in the skin of the frog, *Rana rugosa* that promotes mast cell degranulation.

granulomas; granulomata; nodular lesions, formed during chronic inflammatory responses to infectious agents, neoplastic cells, or foreign bodies. They contain aggregates of mononuclear and epithelioid (modified macrophage) cells. Some also have multinucleated giant cells, plasma cells and eosinophils.

granulopoiesis: granulocytopoiesis; normal maturation of granular leukocytes in bone marrow, and release of mature cells to the bloodstream.

granulosa cells: epithelial cells that surround the oocytes of developing **ovarian follicles** (*q.v.*), derived from pregranulosa cells. Follicle stimulating hormone (FSH) is the major regulator of proliferation, growth, and maturation.

granum: *see* **grana**.

granzymes: at least eight kinds of serine proteases in the granules of cytotoxic T lymphocytes, distinguished from each other by letters A through H.

Graves' disease: thyroid gland disorders associated with two or three of the following: goiter, hyperthyroidism, and exophthalmos. They are caused by immunoglobulins that interact with thyroid gland receptors for thyroid stimulating hormone (TSH), but are not regulated by the negative feedback controls exerted over the pituitary gland hormone.

gravid: pregnant.

gravida: a pregnant woman. Gravida-1, 2, etc. indicate, respectively, first, second, and successive pregnancies. Prefixes are also used, as in primigravida (pregnant for the first time), and multigravida (having had several pregnancies).

gravitaxis: locomotion in response to a gravitational field.

gravitropism: growth directed by a gravitational field, a term usually applied to plants. It accounts, in part, for downward growth of roots, and upward growth of stems.

gravity sedimentation: methods for separating components of a solution by application of strong gravitational forces in ultracentrifuges. The rate of sedimentation is directly related to the weight of the particle and the force of the field, but is also affected by particle size, viscosity, and other factors. *See* **sedimentation coefficient**, **sedimentation velocity**, and **Svedberg units**.

gray crescent: a gray or yellowish-gray region on the surface of the equatorial region of a fertilized amphibian egg. It contains regulators that direct morphogenesis.

gray matter: components of the central nervous system composed mostly of cell bodies and unmyelinated axons; *cf* **white matter**.

GRGDSP: Gly-Arg-Gly-Asp-Ser-Pro; a peptide used to study integrin binding.

GRF: GRF-44; GRF-43; *see* **growth hormone releasing hormone**.

GRH: growth hormone releasing hormone.

griseofulvin: 7-chloro-4,6-dimethoxycoumaran-3-one-2-spiro-1′-(2′-methoxy-6′-methylcyclohex-2′-en-4′-one); an antibiotic made by *Penicillium griseofulvum* that arrests the growth of several kinds of fungi (but is not bactericidal). It disrupts mitotic spindles by interacting with polymerized microtubules at sites different from ones that bind colchicine.

GRO: *MGSA*: three closely linked genes (α, β, and γ) that code for growth-promoting cytokines. They are members of a gene superfamily that also directs the formation of other cytokines with similar amino acid sequences. The products (which include platelet factor-4, platelet basic protein, β-thromboglobulin, interleukin-8, and macrophage inflammatory protein 2), contribute to inflammatory reactions. A related gene has been identified in *v-src* transformed chicken cells. *GRO* expression is regulated in a tissue-specific manner by interleukin-1 and tumor necrosis factor-α (TNFα), both of which bind nuclear factor NF-kB, and also by growth factors in serum.

groES: chaperonin 10; a polypeptide made by *E. coli* that regulates protein folding. A related peptide has been identified in mitochondria of mammalian species.

growth: increase in size associated with accretion of components similar to the types initially present. The term can describe processes that contribute to normal development and the attainment of adult body size, or to abnormal ones that lead to excessive enlargement of the body as a whole, or of one or more components. It can also refer to tumors. When applied to the cells of complex organisms, some authors restrict its use to normal enlargement and hypertrophy; but others include cell proliferation. For microorganisms and cultured animal or plant cells, it usually means increases in cell numbers.

growth factors: a term applied to numerous regulators (including epidermal, fibroblast, platelet-derived, nerve, and insulin-like growth factors (EGF, FGFs, PDGF NGF and IGFs) and related peptides, thrombin, bradykinin, several hematopoietic and immune system stimulants, some peptides that act locally on bone and other tissues, and some unidentified components of serum, all of which stimulate cell growth and proliferation. It is also used for some regulators that additionally promote differentiation (although specialization often diminishes or abolishes the ability to divide). Many types act via paracrine, autocrine, and/or intracrine mechanisms. The various kinds display both overlapping properties and complex interactions.

growth hormone: GH; somatotropin; somatotrophic hormone; STH; species-specific proteins secreted by somatotropes (and related proteins made in the placenta and at some other sites), that promote growth of immature long bones and of other body components, contribute to the regulation of carbohydrate, lipid, protein, nucleic acid and mineral metabolism, and affect inflammatory reactions, immune system processes, and other functions. Under normal conditions, GH accounts for almost 10% of pituitary gland dry weight. The major human type, hGH-N, is a linear, 22K, 191 amino acid single-chain protein with two disulfide bonds, cleaved from a 26K precursor. Approximately 10% of circulating GH is a 20K protein that lacks amino acid moieties 32-46, and is a stronger lactogen, but does not bind to hepatic receptors for the 22K type. Several other forms generated by differential processing of the messenger RNA and posttranslational processing (that can include glycosylation, phosphorylation, and/or amidation), have also been identified; and a 17K type may be the pituitary "diabetogenic factor". "Big" GH is a dimer with intermolecular disulfide bonds; and "big-big" types appear to be growth hormones associated with other proteins. A different gene, expressed only in the placenta, codes for a variant form, hGH-V, that differs in 13 amino acid moieties and has comparable growth promoting (but less lactogenic) potency. Excessive accumulation in maternal blood may account for the diabetes mellitus symptoms that develop during pregnancy in some women, and subside after parturition. Although the lactogenic potency of pituitary 22K is low, 161 of the amino acids are identical with those of human chorionic somatomammotropin, whose synthesis appears to be directed by two genes, hCS-A (*CSH1*), and hCS-B (*CSH2*). The gene family also includes hCS-L (*CSHP*), which appears to be a non-functions pseudogene. Growth hormones of non-primates, and their receptors, differ substantially from primate types. Some display potent prolactin-like properties. Recombinant hGHs made by bacteria (Humatrope, Protropin) have an additional *N*-terminal methionyl group that does not affect potency but can be antigenic. The genes that direct GH synthesis in pituitary glands contain response elements for several hormones. Triiodothyronine (T_3) is required for production of adequate amounts. Glucocorticoids synergize with T_3 (but oppose many effects of GH on target cells). **Growth hormone releasing hormone** (*q.v.*) is the major regulator of somatotrope structure and function. Its release is regulated by neurotransmitters and other factors, and is usually maximal during slow-wave sleep. Potent stimuli for normal cells include dopamine, arginine, and hypoglycemia (but tumor cells of individuals with acromegaly can display different responses). L-DOPA, which is converted in the brain to dopamine, is used in the diagnosis of growth hormone deficiency states. Somatostatin (SS) is the major inhibitor. In various cell types, GH stimulates amino acid uptake, protein, RNA, and DNA synthesis, and lipolysis. High levels in adults cause **acromegaly** (*q.v.*) and insulin resistance. Excessive amounts in juveniles usually have less pronounced effects on intermediary metabolism, but lead to gigantism. Although GH promotes glycogenolysis in the liver, it is glycostatic for skeletal muscle. Some actions are exerted directly on specific receptors. Others, especially on skeletal system components, are mediated in part via peptides that were initially called somatomedins; *see* **insulin-like growth factors**. When nutrition is adequate, GH stimulates the synthesis of insulin-like growth factor-I (IGF-I) in the liver, and its release to the bloodstream. (During times of food deprivation, very little IGF-I is produced in the liver, although GH levels are often elevated. Proteins that oppose IGF-I actions are also made during starvation.) Since growth is metabolically demanding, the inhibitory mechanisms can prolong life when food is not available. GH additionally promotes localized production of IGFs in many target cells. In some types, early direct effects of GH are essential for subsequent responses to IGF-I. High IGF-I concentrations exert negative feedback control over GH secretion by promoting somtatostain release. High circulating fatty acid levels also inhibit. *See* also **growth hormone receptors**.

growth hormone binding proteins: plasma proteins made in the liver that contribute to growth hormone transport, protect against GH loss to glomerular filtrate, and affect hormone-receptor interactions. An acidic, 60K high-affinity type in humans may be a fragment shed from the GH receptor. The concentrations of low affinity 100K forms, identified in many species, are similar in male and female juveniles; but they decline during adolescence in boys, are generally higher in women than in men, and rise during pregnancy.

growth hormone inhibiting hormone: *see* **somatostatins**.

growth hormone receptors: the major form is a large, single chain transmembrane protein (with 620 amino acid moieties in humans and some other species). It is a member of the **cytokine receptor superfamily** (*q.v.*), which includes receptors for prolactin, and for several regulators of hematopoietic functions. High affinity ligand binding and growth hormone actions require that the two sites at opposite ends each hormone molecule bind simultaneously to components of two adjacent receptor molecules. Some of the described biphasic effects of growth hormone may result from ineffective binding, in which just one site on each ligand binds to a receptor monomer.

growth hormone releasing hormone: GRH; GHRH; somatocrinin; a hormone best known for its synthesis in hypothalamic neurons, and for its roles in maintaining somatotrope structure, and promoting growth hormone synthesis and release. The activities of the neurons are controlled by neurotransmitters, hormones, and other factors; *see* **growth hormone**. However, broader functions are suggested by the high concentrations of GRH in lactotropes, corticotropes, and gonadotropes. Moreover, the levels in both exocrine and endocrine pancreas are equivalent to those of the hypothalamus; and substantial amounts are made by the placenta. Smaller ones have additionally been identified in the cerebral cortex, neural

lobe, intestine, testis, and adrenal medulla. Bronchial carcinoid tumors can produce enough to invoke acromegaly. Although the functions outside the hypothalamus have not been defined, GRH is known to affect locomotor activity and to exert influences on the gut. Human GRH is cleaved from a 107 amino acid precursor that contains a 31 amino acid signal sequence. The major form (GRF-44) is H_2N-Tyr-Ala-Asp-Ala-Ile-Phe-Thr-Asn-Ser-Tyr-Arg-Lys-Val-Leu-Gly-Gln-Leu-Ser-Ala-Arg-Lys-Leu-Leu-Gln-Asp-Ile-Met-Ser-Arg-Gln-Gln-Gly-Glu-Ser-Asn-Gln-Glu-Arg-Gly-Ala-Arg-Ala-Arg-Leu-$CONH_2$. GRF-40 is present in the brain and pituitary gland, and GRF (3-44), which is biologically inactive, circulates. Chemically related GRF-44 molecules are made by several mammalian species, but the predominant form in rats has 43 amino acid moieties.

GRP: (1) gastrin releasing peptide; (2) glucose regulated proteins.

GRPP: glicentin-related pancreatic polypeptide: *see* **glicentin**.

GSH: the reduced form of glutathione.

GSH redox cycle: *see* **glutathione**.

GSSG: glutathione disulfide; the oxidized form of glutathione.

GST: glutathione-*S*-transferase.

G_T: *see* **G proteins** and **transducins**.

GTG: gold thioglucose.

GTP: guanosine triphosphate.

GTPase[s]: enzymes that catalyze hydrolysis of guanosine triphosphate (GTP) to guanosine diphopshate (GDP), and in some cases to the monophosphate (GMP), with release of Pi. *See* **GTP binding proteins**.

GTPase activating proteins: GAPs; proteins that augment the GTPase activities of *ras* and related small GTP-binding proteins, and thereby accelerate their deactivation. *See* also **GTP binding proteins**.

GTP binding proteins: a protein superfamily in all eukaryotic cells, whose members bind guanine nucleotides, display GTPase activity, and interact with other cell components in a manner affected by GDP/GTP exchange and GTP hydrolysis. They participate in signal transduction and the functions of hormones and neurotransmitters, intracellular vesicle translocation, exocytosis, and transport across plasma membranes, control of enzyme activities, protein synthesis, cell growth, proliferation and differentiation, and other processes. The group includes trimeric **G proteins** (*q.v.*), smaller, monomeric p21 proteins encoded by *ras* genes, initiation and elongation factors, tubulins, and Golgi factors. The proteins are "inactive" when linked to GDP, but display high affinities for specific ligands. Association with the ligands leads to exchange of GDP for GTP. In most cases, the GTP-bound forms then transiently attach to enzymes or other targets and carry out the functions, but lose their affinities for the initial ligands. When the GTPase component promotes hydrolysis of GTP to GDP + Pi, the "inactive" state is restored. The processes are closely regulated by numerous factors that, for various types, include guanine nucleotide exchange factors (GEFs) which facilitate replacement of GDP by GTP, and GTPase activating proteins (GAPs). Guanine nucleotide release proteins (GNRPs, guanine nucleotide release factors, GNRFs) that promote dissociation from GDP, and thereby indirectly facilitate GTP binding, have also been described. Some small GTP-binding proteins associate with guanine nucleotide inhibitory factors when they hold GDP. Those factors transiently block the GDP/GTP exchange, but dissociate when the ligands bind. Dysregulation severely disrupts cell functions. GTP analogs that resist hydrolysis maintain G proteins in persistently active forms; and some mutant proteins with little or no GTPase activity transform cells and promote tumorigenesis. Some small GTP-binding proteins catalyze ADP-ribosylation of other proteins. Those reactions must also be tightly controlled, since the substrates include other G proteins. *See* also **cholera** and **pertussis toxins**.

GTP-thio-triphosphates: guanosine-triphosphate analogs that resists hydrolysis. They can attach to GTP-binding proteins, and invoke persistent effects of the kinds stimulated more transiently in the presence of GTP. The structure of GTPγS is shown, along with the α and β positions for the sulfur atoms of the other forms. The various types differ somewhat in affinities for target proteins. It has been observed, for example, that GTPαS and GTPγS promote persistent elevation of cytosolic Ca^{2+}, and degranulation in mast cells, presumably by activating G_ϵ (*see* **G proteins**). In contrast, GTPβS induces repetitive Ca^{2+} spikes, an effect attributed to activation of G_p.

guanethidine: Octatensine; [2-hexahydro-1(2*H*)-azocinyl)ethyl]guanidine; a postganglionic sympathetic neuron depressant, used to treat hypertension. Although it is taken up by synaptic vesicles via mechanisms for norepinephrine transport, and can transiently release some norepinephrine, its major early effect is inhibition of neurotransmitter release. Chronic administration depletes norepinephrine stores, but increases target cell sensitivity to the regulator.

guanidine hydrochloride: a reagent used to denature and dissolve proteins by breaking noncovalent bonds.

guanidoacetic acid: glycocyamine; an intermediate in the pathway for creatine synthesis. A mitochondrial en-

guanethidine

guanidine hydrochloride

zyme catalyzes the reaction: arginine + glycine → ornithine + guanidoacetic acid. S-adenosylmethionine: guanidoacetate-*N*-methyltransferase then catalyzes *S*-adenosylmethionine + guanidoacetic acid → *S*-adenosylhomocysteine + creatine.

guanine: G; 2-amino-6-oxypurine; 2-aminohypoxanthine; a nitrogenous base of DNAs and RNAs that pairs with cytosine, and a component of guanosine triphosphate (GTP), cyclic guanosine-3′5′-monophosphate (cGMP), guanophore white pigments, and other cellular compounds. Derivatives that occur in transfer RNAs include 1-methylguanine and N^2-dimethylguanine. *See* also **guanine deaminase** and **guanosine triphosphate**.

guanine deaminase: an enzyme in liver, spleen, and other organs that catalyzes the reaction: guanine + H_2O → hypoxanthine + NH_3, and thereby protects against accumulation of excessive amounts of that nitrogenous base. (The high incidence of a form of gout in pigs, in which guanine accumulates in joints, is attributed to very low levels of the enzyme.)

guanine nucleotide exchange factors: GEFs: regulators that promote exchange of protein bound GDP for GTP, and thereby contribute to the activation of some **GTP binding proteins** (*q.v.*).

guanine nucleotide release proteins: GNRPs; guanine nucleotide release factors: GNRFs: cell components that accelerate dissociation of GDP from **GTP binding proteins** (*q.v.*), and thereby facilitate GTP binding.

guano: the dried, nitrogenous excrement of birds and bats. It contains large amounts of uric acid, and is used as a fertilizer. *See* also **uricotelic**.

guanophore: a pigment cell type of fishes and some other vertebrates that contains guanine crystals which impart a white or silvery appearance.

guanine

1-methyl-guanine

N^2-dimethylguanine

guanosine: guanine riboside; a nucleoside component of ribonucleic acids, made from guanine + ribose-1-phosphate, and phosphorylated by ATP to **guanosine-triphosphate** (GTP, *q.v.*). *See* also **guanosine monophosphate** (GMP), **guanosine diphosphate** (GDP), and **cyclic GMP** (cyclic guanosine 3′5′-monophosphate, cGMP).

cyclic guanosine 3′,5′-cyclic monophosphate: *see* **cyclic GMP** and **guanylate cyclase**.

guanosine deoxyriboside: guanine-2-deoxyribose; a nucleoside that is phosphorylated by ATP to guanosine deoxyribonucleotide triphosphate, and used for DNA biosynthesis. *See* also **guanine**.

guanosine 5′-diphosphate: GDP: guanine-ribose-5′-P-P; a nucleotide that exchanges high energy phosphate groups, for example in reactions such as ATP + GDP $\rightleftarrows$ ADP + GTP. It is formed from GTP in energy releasing reactions, such as oxaloacetate + GTP $\rightarrow$ phosphoenolpyruvate + GDP, and is converted to GTP in some others (for example succinyl-coenzyme A + GDP + Pi $\rightarrow$ succinate + GTP + CoA). *See* also **guanosine triphosphate**, **G proteins**, and **GTPases**.

guanosine 5′[β,γ-imido]triphosphate: *see* **Gpp(NH$_p$)**.

guanosine 3′-monophosphate: guanine riboside-3′ phosphoric acid; 3′-guanylic acid; a nucleotide released during RNA degradation.

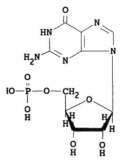

guanosine 5′-monophosphate

pathways for biosynthesis of some sugars and oligosaccharides, via reactions such as: mannose + GTP $\rightleftarrows$ GDP-mannose + P-P and GDP-mannose $\rightleftarrows$ GDP-fucose, and is an inhibitor of glutamate dehydrogenase. *See* also **G proteins** and **cyclic GMP**.

7-methyl-**guanosine triphosphate**: the first nucleotide (5′ cap) of transcribed messenger RNAs.

guanosine 5′-monophosphate: GMP: 5′guanylic acid; guanylate; guanine-ribose-phosphate; a nucleotide synthesized in the reactions: xanthosine-5-phosphate + ATP + glutamine $\rightarrow$ guanosine 5′-monophosphate + AMP + P-P + glutamate, and guanine + 5-phosphoribosyl-1-pyrophosphate $\rightarrow$ guanosine 5′-monophosphate + P-P. It is also formed when phosphodiesterases catalyze cyclic GMP hydrolysis.

guanosine triphosphatase: an enzyme that catalyzes hydrolysis of GTP to GDP + Pi. *See* **GTP binding proteins** and **guanosine 5′-diphosphate**.

guanosine triphosphate: GTP: a term that can designate guanine-deoxyribose-P-P-P, one of the nucleotides used for DNA synthesis, but is more commonly applied to guanine-ribose-P-P-P, which is used for RNA synthesis. When hydrolyzed to GDP + Pi, it releases energy that drives reactions used for gluconeogenesis, protein synthesis, and other processes. It is an intermediate in

guanyl nucleotide regulatory protein: *see* **GTP binding proteins**.

guanylate: guanosine 5′-monophosphate.

guanylate cyclases: guanylyl cyclases; G-cyclases; enzymes that catalyze the reaction: GTP $\rightarrow$ **cyclic GMP** (*q.v.*) + P-P. *Soluble* forms are heterodimers with α and β subunit isoforms of approximately 77.5K and 70.5K, respectively, both of which display catalytic activity. They require heme cofactors, and are activated by nitric oxide, nitrosothiols, free radicals, and other heme-binding substances made by cells. Ca^{2+} activates in some cell types, but inhibits in others. In contrast, *membrane bound* (particulate) types are transmembrane glycoproteins, insensitive to nitric oxide and related regulators, but with intracellular tyrosine kinase-like, as well as cyclase domains. (Early reports that they do respond to NO are now attributed to attachment of soluble types to membranes.) The apparent molecular weights for subtypes GC-A, GC-B, and GC-C are, respectively, 130K, 135-140K, and 140-160K. GC-A appears to be the primary functional receptor for **atrial natriuretic hormones** (*q.v.*), and it is also activated by high levels of brain natriuretic peptide. GC-B may be the receptor for a related C type natriuretic peptide, whereas GC-C is activated by STa (a heat stable enterotoxin made *E.coli* and some other bacteria), and possibly also by **guanylin** (*q.v.*). A different protein, *atrial natriuretic clearance receptor*, also binds the peptides, but is not a G-cyclase. In nonmammalian species, membrane bound G-cyclases are receptors for **speract** (*q.v.*), resact, mosact, and other sperm proteins. Activation of the tyrosine kinase domains may require receptor dimerization and autophosphorylation. The cyclases are substrates for kinase C isozymes, and for protein phosphatase 2A. *See also* **recoverin**.

guanylic acid: *see* **guanosine 3′-monophosphate** and **guanosine 5′-monophosphate**.

guanylyl cyclase: guanylate cyclase.

guanylin: Pro-Asp-Thr-Cys-Glu-Ile-Cys-Ala-Tyr-Ala-Ala-Cys-Thr-Gly-Cys; an acidic peptide made in intestinal and some other epithelial cells of fetuses and adults, chemically related to STa (a bacterial enterotoxin), and capable of displacing that peptide from its receptors (*see* also **guanylate cyclases**). It acts via cyclic guanosine-3′,5′-monophosphate (cGMP) to increase chloride secretion and decrease sodium and water absorption in the small intestine, and is implicated as a factor that causes the diarrhea associated with some infections. It may additionally regulate epithelial transport by acting on receptors that do not bind STa.

gubernaculum: a fibrous cord that directs the movement of the structure to which it is attached. The term is most commonly applied to the fibromuscular strand that connects the lower pole of the embryonic mesonephros to the inguinal peritoneum, and later contributes to descent of the testis.

Guillain-Barré syndrome: idiopathic polyneuritis; an autoimmune disorder that develops following vaccination with attenuated influenza and some other viruses, or during infections (for example by cytomegalovirus), in which lymphocytes and macrophages migrate into peripheral nerves, a form of IgG type immunoglobulin accumulates in the cerebrospinal fluid, and myelin is destroyed. Skeletal muscle paralysis (which often subsides) is a major manifestation, but sensory disturbances can also occur.

guinea pig: *Cavia porcellus*; a species used in laboratory studies because of its convenient size and special characteristics. It rapidly develops ascorbic acid deficiency when deprived of dietary vitamin C, makes growth hormones, insulins, and other hormones different from those of other rodents, has different receptors, and displays some special kinds of immune system responses. Unlike rats and most other small rodents, it has very large adrenal glands in which the major glucocorticoid made is cortisol. The young are born in a comparatively mature state (with hair, teeth, open eyes and open ears) and can survive with a minimum of maternal care. Some mutant strains are easily identified by their coat colors and textures.

gulose: a glucose isomer. Glucuronate reductase catalyzes the reaction: glucuronate + NADPH → L-gulonate + NADP + H^+. Aldonolactonase then promotes conversion of gulonate to gulonolactone which, in turn, is oxidized in the presence of gulonolactone oxidase to ascorbic acid.

guppy: *Lebistes reticularis*; a small, highly fertile, tropical fish species with a short life cycle that is used for studies of development, sex chromosome patterns, and some hormone responses.

gustaducin: G_{gust}; a trimeric **G protein** (*q.v.*) in taste buds that transduces signals involved in perception of chemicals as sweet or bitter.

gustin: a 37K zinc-containing protein that activates a cAMP-phosphodiesterase, and regulates taste bud growth, nutrition, and sensitivity. It is chemically and biologically related to nerve growth factor (NGF), and can displace that hormone from its receptors. Under normal conditions, it accounts for approximately 3% of the total protein of human parotid gland saliva. The levels are low in individuals with hypogeusia. When the cause is zinc deficiency, administration of the mineral restores both gustin levels and taste perception.

gut: gastrointestinal tract.

gut-associated lymphoid tissue: GALT; Peyer's patches, mesenteric lymph nodes, appendix, bursa of Fabricius (in birds), and other lymphoid tissue associated with the gastrointestinal tract.

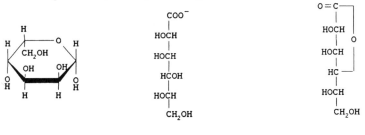

L-gulose   L-gulonate   L-gulonolactone

gut endocrine tissue: the hormone-secreting components of the gastrointestinal tract, including autonomic system nerve endings as well as neuroendocrine (enteroendocrine) cells. Most of the peptide products are similar to or identical with regulators made in the central nervous system.

gut-islet-gut axis: control systems mediated via communication between the gastrointestinal tract and the endocrine pancreas. For example, food intake and the associated changes in the gut lumen promote somatostatin (SS) secretion by gastrointestinal cells, and insulin secretion by pancreatic β cells. In addition to acting locally to slow gut motility and nutrient absorption, SS protects against postprandial hyperglycemia by inhibiting glucagon release from pancreatic islet α cells. Insulin facilitates food absorption, and the uptake of glucose and amino acids by several cell types. When the food is protein-rich, but contains very little carbohydrate, excessive amounts of insulin can (if unopposed) invoke hypoglycemia. Amino acids released from food stimulate secretion of pancreatic glucagon in amounts sufficient to protect against it.

guvacine: 1,2,5,6-tetrahydronicotinic acid; an agent obtained from betel nuts (the seeds of *Areca catechu*). It prolongs the effects of gamma-aminobutyric acid by inhibiting GABA uptake and sequestration.

GVBD: germinal vesicle breakdown.

GVG: γ-vinyl-**GABA**.

GVH reactions: graft versus host reactions.

GYKI 52466: 1-(4-aminophenyl)-4-methyl-7,8-methylenedioxy-5*H*-2,3-benzodiazepine; the hydrochloride is a selectitve, noncompetitive antagonist for AMPA/kainate type excitatory amino acid receptors. It is an anti-convulsant that can protect against brain damage initiated by ischemia.

GYK1 52895: 1-(4-aminophenyl)-4-methyl-7,8-methylenedioxy-3,4-dihydro-5*H*-2,3-benzodiazepine; a selective inhibitor of dopamine uptake into nerve terminals

GYKI 52466

that can counteract psychic depression and parkinsonionism.

gyn-, gyneco-: a prefix meaning female or woman.

gynandromorph: an individual with some male and some female phenotypic characteristics. The term is commonly applied to insects, whereas *hermaphrodite* is preferred for vertebrates.

gynecomastia: breast enlargement in males. It occurs in individuals with Klinefelter's syndrome, prolactin-secreting tumors, thyrotoxicosis, liver diseases that impair steroid hormone metabolism, and conditions associated with excessive production of estrogens. A mild, transient form often develops during puberty in normal males.

gynogenesis: a type of sexual reproduction, in which spermatozoa activate oocytes, but do not contribute genetic components to the embryos; *cf* **parthenogenesis**.

gyrase: the type II topoisomerase made by *E. coli*.

gyrus [gyri]: a circle, circuit, or ring. The term describes brain regions (convolutions) separated from each other by fissures or sulci.

H

H: (1) hydrogen; (2) histidine; (3) enthalpy.

[2]H: deuterium; *see* **hydrogen**.

[3]H: tritium; *see* **hydrogen**.

h: human, as in hCG or hGH.

H1, **H2A**, **H2B**, **H3**, **H4**: *see* **histones**.

H₁, **H₂**: *see* **histamine receptors**.

H-2: the major histocompatibility complex of the mouse.

H-7, **H-8**, **H-9**: three chemically related agents {1-(5-iso-quinolinesulfonyl)-2-methylpiperazine dihydrochloride, N-[2-(methylamino)-ethyl]-5-isoquinoline sulfonamide dihydrochloride, and N-[2-aminoethyl)-5-isoquinoline sulfonamide dihydrochloride} that inhibit, respectively, kinases A, C, and G by competing with ATP for active sites on the enzymes. High concentrations also inhibit myosin light chain kinase.

HA-966: 3-amino-1-hydroxy-2-pyrrolidone; an NMDA receptor antagonist, believed to inhibit neurotransmitter release by acting at the glycine binding site. The $R(+)$ isomer is more potent; but the $S(-)$ counterpart is a more effective sedative and muscle relaxant.

HA-1004: N-(2-guanidoethyl)-5-isoquinolinesulfona-mide hydrochloride; a calcium antagonist that potently inhibits protein kinases A and G, but has little influence on kinase C types.

HAA: a lectin obtained from *Helix aspersa* (*q.v.*).

habenula: (1) a small, straplike fibrous structure; (2) a cluster of caudal, dorsal thalamic neurons derived from the epithalamus that borders the third ventricle and, in many species forms the pineal gland peduncle.

HA-1004

habitat: the conditions under which an organism lives.

habituation: (1) gradual adaptation to an agent or environment; (2) psychological dependence on an agent repeatedly taken; *cf* **addiction**.

habitus: the physical appearance of an individual.

haem-, **haemo-**: a prefix meaning blood.

Haeckel's law: biogenetic law; recapitulation theory; the concept that embryonic and fetal development involves passage through a series of stages in which the individual closely resembles its evolutionary precursors. Although embryos do transiently acquire some characteristics of those types, the concept is no longer accepted in its original form.

Hageman factor: factor XII; an 80K glycoprotein of the cascade for blood **coagulation**, (*q.v.*).

hair: (1) a threadlike appendage; (2) the nonliving, keratinized skin appendages that cover body surfaces, each comprising an externally visible shaft (with medulla, cortex and cuticle), that is continuous with a root which extends below the surface and is surrounded by a hair follicle. Root matrix epithelial cells, nourished by capillaries, divide by mitosis and account for the growth. There are regional differences in responses to regulatory factors that affect hair formation, and in the durations of the anagen (growth), telogen (terminal differentiation) and catagen (involution) phases. The quantity, color, texture, and distribution are determined by genetic factors whose expression is affected by several hormones Tri-

H-7

H-8

H-9

iodothyronine (T_3) influences all of the parameters. 5α-dihydrotestosterone (DHT) is a major stimulant for the growth of facial, chest, axillary, and pubic hair; but it contributes to loss of scalp hair in susceptible individuals. Epidermal growth factor (EGF) and transforming growth factor-β (TGFβ) are among the regulators that inhibit growth. Glucocorticoids inhibit scalp hair growth and the secretion of melanocyte stimulating hormones (which promote melanin and phaeomelanin synthesis). However, they can be metabolically converted to androgens, which stimulate growth on the face and trunk. Melatonin mediates lightening of the fur of animals that undergo seasonal changes, via mechanisms not directly related to its influences on the reproductive system. Minoxidil is one of the pharmacological agents believed to stimulate hair growth by increasing cutaneous blood flow; (3) sensory cell extensions, such as the elongated microvilli of taste buds, or the stereocilia of the inner ear and olfactory mucosa.

hairpin loop: a structure composed of two parallel strands joined at one end, for example a nucleic acid segment formed when a single-stranded nucleotide chain hydrogen bonds at one end to the complementary bases on another strand, or a polypeptide composed of two chains covalently linked at one end. *See* also **zinc fingers** and **Henle loops**.

halazepam: 7-chloro-1,3-dihydro-5-phenyl-1-(2,2,2-tri-fluoroethyl)-2*H*-1,4-benzodiazepin-2-one; a benzodiazepine type sedative and tranquilizer.

Halcyon: a trade name for triazolam.

half-life: $t/2$; $t/\frac{1}{2}$; the time required to decline to half the initial value, a term applied to radioactivity, concentrations, and biological responses. The concentration of a compound in the bloodstream falls at a rate related to those for excretion, degradation (or conversion to other compounds), and sequestration (by blood components, or via cellular uptake). The $t/2$ can differ markedly from the *biological* half-life (time during which *activity* declines by 50%), because cells retain some compounds for extended time periods, and actions initiated by a regulator can continue long after the initiator has disappeared. The half-time for radioactive decay depends mostly on the nature of the atom. It can range from fractions of second to thousands of years.

halide: any fluoride, chloride, bromide, or iodide salt.

halisteresis: movement of minerals, for example of calcium and phosphorus from bone to bulk extracellular fluid. Factors that affect it include pH, and ions such as citrate that combine with calcium.

hallucination: a false perception, usually auditory or visual, that is unrelated to an environmental stimulus. It can be by invoked by some pharmacological agents, and occurs spontaneously in some individuals with schizophrenia and other mental disorders.

hallucinogens: agents that invoke hallucinations.

haloperidol: 4-[4-(4-chlorophenyl)-4-hydroxy-1-piperidinyl]-1-(4-fluorophenyl)-1-butanone; a D_2-type dopamine receptor antagonist, used as a neuroleptic and "antipsychotic" agent. It also interacts with α-type adrenergic receptors, and blocks the psychotomimetic effects of *N*-allyl normetazocine. Prolonged use can cause tardive dyskinesia and hyperprolactinemia.

halophilic: capable of surviving in environments of high ionic strength.

hamartomas: benign tumors composed of excessive numbers of mature cells of the kinds normally found in the region.

hamsters: several small rodents used in laboratory studies, including golden or Syrian (*Mesocricetus auratus*), Turkish (*Mesocricetus brandti*), and Djungarian or Siberian (*Phodopus sungorus*) species. All are seasonal breeders under natural conditions, but only some hibernate. Differences in pineal gland functions are used to study biological rhythms and melatonin actions; and the cheek pouches are convenient sites for implantations. The Chinese hamster (*Cricetulus griseus*) has only 11 pairs of chromosomes, and therefore provides special advantages for some genetics studies. Its ovary cells are cultured for investigation of gonadotropin effects.

hand: *see* **EF hand**.

H antigen: (1) an oligosaccharide expressed at high levels on type O blood erythrocytes, and processed by genetically controlled factors to yield A and B blood antigens; (2) a flagellum antigen of motile gram negative bacteria.

haploid: describes (1) a gamete or other cell with one allele of each type characteristic for the sex and species, on one-half the numbers of chromosomes for a typical somatic cell; (2) an individual with a haploid genome; (3) a microorganism that possesses a single chromosome.

haplotype: a specific combination of linked alleles in a gene cluster.

hapten: an incomplete antigen; a small molecule that stimulates the production of specific antibodies only when it is attached to a protein carrier or other larger molecule.

haptoglobins: α_2-globulins that modulate lymphocyte responsiveness to antigens. Since the blood levels are usually low, but can rise rapidly in response to some forms of stress, they are classified as acute phase proteins. They contribute to iron conservation by binding hemoglobin released from erythrocytes, and can localize in invasive breast cancer tissue.

haptotaxis: accelerated, directed cell movement in response to adhesion factor gradients.

HAR: heterotypic adhesion receptors.

Harderian glands: accessory lacrimal glands in animals with nictitating membranes. They secrete lubricants, and contain melatonin-secreting cells that resemble some pineal gland types. Rudimentary, nonfunctioning structures occur in humans and other species.

Hardy-Weinberg law: the concept that gene and genotype frequencies remain constant in an infinitely large, interbreeding population, in which mating is random and there is no migration or mutation.

harmaline: 1-methyl-7-methoxy-3,4-dihydro-β-carboline; 3,4-dihydrokarmine; an alkaloid in the seeds of *Peganum harmala*, initially observed to stimulate the myocardium, but now used as a monoamine oxidase inhibitor. It is a central nervous system stimulant that acts acts preferentially on type A enzymes; but it also affects diamine oxidases.

harmine: 7-methoxy-1-methyl-9H-pyridol[3,4-b]-indole; an alkaloid in the seeds of *Peganum harmala* with properties similar to those of harmaline.

Hartnup disease: a rare, inherited disorder in which impaired renal reabsorption of some monocarboxylic amino acids leads to development of pellagra-like symptoms. It can be alleviated with nicotinic acid.

Harvey murine sarcoma virus: a virus that carries the *H-ras* oncogene; *see ras*.

Hashimoto's thyroiditis: autoimmune thyroiditis; lymphadenoid goiter; thyroid gland inflammation with lymphocyte infiltration, attributed to production of abnormal circulating antithyroid antibodies and excessive amounts of some lymphokines. Initially, acute release of iodinated thyroid hormones can invoke transient hyperthyroidism; but cell destruction commonly leads to thyroid hormone deficiency. The disease is more common in women than in men.

hashish: a resin secreted by the flowering tops of female *Cannabis sativa* plants. The major active ingredients are tetrahydro-**cannabinols** (*q.v.*).

Hassall's corpuscles: spherical or ovoid clusters of concentrically arranged, degenerating epithelial cells that contain keratohyalin and cytoplasmic filaments, and surround extracellular colloid. They form in thymus gland medullas of many species.

hatching: (1) emergence of an immature organism from a protective coating (such as an egg shell); (2) the shedding of a zona pellucida by a blastocyst that usually occurs shortly before implantation.

HAT medium: a tissue culture medium that contains hypoxanthine, aminopterin, and thymidine. It is used to promote selective survival of hybridoma cells for monoclonal antibody assays. When aminopterin blocks *de novo* synthesis of purines and pyrimidines, normal cells use a salvage pathway to make nucleotides from the hypoxanthine and thymidine. Cells deficient in either hypoxanthine-guanine phosphoribosyltransferase (HGPRT) or thymidine kinase (TK) die. TK$^+$HGPRT$^-$ myeloma cells hybridized with antigen-stimulated TK$^-$ HGPRT$^+$ spleen cells survive.

H$^+$-ATPase: *see* **F$_1$F$_2$-ATPase**.

HAVA: α-hydrazino-δ-amino valeric acid: a competitive inhibitor of ornithine decarboxylase.

Haversian system: osteon; a structural unit of compact bone, comprising a central (Haversian) canal that houses a blood capillary, surrounded by concentric lamellae formed by osteocytes and the matrix they produce. Cytoplasmic extensions pass through canaliculi in the matrix and connect one cell with another.

Hayflick limit: the number of times a normal can divide. Cultured human and mouse cells have been observed to undergo 50, and 30 divisions, respectively.

Hb: (1) hemoglobin; (2) the unoxygenated form of hemoglobin.

HB-EGF: heparin binding EGF-like growth factor.

HbO$_2$, KHbO$_2$: oxygenated hemoglobin.

HC: the constant region of an immunoglobulin heavy chain.

H cells: gastrointestinal cells that secrete vasoactive intestinal peptide (VIP).

HCF: hypercalcemic factors.

hCG: *see* **human chorionic gonadotropin**.

H chains: immunoglobulin heavy chains.

HCHWA-D: human cerebral hemorrhage with amyloidosis-Dutch type; *see* **amyloid precursor protein**.

HCl: *see* **hydrochloric acid**.

hCLRF: human type **chorionic luteinizing hormone release factor** (*q.v.*).

HCMV: human cytomegalovirus.

hCS: human **chorionic somatomammotropin** (*q.v.*).

hCT: human **chorionic thyrotropin** (*q.v.*).

HDC: histamine decarboxylase.

HDLs: high density lipoproteins; *see* **lipoproteins**.

HDL receptors: high density lipoprotein receptors; *see* **lipoprotein receptors**.

head protein: *see* **Hydra**.

heart: in mammals, a hollow, four-chambered organ in the thoracic cavity, composed mostly of myocardium (*see* **cardiac muscle**), lined by endocardium, and coverd with visceral (fibrous) pericardium. It is richly supplied with autonomic nerves and is nourished by coronary arteries. Although its most obvious function is collecting blood from the vena cavae and pulmonary veins, and pumping it into the pulmonary arteries and aorta, the heart is also the major source of circulating atrial natriuretic peptides; and its nerve endings release catecholamines to the bloodstream. The cells also makes some angiotensin converting enzyme. Under normal conditions, the intrinsic contraction rhythmicity is synchronized by the sino-atrial (S-A) node, but the atrio-ventricular (A-V) node can assume limited function when the primary pacemaker is severely damaged; *see* also **intercalated disks** and **Purkinje fibers**. Contractile force is affected by factors such as stretch (related to filling) and temperature, but also by the stimulatory and inhibitory influences, respectively, of sympathetic and parasympathetic neurons, and by circulating catecholamines, triiodothyronine (which acts in part via influences on responses to catecholamines), glucocorticoids, and regulators that act indirectly through reflexes. Insulin stimulates glucose uptake and other metabolic processes, and aldosterone contributes to the control of ion transport. The two-chambered hearts of fishes pump blood to gills. Amphibian and most reptile hearts have three chambers.

heat of fusion: heat energy exchange required for association. In physical chemistry, the term usually designates the heat loss that occurs when a specific quantity of a liquid is converted to a solid at the same temperature under standardized conditions. Conversion of 1 gram of water at 0° C to one gram of ice at a pressure of 1 atmosphere releases 79 calories, mostly because hydrogen bonds are formed. The high specific heat of water protects cells against rapid changes in temperature when they are exposed to environmental fluctuations. During winter months, ice formation on the surface of a pond can release sufficient heat to warm the water below to a temperature compatible with survival for some aquatic animals.

heat of vaporization: the amount of heat required to convert a given volume of a liquid to a gas at the same temperature. Evaporation of sweat is an efficient mechanism for body cooling in mammals, because water has a high heat of vaporization. Conversion of 1 gram to water vapor at 100° C and 1 atmosphere absorbs 540 calories, mostly because hydrogen bonds are broken.

heat shock elements: HSEs: DNA segments in the promoter regions of genes that bind heat shock transcription factors and code for heat shock proteins.

heat shock factors: *see* **heat shock transcription factors**.

heat shock proteins: HSPs: a superfamily of proteins made by many cell types, whose synthesis is preferentially augmented by exposure to excessive heat or cold (without generalized increases in overall protein synthesis). The proteins are highly conserved across the species (including microorganisms). Many of them are called *stress* proteins, since their synthesis is also stimulated by glucose or oxygen deprivation, viral infections, and/or other adverse conditions. The families are distinguished by numbers that relate to their molecular weights (as in HSP70). Various types provide short term resistance to the deleterious effects of stress and accelerate cell recovery, by protecting against chromatin damage, activating specific genes that code for vital factors, binding to abnormal or denatured proteins in a manner that facilitates degradation, and directing protein folding, unfolding, and translocation. Some forms of stress enhance activation and/or production of heat shock transcription factors that accelerate HSP gene expression. Others that act via different mechanisms may require the presence of those proteins. Age-related decreases in production of HSP70 types (which regulate protein transport across endoplasmic reticulum and mitochondrial membranes, and promote the ubiquitin binding that marks some for degradation), have been linked with declining resistance to stress. Different HSPs are implicated as mediators of immune system functions and tumor regression, and as factors involved in the etiology of some autoimmune diseases. Several types made by unstimulated cells translocate to nuclei during specific stages of cell cycles, and have roles in cell growth and proliferation. HSP90 proteins are among the types that complex with unoccupied steroid hormone receptors, and are released following ligand binding; *see*, for example **glucocorticoid receptors**. They are believed to protect unoccupied receptors against degradation, and to contribute in other ways to steroid hormone actions.

heat shock puffs: enlarged regions at specific sites on polytene chromosomes that form in response to excessive heat, and are associated with increased transcription of heat shock proteins.

heat shock transcription factors: HSTFs; highly conserved proteins that bind to heat shock elements and accelerate transcription of heat shock proteins. High temperatures, hypoxia, and some other kinds of stress accelerate HSTF synthesis, and exert other influences that augment their abilities to interact with DNA. It has been speculated that heat, ATP depletion, changes in H⁺ and Ca^{2+} concentrations, and changes in redox potentials, directly affect their configurations, and/or the configurations of proteins that complex with them. Various kinds of HSTFs are substrates for protein kinases and protein phosphatases.

heavy chain: the largest polypeptide chain of a dimeric or multimeric protein. *See also* **immunoglobulins**.

heavy chain class switching: changing from production of one type of immunoglobulin (such as IgM) to another (often IgG), with the same antigen specificity.

heavy meromyosin: HMM; *see* **myosin**.

heavy water: deuterium oxide; [2]H_2O. *See* **deuterium**.

Hebbian modulation: phenomena studied *in vitro* as models for some aspects of synaptic plasticity, long-term potentiation, and learning. According to the initial postulate, synchronous presynaptic and postsynaptic stimulation potentiates or stabilizes synaptic efficiency, whereas asynchronous stimulation at the two sites weakens it. The concept is partially supported by observations that repetitive iontophoretic postsynaptic presentation of acetylcholine to myocytes, with either asynchronous or no presynaptic stimuli, promptly invokes prolonged synaptic depression, whereas synchronous stimulation does not. The depression is linked with elevation of cytosolic Ca^{2+} levels, which may lead to release of a retrograde factor that mediates the effects.

HeLa cells: an undifferentiated, aneuploid cell line derived from a human squamous epithelium type uterine cervix carcinoma. It is used to culture viruses, to study DNA replication, gene transcription, translation, and transformation, and as a source of nucleic acids. Expression of a glycosylated phosphoprotein (p75/150) that is biologically similar to intestinal-type alkaline phosphatase, correlates with tumorigenicity. Over-expression of an initiation factor (EIF-4E) is associated with tumor progression.

helicases: enzymes that promote unwinding of double-stranded DNA helix segments.

heliotropin: piperonal.

heliotropism: tendency to grow towards the sun (or towards a source of light).

helix [helices]: a spring-like structure with evenly spaced, snail-like coils. Hydrogen bonds maintain nucleic acids and many peptides and proteins in such configurations. The most common types are right handed (α-helices). B-DNA (the most abundant form of double-stranded DNA) has two right-handed helices, with 10 nucleotides per turn, that are wound about each other. In proteins, the numbers of moieties per turn are affected by the kinds of amino acid types. Some have two or more coils, separated by linear segments. Two or more protein helices can entwine to form cables.

Helix aspersa: the garden snail. It makes a lectin (HAA), specific for *N*-acetyl-α-D-galactosamyl groups, that promotes agglutination of A type erythrocytes.

Helix pomatia: the edible snail, from which a lectin (HPA), similar to the one from *Helix aspersa*, is obtained.

helix-turn-helix: a configuration common to several DNA-binding proteins. The coils fit into neighboring DNA dimer helices.

helminths: round worms, including cestodes, nematodes, and trematodes. Some are free living; others are parasites.

Heloderma: a genus of lizards whose members include *H. suspectum* (the Gila monster), and *H. horridum* (the beaded lizard). *See* **helodermin**.

helodermin: helospectrin: H-His-Ser-Asp-Ala-Ile-Phe-Thr-Glu-Glu-Tyr-Ser-Lys-Leu-Leu-Ala-Lys-Leu-Ala-Leu-Gln-Lys-Tyr-Leu-Ala-Ser-Ile-Leu-Gly-Ser-Arg-Thr-Ser-Pro-Pro-Pro-NH_2; a venom made by the salivary glands of *Heloderma suspectum* (the Gila monster) that is chemically and biologically related to vasoactive intestinal peptide (VIP) and secretin. It stimulates cAMP formation, pancreatic amylase secretion, and thyroid hormone secretion; and it inhibits calcium incorporation into bone matrix. A peptide that cross-reacts with antibodies directed against it co-exists with calcitonin in ultimobranchial bodies, thyroid gland parafollicular cells, and medullary carcinomas; and small amounts are found in salivary glands, brains, intestines, and other mammalian organs.

helper cells: *see* **T lymphocytes**.

helper virus: a virus that supplies factors a defective virus requires for replication.

hemagglutinins: antibodies, lectins, viruses, or other entities on cell surfaces that promote erythrocyte agglutination. Some cell types infected with viruses produce specific kinds that are used in diagnosis. Cold agglutinins (active only at temperatures lower than 37°C) display low affinities and are usually of the IgM immunoglobulin type, whereas most warm agglutinins are IgGs.

hemangioblast[s]: embryonic cells that can give rise to both blood cells and blood vessels.

hemangioblastomas: vascular tumors of the central nervous system, composed of blood capillaries and stromal cells.

hemangiomas: benign tumors composed mostly of proliferating blood vessels.

hemapheresis: separation of blood into its constituents, with return of some of the components to the donor. When used to obtain plasma, leukocytes, or platelets, the erythrocytes are usually returned (to avoid the development of anemia).

hematin: *see* **heme**.

hematocytopoiesis: hematopoiesis.

hematocrit: the per cent of the volume occupied by erythrocytes when a fresh venous blood sample is treated with an anticoagulant and subjected to centrifugation under standardized conditions. Values are in the general range of 40-54% and 38-46%, respectively, for healthy men and healthy, nonpregnant women. Leukocytes and blood platelets form a "buffy coat" between the erythrocyte and plasma layers.

hematomas: localized accumulations of blood in tissue or extracellular spaces. They form during the early stages of bone fracture repair, following trauma, and under pathological conditions that include blood coagulation defects and the presence of some kinds of cancer cells.

hematopoiesis: hematocytopoiesis: blood cell formation, development, and release to the bloodstream. *See also* **erythropoiesis**, **leukopoiesis**, and **thrombopoiesis**.

hematopoietic stem cells: pluripotential bone marrow cells; the "uncommitted" progenitors of cells that can give rise to erythrocytes, leukocytes, and thrombocytes.

hematoporphyrin: 1,3,5,8-tetramethyl-2,4-bis(α-hydroxyethyl)porphine-6,7-dipropionic acid; a hemoglobin degradation product.

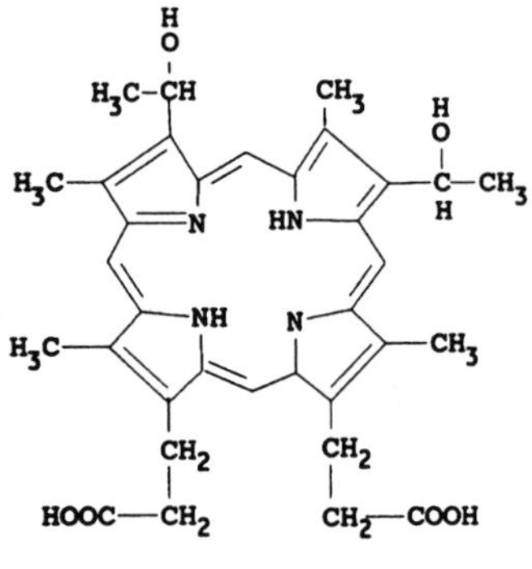

hematoxylin: 7,11b-dihydrobenzideno[1,2-*d*]pyran-3,4, 6α,9,10(6*H*)-pentol; a basic dye used as a biological stain, often with an eosin counterstain.

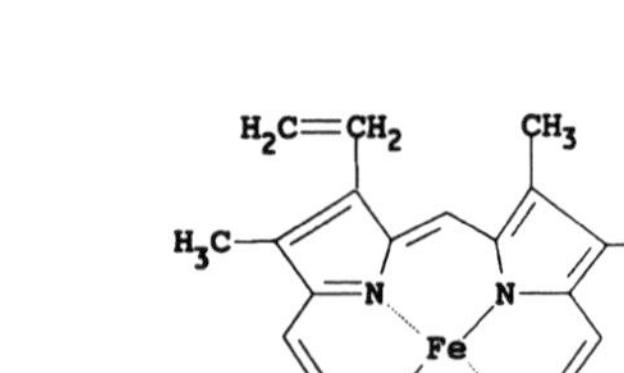

hematoxylin-eosin: a stain used to identify cell types and secretory granules under light microscopy. Acidophilic components appear red, and basophilic ones blue.

heme: 1,3,5,8-tetramethyl-8,13-divinylporphine-6,7-dipropionic acid ferrous complex; the prosthetic group of hemoglobins, myoglobins, cytochrome b, and some catalases and peroxidases (and also of invertebrate erythrocruorins). In addition to its roles in respiratory gas transport (*see* **hemoglobins**), heme is a cofactor for fatty acid oxidation (*see* **prostaglandins**), soluble guanylate cyclases, and other enzymes, and it accelerates the synthesis of some P450 types by modulating transcription factor associations with some genes. It affects several other functions by binding nitric oxide and other biologically active substances, and also binds cyanide. Hematin is an oxidation product prepared for chemical estimation of hemoglobin content, and made by some individuals with pernicious anemia or exposed to certain environmental toxins. *See also* **porphyrins, heme oxygenase, and iron response elements**.

hementin: a calcium-dependent protease made by the salivary glands of the South American giant leech, *Haementeria ghiliarii*. It lyses both fibrinogen and fibrin, and is used as anticoagulant.

hemerythrins: non-heme, high molecular weight (approximately 180K) oxygen carrying proteins that circulate in polychaete worms, brachiopods, and some other invertebrates. Each of the eight subunits of a hemerythrin molecule carries two ferrous ions. The proteins are colorless, but appear pink to violet when they take up oxygen and become oxyhemerythrins.

heme oxygenases: heme oxygenase-1 is a 32K enzyme abundant in liver and spleen, that catalyzes heme degradation to biliverdin (which is then converted to bilirubin), and acts on other porphyrins. Since it is induced by ultraviolet radiation, hydrogen peroxide, heavy metals, and sodium arsenite, and high temperatures promote formation of small amounts in glial cells and a few neuron types, it is classified as a stress protein. The bilirubin product is a scavenger that defends against free radical accumulation. Heme oxygenase-2 is a noninducible enzyme made in discrete brain regions. Its major function there may be generation of **carbon monoxide**

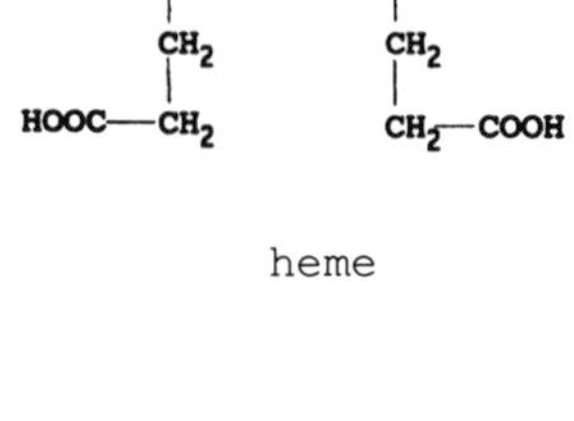

heme

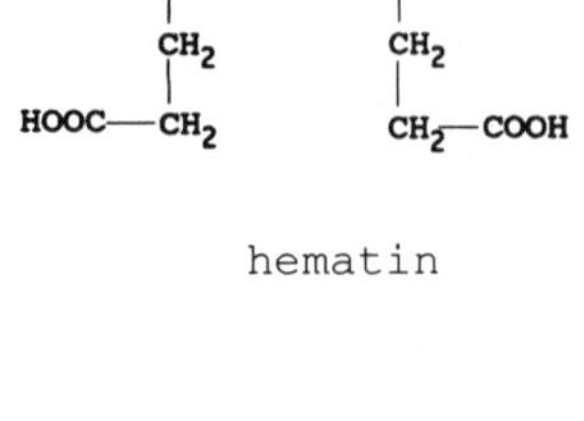

hematin

(*q.v.*), a gas implicated as a neurotransmitter involved in olfaction and long-term potentiation.

hemiacetals: compounds that contain the chemical group shown on the left, formed by reversible combination of an alcoholic with a ketone group. Compounds that contain it include pyranose and furanose sugars, and aldosterone.

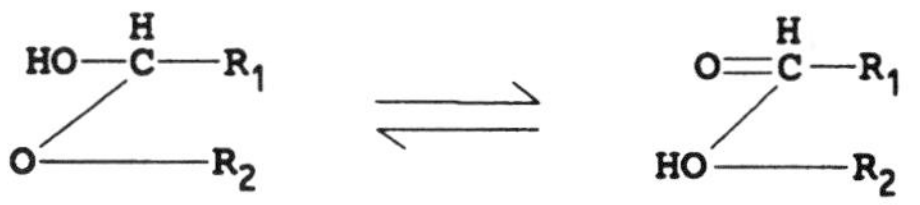

hemicastration: removal of one testicle or ovary, performed if the organ is diseased, or in laboratory animals to study compensatory hypertrophy of the remaining organ, or effects of the loss on gametogenesis, and to transiently lower gonadal hormone levels.

hemicholinium-3: 2,2'-[1,1'-biphenyl]-4,4-dimethyl-morpholinium bromide; a potent, selective inhibitor of choline uptake.

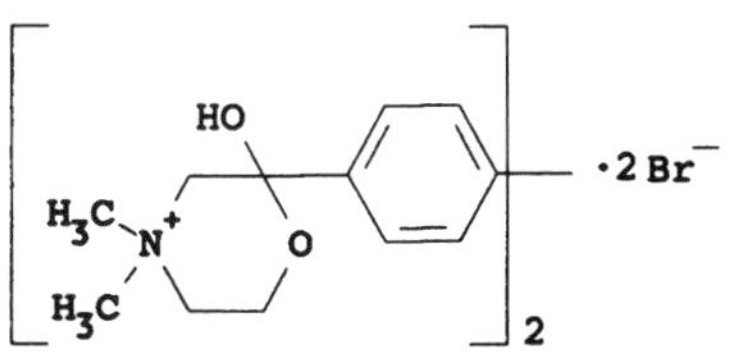

hemidesmosome: a specialization of the plasma membrane of a stratified epithelium basal cell that anchors the cell to the basal lamina. Integrin $\alpha_6\beta_4$ is essential for its assembly and maintenance. *See also* **desmosome**.

hemiplegia: loss of sensation and voluntary function on one side of the body; *cf* **quadriplegia** and **paraplegia**.

hemizygote: a cell or organism of a diploid species with a single copy of a specified gene, chromosome segment, or chromosome type. The term can refer to a gamete or to a normal male with just one X chromosome.

hemo-: a prefix meaning blood. The British form is haemo-.

hemochorial: describes the kind of **placenta** (*q.v.*), in which trophoblast invasion of maternal tissue is extensive, with destruction of maternal blood vessels, and rupture of larger ones during parturition. *Cf* **epitheliochorial** and **syndesmochorial**.

hemochromatosis: hemachromatosis; chronic, progressive disorders caused by autosomal defects that impair iron metabolism, ingestion of excessive amounts of the metal, or repeated blood transfusions. Chronic elevation of the blood levels leads to deposition of iron in tissues, discolors the skin, and can cause cirrhosis of the liver, joint disease, pituitary insufficiency, a diabetes mellitus-like syndrome, and cardiac failure.

hemochrome: hemoglobin, hemocyanin, hemerythrin, erythrocruorin, chlorocruorin, or any other oxygen-carrying blood pigment.

hemocyanins: 450K-13,000K non-heme, copper-containing oxygen-transporting proteins in arthropod and mollusc hemolymph. Keyhole-limpet hemocyanin (KLH), and some others are used as antigens in laboratory studies. Oxyhemocyanin, which is blue, contains one oxygen bound to two copper atoms. Deoxyhemocyanin is colorless.

hemocyte: any formed element of the blood.

hemocytoblast: hematoblast; hemoblast; a totipotential stem cell that can give rise to any of the formed elements of the blood.

hemocytoblastoma: hematocytoblastoma; leukemia.

hemocytometers: instruments used to count blood cells.

hemocytopoiesis: hematopoiesis.

hemodialysis: procedures used to change the composition of blood plasma, for example in individuals with impaired kidney function. Blood is sent through tubing that permits passive (diffusional) exchange of small molecules and ions with a surrounding fluid of controlled composition. Concentration gradients drive removal of nitrogenous wastes, adjustment of electrolyte balance, and, in some cases, uptake of specific nutrients.

hemodiapedesis: passage of blood cells through capillary walls; *see* also **diapedesis**.

hemodilution: accumulation of excessive amounts of water in blood. It can increase the demand on cardiac muscle (since larger amounts of blood must be pumped to achieve adequate oxygenation), disrupt osmotic balance, and invoke edema. The causes include renal dysfunctions and endocrine imbalances that impair water excretion. Vasopressin directly promotes water retention by kidney cells. Aldosterone acts indirectly by augmenting sodium reabsorption.

hemoglobins: Hb: ferrohemoglobins; the pigments that carry respiratory gases in most vertebrates, and account for most of the erythrocyte mass. In mammals, the molecules are tetramers with molecular weights of approximately 64.5K. Each subunit is a globin polypeptide chain linked to a heme. A single iron atom in the ferrous state associates with all four heme groups. The predominant type in human adults is hemoglobin A_1, which contains two α and two β type globin chains. Chronic hyperglycemia causes conversion of some of it to hemoglobin$_{A1c}$ via **nonenzymatic glycosylation** (*q.v.*) of -lysyl moieties. Normal human blood also contains 1.5-3% hemoglobin A_2, with two α and two δ chains. Hemoglobin F, with two α and two γ chains, and a somewhat higher affinity for oxygen, is the major fetal type. In β-thalassemia, A_2 is made in much larger amounts, whereas hemoglobin H, which contains only γ chains, predominates in α-thalassemias. Hemoglobin S is the mutant form that characterizes sickle cell anemia. With the exception of some fishes that live in very cold water, other vertebrates make tetramers similar to mammalian types. Leghemoglobins are related proteins made by some plants. The hemoglobin Fe-heme component reversibly binds oxygen and transports it from the lungs to tissue cells. The amounts carried vary directly with the oxygen tension of the environment (high in the lungs and low in tissues supplied by systemic capillaries); but high H^+ and CO_2 levels, and high temperatures lower the affinity for oxygen, as does bisphosphoglycerate binding to the hemoglobin. Since oxygenated Hb associates with potassium in erythrocytes, whereas unoxygenated Hb binds hydrogen ions, the pigment also performs buffer functions, and contributes to the control of acid-base balance. The exchange can be represented as: $KHbO_2 + H^+ \rightarrow HHb + K^+ + O_2$. Small amounts of circulating carbon dioxide attach to globin amino groups, to form carbaminohemoglobin; but most blood CO_2 is carried as bicarbonate, formed in reactions catalyzed by erythrocyte carbonic anhydrase; see **chloride shift**. Carbon monoxide can displace oxygen and cause formation of carbon monoxide-hemoglobin (HbCO), which does not take up oxygen. The oxygen carrying capacity is also abolished by oxidation of the iron to the ferric state. The resulting product is methemoglobin, hemoglobin M). *See* also **heme, erythropoietin** and **bilirubin**.

hemolymph: the extracellular fluid of invertebrates that performs functions analogous to those of vertebrate blood. It contains high molecular weight oxygen carrying pigments (such as hemocyanin), but no erythrocytes or comparable cell types.

hemolysins: antibodies, toxins made by microorganisms, and other agents that destroy erythrocyte membranes by activating the complement system.

hemolysis: erythrocyte membrane rupture, with discharge of hemoglobin. It occurs when the cells are exposed to hypo-osmotic environments, and take up excessive quantities of fluid (*see* also **ghosts**), and when hemolysins, detergents, or other agents damage the membranes. Although some enters the urine, hemoglobin filtered by renal glomeruli can plug renal tubules and severely disrupt kidney functions.

hemolytic anemias: erythrocyte deficiencies caused by excessively rapid red blood cell destruction. They can be invoked by genetic defects that lead to production of abnormal hemoglobins and red blood cell fragility, autoimmune processes, phagocytic cell dysfunctions, malaria parasites, some bacterial toxins, and some pharmacological agents. *See* also **Rh factor**.

hemolytic plaque assays: sensitive techniques for detecting specific kinds of proteins released by or expressed on the surfaces of cells, in which antibodies applied to erythrocyte surfaces form complement-activating complexes with those proteins, and promote hemoglobin release. Since minute amounts of hemoglobin are easily detected, the assays are especially useful for identifying compounds made in very small amounts, and specific cell types within tissues that contain many other kinds. They are used to determine which secretory products are made by various cell types in pituitary gland preparations, and the effects of regulators on hormone release, and also to identify lymphocyte subsets that make specific kinds of immunoglobulins.

hemonectin: a bone marrow stromal protein that mediates cell adhesion.

hemopexin: an acute phase protein made in the liver and activated by interleukin-6.

hemophilias: inherited diseases in which blood **coagulation** (*q.v.*) is impaired. Hemophilia A (classic hemophilia) is an X-linked recessive disorder that affects the synthesis of factor VIII. In hemophilia B (Christmas disease), which is also X-linked, the missing component is factor IX. Hemophilia C is a rarer autosomal defect that impairs synthesis of factor XI.

hemopoietins: mitogens that increase the sensitivities of hematopoietic stem cells to other regulators. Hemopoietin-1, which synergizes with macrophage colony stimulating factor (M-CSF) to stimulate stem cells that do not respond to M-CSF alone, may be identical with interleukin-1α.

hemosiderins: iron-rich proteins that deposit in body tissues. The predominant type is ferritin, or a closely related substance. *See* also **hemochromatosis**.

hemostasis: bleeding arrest. It is initiated under physiological conditions by localized vasoconstriction and formation of a platelet plug at the site of a blood vessel injury. This is sufficient to control the very small breaks in blood vessel walls that occur frequently under normal conditions. Coagulation follows when plugging does not control the problem.

henbane: the dried leaves and seeds of *Hyoscyamus niger*. *See* **hyoscyamine**.

Henderson-Hasselbalch equation: a mathematical statement that relates the relative concentration of a weak acid [HA] and its salt [A⁻] to the dissociation constant (K) and the pH: $pH = pK + \log \frac{[A^-]}{[HA]}$. It is used to calculate the amounts of acid and salt required to obtain a buffer solution of specified pH.

Henle loop: a U-shaped nephron segment, comprising a descending limb that is continuous with, and receives processed glomerular filtrate from the proximal convoluted tubule, a hairpin turn region, and an ascending limb that delivers fluid to the distal convoluted tubule. Most of the cells of the descending, hairpin, and lower ascending portions are flattened and highly permeable to water and salts. In long Henle loops, the upper part of the ascending limb (the thick segment) contains larger cells that actively pump chloride ions to the extracellular fluid, resist inward diffusion of water and salts, and create a hypertonic interstitial fluid in the renal medulla. The fluid, which is rich in NaCl and urea, is essential for vasopressin mediated water conservation. There are controversies concerning whether sodium ions exit passively down electrical gradients created by the chloride transport, or are actively extruded. *See* also **loop diuretics**.

Hensen's node: primitive knot; a small pit surrounded by an elevated region at the cephalic end of the primitive streak of a vertebrate embryo, visible in humans around

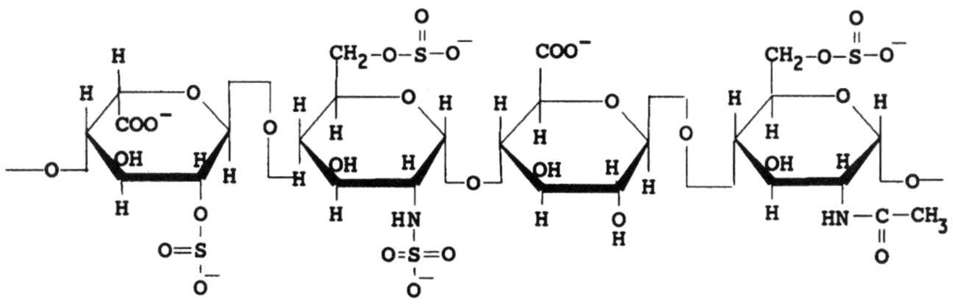

heparan sulfate

the 16th day after conception. During gastrulation, cells migrate through this region, and the node marks the origin of the central canal of the developing notochord.

heparan sulfate: heparitin sulfate: 5-12K glycosaminoglycans of variable composition that contain D-glucuronic acid, L-iduronic acid, and *N*-acetyl-D-glucosamine moieties, most of which are sulfated at one or two positions, along with small amounts of D-galactose and D-xylose. A typical tetrasaccharide fragment is shown. They are components of extracellular matrices, and of cell surface proteoglycans, some of which function as low affinity receptors for basic fibroblast growth factors (bFGFs), a few other growth factors, and some cell adhesion molecules (including N-CAM). Some are heparin precursors that exert heparin-like effects on blood coagulation and cell proliferation. Production accelerates in cultured endothelial cells when confluence is attained.

heparin[s]: linear acidic glycosaminoglycans of variable size and composition, composed mostly of alternating glucuronic acid or iduronic acid, and glucosamine moieties, many of which are sulfated. Most are covalently linked to proteins in 600-100K complexes. Heparins are synthesized in liver, lung, mast cells, basophilic leukocytes, endothelial cells, and at other sites, and are components of cell surface and extracellular matrix proteoglycans that attach to numerous regulatory molecules. They bind and affect the actions of fibroblast growth factors, and are cofactors for lipoprotein lipases. The anticoagulant activity is attributed to their ability to bind thrombin and anti-thrombin III, and thereby augment antithrombin activity. A component with an anti-thrombin binding site is shown, in which R_1 can be either H or SO_3^-, and R_2 can be either SO_3^- or $COCH_3$. High concentrations also block platelet aggregation. 12K-30K protein-free fragments are used to protect against the formation of intravascular blood clots. Smaller ones that lack anti-coagulant properties can block proliferation of

fibroblasts, vascular smooth muscle, mesangial, some epithelial, and some other cell types, by inhibiting a kinase-C dependent pathway that leads to induction of *c-fos* and *c-myc* proteins. They additionally suppress formation of epidermal growth factor (EGF) receptors. Since heparins can inhibit the binding of inositol-1,4,5-triphosphate (IP_3) binding to its receptors, some actions are mediated (or augmented) by influences on Ca^{2+} metabolism.

heparin binding EGF-like growth factor: HB-EGF; a heat resistant, 20K protein with intramolecular disulfide bonds, chemically and structurally related to amphiregulin, and more distantly to epidermal growth factor and transforming growth factor-α (TGF-α). It is secreted by activated macrophages, and acts on EGF receptors (where it displaces EGF), but is a much more potent smooth muscle mitogen. It also stimulates proliferation of fibroblasts and keratinocytes (but not capillary endothelium). Roles in wound repair and contributions to the development of atherosclerosis are mediated by the receptors, and also via binding to cell surface and extracellular matrix heparin.

heparinases: enzymes that degrade heparin, now more commonly called heparin lyases.

heparin binding growth factors: mitogens and related regulators whose activities are affected by heparin binding; *see* α-**fibroblast growth factors** and β-**fibroblast growth factors** for types I and II, respectively.

heparin lyases: heparinases; the major heparin degrading enzymes. They cleave hexosamine groups.

hepatectomy: surgical removal of the liver. Total removal is not compatible with survival, but partial hepatectomy is performed on laboratory animals to study liver functions and regeneration. Since the surgery inflicts severe trauma, hepatotoxic agents such as carbon tetrachloride are more commonly used.

hepatic: related to the liver.

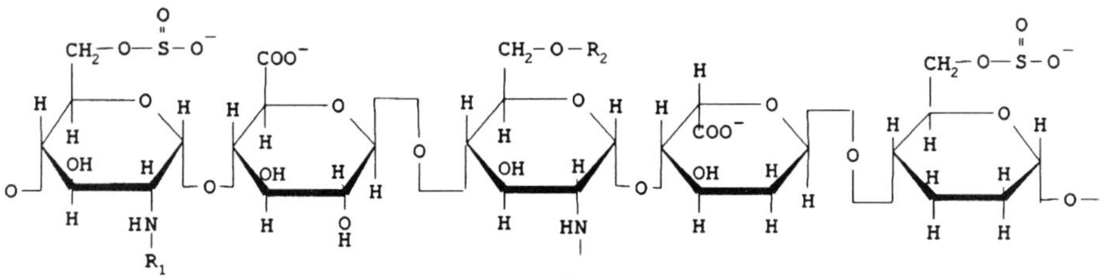

heparins

hepatic portal system: the blood vessels that transport nutrients, hormones and other substances from the small intestine, pancreas, and associated structures to the liver. *See* also **portal systems**.

hepatocyte[s]: the parenchymal cells of the **liver** *(q.v.)*. When mature, they display regional differences in enzyme content. Most do not divide under normal conditions, but *see* **hepatocyte growth factors** and **hepatopoietins**. Formation of similar cells in the exocrine pancreas can be induced with agents that deplete copper.

hepatocyte growth factor[s]: HGFs; regulators, initially identified as mitogens for liver parenchymal cells, that mediate regeneration after injury, and may be identical with scatter factor. A 28K protein (p28) similar to plasminogen activator, and some other serine proteases with such activity have been isolated from blood plasma, platelets, and stromal fibroblast conditioned media. HGF is also a paracrine stimulant for proliferation of melanocytes, endothelial cells, and some epithelium-derived cell types. *See* also **hepatocyte growth factor receptors**, **hepatopoietins** and **basic fibroblast growth factors**.

hepatocyte growth factor antagonist: a 28K protein derived from the messenger RNA that directs the synthesis of hepatocyte growth factor. It binds to the same receptors, competes with HGF when present in high concentrations, and directly inhibits fibroblast mitogenesis. It is made in larger amounts in quiescent than in activated fibroblasts, and is believed to contribute to reestablishment of the resting state following regeneration and wound repair.

hepatocyte growth factor receptor: a 145K protein whose synthesis is directed by the *c-met* proto-oncogene. It displays ligand-activated tyrosine kinase activity, undergoes autophosphorylation, and mediates the effects of both hepatocyte growth factor and hepatocyte growth factor inhibitor.

hepatocyte nuclear factor: HNF-1; a protein of the steroid receptor superfamily that regulates transcription in the liver.

hepatocyte stimulating factor: HSF; *see* **interleukin-6**.

hepatoma growth factor: *see* **fibroblast growth factors** and **scatter factor**.

hepatopoietins: HPTs; proteins that promote DNA synthesis and mitosis in mature hepatocytes. Hepatopoietin A is an acidic glycoprotein composed of 69-70K α and 34-35K β subunits held together by disulfide bonds, produced in acinar cells of the exocrine pancreas, that

may be identical with **hepatocyte growth factor** *(q.v.)*. It travels to the liver via the hepatic portal system, and contributes to regeneration and repair. The blood levels rise after chemical injury (for example with carbon tetrachloride), following partial hepatectomy, and in humans with severe hepatitis. HPTs are also made by submaxillary and parotid glands, by neurons, and possibly also by hepatocytes, and are present in blood platelets, megakaryocytes, kidney, heart, lung, and small intestine. The actions are antagonized by transforming growth factor-β (TGFβ), which is made by hepatocytes. Insulin synergizes with HPT-A, and norepinephrine acts via α_1-type receptors to augment HPT-A and diminish TGFβ effects. Hepatopoietin B (HPT-B) is an as yet uncharacterized growth factor with a molecular weight of less than 500.

hepatotoxic agents: chemicals that invoke liver injury. Since the liver is a major site for uptake, accumulation, and detoxification of foreign substances, it is easily damaged. Carbon tetrachloride and galactosamine are used to study liver functions and regeneration.

HEPES: 4-(2-hydroxyethyl)-1-piperazine-ethanesulfonic acid; a buffer in the physiological pH range, used for cell cultures and in chromatography. It does not cross plasma membranes.

heptoses: 7-carbon sugars, for example seduloheptose; *see* **hexose monophosphate shunt**.

HER: *HER2 (erbB2)* is a human gene that codes for p185^erbB2, a protein that is overexpressed in, and is implicated in the etiology of some breast cancers and other neoplasms. It resembles the epidermal growth factor receptor, but neither EGF (nor transforming factor-α, TGFα) binds with high affinity and activates. The rat counterparts are *neu* gene and p185^c-neu protein. HER3 (c-erb3) is a closely related protein. Heregulins are 228 to 241 amino-acid proteins made in small amounts by normal cells, and in larger ones by malignant types, that activate HER receptors and may be the natural ligands.

herbimycin A: an antibiotic made by several *Streptomyces* species that blocks tyrosine phosphorylation.

Hercules: a term used with numbers for trade names of several agents that kill insects and/or worms. Some are acetylcholinesterase inhibitors. Hercules 528, dioxathion, is phosphorodithioic acid *S,S*-1,4-dioxane-2,3-diyl *O,O,O,O*-tetraethyl ester. Hercules 14503, dialifor, is

Hercules 528

Hercules 14503

phosphorodithioic acid *S*-[2-chloro-1-(1,3-dihydro-1,3-dioxo-2*H*-isoindol-2-yl)ethyl] *O,O*-diethyl ester.

herculin gene: a member of the *MyoD* gene family that resembles *Myf-5* (to which it is linked), *Myo-D*, and the myogenin gene, but is expressed at higher levels than the others. Its product enhanced expression of all three types, and promotes differentiation of fibroblasts to skeletal muscle cells.

heregulins: *see* **HER**.

Her **genes**: *see* **HER** and *erbB-2*.

hermaphrodite: an individual with gonads that produce both male and female type gametes (or resemble ones that make them). In some cases, there is one ovary and one testis, and in others two ovotestes, or an ovotestis plus one ovary or one testis. Hermaphroditism is a normal condition in earthworms, tapeworms, some fish species, and a few other animal types. In most vertebrates, it is caused by sex chromosome aberrations, problems that arise during fertilization or cleavage, or deleterious prenatal influences. *See* **sex determination**, **sequential hermaphroditism**, **protandry**, **protogyny**, **chimeras**, and **freemartin**; and *cf* **pseudohermaphrodite**.

hereditary angioneurotic edema: two or more autosomal dominant diseases attributed to defective production of the C1 inhibitor of the complement pathway, with consequent generation of a kinin-like peptide from C2b that augments capillary permeability. The major manifestations are recurrent episodes of subcutaneous, intestinal, and/or laryngeal swelling.

heritable: transmitted from one generation to the next via cell components. The term does not necessarily imply transmission via nuclear chromosomes (*see* **cytoplasmic inheritance**).

Hermes antigen: CD-44.

heroin: diacetylmorphine; a derivative of **morphine** *(q.v.)* that exerts similar effects but invokes stronger euphoria and is more addictive.

Herpes **viruses**: double-stranded DNA viruses with 80-200 linear genes that infect humans, and related viruses that inhabit other species. *Herpes simplex Type I* (HSV-1) is ubiquitous in humans and is activated by heat. During fevers, it causes cold sores around the lips (which lack sweat glands). *Herpes simplex Type II* (HSV-2, genital herpes) causes reproductive system lesions, and is sexually transmitted. Both types are implicated in the etiology of some forms of cancer. Thymidine kinases

(HSV-TKB) derived from them are used in several kinds of studies (*see*, for example **HAT medium**). *Herpes zoster* (varicella zoster) causes chicken pox and shingles. Other members of the group include cytomegalovirus and Epstein-Barr virus. All types can establish latent infections that become activated when immune system functions are impaired.

Herring bodies: secretory granules of magnocellular neurohypophysial neurons. They contain neurophysins and peptide hormones.

Hers disease: glycogen storage disease VI; an autosomal recessive disorder in which the synthesis of hepatic glycogen phosphorylase is impaired. It is usually a milder condition that von Gierke's disease (glycogen storage disease I), but invokes hypoglycemia, and in some cases gout, and can retard growth in children.

HETEs: hydroxyeicosatetraenoic acids.

heteroalleles: a gene pair on homologous chromosomes of a diploid cell whose members differ from each other in that one carries a mutation at a site different from the mutation on the other; *cf* **homoalleles**.

heterocaryon: heterokaryon.

heterochromatin: transcriptionally inactive chromosome regions with large segments of repetitive base sequences. They condense during interphase, and replicate later than euchromatin. *See* also **X inactivation**.

heteroclitic antibody: an antibody with higher affinity for a heterologous antigen (or antigenic determinant) than for the antigen that stimulated its production.

heterocyclic: describes (1) single rings with more than one kind of atom (as in pyrimidines, imidazoles, and thiophenes); (2) organic compounds with two or more different ring types, such as indoles, quinoles, and steroids.

heterocytotropic: having affinity for cells of other species.

heterocytotropic antibodies: antibodies made by a different species that bind to host components. They can activate mast cells and invoke anaphylactic reactions. *Cf* **homocytotropic antibodies**.

heterodimers: molecules (usually polypeptides or proteins) with two different kinds of **subunits**; *cf* **homodimers**.

heteroduplex: a structure formed by annealing two nucleic acid strands that contain complementary base sequences. It can comprise two DNA segments, one DNA and one RNA, or two RNA strands.

heterogametic: producing two different kinds of gametes, for example X and Y type spermatozoa, or W and Z type ova.

heterogeneic, heterogenic; having two or more different mutations (at the same or different loci) that affect the same phenotypic characteristic.

heterogenous nuclear RNA: hnRNA; primary transcripts that undergo processing to yield mature messenger RNAs.

heterogenous nuclear ribonucleoprotein: hnRNP; a bead-like particle composed of heterogenous nuclear RNA (hnRNA) wrapped around a core that contains at least eight 34K-120K proteins. The particles form when transcription is completed, and are essential for hnRNA processing.

heterografts: xenografts; *see* **grafts**.

heterokaryon: heterocaryon: a cell that contains two or more different kinds of nuclei, formed under normal conditions by some molds, or artificially via hybridization.

heterolecithal: describes an oocyte or ovum with unevenly distributed yolk components.

heterologous: derived from a different source; *see* also **desensitization**.

heteromorphous: having an unusual shape or form.

heterophile antigen: a substance that stimulates production of antibodies capable of binding with high affinity to cells of (or substances made by) other species.

heterophilic: capable of binding to more than one kind of entity.

heterosis: *see* **hybrid vigor**.

heterotherms: poikilotherms; organisms whose body temperatures vary with environmental factors such as temperature and ultraviolet radiation; *cf* **homeotherms**.

heterotopic: describes (1) a cell, tissue, or organ at a site it does not normally occupy. The term can apply to a graft, tumor, or set of cells that has migrated from its usual location; (2) the effects of two different ligands on an enzyme, receptor, or other molecule; *cf* **homotopic**.

heterotrophs: organisms that require organic nutrients made by other organisms; *cf* **autotrophs**.

heterotypic: of a different type.

heterotypic adhesion: adhesion of one cell type to a different cell type, or of one molecular species to another; *cf* **homotypic adhesion**.

heterotypic adhesion receptors: HAR; molecules that mediate adhesion of two or more different cell types, for example of leukocytes to endothelial cells. *See* also **homing receptors**.

heterozygous: possessing two different alleles for one or more genes; *cf* **homozygous**.

HETP: hexaethyl tetraphosphate.

HEV: high endothelial venules.

hexabrachion: a 6-armed structure. Cytotactin, tenascin, and some other extracellular matrix proteins are composed of six disulfide-linked polypeptide chains arranged like the spokes of a wheel.

hexaethyl tetraphosphate: HETP; an acetylcholinesterase inhibitor that is used as an insecticide.

hexaethyl tetraphosphate

hexamethonium: an agent that blocks acetylcholine-mediated ganglionic transmission. It is used under special conditions to treat some forms of hypertension, and as a laboratory tool.

hexestrol: 4,4′-(1,2-diethylethylene)*bis*phenol; dihydrodiethylstilbestrol; a non-steroidal estrogen receptor agonist, used orally and parenterally to treat estrogen deficiency and some conditions (such as postmenopausal osteoporosis) in which estrogens are believed to exert beneficial effects.

hexobarbital: hexobarbitone; Evipal; 5-cyclohexenyl-3,5-dimethylbarbituric acid; a short-acting, orally effective hypnotic and sedative. The sodium salt is used intravenously as a general anesthetic.

hexokinases: Mg^{2+}-dependent enzymes that catalyze the reaction essential for glucose entry into glycolysis, glycogenesis, and most other metabolic pathways: glucose + ATP $\rightarrow$ glucose-6-P + ADP. (They also act on mannose, but differ from fructokinase and galactokinase). Four major isozymes vary in distributions, substrate affinities, and sensitivities to feedback inhibition by glucose-6-phosphate. *Type I*, constitutively expressed in all cells, functions at low glucose concentrations, and is easily inhibited. *Type II*, induced by insulin and also rapidly activated by it in some cell types, has lower affinity for the substrate, and acts best at blood glucose concentrations closer to the upper limit of the physiological range in systemic blood. Elevation of the II:I ratio accelerates glucose uptake. *Hexokinase IV* (glucokinase), also induced by insulin, has the lowest affinity for glucose, is least affected by negative feedback, and functions efficiently at high glucose levels. The large amounts made in the liver facilitate rapid use of sugar delivered by the hepatic portal system during meal absorption. The pancreatic islet β cell isozyme contributes to glucose control over insulin secretion. *Type III* in liver functions at the lowest glucose concentrations, and supports the minimal glucose requirements of those cells during times of fasting. (Fatty acids are major energy sources for hepatocytes.)

hexosamines: sugars in which an —NH$_2$ group replaces one of the side-chain —OH groups, as in glucosamine and galactosamine. They are components (as such, or in forms that are phosphorylated or *N*-acetylated) of glycosaminoglycans, glycolipids, glycoproteins, and some other molecules.

hexosaminidases: enzymes that hydrolyze glycoside bonds of hexosamines and *N*-acetylhexosamines. A negatively charged isozyme (Type A) acts on glycolipids and protects against accumulation of excessive amounts of gangliosides (*see* **Tay Sachs disease**).

hexose: any 6-carbon sugar, such as glucose, fructose, mannose, galactose or fucose.

hexose monophosphate shunt: HMS; pentose pathway: a metabolic pathway especially active in adipose tissue and liver that generates NADPH and pentose sugars.

Some of the reactions are used in photosynthesis. Glucose-6-phosphate dehydrogenase catalyzes: glucose-6-P + NADP$^+$ → 6-phosphoglucono-δ-lactone + NADPH + H$^+$. The lactone rapidly hydrolyzes to 6-phosphogluconate, which reacts with a second molecule of NADP$^+$ to yield ribulose-5-phosphate + CO$_2$ + NADPH + H$^+$. The pentose phosphate can be converted to ribose-5-P via a reaction catalyzed by phosphopentose isomerase. A phosphopentose epimerase converts the product to xylulose-5-P, and a transketolase catalyzes a reaction in which one ribose-P and one xylulose-P combine to yield glyceraldehyde-3-P + sedulose-7-P. The glyceraldehyde-3-P can directly enter the glycolysis pathway, or be used in a reaction catalyzed by a transaldolase which provides fructose-6-P + erythrose-4-P. Transketolase also catalyzes xylulose-5-P + erythrose-P → glyceraldehyde-3-P + fructose-6-P.

hfr cells: bacterial cells that display high recombination frequencies and use F factors to integrate into chromosomes.

HGA: homogentisic acid.

H genes: DNA segments that code for constant and variable regions of immunoglobulin heavy chains.

HGFs: *see* **hepatocyte growth factors** and **hepatopoietins**.

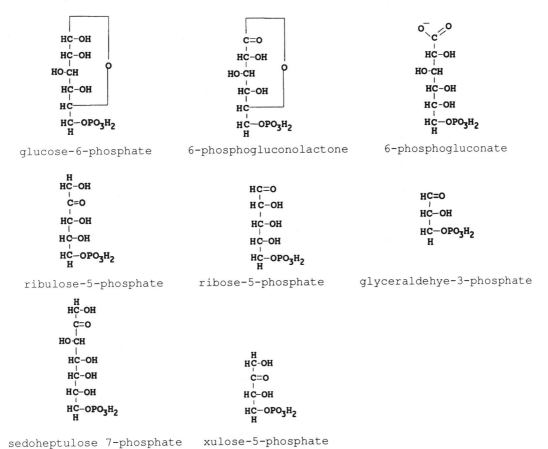

hexose monophosphate shunt

325

hGH: human growth hormone.

HGPRT: HPRT; hypoxanthine-guanine phosphoribosyltransferase.

HHM: (1) humoral hypercalcemia of malignancy; (2) heavy meromyosin; *see* **myosin**.

HHPS: hypothalamo-hypophysial portal system.

HHT: hydroxyhepatanoic acid.

HIAA: 5-HIAA; 5-hydroxyindole acetic acid.

hibernation: narcosis-like winter dormancy, associated with low metabolic rate and body temperature, from which arousal cannot be achieved with most stimuli that interrupt ordinary sleep; *cf* **torpor** and **estivation**. Hamsters, ground squirrels, and many other small mammals, and some poikilotherms, enter this state under natural conditions. Most undergo spontaneous, periodic, transient, partial rewarming and arousal, during which they hyperventilate and may excrete some urine. In males of some species, testosterone levels determine whether arousal will lead to full resumption of waking activity. Pineal gland hormones, and especially melatonin, are implicated as mediators of both hibernation and the physiological preparations that precede it (which include accumulation of fat stores, and replacement of some saturated fatty acids of membrane phospholipids with unsaturated types). The metabolic adjustments that permit long-term food deprivation with no ketosis are under investigation for possible application to the treatment of obesity and some metabolic derangements.

hibernomas: tumors derived from brown adipose tissue.

hidro-: a prefix that refers to sweat glands.

hidrosis: sweating.

high ceiling diuretics: loop diuretics; agents that rapidly invoke large increases in urine volume; *see*, for example **furosemide** and **ethacrynic acid**.

high density lipoproteins: HDLs: lipoprotein particles with diameters in the range of 100-150Å, and densities of 1.063-1.210. They sediment more rapidly than intermediate, low, and very low types (IDLs, LDLs and VLDLs), and transfer cholesterol esters to other **lipoproteins** *(q.v.)*.

high endothelium venules: HEV; lymphatic tissue venules with specialized columnar endothelial cells. Endothelial-leukocyte adhesion molecule-1 (ELAM-1) on the plasma membranes of mesenteric and peripheral lymph node cells binds lymphocyte homing receptors.

high energy bonds: chemical bonds that release substantial amounts of free energy when hydrolyzed. Phosphoenolpyruvate conversion to pyruvate yields 14.8 Calories per mole. Hydrolysis of either acetyl phosphate, or creatine phosphate yields 10.3, and ATP→ ADP + Pi 7.3. Other high energy compounds include GTP, ADP, and carbamyl phosphate. Some of the free energy is used to drive endergonic reactions.

high mobility group proteins: HMGs; acidic nuclear proteins, approximately 1/30 as abundant as histones, classified on the basis of electrophoretic mobility. They bind to 3′-untranslated DNA regions, and contribute to chromosome organization. Preferential association with actively transcribed genes, and extensive posttranslational modifications that alter their binding affinities (including glycosylation, poly ADP-ribosylation, methylation, phosphorylation by cdc2 kinase, acetylation, and methylation) are consistent with major roles in transcription regulation and other nuclear functions. Some effects of triiodothyronine (T_3) are attributed to cAMP-mediated phosphorylations at specific sites. HMG1 and HMG2 types associate with linker DNA and histone H1, and can promote DNA unwinding. HMG1 binds preferentially to A-T rich regions, and also selectively recognizes cruciform DNA. Its levels rise substantially in proliferating cells. HMG14 and HMG17, the most abundant types, associate preferentially with nucleosome cores that contain actively transcribed base sequences. Digestion with DNAase I releases them, and thereby abolishes additional degradation of the DNA by the enzyme. Excessive amounts of HMG14, encoded by human chromosome 21, are made by individuals with Down's syndrome.

high performance liquid chromatography: HPLC: *see* **chromatography**.

Hill coefficient: a measure of binding cooperativity, initially derived from the relationship between hemoglobin oxygenation and the partial pressure of the gas, but now more widely applied. For a reaction of the type A + B $\rightleftarrows$ AB, where [B] is the concentration of free ligand, [AB] the concentration of bound ligand, and Y = [AB]/[AB + [B], it is the value of the slope at midpoint, obtained when Log (Y/1-Y) is plotted on the Y axis and Log[B] on the X. Coefficients of 1, > 1, and < 1 indicate, respectively, no cooperativity, positive cooperativity, and negative cooperativity.

Hill reaction: the reaction in illuminated chloroplasts: 2 H_2O + 2 $NADP^+$ → O_2 + 2 NADPH + $2H^+$. It can be demonstrated with nonbiological electron acceptors such as ferricyanide (which is reduced to ferrocyanide), and with the Hill reagent, 2,6-dichlorindophenol (shown below) which changes from blue when oxidized to colorless when reduced.

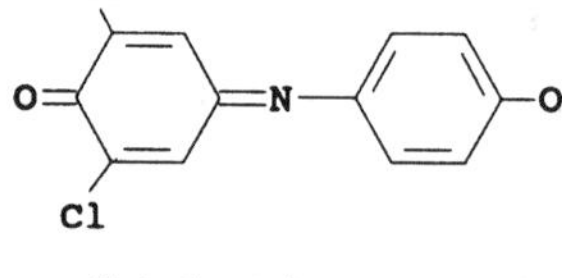

hilum: (1) a small indentation, gap, or hollow region of an organ (such as a lymph node or kidney) that provides an entry site for blood vessels, nerves, and, in some cases, ducts; (2) the scar on a plant seed coat that marks the former attachment site for the ovule stalk.

Himalayan: a mutant allele identified in some mice, rats, guinea pigs, hamsters, and cats that directs synthesis of a tyrosinase whose activity rises at low body temperatures. (It accounts for the dark color of the ear tips and other cool regions in Siamese cats.)

Hind III: a restriction endonuclease derived from *Hemophilus influenzae Rd*, used to generate sticky ends. It catalyzes cleavage of double stranded DNA segments between adenine components:

$$\downarrow$$

5'-A-A-G-C-T-T-3'

3'-T-T-C-G-A-A-5'

$$\uparrow$$

hindbrain: the most posterior of the three brain vesicles of a vertebrate embryo. It gives rise to the metencephalon (the forerunner of the medulla oblongata) and the rhomb-encephalon (which forms the cerebellum).

hindgut: the posterior segment of the embryonic intestine that terminates in the cloaca. It is the precursor of the sigmoid colon and rectum.

hinge region: a protein domain that imparts flexibility and permits changes in the relative positions of the CH_1 and CH_2 chains of IgG, IgA, and IgD type immunoglobulins (*q.v.*), and of components of steroid hormone receptors and some other compounds. Hinge regions of immunoglobulins are sites for cleavage between F(ab)' and Fab fragments.

HIOMT: hydroxyindole-*O*-methyltransferase.

hippocampus: an arched region of the temporal lobe of the cerebrum that borders the floor of the lateral ventricle, and includes Ammon's horn (the hippocampus proper) and the dentate gyrus. It receives afferent innervation from the enterorhinal cortex, and gives rise to the fornix. The hippocampus is a component of the limbic system (Papez circuit), and a major site involved in learning and memory. Some cells respond to glucocorticoids, contribute to the regulation of glucocorticoid and growth hormone secretion, and can be damaged by high levels of the steroid.

hippuric acid: *N*-benzoylglycine; benzoic acid conjugated with glycine, a compound initially identified in the urine of horses, to which it imparts a characteristic odor. Humans normally excrete minute amounts, but more is made when cranberries, asparagus, other foods rich in benzoic acid are eaten or pharmaceutical agents that contain benzoic acid are ingested. Hippuric acid is filtered by glomeruli and is actively secreted by distal convoluted tubule cells; and an analog (para-aminohippuric acid) is used in renal function tests. Several small hippuric acid peptides are substrates for enzyme assays. Hippuryl-phenylalanine is used for carboxypeptidase A, and both Hip-His-Leu-OH and Hip-Gly-Gly-OH for angiotensin converting enzyme.

hirsutism: excessive hair growth, usually with male-type distribution in girls or women. The causes include excessive androgen production (for example by adrenocortical

or ovarian tumors), aberrant androgen metabolism, or formation of abnormal or excessive numbers of androgen receptors. *See* also **adrenogenital syndrome**.

hirudin: an approximately 10.8K polypeptide made by the salivary glands of *Hirudo medicinalis* and some other leeches. It exerts antithrombin activity and is used as an anticoagulant. Hirudin [54-65] (H_2N-Gly-Asp-Phe-Glu-Glu-Ile-Pro-Glu-Glu-Tyr-Leu-Gln-OH), hirudin [54-65] sulfated on the tyrosyl moiety, and *N*-acetyl-hirudin [54-65] are used in assays.

Hirudo: a genus of leeches. They make **hirudin** (*q.v.*), and are used to remove extravasated blood.

His: H; histidine.

His bundle: Bundle of His; A-V bundle: a strip of tissue within the heart specialized for transmission of electrical stimuli from the atrioventricular (A-V) node to the Purkinje fibers of the ventricle.

Hismanal: a trade name for astemizole.

histaminase: histamine deaminase; histidine oxidase; diamine oxidase; a copper-containing enzyme made by kidney, intestinal mucosa, activated mast, and some other cell types, that catalyzes conversion of histamine to imidazoleacetic acid.

histamine: a hormone and neurotransmitter made from histidine via a reaction catalyzed by histidine decarboxylase, in cells of the lungs, spleen, brain, uterus, gastrointestinal tract, and elsewhere, and a component of venoms, microorganisms, and plants. In mast cells and basophilic leukocytes, it co-exists with, and is co-released with heparin, eosinophil chemotactic factor, neutrophil chemotactic factor, and several enzymes (including neutral proteinases, superoxide dismutase, and peroxidase). The mast cells are abundant in skin, and in bronchial and intestinal mucosa; and many physiological, pharmacological, and environmental factors promote their degranulation. They have receptors for IgE type immunoglobulins, and are major sites for the release that contributes in several ways to inflammatory and allergic reactions. Histamine augments the permeability of postcapillary venules and promotes transudation of blood components, stimulates contraction of respiratory tract smooth muscle, accelerates neutrophilic leukocyte chemotaxis and degranulation, dilates small blood vessels, and can cause pain, itching, burning sensations, and skin eruptions. The effects of low concentrations vary widely with the species. Whereas minute amounts invoke lethal bronchospasm in guinea pigs, quantities 100-fold greater are easily tolerated by rats. In humans, histamine contributes to asthmatic attacks, but is less important than leukotrienes. Injection of small amounts rapidly invokes flushing, hypotension, headache, and nasal stuffiness. Histamine also promotes platelet aggregation, stimulates intestinal and uterine smooth muscle sufficiently to cause pain, augments hydrochloric acid production in the stomach, affects gastric emptying, acts on other exocrine glands, and contributes to ovulation and implantation. It additionally promotes the release of norepinephrine, epinephrine, adrenocorticotropic hormone (ACTH), aldosterone, prolactin and some other hormones. Influences are exerted in different ways on the cell proliferation associated with wound healing and tumor growth. In the central nervous system, the highest concentrations are in the hypothalamus; and the levels in cerebrospinal fluid exceed by far the ones in circulating blood. Smaller amounts are in the thalamus, cerebrum, and cerebellum. The receptors are located on glial cells and blood vessels as well as neurons. The central effects include stimulation of prandial drinking and vasopressin release, contributions to arousal and pain perception, acceleration of cerebral blood flow, and influences on body temperature and on some cardiovascular reflexes. Histamine injection can invoke restlessness, anxiety, and insomnia, and in some cases, convulsions, and is implicated as a mediator of motion sickness. Histamine released by neurons in the hippocampus augments NMDA-mediated synaptic transmission, and may contribute to long-term potentiation. *See* also **histamine receptors**.

```
HC═══C─CH₂─CH₂─NH₂
 |     |
HN     N
   \ C /
     |
     H
```

α-methyl-**histamine**: α-MH: the *R* stereoisomer is a selective, potent agonist for H_3 histamine receptors, with limited affinity for H_1 and H_2 types. The *S* isomer is a very weak agonist for all three receptor types.

2-methyl-**histamine**: an H_1 type histamine receptor agonist.

```
HC═══C─CH₂─CH₂─NH₂
 |     |
HN     N
   \ C /
     |
     CH₃
```

3-methyl-**histamine**; *N*-methyl-histamine: a histamine degradation product, made mostly in the central nervous system via a reaction catalyzed by histamine *N*-methyltransferase.

```
HC═══C─CH₂─CH₂─NH₂
 |     |
 N     N
H₃C \ C /
     |
     H
```

4-methyl-**histamine**: an H_2 type histamine receptor agonist.

```
H₃C─C═══C─CH₂─CH₂─NH₂
    |     |
   HN     N
      \ C /
        |
        H
```

histamine *N*-methyltransferase: HNMT: an enzyme prevalent in the central nervous system that catalyzes conversion of histamine to 3-methyl-histamine. Small amounts of the product are directly excreted to the urine. Larger ones are oxidized by monoamine oxidase B to methylimadazole acetic acid.

histaminergic: describes (1) neurons that release histamine; (2) responses invoked by histamine (including ones initiated by release of other mediators).

histamine receptors: widely distributed proteins that mediate histamine actions. Two or three kinds can co-exist in the same cell and undergo simultaneous activation. H_1 subtypes play major roles in inflammation, allergic reactions, and smooth muscle contraction. Ligand binding leads to the generation of inositol phosphates and activation of kinase C isozymes. H_2 subtypes are coupled to G proteins that augment adenylate cyclase activity. They mediate gastric acid secretion and the release of several hormones. H_3 subtypes inhibit both histidine decarboxylase activity and histamine release. The highest levels are in the basal ganglia and olfactory regions. *See* also **histamine receptor antagonists**.

histamine receptor antagonists: H_1-type antagonists (such as diphenhydramine) are used to alleviate allergic reactions. Most cross blood brain barriers. Drowsiness is a major side-effect; and some are components of non-prescription preparations used to promote sleep. (The ones that do not cross the barriers are effective on brain cells when presented *in vitro*.) H_2 antagonists inhibit hydrochloric acid production by gastric parietal cells, and some additionally inhibit pepsinogen release. In order of decreasing potency, the ones most commonly used to treat gastric ulcers include famotidine (Pepcid), nizatidine (Axid), ranitidine (Zantac), and cimetidine (Tagamet). *See* also **burimamide**, **metiamide**, and **tiotidine**. Some of the side-effects (for example on intestinal absorption) are attributed to changes in cell and extracellular fluid pH. Although used for its effectiveness in treating ulcers, cimetidine suppresses immune system responses, inhibits P450-dependent hepatic enzymes, aldosterone release, adrenocorticotropic hormone (ACTH)-stimulated cortisol secretion, and dihydrotestosterone (DHT) binding to androgen receptors, and stimulates prolactin release. Omeprazole and related agents block HCl production by directly inhibiting gastric H^+/K^+-ATPase.

histaminocytes: mast-like gastrointestinal tract cells that release histamine.

histidine: His; H: an essential glucogenic amino acid. It is the direct precursor of histamine, and can also be metabolized to glutamate. Histidine is also a component of many proteins, including hemoglobin, and a constituent of the active sites of chymotrypsin and related

```
                H
HC═══C─CH₂─C─NH₂
 |     |    |
HN     N    H
   \ C /   CH₃
     |
     H
```
R-form

```
                H
HC═══C─CH₂─C─NH₂
 |     |    |
HN     N    H
   \ C /   CH₃
     |
     H
```
S-form

α-methyl-histamine

enzymes. Collagens contain small amounts. Since the amino acid is positively charged at physiological pH, it and can perform buffer functions. Degradation occurs mostly in the liver; *see* **histidine-ammonia lyase**. Long-term deficiency impairs hemoglobin synthesis. *See also* **histidinemia**.

α-fluoromethyl-**histidine**: an irreversible inhibitor of histidine decarboxylase.

histidine-ammonia lyase: the major enzyme for histidine degradation. It catalyzes: histidine → urocanate + NH_4^+. Inability to make sufficient enzyme is a major cause of histidinemia. Urocanic dehydratase catalyzes conversion of urocanate to 4-imidazolone-5-propionate, which is, in turn, converted (via an *N*-formiminoglutamic intermediate) to glutamate.

histidine decarboxylase: an enzyme that catalyzes the rate-limiting reaction for histamine biosynthesis: histidine → histamine + CO_2. Glucocorticoids and other inhibitors are used to treat allergic reactions and some other conditions associated with histamine excess.

histidinemia: an autosomal recessive disorder in which impaired production of histidine-ammonia lyase causes histidine accumulation (and increased urinary excretion of the amino acid and its imidazole metabolites). The manifestations include mental retardation.

histiocytes: long-lived, motile connective tissue macrophages.

histochemistry: use of specific staining procedures to identify cell and tissue components under light or electron microscopy.

histocompatibility: describes similarities between cells or tissues of different individuals of the same species that permit graft acceptance; *see* **histocompatibility antigens.**

histocompatibility antigens: cell surface molecules involved in immune cell recognition and graft rejection. The term usually refers to class 1 and class 2 cell surface proteins whose synthesis is controlled by the major histocompatibility complex. *See also* **minor histocompatibility antigens.**

histocompatibility complex: HMC; usually, the **major histocompatibility complex** (MHC, *q.v.*), a set of genes that codes for MHC antigens, and also for some complement factors, and some other cell proteins (including steroid 21-hydroxylase). *See also* **minor histocompatibility antigens**.

histogenesis: tissue formation and differentiation.

histograms: bar graphs.

histology: (1) microscopic anatomy; (2) the study of tissues.

histones: a family of small, highly conserved, basic, arginine and lysine rich DNA-binding eukaryote proteins, synthesized on cytoplasmic ribosomes and transported to the nuclei, that account for approximately half the chromosome mass. (The chromatin of all eukaryote cells except spermatozoa and their precursors is mostly histone + DNA; *see* also **protamines**.) Histones are essential for maintaining chromatin structure, and they contribute to transcription control. Their affinities for DNA are affected by posttranslational modifications that can include acetylation, methylation, phosphorylation, and ADP-ribosylation. A nucleosome core comprises 140 DNA base pairs wound about an octamer composed of two copies each of histones H2A (14.5K), H2B (13.8K), H3 (15.3K) and H4 (11.3K). A single molecule of histone H1 (21K) binds to H2A on the outside of the core particle, and to linker segments of both DNA strands. It is not essential for nucleosome formation (and little or no H1 is made by yeast cells that have numerous nucleosomes). However, in animals with complex genomes, it contributes to tight coiling of the structures into fibers with diameters of approximately 30 nm. Histones repress transcription by indirectly masking nucleosome TATA sites, by attaching to them directly, by competing with other proteins for binding (and in some cases displacing those proteins), and interfering with transcription factor interactions with upstream promotors.

histone kinases: enzymes that catalyzes histone phosphorylation, and thereby affect the surface charges and DNA binding properties. *See also* **maturation promoting factor**.

histotrophe: histotroph; histiotroph; a mixture of uterine secretions and cell debris, used to nourish the preimplantation embryos of some species.

histrelin: 5-oxo-Pro-His-Trp-Ser-Gly-D-(*N*-benzyl)-His-Arg-Pro-Gly-ethylamide; a potent gonadotropin hormone releasing hormone analog that suppresses gonadotropin secretion by desensitizing gonadotropes, and can also exert gonadocrinin-like effects on the gonads.

urocanate

imidazole-propionate

N-formiminoglutamate

histidine-ammonia lyase

HIV: retroviruses of the lentivirus family; *see* **human immunodeficiency viruses**.

H⁺/K⁺-ATPases: enzymes that use energy derived from ATP hydrolysis to drive electroneutral H^+ and K^+ exchanges across membranes. The enzyme in stomach parietal cells is essential for hydrochloric acid production. Its activity is augmented by acetylcholine acting on muscarinic receptors, and by gastrin. Both regulators elevate cytosolic Ca^{2+}. Histamine stimulates via H_2-type receptors and cAMP generation. In addition to acting directly (via protein kinase A), cAMP contributes to elevation of the Ca^{2+} levels. In some other cell types, the ATPases contribute to cell alkalinization (although most growth factors alkalinize by increasing Na^+/H^+ exchange). *See* also **histamine receptor antagonists**.

HLAs: human lymphocytic antigens; human leukocyte system A; *see* **major histocompatibility complex**.

HLC-60: a promyelocyte cell line that overexpresses *c-myc*. It is used to study hemopoietic growth factors and proto-oncogene functions.

HLH: helix-loop-helix.

H locus: a DNA segment that directs production of a fucosyl transferase needed for the biosynthesis of human ABO blood group antigens.

HMG: (1) human menopausal gonadotropin; (2) high mobility group proteins.

HMG-CoA reductase: hydroxymethyl glutaryl-coenzyme A reductase.

HMM: heavy meromyosin; *see* **myosin**.

HMP: hexose monophosphate shunt.

HMW-K: high molecular weight kininogen, a component of the blood coagulation cascade; *see* **kininogens**.

HMW-NCF: high molecular weight neutrophilic chemotactic factors; seven or more proteins released during allergic reactions that attract neutrophilic leukocytes and are implicated as mediators of tissue damage associated with those reactions.

HNF-1: hepatocyte nuclear factor.

HNMT: histamine *N*-methyltransferase.

hnRNAs: heterogeneous nuclear ribonucleic acids; primary RNA transcripts that are processed to yield mature messenger RNAs.

hnRNPs: *see* **heterogenous nuclear ribonucleoproteins**.

Hodgkin cycle: the electrical changes that follow stimulation of excitable cells. Depolarization begins with the opening of limited numbers of Na^+ channels. Because of the large concentration gradient (high Na^+ outside, low Na^+ inside), the ions rapidly enter the cells. When a threshold level of intracellular Na^+ is attained, the ions exert positive feedback effects on additional voltage-gated Na^+ channels, and the electrical potential rapidly approaches a level of around 100 mv more positive than the resting potential (which is approximately -70 mv for most excitable cells). The Na^+ channels then spontaneously close (but potassium and chloride channels open). A brief period of hyperpolarization characteristically precedes re-establishment of the resting potential. The excess intracellular Na^+ is extruded by Na^+/K^+-ATPases.

Hodgkin's disease: several closely related human diseases in which malignant lymphomas originate in lymph nodes and then spread to the spleen, bone marrow, and other organs (most commonly the liver but in some cases the lungs). The affected tissues contain giant Sternberg-Reed cells, and are infiltrated by lymphocytes, plasma cells, monocytes, histiocytes, eosinophils, and fibroblasts. Cellular immunity is usually severely impaired.

Hoechst 33258 dye: *p*-[5-[5-(4-methyl-1-piperazinyl)-2-benzimidazolyl]-2-benzimidazolyl]phenol; a fluorescent dye used to stain DNA and identify chromosomes. It enhances the photosensitivities of proliferating cells that have incorporated 5-bromodeoxyuridine.

Hoechst 33342: 2′(4-ethoxyphenyl)-5-(4-methyl-1-piperazinyl)-2,5′-*bi*-1*H*-benzimidazole trihydrochloride; a fluorescent dye that binds reversibly to erythroleukemia cells.

Hogben index: *see* **melanophore index**.

Hogben substance of whitening: *see* **W substance**.

Hogben test for pregnancy: a test based on the ability of human chorionic gonadotropin (hCG) in the urine of pregnant women to stimulate ovulation in *Xenopus* females. It is no longer used.

Hogness box: *see* **TATA box**.

holandric: appearing only in males, a term that usually refers to traits carried by Y chromosomes; *cf* **hologynic**.

Hoechst 33258 dye

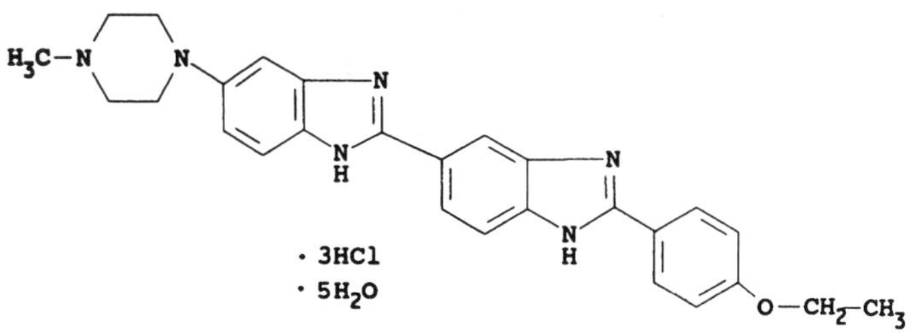

Hoechst 33342

• 3HCl
• 5H$_2$O

Holliday intermediate: Holliday junction: a four-way association of the segments of two homologous chromosomes. Its formation is an intermediate step in the crossing over process that occurs during meiosis, and in gene conversion and phage recombination.

holoblastic cleavage: cell division that leads to formation of two daughter cells of approximately equal size.

holocentric: describes the chromosomes of some species that have diffuse (not sharply localized) centromeres.

holocrine: describes sebaceous and exocrine glands whose secretions are composed mostly of disintegrated cells. *Cf* **apocrine** and **merocrine**.

holoenzyme: an enzyme and its associated prosthetic group; *cf* **apoenzyme**.

hologamy: formation of gametes that are morphologically indistinguishable from somatic cells. Some unicellular organisms reproduce in this way.

hologynic: describes traits (usually inheritable) that appear only in females; *cf* **holoandric**.

holometabolous: characterized by complete metamorphosis, with distinct larval, pupal, and imago stages, a term applied to the development of some insect species.

holophytic: describes organisms (usually protozoa) that require only inorganic nutrients; *cf* **holozoic**.

holotopy: the position of a body part with respect to the whole body.

holotype: an individual that displays the typical characteristics of a species.

holozoic: describes organisms (usually protozoa) that require organic nutrients made by other organisms; *cf* **holophytic**.

homatropine: tropine mandelate; an atropine derivative, more potent than the parent compound for blocking ganglionic transmission, but a less potent muscarinic type acetylcholine receptor antagonist. The hydrobromide salt is used topically to dilate the pupils for eye examinations. The methyl bromide is an orally effective gastrointestinal antispasmodic.

homeobox: DNA segments, in all **homeotic genes** (*q.v.*) and some related ones, that code for homeodomains and play essential roles in development. The base sequences are conserved across species as diverse as yeasts, worms, amphibians, and mammals, and are believed to have arisen from a common ancestral type. Similar genes func-

homatropine

tion in higher plants. Numerous mutations in *Drosophila* and other species have provided information on specific functions of the various types.

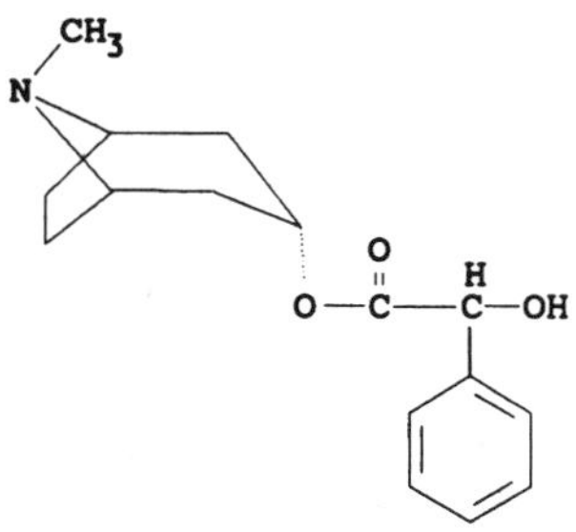

homeodomains: 160-161 amino acid segments of proteins whose synthesis is directed by homeoboxes. Most are nuclear proteins that bind to specific DNA base sequences and control the transcription of specific gene types during defined stages of development. *See also* **homeotic genes**.

homeopathy: the system of treating diseases with highly dilute preparations that contain minute quantities of substances which, in higher concentrations invoke the symptoms.

homeostasis: (1) establishment and maintenance of physiological conditions, a term that can be used with qualifiers such as glucose or mineral. It usually refers to processes that provide internal environments with optimal pHs, osmotic pressures, electrolyte balances, nutrient components, and related chemical properties, but is also used for blood pressure and other parameters. Since small variations around set points occur under normal conditions, and adjustments are continuously made, *homeodynamics* is probably a more appropriate term; (2) conditions in normal animals in which immune responses are mounted against foreign antigens, but not against body constituents; (3) describes factors that sustain a stable genotype in a breeding population.

homeotherms: endotherms; animals that maintain body temperatures within a very restricted range, despite changes in the temperatures of their environments and/or exposure to sun and other sources of radiant heat. Since the body temperatures are usually higher than those of surrounding environments, homeotherms are said to be "warm-blooded". *Cf* **ectotherms**.

331

homeotic genes: genes that contain homeoboxes and additional DNA segments, initially identified as regulators of segmentation differentiation in *Drosophila*. They play broad roles in the development of eukaryote limbs and other organs. Various members of the superfamily direct formation of DNA-binding proteins, some of which are transcription factors for DNA segments that direct the synthesis of extracellular components, and of other regulators. The genes are said to function as molecular switches that interact with other factors to promote differentiation and regulate the activities of mature cells. Their expression varies with the cell type and stage of development. In complex organisms, they occur in tightly linked clusters on several chromosomes. During embryogenesis, they function sequentially. Ones used during early stages can activate others that are needed later, and some late-acting genes repress ones previously activated. Retinoic acid gradients, bone morphogenetic protein-2, transforming growth factor-β (TGFβ), and peptides related to TGFβ are among the factors that affect their functions. Mammalian homologs of *Drosophila* genes are made on at least five different chromosomes, and are assigned numbers that refer to the chromosome group and locus. For example, Hox-1.1, Hox-1.2, and Hox-1.3 are clustered on one chromosome, and members of Hox-2 (and of Hox-3, Hox-4, and Hox-5) groups are on different chromosomes. *See* also **pou domains**, and specific members of the group (for example *int*, *oct*, and *pit-1*).

homeotic mutations: homeobox gene aberrations that impair development of specific embryonic body segments, or cause them to differentiate along pathways appropriate for other (usually adjacent) segments. *See*, for example *fushi tarazu*.

homing receptors: plasma membrane glycoproteins on the surfaces of T lymphocytes and some other mobile cell types, that mediate adhesive interactions with selectins such as endothelial-leukocyte adhesion molecule-1 (ELAM-1) on the high endothelium venules of mesenteric and peripheral lymph nodes. They facilitate accumulation of various cell types at specific sites (for example of memory cells in lymph nodes, and neutrophilic leukocytes in inflammatory lesions). *See* also **gp90**[MEL-14].

hominoids: chimpanzees, organ-utans, gorillas, gibbons, and other members of the *Hominidae* family of primates.

homoactinin A: a component of actin/myosin filaments that is released without degradation, and is used as a marker for filament breakdown.

homoactivin: *see* **activins**.

homoalleles: a gene pair (set of alleles) on two homologous chromosomes, whose members have different kinds of mutations at the same locus. *cf* **heteroalleles**.

homocysteine: an non-essential amino acid that participates in metabolic reactions, but is not incorporated into peptides or proteins. It is generated in three steps. Methionine reacts with ATP to form ADP + *S*-adenosylmethionine. The *S*-adenosylmethionine then donates methyl groups to various acceptor compounds (X-) to form *S*-adenosylhomocysteine + X-CH$_3$. Finally, *S*-adenosylhomocysteine is hydrolyzed to adenosine + homocysteine. Methionine can be regenerated via a reaction catalyzed by homocysteine methyltransferase: homocysteine + N^5-methyltetrahydrofolate $\rightarrow$ methionine + tetrahydrofolate. Homocysteine can also react with serine to form cystathione, via a reaction catalyzed by cystathione synthetase. Cystathionase converts the product to cysteine + α-ketobutyrate. *See* also **homocystinuria**.

homocysteine methyltransferase: *see* **homocysteine**.

homocystine: a non-essential amino acid formed by condensation of two molecules of **homocysteine** (*q.v.*).

$$S-CH_2-CH_2-\overset{NH_2}{\underset{H}{C}}-COOH$$

$$S-CH_2-CH_2-\overset{H}{\underset{NH_2}{C}}-COOH$$

homocystinuria: several conditions in which **homocysteine** (*q.v.*) or homocystine accumulates and is excreted to the urine. An autosomal recessive defect that impairs synthesis of cystathione β-synthase can cause neural tube malformation, mental retardation, and eye defects. Other manifestations can include osteoporosis and thrombosis. Large doses of pyridoxine or folic acid increase activity of the enzyme, and can often prevent the complications. Other causes include serine dehydrase deficiency and some pharmacological agents.

homocytropic antibodies: antibodies that bind to mast cells of the species that make them, and mediate anaphylaxis if the associated antigens are presented; *cf* **heterocytotropic antibodies**.

homodimers: molecules composed of to two identical subunits; *cf* **monomers** and **heterodimers**.

COO⁻	COO⁻	COO⁻
HC-NH$_2$	HC-NH$_2$	HC-NH$_2$
CH$_2$	CH$_2$	CH$_2$
CH$_2$	CH$_2$	CH$_2$
H$_3$C-S-adenosyl	HS-adenosyl	SH$_2$
S-adenosylmethione	*S*-adenosylhomocysteine	homocysteine

p-hydroxyphenylpyruvate   **homogentisate**   **4-maleylacetoacetate**

homogametic: producing just one kind of gamete. XX females and ZZ males are homogametic, since they make only X-type ova and Z-type spermatozoa, respectively, whereas XY males and WZ females are heterogametic.

homogamy: mating preference for other members of the species that share a common genotype or some common phenotypic characteristics.

homogentisic acid: HGA: 2,5-dihydroxyphenylacetic acid; a tyrosine metabolite formed when tyrosine is de-aminated to yield *p*-hydroxypyruvate, and a dioxygenase (*p*-hydroxyphenyl pyruvate hydroxylase) catalyzes decarboxylation. Under normal conditions, homogentisate is further metabolized (via 4-maleylacetoacetate and 4-fumarylacetoacetate intermediates) to fumarate + acetoacetate. Alcaptonuria is an autosomal recessive disorder that impairs production of homogentisate oxidase (which catalyzes formation of the 4-maleylacetoacetate.) After excretion to the urine, homogentisic acid polymerizes to black melanin-like molecules. The condition is often benign, but black pigments that deposit in connective tissues can cause arthritis or aortic valve defects. In plants, homogentisic acid is a precursor of tocopherols.

homograft: a transplant of tissue obtained from a member of the same species. It can be an isograft or allograft. *See* **grafts** and *cf* **heterograft**.

homokaryon: a cell that contains two genetically identical nuclei; *cf* **heterokaryon**.

homologous: describes (1) compounds that share common chemical groups (such as amino acid sequences); (2) organs or organ parts of different species that develop from similar embryonic precursor structures; *cf* **analogous**; (3) antigens and their specific antibodies. *See* also **homologous chromosomes**, and **homologous desensitization**.

homologous chromosomes: chromosome pairs that associate during cell division, and engage in crossing over during meiosis. Usually, the term refers to types whose members are morphologically identical and carry alleles of common genes; but it is sometimes applied to sex chromosomes which share only limited numbers of alleles.

homologous desensitization: rapidly developing loss of sensitivity to an agent that is continuously presented, without concomitant loss of sensitivity to others that act on the same cell type (and, in some cases, via the same transducer); *cf* **heterologous desensitization**. It usually involves covalent modification and/or translocation (but not destruction) of the receptors, and is usually reversed when the initiating agent is withdrawn. *Cf* **down regulation**.

homologous recombination: exchange of corresponding DNA segments (alleles) on homologous chromosomes.

homophilic adhesion: adhesion of one molecule to another of the same kind, or of one cell type to another of the same kind. *See* also **homotypic adhesion**, and *cf* **heterophilic adhesion**.

homopolymers: macromolecules (such as starch, or polyadenylate), composed of identical repeating moieties.

homotypic adhesion: adhesion of one component of an organism to another that does not involve immune interactions.

homovanillic acid: HVA: 3-methoxy-4-hydroxy mandelic acid; a major urinary metabolite of norepinephrine and epinephrine released outside the central nervous system. It is formed in three reactions. Methylation, catalyzed by catecholamine-*O*-methyltransferase (COMT) can precede or follow oxidative deamination, catalyzed by a monoamine oxidase (MAO). The MAO reaction yields an aldehyde that is rapidly oxidized. (In the central nervous system, most of the aldehyde is reduced; *see* 3-**methoxyphenylethylglycol**.)

homozygote: a diploid nucleus, cell, or organism with identical alleles at a specific locus; *cf* **heterozygote**.

horizontal cell: a neuron type in the retina that contributes to processing of visual stimuli. It communicates with two or more adjacent photoreceptors.

horizontal evolution: separation of a population into two or more subgroups, each of which develops into a new species; *cf* **vertical evolution**.

horizontal transmission: passage (of genetic information or an infection) from one individual of a population to another; *cf* **vertical transmission**.

hormonad: an enzyme complex that catalyzes synthesis of a hormone from a precursor molecule without releasing metabolic intermediates.

hormones: a term initially applied to specialized organic molecules synthesized in endocrine glands, and transported via the bloodstream to distantly located target organs. The term is now more commonly applied to all chemical messengers synthesized by organisms that initiate responses by binding with high affinity and specificity to target cell receptors within the same individual. Many are synthesized by neurons and other cell types, and a few (for example angiotensin II) are made extracellularly. Nitric oxide and carbon monoxide are examples of simple molecules that perform regulatory functions; and prostaglandins are among the kinds made by numerous cell types. Some act via paracrine, autocrine, or intracrine mechanisms; and a regulator that travels through the bloodstream can be chemically identical with one that acts locally. Some authors include *ectohormones* (pheromones and other regulators that act on other individuals).

hormone receptors: molecules within or on the surfaces of target cells that bind hormones with high affinity and specificity, and thereby initiate or mediate biological responses.

hormone response elements: HREs; DNA base sequences that bind hormone-receptor complexes and mediate their influences on gene transcription; *see*, for example **glucocorticoid** and **estrogen response elements**.

hormonogens: compounds that can be processed to yield hormones; *see*, for example **renin substrate** and **kininogens**.

horror autotoxicus: self-tolerance; the concept that the immune system does not mount attacks against components of the individual in which it resides. Some autoantibodies are, in fact, made under normal conditions. *See* also **autoimmune disease**.

horseradish peroxidase: HRP; a high molecular weight enzyme that is easily detected in the presence of substrate. It generates hydrogen peroxide, which oxidizes benzidine dyes to dark blue derivatives. The enzyme is taken up by lysosomes of living cells and is used to identify those organelles. Since neurons take it up by retrograde transport, and can thereby be distinguished them from surrounding glial cells, it is a tool for tracing connections to other neurons and to muscle fibers. HRP is linked to secondary antibodies for ELISA assays. Its ability to accelerate iodine incorporation into thyroglobulin can be followed with radioactive markers.

host: (1) a transplant recipient; (2) an organism that provides nutrients or in other ways supports the survival (totally, or during a phase of the life cycle) of another organism.

host versus graft reactions: lymphocyte-mediated responses to foreign cells or tissues; graft rejection. *Cf* **graft vs host reaction**.

hot flashes: irregular episodes of skin blood vessel dilation that occur after estrogen withdrawal (for example after ovariectomy and during normal menopause), attributed to transient disturbances in autonomic system controls. The causes are not known, but may involve changes in dopamine metabolism. They often coincide with, but are not invoked by gonadotropin releasing hormone (LRH) pulses.

hot spot: a DNA site at which recombination is frequent.

housekeeping genes: genes that are constitutively expressed in all nucleated cell types of an organism, whose products are essential for survival. They are among the first to replicate during cell cycle S phases.

Howship's lacunae: rounded pits at bone resorption site surfaces. They usually contain osteoclasts.

HPETEs: hydroperoxyeicosanoic acids.

hPL: human placental lactogen; hCS; *see* **human chorionic somatomammotropin**.

HPLC: high performance (high pressure) liquid chromatography; *see* **chromatography**.

HPRT: HPGRT; hypoxanthine-phosphoribosyltransferase; *see* **hypoxanthine-guanine-phosphoribosyltransferase**.

HPTs: hepatopoietins.

hPUTH: human placental uterotropic hormone.

HR: *see* **hypersensitive response**.

HRP: horse radish peroxidase.

HSA: human serum albumin.

HSD: hydroxysteroid dehydrogenase.

HSEs: heat shock elements.

HSPs: heat shock proteins.

hst: an oncogene that directs production of a secretory protein (FGF-4, FGF/Kaposi), a member of the fibroblast growth factor superfamily implicated in the etiology of Kaposi and other skin tumors. Unlike some others growth factors, it is made from a precursor that contains a signal sequence.

H subunits: *see* **lactate dehydrogenase**.

H substance: a polysaccharide component of type O erythrocytes, and a precursor of A and B type erythrocyte antigens.

HSVs: *Herpes simplex* viruses.

HSV-TK: *Herpes* virus thymidine kinases.

5-HT: 5-hydroxytryptamine: *see* **serotonin**.

HTA: hypophysiotropic area.

HTLVs: human T-cell lymphotropic viruses.

hTG: human type thyroglobulin.

5-HTOL: *see* 5-**hydroxytryptophol**.

5-HTP: *see* 5-**hydroxytryptophan**.

human chorionic gonadotropin: hCG: glycoprotein hormones with α subunits similar to or identical with those of thyroid stimulating, follicle stimulating, and luteinizing hormones (TSH, FSH, and LH), and encoded by the same gene, plus β subunits that share sequences with LH β types, but have additional 24-amino acid *C*-terminal extensions. Although at least six genes that code for the β components are known, the isoforms differ mostly in sugar content. (All are heavily glycosylated.) A pseudogene has also been identified. hCG made by trophoblast cells of pre-implantation blastocysts is needed to convert corpora lutea formed during ovarian cycles to corpora lutea of pregnancy. It appears to be essential for implantation, and for maintaining progesterone and relaxin secretion and other functions of the maternal corpus luteum during the first trimester of human pregnancy. Larger amounts are made by placental syncytiotrophoblast cells as the conceptus matures, and some free subunits are also released. The hormone is taken up by the maternal blood, is excreted to maternal urine, and is the urinary component (detectable within nine days post-fertilization) that reacts positively in pregnancy tests. Roles in protection of the conceptus against immunological rejection, and in suppression of maternal secretion of gonadotropins have been suggested. (However, the levels peak at 8-9 weeks, and decline rapidly thereafter, as the feto-placental unit prepares to take over production of the estrogens and progestins that sustain the pregnancy). In male fetuses, it stimulates testosterone production by developing gonads. Unlike LH, it is not stored in secretory granules. The proposed controls during pregnancy include stimulation by chorionic GnRH (made in cytotrophoblast cells), and a localized negative feedback system in which hCG acts on the cytotrophoblast to promote production of an inhibin-like peptide that depresses hCG synthesis. Supplementary controls may be exerted by epidermal growth factor (EGF), which stimulates, tumor necrosis factor-β (TNFβ), which inhibits, and other regulators. Minute amounts of hCG are made by some adenohypophysial and other cell types of males and nonpregnant females, and some is present in testes. Many kinds of tumor cells (possibly all malignant types) secrete subunits and/or whole hormone (which in some cases differs in structure from the placental type). *See* also **hydatidiform mole**. Related chorionic gonadotropins are made by other mammals. hCG acts on LH receptors, but has a longer biological half-life than the pituitary hormone. It also displays some FSH-like activity. Antibodies raised against the amino acid component that is not contained in LH are under investigation for use in fertility control (*see* **interception**). hCG is used to treat some forms of androgen deficiency, and to promote ovulation (*see* also *in vitro* **fertilization**).

human chorionic somatomammotropin: hCS; human placental lactogen; hPL; a hormone chemically related to growth hormone and prolactin, made by human syncytiotrophoblast cells and released mostly to the maternal blood. Since the levels rise gradually, in parallel with placenta growth, and are high during the second and third trimesters of pregnancy, it has been proposed that measurements can be used as indicators of fetal age. hCS is implicated as a stimulant for maternal mammary gland growth and maturation, and it may indirectly affect some aspects of fetal development. It is a weak agonist for prolactin receptors, can compete for binding, and may in that way inhibit milk production during pregnancy. Observations that the levels rise during fasting, that the hormone can then inhibit nonessential glucose oxidation and promote ketosis (and thereby enhance sugar delivery to the fetus), and can promote maternal fat storage after feeding, are consistent with functions in poorly nourished mothers. Since it can confer insulin resistance, it may also contribute to development of a transient diabetes mellitus-like condition that develops in some women and subsides after parturition. Some observers believe it does not perform essential functions; and well-nourished women who do not make detectable amounts can support the development of healthy infants.

human immune deficiency viruses: HIVs; retroviruses of the lentivirus family. HIV-1 is believed to be the major causative agent for acquired immune deficiency syndrome (AIDS) in humans, and may be identical with a virus previously known as human lymphotrophic virus type III (HTLV-III) and lymphadenopathy associated virus (LAV). It also infects chimpanzees, but does not invoke immunosuppression in those animals. HIV-II, a similar virus that can also cause AIDS, assumes greater importance in some locales. It acts on a broader range of hosts, but appears to be spread more slowly in humans, and to be somewhat less pathogenic. Related types that affect other species include simian immunodeficiency virus (SIV), which invokes AIDS-like symptoms in chimpanzees, equine infectious anemia virus, infectious arthritis virus of goats, and sheep visna virus. In addition to *gag*, *pol*, and *env* (in all retroviruses), HIV possesses at least 6 special genes. The major antigen is the gp120 envelope protein, which is noncovalently linked to transmembrane gp40, and binds with high affinity to T cell CD4. It causes CD4$^+$ cells to coalesce and form syncytia, severely impairs cellular immunity, and binds with lower affinity to monocytes, glial cells, gastrointestinal epithelium, bone marrow progenitor, and other cell types. Internalization by macrophages may preserve the virus for later release. After entering cells, the virus sheds its envelope, and the reverse transcriptase (encoded by *gag-pol*) promotes formation of the first DNA strand. A second *pol* product, ribonuclease H, is required for formation of the second strand. An integrase then facilitates incorporation into the host DNA and use of host RNA polymerase. Some DNA can be retained in latent, unintegrated form, and await activation by other cell components such as host transcription factors, antigens, mitogens, and other viruses. The *tat* gene directs formation of a diffusible protein that interacts with a responsive element, *tar* to enhance transcription. Other gene products are needed for virion packaging and infection of new cells, and as control factors.

human menopausal gonadotropin: HMG; a concentrated, partially purified preparation of urine from postmenopausal women, used mostly for its FSH-like content (for example to promote ovarian follicle maturation). It also displays limited LH-like activity.

human placenta purified factor: *see* β-**fibroblast growth factors**.

human placental lactogen: hPL; hCS; *see* **human chorionic somatomamotropin**.

human placental uterotropic hormone: hPUTH: a hormone that circulates in pregnant women and promotes uterine growth. It also stimulates mammary gland cell proliferation in rodents.

human skeletal growth factor: hSGF; a protein isolated from human bone that stimulates growth of human and chick embryo bone, and is implicated as a factor that couples bone formation with bone resorption.

human T cell lymphotrophic viruses: HTLVs; retroviruses that infect T lymphocytes. HTLV-I is implicated in the etiology of some forms of leukemia, and possibly also some immunodeficiency diseases. HTLV-II is a related virus identified in some humans with leukemia. HTLV-III is probably identical with HIV-1.

human umbilical vein endothelial cells: HUVEC: specialized vascular cells in human placentas. They are used to study homing receptors, cell adhesion molecules, and the functions of some species specific regulators.

human vascular permeability factor: glioma-derived vascular endothelial growth factor.

humoral: describes factors released to blood and other body fluids.

humoral hypercalcemia of malignancy: HHM; elevated blood calcium levels attributed to circulating factors released by tumor or activated immune system cells. See **parathyroid hormone-like peptide** and **osteoclast activating factor**.

humoral hypocalcemic factor of malignancy: *see* **parathyroid hormone-like peptide**.

humoral immunity: protection against specific pathogens mediated by B lymphocytes that release circulating antibodies; *cf* **cellular immunity**.

Hunter syndrome: mucopolysaccharidosis II; several X-linked recessive disorders in which synthesis of iduronate-sulfate sulfatase (a lysosomal enzyme) is impaired. The manifestations can be similar to those of Hurler's syndrome; but mild forms are known, and the inheritance pattern is different.

Huntington's disease: Huntington's chorea; a chronic, progressive, dominant autosomal human disorder whose manifestations in heterozygotes usually begin in the fourth or fifth decade, and include mental deterioration and severe pyramidal system dysfunction associated with irregular, involuntary spasmodic movements and paresis. Excessive activity of excitatory amino acids acting on NMDA type receptors is believed to invoke loss of neurons that release gamma aminobutyric acid (GABA), substance P, and enkephalins in the palladium and substantia nigra. Acetylcholine and somatostatin releasing neurons do not seem to be affected.

Hurler's syndrome: mucopolysaccharidosis IH; autosomal recessive disorders, often fatal by age 10, in which α-iduronidase deficiency leads to glycosaminoglycan accumulation. The manifestations include short stature, progressive mental retardation, facial deformities, restricted joint mobility, cardiovascular or pulmonary dysfunction, corneal opacity, and deafness.

HUVEC: human umbilical vein endothelial cells.

Hv: the variable region of an immunoglobulin heavy chain.

hv sites: *see* **hypervariable sites**.

HX: hypophysectomy.

Hya: the gene on the short arm of the Y chromosome that codes for H-Y antigen.

hyaline: clear; transparent or semitransparent.

hyalinization: hyalinosis; acquisition of a homogeneous, glassy appearance. It can be a sign of cell deterioration.

hyalinosis: extensive hyalinization.

hyalomere: the clear peripheral zone of blood platelet cytoplasm that does not contain granules.

hyalomucoid: hyaluronic acid.

hyaluronectin: an adhesion protein associated with myelinated nerve fibers in the brain, believed to be synthesized by astrocytes.

hyaluronic acid {**hyaluronate**}: hyalomucoid; high molecular weight (up to 8,000 K) polymers of non-sulfated glucuronic acid/N-acetylglucosamine dimers. The ones in basement membranes form long filaments, attached by linker proteins to the cores of some extracellular matrix proteoglycans. Others confer viscosity to ovarian follicle fluid, and form layers around mature oocytes that must be degraded by sperm hyaluronidase to accomplish fertilization. Their presence in fibrinoid layers surrounding trophoblasts probably contributes to protection against immunological rejection. The large amounts in young embryos are involved in control of cell migrations associated with morphogenesis. Postnatally, they are most abundant in the skin dermis, in which they contribute to wound healing, but cartilage contains substantial amounts. They are also major constituents of eye vitreous bodies, and they function as lubricants in synovial fluid. Growth hormone augments hyaluronic acid synthesis; and excessive amounts accumulate in acromegaly. Localized overproduction can be stimulated by immune system factors and contribute to conditions such as exophthalmos. Thyroid hormones accelerate its degradation (*see* also **myxedema**).

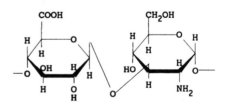

hyaluronidase: spreading factor; enzymes that catalyze hyaluronic acid hydrolysis and additionally act on glycoside bonds of some other polymers. Preparations are administered with some parenteral agents to accelerate absorption and distribution. The enzymes facilitate cell migration in embryos; and the levels fall as the processes approach completion. Later, release by spermatozoa is essential for fertilization; and inhibitors are under investigation for use in contraception. The activity is augmented by glucocorticoids and triiodothyronine (T_3); *see also* **myxedema**. Hyaluronidases are also active components of some snake venoms; and ones released by some microorganisms mediate the spread of infections.

H-Y antigen: a plasma membrane glycoprotein that is required for spermatogenesis. It is a minor histocompatibility antigen whose synthesis in mammals is directed by the *Hya* gene on the short arm of the Y chromosome. It is expressed on the surfaces of mammalian male blastocysts, and on most male cells at later stages of development. The antigen was initially believed to promote conversion of indifferent gonads to embryonic testes; but *see* **testis determining antigen**. In females of highly inbred mouse strains, it initiates T lymphocyte attacks against male cells, and promotes rejection of skin grafts from conspecific male donors. In birds and other species with WZ/ZZ chromosome patterns, it is made by the females.

hybrid: an entity composed of parts derived from two or more sources. The term can describe (1) an offspring of parents of the same species with different alleles (*see* **heterozygous**); (2) an organism produced by the union of gametes (or other sources of genetic components) from two or more different species or strains; (3) a cell that contains genetic components from two or more sources, formed by cell fusion, transfection, or microinjection (*see* **hybrid cells** and **hybridomas**); (4) a heterokaryon; (5) a hybrid antibody; (6) a double stranded molecule composed of DNA from two different sources; or (7) a double stranded nucleic acid complex composed of one DNA and one complementary RNA strand. *See also* **hybridization**.

hybrid antibody: an artificially constructed antibody with two different kinds of combining sites (monovalent for each type.) Cell surface antigens can be visualized with molecules that attach at one site to a cell surface component, and at the other that to a marker (such as ferritin, or an enzyme that produces an identifiable product).

hybrid cell: a single cell formed by the fusing two different kinds, or by microinjecting foreign DNA. Most hybrids derived from different species have unstable genomes that undergo random chromosome loss when they divide. Various kinds of daughter cells can then be cloned and used for gene mapping. Specific functions of some human chromosomes can be studied (without interference from others present in normal cells), when human:mouse hybrids lose most of the human types.

hybrid dysgenesis: germ line defects that arise when heterozygotes acquire certain allele combinations, for example in *Drosophila* progeny of M strain females and P strain males. The manifestations can include chromosomal aberrations, high mutation frequencies (some of which are lethal), and sterility. *See also* **P elements**.

hybridization: formation of molecular hybrids. Since two denatured, single-stranded nucleic acid molecules hybridize only at sites that contain complementary base sequences, the processes yield probes for identifying DNA base sequences common to different species, and for determining chromosomal loci that direct formation of specific kinds of messenger RNAs.

hybridomas: hybrid cell tumors. A cell type that proliferates rapidly can be fused to another that makes large quantities of a desired substance. Myeloma cells are fused with B lymphocytes to produce large quantities of specific kinds of monoclonal antibodies, and with T lymphocytes to obtain lymphokines.

hybridoma-plasmacytoma growth factor: interleukin-6.

hybrid resistance: protective mechanisms conferred by the presence of two histocompatible genotypes. Some heterozygotes are highly resistant to certain microorganisms and environmental toxins; and some more successfully combat the growth of tumors than their homozygous counterparts.

hybrid sterility: inability of some hybrids of different species to produce viable progeny.

hybrid vigor: heterosis; the tendency of heterozygotes to display characteristics superior to those of homozygotes of the same species, such as more rapid growth, larger size, increased longevity, greater resistance to unfavorable environmental factors, and/or higher fertility.

hydantoin: 2,4-imidazolidinedione. Small amounts of hydantoin-5-propionate are formed during histidine degradation. Phenytoin and some other derivatives are used to treat epilepsy.

hydatidiform moles: vesicular cell clusters formed following fertilization of defective ova, in which chorionic villi deteriorate, embryoblasts fail to develop, and paternally derived trophoblast proliferates. They can persist as benign, edematous, grape-like structures that remain localized, or spread to surrounding tissues. Some develop into chorioadenomas, and a few become highly malignant, massively invasive chorioepitheliomas that secrete large quantities of human chorionic gonadotropin (hCG). Some additionally make a factor that differs from thyrotropin (TSH) but stimulates thyroid glands. Although the moles occur most often in women, trophoblastic tissue can persist postnatally and cause tumors in men.

Hydra: a genus of freshwater, radially symmetric coelenterates, used to study regeneration and morphogenesis. They make head activator neuropeptide (head protein), a morphogen with the amino acid sequence *p*Glu-Pro-Pro-Gly-Gly-Ser-Lys-Val-Ile-Leu-Phe.

hydralazine: Apresoline; 1-hydrazinophthalazine; an orally effective agent that relaxes vascular smooth muscle and is used (often in conjunction with others), to treat some forms of hypertension. Some of the effects are attributed to interactions with endothelium and consequent release of nitric oxide.

hydralazine

hydramnios: the presence of excessive amounts of amniotic fluid, often associated with fetal abnormality. It occurs in fetuses nurtured by mothers with diabetes mellitus and some other illnesses.

β-hydrastine:[R-(R^*,S^*)]-6,7-dimethoxy-3-(5,6,7,8-tetrahydro-6-methyl-1,3-dioxolo[4,5g]isoquinolin-5-yl)-1 (3H)- isobenzofuranone; a potent, competitive GABA$_A$ receptor antagonist made by *Corydalis stricta*.

hydratases: enzymes that catalyzes addition of water to compounds, in reactions of the general type:

hydrates: compounds that contain water, usually in easily dissociated forms.

hydration: addition of water, for example when crystals form. *See* also **hydratases**.

hydrazine: a proton acceptor used in amino acid sequence analysis.

hydremia: hemodilution; excessive amounts of water in the bloodstream that is not associated with increased numbers of formed elements or quantities of proteins and small solutes. The causes include renal dysfunctions and impaired negative controls over vasopressin release.

hydrides: compounds, such as CaH_2 and SH_4, composed of elements or radicals linked to hydrogen atoms. (The term is not usually applied to acids, in which hydrogen is the electropositive element.)

hydrocarbons: organic compounds composed of covalently linked carbon and hydrogen atoms, for example CH_4 or C_2H_6.

hydrochloric acid: HCl: the strong acid made by stomach parietal cells that provides the very low pH required to initiate pepsinogen conversion to pepsin, and to support pepsin actions. It also stimulates bile flow and pancreatic juice production, kills ingested microorganisms, and facilitates absorption of iron and some other nutrients. An H^+/K^+-ATPase on the mucosal surfaces of the parietal cells actively transports hydrogen ions to the stomach lumen. The H^+ ions are obtained from water, and a cytoplasmic carbonic anhydrase catalyzes formation of carbonic acid ($HHCO_3$) from $CO_2 + H_2O$, which neutralizes the OH^- ions. The bicarbonate ions formed during the neutralization are transported to the serosal surface, where HCO_3^-/Cl^- exchange provides the chloride ions for active transport to the lumen. (When large amounts of acid are made, bicarbonate released at the serosal surface can transiently increase blood alkalinity; but this is soon followed by excretion of the excess HCO_3^- to urine.) Stimuli associated with eating, and others initiated by food in the stomach, promote the release of regulators that accelerate acid production. Acetylcholine from vagus nerve endings acts on M_1 type muscarinic receptors and elevates Ca^{2+}. Vagal stimulation also elevates the levels of gastrin releasing peptide (GRP), a tachykinin that augments the secretion of gastrin and several other peptides. Gastrin acts via cAMP when it binds to its own receptors, and it also causes release of histamine, which generates cAMP after interacting with H_2 receptors. Gastrin additionally stimulates gastric motility; and the larger forms exert tropic influences on the gastric mucosa. Other stimuli for acid production include ethyl alcohol (and caffeine in individuals who do not become desensitized to it by drinking large amounts of coffee or tea). Positive feedback mechanisms provide for rapid acid accumulation in response to meals; and negative feedback controls prevent overproduction. Very high acidity inhibits gastrin secretion. Other inhibitors include norepinephrine, somatostatin, prostaglandins, and, to a lesser extent, glucose-dependent insulinotropic peptide (GIP). In some individuals, stress acts via the autonomic system to invoke gastric hyperemia and hyperacidity; but in others it promotes release of sufficient norepinephrine to inhibit. Healthy stomach cells maintain a cytoplasmic pH of 7.0 - 7.2 when the pH of gastric juice falls to 1.0 or lower, and are protected against gastric juice acidity and pepsin by mucus released from neck and surface glands. However, because of the external environment, the cells are short-lived, and require continuous replacement. Gastric ulcers can form when dysregulation affects cell renewal, mucus secretion, or negative feedback controls over acid and enzyme production; see also **Zollinger-Ellison syndrome**. Recent evidence suggests, however, that bacterial infections cause at least some of the ulcers. Nonsteroidal anti-inflammatory agents can cause ulceration by affecting the mucus, and by inhibiting production of prostaglandins (which decrease acidity and contribute to cell renewal). Parietal cells also make intrinsic factor, which is required for absorption of vitamin B_{12} (*see* **pernicious anemia**). Small amounts of dilute HCl have been administered (with drinking straws to avoid damage to the mouth and teeth) to individuals with achlorhydria, but beneficial effects have not been unequivocally demonstrated. Severe or repeated vomiting can deplete HCl, cause alkalosis and potassium deficiency, and injure the esophagus, pharynx, mouth, and teeth. Pepsinogen is made by the chief cells. Pepsin is not absolutely essential for protein digestion, but chief cell atrophy can impair digestion.

hydrocinnamic acid: 3-phenylpropionic acid; an agent used to inhibit carboxypeptidases.

hydrocortisone: *see* **cortisol**.

hydrogen: H; the lightest and most abundant element in organic compounds (atomic number 1, atomic weight 1.008). Since the ions are protons, they attract negative charges and form **hydrogen bonds** (*q.v.*). *See* also **pH, acidosis, hydrochloric acid, deuterium** and **tritium**.

hydrogen bonds: weak electrostatic (nonionic, non-covalent) bonds that link hydrogen atoms (protons) with negatively charged components of the same or other molecules. They are major determinants of the three-dimensional configurations of proteins, nucleic acids, some lipids, and other compounds, and mediators of intermolecular associations (for example between two nucleic acid strands, and between some enzymes and their substrates). They also account for many of the special properties of water. Heat is released when they form, and taken up when they break.

hydrogen iodide: HI; hydroiodic acid. *See* **iodine**.

hydrogen peroxide: H_2O_2; a highly reactive compound that mediates some of the bactericidal functions of neutrophilic leukocytes and macrophages, but can damage normal tissues by oxidizing iron, sulfur, and other components of cell molecules, and abolishing the activities of cytochromes and other enzymes. Protection against excess accumulation is provided by catalases, peroxidases, and glutathione. Flavoprotein enzymes and some other oxidases catalyze reactions of the general type: $RH_2 + O_2 \rightarrow R + H_2O_2$. Some hydrogen peroxide is a by-product of other processes. H_2O_2 made by subjecting water to ionizing radiation is used as a topical antiseptic. It rapidly decomposes *in vitro*, especially in the presence of light, via $2H_2O_2 \rightarrow 2H_2O + O_2$. *See* also **myeloperoxidase, thyroid peroxidase, superoxide anions, hydroperoxyl radicals**, and **superoxide dismutase**.

hydroiodic acid: hydrogen iodide; *see* **iodine**.

hydrogenases: enzymes that catalyze reactions in which hydrogen is the reductant. Some microorganisms use them to reduce ferrodoxin and transfer electrons to flavoproteins. *Cf* **hydratases** and **dehydrogenases**.

hydrolases: gastrointestinal, lysosomal, and other enzymes that catalyze cleavage of large molecules to smaller ones,

by adding OH from water to one product, and H to the other, via reactions of the general type: $R_1—R_2 \rightarrow R_1—OH + R_2—H$. *See* also **hydrolysis** and **hydrolysates**.

hydrolysates: products generated by hydrolysis. Amino acids released in that way from proteins are used for numerous purposes, including parenteral nutrition and preparation of defined media. Mixtures that contain only certain types in known concentrations are used for metabolic studies.

hydrolysis: digestion; reactions catalyzed by **hydrolases** (*q.v.*). It is the major mechanism for converting large molecules to smaller ones (for example polysaccharides to oligosaccharides, disaccharides to simple sugars, proteins to peptides and amino acids, fats to fatty acids and glycerol, and nucleic acids to oligonucleotides). *Cf* **dehydration synthesis**.

hydrometers: instruments for measuring the specific gravities of fluids.

Hydromox: a trade name for quinethazone.

hydronephrosis: dilation of the renal pelvis and calices, and sometimes also the collecting ducts, usually caused by obstruction of the ureters.

hydronium ion: H_3O^+; an ion type formed rapidly when hydrogen ions associate with water molecules. Most "H^+" in biological fluids is in this form.

hydroorotic acid: hexahydro-2,6-dioxo-4-pyrimidine-carboxylic acid; an intermediate of bacterial pathways for the biosynthesis of thymine, cytosine, and uracil. High concentrations inhibit the growth of microorganisms that require orotic acid.

hydroperoxyeicosatetrenoic acids: HPETEs; 20-carbon arachidonic acid metabolites with four double bonds, formed in reactions catalyzed by lipoxygenases and epoxygenases, including 5-HPETE (5-hydroperoxy-6,8,11,14-eicosatetraenoic acid, a leukotriene precursor), 12-HPETE, which is converted to 12-HETE (a neutrophil and eosinophil chemotactin), and 15-HPETE (an inhibitor of prostacyclin synthesis).

hydroperoxyl radical: $HO_2\bullet$; a cytotoxic free radical produced when hydrogen attaches to superoxide anions. It is formed during some reactions catalyzed by oxidases, and can react spontaneously with a second hydroperoxyl radical to yield hydrogen peroxide.

5-HPETE   12-HPETE   15-HPETE

hydroperoxyeicosatetrenoic acids

hydrophilic: having a strong affinity for, or tending to dissolve in water. *Cf* **hydrophobic**.

hydrophobic: having low affinity for water; *cf* **hydrophilic**. Many lipids are hydrophobic; but *see* **amphipathic**.

hydrostatic pressure: usually, the blood pressure within a vessel.

3-hydroxyacyl-CoA dehydrogenase: L-3-hydroxyacyl-CoA dehydrogenase; an enzyme of the fatty acid oxidation pathway that catalyzes the reaction: 3-hydroxyacyl-CoA + NAD$^+$ → 3-ketoacyl-CoA + NADH + H$^+$.

hydroxyallysine: *see* **hydroxylysine**.

11β-hydroxy-androstenedione: Δ^4-11β-hydroxy-4-androstene-3,17-dione; a steroid made in the adrenal cortex of many species. It is a weak androgen, and a urinary 17-ketosteroid.

hydroxyapatites: hydroxylapatites: the most abundant inorganic components of bone and dentine extracellular matrices. Small amounts are deposited at other sites, for example in pineal gland psammoma bodies. $Ca_{10}(PO_4)_6(OH)_2$ is a formula proposed for the major biological form. Hydroxyapatites can also be obtained from some rocks. Since they are good adsorbents, preparations containing them are used in chromatography (for example to separate double-stranded from single-stranded DNA), and for purifying steroids, proteins, plasmids, and viruses.

3-β-hydroxybutyric acid {3-**hydroxybutyrate**}: *see* **ketones**.

γ-hydroxybutyrate: a glutamic acid metabolite. High concentrations reversibly block dopaminergic functions.

$$HO-CH_2-CH_2-CH_2-COO^-$$

hydroxycholecalciferols: *see* 1α-hydroxy, 25-hydroxy, 1,25-dihydroxy, 24,25-dihydroxy, and 1,24,25-trihydroxy-**cholecalciferols**.

7α-hydroxycholesterol: an intermediate in the pathway for conversion of cholesterol to bile acids.

25-hydroxycholesterol: *see* 25-hydroxy-**cholesterol**.

3-hydroxy-4,5-dimethoxybenzoic acid: an agent used to inhibit catecholamine-*O*-methyltransferases.

6-hydroxydopamine: 6-OH-DA: *see* 6-OH-**dopamine**.

hydroxyeicosatetraneoic acids: HETEs: several 20-carbon arachidonic acid metabolites formed from hydroperoxyeicosatetraenoic acids and some leukotrienes. The monohydroxylated forms include 5-HETE, 12-HETE and 15-HETE, and the dihydroxylated types 5,6-diHETE (5,6-DHETE), 5,12-DHETE (LTB$_4$), 8,15-DHETE, and 14,15-DHETE. 12-HETE, 5,12-DHETE, and some others are chemotaxins for neutrophils and eosinophils.

hydroxyestrogens: *see* **catechol estrogens**.

hydroxyflutamide: a nonsteroidal antiandrogen with properties and uses similar to those described for **flutamide** (*q.v.*).

hydroxyheptadecanoic acid: HHT; an arachidonic acid metabolite formed from prostaglandin H$_2$ in the reaction: PGH$_2$ → HHT + malonyl dialdehyde.

5-hydroxyindolacetaldehyde: a metabolite formed when a monoamine oxidase catalyzes serotonin degradation. Most of the product is oxidized to 5-hydroxyindole acetic acid, but some in the central nervous system is reduced to the corresponding alcohol.

5-hydroxyindole-3-acetic acid: 5-HIAA; a serotonin metabolite normally made in neurons and in pineal glands, via reactions catalyzed by monoamine oxidases and alcohol dehydrogenases. Carcinoid tumors derived from midgut embryonic cells release large amounts. 5-HIAA is a major end-product that is released to urine, but small amounts are methylated to 5-methoxyindole acetic acid.

hydroxyindole-*O*-methyltransferase: HIOMT: an enzyme that catalyzes the reaction: *N*-acetylserotonin + *S*-adenosylmethionine → melatonin + *S*-adenosylhomocysteine. Its activity in pineal glands rises during dark-

5-HETE   12-HETE   15-HETE

5,6-DHETE   5,12-DHETE

8,15-DHETE   14,15-DHETE

hydroxyeicosatetraneoic acids

ness, and is rate-limiting for melatonin biosynthesis in many (but not all) species.

hydroxylamines: compounds with the general formula R—N—OH. They are used as reducing agents and anti-oxidants, in assays for thioesters, to cleave asparagine-lysine bonds, and to inhibit GABA-transaminase. They are also mutagens that act on amino groups of DNA cytosine bases to yield products that pair with adenine (rather than guanine).

hydroxylapatite: *see* **hydroxyapatites**.

hydroxylases: enzymes that catalyze reactions of the general type shown. The ones that act on steroids and related compounds are named for the carbon positions affected; *see* for example 1α-, 11β- 17α- and 21-hydroxylases. *See* also **cytochrome P$_{450}$**.

$$-CH + O \longrightarrow -C-OH$$

1α-hydroxylases: enzymes made in largest amounts in kidneys that catalyze reduction of ketone groups on secosteroids and related molecules. The activity of **cholecalciferol 1α-hydroxylase** (*q.v.*) is rate-limiting for production of 1,25-dihydroxy-cholecalciferol.

6α-hydroxylase: an enzyme that acts on corticosterone and cortisol. Its products promote Na$^+$ retention, but do not activate type I or type II glucocorticoid receptors.

7α-hydroxylase: a hepatic hydroxylase that catalyzes conversion of cholesterol to its 7α-OH derivative (a step in the pathway for formation of bile acids), and con-tributes to the degradation of progesterone, testosterone, and other steroid hormones.

11β-hydroxylase: an adrenocortical enzyme essential for glucocorticoid synthesis that catalyzes conversion of 11-deoxycorticosterone and 11-deoxycortisol to cor-ticosterone and cortisol, respectively. It also acts on pregnenolone, progesterone, and some other steroids. Adrenocorticotropic hormone (ACTH) and cAMP induce

the enzyme, and seem to essential for maintaining normal activity.

15α-hydroxylase: an enzyme in fetal liver that acts on dehydroepiandrosterone (DHA) and 16-OH-DHA to form 15,16-DHAS, which is then converted to estetrol.

16α-hydroxylase: an enzyme in fetal liver that catalyzes addition of oxygen groups on carbons 16 of dehydro-epiandrosterone (DHEA, DHA) and DHAS. The products are substrates for 15α-hydroxylase.

17α-hydroxylase: an enzyme that acts on pregnenolone, progesterone, and some other steroids, and is essential for the biosynthesis of cortisol, androgens, and estrogens. Luteinizing hormone (LH) promotes its synthesis in the gonads. It is induced by adrenocorticotropic hormone (ACTH) in adrenal glands of cortisol secretors, but is inactive there in species in which corticosterone is the primary glucocorticoid.

18-hydroxylase: an adrenocortical enzyme that acts on several steroids, and is essential for aldosterone biosyn-thesis.

20-hydroxylase: *see* **20α-hydroxysteroid dehydro-genase**.

21-hydroxylase: an adrenocortical enzyme that acts on progesterone, 17α-hydroxyprogesterone, pregnenolone and some other steroids, and is essential for the biosyn-thesis of glucocorticoids and mineralocorticoids. *See* also **adrenogenital syndrome**.

C20,C22-hydroxylase: *see* **side chain cleavage**.

24-hydroxylase: *see* **cholecalciferol 24-hydroxylase**.

5-hydroxylysine: a collagen component, formed after lysine is incorporated into procollagen, via a reaction catalyzed by a peptidyl lysyl hydroxylase. The amounts made vary with the collagen types. Sequential actions of galactosyltransferase and glucosyltransferase incorporate some of the moieties into glucosyl-galactosyl-lysyl derivatives. Lysyl oxidases act on terminal non-glycosy-lated lysyl and hydroxylysyl groups of collagen chains to

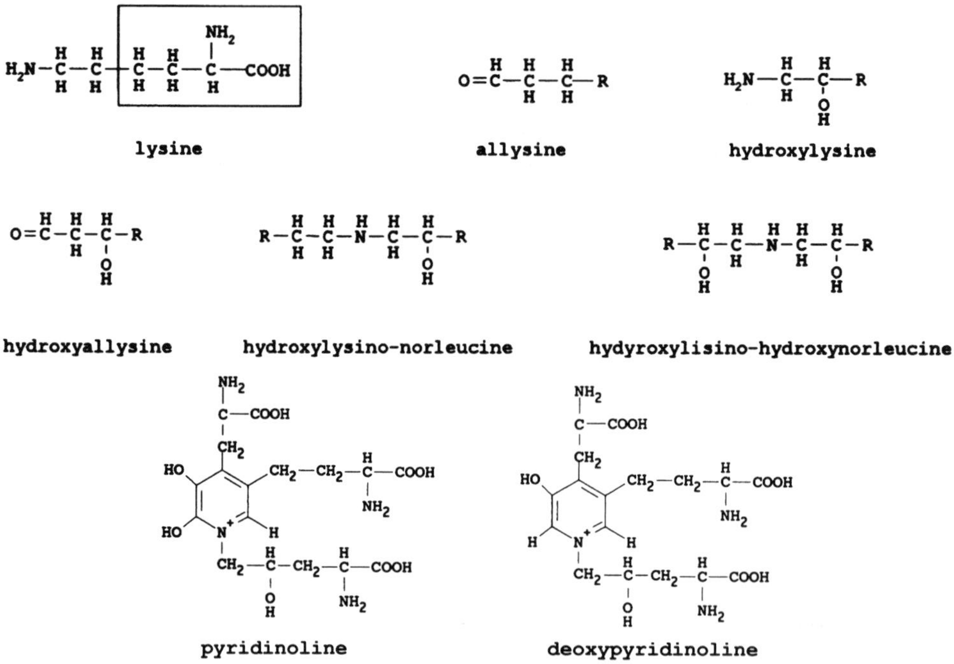

lysine

allysine

hydroxylysine

hydroxyallysine

hydroxylysino-norleucine

hydyroxylisino-hydroxynorleucine

pyridinoline

deoxypyridinoline

5-hydroxylysine

form the aldehydes, allysine (α-aminoadipic acid semial-dehyde) and hydroxyallysine (5α-hydroxy-α-amino-adipic acid semialdehyde), respectively. Interchain cross linkages are then formed by the reactions in which an allysine at the end of one collagen chain reacts with a hydroxylysine in the helical region of another to form a hydroxylysino-norleucine derivative. The same product is formed if a terminal hydroxyallysine combines with a helical hydroxylysine. When hydroxyallysine combines with hydroxylysine, the product is hydroxylysino-hydroxynorleucine. Intrachain cross linkages also form in bone and cartilage when hydroxyallysine groups are converted to pyridiniums via keto-amine intermediates, and when allysines are converted to Schiff bases that react with histidine groups. The lysine component en-closed in the box is represented by R in five of the structures shown. When bone and cartilage are degraded, pyridinoline (PYD) and deoxypyridinoline (DPD) are ex-creted to the urine. The amounts are better indicators of degradation rates than hydroxyproline, since collagens in skin and at other sites do not release such compounds. Small amounts of hydroxylysine are also found in elastin.

p-**hydroxymercuribenzoate**: an agent that binds to sulf-hydryl groups and thereby inactivates aspartate transcarb-amoylase and some other enzymes.

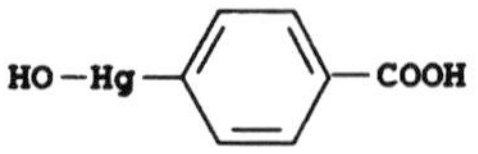

3-**hydroxy-4-methoxy mandelic acid**: *see* **vanillyl mandelic acid**.

5-**hydroxymethyl cytosine**: a pyrimidine that base pairs with guanine. It replaces cytosine in the DNA of T-even

coliphages. A phage DNAse that recognizes cytosine nucleotides degrades the DNA in infected hosts.

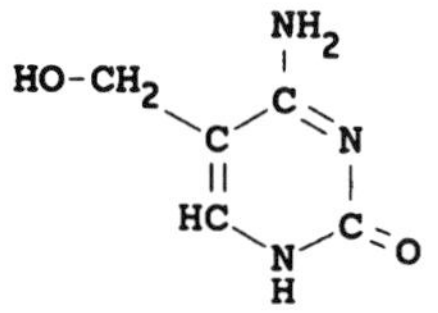

3-**hydroxy,3-methyl glutaryl coenzyme A**: HMG-CoA; an intermediate in the pathway for cholesterol biosynthe-sis, made from the reaction catalyzed by hydroxymethyl glutaryl-CoA synthetase: acetyl-CoA + acetoacetyl-CoA → HMG-CoA + CoA. *See* also **hydroxymethyl glutaryl-coenzyme A reductase**.

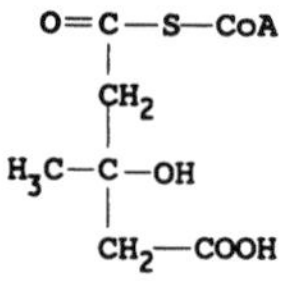

hydroxymethyl glutaryl-coenzyme A reductase: HMG-CoA reductase; an enzyme that catalyzes conver-sion of 3-hydroxy,3-methyl glutaryl coenzyme A to dihydroxymethylvalerate (mevalonate). It is the major rate-limiting step for cholesterol biosynthesis, and is regulated in part by insulin, glucagon, and other hor-mones. Cholesterol or a related metabolite exerts nega-tive feedback control.

4-**hydroxyphenylpyruvate**: an intermediate in the path-way for phenylalanine and tyrosine degradation. Tyrosine transaminase catalyzes the reaction: tyrosine + α-keto-glutarate → 4-hydroxyphenylpyruvate + glutamate.

4-Hydroxyphenylpyruvate dioxygenase then catalyzes
4-hydroxyphenylpyruvate + O_2 → homogentisate +
CO_2.

4-hydroxyphenylpyruvate dioxygenase: *see* **4-hydrox-
yphenylpyruvate**.

hydroxypindolol: *see* **pindolol**.

17α-hydroxypregnenolone: a cholesterol metabolite
made in steroid hormone secreting cells, and released in
small amounts. It is a precursor of 17α-hydroxypro-
gesterone, dehydroepiandrosterone, cortisol, androgens,
and estrogens.

16α-hydroxyprogesterone: a progesterone metabolite
made in the placenta.

17α-hydroxyprogesterone: a cholesterol metabolite
made from 17α-hydroxypregnenolone or progesterone in
steroid hormone secreting cells, and released in small
amounts. It is a precursor of androgens and estrogens.

hydroxyprolines: collagen components, formed after
proline is incorporated into procollagen via reactions
catalyzed by prolyl hydroxylases. Usually, much more
4-OH-proline than 3-hydroxyproline is made, but the
relative amounts vary with the collagen types. Some are
released to blood and urine when collagen is degraded.
Since bone contains the largest amounts, and degrades
collagens more rapidly than the other tissues, the urinary
levels provide rough estimates of bone resorption rates
under most conditions; but *see* 5-**hydroxylysine**.

2-**hydroxysaclofen**: 3-amino-2-(4-chlorophenyl)-2-hy-
droxy-propylsulfonic acid; a selective GABA$_B$ receptor
antagonist.

3α-**hydroxysteroid dehydrogenases**: 3α-HSD; oxo-
reductases most abundant in liver that catalyze reduction
of 5α-dihydrotestosterone (DHT) to 5α-androstane-3α,
17β-diol, and of dihydrocortisone and dihydropro-
gesterone to their tetrahydro derivatives. They also act on
androsterone and some other steroids, and promote conversion of 7α-hydroxy- and 7α,12α-dihydroxy-5β-
cholestane-3-ones to bile acids, and of prostaglandin $F_{2α}$
to prostaglandins E_2 and B_2. Additionally, they change
benzopyrene mutagens to forms that can be detoxified by
glutathione. The enzymes are strongly inhibited by nonsteroidal anti-inflammatory agents such as indomethacin
and aspirin.

3β-**hydroxysteroid dehydrogenase**, 3β-HSD: an enzyme essential for the biosynthesis of progesterone
and its derivatives. It directly catalyzes oxidation of
alcoholic groups on carbon 3 positions of steroids to
ketones, and is a component of a complex with isomerase activity that promotes shifting of A ring double
bonds from the 5,6 to 4,5 positions. Its activity is
increased by luteinizing hormone (LH), human
chorionic gonadotropin (hCG), prolactin, and progesterone, and is decreased by estrogens.

17β-**hydroxysteroid dehydrogenase**: an enzyme that
catalyzes conversion of Δ^4-3,17-androstenedione to
testosterone, of 5α-dihydrotestosterone to 5α-andros-
tanedione, and of 5α-androstane-3α-17β-diol to an-
drenosterone, and also acts on some other steroids
oxygenated at position 17.

20α-**hydroxysteroid dehydrogenases**: 20-hydroxy-
steroid oxoreductases: enzymes that catalyze reversible
addition (or removal) of hydrogen atoms at carbon 20
positions of steroids with 21 carbon atoms. The substrates include pregnenolone, progesterone, and 17α-
progesterone. Various types occur in placenta, amniotic
fluid, gonads, and spermatozoa, and some lymphocytes.
Interleukin-3 induces the enzyme in the thymus gland,
spleen, and bone marrow. Progesterone inhibits at some
sites.

hydroxysteroid oxoreductases: enzymes that catalyze
reversible interconversion of alcoholic and ketone groups
attached to steroid carbons. The term is appropriate for
the ones that act in both directions, but is also applied to
an enzyme that acts at 17α positions whose effects are
reversed by a dehydrogenase.

3-hydroxyproline   4-hydroxyproline

hydroxyprolines

5-hydroxytryptamine: serotonin.

2-methyl-5-hydroxytryptamine: a 5-HT$_3$ type serotonin receptor antagonist.

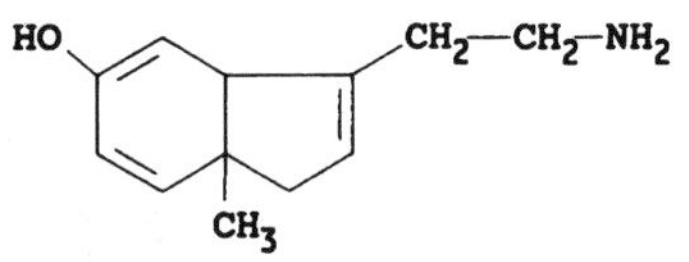

5-hydroxytryptophan; 5-HTP: a tryptophan metabolite formed in the reaction catalyzed by tryptophan hydroxylase: tryptophan + O → 5-hydroxytryptophan. It is a precursor of serotonin, and of serotonin derivatives that include melatonin, 5-hydroxytryptophol, bufotenine, and psilocybin. 5-HTP is used to treat some forms of epilepsy and some neuromuscular disorders, and as an antidepressant and analeptic.

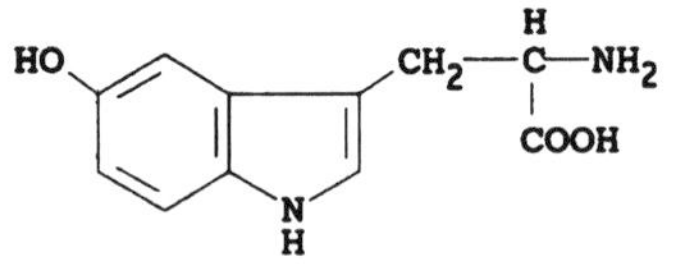

5-hydroxytryptophol: a serotonin metabolite made in pineal glands and implicated as a regulator of gonadotropin secretion. Hydroxindole-O-methyltransferase (HIOMT) converts it to 5-methoxytryptophol.

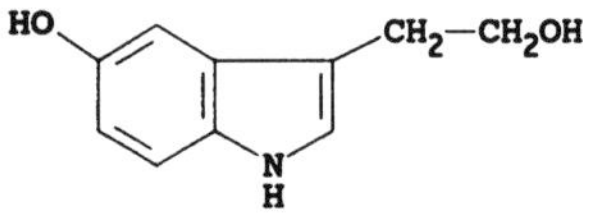

hydroxyurea: an agent that inhibits ribonucleotide reductase, and thereby semi-conservative DNA replication (but not DNA repair). It is used to treat melanoma, chronic granulocytic leukemia, and some ovarian cancers. Although high levels are myelotoxic, moderate ones, used in combination with erythropoietin and iron supplements, confer beneficial effects in individuals with sickle cell anemia and some thalassemias by accelerating production of fetal type hemoglobin. Fetal hemoglobin inhibits polymerization of hemoglobin S (the sickle cell type), and thereby decreases vascular occlusion and hemolysis.

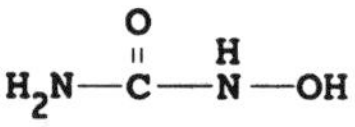

hydroxyzine: N-(4-chlorobenzhydryl)-N'(hydroxyethoxyethyl)-piperazine; an H$_1$-type histamine receptor antagonist with antiemetic and anxiolytic properties. It is used for preoperative and postoperative sedation.

hygromycin B: O-6-amino-6-deoxy-L-glycero-D-galacto-heptopyranosylidene-(1→2,3)-O-β-D-talopyranosyl(1→5)-2-deoxy-N^3-methyl-D-streptamine; an antibiotic made by *Streptomyces hygroscopicus* that acts on DNAs and inhibits the growth of both prokaryotes and eukaryotes that infect mammals. It used in veterinary medicine as an antihelminthic. An *E. coli* gene that confers resistance is used to identify and select recombinant clones.

Hymenoptera: an order of insects that includes bees, ants, and wasps.

hyoscine: scopolamine.

hyoscyamine: α-(hydroxymethyl)benzeneacetic acid 8-methyl-8-azabicyclo[3,2,1]-oct3-yl ester; an alkaloid made by several *Solanaceae* species, and a major active component of henbane. It is a muscarinic type acetylcholine receptor antagonist with properties similar to those of atropine.

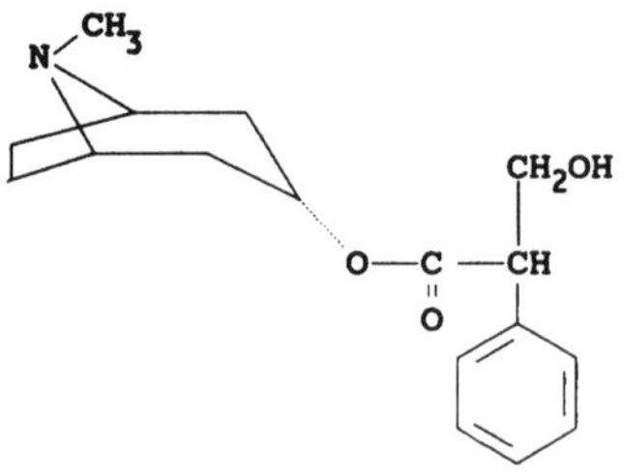

hyp-: hypo-.

Hyp: hydroxyproline.

hypalgesia: diminished sensitivity to pain.

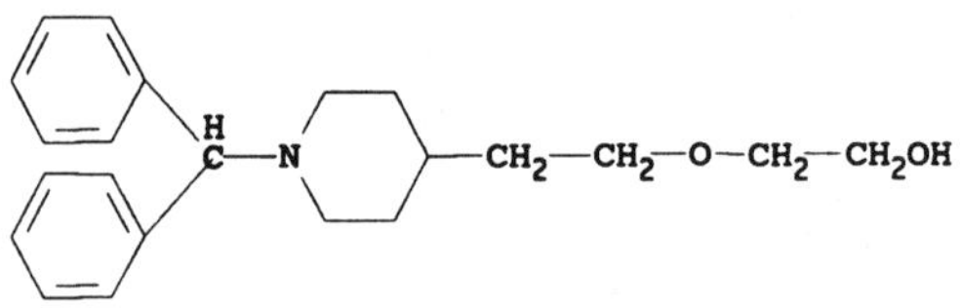

hydroxyzine

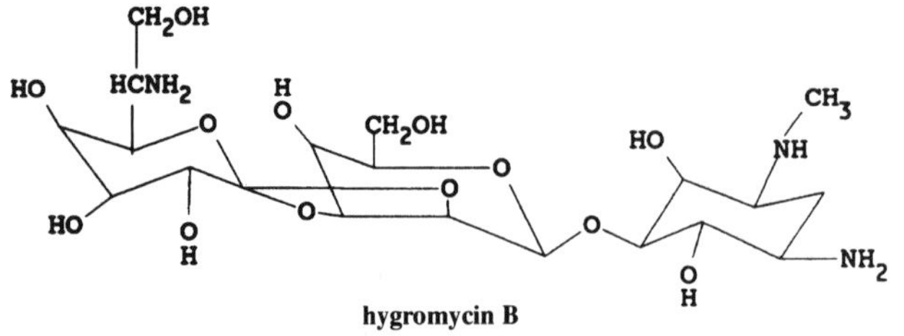

hygromycin B

hyper-: a prefix meaning excess (too much or too many).

hyperbaric: at a pressure of more than 1 atmosphere. Although oxygen is delivered under high pressure to alleviate severe hypoxia cause by damaged pulmonary membranes, and to treat decompression sickness, it can damage the lungs.

hypercalcemia: excessively high blood calcium concentrations. It acutely depresses excitablility in peripheral neurons and skeletal muscle, by decreasing the permeability to Na^+ ions, but accelerates Ca^{2+} entry in the myocardium, increases contractile force, and can cause systolic arrest. Chronic elevation leads to metastatic calcification, especially when phosphate levels are also high. *See* also **calcium**, 1,25-**cholecalciferol, humoral hypercalcemic factor of malignancy**, and **parathyroid hormone**.

hypercalcemic factors: *see* **hypercalcin** and **humoral hypercalcemia of malignancy**.

hypercalcin: a component of amphibian and fish pituitary glands that elevates blood calcium levels. It may be chemically and biologically related to parathyroid hormone (which is not made by fishes).

hypercalciuria: excessively high urine calcium levels, usually associated with hypercalcemia. The excess calcium can deposit in and damage the kidneys, ureters, and urinary bladder.

hypercapnia: excessively high blood carbon dioxide. The most common cause is impaired pulmonary ventilation.

hyperdiploid: possessing more chromosomes than the diploid number characteristic of the species.

hyperglycemia: excessively high blood glucose concentrations. It leads to glycosuria, dehydration, and other metabolic dysfunctions. The most common cause is insulin deficiency (*see* **diabetes mellitus** and **glucose**), but it can also be invoked by excessive amounts of glucocorticoids, growth hormone, and/or glucagon. The amounts of epinephrine released during severe stress can cause transient hyperglycemia, which soon subsides.

hypergonadotropic hypogonadism: impaired development and/or functions of the gonads, caused by genetic defects that affect differentiation, production of gonadal hormones, and/or ability to respond to gonadotropins. Excessive amounts of gonadotropins are then secreted because of loss of the negative feedback controls normally exerted on the gonadotropes. *Cf* **hypogonadotropic hypogonadism**.

hypergyny: mating that improves the social standing or rank of a female.

hyperkalemia: excessively high blood potassium concentrations. It lowers blood pressure by promoting vasodilation, and by depressing cardiac contractile force and slowing conduction, and can also indirectly invoke metabolic alkalosis. The causes include aldosterone deficiency and renal dysfunction.

hypermorphs: individuals with mutant genes whose effects are more powerful than those of wild types.

hypernatremia: excessively high blood sodium concentrations. The consequences include water retention, expansion of extracellular fluid volume, and metabolic alkalosis. *See* also **aldosterone**.

hyperosmolar: describes a solution that contains larger numbers of solute particles per unit volume than a reference solution, and thereby exerts a higher osmotic pressure. If the solute does not diffuse across plasma membranes, a solution hyperosmolar to cytoplasm is also hypertonic. (However, if the solute rapidly enters cells, it draws in water, and is therefore hypotonic).

hyperparathyroidism: conditions caused by excessive secretion of **parathyroid hormone** (*q.v.*). The most obvious consequences result from hypercalcemia, but other effects include bone abnormalities and phosphate metabolism derangements.

hyperphagia: excessive food intake. The term usually refers to abnormal conditions, caused, for example by hypothalamic lesions, endocrine imbalances, genetic defects that affect enzyme production, and/or psychological disorders. Previously healthy laboratory animals often increase their food intake above levels required to maintain body weight when exposed to some forms of stress. *See* also **cafeteria diets**.

hyperplasia: increased growth of a tissue or organ by proliferation of the cell types normally present at that location; *cf* **hypertrophy** and **metaplasia**.

hypersensitive responses: HR; rapidly developing reactions of plants to injury inflicted by pathogenic viruses, bacteria, fungi, insects, other invertebrate pests, or mechanical assault. A major component is localized necrosis that blocks the spread of infections and toxins to healthy parts of the plant, and provides some protection against future attacks to the region. The injury initiates **systemic acquired resistance** (*q.v.*), mediated in part by cell wall oligogalacturonide fragments. The plants then synthesize several kinds of protective factors, collectively called pathogen related proteins. These include phytoalexins, proteinases that injure predators and disrupt the functions of insect digestive systems, and factors that promote strengthening of cell walls and cuticles. One of the early responses is synthesis of prosystemin at wound sites and other parts of the plant. It is cleaved to systemin, a hormone that induces at least two serine protease inhibitors (an 8.1K inhibitor I and a 12.3K inhibitor II), both of which decrease the digestibility and nutritional quality of leaf proteins. Lipases that release α-linolenic acid are also activated, and the fatty acid is converted to **jasmonic acid** (*q.v.*) and its more volatile, methylated derivative. *See* also **ethylene**.

hypersensitivity: excessive responsivity, a term that usually refers to exaggerated and potentially damaging immune system responses to one or more antigens. The manifestations of *immediate hypersensitivity type I* are caused mostly by antigen interactions with IgE type immunoglobulins, and consequent release of histamine and other regulators (*see* **allergy**, **anaphylaxis**, and **urticaria**). *Immediate hypersensitivity type II* follows antigen interactions with circulating antibodies (produced by B lymphocytes), and usually involves complement fixation. *Immediate type III* responses are invoked by antigen-antibody complexes that attach to, and can damage tissues. *Delayed hypersensitivity* is mediated by T lymphocytes.

hypertensin: an obsolete term for angiotensin II.

hypertensinogen: an obsolete term for renin substrate.

hypertension: excessively high blood pressure. The known causes include excessive production of vasoconstrictors, inadequate levels of vasodilators, electrolyte imbalances, pathological changes in blood vessels, and pharmacological agents. For some of the factors known to affect blood pressure, *see* **angiotensin II**, **norepinephrine**, **glucocorticoids**, **aldosterone**, **vasopressin**, **atrial natriuretic peptides**, **endothelins**, **nitric oxide**, **potassium**, and **arteriosclerosis**. The term *essential* is applied when no cause is known.

hyperthermia: excessively high body temperature. The major cause is hypothalamic dysfunction. It can follow head injury, or excessive exposure to ultraviolet radiation (which damages thermoregulatory components). Other causes include severe dehydration and some toxins.

hyperthyroidism: conditions in which excessive amounts of iodinated thyroid hormones are secreted; *see* also **triiodothyronine**. The causes include autoimmune diseases in which thyroid stimulating antibodies are made (*see* **Graves' disease**), thyroid gland tumors that do not require high thyroid stimulating hormone (TSH) levels to secrete excessive amounts, and TSH-secreting tumors that are not regulated by the usual feedback controls.

hypertonic: describes environments that cause water to be osmotically drawn from cells. They are usually aqueous solutions with high concentrations of solutes that do not diffuse across plasma membranes. Concentrations hypertonic for one cell type may not be for another. For example, although sodium ions do not rapidly diffuse into either type, 0.9% NaCl is hypertonic for amphibian erythrocytes (and will cause them to shrink), whereas it is approximately isotonic for mammalian red cells. Cf **hyperosmotic** and **hypotonic**.

hypertrophy: excessive growth via enlargement (but not proliferation) of the cells of an organ or tissue; *cf* **hyperplasia**.

hypervariable site: hv site: a domain that can take several forms in members of the same species. The term usually refers to the variable regions of immunoglobulin light and heavy chains involved in antigen recognition.

hypha: a fungus thallus filament.

hypnotics: agents that induce sleep; *cf* **sedatives**.

hypo-: a prefix (1) meaning too little, too few, or subnormal, or under; most terms modified by the prefix hyper-, can also be modified by hypo-; (2) applied to acids with fewer oxygen atoms than reference compounds, and to their salts and ions. For example, H_3PO_3 and H_3PO_2 are, respectively, phosphorus and hypophosphorus acids. Similarly, sodium chlorite is $NaClO_2$, whereas sodium hypochlorite is $NaClO$.

hypobaric: at a pressure of less than 1 atmosphere.

hypoblast: the embryonic tissue that lies below the epiblast. It is the site for mesoderm induction.

hypocapnia: excessively low blood carbon dioxide concentration. One cause is hyperventilation, which occurs during "panic attacks" (and in individuals learning to play wind instruments). Since CO_2 conversion to carbonic acid provides the major stimulant for respiratory center neurons in the medulla oblongata (and is a physiological dilator when acting locally), hypocapnia can lead to hypoxia and constriction of cerebral blood vessels with manifestations that include dizziness and paresthesias. Although some other blood vessels constrict, and cardiac activity is stimulated, the vasomotor center is depressed. Chronic hypocapnia invokes respiratory alkalosis, which decreases the fraction of blood calcium present as free Ca^{2+} ion; and severe conditions can invoke tetany.

hypodermis: subcutaneous tissue.

hypogeusia: diminished taste perception. Taste bud renewal rates decline with advancing age in normal humans, but taste perception is usually affected to a lesser extent than olfaction.

hypoglycemia: excessively low blood glucose levels. The earliest manifestations are anxiety, restlessness, irritability, and inability to perform demanding mental activities. Further decreases in the sugar levels invoke what has been described as a "sense of impending doom". Somewhat more severe hypoglycemia causes tremors. If the condition progresses, it can lead to convulsions and coma. The most common cause is insulin excess. It can occur when overreactive or increased numbers of pancreatic β cells (or tumors derived from them) release too much, or when an overdose is inadvertently administered to an individual with insulin-dependent diabetes mellitus. Small numbers of humans respond to stress by releasing excessive amounts. In fewer individuals than is suggested by some lay "health" magazines, ingestion of sugar can lead acutely to release of sufficient insulin to cause a mild form of hypoglycemia. Such conditions are best treated with carbohydrate-restricted diets (which lead, over time, to some reduction in the numbers of insulin-secreting cells). Although short periods of fasting lower the glucose levels, they usually do not lead to true hypoglycemia, because adrenocortical hormones (released in larger amounts at such times), promote gluconeogenesis; and glucagon promotes glycogenolysis. Growth hormone levels also rise during fasting; and epinephrine secretion is stimulated if the sugar levels are not maintained. Severe fasting hypoglycemia can occur in individuals with adrenocortical insufficiency (which impairs appetite and as well as hepatic gluconeogenesis and glycogen storage).

hypoglossal: below the tongue.

hypoglycorrhachia: subnormal glucose levels in cerebrospinal fluid. A major cause is impaired production of the GLUT-1 type glucose transport carrier.

hypogonadotropic hypogonadism: impaired development and/or inadequate function of the gonads caused by gonadotropin deficiency. Although the problem can originate in the adenohypophysis, it is more commonly caused by hypothalamic dysfunctions that affect the synthesis and/or release patterns for gonadotropin releasing hormone (GnRH). *See* also **Kallmann's syndrome**, and *cf* **hypergonadotropic hypogonadism**.

hypoosmotic: describes a solution that contains fewer solute particles per unit volume than a reference solution, and thereby exerts less osmotic pressure; *cf* **hyperosmotic** and **hypotonic**.

hypophysial cleft: residual cleft; the remnant of the lumen of Rathke's pouch that persists in a mature pituitary gland. When the ventral surfaces of pituitary glands of rats and some other laboratory animals are exposed, and the **anterior pituitary** (*q.v.*) is removed, the break occurs in the cleft region.

hypophysis: the pituitary gland; *see* **adenohypophysis** and **neurohypophysis**.

hypophysiotropic area: HTA; the hypothalamic region that contains the neurons essential for maintaining adenohypophysial functions. *See* **hypothalamic releasing hormones**.

hypophysectomy: HX; removal of (1) the entire pituitary gland; (2) the adenohypophysis.

hypoploid: having fewer chromosomes than the number characteristic of the species.

hypospadias: sex differentiation defects in males, in which the urethral folds fail to unite, and the urethral orifice assumes a position on the under surface of a poorly developed penis. It can be caused by androgen receptor defects, 5α reductase deficiency, or inability to secrete adequate amounts of testosterone during critical stages of embryonic and early fetal development.

hypostatic gene: a gene whose phenotypic manifestation is blocked by a nonallelic (epistatic) gene.

hyposthenuria: inability to produce concentrated urine, usually because of vasopressin deficiency. Other causes include too few, or abnormal vasopressin receptors, and nephron defects.

hypothalamic: within, associated with, or affected by the hypothalamus.

hypothalamic "areas": neuron clusters within the hypothalamus implicated in the regulation of specific functions. The existence of circumscribed, morphologically distinct entities such as "feeding centers", "drinking centers", or "pleasure-reward centers" has been questioned; but *see* **hypophysiotropic area**.

hypothalamic "centers": *see* **hypothalamic "areas"**.

hypothalamic inhibitory hormones: hormones secreted by neurons within the hypothalamus that exert inhibitory influences on adenohypophysial cells. *See*, for example **prolactin inhibitory factor** (PIF).

hypothalamic nuclei: neuron clusters within the hypothalamus associated with specific functions; *see* for example **supraoptic**, **paraventricular**, **arcuate**, **ventromedial**, **lateral**, **suprachiasmatic**, and **periventricular nuclei**. *See* also **magnocellular** and **parvocellular nuclei**.

hypothalamic obesity: body weight gain associated with hyperphagia, excessive insulin secretion, lipid metabolism defects, and "finickiness", invoked by large brain lesions that include ventral hypothalamic regions, and related syndromes caused by development defects or hypothalamic injury. The paraventricular nuclei are among the sites known to contribute to the control of food intake and fat accumulation.

hypothalamic release factors: *see* **hypothalamic releasing hormones**.

hypothalamic releasing hormones: hormones made by hypothalamic neurons and released to hypothalamo-hypophysial blood vessels, that are essential for maintaining normal structures and functions of adenohypophysial cells. The group includes thyrotropin, corticotropin, growth hormone, and gonadotropin hormone releasing hormones (TRH, CRH, GRH, and GnRH). The regulators were called hypothalamic release factors when the biological activities could be demonstrated but the chemical identities had not yet been established. The same (and/or closely related) molecular species are made in other parts of the brain, and outside the central nervous system.

hypothalamo-hypophysial nerve tracts: bilateral axon bundles that originate in **magnocellular** hypothalamic nuclei (*q.v.*), and descend the infundibulum. Most terminate in the neurohypophysis, but some end in the median eminence or pars intermedia. Hormones transported by the axons include vasopressin and oxytocin. *See* also **supraoptic** and **paraventricular nuclei**.

hypothalamo-hypophysial portal system: HHPS; small blood vessels that link the hypothalamus with the hypophysis; venules that drain the regions supplied mostly by superior hypophysial arteries (anterior hypophysial arteries in tetrapods), and the capillaries that branch from them. The major function is transport of hypothalamic releasing hormones to adenohypophysial cells; but some blood flows in the opposite direction and carries regulators involved in negative feedback controls. There is also some exchange of blood with neurohypophysial vessels.

hypothalamus: the brain region that forms the floor and lower lateral walls of the third ventricle, and is bounded by the hypothalamic sulcus, cerebral ganglia, optic tracts, and subthalamus. Various neuron groups within the hypothalamus are major sites for the synthesis of hypothalamic releasing hormones, vasopressin, oxytocin, and other regulators. Different neuron clusters are more directly involved in thermoregulation, autonomic system controls, emotional expression, and other functions.

hypothesis: a tentative conclusion based on limited information, used to design experiments and/or interpret data; *cf* **theory**.

hypotonic: describes solutions or environments that cause cells to take up water by osmosis; *cf* **hypertonic** and **hypoosmotic**. Erythrocytes exposed to hypotonic solutions undergo hemolysis.

hypovolemia: abnormally low blood volume. The causes include vasopressin or aldosterone deficiency, receptor defects, some renal disorders, and severe dehydration.

hypoxanthine: 6-oxypurine; a metabolite produced by deamination of adenine. Much of it is degraded to uric acid and excreted to urine. It can, however, enter a "salvage pathway" via the reaction catalyzed by hypoxanthine-guanine phosphoribosyl transferase: hypoxanthine + PRPP → inosinate + P-P. Inosinate is then used to make guanylate.

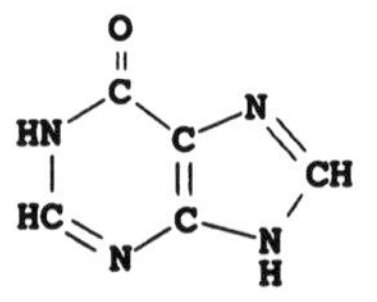

hypoxanthine guanine phosphoribosyltransferase: HPRT; HGPRT; an enzyme of the "salvage" pathway for purine nucleotide recycling, in which guanine is converted to guanosine monophosphate (GMP), and hypoxanthine to inosine monophosphate (IMP). *See* also **hypoxanthine, HAT medium** and **Lesh-Nyhan syndrome**.

hypoxia: usually, subnormal oxygen content. Conditions in which the circulating blood contains insufficient oxygen are classified on the basis of cause: *anemic* (inadequate hemoglobin content), *circulatory* (impaired delivery to cells, because of excessive vasoconstriction or myocardial insufficiency), *diffusional* (damaged pulmonary membranes), and *hypoxic* (low oxygen tension in the inspired air). Carbon monoxide lowers blood oxygen levels by attaching to hemoglobin and blocking the association with oxygen. In *histotoxic* hypoxias, the blood oxygen content can be in the normal range, but the ability of cells to use it is impaired. Toxins such as cyanide paralyze the cytochrome system.

hypusine: *N*-(4-amino-2-hydroxybutyl)-L-lysine; a component of initiation factor 5A (eIF-5A), made from spermidine via a deoxyhypusine intermediate. It is a component of all eukaryote cells, and is essential for cell replication. The levels increase in parallel with protein synthesis when cells enlarge.

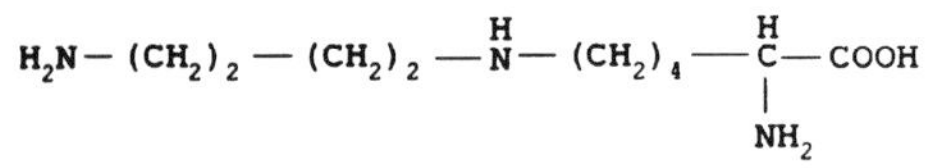

$$H_2N-(CH_2)_2-(CH_2)_2-\underset{H}{N}-(CH_2)_4-\underset{\underset{NH_2}{|}}{\overset{H}{C}}-COOH$$

deoxyhypusine

$$H_2N-(CH_2)_2-\underset{\underset{H}{\overset{|}{O}}}{\overset{H}{C}}-CH_2-\underset{H}{N}-(CH_2)_4-\underset{\underset{NH_2}{|}}{\overset{H}{C}}-COOH$$

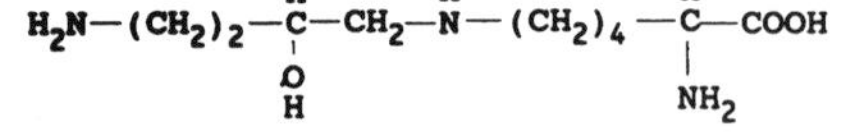

hypusine

hysterectomy: removal of the uterus. It is performed on some laboratory animal species to study the effects of humoral factors released by the cells on processes such as luteolysis (and in humans when the organs are diseased).

hysteresis: describes systems in which one process lags behind (and may be dependent upon) a previous one.

Hystricomorpha: a suborder of rodents that includes guinea pigs, porcupines, and chinchillas. Compared with most other rodents, the young are born after relatively long gestation periods, have body hair at the time of birth, and are in other ways more mature.

hyt/hyt: a mouse strain that carries a mutation which leads to the development of hypothyroidism.

H zone: the part of a skeletal muscle dark band that appears lighter than neighboring regions because it does not contain overlapping actin filaments. It is crossed by an M line.

I

I: (1) isoleucine; (2) iodine.

i: inside or intracellular, used as a subscript, as in Ca_i^{2+}.

Ia antigens: class II cell surface proteins whose synthesis is directed by I regions of murine major histocompatibility complex genes. They are expressed predominantly on B lymphocytes and macrophages, but some are on dendritic cells and thymus gland epithelium.

Ia genes: DNA components of murine chromosomes that direct production of Ia antigens.

IAA: indole acetic acid.

IAP: (1) islet activating protein; *see* **pertussis toxin**; (2) immunosuppressive acidic protein; *see* α_1**-acidic glycoprotein**.

iatric: pertaining to medicine or physicians. It can be a suffix, as in pediatric.

iatrogenic: caused by medical treatment (such as pharmacological agents, surgery, physical therapy, special nutrients, or suggestion).

I band: the isotropic band of a skeletal muscle sarcomere that contains only thin microfilaments; *cf* **A band** and **H zone**.

iberiotoxin: a peptide in the venom of the scorpion, *Buthus tamalus*. It is a highly selective blocker of Ca^{2+}-activated potassium ion channels that constricts arterial smooth muscle and opposes negative feedback controls. In the amino acid sequence shown, cysteine moieties are joined at positions $7 \rightarrow 28$, $13 \rightarrow 33$, and $17 \rightarrow 35$: pGlu-Phe-Thr-Asp-Val-Asp-Cys-Ser-Val-Ser-Lys-Glu-Cys-Trp-Ser-Val-Cys-Lys-Asp-Leu-Phe-Gly-Val-Asp-Arg-Gly-Lys-Cys-Met-Gly-Lys-Lys-Cys-Arg-Cys-Tyr-Gln-OH.

IBMP: 1-isobutyl-3-methoxypyrazine.

IBMX: MIX; *see* **isobutyl methylxanthine**.

ibogaine: 12-methoxyibogamine; an alkaloid made by the African shrub, *Tebernanthe iboga*. It is a central nervous system stimulant, hallucinogen, and anti-convulsant reported to be useful for treating cocaine and morphine addiction.

ibotenic acid {**ibotenate**}: α-amino-2,3-dihydro-3-oxo-5-isoxazoleacetic acid; an excitotoxin made by *Amanita* mushrooms. It is a mixed NMDA receptor agonist-an-tagonist, used to potentiate anesthesia, suppress tremors and emesis in laboratory animals, and as an insecticide.

ibuprofen: α-methyl-4-(2-methylpropyl)benzene acetic acid; an orally effective nonsteroidal analgesic, antipyretic and anti-inflammatory agent that inhibits cyclooxygenase. It is used to treat rheumatoid arthritis and osteoarthritis, and to alleviate non-visceral pain.

IC₅₀: the concentration of an inhibitor that decreases an enzyme activity or response to a regulator by 50%

ICAs: circulating IgG type immunoglobulin antibodies that bind cytoplasmic antigens of pancreatic islet and some other cell types, but are neither species nor organ specific. Small amounts are made by healthy individuals, and larger ones by many with newly diagnosed insulin dependent diabetes mellitus and some other autoimmune diseases. They are believed to either initiate cell destruction or amplify the effects of other deleterious factors. *Cf* **ICSA**.

I₂CA: indole-2-carboxylic acid.

ICABP: intestinal calcium binding protein.

ICAM-1: intercellular adhesion molecule-1.

iC3b: C3Bi; a product formed when complement factor 1 catalyzes cleavage of factor 3. It binds to complement receptor 3 (CR3) on monocytes and neutrophilic leukocytes, and enhances phagocytosis. *See* also **complement** and **mac-1**.

iC4b: C4Bi; the major product formed when complement factor 1 catalyzes cleavage of factor 4.

I cell[s]: (1) gastrointestinal tract cells that secrete cholecystokinin; *see* also **I cell disease**.

I cell disease: inclusion cell disease; mucolipidosis II; a rare autosomal recessive metabolic disorder, usually fatal during childhood, in which the ability to synthesize *N*-acetylglucosaminyl phosphotransferase (an enzyme essential for mannose phosphorylation, and a component of the lysosomes of fibroblasts and some other cell types), is

ICI 198,615

impaired. The manifestations include cartilage maturation defects, coarse faces, severe retardation of somatic growth and brain development, and accumulation of cytoplasmic inclusions.

ICI 174,864: *N*,*N*-diallyl-Tyr-Aib-Aib-Phe-Leu-OH; an opioid receptor antagonist that exerts more potent effects on μ than on δ types.

ICI 198,615: 2-([2-methoxy-4-([phenylsulfonyl)amino] carbonyl)-phenyl]methyl)-1*H*-indazol-6-yl]-carbamic acid cyclopentyl ester; a potent LTE$_4$ type leukotriene receptor antagonist that relaxes bronchiole smooth muscle.

icosanoids: 20-carbon unsaturated fatty acids and their derivatives (including prostaglandins and leukotrienes). *See* **eicosanoids**.

ICS 205-903: (3α-tropanyl)-1*H*-indole-3-carboxylic acid ester; a selective antagonist for 5HT$_3$ type serotonin receptors.

ICSAs: antibodies that bind to pancreatic beta cell surface antigens, detectable in many individuals with insulin dependent diabetes mellitus, and in smaller percentages of first-degree relatives. They are believed to either initiate cell destruction or amplify the effects of other factors.

ICSH: interstitial cell stimulating hormone; *see* **luteinizing hormone**.

ichthyo-: a prefix meaning fish.

ichthyotocin: IT; isotocin.

icterus: jaundice.

icv: intracerebroventricular.

[125I]CYP: radioactively labeled cyanopindolol; a β-type adrenergic receptor antagonist, used as a ligand to identify the receptors. Serotonin competes to some extent for the binding sites. *See* also **pindolol**.

ID$_{50}$: (1) minimal infective dose; (2) median infective dose.

idazoxan hydrochloride: 2-(1,4-benzodioxan-2-yl)-imidazoline hydrochloride; a selective α$_2$ type adrenergic receptor antagonist.

IDCs: interdigitating cells.

IDDM: insulin-dependent diabetes mellitus.

identical twins: *see* **monozygotic twins**.

idiogram: a diagram that represents the DNA components of a single chromosome, or of a karyotype.

idiopathic: self-originating; an abnormal condition caused by endogenous factors, for which no cause has been established.

idiotope: (1) an antigenic determinant on the variable region of a specific kind of immunoglobulin molecule. (An immunoglobulin molecule can have more than one idiotope); (2) an epitope on the variable region of an antibody recognized by combining sites of other antibodies of the same individual; *see* also **idiotype**.

idiotope anti-idiotope networks: proposed self-regulating immune system mechanisms, in which idiotopes made by one set of B lymphocytes promote the synthesis of, and bind to anti-idiotopes (antibodies) on the surfaces of others. Depending on conditions that include the levels of idiotopes and the kinds and amounts of modifying factors, anti-idiotopes can limit or augment synthesis of the initiating types, and can also act as antigens that direct formation of anti-anti-idiotopes (some of which resemble the original idiotopes). The balances change when foreign antigens are presented, and the net effects are influenced by the amounts and the routes of entry.

idiotype: the characteristics of the variable regions of antibodies produced by one B lymphocyte clone, or of the recognition sites for one kind of T lymphocyte receptor.

IDLs: intermediate density lipoproteins; *see* **lipoproteins**.

idose: aldohexose sugars that differ from glucose in the positions of alcoholic groups attached to carbon atoms at positions 2, 3, and 4. The D form is shown. *See* also L-**iduronic acid**.

idoxuridine: *see* 5-**iodo-5′-deoxyuridine**.

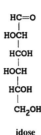

idose

L-**iduronic acid** {**iduronate**}: a sugar acid component of dermatan sulfate, heparan sulfate, and heparins, made from glucose-1-phosphate. Most of the moieties are sulfated at position 2. *See also* **Hurler's syndrome**.

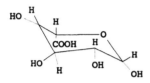

IF: (1) initiation factor; (2) intermediate filament.

IFNs: **interferons** (*q.v.*). The various types are designated by Greek letters, as in IFNα.

Ig: immunoglobulin; *see* specific types.

IgA: immunoglobulin A; immunoglobulins with α type heavy chains. Most are 160K "monomers" (each composed of two identical light and two identical heavy chains). These and some 320K "dimers" account for 10-15% of the immunoglobulins of human blood. 415K molecules with two additional chains are secreted to saliva, tears, milk, and the fluids on the surfaces of gastrointestinal, respiratory, and genitourinary epithelium, where they contribute to defenses against bacterial and some viral infections. The molecules do not cross the placenta, but are present in colostrum. Two subclasses have been identified, with IgA1 predominating in blood and IgA2 in secretions.

IgA enhancing factor: interleukin-5.

IgD: immunoglobulin D; immunoglobulins with δ type heavy chains. 175K monomers are co-expressed with IgMs on the surfaces of mature B lymphocytes, with highest levels on memory cells. Only minute amounts circulate.

IgE: immunoglobulins with ε type heavy chains. 190K monomers complex with antigens that bind to Fcε receptors on mast cells and basophilic leukocytes. They trigger the release of histamine, serotonin, and other mediators of allergic reactions.

IGF[s]: insulin-like growth factors; *see* **insulin-like growth factor-1** and **insulin-like growth factor-2**.

IGF-I: somatomedin C; *see* **insulin-like growth factor-I**.

IGF-II: somatomedin A; *see* **insulin-like growth factor-II**.

IGF-BPs: insulin-like growth factor binding proteins.

IGFRcs: insulin-like growth factor receptors.

IgG: immunoglobulins with γ type heavy chains. In humans, subclasses, IgG1, IgG2, IgG3, and IgG4 have been identified. 50K monomers predominate in circulating blood, 70% of which are usually IgG1. They bind complement, and are essential for secondary immune responses. IgGs transported across the placenta contribute to protection of fetuses and very young infants against infections.

IgM: immunoglobulins with μ type heavy chains. They avidly bind antigens, fix complement, and can promote cell agglutination, but do not cross the placenta. IgMs are the first immunoglobulins to appear on the surfaces of immature B cells, and the major types secreted by most antigen-activated B cells during primary immune responses. They are 955K pentamers in humans, and tetramers in some other species. Some form of IgM is synthesized by all vertebrates; and most fishes make only this class of immunoglobulins.

IL-1, IL-2....IL-13: *see* **interleukins** and specific types.

ILA: insulin-like activity.

Ile: I; isoleucine.

ileum: the distal 3/5 of the small intestine that extends from the end of the jejunum to the opening of the cecum (approximately 12 feet long in humans). It is the major site for nutrient absorption, and contains many lymph follicles.

ilium: usually, the broad, flaring portion of the hip bone, fused when mature with the ischium and pubis.

iloprost: a chemically stable prostacyclin analog used to inhibit platelet aggregation and protect against damage caused by ischemia.

imaginal discs: epithelial folds in the larvae of *Drosophila* and many other insect species that develop into adult appendages (legs, wings, or antennae).

imago: the adult, sexually mature stage of the life cycle of an insect.

IM, im: intramuscularly.

IM-9 cells: a lymphoblastoid cell line derived from a patient with multiple myeloma.

imbibition: absorption, without chemical change, of vapors and liquids into submicroscopic pores of a gel or solid substance.

IMCal: a **calcium binding protein** (*q.v.*) in brush border membranes of small intestine cells, believed to contribute to calciferol-regulated calcium absorption. It does not directly mediate ion uptake.

imetit dihydrobromide: *S*[2-(imidazol-4-yl)ethyl]isothiourea dihydrobromide; a potent, selective agonist for H₃ type histamine receptors.

imidazole: 1,3-diazole; a heterocyclic aromatic base used to activate cyclic nucleotide phosphodiesterases and inhibit thromboxane synthesis, and as a buffer. Several derivatives are used to combat fungus infections.

imetit dihydrobromide

imidazole

imino acids: acids that contain an —NH— group. Proline and hydroxyproline are imino acids, but are included among the "amino" acids.

L-N^5-(1-**iminoethyl**) **ornithine**: L-NIO; a potent, irreversible inhibitor of nitric oxide synthetase.

iminoglycinuria: the loss of glycine and imino acids (proline and hydroxyproline) to the urine. It can occur in normal infants whose renal transport mechanisms have not fully matured, when blood contains excessively high concentrations of the compounds, and in individuals with autosomal recessive disorders that impair transport. In severe cases, it is associated with seizures and/or mental retardation. *See* also **Fanconi syndrome** and **Hartnup** disease.

imipramine: 10,11-dihydro-*N,N*-dimethyl-5H-dibenz-[*b,f*]-azepine; the hydrochloride is an orally effective tricyclic antidepressant that inhibits catecholamine uptake by synaptic vesicles, and is used to treat enuresis and compulsive disorders.

immediate early genes: *c-fos*, *c-jun*, and other genes rapidly activated by growth factors.

immediate hypersensitivity: *see* **hypersensitivity**.

immortalization: cell transformation that blocks progression to senescence, and causes cells to survive and proliferate long after the time when their normal counterparts would have died. The changes can develop spontaneously in cell cultures, and can be induced with mutagens, or by transfection.

immune complexes: large antigen-antibody aggregates. Most contain IgG type immunoglobulins, some of which may by directed against self-antigens. They can cause damage by fixing complement, invoking inflammatory reactions, and/or depositing in vascular tissue, in glomerular basement membranes, and at other sites. Circulating complexes contribute directly to serum sickness and Arthus reactions.

immune deficiency diseases: disorders in which the ability to mount effective immune responses against foreign antigens is impaired. The causes include congenital absence or deficiencies of B and/or T cells, and lymphocyte destruction by viruses. In some cases, only certain aspects of immune system functions are lost. *See* also **agammaglobulinemia**, **Di George syndrome**, **severe combined immunodeficiency disease** (SCID), and **acquired immune deficiency syndrome** (AIDS).

immune hemolysis: erythrocyte destruction by antibodies and complement.

immune interferon: *see* γ-**interferons**.

immune networks: *see* **idiotope-anti-idiotope networks**.

immune rejection: destruction of cells, tissues, or organs by immune system cells that recognize them as "foreign". *See* also **graft rejection**.

immune response genes: Ir genes; major histocompatibility complex components that code for class II proteins involved in the functions of helper and suppressor T lymphocytes. *Cf* **Ia** (immune associated) **genes**.

immune serum: blood serum prepared from individuals who have produced specific kinds of circulating antibodies. Some types are used to protect recipients against infections. *See* **immunity**; and *see* also **immunoassays**.

immune systems: networks of interacting cells and cell products that confer resistance to specific pathogens and toxins, and destroy tumor and virus-infected cells (but *see* also **autoimmune disease** and **natural killer cells**).

immunity: enhanced resistance to the effects of *specific* foreign substances (antigens), conferred by immune system cells and their products; *cf* **nonspecific defenses**. The antigens can be microorganisms and their products, vaccines prepared from them, substances made by virus-infected or tumor cells of the same individual, or components of grafts from individuals who are not genetically identical; but *see* also **hypersensitivity** and **autoimmune disease**. *Active* (acquired) immunity is initiated by exposure to the antigens. It can be *humoral*, mediated by B-lymphocyte derived substances that circulate, and usually directed against microorganisms and toxins. Each B lymphocyte subset expresses a specific kind of antibody on its surface that serves as an antigen receptor. When the antigen is presented, the subsets activated by it proliferate, and the progeny modulate to plasma cells that produce and secrete very large quantities of the specific kinds of antibodies. Various types function as anti-toxins, opsins, or precipitins, or form antigen-antibody complexes that activate the complement system. Some are stimulants for eosinophils, mast cells, and other cell types that release mediators. In contrast, *cellular* active immunity involves direct destuction of virus-infected, transformed, and other cell types perceived as "foreign". It is initiated when antigen presenting cells ingest and process antigens, and present the derivatives, along with class 1 proteins, to cytotoxic T lymphocytes that bear specific kinds of receptors. Activated T lymphocytes attach to the offending cells, undergo talin-mediated actin filament reorganization, and changes in microtubule orientation that facilitate injection of perforins, which polymerize in target cell plasma membranes and form channels that cause leakage of the cytoplasmic components. T lymphocyte subsets also release lymphokines, some of which contribute directly to cell destruction. Others activate and promote proliferation of different kinds of T cells. (Some helper type T cells release mediators that contribute to B cell functions.) *Passive* immunity is conferred by immune system products from other individuals, such as sera that contain antibodies. Fetuses receive maternal immunoglobulins that cross the placenta. Young infants absorb antibodies from colostrum and milk; but mature gastrointestinal tracts secrete enzymes that degrade ingested immunoglobulins. *Natural* immunity is a passive type, mediated by constitutive production of specific substances, that does not require prior antigen presentation or cell activation. Natural killer (NK) and some other cell types contribute to defenses against foreign cells, but differ from "true" immune system types, because their activation is not antigen-specific. *See also* **lymphocytes** and **memory cells**. For plant responses to pathogens that lead to acquired resistance, *see* **hypersensitive response**, **systemic acquired resistance** and **phytoalexins**.

immunoassays: sensitive techniques in which labeled antibodies are used to measure the concentrations of specific substances in body fluids, cells, or cell homogenates. Since the chemical groups of the substances identified by the antibodies are usually not the biologically active sites, the values obtained do not necessarily parallel those derived from bioassays. *See* also **radioimmunometric**, **radioreceptor**, and **enzyme-linked immunosorbent assays**.

immunization: administration of an antigen for the purpose of stimulating immune system responses against the same, and/or closely related antigens. Killed or attenuated bacteria can promote resistance to virulent microorganisms without invoking the consequences of infection. Specific kinds of antigens are injected into laboratory animals to study immune system responses, to combine with and thereby block the effects of specific kinds of regulators, or to obtain antibodies for immunoassays. Most antibodies obtained by antigen injection are polyclonal (and therefore capable of reacting with more than one kind of cell or body fluid component). Monoclonal types acquired from transfected microorganisms and cell hybrids are preferable for many purposes.

immunoabsorption: techniques for isolating proteins or glycoproteins from liquid mixtures, based on their high affinities for substances attached to solid phases. Test mixture components that adhere to the solid phases can be eluted for further purification, analysis, and use.

immunoblotting: techniques in which small quantities of proteins, glycoproteins, or other substances are transferred from gels to solid supports such as nitrocellulose sheets, and identified by their abilities to engage in antigen-antibody reactions with molecules on the supports. The agents on the supports are usually labeled with markers (such as radioactive atoms or enzymes) that facilitate identification and analysis of the transferred substances.

immunocompetence: ability to mount an effective immune response against a foreign antigen.

immunoconglutinin: antibodies that react with fixed complement components (usually C3b or C4). High levels are present in some individuals with rheumatoid arthritis.

immunocytochemistry: techniques for identifying and localizing small amounts of cell and/or tissue proteins or glycoproteins, based on their abilities to bind to specific antibodies. Most methods employ one antibody that directly binds to the test substance, and a second that attaches at one end to the first antibody, and at the other to a fluorescent marker, gold bead, or enzyme (such as horseradish peroxidase) which can be used for visualization in micrographs.

immunodiffusion: techniques for identifying and quantifying immune system substances, in which antigens and antibodies diffuse through gels and produce lines at sites where the concentrations are optimal for precipitation of insoluble complexes. In *radial* immunodiffusion, a measured quantity of an antigen solution is placed in a well on an agar plate that contains uniformly distributed antibody. The radius of the precipitin ring formed is directly related to the antigen concentration. *See* also **Ouchterlony plates** and **immunoelectrophoresis**.

immunodominant: describes the component of a complex antigen that binds the largest numbers of antibody types, or invokes production of the highest antibody titers.

immunoelectrophoresis: techniques for separating electrically charged molecules in gels by subjecting them to electrophoresis, and then purifying the fractions by immunodiffusion.

immunofluorescence: techniques used to visualize the distributions of specific molecular species (in cells or extracellular matrices), based on their abilities to engage in antigen-antibody reactions with substances linked to markers such as fluorescein or rhodamine.

immunogen: any substance that can initiate an immune response. It can (but need not be) an antigen. *See* also **haptens**.

immunogenicity: antigenicity; the capacity of an antigen to invoke immune responses.

immunoglobulins: glycoproteins made by lymphocytes and plasma cells. Humans make $10^6 - 10^8$ different kinds, and the ones released to the bloodstream normally account for approximately 20% of the total plasma protein. Each molecule contains two identical glycosylated heavy (H) chains, cross-linked by disulfide bonds to two identical light (L) chains. Both chain types contain *C*-terminal constant (C) domains (amino acid sequences common to all members of the immunoglobulin class), and *N*-terminal variable (V) domains (specific for each type) that recognize antigens. The positions of the multiple C domain copies are designated by subscripts (C_{H1}, C_{H2}, C_{H3}, C_{H4}). The classes are named for the kinds of 50-70K globular polypeptides contained within their heavy chain constant domains: alpha-1 and alpha-2 (α_1 and α_2) in IgA_1s and IgA_2s, respectively; delta (δ) in IgDs; epsilon (ϵ) in IgEs; gamma-1, gamma-2, gamma-3, or gamma-4 (γ_1, γ_2, γ_3, γ_4) in the various IgG subtypes (IgG_1, IgG_2, IgG_3, and IgG_4); and mu (μ) in IgMs. The C and V domains are linked by joining (J_H or J_L) segments. A hinge region between C_{H1} and C_{H2} confers flexibility, and is more susceptible to proteolytic degradation than other parts of the molecule (*see* **Fab** and **Fc** fragments). Each heavy chain additionally contains a small diversity segment (D_H) located between the variable (V_H) and joining (J_H) segments. Four subtypes of the two major light chain types, kappa (κ) and lambda (λ) have been identified. A single immunoglobulin molecule contains just one kind (designated, for example as C_k and V_k for a molecule with the kappa subtype). Light chains do not have diversity segments. The entire unit is called a monomer; and both IgGs and IgEs are said to be monomers. IgMs of humans and many other species are called pentamers (since each molecule is composed of five identical monomers). They are united by a J chain polypeptide (different from the J segment described above). A secretory form of IgA, which is a dimer, has an extra component (not present in the other classes) located between the J chain and one of the monomers. The configuration formed by the *N*-terminal region of one heavy and one light chain constitutes a paratope (an epitope recognizing region). There are two identical antigen binding sites per monomer. Each chain type is encoded by a separate gene. An isotype is a single kind of molecule with a specific combination of H and L chain types. An idiotype is an antigenic determinant that distinguishes one V from other V domains. Allotypes are allelic forms of H and L chains. Each individual inherits a characteristic set. In an undifferentiated B cell, a gene that codes for light chains contains DNA segments that specify various allelic forms (for example V_K1, V_K2, V_K3) in tandem, followed by segments that specify J segments (J_1 through J_5), followed by an intervening segment and a gene for the constant region (C_K). The DNA undergoes processing to yield a smaller sequence that contains just one V_K type, three J components, and one C_K. During transcriptional processing, two more J segments are deleted. The protein that is finally translated has the form V_K-J_3-C_K. Heavy chain assembly follows a similar pattern, but includes insertion of diversity segments. Antibody diversity is achieved by various combinations of H and V chain subtypes, and by spontaneous mutations that affect them. In "resting" B cells, immunoglobulins are integral membrane proteins whose exposed regions function as antigen receptors. When activated by an appropriate antigen, a B cell undergoes changes that lead to formation of many more cells of the same kind. Most of the progeny become plasma cells that make very large quantities of one specific immunoglobulin type. The molecules are secreted and then serve as circulating antibodies (*see also* **immunity** and **memory cells**). The immunoglobulin *superfamily* includes some structurally related proteins with different functions; *see*, for example **T cell receptors** and **intercellular adhesion molecules**. *See also* **IgA**, **IgD**, **IgE**, **IgGs**, and **IgM**.

immunological memory: persistent immune system effects invoked by transient exposure to antigens that support rapid, vigorous responses if the same antigens are presented at a later time; *see* **memory cells**.

immunological suppression: diminution or elimination of the ability to mount effective immune system responses to one or more antigens. Generalized suppression can be invoked by X-rays, some viruses and toxins, high levels of glucocorticoids, and pharmacological immunosuppressants. It decreases the probability of graft rejection, and can attenuate autoimmune processes. In laboratory animals, hematopoietic tissues are radiated to study immune system processes, or to promote acceptance and survival of tissues and organs that would otherwise be rejected. *See also* **immunological tolerance**.

immunological surveillance: continuous search for, and destruction of foreign antigens (for example ones expressed on the surfaces of microorganisms, or on virus infected or transformed cells), by lymphocytes, natural killer, and killer cells.

immunological tolerance: failure to mount immune system responses against specific antigen types. Most immature lymphocytes that recognize self-antigens are destroyed during early stages of development. Small numbers persist, but do not respond to ordinary levels of the antigens, possibly because they encounter them in the absence of co-stimulants before acquiring the ability to express CD28. Tolerance can be induced in mature immune systems by administering antigens in quantities too small to stimulate T helper lymphocytes, and following this with repeated doses of gradually increasing size. The procedures are used to desensitize individuals to allergens. A single massive dose is also sometimes effective. The molecules are then believed to "overwhelm" the antibody binding capability, or to promote formation of large amounts of anti-idiotopes (*see* **idiotope-anti-idiotope networks**). There are controversies concerning contributions of certain T lymphocyte subsets (suppressor cells) to the development of tolerance.

immunoperoxidase: staining techniques used to identify the presence and locations of specific kinds of molecules (especially proteins and glycoproteins), and in some cases to determine their levels. Peroxidase linked to a specific immunoglobulin type binds to the cell component (antigen), and, in the presence of a chromogen such as benzidine, imparts a color that is easily detected. *See also* **immunocytochemistry**.

immunophilins: a family of phylogenetically conserved proteins, initially identified as cell components that mediate the effects of potent immunosuppressants, including cyclophilins that bind cyclosporin A (CsA), and several FK 506 binding proteins (FKBPs) that attach to rapamycin as well as to FK 506. CsA-cyclophilin and some FK 506-FKBP complexes are potent inhibitors of calcineurin isozymes (calcium and calmodulin dependent serine-threonine phosphatases essential for T lymphocyte signal transduction). The lymphocyte enzyme is a rate-limiting determinant for induction of NF-AT, NF-IL2A, and other transcription factors that activate genes for interleukin-2 and other lymphokines during G1 phases of cell cycles. In contrast, complexes formed with rapamycin act at later stages to inhibit hematopoietic cell proliferation mediated by interleukins 2, 3, and 4, and by erythropoietin and granulocyte-macrophage colony stimulating factor (GM-CSF). Some of the complexes additionally affect rotamase activity and are therefore implicated in the control of protein folding. A few that are chemotactic for eosinophils and neutrophilic leukocytes can augment peroxidase activity and accelerate tyrosine phoshorylation of specific proteins. FK 506 bound to FKBP-59 (p59), and some other FKBP complexes, attach to heat shock proteins hsp70 and hsp90, and are components of unoccupied receptor complexes for steroid hormones; and influences on steroid hormone mediated transcription have been described. Estrogen receptor binding cyclophilin (ERBC) is a 40K protein related to CsA cyclophilin. FKBP-52 is a mouse immunophilin with an ATP/GTP binding site that promotes phosphorylation of a 59K lymphocyte nuclear protein implicated in signal transduction. *See* also **cyclosporin A**, **FK 506** and **rapamycin**.

immunoprecipitation: precipitation that occurs when a specific kind of antibody is added to a solution that contains the corresponding antigen, and both components are present in appropriate concentration ranges.

immunoradiometric assay: IRMA; *see* **radioimmunometric assays**.

immunoreactivity: (1) a measure of the ability to mount an immune response to an antigen; (2) describes substances that bind to specific kinds of antibodies; for example the term glucagon-like immunoreactivity is applied to all molecules with domains that confer high affinity for antibodies directed against glucagon.

immunoselection: usually, (1) procedures for isolating specific cell types from mixed cultures, based on differences in vulnerability to cytotoxic and other immunological factors; (2) selective survival (or death) of fetuses, based on genotypic characteristics that affect immunological compatibility with the maternal system.

immunosenescence: the decline in immune system functions that occurs with advancing age, mediated in part by involutional changes in thymus glands.

immunosuppressants: agents that diminish or abolish certain immune system responses, by destroying the cells that mediate them, or by interfering with their functions. Pharmacological immunosuppressants, such as cyclosporin A and rapamycin are used to block transplant rejection, to arrest the progression of some autoimmune diseases, and as laboratory tools. Naturally occurring

types may contribute to special functions, such as protection of conceptuses against immunological rejection by maternal immune systems. Components of seminal plasma that protect spermatozoa against antigens in female reproductive system tracts have been described.

immunosympathectomy: selective destruction of sympathetic system neurons with specific kinds of antibodies, usually to study the functions of the system. Antibodies directed against nerve growth factor (NGF) permanently block development of the neurons when presented early in life, and inflict severe, only partially reversible damage at later times. Ones directed against dopamine-β-hydroxylase (which catalyzes dopamine conversion to norepinephrine) invoke milder impairment, because large amounts of the enzyme are made, and not all is accessible to the antibody.

immunotoxins: agents that bind to and inactivate antibodies, destroy lymphocytes, or in other ways impair immune system functions. Toxins bound to immunoglobulins and Fab fragments can selectively destroy tumors that express antigens not made by normal body cells.

IMP: inosine monophosphate.

impedance: opposition to flow.

implant: something embedded in an organism, such as a cardiac pacemaker, an electrode that restores some function in a defective ear, or a dental type. Capsules that release substances at controlled rates can be inserted at appropriate sites, to directly deliver their products where desired, and to maintain constant concentrations over pre-selected time periods. They are used to study the effects hormones and other regulators, correct deficiencies, deliver therapeutic agents, and achieve contraception. Many problems associated with other forms of delivery (including stress to the recipient, the inconvenience associated with the need for repeated injections, uncertain absorption rates, widely fluctuating blood levels, and degradation by hepatic and other enzymes) are thereby averted. Implanted tumors can be grown in specially treated hosts, and internal organs can be implanted at superficial sites for manipulation and observation.

implantation: usually (1) nidation; blastocyst penetration into, and interaction with endometrial cells. The uterus is receptive during just a brief phase of the ovarian cycle. Its preparation requires exposure to follicular phase estrogen (which stimulates endometrial cell proliferation and induction of progesterone receptors), followed by luteal phase progesterone (which promotes cell specialization and increases the blood supply). Additional estrogen must then be presented, one function of which appears to be induction of LIF (*see* **differentiation inducing factor**). In humans, nidation begins approximately 8 days after conception (which coincides with the mid-luteal phase). The events must be synchronized with blastocyst development, and preceded by blastocyst "hatching", which occurs in the uterine lumen. The blastocyst makes stromelysin, type IV collagenase, and other proteolytic enzymes that are essential for migration across the basement membranes of uterine epithelium and vascular endothelium. The invasion is localized to the leading edge of blastocyst cells, in part via urokinase type plasminogen activator receptors on trophoblast surfaces that bind to and activate plasminogen, and also by several protease inhibitors. Proteins related to receptors for low density lipoproteins (LDLs) appear to be important for internalizing protease-inhibitor complexes. (The inhibitors protect the endometrium against excessive destruction.) Endometrial cells also releases colony stimulating factor-1 (CSF-1, M-CSF) and transforming growth factor-β (TGFβ) that accelerate maturation of invasive trophoblast cell types to noninvasive syncytiotrophoblast.) *See* also **diapause**, **ectopic pregnancy**, and **placenta**; (2) placement of an implant.

impotence: impotency; inability to achieve penile erection and ejaculation. Declining activities of hypothalamic neurons that secrete gonadotropin releasing hormone (GnRH) may account for some of the impotency that occurs in aging men; but circulatory problems such as atherosclerosis, obliteration of cavernous blood vessels, and cardiac dysfunction are more common; and agents used to lower blood pressure have adverse effects; *see* also **nitric oxide**. Testosterone synthesis diminishes with advancing age; and lower levels of hormone available for local actions on the testis, and for delivery to the epididymis, may contribute. (Blood testosterone levels may not fall, since degradation and clearance rates also decline.) Other factors include excessive prolactin secretion, hepatic and renal dysfunctions that alter the metabolism of various hormones, neurological defects, psychological influences, and diabetes mellitus (which impairs both vascular and neural functions).

impregnation: (1) the act of making pregnant; (2) fertilization; (3) saturation of one substance with another.

imprinting: (1) imposition of a persistent behavior pattern, by subjecting a young individual (for example a recently hatched bird) to one or a specific set of stimuli; (2) an organizational influence exerted early in life that affects subsequent responses to hormones and other factors; *see*, for example **defeminization**.

Imuran: a trade name for azathioprine.

ImuVert: a ribosomal preparation from *Serratia marcescens* (a species of gram positive bacteria) that exerts interferon-α (IFNα)-like stimulation of NK cells. It can protect against alopecia and certain other side effects invoked by cyclophosphamide, doxorubicin, cytosine-arabinoside, and other chemotherapeutic agents without blocking the beneficial effects.

inactive X chromosome: usually, the X chromosome in normal female mammals that undergoes condensation and selective transcriptional inactivation. (In XXX females, XXY and XXYY males, and other individuals with abnormal patterns, all of the supernumerary X chromosomes can undergo inactivation; *see* also **Barr bodies**). In normal females, both X chromosomes function during oogenesis and the earliest stages of embryonic development. The inactivation in somatic cells begins in older embryos, affects most of the genes, and persists postnatally. In proliferating cells, the affected chromosome replicates later than the others. The processes are initiated randomly; some cell types express maternal, and others paternal genes. However, once established, all progeny acquire the patterns established by the parent cells. *See* also **Turner's syndrome**.

inanition: inadequate intake of one or more nutrients.

inborn errors: genetically determined defects that impair production of one or more enzymes or other substances essential for normal development and/or functions.

inbred strain: a population of organisms produced by repeated sibling-sibling and/or parent-progeny matings. The members are homozygous for most traits, but male mammals (with Y chromosomes) have genes not present in females. They are used for studies in which it is desirable to eliminate the effects of genetic differences on responses to experimental procedures. Homozygosity can be associated with shorter life spans, smaller sizes, and/or lower fertility; *cf* **hybrid vigor**.

INCAM-110: a 110K glycoprotein induced by cytokines, and expressed on the surfaces of vascular endothelial cells at sites of injury. It facilitates migration of circulating leukocytes to those sites, and mediates heterotypic adhesion of leuokocytes to activated endothelial cells (and homotypic adhesions of melanoma and some other cell types).

inclusions: aggregations of pigments, metabolic products, or other substance within cells that are not enclosed by membranes; *cf* **organelles**.

inclusion bodies: aggregations of cytoplasmic or nuclear components with characteristic staining properties. Some occur at sites of virus replication.

incompatibility: describes (1) genetic or antigenic differences between donor and recipient cells, or between individuals, that invoke immunological rejection; (2) properties of pharmacological agents that render them unsuitable for administration in combination (because of antagonistic, excessively synergistic, or toxic effects); (3) immiscible substances, such as oils and aqueous solutions.

incomplete Freund's adjuvant: a water-in-oil emulsion used to augment responses to administered antigens. Since it does not contain the *Mycobacteria* present in complete Freund's adjuvant, it is a weaker, but less toxic stimulant.

incomplete dominance: describes an allele of a heterozygote that exerts the major effects on a phenotypic trait, whose influences are modified by expression of a recessive allele for the same trait; *cf* **dominant**, **codominant**, and **recessive**.

incompletely linked genes: contiguous genes on a chromosome that are often inherited together, but can engage separately in crossing over during meiosis.

incretins: incompletely characterized gastrointestinal tract hormones that stimulate insulin secretion in response to food ingestion. Glucose-dependent insulinotropic peptide (GIP) displays such activity, but GLP-I (*see* **glucagon-like peptides**) is more potent.

incross: mating of organisms homozygous for an allele.

independent assortment: the Mendelian concept that inheritance of an allele for one trait is not affected by inheritance of alleles for different traits. Although it holds for certain genes, *see* **linked genes** and **linkage disequilibrium**. *See* also **incomplete dominance** and **codominance**.

Inderal: a trade name for propranolol.

indican: "animal" indican is indol-3-yl sulfate, a tryptophan metabolite excreted to the urine, usually as the potassium salt. "Plant indican" is indoyl-3-β-D-glucoside. *See* also **indigo blue**.

indicator: (1) a substance used to identify certain properties, or to follow the progress of a reaction, for example an agent whose color is affected by pH or oxidation-reduction potential, one that fluoresces when it binds calcium, or a radioactive marker; (2) a strain of microorganisms used to test the presence of a specific component. *See* also **indicator gene**.

indicator gene: a gene that is easily identified (directly, or via an effect it exerts) that is linked to another gene, and can be used to detect the presence of that other gene.

indifferent external genitalia: the precursors of the externally visible reproductive system organs that are morphologically similar in young male and female embryos. *See* **genital tubercle**, **genital swellings**, **genital folds**, and **urogenital sinus**.

indifferent gonads: the progenitors of testes and ovaries. They develop from genital (urogenital) ridges, and are initially morphologically similar in XX and XY conceptuses. In both sexes, they contain gonocytes, epithelial, and mesenchymal cells. *See* also **indifferent stage**.

indifferent stage: the phase of embryonic development during which the reproductive system organ precursors appear similar in XX and XY type mammalian conceptuses. At approximately 5½ weeks after conception in humans, both male and female embryos have indifferent gonads, Müllerian ducts, Wolffian ducts and indifferent external genitalia. *See* also **testis determining antigen** and **sex differentiation**.

indigo blue: indigo; 2-(1,3-dihydro-3-oxo-2*H*-indol-2-ylidene)-1,2-dihydro-3*H*-indole-3-one; a dye obtained as a glucoside from *Indigofera* and some other plants, and used as a counterstain in histology and cytology. Two indican molecules fuse to form one of the dye when urine that holds large amounts is treated with Obermayer's

reagent (which contains hydrochloric acid and ferric chloride).

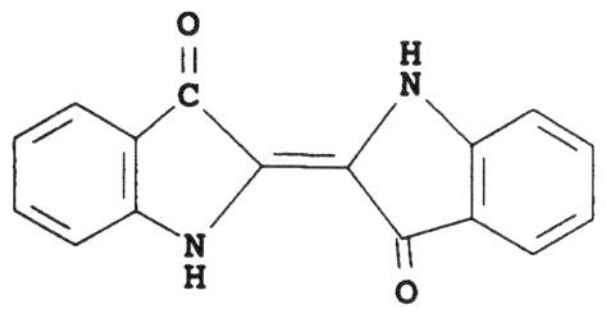

indigo carmine: acid blue; 2-(1-dihydro-3-oxo-5-sulfo-2*H*-indol-2-ylidene)-2,3-dihydro-3-oxo-1*H*-indole-5-sulfonic acid disodium salt; a reagent used to detect nitrate and chlorate, and for renal function tests.

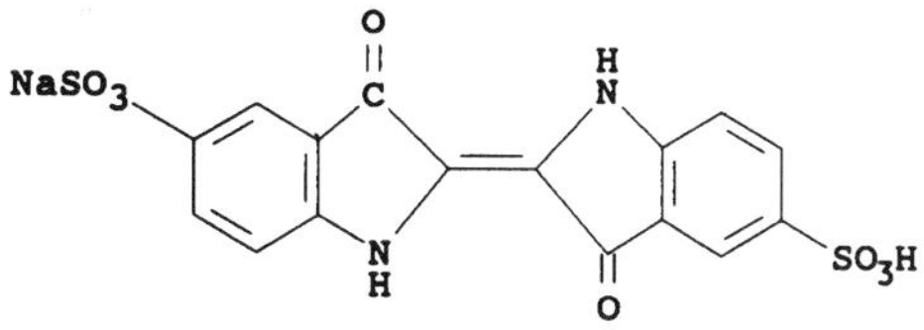

Indocin: a trade name for indomethacin.

indole: 2,3-benzopyrrole; a tryptophan metabolite produced by intestinal bacteria and excreted with feces. Small amounts are absorbed and converted in the liver to indican. Many microorganisms use it to make tryptophan, via the reaction: indole + serine → tryptophan + H_2O.

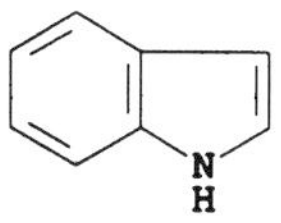

5-hydroxy-**indoleacetaldehyde**: an intermediate in the pathway that degrades serotonin and related amines, formed by a reaction catalzyed by monoamine oxidases. Most of it is the converted by alcohol dehydrogenases to 5-OH-indole acetic acid; *see* also 5-**hydroxindol-3-acetic acid**.

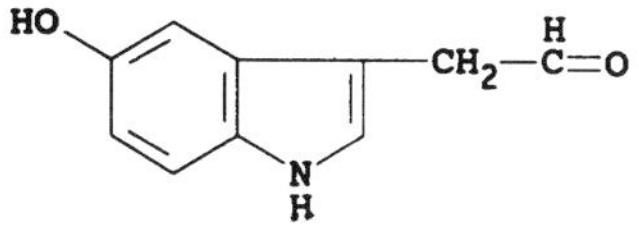

indole-3-acetic acid: IAA: a tryptophan metabolite made in pineal glands and excreted to urine. No function has been identified in animals, but IAA is a major growth-promoting hormone (auxin) in plants.

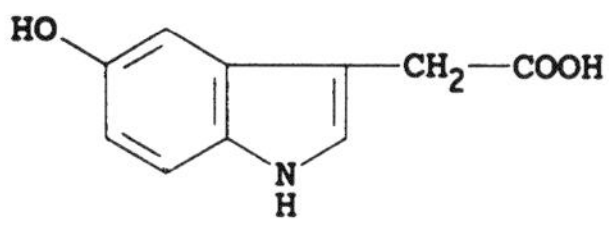

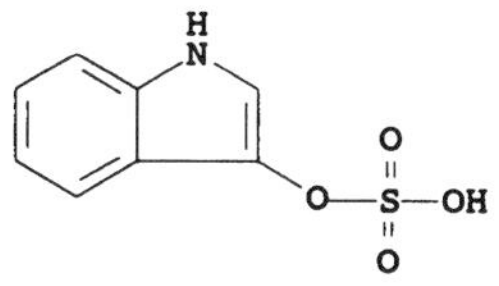

"animal" indican

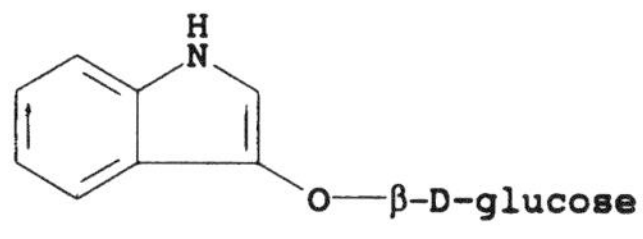

"plant" indican

5-OH-indole acetic acid: 5-HIAA; a serotonin metabolite formed in reactions catalyzed by monoamine oxidases and alcohol dehydrogenases, and excreted to the urine. *See also* 5-**hydroxyindole-3-acetic acid**.

indoleamines: serotonin, melatonin, some other tryptophan derivatives, and chemically related amines.

indolamine-2,3-dioxygenase: an enzyme that catalyzes tryptophan conversion to kynurenine, and oxidation of the pyrrol rings of other compounds. Since it is induced by interferon-γ (IFNγ), and the reactions use superoxide anions, it can protect against oxidative damage during inflammation. It may also contribute to the destruction of tumor cells and microorganisms by depleting their tryptophan supplies.

indole blocking factor: an inhibitor of indole conversion factor, made by cells that synthesize melanins. Its activity is regulated by melanocyte stimulating hormone (MSH) and melatonin.

indole-2-carboxylic acid: I2CA; a competitive antagonist for NMDA receptors.

indole conversion factor: an enzyme that catalyzes formation of indole 5,6-quinone (an intermediate in the pathway for biosynthesis of melanins from tyrosine).

indomethacin: Inderal; 1-(4-chlorobenzoyl)-5-methoxy-2-methyl-1H-indole-3-acetic acid; an orally effective, nonsteroidal cyclooxygenase inhibitor, used for its anti-inflammatory, antipyretic, and analgesic effects, to treat Hodgkin's disease, rheumatoid arthritis, osteoarthritis, gout, Bartter's syndrome, and some other diseases. It is more potent than salicylates, but the toxic effects of long-term use can include renal failure and thrombocytopenia. Indomethacin also inhibits 3α-hydroxysteroid dehydrogenase and insulin receptor tyrosine kinase.

induced enzymes: enzymes whose synthesis is accelerated by hormones or other regulators. Some types are made constitutively in smaller amounts, whereas others cannot be detected in unstimulated cells.

induced mutations: changes in nucleic acids (usually DNAs) invoked by mutagens.

induced ovulators: reflex ovulators: mammals in which ovarian follicles mature, but ovulation is delayed until stimulation of the vulval region (usually during mating) initiates a neuroendocrine reflex that promotes the LH (luteinizing hormone) surge. Since the estrus period is prolonged, and release of mature oocytes follows soon after mating, fertility is generally high. The reflex can be invoked by stimulating the region with a glass rod. Rabbits and ferrets are among the animal types used to study the mechanisms. *Cf* **spontaneous ovulators**.

induced proteins: proteins synthesized in larger amounts when hormones or other regulators accelerate transcription of their messenger RNAs. Small amounts of some types are made by unstimulated cells.

inducer: usually, an agent that accelerates gene transcription. *See also* **embryonic inducers**.

inducer cells: *see* **T lymphocytes**.

induction: usually (1) processes whereby the production of specific kinds of messenger RNAs is accelerated; (2) stimulation of a process or response; (3) the effects of inducers made by certain embryonic cell types that determine the developmental patterns for other cells.

infarct: a necrotic area formed following interruption of the blood supply to the region.

infection: processes whereby pathogenic organisms invade a host, become established, multiply, and exert their effects.

infectious mononucleosis: a disease caused by Epstein-Barr virus infection, most prevalent in adolescents and young adults. The acute manifestations include fever, malaise, fatigue, sore throat, and swollen lymph glands, accompanied by neutropenia, thrombocytopenia, and lymphocytosis, as well as markedly increased numbers of circulating moncytes. The recovery phase is prolonged, and is associated with the appearance of heterophile antibodies, and possibly also with transient activation of suppressor type T lymphocytes. The concept that otherwise unexplained chronic fatigue is commonly caused by Epstein-Barr virus infections has not been substantiated.

infestation: a term sometimes used synonymously with infection, especially when the pathogenic organism is a protozoan or larger parasite, but more commonly applied to the attachment of surface parasites such as lice or ticks.

inflammation: complex responses to irritation, injury, or infection that provide the first line of defense against microorganisms and their toxins, small parasites, and other noxious agents, and impede their spread to other parts of the body, but are not specific for the offending agents; *cf* **immunity**. They involve activation of vascular endothelium, leukocytes, mast cells, macrophages, fibroblasts, neurons, endocrine, and other cell types, the release of numerous mediators, and intricate interactions which include cascades and positive feedback systems, as well as cell:cell and cell:matrix communication. The "classical" description of localized manifestations includes *rubor* (erythema), *calor* (rise in temperature), *tumor* (localized edema), and *dolor* (pain). Under normal conditions, negative feedbacks and other mechanisms limit the potential for cell injury, terminate the responses when appropriate, and initiate healing. However, tissue damage can be extensive when the controls are defective and the responses persist long after they have served their purposes. Initially, histamine, prostaglandins, bradykinin, and other secretory products promote vasodilation and facilitate transport of blood cells and other blood components to the site. Soon afterward, histamine and other regulators constrict postcapillary venules, invoke stagnation, and increase capillary permeability. Proteins then leach out, osmotically draw fluid from the blood, and cause swelling. Extravasation of leukocytes is facilitated by the leakage, and by endothelium-leukocyte adhesion molecule-1 (ELAM-1) and other endothelial cell products. Isolation of the region is initiated by fibrinogen, which (in the presence of thrombin) forms fibrin clots. Somewhat later, a stronger wall is formed by collagen released from fibroblasts. Pain is caused by pressure exerted on nerve endings, and the presence of histamine, serotonin, eicosanoids, bradykinin, platelet activating factor (PAF), and other mediators. Chemotaxins attract neutrophilic leukocytes, macrophages, and other cells to the site. The neutrophils ingest bacteria and toxins, and they kill microorganisms by releasing proteolytic enzymes and producing hydrogen peroxide and free radicals. Some of the cells are killed in the processes. Macrophages ingest the dead leukocytes, as well as dead bacteria and debris, and they release additional mediators, including interleukin-1 (which is also made by endothelial cells). IL-1 is pyrogenic, and can cause fever if sufficient amounts enter the bloodstream. It also a stimulant for immune system and some endocrine cells. Interleukins additionally promote the release of glucocorticoids and opioid peptides (physiological factors that limit excessive reactivity, in part by decreasing mediator release). Enzymes such as indoleamine 2,3-dioxygenase that use superoxide anion, catalases, and a variety of antioxidants (such as reduced glutathione, ascorbic acid, vitamin C and bilirubin) protect against oxidative damage. Prostacyclin, fibroblast growth factors, and other mediators then contribute to tissue repair. The acute phase can progress to a chronic condition that involves lymphocyte infiltration, and can lead to complement activation and immune system responses that damage previously healthy cells.

informosomes: messenger RNA molecules enclosed in protein coats that protect them against degradation by ribonucleases, and facilitate their transport from nuclei to cytoplasm.

infradian rhythms: cyclical events with periodicities of more than 24 hours, such as ovarian cycles, and seasonal variations in reproductive system functions. *Cf* **circadian** and **ultradian rhythms**.

infundibular nucleus: *see* **arcuate nucleus**.

infundibular process: pars nervosa; the neural lobe of the neurohypophysis.

infundibular recess: hypophysial recess; the part of the third ventricle of the brain that extends into the neurohypophysis.

infundibular stalk: *see* **infundibulum**, definition 2.

infundibular stem: the neural component of the infundibulum that extends from the tuber cinereum to the neural lobe. Hypothalamo-hypophysial nerve tracts pass through this region.

infundibulum: (1) a funnel-shaped passage; (2) the structure that forms part of the floor of the third ventricle of the brain, and extends downward to connect the hypothalamus with the hypophysis. The connecting region is also known as the infundibular stalk. *See* also **median eminence**; (3) the region of a Fallopian tube with the largest diameter. It receives oocytes that enter the ostium, and transports them downward to the fertilization site (or to the uterus if fertilization does not occur).

ingestion: eating; in complex animals, taking substances into the mouth and passing them on to the gastrointestinal tract. In unicellular organisms, taking substances from the environment (usually via phagocytosis) and passing them to food vacuoles.

inheritance: acquisition of the components of parent cells that can be transmitted to progeny. Gamete DNAs are the primary vectors, but *see* **cytoplasmic** and **maternal inheritance**, and *see* also **sex-linked inheritance**.

inhibins: dimeric glycoproteins initially identified in ovarian follicular and seminal fluids, and implicated as hormones that exert negative feedback control over follicle stimulating hormone (FSH) release. They also decrease FSH synthesis, the numbers of gonadotropin releasing hormone (GnRH) receptors on gonadotropes, the amount of luteinizing hormone (LH) secreted in response to GnRH, and the release of oxytocin; and they exert numerous autocrine and/or paracrine effects on reproductive system structures. For example, they contribute to ovarian follicle maturation and spermatogenesis, enhance LH-stimulated androgen production, and antagonize LH-stimulated progesterone synthesis. Although granulosa and Sertoli cells are the major sources of circulating hormone, inhibins have been identified in Leydig cells, prostate gland, spermatozoa, placenta, adrenal cortex, bone marrow, hypothalamus, adenohypophysis, kidney, spleen, lymphocytes, and gastric juice. In embryos they are implicated as regulators of nervous system development. Many of the actions oppose those of activins. The peptides are members of a superfamily that includes activins, transforming growth factor-β (TGFβ), Müllerian duct inhibitor, some bone morphogenetic proteins, the products of the *Drosophila* decapentaplegic complex and amphibian *Vg-1* genes. They also share amino acid sequences with androgen binding proteins. Several forms that differ in molecular weights and surface charges have been identified, and there are species variations. Each molecule is composed of a glycosylated α subunit (which contains an unusual carbohydrate component), linked by disulfide bonds to a smaller β-subunit. Heterogeneity results from differences in amino acid composition, glycosylation, and other factors such as aggregation, association with other proteins, and phosphorylation. The three known precursors of inhibin and related hormones are preproinhibin α, preproinhibin $β_A$ and preproinhibin $β_B$, each of which is cleaved to yield a corresponding subunit. Inhibin A is α-$β_A$ (a dimer composed of one α and one $β_A$ type subunit), and inhibin B is α-$β_B$. All differ from the single-chain polypeptide, folliculostatin, which also inhibits FSH release (at least in part by binding activins). The effects of various hormones on the synthesis of α and β the subunits vary with the cell types, and with the stages of cell maturation. FSH is a major stimulant in ovaries and immature testes, but has little effect on mature testes. Adrenocorticotropic hormone (ACTH) stimulates in the adrenal cortex. Additional regulators include androstenedione and other gonadal steroids, insulin-like growth factor-1 (IGF-1), and epidermal growth factor (EGF).

inhibin A, **inhibin B**: *see* **inhibins**.

inhibition: partial or complete suppression of a reaction or other process. *See* also **competitive**, **noncompetitive**, **uncompetitive**, **presynaptic**, and **contact inhibition**.

inhibitory neurotransmitters: chemical messengers made by neurons that block or attenuate responses, usually by promoting hyperpolarization and thereby diminishing target cell sensitivities to stimulants. *See*, for example **gamma aminobutyric acid** (GABA).

inhibitory postsynaptic potential: IPSP: an electrical change in a target cell invoked by an inhibitory neurotransmitter that raises the threshold for stimulation; *cf* **excitatory postsynaptic potential**.

inhibitory synapses: functional connections between neurons, or between neurons and other target cells, in which inhibitory neurotransmitters are released.

initiation codon: *see* **initiation complex** and **AUG**.

initiation complex: a unit that must be assembled before protein synthesis on a ribosome can begin, composed of an initiation codon (AUG), guanosine triphosphate (GTP), a small ribosomal subunit, and a messenger RNA molecule. In eukaryotes, the assembly requires at least nine initiation factors and several cofactors. The first step is formation of a ternary complex composed of one molecule each of initiation factor eIF2, methionine linked to its transfer RNA (Met-tRNA), and GTP. EIF2 mediates attachment of the complex to a small (40S) ribosome subunit, and cap-binding proteins promote addition of 5′-mRNA. EIF1 and eIF3 stabilize the binding. Subsequent association with an mRNA (with the met-tRNA correctly positioned at the initiation codon), requires initiation factors 4A, 4B, 4C, and 4D, and the energy released by IF4E-mediated ATP hydrolysis. After assembly, the met-tRNA•eIF2•GTP•40S•mRNA attaches to a large (60S) ribosomal subunit, eIF5 promotes GTP hydrolysis, and GDP and eIF2 are released. In prokaryotes, a similar process is required, but *N*-formyl-Met-tRNA takes the place of Met-tRNA, the ribosomal

subunits are smaller (30S and 50S), and the initiation factors are IF2, IF2, and IF3.

initiation factors: IFs: several catalytic proteins required for formation of **initiation complexes** (*q.v.*). There are at least nine in eukaryotes (eIFs 1, 2, 3, 4A, 4B, 4C, 4D, 4E, and 5) along with subtypes, and at least three (IFs 1, 2, and 3) in prokaryotes.

initiation site: usually (1) a nucleic acid locus where transcription begins; (2) a ribosomal or messenger RNA site where protein synthesis begins.

innate: inborn; inherited; occurring without learning or conditioning.

inner cell mass: embryoblast; the blastocyst cells that give rise to the structures of the new individual, and to some extra-embryonic tissue; *cf* **trophoblast**.

inner mitochondrial membrane: the part of a mitochondrion that borders the matrix and is separated from the outer mitochondrial membrane by an intramembranous space. It holds enzymes for oxidative phosphorylation and for oxidation of pyruvate and fatty acids.

innominate: unnamed or nameless; a term applied to some anatomic structures, as in innominate vein or artery.

inoculum: a substance introduced into an organism or cell culture, artificially, or under natural conditions (for example by an insect bite).

inorganic: describes all chemical compounds that do not contain carbon atoms, and most that do not have carbon atoms covalently linked to other carbons or to oxygen, or nitrogen atoms. Some authors include simple molecules such as CO and CO_2. *Cf* **organic**.

inosinate: *see* **inosine monophosphate**.

inosine: hypoxanthine riboside; a purine nucleoside made from adenosine via a reaction catalyzed by adenosine deaminase. It inhibits nucleoside transport, and its neurotropic effects include stimulation of protein and catecholamine (but not acetylcholine) synthesis. *See* **inosine monophosphate**.

inosine monophosphate: IMP; inosine 5′-phosphate; inosinic acid {inosinate}: a hypoxanthine nucleotide made from adenosine monophosphate, in the reaction: hypoxanthine + 5-phosphoribosyl-1-pyrophosphate → IMP + P-P. It is convertible to AMP and GMP, is a component of transfer RNAs, and can base pair with adenine, cytidine, and uridine nucleotides.

inosinic acid: inosine monophosphate.

inositol: a term often used synonymously with *myo*-inositol (*cis*-1,2,3-*trans*-4,6-cyclohexanol, shown); but nine inositol isomers are known, several of which occur in biological tissues. Myoinositol is a lipotropic component of the vitamin B complex, known under other names that include meat sugar, rat antispectacle eye factor, and mouse antialopecia factor. It is also a growth factor for microorganisms. In eukaryotes, it is a component of many lipids and biological regulators. *See* also **phospha-**

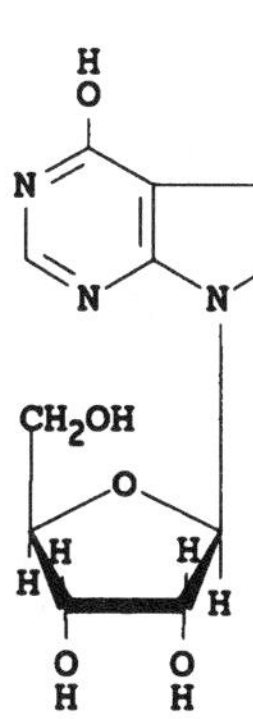

inosine

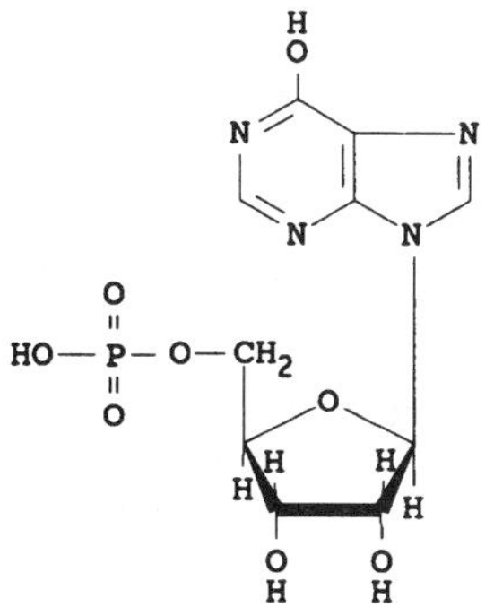

inosine-5′-monophosphate

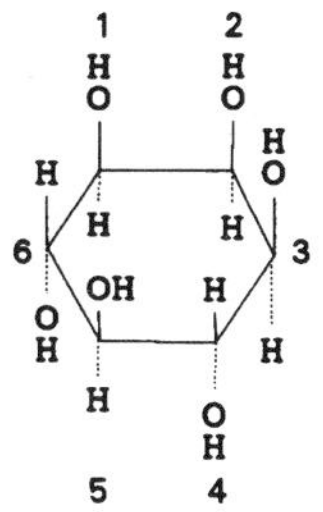

inositol

tidylinositols, **phosphatidylinositol phosphates**, **inositol phosphate glycans**, and **inositol phosphates**.

inositol kinases: enzymes that catalyze phosphorylation of inositol and inositol phosphates. Some are components of complex cascades involved in the control of cell proliferation. They are activated by numerous mitogen ligands for tyrosine kinase type receptors, and by thrombin, f-Met-Leu-Phe, and some others that use G protein transducers. Inositol-3-phosphate kinases catalyze conversion of inositol-1,4,5-triphosphate (IP$_{1,4,5}$) to inositol 1,3,4,5 tetrakisphosphate (IP$_{1,3,4,5}$). The product is a substrate for an inositol phosphate phosphatase that converts it to inositol 1,3,4 triphosphate (IP$_{1,3,4}$, the most abundant of cellular inositol phosphates), and for others that yield IP$_{3,4}$ and IP$_3$. **Phosphatidylinositol kinases** ($q.v.$) are different enzymes. The products of some of the reactions catalyzed are inositol-phosphate precursors.

inositol lipid kinases: a term loosely applied to phosphatidylinositol kinases and other enzymes that act on inositol-containing lipids.

inositol phosphate[s]: molecules composed of inositols conjugated at various positions to one or more phosphate groups. The names commonly applied do not fully conform with standard chemical terminology. The most intensively studied member of the group is inositol 1,4,5-triphosphate (usually called IP$_{1,4,5}$, but also known as IP$_3$, Ins(1,4,5)P$_3$, and D-myo-inositol 1,4,5-triphosphate). It is formed when certain phospholipase C isozymes (phosphoinositide Cs) catalyze hydrolysis of phosphatidylinositol-4,5-biphosphates (PIP$_2$s) and is a substrate for **inositol kinases** and **inositol phosphate phosphatases** ($q.v.$). Phosphoinositidase C isozymes are activated by many hormones and neurotransmitters; and the reactions simultaneously release **diacyl glycerols** ($q.v.$). IP$_{1,4,5}$ promotes release of calcium ions from intracellular sequestration sites (endoplasmic reticulum and/or calciosomes). Proteins with molecular weights in the 250-260K range implicated as IP$_3$ receptors have been identified on endoplasmic reticulum membranes that border nuclei, and are known to be induced by IP$_{1,4,5}$. Regulators of the functions include heparin, which inhibits binding to receptors and calcium release, and calmedin, which exerts opposing effects in the brain. In the presence of IP$_{3,4,5}$, IP$_{1,3,4,5}$-tetrakisphosphate acts on calcium ion channels, accelerates Ca^{2+} uptake from extracellular fluids and increases the availability of intracellular calcium pools for recruitment by IP$_{1,4,5}$. IP$_3$ activates neutrophilic leukocytes and fibroblasts, and is a component of cascades involved in mitogenesis. It is also part of a positive feedback system, in which elevation of cytosolic Ca^{2+} augments phosphoinositide activity and IP$_{1,4,5}$ formation. There are 61 other possible myo-inositol phosphate isomers, half of which have been identified in animal cells. Several are known to be biologically active.

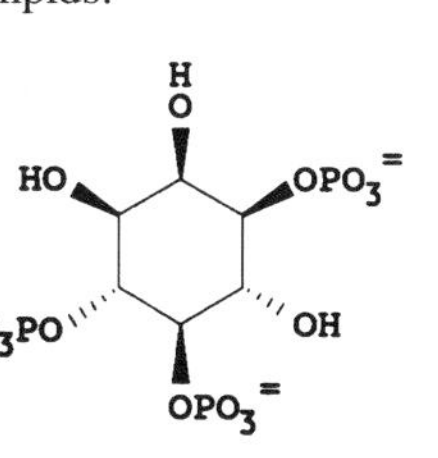

inositol-1,4,5-triphosphate

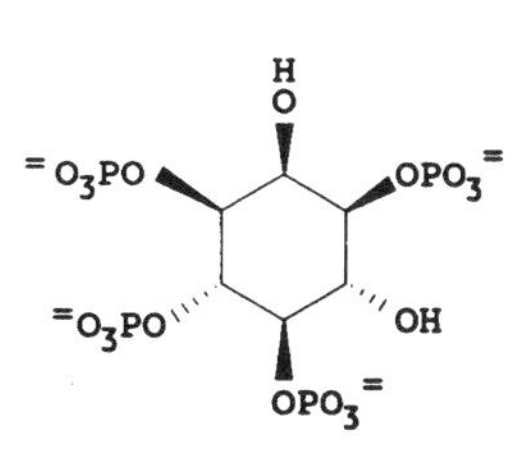

inositol-1,3,4,5-tetrakisphosphate

Certain others initially believed to be degradation products may perform special functions, since cells accumulate them in micromolar concentrations. Inositol 2,4,5-triphosphate ($IP_{2,4,5}$) seems to exert effects similar those described for $IP_{1,4,5}$. $IP_{1,4}$ can activate a DNA polymerase; and inositol hexakisphosphate, which accumulates in large amounts in plant cells, serves as a precursor for other compounds, and has anti-oxidant properties. The acronym IP_6 is used for both the hexakisphosphate ($IP_{1,2,3,4,5,6}$), and for inositols with a single phosphorylation at position 6. Other members of the group include pentakisinositol phosphates (IP_5s) and some cyclic compounds in which bonds link phosphate group atoms.

inositol phosphate phosphatases: enzymes that catalyze dephosphorylation of inositol phosphates. Some are inhibited by **lithium** (*q.v.*).

inositol phosphate glycans: glycosyl-inositol-phosphates linked to oligosaccharides. In cell membranes, they are covalently linked to enzymes, cell adhesion molecules, and other compounds that have extracellular domains, and serve as anchors that retain the ends of those compounds within the lipid bilayers and maintain their orientations. Phosphatidylinositol-specific phospholipases that catalyze release of the ligands can provide activated molecules for other functions. Their activities are regulated by cytoplasmic factors, and substrate specificities depend in part on the fatty acid moieties. Insulin promotes liberation of two inositol glycans from membrane-bound proteins that are implicated as second messengers and/or modifiers of the activities of several insulin-induced enzymes.

inotropic: affecting muscle contractility; *cf* **ionotropic**.

insects: a very large class of Arthropods that includes flies, ants, mosquitoes, bees, wasps, fleas, and bugs (but not spiders, ticks, or mites). All have three pairs of jointed legs, and bodies divisible into head, thorax, and abdominal segments. Some species are directly parasitic, and several use humans and other animals as intermediate hosts. A few produce venoms that affect nervous system functions. Insects are used to study development (*see* **homeoboxes**), inheritance, behavior, and pheromone functions. They make many substances that resemble counterparts in vertebrates, including heat shock proteins, glucagon-like molecules, and prothoracicotropic hormone (which has insulin-like properties). *See* also *Drosophila*.

insectivores: animals that feed on insects.

Insectivores: members of the mammalian order Insectivora, which includes anteaters, shrews, moles, and hedgehogs.

insemination: delivery of spermatozoa to female reproductive tracts. Sperm are deposited into the vagina in humans and many other species, and into the uterus of horses, pigs, dogs, guinea pigs, rats, and some others. A single insemination provides gametes for numerous sequential fertilizations in a few. Human sperm have shorter life spans, but limited storage occurs in human vaginal crypts. *See* also **artificial insemination**.

insertional mutations: changes in DNA composition caused by inclusion of additional nucleotides, such as viral genes or transposons. The effects depend on the kinds added, and their positions. Some change open reading frames. Others modulate transcription rates by affecting the functions of promoters and other regulatory elements.

inside-out-patch: a device used to study membrane properties, in which the outer face of a membrane segment covers an electrode, and the inner face is exposed to a solution in a micropipette attached to the electrode. *See* also **patch clamping**.

inside-out-vesicles: structures that form spontaneously when membranes are mechanically disrupted, in which the side that bordered the lumen when it was in the cell faces the external environment. They are used to study membrane transport.

in situ: in position; in the original location.

in situ **hybridization**: techniques for localizing specific DNA segments of chromosomes. The chromosome is squashed on a glass slide, the DNA is denatured, and adhering RNAs and proteins are removed. The product is then incubated with a tritium labeled DNA probe of known composition, to determine regions of the test material with which it can base pair.

instar: a stage in the life cycle of a holometabolous insect that occurs between two successive molts.

instincts: unlearned behavior patterns.

instructive theory: an outmoded concept that the specificity of an antibody is conferred by initial contact with the associated antigen.

insulin: species-specific hormones secreted mostly by pancreatic islet β cells, but also in small amounts in the brain and elsewhere. They promote acquisition, distribution, conservation, and efficient use of nutrients, and protect against hyperglycemia by stimulating glucose uptake in skeletal and cardiac muscle, adipose tissue, and several other cell types, glucose conversion to glycogen (especially in liver and skeletal muscle), and glucose oxidation, and by inhibiting gluconeogenesis and glycogenolysis. The effects on glucose transport include induction of a special class of carriers, and influences on microtubules and microfilaments that promote translocation of the carriers from cell interiors to plasma membranes. They provide cells with fatty acid fuels by activating lipoprotein lipases and accelerating fatty acid synthesis, and protect against ketosis by promoting use of fatty acids for synthesis of triacylglycerols and some other lipids, and by inhibiting fatty acid oxidation and the enzymes used for ketone production. Additionally, they facilitate the uptake of several kinds of amino acids, and the incorporation of amino acids into proteins, inhibit proteolysis, and promote the formation of many kinds of messenger RNAs. In some cell types, insulins are directly mitogenic; and in some others they indirectly support cell proliferation by augmenting localized synthesis of insulin-like growth factor-1 (IGF-I) and other growth factors. High levels also activate IGF-I receptors. The antilipolytic, anti-ketogenic, and lipogenic actions, along with direct influences on the kidneys and on vasopressin release, all contribute to control of acid-base and water balance; and the reactions involved in glucose oxidation provide ATP, NADPH, and other substances for anabolic pathways. Insulin receptors are expressed on neuroglia and on some neurons, and the central actions include neurogenesis in fetuses, appetite control, influences on taste perception and olfaction, and decreased firing rates for some sympathetic system cells. Peripherally, synergisms with numerous regulators affect processes such as ovarian follicle maturation, steroidogenesis, 1,25-dihydroxy-cholecalciferol synthesis, production of insulin-like growth factor-II (IGF-II), and immune system functions. In addition to inducing many enzymes (including glucokinase, glycogen synthase, phosphosphofructokinase, and acetyl-Co A carboxylase), and suppressing synthesis of some others, such as phosphoenolpyruvate carboxykinase (PEPCK), insulins rapidly affect the activities of several by activating specific phosphatases and kinases. In some cell types, they lower cAMP levels by activating cyclic nucleotide phosphodiesterases and/or inhibiting adenylate cyclases. Glucose is the major stimulant for insulin release, and its presence is essential for the actions of most other stimulants. Glucose also promotes insulin synthesis, formation of glucose receptors, and growth of pancreatic islet β cells. The effects include accelerated Ca^{2+} uptake from the surrounding fluids, and the synthesis of **cyclic adenosine diphosphate ribose** *(q.v.)*. Other stimuli for insulin release include glucagon, some amino acids, some gastrointestinal hormones, acetylcholine, and interleukin-1 (IL-1); *see* also **anticipatory controls**. Linoleic and linolenic acids are highly effective in some species. Norepinephrine acting on α_1-type adrenergic receptors inhibits. (The β-type adrenergic receptors mediate release, but their effects are usually masked by the activities of the more numerous α forms.) Most of the symptoms of diabetes mellitus have been linked with insulin deficiency and/or insulin resistance. All insulins are composed of A and B peptide chains linked by disulfide bonds. They are cleaved from proinsulins, via reactions that liberate a connecting C peptide and two dipeptides as well as the active hormone. Proinsulins are stored in secretory granules, are released in small amounts, and display very weak insulin-like activity. In the proinsulin diagram (p. 364), the dark circles represent C-peptide amino acids, the shaded ones the insulin A chain, and the clear ones the insulin B chain.

Circulating C peptide concentrations provide a measure of endogenous insulin production in individuals treated with hormones from other sources (since preparations from other animals do not contain it); but the C-peptides have longer half-lives. Humans make mostly one insulin type, with a molecular weight of 5734. Rats and some others make two or more. The dots in the human insulin diagram indicate sites at which species differences are known. Guinea pigs and a few others make unusual proteins (and have atypical receptors), but insulins of most vertebrate species are effective in a wide variety of animal types.

insulinases: enzymes that degrade insulin but also act on other substrates. Liver and kidney proteases rapidly cleave some of the peptide bonds, and a hepatic glutathione dehydrogenase inactivates by reducing the disulfide bonds and releasing free A and B chains.

insulin-dependent diabetes mellitus: IDDM; Type I diabetes mellitus; forms of **diabetes mellitus** *(q.v.)* in which insufficient insulin is secreted, and in which survival depends on replacement therapy; *cf* **non-insulin dependent diabetes mellitus**.

insulin-like activity: ILA; body fluid components that exert actions similar to those of insulin, but do not bind to anti-insulin antibodies. Insulin-like growth factor-I (IGF-I) accounts for much of the activity in well-nourished individuals; *see* also **nonsuppresible insulin-like activity**.

insulin-like growth factors: IGFs; peptides that exert some insulin-like actions, and mediate many of the effects of growth hormone, but do not bind to antibodies directed against insulin; *see* **insulin-like growth factor-I, insulin-like growth factor-II**, and **somatomedins**.

insulin-like growth factor-I: IGF-I; basic peptides structurally related to proinsulins, that mediate many of the anabolic effects of growth hormone, and also exert some insulin-like actions; *see* also **somatomedin C**. The major circulating form, which is similar in most mammals, originates in the liver. It has 70 amino acids with three intrachain disulfide bridges, and contains sequences similar to those of insulin A and B chains. However, the component analogous to insulin C peptide is retained, and there is an additional *C*-terminal D chain. The human type has the amino acid sequence: H₂N-Gly-Pro-Glu-Thr-Leu-Cys-Gly-Ala-Glu-Leu-Val-Asp-Ala-Leu-Gln-Phe-Val-Cys-Gly-Asp-Arg-Gly-Phe-Tyr-Phe-Asn-Lys-Pro-Thr-Gly-Tyr-Gly-Ser-Ser-Ser-Arg-Arg-Ala-

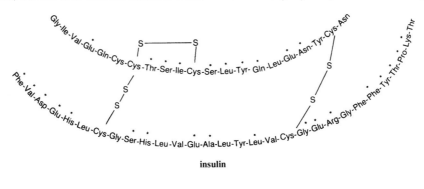

insulin

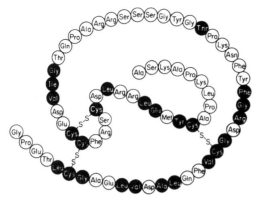

IGF-I

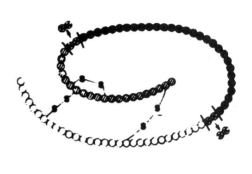

proinsulin

Pro-Gln-Thr-Gly-Ile-Val-Asp-Glu-Cys-Cys-Phe-Arg-Ser-Cys-Asp-Leu-Arg-Arg-Leu-Glu-Met-Tyr-Cys-Ala-Pro-Leu-Lys-Pro-Ala-Lys-Ser-Ala-OH, with disulfide bonds that connect cysteine moieties at position 6 → 48, 18 → 61, and 47 → 52. The black circles in the diagram show moieties identical to those of insulin A and B chains. In well-nourished individuals, the levels are positively regulated by growth hormone. Prolactin exerts similar effects in at least some species. Starvation, carbohydrate deprivation, and liver disease are among the factors that blunt the responses to GH; and glucose levels may contribute to transcriptional control. GH also induces truncated forms that lack an *N*-terminal tripeptide in almost all cell types, and function as paracrine and/or autocrine regulators. The amounts made vary with the cell types, and with the stages of maturation. Their production is affected by steroid hormones and other regulators. Intracellular proteases that process circulating hormone provide additional controls. Most IGF-I actions are modulated by **insulin-like growth factor binding proteins** (IGFBPs, *q.v.*). 1,25-dihydroxyvitamin D inhibits IGF-I release in bone, and it augments production of IGFBP-4. IGF-I peptides are also present in cerebrospinal, amniotic, and other fluids, and in saliva and milk; and large amounts are made by some tumor cells. IGF-I was initially believed to mediate *all* of the anabolic effects of growth hormone on cartilage and bone, a concept supported by observations that some forms of dwarfism are caused by inability to make IGF-I although GH levels are high. It is now recognized that GH influences on cell maturation precede, and invoke responsivity to IGF-I. Insulin is a growth stimulant for many cell types, and is mitogenic for a few. Responses to physiological concentrations are attributed to interactions with insulin receptors; but ones that require very high concentrations evidently involve binding to IFG-I types. IGF-I can directly promote growth in individuals with insulin-dependent diabetes mellitus who do not respond directly to GH, and in some with children with growth retardation caused by failure to make functional GH receptors. Although less potent than insulin for such processes, IGF-I promotes glucose and amino acid uptake, and protein synthesis. It functions as a progression factor in the presence of competence factors such as platelet derived and fibroblast growth factors (PDGF and FGF), accelerates steroidogenesis in gonads, and augments renal blood flow and glomerular filtration. Injury stimulates localized IGF-I production, and the peptide contributes to wound healing and compensatory hypertrophy. Influences on neurotransmitter release have also been described. The ability of IGF-I peptides to inhibit GH secretion appears to be mediated in part via somatostatin. There is evidence for roles in hematopoiesis and embryonic development (but *see* also **insulin-like growth factor II**). Some of the effects have been linked with elevation of cytosolic Ca^{2+}, and with cytosol alkalinization. A few may depend on binding to insulin receptors.

insulin-like growth factor-II, IGF-II: neutral peptides chemically and structurally related to insulin-like growth factor-I; *see* also **somatomedin A** and **multiplication stimulating activity** (MSA). The predominant form has 67 amino acids, with disulfide bridges joining moieties 9 → 47, 21 → 60, and 46 → 51. In embryos and fetuses, the major inducers are placental lactogens. In rats and some other species, only embryos and fetuses have high levels; but in humans and some others, the concentrations are low in fetuses, and rise rapidly during the first postnatal year. Choroid plexuses and leptomeninges are the major sources within the central nervous system. IGF-II peptides contribute to the growth and differentiation of many cell types (including myoblasts, immature neurons, and hematopoietic cells), and they interact with pituitary gland hormones at some sites, (for example thyroid stimulating hormone in thyroid glands and follicle stimulating hormone in the gonads). Their production is, in turn, affected by regulators released by the target organs, and it varies with the stage of development and maturation. Glucose also modulates release; and high levels have been found in newborn infants of mothers with insulin-dependent diabetes mellitus. Retinoic acid is another important inducer, at least at some sites. Specific receptors bind IGF-II with high affinity. However, different loci on the same hormones interact with IGF-I types, and some of the growth-promoting effects are mediated in that way. There are also indications that IGF-IIs antagonize IGF-I at some sites by competing for the receptors and/or accelerating IGF-I degradation. They additionally augment production of IGFBP-2. Rodents with mutations that impair IGF-II synthesis are undersized, but have normal body proportions. Ones that lack IGF-II receptors are of normal size at birth but are edematous and have other defects. The insulin-like actions are generally weaker than those of IGF-I; and IGF-II peptides are less efficient stimulants for bone and cartilage. *See* also **insulin-like growth factor-2 receptors**. The amino acid sequence for the major human type is HN$_2$-Ala-Tyr-Arg-Pro-Ser-Glu-Thr-Leu-Cys-Gly-Gly-Glu-Leu-Val-Asp-Thr-Leu-Gln-Phe-Val-Cys-Gly-Asp-Arg-Gly-Phe-Tyr-Phe-Ser-Arg-Pro-Ala-Ser-Arg-Val-Ser-Arg-Arg-Ser-Arg-Gly-Ile-Val-Glu-Glu-Cys-Cys-Phe-Arg-Ser-Cys-Asp-Leu-Ala-Leu-Leu-Glu-Thr-Tyr-Cys-Ala-Thr-Pro-Ala-Lys-Ser-Glu-OH.

insulin-like growth factor binding proteins: IGF-BPs; at least six classes of chemically related proteins, secreted by many cell types, that bind IGFs with high affinity (but do not bind insulin), each with its characteristic kind of *C*-terminal amino acid sequence. They differ from IGF receptors, but affect IGF functions in various ways that include influences on transport from blood to target cells, circulating half-lives, and interactions with both receptors and extracellular matrices. Heterogeneities within each class are attributed to differential posttranslational processing that includes phosphorylation, dimerization, and (except for types 1 and 2) glycosylation. The kinds and amounts made depend on the cell type and the developmental state. Their abilities to either enhance or suppress IGF actions are related to not only the chemical structures, but also the concentrations (which affect attachments to cell membranes), and the presence of other regulators. Most IGFs within the bloodstream are components of 150K complexes, each of which contains one molecule of an 88K acid-labile peptide, one IGF, and two or more IGFBP-3 molecules. IGFBP-3 proteins are also present in lymph, cerebrospinal and amniotic fluids, and most exocrine secretions. Soluble forms present in low to moderate concentrations sequester IGFs and limit their access to receptors. When present in high concentrations, they attach to plasma membranes, and in some cases augment IGF-receptor binding.

insulin like growth factor binding protein-1: IGFBP-1; IGFBP-28; placental protein-12; 25K-33K, acid-stable, cysteine-rich proteins, devoid of carbohydrate, that bind IGF-I and IGF-II peptides with similar affinity. A major form in rats contains 247 amino acid moieties. The proteins are made in uterine decidua, epithelia and stroma, by hepatocytes, fibroblasts, and neurons, and at other sites. High concentrations occur in amniotic fluid. Phosphorylation enhances the affinities for IGFs, and Arg-Gly-Asp sequences mediate adhesion to cell membranes. Progesterone increases their production. Factors that decrease it include glucose, insulin, glucocorticoids, and growth hormone. Postnatally, feeding rhythms account for some of the variations in body fluid levels.

insulin like growth factor binding protein-2: IGFBP-2; 24-34K proteins made by hepatocytes, smooth muscle, choroid plexus, and decidual, and other cell types, and most abundant in ones that rapidly proliferate. They display somewhat higher affinity for IGF-II than for IGF-I. The major type in rats has 270 amino acids. Secretion is increased at some sites by IGF-I and estrogens, and decreased by growth hormone, glucocorticoids, and insulin.

insulin-like growth factor binding protein-3: IGFBP-3; growth-hormone dependent IGFBP; BP-53; heavily glycosylated 24-54K glycoproteins made by hepatocytes, fibroblasts, and endothelium, and at other sites, and present in highest concentrations in rapidly proliferating cells. The major type in rats has 265 amino acids. IGFBP-3s display higher affinity for IGF-II than for IGF-I, but are components of the 150K complexes in blood plasma that bind both factors (*see* **insulin-like growth factors**), prolong their half-lives in the bloodstream, and serve as reservoirs for growth factor delivery to target organs. IGFBP-3 also attaches to plasma membranes, and it has been proposed that its proteolytic processing by cellular enzymes facilitates IGF binding to receptors (since the products have lower affinities for the growth factors). However, several inhibitory influences of the products, for example on follicle stimulating hormone (FSH) stimulated estrogen and progesterone production are known. Growth hormone is the major positive regulator of IGFBP-3 synthesis (both directly and via IGF-I), but the levels also rise in response to insulin.

insulin-like growth factor binding protein-4: IGFBP-4; 24-26K glycoproteins identified in many cell types, and in cerebrospinal and other fluids. They display especially high affinity for IGF-II. The major form in rats has 233 amino acids. The amounts made depend on the cell types and the maturational stages. High levels are present in ovarian antral follicles undergoing atresia, and roles in dominant follicle selection have been proposed.

insulin-like growth factor binding protein-5: IGFBP-5; approximately 28K glycoproteins that bind IGF-I and IGF-II. The major form in rats has 252 amino acids. The amounts made depend on the cell types. Since high levels are found in ovarian pre-antral follicles undergoing atresia, IGFBP-5 may contribute to species-related restrictions on the numbers of follicles that mature during any given ovarian cycle.

insulin-like growth factor binding protein-6: IGFBP-6; a recently identified 21K protein that binds IGFs. The form in rats has 201 amino acids.

insulin-like growth factor receptors: IGF-Rcs: transmembrane proteins that bind IGFs with high affinities, and mediate their functions; *see* specific types. Most target cells express both IGF-I and IGF-II types, in addition to ones for insulin, or one type plus insulin receptors.

insulin-like growth factor-I receptors: IGF-I Rcs; IGF type I receptors; glycoproteins structurally similar to insulin receptors, composed of two extracellular, disulfide-linked α subunits, each attached via a disulfide bond to a transmembrane β subunit. The major types are 300-350K, with approximately 135K α and 95-98K β components, but smaller α subunits have been identified in the brain. The α subunits bind IGF-Is with high affinity, display somewhat lower affinities for IGF-IIs, and interact with insulin when that hormone is present in high concentrations. Ligand binding activates intracellular tyrosine kinases of β subunits. This leads promptly to autophosphorylation, and soon afterward to phosphorylation of other cellular proteins. Most IGF-I actions are mediated via type I receptors, but IGF-Is present in high concentrations additionally activate insulin types; and a few anabolic influences are attributed to interactions with type II receptors. The numbers of IGF-I receptors are regulated in part by nutritional states, and they increase in parallel with growth rates. They are down regulated, via internalization, by both IGF-I and insulin.

insulin-like growth factor-II receptors: IGF-II Rcs: IGF type II receptors; approximately 250K single-chain transmembrane proteins with large extracellular and very small intracellular domains, that bind IGF-II with high affinity. They display low affinities for IGF-I, and none for insulin. Although avian and amphibian IGF-II receptors lack the property, the extracellular domains in humans, cattle, rodents, and some others mammals bind mannose-6-phosphate at different sites, and are therefore also known as IGFII/mannose-6-phosphate receptors. Both ligands can bind at the same time; and free sugar-phosphate augments the affinity for IGF-II. **Mannose-6-phosphate receptors** (*q.v.*) mediate transport of certain proteins (including some enzymes) from *trans*-Golgi networks to prelysosomes. IGF-II receptors lack intrinsic tyrosine kinase activity, but do undergo phosphorylation. Some IGF-II functions require interactions with IGF-I receptors. IGF-II receptors on some cell types accelerate IGF-I degradation, and interference with the actions of those hormones is attributed in part to IGF-II receptor shedding and release to extracellular fluids. Although membrane bound IGF-II receptors are internalized, and insulin accelerates recycling, they are not down regulated by either insulin or IGF-II. Growth hormone augments the numbers in adipocytes, and it modulates the insulin effects. In most tissues, the numbers in juveniles decline with advancing maturity.

insulin-like immunoreactivity: ILA; substances that interact with antibodies directed against insulin. Most of the antibodies bind proinsulin, and some attach to related proteins. *Cf* **nonsuppressible insulin-like activity**.

insulinomas: insulin-secreting tumors. Most are benign types in pancreatic islets. The major manifestation is **hypoglycemia** (*q.v.*).

insulin receptors: glycoproteins identified in almost all cell types (including erythrocytes) that bind insulin with high affinity and specificity, and mediate the actions of the hormone. Most are in plasma membranes. These are 400K tetramers, each composed of two 130K α- and two 95K β subunits. They display limited affinity for IGF-I (and none for IGF-II). The α subunits project to the cell exterior and contain the insulin-binding sites. They are linked by disulfide bonds to β subunits whose tyrosine kinases are activated by ligand binding. The activation, which is essential for many insulin functions, leads to autophosphorylation of the β subunits, and, soon afterward, to phosphorylation of several other proteins (including some phosphatases). Many effects appear to involve cascades and complex interactions of several second messengers, including Ca^{2+}. A special G protein transducer has been described; and kinase C

isozymes and inositol glycans are important in at least some cell types. Chronically elevated insulin levels invoke insulin resistance, in part by down regulating the receptor numbers.

insulin receptor substrate-1: IRS-1; p185; a 185K protein implicated as a major mediator of signal transduction when insulin binds to its receptors. It is rapidly phosphorylated when the insulin receptor β chain tyrosine kinase is activated, and the phosphorylated form binds to phosphatidylinositol-3-kinase. It may promote translocation of that enzyme to membrane sites, and thereby facilitate substrate binding. There is some evidence that phosphatidylinositols phosphorylated at the 3 positions function as receptors; but no ligands have as yet been identified.

insulin resistance: impaired ability to respond to insulin. The causes include defective or inadequate numbers of insulin receptors, postreceptor dysfunctions related to abnormal or inadequate numbers of glucose transport proteins and/or metabolic enzymes, and excessive amounts of hormones such as glucocorticoids and growth hormone that oppose insulin actions. It has been proposed somatostatin, along with excess glucagon, contributes in some cases, and that severe, chronic insulin deficiency alters receptor functions. Most (possibly all) individuals with type II **diabetes mellitus** (*q.v.*) have some insulin resistance. *See* also **amylin**.

insulitis: inflammation of the pancreatic islets, associated with infiltration of lymphocytes and other leukocytes, and with β-cell destruction. It can be initiated by viral infections; but in most cases the damage is attributed to autoimmune attacks mounted against previously healthy cells. The condition has been detected in many individuals with newly diagnosed insulin-dependent diabetes mellitus.

int-1: a proto-oncogene, now known as ***wnt-1*** (*see* **wnt genes**), expressed in spatially restricted parts of neural tubes and embryonic structures that develop from them. In mammals, it directs formation of a 370 amino acid protein that is processed to a secreted 44K growth factor which attaches to cell membranes and extracellular matrices, affects gap-junction communication, and is essential for development of some parts of the brain. A homologous *wnt-1* (*wingless*) *Drosophila* gene codes for a related, 468-amino acid protein product that directs pattern formation. Mice homozygous for a nonfunctional *wnt-1* mutation have ataxia, along with defective cerebellum and midbrain formation. *Wnt-1* is also expressed in postmeiotic spermatocytes, in which it may contribute to spermiogenesis. Although not transcribed in normal mammary glands, it is activated when mouse mammary tumor virus integrates into the DNA, and it appears to then stimulate tumor growth.

int-2: a proto-oncogene expressed in nervous tissues of young embryos that directs formation of a member of the fibroblast growth factor family. The nucleic acid structure is consistent with production of a 245 amino acid precursor. It has been suggested that both secreted and nuclear forms are made, and that the final products are 27.5K,

31.5K, and 36-44K proteins. Although both types can insert into mammary tumor virus genes, and both are expressed in nervous tissues, *int-1* is not otherwise related to *int-2*; *see* **wnt genes**.

int-3: a gene also known as *irp* in mice that codes for a transmembrane protein essential for normal embryonic development, and is also expressed in adult brain. It is not directly related to either *int-1* or *int-2*; *see* **wnt genes**.

integral membrane proteins: proteins that reside entirely within membranes. The term usually refers to plasma membrane types that lack both extracellular and intracellular domains. *Cf* **transmembrane** and **peripheral proteins**.

integrases: viral enzymes that catalyze processes which lead to insertion of nucleic acid segments into host DNA. They recognize specific base sequences on both viral and host nucleic acids, and usually act in conjunction with other factors to promote cleavage at specific sites and establish new molecular links.

integration: (1) incorporation of a new nucleic acid segment into a preexisting molecule; *see* **integrases**; (2) neuronal interactions that achieve a coordinated response to a stimulus.

integrins: at least twenty adhesion glycoproteins composed of 120-180K α subunits non-covalently associated with 90-110K β subunits. All are receptors for cell surface and extracellular matrix molecules. Many additionally bind (in some cases indirectly) to cytoskeleton proteins. Both subunits traverse plasma membranes and participate in the binding. Fourteen α, and eight β types have thus far been identified; but only limited numbers of α and β combinations have been found. One classification system is based on the presence of a common subtype. For example, all integrins with a 95K β_2 subunit are included in the leucocyte adhesion group. However, letters that refer to ligands or locations are also used; and both the subunits and dimers are known under different names. α_v was named for its affinity for vitronectin, and α_E (also known as α_6) for its presence on epithelial cells. CD18 is β_2, and CD11s are α types. Integrin $\alpha_{IIb}\beta_3$ is also called platelet-specific integrin and GPIIb/IIIa; and the leucocyte adhesion group includes LFA-1 (α_L,β_2), p150,95 ($\alpha_x\beta_2$), and Mac-1 (α_m,β_2, also known as CR3 and as Mo-1). Most cells constitutively express several varieties, some of which are cytoplasmic in resting states, but translocated to membranes in response to activators. Some forms are expressed on just one or a few cells types, whereas others occur more universally. The extracellular ligands include fibronectin, hemonectin, type I collagen, elastin, proteoglycans, hyaluronic acid, fibrinogen, fibrin, thrombospondin, osteopontin, von Willebrand factor, complement fragment iCb3, laminins, at least 6 very late activated antigens (VLA-1 through VLA-6), LFA-1, cranins, and CSAT (a chicken embryo fibroblast cell surface attachment glycoprotein complex), as well as position-specific molecules identified in *Drosophila*, bacterial and phage components, and some chemically related molecules made by amphibians and nematodes. The cytoskeletal ligands include actin, talin,

vinculin, tensin, and tropomyosin. Most (but not all) ligands contain Arg-Gly-Asp (RGD) amino acid sequences that are recognized by integrins, and a few have immunoglobulin-like structures. Amino acid sequences recognized on specific ligands include Lys-Gln-Ala-Gly-Asp-Val (KQAGDV) on fibrin, and Asp-Gly-Glu-Ala (DGEA) on type I collagen. The α subunits additionally contain domains for Ca^{2+} and/or Mg^{2+}. Binding specificity is attributed to simultaneous attachments to two or more ligand domains, and/or recognition of RGD sequences in special contexts. Gangliosides that co-localize with integrins may play regulatory roles, and tyrosine phosphorylations of β subunits affect the properties. (Increased phosphorylation has been observed for some transformed and malignant tumor cells; but metastatic potential is also related to failure of those cells to produce extracellular matrix components.) By mediating cell-cell, cell-matrix, an cell surface-cell interior interactions, integrins maintain tissue integrity, regulate cell differentiation, shape, migration, and activation, and contribute to signal transduction. Some effects have been linked with activation of kinase C isozymes, and/or influences on ion channels. They play roles in morphogenesis, hemostasis, platelet aggregation, wound healing, host-parasite interactions, phagocytosis of microorganisms and debris, inflammation, immune system functions, and metastasis. *See* also **disintegrins**.

integument: (1) the skin; (2) an outer coat or envelope.

interband: the region between two chromosome bands.

interbrain: the diencephalon.

intercalated cells: a population of mitochondria-rich "dark" renal collecting duct cells, more abundant in the cortex than in the medulla. They are fewer in number than the light, vasopressin-regulated cells, and display lower Na^+-K^+-ATPase activity, but are rich in carbonic anhydrase. An E^+ subtype predominates in the medulla, engages in endocytosis of macromolecules presented in the lumen, and contributes to sodium and bicarbonate reabsorption. The E^- subtype predominates in the cortex and secretes bicarbonate.

intercalated discs: electron-dense complexes that contain gap junctions and desmosomes, and provide avenues of communication between cardiac myocytes essential for coordinated contraction.

intercalating agent: a substance that inserts into a preexisting macromolecule, membrane, or other structure. When acridine orange and actinomycin D insert between DNA base pairs, they disrupt the complementary strand associations that normally occur during replication, and invoke mutations by facilitating base additions, deletions, and/or substitutions. Actinomycin D is used over a limited concentration range to block DNA-directed premessenger RNA synthesis.

intercellular: between cells; *cf* **intracellular**.

intercellular adhesion molecules: ICAMs; CAMs: cell surface glycoproteins that interact with integrins and other cell surface components involved in cell adherence, inflammation, and immune system functions. Most are members of the immunoglobulin superfamily, and are chemically most closely related to IgMs. In addition to **ICAM-1** (*q.v.*), the group includes N-CAMs (neural cell adhesion molecules), L-CAMs (liver cell adhesion molecules), myelin associated glycoprotein (MAG), lymphocyte function associated antigen-3 (LFA-3) and the CD2 antigens on lymphocyte surfaces. *See* **INCAM-110** and **selectins**, and *see* also **cell adhesion molecules**.

intercellular adhesion molecule-1: ICAM-1; CD54; an inducible 95K glycoprotein chemically related to neural cell adhesion molecule (N-CAM), myelin-associated glycoprotein (MAG), and immunoglobulins, but different from cadherins and devoid of an RGD sequence. It is expressed on endothelial cell, lymphocyte, fibroblast, and monocyte cell surfaces, and participates in adhesion that is associated with immunological and inflammatory reactions by engaging in heterophilic binding to T lymphocyte, B lymphocyte, monocyte, and myeloid cell membrane glycoproteins, including LFA-1. Some of its functions are related to physical associations with high-affinity interleukin-2 (IL-2) receptors. Transforming growth factor-β (TGFβ) decreases its production.

intercellular retinol binding protein: a 140K protein made in the retina, that binds retinol and is believed to contribute to photoreceptor functions.

interception: (1) interruption of a pregnancy; (2) fertility control by agents that act soon after conception, but after implantation has been initiated; *cf* **contraception** and **abortion**.

intercross: mating of two diploid individuals, both heterozygous at a specified locus.

interdigitating cells: IDCs; large, non-phagocytic, non-lymphocytic, irregularly shaped mononuclear cells of the thymus gland reticulum that derive from bone marrow, express class II surface antigens, and are implicated in thymocyte maturation. They are members of a larger group of antigen-presenting cells collectively known as dendritic cells, which includes skin Langerhans cells and the veiled cells of lymph nodes.

interface: the boundary between two phases of a heterogenous system, for example between two immiscible liquids.

interference microscopy: *see* **microscopy**.

interferons: IFNs; three classes of species-specific 16-27K cytokines, initially identified by their abilities to inhibit viral replication, but now known to exert major influences on the proliferation and differentiation of many cell types, and to provide protection against the growth of malignant ones. They are homodimers, produced constitutively in small amounts, and rapidly made in larger ones in response to viruses and some bacterial components, bacterial toxins, protozoa, and growth factors. Most are glycosylated. Double stranded RNAs are especially potent stimulants; and much of the antiviral and antiproliferative activity is attributed to IFN stimulation of dsRNA protein kinase synthesis. The enzyme is a serine-threonine kinase activated by autophosphorylation, that inhibits protein synthesis by catalyzing phosphorylation of the α subunits of eukaryote translation initiation factor eIF-2. IFNs are secreted, and most of their effects require interactions with target cell interferon response elements that affect the transcription of specific genes. The actions are modulated by several cytokines, some of which are induced by IFNs (*see* also **interferon regulatory factors 1** and **2**); and one kind of IFN influences the actions of others. Some endogenous factors, and some viral components suppress IFN production, and gangliosides are implicated as type I IFN antagonists. After binding to their receptors, IFNs are rapidly internalized. Although the processes lead to IFN degradation, they also facilitate IFN translocation to nuclei, in which direct effects may be exerted. (IFNβs bind strongly to nuclear membranes and nucleoplasm components). The α and β IFNs bind to common receptors, and are collectively known as type I IFNs. Some of their effects, for example growth inhibition (but not antiviral potency) are attributed to cAMP generation; but dsRNA additionally directly augments adenylate cyclase activity and inhibits growth. The γ (type II) IFNs act on different receptors. They promote phosphatidylcholine hydrolysis, diacylglycerol generation, and activation of specific protein kinase C isozymes (including calcium independent PKC ε forms in some cell types), but are not known to affect phosphatidylinositol turnover, inositol triphosphate generation, or elevation of cytosolic Ca^{2+}. The γ types also affect the secretion of several pituitary hormones. Functions affected by IFNs include cell cycle regulation, selective expression of major histocompatibility complex antigens, antibody production, antibody switching, macrophage and natural killer cell stimulation, and the killing of parasites and tumor cells. They contribute to both immediate and delayed hypersensitivity and inflammatory responses, elevate body temperature, and promote sleep. Although overproduction can invoke autoimmune diseases (including some endocrine system disorders), the cytokines indirectly protect normal cells by stimulating the release of growth factors which oppose the attacks (but do not diminish the antiviral potency). IFNs additionally play roles in embryonic development and hematopoiesis. They are used to treat of some forms of leukemia and other malignant diseases, and some viral infections, but invoke serious side effects. *See* specific types.

interferon α: IFNα; leukocyte interferon: a family of acid-stable, chemically and biologically related cytokines made in largest amounts by activated circulating leukocytes and lymphoblastoid cells exposed to live or inactivated viruses or double-stranded RNAs, or to endotoxin and some other bacterial products. Most other nucleated cells make small amounts, but do not secrete them. Transforming growth factor-β (TGFβ) inhibits the synthesis. Several genes contribute to the production of a variety of α subtypes, most with 165 or 166 amino acid moieties, that vary in affinities for the same receptors. Chemically related trophoblast protein-1, made by sheep and cattle during early pregnancy, displays similar antiviral potency and may contribute to protection against maternal rejection of conceptuses (but is also anti-luteolytic). IFNαs act on receptors that also bind IFNβs; and both are included in the term type I interferons. IFNαs can raise body temperature, augment production of colony-stimulating factor-I (M-CSF), interleukin-1, and interleukin-6, antagonize platelet derived growth factor (PDGF) actions, and decrease the numbers of epidermal growth factor (EGF) receptors. They play roles in embryonic development and hematopoiesis. Some effects involve synergism with tumor necrosis factor-α (TNFα) and other regulators. An essential component of their antiviral actions involves translocation and activation of kinase $C_β$-type isoforms, phosphorylation of initiation factor eIF2, and dephosphorylation of some other proteins. The kinase is activated by diacylglycerols liberated from phosphatidylcholines (but not phosphatidylinositols). IFNα can also accelerate degradation of messenger RNAs for *c-myc* and *c-fos*, and slow formation of *ras* mRNAs and proteins in some cell types. Mutations that impair their synthesis have been linked with the development of gliomas and some forms of leukemia. IFNα is used to treat Kaposi's sarcoma and some other tumors. *See* also **interferon stimulated gene factor 3.**

interferon β: IFNβ; fibroblast interferon; betaferon; acid-stable cytokines chemically related to IFNαs, and included with them in the term type-I interferon. They are similar in size (most with 166 amino acids), interact with the same receptors, and exert some similar effects, for example on macrophages, natural killer cells, body temperature, colony stimulating factor-1 induction, expression of class I major histocompatibility complex antigens, hematopoiesis, and platelet derived growth factor (PDGF) antagonism. Activated fibroblasts produce the largest amounts; but other cell types make IFNβ, and fibroblasts make other IFNs. There are fewer β than α subtypes, but some clear differences between $IFNβ_1$ and $IFNβ_2$ (which is identical with interleukin-6). Endotoxin, platelet-derived growth factor, tumor necrosis factor-α, and interleukins 1 and 2 stimulate the production. Some growth inhibiting effects have been linked with negative control over the expression of *c-myc, c-fos*, β-actin, ornithine decarboxylase, and other PDGF-regulated genes.

interferon γ: IFNγ; gamma interferon; immune interferon; type II interferon: a family of acid-labile cytokines with antiviral properties, whose members differ chemically from type α and β interferons, and interact with different receptors (expressed on macrophages, astrocytes, endothelial, and other antigen presenting cells). The human types have 143 amino acid moieties, with molecular weights affected by glycosylations and aggregations. They are produced in largest amounts by natural killer cells and a subset of activated helper type T lymphocytes. Interleukins 1 and 2 are major stimulants; and IFNγ augments interleukin-1 production. Interleukin 10 inhibits; and IFNγ down regulates its own receptors. IFNγ stimulates the synthesis of tumor necrosis factors α and β (TNFα and TNFβ), and the selective expression of class II major histocompatibility antigens (as well as the class I types affected by type I IFNs), but inhibits IL-4 synthesis. In addition to influences on macrophage and natural killer cell functions, it regulates collagen synthesis and mast cell activity, and exerts selective effects on immunoglobulin secretion. (It augments IgG_{2a} syn-

thesis, but blocks interleukin-4 mediated switching to IgG1 and IgE.) It also induces Fc receptors for IgG, enhances inflammatory responses in several ways, and contributes to the cytotoxicity by increasing superoxide anion production. It is more potent than type I IFNs for inhibiting malignant cell proliferation. Some effects on protein synthesis have been linked with tryptophan depletion, since it induces indoleamine 2,3-dioxygenase. Its ability to promote astrocyte proliferation contributes to repair following central nervous system injury; but excessive amounts invoke gliosis. Additionally, IFNγ functions in embryonic development, and promotes production of some platelet proteins. Roles in hematopoiesis include influences on interleukin-7-sensitive pre-B cells that lower B lymphocyte numbers. The many interactions with endocrine and immune system cells include a feedback loop in which the cytokine stimulates synthesis of 1,25-dihydroxy-cholecalciferol (an inhibitor of IFNγ synthesis). In pituitary glands, IFNγ activates folliculo-stellate cells and thereby indirectly diminishes (but does not totally suppress) the release of prolactin and the stimulated release of adrenocorticotropic and growth hormones (ACTH and GH). It also decreases the sensitivity of thyroid gland cells to thyroid stimulating hormone (TSH), and of pancreatic β cells to glucose. Its ability to invoke insulin-dependent diabetes mellitus in laboratory animals appears to be lymphocyte mediated.

interferon gene regulatory elements: IREs; DNA regions with sequences that bind interferon regulatory factors 1 and 2 and control interferon synthesis.

interferon regulatory factor-1: IRF-1: a transcription activator protein induced by viruses and interferons that binds to upstream *cis* regulatory components of interferon genes. By augmenting interferon synthesis, it indirectly inhibits the growth of malignant and some normal cell types (including pre-B lymphocytes).

interferon regulatory factor-2: a protein that antagonizes the effects of interferon regulatory factor-1 by competing with it for DNA binding. It is one of the factors that protects against overproduction of the cytokines.

interferon stimulated gene[s]: ISGs; genes activated by interferons.

interferon stimulated gene factor 3: ISGF3; a transcription regulator induced by interferon-α that binds to interferon stimulated regulatory elements.

interferon stimulated regulatory elements: ISREs; DNA regions that bind interferon regulatory factors and control the expression of interferon stimulated genes.

intergenic: describes (1) a chromosome segment located between two genetic loci that is not necessarily involved in the expression of either; (2) a mutation in a region between two genetic loci.

interkinesis: usually, (1) the interval between meiosis I and meiosis II; (2) the interval between two successive mitotic divisions; *see* also **cell cycles** (G_o phase), and *cf* **interphase.**

interleukins: ILs: species-specific cytokines that regulate hematopoietic and immune system functions, and provide major links between the immune and endocrine systems. The functions affected include embryonic development, neurotransmission, body temperature, sleep, acute phase reactions, inflammation, tumor cell killing, and apoptosis, as well as the secretion of hypothalamic, pituitary, and other hormones. There are at least fourteen different subtypes, some of which exist in multiple forms that include biologically active precursors, large membrane-bound mature forms, small secreted peptides, and truncated derivatives. Most are known under several names. All share similar three-dimensional structures, but the subtypes vary in amino acid composition, size, and glycosylation; and their synthesis is directed by separate genes which are differentially regulated. (The carbohydrate components do not seem to be major determinants of activity, but can affect the half-lives.) Although each subtype invokes it own spectrum of responses, the biological activities vary with the cell types and states of maturation, and with the presence of other kinds of molecules (different interleukins, interferons, other growth factors, "classical" hormones, and nonhormonal proteins). The interactions include overlapping functions, additive effects, synergisms, and antagonisms. Some effects are exerted directly on the target cells; but many are achieved via influences on the secretion or functions of other regulators. The genes that direct their synthesis have structures which resemble those coding for oncostatin M, granulocyte-macrophage colony stimulating factor (GM-CSF), and other hemopoietic modulators.

interleukin-1: IL-1: interleukins 1α and 1β were formerly collectively called *endogenous pyrogen* (although the effects on body temperature are mediated via prostaglandins, and many other regulators invoke fever), and also *catabolin* (although many other cytokines are catabolic). IL-1α is identical with hemopoietin-1, and IL-1β with lymphocyte activating factor (LAF). Terms introduced before it was recognized that there are two distinct forms, but now seldom used because of possible confusion with other mediators include serum A amyloid inducer (SAA-inducer), and mitogenic protein (MP). Other terms discarded when additional interleukins were discovered include B cell activating factor (BAF), and B cell differentiation factor (BDF), since both B cell stimulation factor I and B cell differentiation factor I have been applied to interleukin-4, and both B cell stimulation factor II and B cell differentiation factor II to interleukin-6. (Interleukin-2 has been called thymocyte mitogenic factor, and T cell growth factor, whereas T cell growth factor II applies to interleukin-4). T cell replacing factor III (TRF-III) is disliked by endocrinologists, not only because it has been applied to interleukin-5, but also because TRF is an acronym for thyrotropin release factor. Most cell types that secrete interleukin-1 make both α and β forms, which differ in amino acid sequences and surface charges, and whose synthesis is directed by different genes. The two cytokines act on common receptors, including 80K glycoproteins on fibroblasts, endothelial cells, hepatocytes and some other cell types, and 68-70K types on

macrophages and neutrophilic leukocytes. The predominant secreted forms are 16K-17K peptides, made from 31-32K precursors that are processed at the time of release. IL-1α precursors, as well as shortened forms are secreted; and all types (including ones bound to plasma membranes) are biologically active. In contrast, IL-1β is usually released as an inactive precursor under most conditions (including cell necrosis), and undergoes extracellular processing. (However, intracellular processing of both IL-1α and IL-1β can be activated by apoptotic stimuli.) Some smaller (10K) secreted forms, which may be fragments, are also active. Monocytes, macrophages, and B lymphocytes are the major sources, but fibroblasts, natural killer cells, neutrophilic leukocytes, endothelium, renal mesangial cells, astrocytes, placenta cells and some others make IL-1s in response to infection, injury, interferon-γ (IFNγ), lipopolysaccharide, complement components C3a and C5a, and/or antigen-antibody-complement complexes. Activated T_H cells are potent stimulants for production by macrophages. Keratinocytes make considerable quantities, but they are among the cell types that contain substantial amounts of an interleukin-1 receptor antagonist. Both IL-1 types are major mediators of inflammation and immune system functions. Their influences on hematopoiesis involve stimulation of the secretion of other growth factors, and both synergistic and permissive type interactions with those regulators. IL-1s display homologies to, interact with, and exert some actions similar to those of tumor necrosis factors (TNFs) and IL-6. Each class of regulators promotes release of the others, and although different receptors are involved, overlapping functions include stimulation of T (and especially T_H), and B lymphocyte maturation and proliferation, induction of both IL-2 and IL-2 receptors, activation of mature T and B lymphocytes, natural killer cells, dendritic cells, monocytes, macrophages, eosinophils, endothelial cells, and synoviocytes, stimulation of fibroblast, endothelial cell, astroglia, and mesangial cell proliferation, and production of acute phase proteins (including fibrinogen, haptoglobin, and C-reactive protein). They are also chemotactic for neutrophilic leukocytes and macrophages. Some of the effects on T lymphocytes have been linked with tyrosine kinase activation. Neither the cytokines nor the receptors possess such activity, but IL-1s activate p57^{lck} (a kinase that associates with CD2, CD4 and CD8) via processes believed to involve CD45-mediated dephosphorylation of the enzyme. Excessive IL-1 production is implicated in the etiology of several diseases. For example, the effects on neovascularization, mediated in part via induction of basic fibroblast growth factors in smooth muscle cells, can contribute to the development of atherosclerosis, effects on keratinocytes are believed to facilitate development of psoriasis, and the cytotoxicity contributes in major ways to the tissue destruction associated with rheumatoid arthritis. Skeletal muscle atrophy can occur when the secretion is prolonged, and appetite depression exacerbates the consequences of proteolytic enzyme activation. However, in the presence of other regulators, IL-1α can inhibit excessive epithelial cell proliferation and promote prostacyclin synthesis. IL-1β can, under some conditions, invoke destruction of pancreatic islet and ovarian cells, but exogenous IL-α has been observed to be protective in some animal models. IL-1β also exerts several effects on cell-matrix interactions, cell shape, and associated changes in protein synthesis, in part by promoting phosphorylation and redistribution of talin. Its ability to cause loss of focal contacts may contribute to metastasis. Both IL-1 types can invoke bone resorption and hypercalcemia, by stimulating prostaglandin synthesis, recruiting osteoclasts, and exerting influences on osteoblasts that lead to osteoclast activation and augmented collagenase synthesis. The effects on bone are implicated in the etiology of postmenopausal osteoporosis, and are antagonized by estrogens. Interactions with other regulators probably account for some seemingly contradictory effects, such as stimulation of collagen and glycosaminoglycan synthesis in osteoblasts. Both IL-1 types also accelerate the synthesis of thromboxanes, cell adhesion molecules, platelet activating factor (PAF), interleukin-6, granulocyte-macrophage colony stimulating factor (GM-CSF), some immunoglobulins, and receptors for epidermal growth factor and complement component C3b; and both can invoke natriuresis. They promote expression of some proto-oncogenes (including *c-fos* and *c-myc*), facilitate blood coagulation, and exert a wide variety of inhibitory influences (for example on albumin and proteoglycan synthesis, and on lipoprotein lipase activity). Some differences between IL-1α and IL-1β influences on neuroendocrine responses to infections and other forms of stress have been described; but both can promote thyroid gland growth, enhance nerve growth factor (NGF) production, and act on both the hypothalamus and adenohypophysis to augment release of corticotropin releasing hormone (CRH), adrenocorticotropic hormone (ACTH), and β-endorphin, all of which dampen immune system responses. IL-1s also inhibit human chorionic gonadotropin (hCG) binding to target cells, hCG-mediated cAMP generation and androgen synthesis, and also $P450_{scc}$ synthesis, actions enhanced by TNFα (although TNFα acting alone is ineffective). IL-1β is additionally reported to suppress insulin-like growth factor-1 (IGF-1) formation in the testis, and to promote the release of thyroid stimulating and growth hormones (TSH and GH), but inhibit thyronine binding globulin and transthyretin synthesis. In the hypothalamus, the cytokines decrease gonadotropin releasing hormone (GnRH) pulse frequency, and thereby rapidly lower luteinizing hormone (LH) levels, but do not affect follicle stimulating hormone (FSH) pulses, and can augment FSH pulse amplitude. In olfactory bulbs, they modulate sensory inputs, in hippocampus they affect memory, and in other brain regions they invoke slow-wave sleep. Nerve growth factor (NGF) induces ILα in peripheral neurons, and the cytokine, in turn can induce substance P in sympathetic ganglion Schwann cells, and promote glial cell proliferation. It is released from noradrenergic sympathetic and adrenomedullary cells in response to acetylcholine.

interleukin-2: IL-2; T cell growth factor-1; thymocyte dependent growth factor-1; TCGF-1; thymocyte stimulating factor; 15-30K cytokines secreted by a subset of activated helper type T lymphocytes (T_{H1}, but not T_{H2} subtypes). Older terms include killer cell helper factor (KHF) and thymocyte mitogenic factor (TMF). Interleukin-1 (IL-1) is a major stimulant for expression of IL-2 receptors, as well a for IL-2 production by cells exposed to antigens and major histocompatibility complex (MHC) proteins. Production of IL-2 initiated by CD2 and the CD3 T lymphocyte receptor complex requires the activity of CD45 (a tyrosine phosphatase; *see* also **interleukin-1**), and signal transduction has been linked with activation of *ras* proteins. The high affinity IL-2 receptors are dimers, composed of p70 α, and p55 β subunits, associated with ICAM-1 and other proteins. (The β subunits are recognized by anti-Tac antibodies). Each of the uncombined subunit types can independently bind IL-2s, but with low affinity. IL-2 augments the activities of antigen-primed cytotoxic and helper type T lymphocytes and promotes their proliferation, an effect that requires the presence of prolactin within the nuclei. It also enhances the activities of some natural killer cells, stimulates synthesis of interferon γ (INFγ) and granulocyte-macrophage colony stimulating factor (GM-CSF), with which it synergizes, and can promote fluid retention. It induces ICAM-I expression in mast cells and monocytic macrophages, and may thereby contribute to their accumulation at sites of inflammation, and to other processes that require cell:cell adhesion (but does not affect ICAM expression in basophilic leukocytes or fibroblasts). Picomolar concentrations (which may originate in resident lymphocytes) act directly on adenohypophysial cells to augment the release of prolactin, adrenocorticotropin (ACTH), and thyroid stimulating hormone (TSH), and to inhibit the release of luteinizing, follicle stimulating, and growth hormones (LH, FSH, and GH). Glucocorticoids are major inhibitors of IL-2 secretion, and are probably components of feedback control loops (since ACTH augments glucocorticoid secretion). A transglutaminase promotes IL-2 dimerization, and appears to convert it to a cytokine that attacks oligodendrocytes. The enzyme may thereby facilitate nerve regeneration (since oligodendrocytes inhibit nerve growth).

interleukin-3: IL-3; multilineage colony stimulating factor, multi-CSF; hemopoietic growth factor-2; mast cell growth factor-1, MCGF-1; megakaryocyte cell stimulating factor, MK-CSF; P cell stimulating factor, persisting cell stimulating factor, PCGF; burst promoting activity, BP; 14-28K lymphokines secreted by activated T_{H2} and some other T lymphocytes that are identical with several regulators known as colony-forming unit (CFU) stimulants. They promote proliferation and differentiation of hematopoietic stem cells and their progeny (neutrophils, eosinophils, lymphocytes, mast cells, megakaryocytes, macrophages, and erythrocyte precursors), and may be essential for responses to granulocyte colony and granulocyte-macrophage colony stimulating factors (G-CSF and GM-CSF). They also stimulate spleen growth and reticulocytosis, induce 20α-hydroxysteroid dehydrogenase in some of the spleen cells (and augment its activity in T cells), and increase the numbers of blood platelets. Some actions, including influences on the growth of myelogenous leukemia cells, have been linked with increased *c-fos* and *c-myc* expression. IL-3s additionally promote histamine release, and induce some T lymphocyte antigens.

interleukin-4: IL-4; B cell growth factor I, BCGF-I; B cell stimulating factor-I, BSF-1; B cell differentiating factors 1, γ and ε (BCDF-1, BCDFγ and BCDFε); IgGI induction factor; T cell growth factor-2, TCGF-2; mast cell growth factor-2, MCGF-2; macrophage fusion factor; MFF; several approximately 20K T cell cytokines secreted by a subset of activated helper type T lymphocytes (T$_{H2}$, but not T$_{H1}$ subtypes), basophilic leukocytes, and some spleen and bone marrow cells. The major forms in humans and mice have 153 and 141 amino acids, respectively. IL-1 stimulates IL-4 production, but IL-4 itself is the major factor for promoting T$_{H2}$ subset differentiation and acquisition of the abilities to produce interleukins 5, 9, and 10, as well as additional interleukin-4. The other interleukins, in turn, affect T$_{H2}$ functions. IL-4 interacts with them as a costimulant for differentiation, proliferation, and activation of B lymphocytes, and for accelerating immunoglobulin class switching (from IgG1 to IgE). The lymphokines also potentiate lipopolysaccharide influences on switching from IgM, IgG3 and IgG2b to IgG1 and IgA, promote differentiation of thymocytes, and appear to facilitate formation of T lymphocytes types with γδ receptors. Additionally, IL-4 supports differentiation of the precursors of B lymphocyte, erythroid, and mast cells, and acts in conjunction with antigens to promote proliferation of the mature types; and it augments the activities of peripheral blood lymphocytes. In macrophages, it stimulates phagocytic activity and the expression of class I and class II major histocompatibility complex antigens. IL-4 deficiency seriously impairs production of IgG1 type immunoglobulins, and can totally block IgE formation. Reported effects of IL-4 on macrophage fusion have been linked with roles in granuloma formation. In mast cells, it heightens cytotoxicity. Although several effects are enhanced by IL-5, IL-4 is required for IL-5 release in response to some parasites. The genes coding for IL-4 are similar to those for granulocyte-macrophage colony stimulating factor. The activities may be controlled in part by shedding of IL-4 receptors.

interleukin-5: IL-5; B cell growth factor-2, BCGF-2, BCGF-II; IgA enhancing factor; high molecular weight (50-60K) lymphokines, formerly known as T cell replacing factor (TRF-I), eosinophil differentiation factor (EDF), and eosinophil colony stimulating factor (Eo-CSF). Human and mouse types have 112 and 111 amino acid moieties, respectively. IL-5 is made mostly by T$_{H2}$ cells. It stimulates growth and differentiation of T lymphocytes, B lymphocytes and eosinophils, enhances IgA production, and induces IgE and CD23 (FCRII). Interleukin-4 is essential for supporting its roles in parasite killing and in delayed hypersensitivity responses.

interleukin-6: IL-6; interferon β$_2$; IFNβ$_2$; B cell stimulating factor-2, BSF-2, BSF II; B cell differentiating factor-2, BCDF-2, BCDF-II; hybridoma growth factor; hybridoma/plasmacytoma growth factor, HPGF; hepatocyte stimulating factor, HSF; T cell activating factor, TAF; cytolytic T cell differentiating factor; macrophage-granulocyte inducer-2, MGI-2; 21-26K peptides made by fibroblasts, bone marrow stromal cells, T lymphocytes, macrophages and keratinocytes, and also by astrocytes and endothelial, pituitary, some tumor, and some other cell types. Especially high concentrations are present in the zona glomerulosa of the adrenal cortex, in synovial fluids of some patients with rheumatoid arthritis, and in conditioned media from several kinds of cancer cells. A human type with 184 amino acid moieties has been identified. Potent stimuli for IL-6 release at several sites include IL-1α, IL-1β, and lipopolysaccharide (endotoxin), which act via protein kinase C, and vasoactive intestinal peptide (VIP) which acts via cAMP. Glucocorticoids inhibit at most of them; but not in the zona glomerulosa (in which IL-6 synthesis is augmented by ACTH and angiotensin II). The three-dimensional structures resemble that of granulocyte colony stimulating factor (G-CSF), and genes coding for the two regulator types are similar. The proteins are also chemically related to oncostatin M and leukocyte inhibitory factor (LIF); and occupied receptors for all of the regulators associate with glycoprotein gp130 in a manner that leads to tyrosine phosphorylation of other proteins. IL-6 contributes to growth and tissue repair. Overexpression stimulates malignant tumor cells, and inhibition of cell:cell adhesion facilitates metastasis. Cardiac myomas, cervical cancers, bladder cancers, and myelomas are among the transformation sites known to produce substantial amounts. Some effects are antagonized by p53, which suppresses IL-6 gene activation. IL-6 acts directly and also synergizes with IL-3 to support growth of hemopoietic stem cells and megakaryocyte maturation, and it promotes terminal differentiation of B lymphocytes and IgG production. It also augments spleen cell responses to concanavalin A, enhances T cell cytotoxicity, elevates blood thymulin levels, stimulates keratinocyte proliferation and the synthesis of acute phase proteins, and augments osteoclastic bone resorption in a manner antagonized by estrogens. IL-6 synthesized in adenohypophysial folliculate-stellate cells may be an important regulator of hormone secretion with special roles during stress and infection. It is a potent stimulant for neurons that secrete corticotropin releasing hormone (CRH), and it thereby slowly elevates adrenocorticotropic hormone (ACTH), β-endorphin, and glucocorticoid levels. It also acts in a concentration-dependent manner to augment the release of luteinizing hormone (LH), prolactin (PRL), and growth hormone. Glucocorticoids, β-endorphin, GH, and PRL are all known to affect immune system responses; and the immune system suppression that follows hypophysectomy can be partially reversed with PRL. Moreover, there is a positive feedback loop in which IL-6 stimulates IL-1 production. Roles in nervous system development have been proposed, since IL-6 acting on its own receptors exerts actions similar to those of nerve growth factor on chromaffin cells.

interleukin-7: IL-7; T cell growth factor; lymphopoietin 1; 25K glycoproteins made by bone marrow and thymus gland epithelial stromal cells that promote proliferation of pre-B cells (B lymphocyte precursors which have not yet expressed cell surface immunoglobulins, but display some surface antigens not found on less mature progenitors). IL-7 is a cofactor for expression of T cell receptor β genes, but it does not stimulate immunoglobulin production or the proliferation of mature B cells. Two types have been identified in the spleen, along with two kinds of receptors, one of which is secreted. One receptor type shows homology with prolactin receptors. Ligand binding leads to tyrosine phosphorylation of several cytosolic proteins. IL-7 appears to be important for supporting the growth of thymocytes, and is especially effective for $CD4^-8^-$ cells. It also activates resting T lymphocytes via an IL-2-independent mechanism, promotes IL-2 synthesis, synergizes with other T cell stimulants, and functions as a competence factor that induces responsivity to IL-2 and IL-4.

interleukin 8: IL-8; neutrophilin; neutrophil activating peptide, NAP; neutrophil-activating factor, NAF; monocyte-derived neutrophil chemotactic factor, MDCNF; leukocyte adhesion inhibitor, LAI; a 72-amino acid, heat and acid stable peptide initially described as a regulator made by activated T cells and monocytes that is chemotactic for, and activates neutrophilic leukocytes, and promotes lymphocyte accumulation at sites of injury. It is almost identical with a peptide released by cytokine activated endothelial cells, and it shares the ability to oppose endothelial leukocyte adhesion molecule-1 (ELAM-1)-mediated adhesion of neutrophilic leukocytes to blood vessel walls, decrease leukocyte extravasation to sites of inflammation, and protect blood vessels walls against inflammation-associated injury and its potential consequences (such as septic shock).

interleukin 9: IL-9; mast cell growth enhancing activity, MEA; T cell growth factor III, TCGF-III; P40; a cytokine made by a subset of helper type T lymphocytes (T_{H2} subtypes) that contributes to the maturation of erythroid and T lymphocyte precursor cells, and can promote antigen-independent proliferation of mature T_H cells.

interleukin 10: IL-10; cytokine synthesis inhibitory factor, CSIF: a 160-amino acid cytokine made by a subset of helper type T lymphocytes that acts on a different helper subset to inhibit formation of messenger RNAs for interferon γ and IL-2. It suppresses macrophage-mediated activation during delayed type hypersensitivity responses, but acts in conjunction with other regulators to promote thymocyte growth and induction of class II histocompatibility antigens. IL-10 also stimulates mast cells, and

may additionally act on natural killer (NK) types. It is induced by Epstein-Barr virus infection and displays 78% homology with the BCRF-1 viral protein (which suppresses host immune system responses by mimicking IL-10 effects on cytokine production).

interleukin 11: IL-11; a 23K, 199 amino acid cytokine made by bone marrow stromal cells, and identified as a factor that promotes proliferation of an IL-6 dependent plasmacytoma cell line. It directly promotes maturation of cells committed to macrophage formation, and enhances megakaryopoiesis and thrombopoiesis. In common with IL-6, it also shortens the times pluripotential hematopoietic precursor cells spend in G_o phases of cell cycles, and synergizes with IL-3 to enhance formation of granulocyte-macrophage colonies. It additionally stimulates T-cell dependent maturation of B lymphocytes that make IgG immunoglobulins.

interleukin 12: cytotoxic lymphocyte maturation factor; CLMF; a 75K glycoprotein made by peripheral B lymphocytes activated by phorbol esters, calcium ionophores, and other stimulants. It is a dimer composed of 40K and 35K subunits, each type encoded by its own gene. IL-12 directly promotes proliferation of cytotoxic T lymphocytes, augments interferon γ (IFNγ) production by "resting" lymphocytes, and synergizes with IL-2 to induce lymphokine activated killer (LAK) cells.

interleukin 13: IL-13; a cytokine that inhibits lipopolysaccharide-stimulated production of inflammatory cytokines by peripheral blood monocytes, synergizes with interleukin-2 to regulate interferon-γ (IFNγ) synthesis by large granular lymphocytes, and promotes B lymphocyte proliferation and expression of CD23. It is synthesized by T lymphocytes that make interleukins 3, 4, and 10, and granulocyte-macrophage colony stimulating factor (T_{H2} subtypes), and may be a multipotent suppressant that protects against excessive inflammatory responses. A recombinant protein decreases the levels of interleukins 1β, 6, and 8, and of tumor necrosis factor-α (TNFα); and it inhibits human immunotropic virus (HIV) replication in macrophages. In humans, IL-13 synthesis is directed by a gene closely linked to the one for interleukin-4, but the protein products have very limited sequence homology. CD28 is an inhibitor. At least some IL-13 is membrane bound, but a heavily glycosylated, 12.4 K form is secreted.

interleukin receptor antagonist: IRAP; 80K intracellular proteins chemically similar to interleukin-1β that bind to IL-1 receptors, and block the actions of both IL-1α and IL-1β. They are induced by endotoxin; but unlike IL-1s, the synthesis is controlled at the level of transcription. One type made by monocytes is believed to protect against overactivity and consequent tissue damage. Another, derived by alternate splicing of the same RNA, has been identified in keratinocytes; and deficiencies have been linked with the development of psoriasis.

intermediary metabolism: chemical reactions for conversion of nutrients and their derivatives to cellular and extracellular components, to forms that release energy, and to waste products.

intermediate density lipoproteins: ILDLs; circulating particles with weights intermediate between those of very low and low density lipoproteins (VLDLs and LDLs), formed when triacylglycerols are released from VLDLs. They contain apoproteins B-100 and E, and are rich in cholesterol esters. Hepatocytes take them up via receptor-mediated endocytosis and convert them to VLDLs. *See* also **lipoproteins**.

intermediate filaments: IFs; at least 30 tough, fibrous, insoluble 40-130K proteins that aggregate to form 7-11 nm diameter strands finer than microtubules, but coarser than microfilaments. By binding to numerous proteins, they support and maintain the morphologies and positions of cell components, regulate nuclear pore functions, and provide mechanisms for communication between nuclei and cell surfaces, and between cell surfaces and extracellular matrix components. The levels of some that persist for long time periods are regulated mostly by factors which affect transcription and messenger RNA stability. Phosphorylation and dephosphorylation promote rapid disassembly and reassembly, respectively, of other types. Acetylation, and possibly also glycosylation are additional forms of posttranslational control. The sizes, amino acid compositions, and functions vary with the cell types; but all IFs are polypeptide ropes that share structurally similar α-helix cores composed (in most types) of domains with similar numbers of amino acids. The genes that direct their synthesis are heterogeneous, but members of a single family. A single IF type can perform more than one function. For example, some laminins form basket-like structures around nuclei, whereas others extend from the nucleus to the plasma membrane. The proteins are classified on the basis of shared *N*- and *C*-terminal amino acid sequences. Type I filaments (keratins made by epithelial cells) are major hair and skin structural proteins. Type II filaments include vimentin (a structural protein of fibroblasts, adipocytes, and other cell types derived from mesoderm), desmin (which forms skeletal muscle scaffolds that hold Z disks and myofilaments in place, and is made in smooth muscle), and glial fibrillary acidic protein (made by astrocytes and Schwann cells). Type III IFs are the neurofilament proteins of axons and dendrites; and Type IV IFs are nuclear lamins. Microorganisms and plants make molecules similar to the vertebrate types.

intermediate filament associated proteins: IFAPs; several classes of proteins that bind to, and affect the functions of intermediate filaments. The group includes spectrin, ankyrin, desmoplakin, internexins, filaggrins, plectin (which may be identical with β-internexin), and some microtubule associated proteins.

intermediate junctions: sites of attachments for adjacent cells, composed mostly of glycoproteins, and often located beneath tight junctions. Some contain mats of fine filaments. They strengthen tissues and permit water passage between cells, but block exchanges of ions and molecules; *cf* **gap junctions**.

intermediate lobe: pars intermedia: PI; a component of the adenohypophysis of many vertebrate species, in which proopiomelanocortin (POMC) is cleaved to α-melanocyte stimulating hormone (α-MSH), corticotropin-like intermediate peptide (CLIP), and endorphins. Unlike pars distalis cells, they have limited blood supplies, receive most of their nutrients via diffusion, and are regulated mostly by neurotransmitters that originate in the hypothalamus. The PI is large in camels, llamas, and other mammals highly resistant to water deprivation. Reptiles, amphibians, and elasmobranch fishes incorporate similar cell types into neurointermediate lobes. A pars intermedia develops in human fetuses, but it degenerates as the hypophysis matures, and only scattered cells persist. The structure never forms in whales, most birds, and other animal types in which the embryonic adenohypophysis does not directly contact the developing neurohypophysis.

intermedins: melanocyte stimulating hormones, made mostly in pars intermedia cells, and neurointermediate lobes.

internalization: translocation of hormones, hormone receptors, hormone-receptor complexes, lipoproteins, ferritin, and other molecules from cell surfaces to cell interiors, via endocytosis. The processes are usually initiated by ligand binding to cell surface receptors (some of which are located in coated pits). Receptosomes then form via fusion of plasma membrane fragments that surround the complexes, and are translocated to the endoplasmic reticulum for subsequent distribution (in many cases to lysosomes). Internalization is used for nutrient acquisition, regulation of receptor numbers (*see* **down regulation**), and translocation of regulators to intracellular target sites.

interneuron: internuncial neuron; a neuron within the central nervous system that receives afferents from one or more others, and conveys messages (via synapses) to two or more different neurons.

internexins: a class of intermediate filament associated proteins. α subtypes are components of neural tissues. β types associate with heat shock proteins and with vimentin networks.

internode: a structure situated between two nodes; *see*, for example **nodes of Ranvier**.

internuncial neuron: *see* **interneuron**.

interoceptors: structures that receive sensory inputs from visceral, joint, muscle, or other internal body components; *cf* **exteroceptors**.

interphase: usually, the interval between successive mitotic cell divisions, which includes the G_1 and S phases of the cell cycle; *cf* **interkinesis**.

interrenal glands: usually, endocrine organs of fishes situated between the kidneys that produce adrenocortical type steroid hormones. (*Suprarenal* is used for analogous organs that lie above the kidneys.)

intersex: an individual of a bisexual species that has characteristics intermediate between those of a female and a male. *See also* **pseudohermaphroditism**.

interstitial: located in spaces between organs or other cells (as in interstitial fluid).

interstitial cells: cells located between (or adjacent to) other cell types. The interstitial (Leydig) cells of the testis (located outside the seminiferous tubules) are the major sites for androgen production in males.

interstitial cell stimulating hormone: ICSH: *see* **luteinizing hormone**.

interstitial fluid: fluid that surrounds cells. *See also* **bulk extracellular fluid** and special types, such as **cerebrospinal fluid**, **bone fluid**, and **aqueous humor**.

interstitial ovarian glands: cords or clumps of cells located outside the ovarian follicles of some species that secrete steroid hormones.

interstitiotropes: adenohypophysial cells that secrete luteinizing hormone (interstitial cell stimulating hormone). Most **gonadotropes** (*q.v.*) also secrete follicle stimulating hormone and other regulators.

intervening sequences: *see* **introns**.

intestine: usually (1) the tubular part of the gastrointestinal system that extends from the pylorus of the stomach to the anus, and includes the small intestine (long but narrow in diameter, composed of duodenum, jejunum and ileum) and the large intestine (shorter, but with a larger diameter, composed of cecum, colon, rectum, and anal canal). Both divisions are lined with mucosa, and have submucosa, muscularis, and serosa layers. (2) the **small intestine** (*q.v.*). *See also* **large intestine**, and the component parts of both segments.

intestinal calcium binding proteins: ICaBPs; several proteins made by cells of the small intestine that bind avidly to calcium, and are induced by 1,25-dihydroxycholecalciferol (1,25-dihydroxyvitamin D), including a 7K member of the S 100 family and a 28K form. They are believed to facilitate absorption of dietary calcium by increasing the free Ca^{2+} ion gradient across the plasma membranes, and to protect the cells against accumulation of excessive amounts of free cytoplasmic Ca^{2+}.

intestinal trefoil factor: ITF; *see* **trefoil proteins**.

intima: tunica intima; usually, the innermost layer of an arteriole, artery, venule, or vein, composed of endothelial cells, a basement membrane, and some connective tissue, surrounded by the tunica media. The endothelial cells provide a smooth surface that minimizes mechanical damage to erythrocytes, blocks their egress from the bloodstream, and protects formed elements of blood against exposure to collagen and other connective tissue components.

Intocostrin: a trade name for tubocurarine chloride.

intra-: a prefix meaning within, as in intradermal, intragastric, or intravenous.

intracellular: within a cell; *cf* **extracellular**.

intracrine: describes actions of a regulator made by a cell that are initiated by binding to receptors within (or on the surface of) the same cell. *Cf* **autocrine** and **paracrine**.

intramembranous ossification: bone growth, not preceded by cartilage formation, in the skull, clavicles, and some other parts of the fetal skeleton. Osteoprogenitor cell clusters within fibrous membranes differentiate to osteoblasts, organize into ossification centers, and secrete collagenous matrix which soon becomes mineralized to form trabeculae. The membrane becomes periosteum, the osteoblasts transmodulate to osteocytes, and the trabeculae, which fuse, are invaded by blood vessels that carry osteoclast precursors. Spongy bone forms when endosteum organizes and carves out marrow cavities. Remodeling at some sites replaces it with compact bone. *Cf* **intrachondral ossification**.

intrathecal: usually (1) within the subarachnoid space; (2) within the theca.

intrauterine devices: IUDs; loops, rings, or similar objects inserted into the uterus to prevent fertilization, implantation, and/or the progression of very early pregnancy. They do not block sperm entry or directly kill gametes, but invoke sterile inflammatory reactions and associated production of prostaglandins. PGF2α is a potent stimulant for reproductive tract smooth muscle that can promote expulsion of oocytes and very young conceptuses, and interfere with implantation. IUDs, especially ones that contain and release progestins or copper, can be effective for long time-periods. The drawbacks include pain at the time of insertion and often afterward. In some women, IUDs cause excessive blood loss during menstruation, or bleeding at other ovarian cycle phases; and they may increase the susceptibility to reproductive tract infections. Stiff devices carry the risk for perforation of uterine walls, and soft ones are more likely to by expelled. There are controversies concerning whether IUDs increase the incidence of ectopic pregnancies.

intravital staining: staining of living cells within an organism; *cf* **supravital staining**.

intrinsic clotting pathway: *see* **coagulation**.

intrinsic factor: a 59K glycoprotein secreted by gastric mucosa parietal cells that forms a complex with, and is essential for absorption of vitamin B_{12} (extrinsic factor). A releasing factor in the ileum promotes dissociation of the complex and facilitates active transport of the vitamin. Inadequate production of intrinsic factor is the major cause of vitamin B-12 deficiency. The consequences include pernicious anemia and neurological defects.

intromission: ejaculation of sperm within the female reproductive tract.

introns: intervening sequences; gene or premessenger RNA (hnRNA) segments that do not contribute to mature messenger RNAs, and are therefore not represented in the translation products. Most, but not all eukaryote genes have introns. *See also* **split genes**, and *cf* **exons**.

intussception: usually (1) growth that takes place within established tissue, via enlargement and division of pre-existing cells, and/or formation of additional extracellular matrix. It occurs, for example in newly forming cartilage; *cf* **apposition**; (2) invasion of one structure by another, such as invagination of one part of the intestine into a neighboring part.

inulin: approximately 5K edible fructofuranose polysaccharides obtained from Jerusalem artichoke tubers that diffuse very slowly across capillary endothelium, but do not cross the plasma membranes of most cell types. Since they are filtered by renal glomeruli, but are neither reabsorbed nor secreted by nephron tubules, they are used for renal function tests, and as markers for extracellular fluids.

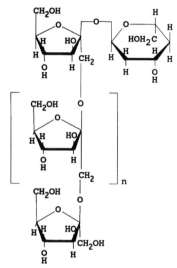

invagination: folding inward; formation of a pocket; a term applied to cell movements during gastrulation.

invasion: (1) movement of one cell type (such as a metastasizing cancer type, or an infecting microorganism) into territory usually occupied by another.

inversion: (1) in molecular biology, cleavage, rotation, and reinsertion of a DNA segment; (2) turning inward; (3) change to an upside down, or inside out arrangement.

invertase: invertin; an old term for sucrase (whose action changes the optical rotation of the solution). The products (glucose + fructose) are collectively called invert sugar.

invertebrate: describes metazoic animals that never acquire a vertebral column. The term is sometimes applied to Urochordates and Hemichordates, but is more commonly used for arthropods, molluscs, worms, and other animal types that do not form a notochord.

inverted repeat: IR; two copies of the same DNA sequence oriented in opposite directions within the same molecule. They occur on opposite ends of transposons; *see* also **palindromes**.

in vitro: occurring outside the body, for example in a test tube or cell culture. Since they are simpler than *in vivo* types, and are more easily controlled, *in vitro* systems are preferred to study enzyme properties, define metabolic pathways, determine the specific cell types of a complex tissue that engage in a function, or examine the effects of specific regulators and other environmental factors. Agents too toxic for whole animals can be administered, and some problems, such as the influences of substances released from other cell types, can be averted. The information obtained does not always agree with data obtained *in vivo*, since most systems do not provide truly physiological environments or the usual interactions with other body components.

in vitro **fertilization**: IVF; fertilization of oocytes outside the female body. The techniques are used to achieve pregnancy in women with obstructed Fallopian tubes (*see* **GIFT**), acquire zygotes with desired genetic characteristics for experimental purposes, and study early embryo development. Young embryos can be nurtured in surrogate mothers, in some cases when a women who donates the oocytes cannot support a pregnancy, but more commonly to increase the populations of rare and endangered species, or expensive animal breeds. The recipients are usually farm animals for larger types, and laboratory species for smaller ones.

in vivo: occurring within the living body; *cf in vitro*.

involucrin: a specialized fibrous membrane protein made by terminally differentiated squamous epithelial cells. In skin it appears first in the spinous layers, and is the major precursor of cornified epidermis cell envelopes.

involution: (1) progressive degeneration or diminution in size, for example in aging thymus glands, in the uterus after parturition, or in mammary glands when lactation is terminated; (2) turning or rolling inward, a term applied to processes such as cell migrations during gastrulation.

iodalbumin: albumin that contains tyrosine-linked iodine. It displays weak, thyroglobulin-like properties, and can release iodine for use by thyroid glands. Very small amounts circulate in blood.

iodinated thyroglobulin: *see* **thyroglobulin**.

iodinated thyroid hormones: *see* **thyroxine** and **triiodothyronine**.

iodine: I; an element (atomic number 53, atomic weight 129.904). Iodide ion is avidly taken up and concentrated by thyroid gland cells, and is an essential component of thyroxine and triiodothyronine. However, excessive amounts impair thyroid gland functions; *see* also **Lugol's solution**. Smaller amounts are concentrated in respiratory system mucosa; but it is not known if iodides in expectorants are effective because they draw water into cells or, alternatively, act as irritants. Tracer doses of radioactive isotopes with short half-lives (^{131}I, ^{125}I, and ^{123}I) are used to diagnose thyroid gland functions, and larger amounts of [131]I (which release gamma rays) to selectively destroy thyroid tissue in individuals with excessive numbers of functioning follicular cells. (The isotopes do not kill thyroid cancer cells that lack the ability to actively transport the ion.) Radioactive iodine is also incorporated into organic compounds for imaging procedures, and to diagnose hepatic and renal disorders; *see* also **iodopyracet**. Both stable ($^{[127]}$I) and radioactive isotopes are attached to hormones to identify receptors and study hormone-receptor interactions, and to other molecules as markers in metabolic studies. Some preparations of the more common iodine type are used as topical antiseptics. *See* also **thyroglobulin, protein bound iodine, butanol extractable iodine, iodine deficiency goiter**, and **iodine number**.

iodine deficiency goiter: thyroid gland enlargement that develops when an inadequate supply of dietary iodine decreases the synthesis of iodinated thyroid hormones, and thereby diminishes negative feedback control over thyroid stimulating hormone (TSH) secretion. The early effects can be reversed by iodine administration; but chronic deficiency invokes pathological changes that impair the ability to concentrate the ion.

iodine number: a measure of the numbers of unsaturated carbon-carbon bonds in fatty acids and related molecules, based on reactions in which the iodine is incorporated into them.

iodoacetamide: an alkylating reagent used to inhibit cysteine proteases. It binds sulfhydryl groups via reactions of the general type: R-SH + iodoacetamide → R-acetamide + HI.

iodoacetamide   R-acetamide

iodoacetate: a reagent that reacts with imino groups, and converts histidine moieties to carboxymethyl derivatives. It is used to determine the locations of histidyl groups in ribonucleases and other proteins. It also binds to sulfhydryl groups, and inhibits many enzymes, including some used in glycolysis.

iodocasein: casein that contains tyrosine-linked iodine. It has weak, triiodothyronine-like properties.

iodoform: triiodomethane; a topical antiseptic.

iodoproteins: iodinated plasma proteins. Normal thyroid gland follicular cells release small amounts to the bloodstream. The levels are high in many individuals with thyroiditis, nontoxic goiters, and thyroid gland cancers.

iodopsin: visual violet; a chicken cone retinal photoreceptor pigment sensitive to red light, composed of 11-*cis*-retinal bound to an opsin different from blue light sensitive cone, and retinal rod proteins. *See* also **opsins** and **rhodopsin**.

iodopyracet: Diodrast; 3,5-diiodo-4-pyridone; an X-ray contrast agent used for diagnostic procedures. It releases iodine, and can thereby interfere with thyroid function studies.

iodothyronines: iodinated thyroid hormones and their degradation products, including thyroxine (T_4), triiodothyronine (T_3), reverse T_3, diiodothyronines, and monoiodothyronines.

iodotyrosines: tyrosine molecules in which iodine atoms replace one or two of the hydrogen atoms; *see* **monoiodotyrosine** and **diiodotyrosines**. They are iodothyronine degradation products that cannot be directly incorporated into thyroglobulins.

2′-deoxy-5-iodouridine: idoxuridine; IDU; IDUR; IUDR; a very potent thymidine kinase and thymidylate synthetase inhibitor that incorporates into viral and mammalian DNAs and renders them susceptible to breakage. It is effective against *Herpes simplex* keratitis, but viral resistance develops rapidly.

ions: electrically charged particles. Atoms become positively charged cations when they lose electrons, and negatively charged anions when they gain them. They form compounds with electrovalent bonds that dissociate in aqueous solutions. *See* also **zwitterions**.

iodoacetate   1-carboxymethylhistidyl derivative   3-carboxymethylhistidyl derivative

ion channels: pores in cell membranes through which ions diffuse. *See* **potassium**, **sodium**, **calcium** and **chloride channels**, and also **voltage gated** and **receptor operated** types.

ion exchange chromatography: *see* **chromatography**.

ion exchange resins: high molecular weight polymers that selectively take up one kind of ion and release another, for example ones that exchanges Na^+ for H^+ or Ca^{2+}, or Cl^- for OH^- or HCO_3^-. They are used to soften water and to purify some compounds.

ionic bonds: electrovalent bonds formed when anions combine with cations.

ionic coupling: electrical coupling.

ionizing radiation: alpha particles, beta particles, positrons, and gamma rays emitted by radioactive compounds.

ionomycin: a polyether antibiotic made by *Streptomyces conglobatus*, effective against gram negative bacteria. It is a divalent cation ionophore that avidly binds calcium ions at pHs of 7 and higher, and can transfer the ions from aqueous to lipid phases. Since it accelerates cell uptake and redistribution of Ca^{2+}, and thereby affects phospholipases and many other enzymes, it is used to study cell activation. It is a more efficient Ca^{2+} carrier than A23187, but does not fluoresce.

β-ionone: 4-(2,6,6-trimethyl-1-cyclohexen-1-yl)-3-buten-2-one; an intermediate in pathways for biosynthesis of vitamin A and carotenoids in plants.

ionophores: agents that facilitate ion transport across cell membranes. Ionomycin, valinomycin, and amphotericin are lipophilic antibiotics that bind ions and diffuse with them across plasma membrane phospholipid bilayers. Monensin more rapidly traverses intracellular types. Gramicidin dimers form ion channels by inserting into membranes. Other kinds inhibit ATP synthesis or other processes that normally limit the transport. Usually, low concentrations are quite selective for a single ion type (with small effects on others with the same charges and valences), whereas high concentrations affect additional ion types of like charges but different valances. A23187

is selective for Ca^{2+} and Mg^{2+} (with some Mn^{2+}) at low concentrations, but high ones also affect Na^+ and K^+. *See* also **monactin**, **nonactin**, and **nigericin**.

ionophoresis: electrophoresis of small, charged particles.

ion selective electrodes: electrodes with membranes (ideally) permeable to a single kind of ion that are used to measure its concentration in solutions which additionally contain other solutes. Proton permeable glass is used for pH electrodes. Ionphores are embedded in the membranes of other types.

iontophoresis: procedures in which electric currents are used to transfer soluble salts from surfaces to interiors.

iopanoic acid: 3-amino-α-ethyl-2,4,6-triiodobenzenepropanoic acid; a radio-opaque agent used to visualize soft tissues during fluoroscopy and X-ray examinations. It also inhibits deiodinases in liver and thyrotropes that catalyze thyroxine conversion to triiodothyronine.

IPs: (1) inositol phosphates; (2) induced proteins.

IP$_3$: (1) inositol triphosphate, and especially inositol$_{1,4,5}$ triphosphate (IP$_{1,4,5}$); (2) inositol-3-phosphate. *See* **inositol phosphates**.

IP-1: a labile 30-40K protein that associates with Fos and Jun proteins and blocks AP-1 binding to gene regulatory regions. It is inactivated by phosphorylation.

ipecac: an emetine-containing preparation made from *Uragoga ipecacuanha* and some other plants, used as an emetic to promote elimination (by vomiting) of ingested, noncorrosive poisons, and as an amebicide. Small amounts are added to some potentially dangerous therapeutic agents to prevent accidental overdosage. Since it stimulates mucosal exocrine glands, minute amounts are contained in some expectorant cough medicines. Although toxic, larger ones are used by some individuals with bulimia to induce vomiting. *See* **emetine**.

ipratropium bromide: Atrovent; 8-isopropyl-noratropine methobromide; a synthetic anticholinergic alkaloid

ionomycin

378

used to dilate the bronchioles in individuals with obstructive pulmonary diseases and bronchial asthma. It is usually administered as an inhalant. Unlike β-adrenergic agonists, its effects develop slowly and can persist for many hours. It invokes fewer systemic side effects than atropine, in part because it does not cross blood brain barriers.

ipratropium bromide

iprindole: 1-(3-dimethylaminopropyl)-2,3-hexamethyleneindol; a tricyclic antidepressant that does not significantly affect norepinephrine uptake by nerve terminals. Some effects may be related to desensitization of β₂-type adrenergic receptors.

iproniazid: Marsilid; 1-methyl-2-(1-methylethyl)-5-nitro-1-*H*-imidazole; an agent related to, and now replaced by isoniazid for combatting tuberculosis. As a monoamine oxidase inhibitor that acts preferentially on A type enzymes, it was used for a time as an antidepressant, but (because of hepatotoxicity) is no longer available in the United States.

ipsilateral: on the same side; *cf* **contralateral**.

IRBP: intracellular retinol binding protein.

IREs: (1) iron response elements; iron regulatory elements; (2) interferon response elements.

IRE-BPs: iron response element binding proteins.

I region: a component of the mouse major histocompatibility gene complex with functions comparable to those of the human D/DR region.

IRFs: interferon regulatory factors.

IRG[s]: immunoreactive glucagon-like molecules; peptides that bind with high affinities to antibodies directed against glucagon. Some exert actions qualitatively similar to those of glucagon. *See* **glucagon-like immunoreactivity**.

Ir genes: immune response genes.

IRI: insulin, proinsulin, and some insulin degradation products that bind with high affinities to antibodies directed against insulins.

iridophores: leukophores; melatonin-regulated chromatophores in the skins of some fishes and other heterotherms with light-reflecting plates (reflectosomes) composed of white purine pigments. They can interfere with melanophore index bioassays.

iris: the externally visible component of the vascular tunic of the eye that contains the pigments for eye color, and the smooth muscle that controls pupil size. Its margins are attached to the ciliary body. The circular muscle, which decreases pupil size when it contracts, is controlled by acetylcholine released from oculomotor nerve endings. The opposing radial muscle is stimulated by norepinephrine from a branch of the superior cervical ganglion.

IRM: interference reflection microscopy.

IRMA: immunoradiometric assays; sensitive techniques in which monoclonal antibodies linked to solid media such as sephacryl 500f are used to determine the concentrations of macromolecules present in small amounts. The procedures are similar to those described for enzyme-linked immunosorbent (ELISA) assays, but the second antibody is labelled with radioactive atoms.

iron: Fe; an element (atomic number 26, atomic weight 55.847). As an essential component of hemoglobins, myoglobins, catalases, peroxidases, lipoxygenases, aconitase, ferredoxins, cytochrome system components and other biologically active molecules, Fe exerts numerous effects on metabolism and cell growth. Both deficiencies and excesses invoke serious effects (*see* **anemia**, **hemosiderin**, and **free radicals**). For mechanisms that control the levels, *see* **ferritin, transferrin**, and **iron response elements**. [55]Fe and ^{59}Fe are radioactive isotopes with half-lives of 2.7 years and 45 days, respectively.

iron regulatory elements: *see* **iron response elements**.

iron response element[s]: iron regulatory elements; IREs; approximately 28-base nucleotide sequences in untranslated terminal repeat regions (UTRs) of several kinds of messenger RNAs that bind cytoplasmic regulators in a manner affected by prevailing Fe levels. The 5′ UTR of ferritin mRNA contains one IRE, and the 3′ UTR of the ferritin receptor RNA has five. IRE-BP (iron response element binding protein) is a 90K iron-sulfur protein that binds to both messengers, and displays aconitase activity. Fe controls its oxidation-reduction state, and high levels lower its affinity for the response elements. When iron levels are low (and more receptor is needed) IRE-BP binds tightly to the receptor mRNA and protects it against degradation. In contrast, less *ferritin* (which sequesters the metal) is needed when Fe is scarce;

and IRE-BP binding to ferritin mRNA inhibits translation. (IRE-BP is also known as ferritin repressor protein, FRP). When iron levels rise, a "ferritin inducer" relieves the translation inhibition, and also destabilizes ferritin receptor mRNA. Since heme binds to, and can inactivate IRE-BP, it was once believed to be the major inducer. However, inorganic iron is effective in the absence of heme; and heme induces heme oxidase (which degrades heme). Inhibitors of heme oxidase synthesis block the heme effects, and inducers of heme oxidase increase heme effectiveness. It is therefore believed that heme functions, at least in part, as an Fe donor.

iron response element binding protein: IRE-BP; ferritin repressor protein; FRP; *see* **iron response elements**.

irp: a mouse gene essential for embryonic development; *see* **wnt genes**.

irradiation: treatment with, or exposure to photons, neutrons, gamma rays, X-rays, ultraviolet rays, or other forms of radiation.

ischemia: inadequate blood delivery to cells or tissues, caused by blood vessel occlusion or excessive constriction. The consequences include oxygen and nutrient deficiency, and metabolic waste accumulation. The pH falls, the activities of several kinds of degrading enzymes increase, and enzyme release from lysosomes accelerates.

sodium **isethionate**: the sodium salt of hydroxyethylsulfonic acid. It is used to inhibit granule lysis. A chlorinated form affects intracellular Ca^{2+} transport.

ISGs: interferon stimulated genes.

islet-1: *see* **LIM**.

islet activating protein: IAP; *see* **pertussis toxin**.

islet cells: *see* **pancreatic islets**.

islets of Langerhans: *see* **pancreatic islets**.

iso-: a prefix meaning (1) same; (2) an isomeric form.

isoagglutinins: antibodies that clump cells from other individuals of the same species. Some are used for blood typing.

isoagglutinogens: antigens that promote production of isoagglutinins.

isoallele: an allele of a heterozygote that affects the phenotype only in the presence of another specific (usually mutant) allele.

isoalloxazine: the component of flavine nucleotides that reversibly accepts and donates electrons; *see* **FAD**.

isoandrosterone: epiandrosterone.

isoantibodies: antibodies induced by antigens from other individuals of the same species.

1-isobutyl-3-methoxypyrazine: IBMP; an odorant used to study the functions of olfactory neurons. It rapidly elevates cyclic guanosine monophosphate (cGMP) levels.

isobutyl methylxanthine: IBMX; MIX; 1-methyl-isobutylxanthine; an agent used to inhibit cyclic nucleotide phosphodiesterases. It also exerts effects unrelated to cAMP accumulation, for example on intracellular Ca^{2+} transport. *See* also **methyl xanthines**.

isocaproyl aldehyde: the side-chain cleaved from cholesterol during the reaction that yields pregnenolone; *see* **side-chain cleavage**. It is rapidly oxidized to caproic acid.

α-keto-**isocaproate**: an intermediate in the pathway for leucine coversion to acetyl-CoA; *see* **isovaleryl-Co A dehydrogenase**. It stimulates insulin secretion.

isochromatid break: breaks in both sister chromatids at the same loci. It can be followed by lateral fusion that yields one dicentric chromatid plus an acentric fragment.

isochromosome: an abnormal chromosome (usually an X or Y type) that lacks a segment present on its normal counterpart, but has two almost identical arms with base sequences oriented in opposite directions. It is formed during cell division. One possibility is transverse (rather than the usual longitudinal) separation of replicated chromatids, with loss of one arm from each. Another is loss of the short-arm segments from two unreplicated chromatids, followed by fusion of the long arms, loss of centric fragments, and duplication of the fused elements.

isocitrate: an intermediate formed from citrate in the tricarboxylic acid cycle; *see* **isocitric dehydrogenase**. *See* also **glyoxylate cycle**.

$$
\begin{array}{c}
\text{COO}^- \\
| \\
\text{CH}_2 \\
| \\
\text{HC}-\text{COO}^- \\
| \\
\text{HO}-\text{CH} \\
| \\
\text{COO}^-
\end{array}
$$

isocitrate

isocitrate lyase: an enzyme that cleaves isocitrate to succinate + glyoxylate; *see* **glyoxylate cycle**.

isocitric dehydrogenase: an enzyme that catalyzes conversion of isocitrate to α-ketoglutarate. Oxalosuccinate (formed via: isocitrate + $NAD^+ \rightarrow$ oxalosuccinate + $NADH + H^+$) is an intermediate in the pathway that is not released from the enzyme-susbtrate complex. When parathyroid hormone inhibits the enzyme in osteoblasts, citrate accumulates, binds Ca^{2+} released during bone resorption, and contributes to mineral translocation to extracellular fluids.

isocoding mutations: point mutations that do not alter the amino acid specificities of the codons. (For example, subsitution of an AAG triplet for AAA changes the messenger RNA codon from UUU to UUG; but both UUU and UUG base pair with the phenylalanine transfer RNA anticodon.)

isoelectric focusing: sensitive electrophoresis techniques in which compounds maintained at stable pHs are separated on the basis of differences in isoelectric points. They can be used in combination with other separation procedures.

isoelectric point: the pH at which a particle (usually a protein molecule) does not move in an electrical field because its net electrical charge is zero.

isoenzymes: isozymes.

isoforms: hormones, enzymes, structural proteins, or other molecules that perform similar functions, and resemble each other sufficiently to be included in a family (or subfamily), but differ in chemical make-up. Some are products of separate, but similar genes. Other variations arise posttranslationally.

isogametic: producing male and female gametes of similar size, shape, and motility. Some simple plants are isogametic.

isogamy: reproduction that involves the fusion of gametes of similar size, shape, and motility; *cf* **heterogamy**.

isogeneic: describes a graft from a donor that is genetically identical to the host (or from another part of the same individual).

isogenic: describes tissue from the same individual, an identical sibling, or another member of the same highly inbred strain which is genetically identical or differs only in characteristics related to sex chromosomes.

isografts: isogeneic (isologous) grafts.

isoguvacine: 1,4,5,6-tetrahydronicotinic acid; a $GABA_A$ receptor agonist, pharmacologically similar to gabacuculline.

isohemagglutinins: antibodies that clump cells of genetically different members of same species (for example, anti-B types in type A blood plasma that agglutinate type B erythrocytes).

isohemolysins: naturally occurring antibodies that destroy erythrocyte membranes when they bind surface antigens on the cells of genetically different members of the same species.

isolabeling: the appearance, during metaphase II of meiosis, of a radioactive marker on both sister chromatids, when tritiated thymidine is administered during the S phase of the cell cycle. It is attributed to crossing over during synapsis. (Commonly, both chromatids are labeled at metaphase I, but just one at metaphase II.)

isolecithal: describes oocytes or eggs in which the yolk is evenly distributed; *cf* **telolecithal**.

isoleucine: Ile; I; 2-amino-3-methyl isovaleric acid; a neutral, essential amino acid that stimulates insulin secretion, and is a component of most proteins. It can be made from threonine, and is metabolized to succinyl coenzyme A, α-keto-isocaproate, and acetyl-coenzyme A.

$$
\begin{array}{c}
\text{COOH} \\
| \\
\text{H}_2\text{N}-\text{CH} \\
| \\
\text{HC}-\text{CH}_3 \\
| \\
\text{CH}_2-\text{CH}_3
\end{array}
$$

isoleucyl-seryl-bradykinin: a T-kinin; *see* **kallikreins**.

isologous: isogeneic; isogenic; homologous.

isomers: chemical compounds with the same overall molecular compositions, but different arrangements of the atoms (usually around asymmetric carbons); *see also* **stereoisomerism**. Some isomers of naturally occurring compounds are used as antimetabolites; *see*, for example **isoriboflavin** and **isonicotinic acid**.

isomerase: an enzyme that catalyzes conversion of a compound to one of its isomers. See, for example **phospohexoseisomerase**. *Cf* **mutase**, and *see* also **anomerase**.

isometric contraction: building up of muscle tension with no change in muscle length. It is used to maintain posture, and to lift weights; *cf* **isotonic contraction**.

isomorphic: having the same form.

isoniazid: 4-pyridinecarboxylic acid hydrazide; isonicotinic acid hydrazide; an agent that inhibits several enzymes, and is especially effective against ones that catalyze elongation of long-chain fatty acids. It kills some microorganisms, and is used to combat tuberculosis infections, but can invoke peripheral neuritis, hematological disorders, arthritis, liver damage, impaired mental functions, and other problems. Host toxicity is partially counteracted with pyridoxine.

isonicotinic acid: pyridine-4-carboxylic acid; an antimetabolite that blocks nicotinic acid dependent reactions, usually used as the hydrazide (*see* **isoniazid**).

isoncotic: exerting the same **oncotic pressure** (*q.v.*).

isoosmotic: isosmotic; exerting the same osmotic pressure; *cf* **isotonic**.

isonipecotic acid: 4-piperidine carboxylic acid; an anticonvulsant GABA receptor agonist.

isopentyl pyrophosphate: an intermediate in the pathway for biosynthesis of farnesyl pyrophosphate, squalene, cholesterol, and chemically related compounds. Mevalonate is converted in two steps to 5-pyrophosphate-mevalonate, and the product reacts with ATP to yield isopentyl pyrophosphate + ADP + Pi + CO_2. The next step is conversion of isopentyl pyrophosphate to dimethylallyl pyrophosphate.

isophan: similar in appearance; *see* **phenocopy**.

Isophane insulin: NPH (neutral protamine Hagedorn) insulin; an intermediate-acting suspension of insulin, protamine sulfate, zinc, and buffers, used to treat diabetes mellitus.

isopotential: having the same (1) electrical charge; (2) potential force or energy; (3) ability to do work.

isoprenaline: isoproterenol.

isoprene: 2-methylbuta-1,3,-diene; a hydrocarbon building block for the biosynthesis of mevalonate and compounds derived from it (including terpenes, cholesterol,

dolichols, ubiquinones, and chlorophyll). *See also* **isoprenylation**.

isoprenylation: posttranslational formation of thioester bonds between isoprene moieties and cysteines (usually located in the fourth positions of protein *C*-termini). The hydrocarbon can derive from farnesyl, hydroxyfarnesyl, geranylgeranyl, dolichol, isopentyladenine, or other precursors. Molecules processed in this way include *ras*-related GTP-binding proteins, some cytoplasmic and nuclear matrix types, G protein γ subunits, lamins, and some fungus pheromones. The processes precede, and are essential for subsequent additional modifications (such as peptide bond cleavage, carboxymethylation, phosphorylation, palmitoylation, or myristoylation), and for achieving correct orientations of some plasma membrane proteins, and/or mediating their regulated release. They also facilitate tight binding of lamins to nuclear membranes and matrices, and may contribute to interactions between cytosolic proteins and endoplasmic reticulum receptors. Roles in signal transduction, cell growth, and maintenance of cell shape, and influences on transformation have been proposed. Specific enzymes are involved, and some inhibitors selectively suppress tumor growth.

isoproterenol: isoprenaline; isopropylarterenol; Isuprel; 3,4-dihydroxy-α-[(isopropylamino)methyl]benzyl alcohol; a nonselective β-type adrenergic receptor agonist that acts on both $β_1$ and $β_2$ subtypes. It is an epinephrine analog, used to study adrenergic functions, and clinically as a bronchodilator and cardiac stimulant. Its effects in laboratory animals include stimulation of melatonin synthesis.

Isoptin: a trade name for verapamil.

isopycnic: isopyknic; having the same density; *see also* **centrifugation**.

isopyrin: 4-isopropylaminoantipyrine; an agent used for its analgesic, antipyretic, and anti-inflammatory properties.

isorenins: proteolytic enzymes that cleave angiotensin-I from renin substrates, but differ from "true" renins in molecular weights and pH optima. They are made in brain, uterus, and adrenal glands, and elsewhere; and large amounts accumulate in the salivary glands of some rodents.

isoriboflavin: 8-dimethyl-6-methyl-riboflavin; an antimetabolite used to invoke riboflavin deficiency in laboratory animals.

isoschizomers: pairs of restriction enzymes that recognize the same nucleic acid base sequences, but cleave the molecules at different sites. Pairs with just one member that acts on methylated sequences are used to study the effects of DNA methylation on gene expression.

isosexual: having characteristics of the same gender.

isosexual precocity: precocious puberty in which development follows normal patterns (consistent with the sex chromosome types), but occurs earlier than usual. Gonadotropin-secreting tumors are the most common causes.

isothermal: describes reactions that proceed at constant temperatures.

isothiocyanates: compounds in mustard oils, some glycosides, and other naturally occurring substances with the general formula: R—N=C=S. They are metabolized to thiocyanates which affect thyroid gland functions.

isotocin: ichthyotocin; IT; a neurohypophysial peptide made by some bony fishes, chemically and biologically related to oxytocin, but only two-thirds as potent for promoting milk ejection in mammals, and one third for stimulating uterine contraction. It lacks significant antidiuretic activity.

isotonic: describes solutions that do not promote net transfers of water into or out of cells. They are not necessarily isosmotic with cytoplasmic constituents, since molecules or ions that penetrate plasma membranes can draw water into cells. Cf **hypertonic** and **hypotonic**.

isotonic contraction: muscle contraction in which constant tension is maintained during shortening, used to move bones and contract the diaphragm; cf **isometric contraction**.

isotopes: elements with the same atomic numbers but different atomic weights (equal numbers of protons and electrons, but different numbers of neutrons). Usually, the form that predominates is assumed if no weight for the element (or its compounds) is given. [1]H is the most prevalent form of hydrogen, [2]H (deuterium) is a stable isotope, and [3]H (tritium) is radioactive. The less common isotopes are used as markers in metabolic and physiological studies. When differences in neutron numbers account for only relatively small differences in atomic sizes, all forms of the element display almost identical chemical properties.

isotopic dilution analysis: methods for determining the concentrations of substances present in small amounts in mixtures. A known quantity of the compound labelled with a radioactive isotope of predetermined activity is added. The labeled and unlabled compound are extracted together, and the change in specific activity is measured.

isotretinoin: Accutane; the 13-*cis* isomer of retinoic acid. It inhibits sebaceous gland activity, and is used to treat psoriasis, some forms of acne, and some other skin diseases. However, it is toxic and can cause fetal defects if used by pregnant women.

isotropic: describes entities that refract, transmit or reflect light to the same extent in all directions, or environments with properties that are the same at all points; cf **anisotropic**.

isotype: (1) an antigenic determinant shared by all members of a species, but not made by other species; cf **idiotype** and **allotype**; (2) a common feature shared by a group of macromolecules (for example by members of an immunoglobulin subclass).

isotype switching: a change in the class or subclass of immunoglobulins made by a B lymphocyte, for example from an IgM to an IgG.

isovaleric acid: delphinic acid; 3-methylbutanoic acid;; *see* **isovalericacidemia**.

isovalericacidemia: Sidbury syndrome; an autosomal recessive disorder in which impaired ability to make isovaleryl-CoA dehydrogenase leads to accumulation of

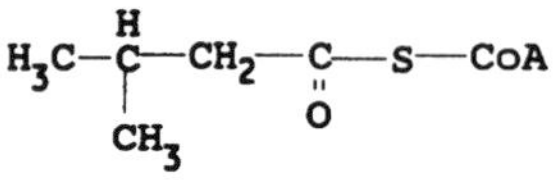

isovaleryl-CoA

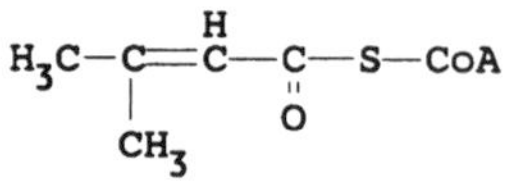

β-methylcrotonyl-CoA

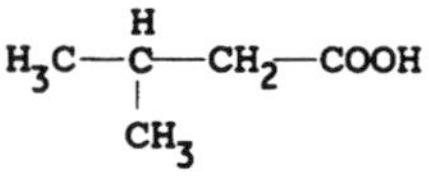

isovaleric acid

isovaleric acid. The manifestations include psychomotor retardation and an objectionable body odor. It occurs in some infants who subsequently develop normally, and can often be alleviated with exogenous biotin (a co-factor for the enzyme) or glycine (which conjugates with and thereby accelerate isovaleric acid excretion).

isovaleryl-CoA dehydrogenase: a biotin-dependent flavoprotein enzyme that catalyzes an essential step in pathways for leucine degradation to acetoacetic acid + coenzyme A. The amino acid is first converted to α-keto-isocaproate, and its product is decarboxylated in the presence of coenzyme A to isovaleryl-CoA. The dehydrogenase then catalyzes formation β-methylcrotonyl-CoA + $2H^+$. *See* also **isovalericacidemia**.

isoxazole: an agent used to inhibit 3ß-hydroxysteroid dehydrogenases.

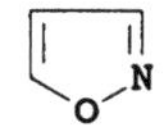

isoxazolyl penicillins: cloxacillin, oxacillin, and other semi-synthetic penicillin derivatives with isoxazole sidechains. They resist degradation by penicillinases, but retain antibiotic potencies similar to those of the parent compounds.

isoxsuprine hydrochloride: 1-(*p*-hydroxyphenyl)-2-(1-methyl-2-phenoxyethylamino)-1-propanol; a β-type adrenergic receptor agonist, used as a vasodilator.

isozymes, isoenzymes: two or more forms of an enzyme that differ somewhat in chemical composition but catalyze the same kinds of reactions. They can differ in substrate affinities and specificities, and distributions within the organism. One can preferentially accelerate a reaction to the right, and the other drive it to the left by tightly binding the product. In some cases, each form is encoded by a separate gene. In others, differential RNA splicing and/or posttranslational processing account for the variations. Mechanisms for controlling the synthesis, processing, activation, and/or degradation of one type may not affect the other. *See*, for example **lactate dehydrogenases**, **kinase C isoforms**, and **pyruvate kinases**.

isradipine: 4-(4-benzofurazanyl)-1,4-dihdyro-2,6-dimethyl-3,5-pyridinecarboxylic acid methyl, isopropyl ester;

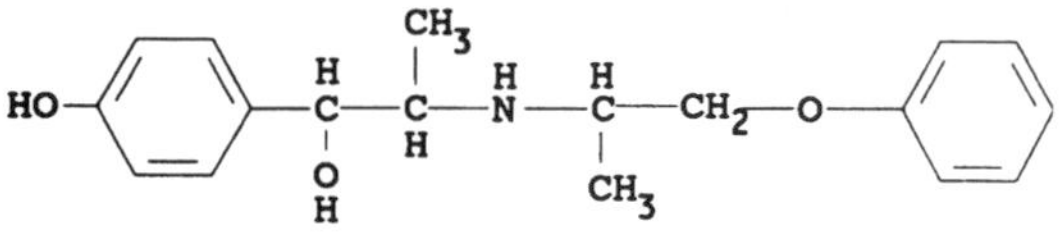

isoxsuprine hydrochloride

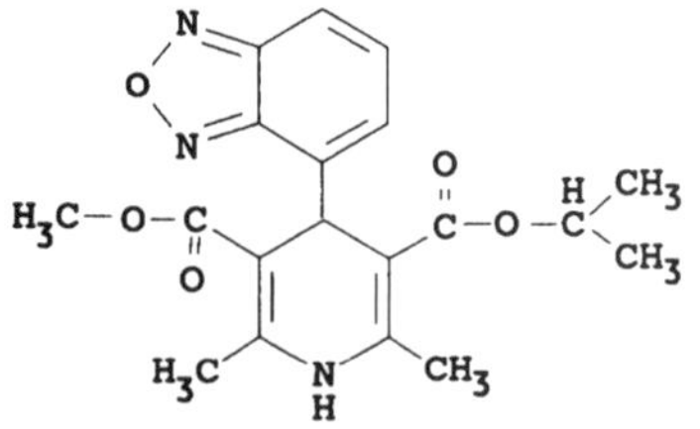

isradipine

a dihydropyridine type Ca^{2+} channel blocker, used to treat angina pectoris and hypertension.

ISRFs: interferon stimulated response factors.

isthmus: (1) a narrow strip of tissue that connects two larger structures (which can be parts of the same organ, as in thyroid glands); (2) a short, narrow passage or constriction between two wider regions of a canal; *see* **Fallopian tubes**.

ITF: intestinal trefoil factors; *see* **trefoil proteins**.

ITP: inosine triphosphate.

ITYA: 5,8,11,14-eicosatetraenoic acid.

IUD: intrauterine device.

IV: intravenously.

i value: the total concentration of DNA termini in a ligation system. It varies with the DNA concentration, and affects the kinds of recombinant molecules formed. *See* also **j value**.

ivermectin: 22,23-dihydroavermectin B_1; a mixture composed mostly of ivermectin B_{1a}, with lesser amounts of ivermectin B_2. The compounds are broad-spectrum antiparasitic agents prepared from avermectins made by *Streptomyces avermitilis*, and used as antihelminths, ascaricides, and insecticides. They act on GABA-mediated interneuon and neuromuscular synapses, and some effects are attributed to $GABA_A$ receptor binding. However, hyperpolarization at other sites involves influences on different kinds of chloride channels. In the structure shown, R = —C_2H_5 for the B1a type, and —CH_3 for the B_{1b}.

ivermectin

IVF: *in vitro* fertilization.

ixodin: a hirudin-like anticoagulant, obtained from *Ixodes ricinus*, *Acari*, and other blood-sucking ticks. It inhibits thrombokinases.

J

J: joule.

JA: jasmonic acid.

jacalin: a lectin of the Jackfruit, *Arotcarpus integrifolia* that specifically binds IgA type immunoglobulins, and is used to separate them from other plasma proteins.

jackbean: a tropical leguminous plant, *Canavalia ensiformis*. It is a major source of concanavalin A, and of urease and some other enzymes.

Jacobson's organ: vomeronasal organ; a chemoreceptor organ that in many primate and some other species comprises several small sacs with pores which open into the nasal or oral cavity and make functional connections with the accessory olfactory tracts, hypothalamus and other components of the limbic system. It senses low volatility pheromones that are sniffed or ingested, but does not mediate conscious perception of odors.

JAK kinases: Janus kinases; several tyrosine kinases that promote dimerization of, bind to, and mediate signal transduction for erythropoietin, growth hormone, prolactin, G-CSF, GM-CSF, interleukins 2, 3, 4, 5, and 6, and other cytokine family receptors.

Janus green B: 3-(dimethylamino)-7-[[4-(dimethylamino)phenyl]azo-5-phenylphenazinium chloride; a dye used to stain cell nuclei.

JAR cells: a choriocarcinoma cell line obtained from human placental tissue that makes large amounts of human chorionic gonadotropin (hCG).

jasmolins: pyrethrum flower compounds used as insecticides; *see* **pyrethrins I and II**.

jasmone: 3-methyl-2-(2-pentenyl)-2-cyclopentene-1-one; a volatile jasmine flower component, used in perfumes.

jasmonic acid: a plant hormone synthesized via a lipoxygenase catalyzed reaction that converts α-linolenic acid to 13(*S*)-hydroperoxy-linolenic acid, followed by a second in which the product is made into the direct

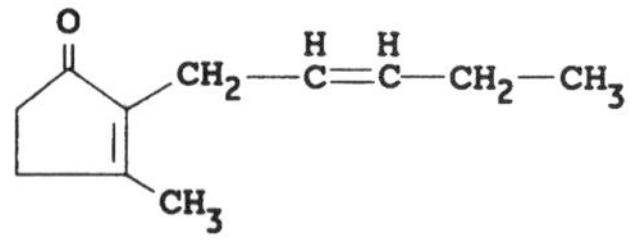

jasmone

precursor, 12-oxo-phytodienoic acid. Positive feedback control over the biosynthesis has been suggested, since the linolenic acid metabolite induces a lipoxygenase. Epijasmonic acid (the + isomer) acts directly, and also after conversion to methyl-jasmonic acid (Me-JA), which is volatile and also biologically active. The effects exerted under normal conditions include acceleration of leaf senescence, stomatal closure, and induction of ethylene and several proteins. Gene expression is constitutive; but much larger amounts of the hormones are made in response to mechanical injury and insect feeding. JA is a component of **systemic acquired resistance** responses (*q.v.*) that contribute to induction of protease inhibitors I and II and other pathogen related proteins.

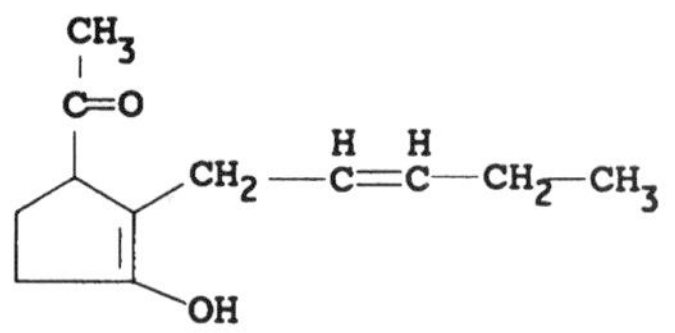

jaundice: conditions caused by biliary obstruction, hepatocellular dysfunction, and hemolytic diseases, in which bilirubin accumulates and deposits in the integument, sclera, and other structures, and imparts a yellow tinge.

J chains: 17.6K glycoproteins that link IgA and IgM immunoglobulin monomers near the Fc ends of their heavy chains, via disulfide bonds. They are synthesized by activated B lymphocytes, and contribute to immunoglobulin production and secretion. Three isoforms that differ in carbohydrate content have been identified. (J chains differ from J segments, whose synthesis is directed by other genes.)

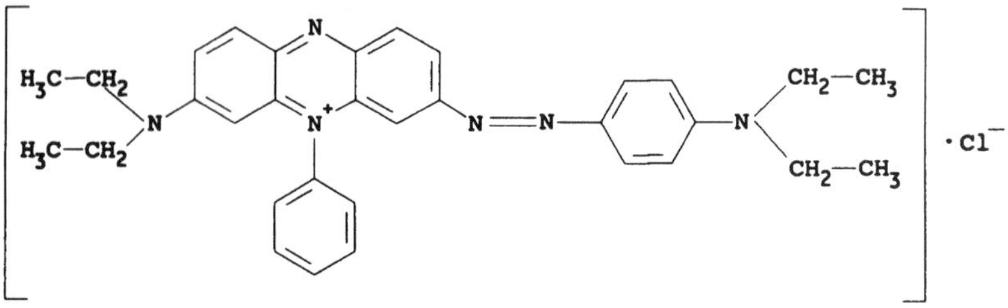

Janus green B

JEG-3 cells: a human choriocarcinoma cell line used to study the synthesis of pregnancy-associated proteins.

Jerusalem artichoke: the edible, carbohydrate-rich subterranean *Helianthus tuberosus* tuber. It is used as a source of inulin.

J gene segments: Five sets of DNA segments, arranged in tandem on genes that direct immunoglobulin synthesis. They code for 12-21 amino acid components of light and heavy chain hypervariable regions, and of T cell receptor α and β chains. *Cf* **J chains**.

J1 glycoprotein: tenascin.

jejunum: the proximal two-fifths of the small intestine, located between the duodenum and the ileum. The cells secrete enterokinase and express aminopeptidases and dipeptidases on their surfaces which act on the digestion products produced by pancreatic juice enzymes. The villi are generally larger and more vascularized than those of the ileum, and are major sites for bile salt dependent lipid absorption. The cells also absorb much of the dietary sugar, amino acids, and Na^+, K^+, and HCO_3^- ions, but are less important for Cl^- and Ca^{2+} than those of the ileum. Substantial amounts of water are taken up with the ions (but *see* **colon**).

jet lag: transient discomfort associated with rapid travel across east-west time zones, attributed to desynchronization of glucocorticoid, melatonin, and other circadian rhythms.

JG22E: an antibody used to detect CSAT (chicken embryo fibroblast cell surface protein).

JGA: juxtaglomerular apparatus.

JG cells: juxtaglomerular cells.

JH: juvenile hormone.

Jimson weed: *see* **strophanthin**.

1-deoxynor-**jirimycin**: dideoxynor-jirimycin: 1,5-dideoxy-1,5-imino-D-glucitol: an agent used to inhibit Golgi enzymes that process oligosaccharides with *N*-linked asparagine moieties, and to slow formation of oligosaccharides. It acts specifically on asparagine-mannose bonds. An *N*-methyl analog affects asparagine-glucose linkages.

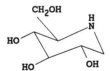

JOD: juvenile onset **diabetes mellitus** (*q.v.*).

JODY: junenile onset **diabetes mellitus** (*q.v.*) in the young.

joints: articulations; structures that connect one bone to another. One classification system is based on the major components (*see* **synostoses, synchondroses, syndesmoses**), and another on the kinds of movement (*see* **synarthroses, amphiarthroses**, and **diarthroses**). Restrictions on movements permitted by synovial joints (diarthroses) are imposed by the shapes of the bone ends, and by ligaments and other structures. Various terms (such as ball and socket, and ellipsoid) refer to the bone shapes, and others (for example monaxial and biaxial) to the numbers of planes in which movement is supported. *See* also **arthritis**.

joule, J: (1) a unit of energy equivalent to one watt-second, one volt-coulomb, 1/4.184 calories, or 10^7 ergs; (2) the heat generated by 1 ampere flowing against a resistance of 1 ohm for one second; (3) the amount of energy required to apply a 1 newton force over a distance of one meter.

J receptor: a receptor type in the lungs (named for its juxtacapillary location) that contributes to Hering Breuer reflexes. It senses deflation, and is also affected by pulmonary congestion. When stimulated, it promotes shallow, rapid breathing.

JTC-12.P3 cells: a monkey kidney cell line.

jumping genes: mobile genetic entities; *see* **transposons**.

jun: genes that code for a set nuclear proteins whose common *C*-terminal domains mediate noncovalent bonding to c-fos and related proteins to form AP-1 transcription factor dimers. Leucine zipper domains of the *C*-terminal regions, homologous to those of proteins encoded by *c-fos, c-myc, c-ros, gro-1, CEBP*, and *GCNA*, mediate dimer binding to TGACTCA and closely related DNA base sequences in the promoter regions of several genes. (Functional differences among the group are related to their *N*-termini.) In common with *c-fos* and some others, *c-jun* is classified as an immediate early response gene, since it is rapidly activated by platelet-derived, epidermal, fibroblast, nerve growth and transforming growth factors (PDGF, EGF, FGF, NGF and TGF), by tumor necrosis factor-α (TNFα), insulin-like growth factor-I (IGF-I), interleukin-1 (IL-1), and some undefined growth stimulants present in serum, by some tumor promoters (including the phorbol ester TPA), and by irradiation, and other factors. TPA and some other stimulants also rapidly enhance the binding of pre-existing c-jun protein to DNA, and they act on TREs (TPA responsive elements) in *c-jun* promotors to accelerate transcription. *C-jun* codes for 39-71K c-jun (Jun-1) proteins essential for growth, normal nervous system development, and germinal cell entry into meiosis. C-jun:c-fos dimers are especially potent stimulants for proliferation of many cell types; and excessive amounts invoke transformation. At least some of the effects involve activation of kinase C isozymes. The proteins are additionally involved in transduction of environmental signals to cell nuclei, and they affect functions such as neurotransmitter mediated depolarization and cardiac myocyte contractile responses to stretch. Cell type specific roles are suggested by observations that estrogens augment c-jun synthesis in the uterus but repress it in oviducts. C-jun homodimers are unstable, but they form when gene expression is stimulated, bind to *c-jun* promoters, and exert positive feedback control over transcription. They also act posttranslationally to augment the activities of the preformed proteins. However, they are negative regulators of *c-fos* transcription. Several control systems that protect against c-jun dimer overactivity have been described. For example, differentiation inducers inhibit c-jun synthesis, cardiac hypertrophy diminishes c-jun mediated responses to stretch, and in many cell types glucocorticoids, progesterone, retinoic acid, and 1-25-dihydroxyvitamin promote differentiation and suppress c-jun mediated proliferation. Moreover, receptors for those hormones block dimer binding to DNA. *Jun-B*, another early immediate response gene that codes for a related 40K product, is preferentially induced in some cell types, for example by human chorionic gonadotropin (hCG) in maturing Sertoli cells. Its heterodimers are less potent mitogens, and in some systems they inhibit c-jun effects. Both proteins have been called third messengers, since their production and abilities to initiate long-term responses to cell stimulation are regulated in part by cAMP and other second messengers. *Jun-D* directs formation of a different 40K protein that is not mitogenic. The gene is not usually not activated until long after c-jun levels have risen, and its product forms homodimers that antagonize the effects of c-jun (and in some cases also of jun-B). *V-jun* is an avian sarcoma virus 17 oncogene whose 55K product was initially identified in chicken fibrosarcomas.

junctions: joining regions; *see* also **gap**, **intermediate**, and **tight junctions**.

junctional transmission: *see* **myoneural junctions**.

"junk DNA": "selfish DNA"; DNA that undergoes replication but does not code for proteins. Some components function as transcription regulators. By incorporating into preexisting genes, they can contribute to mutations and evolutionary changes.

Jurkat: a human T cell leukemia cell line. Strains with special kinds of mutations are used to study T lymphocyte functions.

juvenile hormones: JH; allatum hormones; chemically related sesquiterpenoids secreted by insect corpora allata that antagonize the maturational, but not the molt-promoting actions of ecdysones. In the generalized structure shown, R = —CH$_3$ or —CH$_2$-CH$_3$.

juvenile onset diabetes mellitus: JOD; a term applied to insulin-dependent forms of diabetes mellitus caused by pancreatic beta cell destruction, because the manifestations usually begin during infancy, childhood, or adolescence. However, since the symptoms in some individuals begin later in life, the terms insulin-dependent (IDDM) and type I diabetes mellitus are preferred. Moreover, a somewhat rare disorder, MODY (maturity onset diabetes mellitus in the young) in which insulin resistance rather than hormone deficiency predominates, can develop in young individuals.

juxtacrine: describes regulation mediated by plasma membrane-bound regulators on cell surfaces that bind to receptors on adjacent cells. For example, membrane bound pro-TGFα can stimulate mitogenesis in other cells when it binds to their EGF receptors. *Cf* **autocrine** and **paracrine**.

juxtaglomerular apparatus: JGA; a specialized, innervated structure named for its location, composed of juxtaglomerular, macula densa, lacis, and mesangial cells. It is the major source of circulating renin, and it contributes indirectly (via angiotensin II) to the control of systemic blood pressure, catecholamine release, and aldosterone secretion.

juxtaglomerular cells: JG cells; modified (epithelioid) smooth muscle in the tunica media layers of renal afferent arterioles that synthesize, store, and secrete renin, and have stretch receptors. Most are located near glomeruli, and are components of the juxtaglomerular apparatus. High pressure in the vessels stretches the cell membranes, activates receptors, and inhibits renin release. (Therefore less enzyme is secreted when the blood volume increases, or when hydrostatic pressure rises.) The cells are also regulated by messages from macula densa cells. Catecholamines acting on β$_2$-type adrenergic receptors stimulate enzyme release (presumably by promoting cAMP generation), but can inhibit via α$_1$-type receptors. Other stimulants include prostacyclin, and high blood K$^+$. Inhibitors include vasopressin and atrial natriuretic factors. Although parathyroid hormone (PTH), which acts on adenylate cyclase, can increase renin secretion, high Ca^{2+} is said to inhibit. Changes in extracellular fluid Na$^+$ ion concentrations within a range likely to be encountered *in vivo* have no direct effects, but they promote extracellular fluid volume expansion and may increase cell sensitivities.

juxtamedullary nephrons: nephrons of mammals and birds whose glomeruli are located close to the renal medulla. They have long Henle loops that contribute to water conservation. *Cf* **cortical nephrons**.

j-value: the effective concentration of one end of a DNA molecule in the vicinity of the other ends of the same molecule. It is a function of molecule length (but not concentration), and provides some information on DNA structure. J values are used in conjunction with i values (which are related to the concentrations). Linear molecules have j:i ratios of 1 or less, whereas circular DNAs have values of 2 or more.

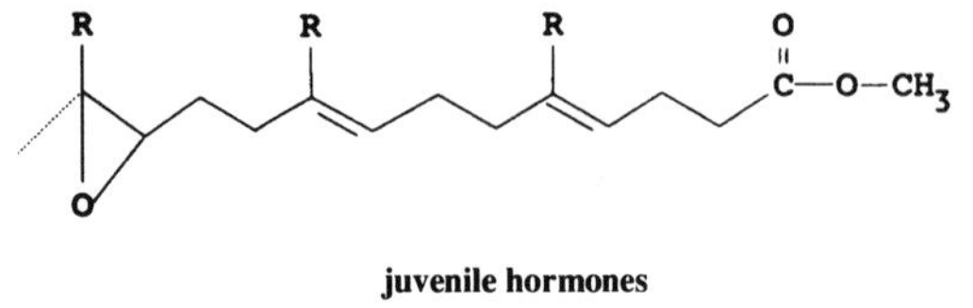

juvenile hormones

K

K: (1) potassium; (2) lysine; (3) equilibrium constant; (4) degrees Kelvin; (5) kilo-, as in Kcal and Kg; (6) kilodaltons (Kd), as in 50K; (7) designates a molecular component, as in K (kappa) chain. *See* also **pK, vitamin K. substance K, neuromedin K**, and **K cells.**

K, k antigens: allelic forms of Kell human blood group antigens, on the erythrocytes of approximately 8% of Caucasians.

4K: *see* **amyloid.**

k: reaction rate; k_1 and k_2 are used for reactions going to the right and left, respectively; k_a and k_d are, respectively, association and dissociation rates.

κ: kappa; a symbol (1) used with other terms to identify one component of a molecule (as in κ chain); when used as a subscript, as in $C_κ$ or $V_κ$, the upper case letter shows the location; (2) for a special kind of molecule (as in κ receptor).

KA: α-kainic acid.

K_a: (1) association constant; (2) acid dissociation constant.

α-kainic acid {kainate}: KA; 2-carboxy-4-(1-methylethenyl)-3-pyrrolidineacetic acid; a glutamate analog initially derived from the red alga, *Digenea simplex*, used to identify a subset of excitatory amino acid receptors. It can severely damage the hippocampus, and invoke the symptoms of Huntington's chorea. Although a more potent neurotoxin than glutamate, it acts mostly on cells with quisqualate type receptors, with little effect on those expressing only *N*-methyl-D-aspartate (NMDA) types. Some actions require the presence of glutamate or other substances that act on different receptor subtypes. KA is taken up by the terminals of some neuron types, and undergoes retrograde transport to the cell bodies (where it acts). In laboratory studies, it is used to selectively kill such neurons. *See* also **kainate receptors.**

kainate receptors: a subpopulation of glutamate receptors activated by kainic acid (KA) and AMPA (α-amino-3-hydroxy-5-methylisoxazole propionic aid), but not by NMDA (*N*-methyl-D-aspartate) or aspartate. The functions are not inhibited by high Mg^{2+} levels. Olfactory bulb, hippocampus, and cerebellar Purkinje cells have the largest numbers. The receptors are dimers; and various combinations of three subunit types (Glu-K1, Glu-K2, and Glu-K3) may explain differences in responses to pharmacological agents. Some have properties that overlap with those of quisqualate receptors, whereas others do not. KA is a more effective ligand than glutamate for all kainate subtypes. When activated, all invoke depolarization by forming Na^+ and K^+ channels. Those with Glu-K2 subunits additionally promote Ca^{2+} uptake. Repeated seizures are reported to down regulate the numbers in medulla oblongata neurons that project to the cerebellum.

kairomones: chemical messengers released by one kind of organism type that act on another type, and are usually beneficial to recipients but not to the donors. *See* also **pheromones**, and *cf* **allomones.**

KAL: *see* **Kallmann's syndome.**

kaliuresis: increased urinary excretion of potassium.

kallidin: lysine-bradykinin; Lys-Arg-Pro-Pro-Gly-Phe-Ser-Pro-Phe-Arg; a kinin cleaved from kininogens by renal and glandular kallikreins. Aminopeptidases catalyze its conversion to bradykinin, which exerts similar effects. However, although three receptor types (B_1, B_2, and B_3), have been identified for bradykinin, most kallidin actions appear to be mediated via the B_2 form. Kallidin lowers blood pressure by dilating renal and other arterioles, inhibiting norepinephrine discharge from sympathetic nerve endings, opposing the Na^+ and water retaining effects of aldosterone and the cardiovascular effects of angiotensin-II, and stimulating release of histamine and possibly also endothelium derived relaxation factor (EDRF; *see* **nitric oxide**). The concept that it is an important regulator is supported by observations that rats with sodium-dependent hypertension, and some humans with essential hypertension make subnormal amounts. Kininase II (which degrades kallidin) is identical to angiotensin converting enzyme; and pharmacological inhibitors that lower blood pressure act in part by slowing kallidin inactivation. Moreover, aldosterone "escape" is attributed in part to increased kallidin production. Kallidin, does, however, stimulate smooth muscle in some large arteries and veins, and it facilitates baroreceptor reflexes that promote adrenomedullary hormone secretion. Some effects have been linked with activation of phospholipase isozymes and consequent production of prostaglandins. Although prostaglandins can prolong the responses by activating kallikreins, they also promote renin release. Kallidin additionally contributes to inflammatory reactions, and it accelerates blood clotting by interacting with coagulation factors.

kallikreins: widely distributed, chemically diverse serine proteases that generate kinins by catalyzing cleavage of kininogen Met-Lys, Lys-Ser, and Ser-Arg bonds. They are encoded by at least 30 genes, and have been identified in hypothalamic nuclei and other brain regions, pineal gland, adenohypophysis, exocrine pancreas, salivary glands, duodenum, and the external surfaces of renal tubular and some other cells types. They are also present in blood plasma, lymph, urine, duodenal fluid, feces, and exocrine secretions (including pancreatic juice and saliva). Plasma types are predominantly high molecular weight (approximately 80K) glycoproteins that release mostly bradykinin and also activate neutrophilic and basophilic leukocytes, coagulation factors VII and XII, plasminogen and fibrinolysin, and additionally interact with factor XI, and affect other substrates. A different enzyme in plasma cleaves T-kininogen and releases isoleucyl-seryl-bradykinin (T-kinin). The tissue types are acidic 24-48K glycoproteins that yield mostly kallidin, but also act on arginine and lysine esters. Some contribute to transcription regulation and hormone processing. In animals with a pars intermedia, dopamine invokes parallel increases in kallikrein and proopiomelanocortin (POMC) synthesis, and estrogens increase kallikrein messenger RNA. Pars distalis lactotropes make the enzyme, and high levels occur in tumors derived from those cells. Estrogens (lactotrope stimulants) raise the levels, but dopamine (which inhibits prolactin release) lowers them. Naturally occurring inhibitors include activated complement component C1, α_2-macroglobulin, α_1-antitrypsin, and antithrombin III; *see* also **aprotinin**. Before activation by prostaglandins and other regulators, the enzymes exist as prekallikreins.

Kallmann's syndrome: olfactogenital dysplasia; hypogonadotropic hypogonadism associated with hyposmia or anosmia; a human disorder, most prevalent in males, in which gonadotropin releasing hormone (GnRH) deficiency is associated with impaired development of the reproductive and olfactory systems. Usually, secondary gonadal hormone deficiency leads to delayed closure of the epiphyses, and acquisition of eunuchoidal body proportions. The severity varies among afflicted individuals. In some cases, the gonads and olfactory bulbs do not develop at all, and there is no pubertal maturation; but in others some gonadal hormones are secreted, puberty is delayed but completed, and limited olfactory perception is acquired. Associated manifestations can include microphallus, severe renal dysgenesis (which can be unilateral) accompanied by water balance dysfunction, hyposmia and excessive thirst, hearing impairment, neurological and musculoskeletal defects, cleft-palate, facial deformities, and abnormal skin pigmentation. In males with just one kidney, the vas deferens does not differentiate on the side of the missing organ. Sporadic, autosomal recessive and dominant forms occur, but X-linked disorders are most common. The aberrations are attributed to inability to synthesize adequate amounts of a neural cell adhesion molecule that regulates cell migrations during embryogenesis. Consequently, GnRH secreting neurons, which originate in embryonic olfactory placodes, do not enter the hypothalamus; and terminalis and vomeronasal nerves fail to establish their connections with the cerebrum. Mutations or deletions of

KAL, a gene in the pseudoautosomal region of the long arm of the X chromosome (which escapes X inactivation in females) have been detected in some individuals. Its counterpart on the Y chromosome appears to be a non-functional pseudogene. The product is believed to be a 679 or 680-amino acid adhesion protein with domains similar to ones in neurophysins and some protease inhibitors, and fibronectin III-like sequences similar to those of known cell adhesion molecules, and of some protein tyrosine kinases and phosphatases.

kanamycin: an aminoglycoside antibiotic complex made by *Streptomyces kanamyceticus*. It contains kanamycins B and C, but the term usually refers to kanamycin A (shown below). It disrupts protein synthesis by acting on 70S ribosomes and causing misreading of the codons. Although effective against aerobic gram positive microorganisms, its clinical use is limited by its high toxicity, which most commonly affects the kidneys and ears.

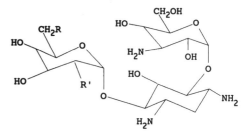

kaolin: China clay; porcelain clay; a hydrated aluminum silicate hydroxide, $H_2Al_2Si_2O_8 \bullet H_2O$, used as an adsorbent to recover some substances from mixtures. When ingested, it takes up many kinds of bacterial toxins and aids in their evacuation. Since it binds morphine, atropine, and other alkaloids, and thereby causes their retention in the intestines, it is used in oral preparations of those agents that alleviate diarrhea and cramps without exerting marked central nervous system effects. It is also used in poultices and other topical preparations.

Kaposi growth factor: fibroblast growth factor-4.

Kaposi's sarcomas: malignant tumors, usually in skin or viscera, composed predomantly of spindle-shaped cells. They occur mostly in individuals afflicted with T cell deficiencies — especially in those infected with the acquired immune deficiency syndrome (AIDS) virus, but also in association with some lymphomas.

kappa: κ; *see* **kappa chain** and **opioid receptors**.

kappa chain: κ, K chain; one of the two kinds of light chains of **immunoglobulins** (*q.v.*).

karyo-: a prefix meaning nucleus.

karyokinesis: nuclear division. It is closely followed in most, but not all cell types by cytokinesis.

karyolysis: cell death that begins with nuclear swelling and chromatin deterioration.

karyolymph: karyoplasm; *see* **nucleoplasm**.

karyon: nucleus.

karyoplasm: nucleoplasm.

karyoplasts: nuclei isolated from eukaryotic cells, surrounded by thin layers of cytoplasm. They are used to study intracellular localizations of hormone receptors and other large molecules, and influences of added cytoplasmic factors on nuclear functions.

karyopyknosis: shrinkage of cell nuclei that is associated with chromosome condensation and deterioration.

karyotype: the complete set of chromosomes of a cell, or characteristic of an organism.

kassinin: H_2N-Asp-Val-Pro-Lys-Ser-Asp-Gln-Phe-Val-Leu-Met-NH_2; an amphibian tachykinin with biological properties similar to those of neurokinin α.

kasugamycin: an antibiotic made by *Streptomyces kasugagaensis* that inhibits protein synthesis by attaching to aminoacyl-tRNA binding sites of bacterial ribosome 30S subunits, and blocking methylation of 16S RNA.

katacalcin: H-Asp-Met-Ser-Ser-Asp-Leu-Glu-Arg-Asp-His-Arg-Pro-His-Val-Ser-Met-Pro-Gln-Asn-Ala-Asn-OH; a peptide cleaved from the *C*-terminal region of pro-calcitonin, and released with calcitonin in equimolecular amounts. It lowers blood calcium levels and augments some CT actions, but does not affect plasma sodium, potassium, or phosphate. *Cf* **calcitonin gene related peptide**.

K^+-ATPases: bacterial enzymes that use energy released by ATP hydrolysis to drive K^+ ion uptake. Mammalian cells use H^+/K^+ and Na^+/K^+ ATPases to exchange K^+ for H^+ and Na^+.

kb: kilobase.

kbp: kilobase pairs.

K cells: (1) killer cells; a subpopulation of peripheral leukocytes that contributes to antibody-dependent cellular cytotoxicity, and provides protection against some forms of malignancy. The cells lack the surface markers that characterize natural killer (NK) cells and "killer lymphocytes", but have receptors for IgG immunoglobulin Fc regions, mediate graft rejection, and are implicated in the etiology of subacute thyroiditis and other autoimmune disorders. Some investigators believe they are special kinds of lymphocytes; but others suggest that at least some K cells are more closely related to monocytes; (2) gastrointestinal cells that secrete glucose dependent insulinotropic peptide (GIP).

Kd: K_d; K; dissociation constant; *see* **equilibrium constant**.

K_{eq}: equilibrium constant.

keloids: scar-like, collagen-rich skin lesions, usually formed in highly pigmented areas during overreactions to injuries.

kemptides: several synthetic substrates for protein kinase A, including H_2N-Leu-Arg-Arg-Ala-Ser-Leu-Gly-OH and H_2N-Arg-Gly-Tyr-Ser-Leu-Gly-OH.

kentsin: Thr-Pro-Arg-Lys; a synthetic peptide with gonadotropin releasing hormone (GnRH)-like activity.

Kendall's compounds: obsolete terms for steroids isolated from adrenocortical tissue. For A, B, C, D, E, F, G, H, Q, and S, *see* listing under **compounds** A, B, etc.

kerasins: brain **cerebrosides** (*q.v.*) that contain galactose, sphingosine, and lignoceric acid moieties.

keratan sulfates: glycosaminoglycans of cornea, cartilage, and spinal cord nucleus pulposus with galactose, *N*-acetylglucosamine-sulfate, fucose, mannose, and sialic acid moieties. *Type II* keratin sulfate differs from *Type I* in carbohydrate content, and it contains *N*-acetylgalactosamine.

keratins: 27 or more 40-70K cysteine-rich, insoluble, protease-resistant acidic and neutral scleroproteins made by differentiated stratified epithelia. Some form **intermediate filaments** (*q.v.*), play roles in desmosome formation, and contribute in others ways to strength and other tissue properties. "Hard" keratins accumulate in epidermal derivatives such as hair, fingernails, horns, wool, and scales, and are also present in tooth enamel and egg shells. "Soft" types (pseudokeratins) are components of differentiated epidermal, vaginal, intestinal, and other epithelia. *See* also **involucrin**.

keratinization: cornification; hardening and desiccation of epithelial tissue, for example in integument outer layers, and in vaginal mucosa.

keratinocytes: the major skin epidermis cell type. The cells originate and proliferate in the basal layers, and gradually undergo differentiation (including changes in keratin synthesis) as they are pushed outward toward the tissue surfaces by newly formed basal cells. Their abilities to perform many functions have been linked with their large numbers, locations (which permit transmission of environmental signals to underlying dermis), responsivity to numerous stimuli, and the synthesis of several regulators. They are the major sites for vitamin D formation, and they convert some of it to 1,25-dihydroxycholecalciferol (1,25-D), which promotes cell differentiation, inhibits mitosis, and exerts negative feedback control over its own synthesis. Many of the products act both peripherally and in an autocrine manner; and keratinocytes additionally interact with underlying fibroblasts and other cell types. Most regulators that promote keratinocyte differentiation inhibit proliferation. Interleukin-1 (IL-1), keratinocyte growth factor, and prostaglandin E_2 (PGE_2) are mitogenic. Transforming growth factor-α and epidermal growth factor (TGFα and EGF) prolong cell survival and may indirectly promote proliferation by affecting cell migration, whereas transforming growth factor-β (TGFβ), pyro-Glu-Glu-Asp-Ser-Gly-OH, and other peptides inhibit. Interferon-γ (IFNγ) may inhibit indirectly by accelerating 1,25-D formation. Keratinocytes also make a deiodinase that converts thyroxine (T_4) to triiodothyronine (T_3, which acts locally on lipid metabolism), and enzymes that catalyze testosterone, androstenedione, and progesterone metabolism. They additionally make thymopoietin, thymulin, PTH-like peptide, and a melanocyte stimulant.

keratinocyte growth factor: a member of the **fibroblast growth factor** family *(q.v.)*.

keratohyalin: a keratin precursor that accumulates in the granular layer of the epidermis, in Hassall's corpuscles, and at some other sites.

keratosis: formation of benign (but potentially precancerous) lesions in skin exposed to excessive ultraviolet radiation.

kernicterus: brain damage attributed to accumulation of excessive amounts of bilirubin (which stains the affected tissue). The lesions occur mostly commonly in the basal ganglia, cerebellum, and brain stem nuclei.

Ketalar: a trade name for ketamine.

Ketalgin hydrochloride: a trade name for methadone hydrochloride.

ketalorphin: a synthetic opioid peptide analog used to inhibit enkephalinases.

ketamine: 2-(2-chlorophenyl)-2-(methylamino)-cyclohexanone; an agent that very rapidly invokes general anesthesia in laboratory animals. It is used in veterinary medicine, and clinically for special purposes, often in combination with diazepam. Unlike most general anesthetics, it acts primarily on phencyclidine (PCP) type receptors in the cerebral cortex and limbic system. Although its ability to rapidly invoke intense analgesia is useful for some purposes, it also causes amnesia and sensations of dissociation from the environment. The recovery period is prolonged, and often associated with unpleasant dreams, delirium, and sometimes also delusions and hallucinations. After-effects recur for days in some individuals. Influences on sympathetic nervous systems vary with the species.

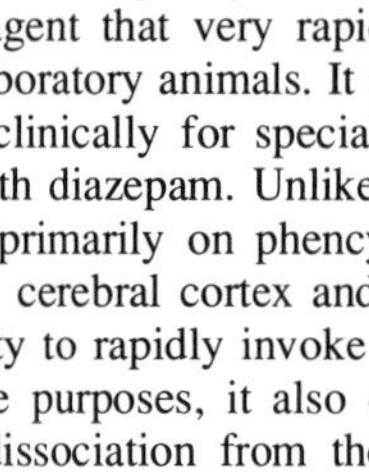

ketanserin: 3-[2-[4-(4-fluorobenzoyl)-1-piperidinyl] ethyl]-2-4[1*H*,3*H*]-quinazolinedione]: a serotonin antagonist that acts preferentially on 5HT$_2$-type receptors, and antagonizes serotonin-mediated stimulation of smooth muscle contraction, blood platelet aggregation, and aldosterone secretion. It exerts some inhibitory influences on α-adrenergic, H$_1$-type histamine, some dopamine, and possibly also a subgroup of 5HT$_{1B}$ receptors. It

is used to treat some forms of hypertension, and as a laboratory tool.

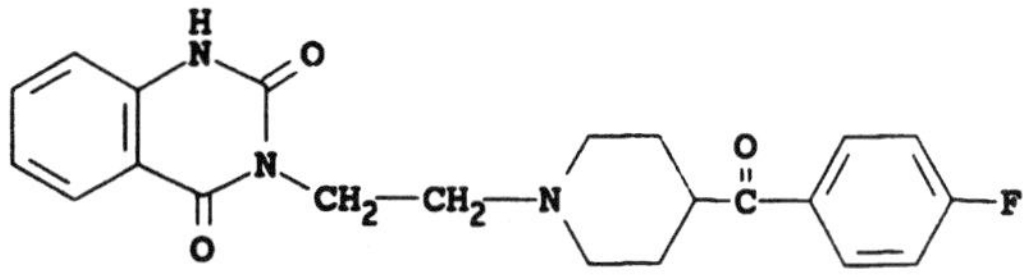

ketazocine: a synthetic morphine derivative chemically related to pentazocine. It is an agonist for, and is used to identify κ type opioid receptors.

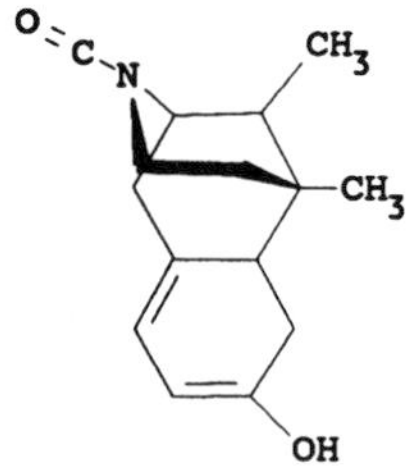

ketimines: compounds formed by replacing oxygens of ketones with imino groups. They are pyridoxamine precursors. Chronic hyperglycemia can lead to formation of large amounts from glucose (via aldimine intermediates) that invoke toxicity by attaching to proteins; *see* **nonenzymatic glycosylation**. The R groups in the structures shown are amino acid components.

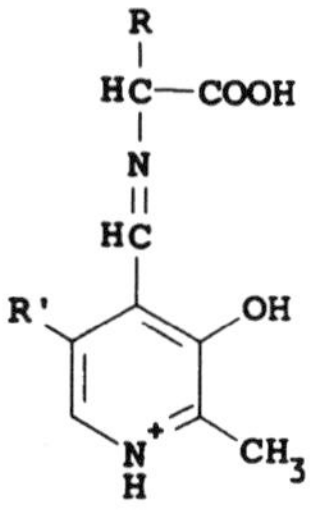

aldimine 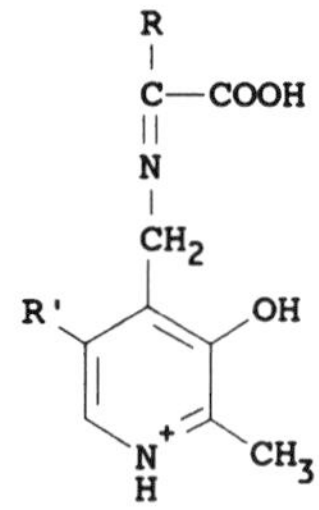   ketamine

keto-: a prefix that designates the presence of a carbonyl (—C=O) group. The location is is usually indicated, as in 17-ketosteroid or α-ketoglutaric acid. For keto- compounds, see under chemical name that follows keto-.

ketoacidosis: metabolic acidosis associated with the accumulation of **ketone bodies** *(q.v.)*.

ketoconazole: KTZ: Nizoral; an imidazole derivative effective against many kinds of fungi. It strongly inhibits lanosterol 32-demethylase, thereby blocks ergosterol and cholesterol biosynthesis, and kills the organisms by augmenting plasma membrane permeability. Preparations that contain it are used topically to treat ringworm, and both topically and orally to kill *Candida* and some other yeasts. It also inhibits some mammalian cytochrome P450 dependent enzymes, and the effects on C17-20 lyase activity (and therefore on androgen biosynthesis) are used to treat prostate gland cancers. The ability of high concentrations to also inhibit 11ß-hydroxysteroid dehydrogenase (and glucocorticoid synthesis) was initially believed to account for the beneficial effects in Cushing's disease, but KTZ additionally antagonizes

ketoconazole

adrenocorticotropic hormone (ACTH) by attaching to adenylate cyclase catalytic subunits. Influences on aromatases have also been described. Some undesirable effects, such as gynecomastia, are caused by inhibition of steroid degrading enzymes. In rare cases, KTZ invokes severe liver damage and allergic reactions.

ketogenic: promoting the formation of **ketone bodies** *(q.v.)*. Glucagon and other hormones that accelerate fatty acid oxidation in the liver augment ketone production; and glucagon additionally increases substrate availability by inhibiting acetyl-coenzyme A co-carboxylase. Under physiological conditions, opposing actions of insulin limit the effects. *See also* **ketogenic amino acids**.

ketogenic amino acids: leucine, lysine, and other amino acids that are metabolized to acetyl-coenzyme A or acetoacetyl-CoA; *cf* **glucogenic amino acids**. Isoleucine, phenylalanine, tryptophan, and tyrosine are both ketogenic and glucogenic.

α-ketoglutaric acid {α-**ketoglutarate**}: 2-oxo-1,5-pentanedioic acid; a metabolite formed in the tricarboxylic acid cycle via: oxalosuccinate + H$^+$ → α-ketoglutarate + CO$_2$. It reacts with NAD$^+$ + coenzyme A to yield succinyl-CoA + CO$_2$ + NADH + H$^+$. Reversible reactions in which it participates include: glutamate + NAD$^+$ ⇄ NH$_4$+ + α-ketoglutarate + NADH + H$^+$, and α-ketoglutarate + aspartate ⇄ pyruvate + glutamate. It is also used for collagen synthesis in the reaction: α-ketoglutarate + prolyl moiety + O$_2$ → 4-hydroxyproly moiety + succinate. The ion is shown; *see* also **glutamic acid**.

```
        COO⁻
        |
        C=O
        |
       HOCH
        |
       HCOH
        |
       HOCH
        |
        COO⁻
```

ketone[s]: organic compounds that contain carbonyl (—C=O) groups, in which the carbon atom is linked to another carbon; (2) any of the ketone bodies.

ketone bodies: three small molecules derived from the fatty acids. Acetoacetic acid can be converted to the other two via the reactions: acetoacetic acid + NADH + H$^+$ ⇄ β-OH-butyric acid + NAD$^+$, and acetoacetic acid - CO$_2$ → acetone. *See* also **ketosis**.

ketonemia: excessively high blood ketone levels; *see* **ketosis**.

ketonuria: high urinary ketone levels; *see* **ketosis**.

ketosis: production and accumulation of excessive quantities of ketone bodies. It occurs when acetyl-coenzyme A oxidation in the tricarboxylic acid cycle does not keep pace with fatty acid degradation to acetyl-Co A. A sudden switch from a balanced to a lipid-rich, carbohydrate poor diet invokes the condition by providing excessive amounts of fatty acids. Some metabolic adaptations follow in healthy individuals, so that ketosis is usually mild if proteins for gluconeogenesis are also eaten. A more severe condition develops during prolonged food deprivation, since liver glycogen reserves are depleted, only limited amounts of body protein are available, insulin levels fall, and there is excessive dependence on fatty acid fuels. Resting skeletal muscle, liver, and some other tissues efficiently oxidize lipid fuels, but neurons and contracting muscle require glucose. Glucose-deprived neurons oxidize some β-hydroxybutyrate, but there are controversies concerning whether normal functions are maintained. High levels of glucocorticoids, glucagon, and some other hormones invoke ketosis by accelerating both lipolysis and ketogenesis; but they also stimulate insulin secretion. The most severe conditions are caused by insulin deficiency, since insulin is needed to oppose excessive influences of lipolytic hormones, and to promote fatty acid incorporation into triacylglycerols. The consequences include metabolic acidosis, dehydration, and, in severe cases, coma. Acetoacetic and β-hydroxybutyric acids directly lower blood pH. They are excreted in combination with Na$^+$, and thereby deplete circulating NaHCO$_3$, and lower blood NaHCO$_3$: HHCO$_3$ ratios; and the excretion draws water to the urine.

17-ketosteroids: 17-KS: adrenosterone, androsterone, epiandrosterone, dehydroepiandrosterone (DHA, DHEA), etiocholanolone, and other steroids with ketone (oxy)

acetoacetate   β-hydroxybutyrate   acetone

ketones

393

groups attached to the carbon atoms at position 17. Most are degradation products of adrenocortical and gondal hormones; but some are biologically active. They circulate and are excreted to the urine. Some tumors make large amounts.

11-ketotestosterone: a major teleost androgen, and a 17α-hydroxyprogesterone metabolite whose production in mammalian testicular cells is augmented by gonadotropins.

β-ketothiolase: acetyl coenzyme A acyltransferase.

***kex*-2**: a yeast gene that codes for subtilisin-like, Ca^{2+}-dependent proteases essential for processing precursor proteins to mature forms. They act on Arg-Arg and Lys-Arg bonds near *C*-termini, and are required for release of mating pheromone α from its precursor, formation of a protective cytotoxin, and other functions. The products of mammalian DNA sequences that code for similar proteases include furins (Golgi localized endoproteinases that act on a wide variety of substrates), and several enzymes in secretory granules, including neuroendocrine cell proteases PC1, PC2, and PC3, with more restricted specificities, that cleave prohormones. Various combinations of enzymes appear to account for cell specific processing such as proopiomelanocortin (POMC) cleavage to α-melanocyte stimulating hormone (α-MSH) and corticotropin-like intermediate peptide (CLIP) in pars intermedia cells, but to adrenocorticotropic hormone (ACTH) in pars distalis cells.

kg: kilogram.

KI: potassium iodide.

kidneys: innervated, bilateral retroperitoneal organs essential for maintaining the normal volume and composition of blood and bulk extracellular fluid; *see* also **nephrons**. In addition to regulating water, electrolyte, and acid base balance via selective excretion and reabsorption of ions, and removing nitrogenous wastes and toxins (via filtration and secretion), they produce renin, kallidin, and other factors that affect systemic blood pressure, convert 25-hydroxyvitamin D to its 1,25- and 24, 25- derivatives, make erythropoietin, synthesize several prostaglandins with diverse functions, degrade some proteins (including insulin), and can produce limited amounts of glucose during times of food deprivation. Vasopressin exerts the major controls over water conservation. Aldosterone accelerates K^+ and H^+ excretion, but indirectly promotes water retention by stimulating Na^+ and bicarbonate reabsorption. Several effects of those and other hormones are opposed by natriuretic peptides. Parathyroid hormone increases phosphate excretion and Ca^{2+} retention. Norepinephrine, dopamine, and eicos-

anoids regulate renal blood flow and pressure. Other hormones that act on the kidneys include glucocorticoids, triiodothyronine, and calcitonin.

killifish: *see Fundulus heraclitus*.

killer cells: usually (1) K cells; (2) cytotoxic cells, including natural killer (NK), and lymphokine activated T_C type lymphocytes, as well as killer cells; (3) single-celled microorganisms (for example some *Paramecia*) that kill other organisms.

kilobase: kb; 1000 nucleic acid bases; a measure of the length of a ribonucleic acid (RNA), or single-stranded deoxyribonucleic acid (DNA) segment.

kilobase pair: kbp; a set of 1000 complementary base pairs of a double stranded nucleic acid segment.

kilocalorie: Calorie; C; the unit most commonly used for heat loss or production by whole organisms, equivalent to one thousand **calories** (*q.v.*).

kilodalton: Kd; K; 1000 daltons; the unit most commonly used for the molecular weights of large molecules. (One dalton is the weight of a hydrogen atom).

kinases: at least 200 enzymes that catalyze transfers of terminal phosphate groups of adenosine triphosphate (ATP), guanosine triphosphate (GTP) and other high energy phosphate compounds to or from specific substrates; *cf* **phosphorylases**. Some affect rate-limiting steps of intermediary metabolism by acting on small molecules such as glucose, fructose-6-phosphate, and phosphoenolpyruvate. Others, such as inositol phosphate kinases, contribute to second messenger generation and metabolism. Creatine kinase facilitates energy storage in chemical bonds for future use. Various **protein kinases** (*q.v.*) act on other enzymes (some of which are activated by phosphorylation and others inactivated), on cytoskeletal components (including microtubules and microfilaments that affect morphology and intracellular translocations), on ion channel proteins that regulate transport, and on ribosomal and nuclear factors. Enzymes affected by phosphorylation are involved in processes as diverse as photoreception, olfaction, lymphocyte and neutrophil functions, embryonic development, and cell division. Specific kinase types regulate DNA replication, gene transcription, or translation, or mediate post-translational modifications (including prohormone processing). Many are components of complex cascades. Ligand-binding activates kinase components of receptors for insulin, insulin-like growth factor-I, nerve growth factor, and several other hormones, and consequent phosphorylations of their substrates mediate hormone actions. In contrast, phosphorylations decrease the effects of some regulators by invoking desensitizations (both homologous and heterologous). Kinases A, C, and G are among the types name for the factors required for activation, whereas casein kinases, hexokinases, pyruvate kinase, histone-1 kinase and myosin light chain kinase are examples of types identified by their substrates. The terms serine-threonine and tyrosine kinases indicate the moieties of the substrates that accept the phosphate groups, whereas names such as mitogen activated kinases

(MAPs) and extracellular signal regulated kinases (ERKs) refer to functions. All protein kinases contain similar domains that mediate binding to the high energy phosphates, and others for substrate binding, catalysis, and control of their activities. Some function at very low levels in "resting" cells, and are activated by covalent modifications such as phosphorylation or dephosphorylation at specific sites, or by Ca^{2+}, Ca-calmodulin, phospholipids, phosphatidic acid, long-chain unsaturated fatty acids, and other cell components. Different typs have regulatory subunits that must be dissociated or modified; and truncated forms that lack the inhibitory components, or defective, mutated ones can invoke transformations. Numerous phosphatases reverse the kinase effects.

kinase I, **kinase II**: type I and type II calcium/calmodulin dependent kinases; *see* **calmodulin**.

kinase A: cAMP-dependent protein kinases; enzymes activated by cyclic adenosine-3′5′-monophosphate that catalyze transfers of high energy phosphate groups from ATP to serine or threonine moieties of other molecules. When cAMP levels are low, the enzymes are present mostly in inactive forms, composed of two catalytic (C) and two regulatory (R) subunits. Elevation of the nucleotide levels (by hormones, neurotransmitters and other factors) releases C* (the active catalytic component) via reactions that can be represented as: R—C—C—R + 4 cAMP → 2 R—cAMP + 2 C*. Mechanisms for inactivation include cAMP degradation by phosphodiesterases, cAMP extrusion, and C* binding to inhibitors. Two major types (I and II) have different cellular distributions, and different regulatory subunits that affect both tendencies to undergo autophosphorylation and the affinities for substrates and cAMP. Glycogen phosphorylase *b* kinase, glycogen phosphorylase *b*, and hormone-sensitive lipases are among the kinds activated by the kinase A-mediated phosphorylation, whereas glycogen synthase is a type that is inactivated. Other substrates include pyruvate dehydrogenase, hydroxymethyl glutaryl coenzyme A (HMG-CoA) reductase, tyrosine hydroxylase, ribosomal protein S-6, rhodopsin, some calcium ion channel proteins, some histones, and some hormone receptors. Several effects of kinase A mediated phosphorylation at certain substrate loci are antagonized by kinase C mediated phosphorylation of different domains within the same molecules. *See* also **adenylate cyclases** and **cyclic nucleotide phosphodiesterases**.

kinase 2α: a kinase induced by interferons α and β (IFNα and IFNβ), and activated by double-stranded RNAs, that contributes to defenses against viral infections.

kinase C: PKC: protein kinase C; several isozymes that catalyze transfers of terminal phosphate groups from ATP to specific serine or threonine moieties of acceptor molecules, so named because the actions of the first ones isolated are calcium (and phospholipid) dependent. C_α, $C_{\beta I}$, $C_{\beta II}$, C_γ, C_δ, C_ε, and C_ζ subtypes have been studied, and there is evidence for the existence of additional forms. A shared Greek letter subscript indicates that the synthesis is directed by a common gene whose transcripts undergo alternate splicings. Most cells contain more than one type; and the relative amounts vary with the stages of

maturation and other factors. Since subtypes δ, ε, ζ, and η are not much affected by Ca^{2+} ion concentrations, they have been called "novel" protein C kinases (nPKC). The isoforms differ in substrate specificities, kinetic properties, intracellular distributions, and responses to physiological regulators and oncogene products. Diacylglycerols (DG), generated by hormones, neurotransmitters and other phospholipase C activators, increase the activities of all subtypes, in some cases by augmenting the sensitivities to Ca^{2+}. Their effects subside when phosphodiesterases degrade them. Tumor promoting phorbol esters are DG analogs that resist degradation and initially invoke sustained activity. However, they slowly "down regulate" PKC activity when presented for long time periods (in part by accelerating enzyme destruction), and are used for this purpose in laboratory studies. Some hormones and neurotransmitters activate kinase C isozymes by generating inositol phosphates that elevate cytosolic Ca^{2+} levels. PKC isozymes affected in this way limit the durations of their own actions at some sites by catalyzing phosphorylation of inositol 1,4,5-triphosphate ($IP_{1,4,5}$, IP_3) receptors. Other limitations result from kinase A-mediated phosphorylation of some target molecules at sites different from the ones affected by kinase C. In contrast, some isozymes are activated by arachidonic, oleic, linoleic, linolenic, docosahexanoic, and other long-chain unsaturated fatty acids, lipoxygenase metabolites, and/or phosphatidic acids; and PKCs sustain some effects by activating phospholipase D isozymes and other enzymes that generate those molecular species (and also diacylglycerols). Factors that promote translocations of cytosolic PKCs to plasma and intracellular membranes stimulate by establishing enzyme contact with membrane components; and two proteins (30K and 33K) that bind PKCs with high affinity are proposed "receptors" (RACKs) that facilitate attachments to membrane phospholipids. Sphingosine, sphingamine, and related bases are physiological inhibitors. Another form of activation is mediated by calpain, which catalyzes limited, calcium-mediated cleavage of specific peptide bonds, removes a negative regulator component, and generates a PKC form that does not require activators (*see* **kinase M**). PKCs are major regulators of cell differentiation and proliferation, and of many other processes. The numerous targets include Na^+/K^+-ATPases (which affect membrane potentials, cell pH and active transport of amino acids and other molecules), microfilaments and microtubules (which affect morphology and intracellular translocations), nuclear receptors for 1,25-dihydroxycholecalciferol (1,25-dihydroxyvitamin D), triiodothyronine (T_3), and other hormones, and T lymphocyte activation mechanisms. They augment neutrophil membrane H^+ permeability and superoxide radical generation, antagonize PKA influences on chloride channels in the lungs, promote the release of aldosterone, growth hormone and insulin, and mediate some insulin actions. They also induce some hormone receptors and hormone-binding proteins, accelerate bone resorption and intestinal transport of Ca^{2+}, promote differentiation of myoblasts and other cell types, and play roles in fertilization. *See* also **phosphatidic acids**. Inhibitory, as well as stimulatory influences have been described, for example on the secretion gonadotropin releasing hormone (GnRH). Some effects oppose those of *ras* gene products.

kinase G: cGMP-dependent kinases; enzymes that catalyze transfers of phosphate groups from ATP to serine or threonine moieties of other molecules when activated by cyclic guanosine-3′5′-monophosphate. The nucleotide binds to the regulatory components and lifts the inhibition otherwise exerted. However, unlike the mechanisms for kinase A activation, the regulatory subunits do not dissociate from the catalytic components. Kinase G acts on some kinase A substrates, but it also catalyzes phosphorylations that oppose kinase A effects. Although several ligands activate **guanylate cyclases** (*q.v.*), and generate **cyclic GMP** (*q.v.*), not all effects of the nucleotide involve G kinase. cGMP acts on some phosphodiesterases, promotes nitric oxide generation, and exerts other direct influences.

kinase-kinases: kinases that catalyze phosphorylations of, and thereby affect the activities of other kinase enzymes. They are components of glycogenolysis, cell cycle control, and other cascades.

kinase M: truncated forms of kinase C that have been activated by proteolysis (catalyzed, for example by calpains), and are no longer dependent on lipids. (Some kinase C isozymes have inhibitory subunits that mask the substrate binding sites.)

kinase N: a serine-threonine protein kinase induced by nerve growth factor (NGF) that is not inhibited by Mn^{2+}, and does not appear to be activated by factors known to regulate other protein kinases. The substrates include histone H1, tyrosine monooxygenase, ribosomal S-6 protein, and MAP-2 kinases. Kinase N may be related to one or more extracellular signal-regulated kinases (ERKs) induced by growth factors that act on similar substrates and couple growth factor mediated tyrosine phosphorylation to activation of serine-threonine kinases.

kinase NII: protein K; *see* **polyamine dependent kinase**.

kinase P: polypeptide dependent protein kinase; serine-threonine kinases activated by basic (usually lysine-rich) polypeptides, identified in blood platelets, placental membranes, yeast cells, and at some other sites. One type associates physically (and co-purifies) with epidermal growth factor (EGF) receptors, enhances the effects of EGF on receptor tyrosine autophosphorylation, and inhibits ligand-receptor influences on serine-threonine phosphorylations. Enzymes of this group contribute to the control of acetylcholine receptor and tubulin phosphorylation. The members share some chemical properties, but have different substrate affinities. They act on acceptor molecules not affected by kinases A and C. Syringomycin and polymyxin B augment their activities (but do not affect kinase A enzymes).

phosphatidic acid activated protein **kinases**: enzymes that catalyze phosphorylations of target proteins on serine and threonine moieties and thereby promote DNA syn-

thesis, platelet aggregation, superoxide generation by neutrophilic leukocytes, and the release of insulin, parathyroid hormone (PTH), and other hormones. They may be kinase C isozymes.

kindling: intermittent changes in central nervous system neuron electrical activity invoked by partial depolarizations that lower stimuli thresholds. The electrical changes spread progressively over wider regions, and can invoke seizures.

kine-: a prefix meaning movement.

kinesin: an elongated protein composed of one 65-70K and two 110K subunits that binds to vesicles and other particles, and to ATP, and uses energy released by microtubule-activated ATPase to generate forces that move particles from minus to plus ends of microtubules; *cf* **dynein**. (It can also promote microtubule movements along glass plates.) Kinesin is abundant in neurons, in which it promotes rapid transport of synaptic vesicles to axon termini. It also binds to non-microtubule components of mitotic spindles, where it mediates spindle elongation and chromosome movement, and to endoplasmic reticula, where it provides forces for maintaining and extending tubulovesicular structures. In macrophages and other cell types, it facilitates lysosome elongation.

kinetensin: Ile-Ala-Arg-Arg-His-Pro-Tyr-Phe-Leu; a peptide related to neurotensin that releases histamine from mast cells. It is obtained from pepsin-treated blood plasma.

kinetin: 6-furfurylaminopurine; a potent cytokine, generated by heating plant and yeast DNA. It is used to promote the growth of microorganisms in cell cultures.

Kinetin : a trade name for a hyaluronidase preparation.

kinetochore: a specialized trilaminar structure on the outer surface of a centromere, comprising an inner plate that overlies the central domain, a middle electron translucent zone, and an outer plate (which is covered with a fibrous corona when no microtubules are attached). It contains some DNA, provides attachment sites for tubulin, dynein, calmodulin, and p34[cdc2], and is essential for chromosome movements during cell division.

kinetosomes: self-replicating centriole-like organelles; *see* **basal bodies**.

kinins: peptides cleaved from kininogens via reactions catalyzed by kininases. **Bradykinin** and **kallidin** are among the types that contribute to inflammatory and allergic responses, in part by activating phospholipases and generating eicosanoids. They promote vasodilation, affect vascular permeability, invoke pain sensations, and stimulate some smooth muscle cells. Kallidin contributes to blood pressure regulation, and bradykinin stimulates salivary gland secretion. Other peptides include T-kinin, and some components of the venoms of wasps and other insects.

kininases: proteolytic enzymes that cleave amino acid sequences from kinins.

kininase I: an aminopeptidase that acts on phenylalanine-arginine bonds of kinins, converts kallidin to bradykinin, and degrades angiotensins.

kininase II: angiotensin converting enzyme (ACE); an enzyme that catalyzes cleavage of dipeptides from the *C*-terminal ends of kinins. It converts angiotensin I to angiotensin II, and bradykinin, kallidin and related kinins to biologically inactive peptides.

kininogens: peptides or proteins that can be cleaved to yield one or more kinins. High molecular weight (100-250K) acidic glycoproteins made in the liver and secreted to the bloodstream are substrates for plasma type kallikreins and other enzymes that generate bradykinin. A lower molecular weight (50-75K) type cleaved by tissue kallikreins generates kallidin.

kininogenases: kallikreins and related enzymes that generate kinins by catalyzing cleavage of kininogen peptide bonds.

kinocilia: motile filaments that extend from the cytoplasm to free cell surfaces.

kirromycin: mocimycin; delvomycin; an antibiotic made by *Streptomyces ramocissimus* that inhibits protein synthesis by altering the configuration of GTP-linked elongation factor EF-Tu. A 5,6-dihydro derivative is added to poultry feed.

Kirsten sarcoma virus: a retrovirus initially isolated from mice that contains a *Ki-ras* oncogene, and induces sarcomas in newborn rats; *see* **ras**.

kistren: a 68K protein made by the Malayan pit viper *Agkistrodonon rhodostoma* that strongly inhibits platelet aggregation by blocking GPIIb/IIIa binding to fibrinogen.

c-kit: proto-oncogenes that code for approximately 145K transmembrane receptors with tyrosine kinase activity which resemble receptors for colony stimulating factor-1 (CSF-1, M-CSF) and platelet-derived growth factor. They are expressed in embryonic cells, placenta, liver, heart, bone marrow, fibroblasts, and gonads. The names given to the primary ligand include mast cell growth factor (MGF, which differs from M-CSF), **stem cell growth factor**, SCF (*q.v.*), kit ligand (KL), and Steel factor. The existence of other growth factor type ligands has been suggested. *C-kit* was initially identified within the *W* (white spotting) mouse locus, as the gene that codes for a receptor that binds the *Steel* (*Sl*) product. Related genes occur in other mammals, including humans. Both *c-kit* and *Steel* genes are semidominant, and essential for normal development of hematopoietic, germinal, mast cell, and melanocyte precursors, and for several postnatal functions. In addition to acting directly, stem cell factor synergizes with granulocyte-macrophage colony stimulating factor (GM-CSF), interleukin-7, erythropoietin, and other regulators; and it supports fibroblast-mediated, interleukin-3 independent proliferation. Several kinds of spontaneous mutations have been identified for both genes. Homozygotes with severe types of either kind die prenatally, usually during midgestation. Heterozygotes, and animals with less damaging mutations suffer severe macrocytic anemia, mast cell depletion, loss of fur pigment, and sterility. A related oncogene, *v-kit*, made by the Hardy-Zuckerman-4 feline sarcoma virus, codes for p80$^{gag-kit}$, which invokes transformation.

Kjeldahl method: *see* **Nessler's reagent**.

KL: *kit* ligand; mast cell growth factor, MGF; mast/stem cell growth factor; *see* **stem cell factor**.

Klinefelter's syndrome: several closely related disorders in human males, in which impaired reproductive system maturation is attributed to the presence of excessive numbers of X chromosome genes. Most individuals have 47-XXY karyotypes, but XXYY, XXXXY, mosaic, and other variants are known (and in rare cases there are two X chromosomes, one of which holds some Y-related genes). The incidence rises in parallel with parental age; and the supernumerary chromosomes are usually contributed by the spermatozoa. The most common manifestations include streak gonads with oligospermia or azoospermia, tall stature, and varying degrees of mental retardation that can be associated with personality disorders. More than half the affected individuals display gynecomastia. Subnormal androgen production accounts for the high gonadotropin levels, but other factors contribute to the growth of long bones (especially obvious in the ankle to knee segments). Some individuals are fertile and enjoy normal intelligence, possibly because of partial X chromosome inactivation or mosaicism.

K$_m$: Michaelis constant.

KN-62: (*S*)-5-isoquinolinesulfonic acid, 4-[2-[(5-isoquinolinyl-sulfonyl)methylamino]-3-oxo-3-(4-phenyl-1-

kirromycin

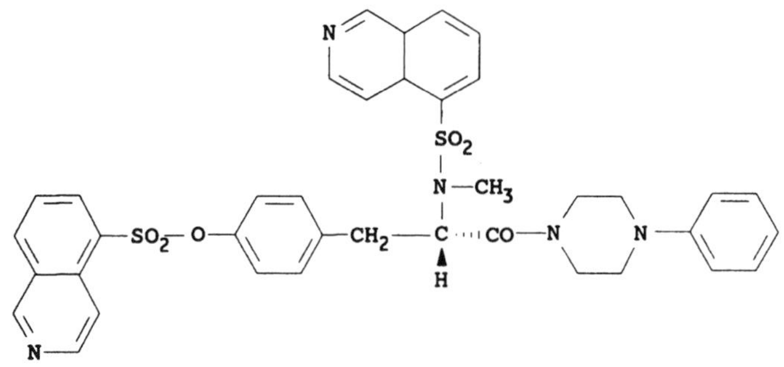

KN-62

piperazinyl)-propylphenyl ester; a selective inhibitor of brain calmodulin-dependent protein kinase II.

knirps: a *Drosophila* gene that directs formation of a gap segmentation protein essential for normal somatic development.

kojic amine hydrobromide: 2-(aminoethyl)-5-hydroxy-4*H*-pyran4-one-hydrobromide; a GABA agonist that inhibits sodium-independent GABA binding to brain membranes. Kojic acid (in which —CH$_2$OH replaces the the —CH$_2$NH$_2$ side-chain) is an antibiotic made by *Aspergillus oryzae*.

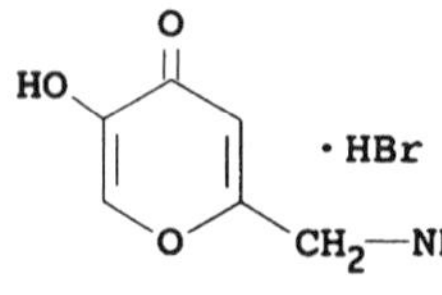

krebiozen: an undefined substance isolated from the blood of fungus-injected horses, once claimed to be a polysaccharide that cures cancers. Its use is now banned by the Food and Drug Administration. Creatine is a major component.

Krebs cycle: citric acid cycle; *see* **tricarboxylic acid cycle**.

Krebs-Henseleit cycle: urea cycle.

Krebs-Ringer solution: a modified **Ringer's solution** (*q.v.*) that contains phosphate buffers and magnesium salts.

kringles: cysteine-rich, pretzel-shaped domains formed by amino acid moieties held together by intramolecular disulfide bonds. Proteins containing them include plasminogen, tissue-type plasminogen activator, prothrombin, and coagulation system serine proteases.

Krox-20: a serum-inducible transcription activator with three zinc fingers that contributes to the regulation of hindbrain development.

17-**KS**: 17-ketosteroids.

KTZ: ketoconazole.

Kupffer cells: von Kupffer cells; liver stellate cells; specialized phagocytic cell components of the reticuloendothelial system that line liver sinusoids and remove dead and degenerating erythrocytes and other debris.

Kurloff cells: cells of undefined function in the peripheral blood and lymphoid systems of guinea pigs that are pregnant, or have been treated with estrogens. Each contains a contain large, PAS positive granule. They may be modified lymphocytes.

kurtosis: describes a statistical distribution curve that is either steeper or more shallow than a normal one for the same parameters.

kuru: a chronic, progressive neurological disorder believed to be caused by a prion related to the agent that causes Creutzfeldt-Jakob disease. It occurs in natives of a restricted locale in New Guinea who practice cannibalism, where transmission is attributed to ingestion of brain tissue. A very long asymptomatic latent period is followed by development of dementia and cerebellar deterioration.

Kv: kilovolt.

kwashiorkor: a severe nutritional disease attributed to deficiency of some essential amino acids, especially lysine. The manifestations include anemia, impaired growth, edema, diarrhea, and scalp hair that is red and brittle. *Cf* **marasmus**.

kymographs: devices for tracing movements on drums that rotate at defined speeds. In one type, the drum is covered with paper marked off in boxes that correspond to increments in time on the horizontal, and amplitude on the vertical axis. A lever attached to an object such as skeletal, smooth, or cardiac muscle, is fitted with a pen that moves with and records contractions. Another type has a calibrated lead sheet with vertical slits. X-rays sent through the object pass through the slits to a photographic plate.

kynurenic acid: 4-hydroxyquinaldic acid: a tryptophan degradation product. The quantities excreted in urine are augmented by deficiencies of vitamins B$_1$, B$_2$, and B$_6$.

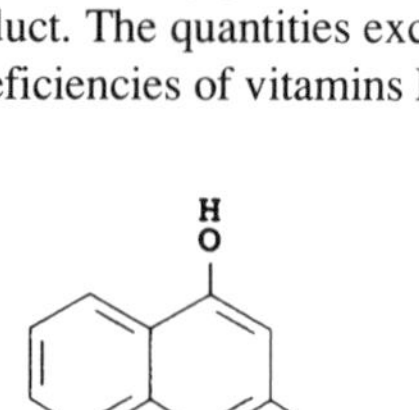

398

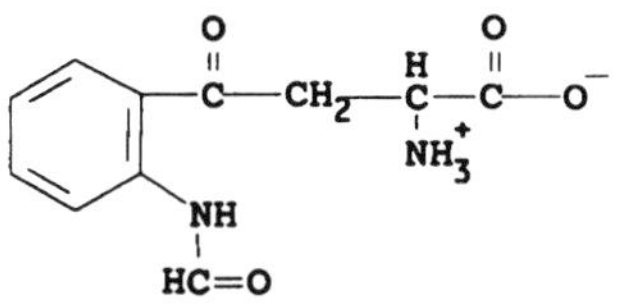

formyl-kynurenine

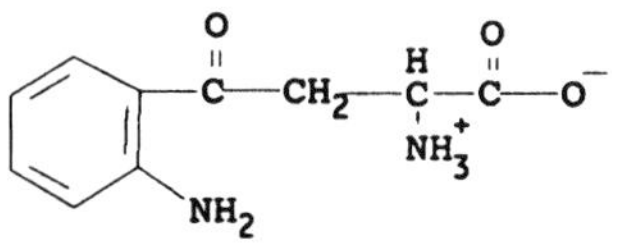

kynurenine

kynurenine: 3-anthranoylalanine acid; an intermediate in one pathway for tryptophan degradation. Tryptophan is oxidized to formylkynurenine via a reaction catalyzed by tryptophan oxidase (TO, tryptophan dioxidase, tryptophan pyrrolase, TP), and the product is converted to kynurenine. Tryptophan oxidase is induced in the liver by glucocorticoids. By depleting tryptophan stores, high levels facilitate gluconeogenesis, since tryptophan-containing proteins cannot be made, and amino acids that would otherwise be used to make them become available for conversion to glucose. Kynurenine can be metabolized to glutaryl-CoA (a carbohydrate precursor) + acetyl-coenzyme A, or to alanine + anthranilic acid (a nicotinic acid precursor).

kyorin: an aldose reductase inhibitor; *see* **ADN-138**.

kyotorphin: Tyr-Arg; an endogenous dipeptide that potentiates enkephalin activity by inhibiting enkephalinases. It does not interact directly with opioid receptors.

L

L: leucine; (2) left-handed configuration; *see* **stereoisomerism**.

l: levorotary; (-); describes molecules that rotate the plane of polarized light to the left; *cf d*.

L.: *Lactobacillus*.

L1: (1) *see* **LINE-1**; (2) a 1241-amino acid member of the immunoglobulin superfamily composed of 80K and 140K subunits, with domains resembling those of fibronectin, the receptors for platelet derived growth factor (PDGF) and macrophage colony stimulating factor (M-CSF), and the tyrosine kinase transforming protein of a feline sarcoma virus. It mediates neuron:neuron adhesion, neurite outgrowth on Schwann cells, neurite fasciculation, cerebellar granule migration, and intestinal crypt epithelial cell interactions.

L6: a myoblast cell line used to study skeletal muscle differentiation.

L34: a tumor cell surface antigen related to mac-1.

L 692,400: a synthetic agent that antagonizes the effects of **L 692,429** (*q.v.*) and GHRP-6, but not of growth hormone releasing hormone (GRH) on the secretion of growth hormone.

L 692,429: 3-amino-3-methyl-*N*-(2,3,4,5-tetrahydro-2-oxo-1-{[2'-(1*H*-tetrazol-5-yl)(1,1,-biphenyl)-4-y]methyl}-1*H*-benzazepin-3(*R*-yl)butanamide; a potent, orally effective growth hormone secretagogue with properties similar to those of GHRP-6. It opposes somatostatin, activates a protein kinase C isozyme, depolarizes somatotropes and elevates cAMP levels. Antagonism by nifedipine, but not ω-conotoxin are consistent with effects on L-type CA^{2+} channels. Potential uses include treatment of children with growth hormone deficiency, anabolic effects in elderly persons and prevention of osteoporosis, acceleration of burn healing, stimulation of T lymphocyte development, synergism with gonadotropins for ovulation induction, and antagonism of the catabolic influences of glucocorticoids.

La: lanthanum.

L 692,429

label: a radioactive isotope, fluorescent compound, enzyme, electron-dense substance, or other marker used to identify macromolecules, metabolites, organelles, or other entities.

labetalol: 2-hydroxy-5-[1-hydroxy-2-[(1-methyl-3-phenylpropyl)amino]ethyl]benzamide; a mixture of four diastereoisomers used to treat hypertension. Its components directly promote vasodilation and inhibit the type 1 pathway for neuronal uptake of norepinephrine. The *R,R* form, which accounts for much of the pharmacological activity, is a potent competitive antagonist for β_1-type adrenergic receptors, a weak α_1 antagonist, and a partial agonist for the β_2-type. The *S,R* isomer is a more effective α_1 antagonist.

labia: plural of labium.

labia majora: the most prominent parts of mammalian female external genitalia, composed of two large cutaneous folds that course downward and backward from the mons pubis. They develop from the embryonic genital swellings (which fuse in males to form the scrotum).

labia minora: two small cutaneous folds that lie between the labia majora and the vaginal orifice. They develop from the embryonic genital folds (which contribute to formation of the shaft of the penis in males).

labium: a lip or liplike structure.

labor: *see* **parturition**.

labyrinth: (1) the acellular fetal part of the placenta of rats and some other mammals; (2) the inner ear chamber, composed of a bony labyrinth (a series of channels in the temporal bone), lined by a membranous labyrinth separated from the bony part by perilymph and divided into compartments filled with endolymph.

lac: *see lac* **operon**.

LAC-I: lipoprotein associated coagulation inhibitor.

LACA: l-azetidine-2-carboxylic acid; a proline analog and antagonist, initially obtained from lily-of-the-valley (*Convallaria majalis*) and some other plants, that promotes formation of abnormal proteins, inhibits the growth of *E. coli*, blocks seed germination in many plant species, and slows collagen synthesis. It is used as a laboratory tool to inhibit laminin and fibronectin deposition, aggregation of immature Sertoli cells into sex cords, Leydig cell differentiation, and other morphogenetic processes.

lacis: a network.

lacis cells: phagocytic mesangial (Goormaghtigh, agranular JG, pseudo-Meisserian) cells of the juxtaglomerular apparatus, located mostly external to the glomeruli, between the afferent and efferent arterioles. They extend intertwining cytoplasmic processes that abut on other cell types, are part of the vascular cuff (Polkissen), and may contribute to blood pressure control. They contain, but are not believed to synthesize renin.

lac **operon**: lactose operon; a cluster of *E. coli* genes (*x*, *y*, and *z*) controlled by a single promoter that directs formation of a messenger RNA which codes for β-galactosidase, galactoside permease, and galactoside transacetylase. In cells supplied with glucose, lactose repressor protein binds to the promoter and inhibits transcription. Bacteria transferred to lactose media synthesize allolactose, a metabolite that binds to the repressor and lifts the inhibition. Glucose deprivation causes accumulation of cyclic adenosine monophosphate, which exerts positive control via CRP (cAMP regulator protein). That protein binds both cAMP and a DNA region contiguous with the *lac* operon.

lac **repressor**: lactose repressor; *lac* repressor protein; a tetrameric protein composed of 37K subunits that binds to *lac* operons and inhibits transcription.

lacrimal glands: lachrymal glands; tear glands.

lactacidosis: metabolic acidosis caused by lactic acid accumulation. Some older oral hypoglycemic agents used to treat diabetes mellitus invoke the condition; *cf* **ketoacidosis**.

lactagogues: galactagogues; agents that stimulate lactation.

lactalbumin: milk albumin; α-lactalbumin, β-lactoglobulin, and some similar milk and colostrum proteins that resemble serum albumin and differ from caseins.

α-**lactalbumin**: *see* **lactose synthetase**.

β-**lactamase**: cephalosporinase; penicillinase; an enzyme made by some bacteria that catalyzes penicillin lactam ring hydrolysis, and thereby confers resistance to the antibiotics.

lactases: enzymes that catalyze: lactose + $H_2O \rightarrow$ glucose + galactose. Substantial amounts are expressed on the surfaces of intestinal cells of healthy infants and children. The synthesis declines with age in many individuals, and leads to development of lactose intolerance. Bacteria make β-galactosidases.

lactate: (1) to secrete milk; (2) the lactic acid ion, made via: pyruvate + NADH + $H^+ \rightleftarrows$ lactate + NAD^+. Large amounts are made during vigorous contraction, because glycolysis provides the substrate, and the skeletal muscle lactate dehydrogenase isozyme (with high affinity for pyruvate) drives the reaction to the right. The reaction diminishes fatigue otherwise caued by low cytosolic pH and fuel shortage, by removing free H^+, and converting NADH to NAD^+ (the form required for glycolysis). Unlike pyruvate, lactate diffuses out of the cells. Much of it travels to the liver (in which it serves as a glucose precursor). Some is used directly as fuel by cardiac myocytes and a few other cell types. Circulating lactate improves oxygenation and hastens CO_2 loss by lowering blood pH, and thereby stimulating the respiratory center in the medulla oblongata. Epinephrine raises blood glucose levels mostly by accelerating glycogenolysis (and thereby glycolysis) in muscle. Some circulating lactate is excreted by the kidneys. Sweat glands can accumulate substantial quantities; and small amounts enter saliva. Parathyroid hormone augments lactate formation in bone, where the ion binds calcium ions and facilitates their transport to extracellular fluids. Lactate is also made by some anaerobic bacteria (*see* ***Lactobacillus***), and by invertebrates.

$$
\begin{array}{c}
COO^- \\
| \\
H\,COH \\
| \\
CH_3
\end{array}
$$

lactate dehydrogenase: L-lactate dehydrogenase; lactic dehydrogenase; LDH; tetrameric cytosolic enzymes that catalyze: lactate + $NAD^+ \rightleftarrows$ pyruvate + NADH. Five isozymes, named for the numbers of M (skeletal muscle) and H (heart) 35K subunits, differ in tissue distributions, and can be used as markers in cell fractionation studies. Skeletal muscle makes mostly M_4, with high affinity for pyruvate that favors lactate production. Liver and heart contain mostly H_4, which binds more tightly to lactate and drives the reverse reaction. (Other kinds are M_3H, M_2H_2, and MH_3.) The amounts of enzyme leaked to the blood stream in conditions such as myocardial infarction, hepatocellular necrosis, infectious mononucleosis, diabetic ketosis, sickle-cell anemia, and malignant lymphoma are used to assess tissue damage.

lactation: milk synthesis and release.

lactic acid: 2-hydroxypropionic acid; *see* **lactate**.

lacteals: central lymph vessels of intestinal villi. They absorb finely dispersed dietary lipids and transport them to larger lymphatic vessels. When filled with chyle, they acquire a milky appearance.

Lactobacillus: a genus of gram positive, lactic acid producing bacilli. Non-pathogenic srains inhabit the normal human mouth, intestine, and vagina, and are ingested with yogurt and other foods. They provide some protection against harmful microorganisms.

lactoferrin: lactotransferrin.

lactoflavin: riboflavin.

lactogenesis: milk synthesis.

lactogens: agents that stimulate mammary gland maturation and/or milk production. *See* also **placental lactogens** and **prolactin**.

lactoglandin: a neurophysin-like protein made in mammary glands.

lactoglobulin: a lactalbumin component, composed of 18K globular proteins that form dimers and larger complexes. It is a major constituent of cow milk whey, but only small amounts occur in the milk of humans and many other species. *See* also **placental protein-14**.

lactonases: enzymes that catalyze hydrolysis of 6-phosphogluconolactone (a metabolite of the hexose monophosphate pathway), and of some other lactones.

lactones: organic compounds with internal ester bonds formed when a —COOH on a carbon chain reacts with a —COH at a different position, water is released, and a ring is formed; *see* for example 6-**phosphogluconolactone**.

lactoperoxidase: a heme-containing milk protein with properties similar to those of thyroperoxidase that acts on most of the same substrates, and may perform bactericidal functions. It is used to generate active iodine atoms for labeling membrane proteins.

lactose: milk sugar; glucose galactoside; 4-*O*-β-D-galactopyranosyl β-D-glucose; a component of dairy foods, digested to glucose + galactose; *see* **lactase** and **lactose synthetase**.

lactose operon: *see lac* operon.

lactose permease: a 47K integral membrane protein that promotes active uptake of lactate across the plasma membranes of some bacteria. Its synthesis in *E. coli* is directed by the *y* gene of the *lac* operon.

lactose repressor: *lac* repressor. *see lac* operon.

lactose synthase: lactose synthetase.

lactose synthetase: a mammary gland enzyme complex composed of galactosyltransferase (A protein) plus α-lactalbumin (B-protein.) During pregnancy, the glands contain mostly A protein, because high progesterone levels inhibit synthesis of B type. The reaction then catalyzed is: UDP-galactose + *N*-acetylglucosamine → *N*-acetyllactosamine + UDP. Following parturition (when progesterone levels fall), prolactin induces B protein. This changes the substrate affinity, so that glucose (rather than *N*-acetylglucosamine) is used. In milk-producing glands the reaction is: UDP-galactose + glucose → lactose + UDP. *See* also **galactosyltransferases**.

lactotransferrins: lactoferrins; iron-transporting glycoproteins chemically related to serum transferrin, but with much higher affinity for Fe, made in mammary glands, liver, oviducts, uterus, vagina, kidneys, lungs, lymph nodes, spleen, and granular leukocytes (but not in testis, seminal vesicles, or epididymis). They are released to milk, saliva, and bile, and to uterine, vaginal, and seminal fluids and some other mucus gland secretions (but are not present in duodenal secretions, cerebrospinal fluid, or sweat). Neutrophilic leukocytes store them in granules, and release them during inflammatory reactions. Lactoferrins arrest bacterial growth by depleting their iron supply. At least two forms (65K and 70K) have different tissue distributions; and mechanisms for regulating the synthesis vary with the cell type. The known stimulants include estrogens in the uterus, prolactin in mammary glands, and interleukin-1 in leukocytes.

lactotropes: lactotrophs; mammotropes; mammotrophs; acidophilic adenohypophysial cells that secrete prolactin (PRL). The subtypes vary in synthetic activities and sensitivities to regulators; *see* also **mammosomatotropes**. Estrogens stimulate cell proliferation and hormone synthesis. PRF (prolactin release factor) is a general term for regulators that promote PRL release. Vasoactive intestinal peptide (VIP) is implicated as a major type during lactation. Thyrotropin releasing hormone (TRH) exerts some effects, but is not generally regarded as a major regulator, in part because thyroid stimulating hormone (TSH) and PRL levels do not rise in parallel. Unlike most adenohypophysial cell types, lactotropes are mostly under inhibitory control. PIF (prolactin inhibitory factor) is a general term for hypothalamic factors that exert the effects. Dopamine is a major type; and most PRL releasers act in part by lowering the dopamine levels. Gonadotropin-associated peptide (GAP) is another physiological inhibitor.

lactotroph: lactotrope.

lactotropic hormone: lactotropin; mammotropin; *see* **prolactin**.

lacuna: (1) a space or gap; (2) a small fluid-filled cavity, for example one that surrounds a chondrocyte or osteocyte. *See* also **Howship's lacunae**.

LAD: leukocyte adhesion deficiency.

laetrile: vitamin B17; a preparation obtained from the pits of apricots, peaches, and bitter almonds. Its major ingredient is amygdalin (D-mandelonitrile-β-glucosido-

6β-D-glucoside, shown below). Claims that it possesses antineoplastic potency have not been substantiated. Its toxicity is attributed mostly to the cyanide generated during amygdalin degradation.

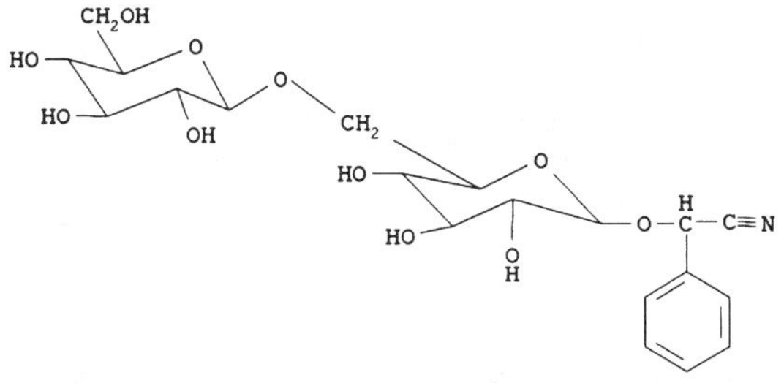

LAF: lymphocyte activating factor; *see* **interleukin-1**.

lagging strand: the nucleic acid chain that forms Okazaki fragments during **DNA replication** (*q.v.*). *Cf* **leading strand**.

Lagomorpha: an order of mammals that includes rabbits, hares, and pikas. Unlike rodents, they have two pairs of upper incisors.

LAI: leukocyte adhesion inhibitor; *see* **interleukin-8**.

LAK: lymphokine activated killer cells.

LAM-1: lymphocyte adhesion molecule-1; *see* **MEL-14**.

Lamarckism: an outmoded concept that acquired characteristics, such as changes caused by use (or disuse) of body parts, can be inherited, and can lead to the formation of new species. (The giraffe did not acquire its long neck by stretching for leaves on tall trees; but certain metabolic adaptations to changes in nutrients and other environmental conditions have been observed to affect traits that are passed on to the daughter cells of some organisms.)

lamban: *see* **phospholamban**.

lambda (λ) bacteriophage: a bacterial DNA virus initially isolated from *E. Coli* that undergoes cycles of lysis and lysogeny. The genome contains 48,502 base pairs and directs formation of 60 or more proteins. It is used as a cloning vector, and for studies of transcription control.

lambda chain: *see* **L chain**.

lamella: a thin layer or sheet, for example of an osteon.

lamellipodia: ruffled edges; layered cytoplasmic projections that mediate attachments to solid surfaces, present for example on some fibroblasts.

lamellocytes: discoidal blood cells that encapsulate foreign objects, and produce melanins. Endoparasitic wasps protect their eggs against host defenses by injecting virus-like particles with lamellolysin activity.

lamins: fibrous proteins that self-assemble into filaments, form continuous networks along the nucleoplasmic faces of the inner layers of somatic cell nuclear envelopes, and complex with nuclear pore components. A single gene directs the synthesis of both A (70K) and C (60K) types, which display homologies to intermediate filament proteins, and contain *C*-terminal domains similar to keratin amino acid sequences. They bind chromatin, and anchor interphase chromosomes to nuclear membranes. Observations that they become hyperphosphorylated, disassemble, and dissociate from membranes during prophase, and then reassemble and re-associate during telophase, are consistent with roles in disintegration and formation of nuclear envelopes. Synthesis of lamin B (67K), which contains thioether linked farnesyl groups, is directed by a different gene that is regulated in part by methylation. It associates with nuclear membrane vesicles and is believed to target the vesicles to chromosome surfaces during telophase. Lamins disappear during spermatogenesis. Oocytes have just one type.

lamina: a thin, flat layer. *See also* **basal lamina** and **nuclear lamin**.

lamina terminalis of the organum vasculosum: *see* **OVLT**.

laminin: an approximately 900K, cruciform matrix glycoprotein, with one long (4000K) A chain shaft, plus two shorter (200K B1 and B2 subunit) arms, linked by disulfide bonds. It appears first in two-celled embryos, and probably contributes to control of cell migrations during early development. Epithelial, endothelial, Schwann, and muscle cells are among the mature types that secrete it to basement membranes. The molecules interact with receptors on cell surfaces, and have binding sites for Type IV collagen, heparan sulfate, entactin, and other extracellular matrix components. They lack the RGD (Arg-Gly-Asp) sequences found in many other extracellular matrix glycoproteins, but have YIGSR (Tyr-Ile-Gly-Ser-Arg) binding domains that mediate epithelial cell adhesion to underlying connective tissues, cell migration, spreading, and chemotaxis. Epidermal growth factor (EGF)-like domains that interact with integrins may account for their abilities to enhance the growth of cultured epidermal and some other cell types, and to affect differentiation. Laminins additionally promote neurite extension, and stimulate production of a metallo-proteinase that cleaves collagen. Roles in metastasis have been suggested. S-laminin is a related glycoprotein restricted to synaptic regions that contains related YTGLR (Tyr-Thr-Gly-Leu-Arg) domains. It promotes formation and/or stabilization of permanent synapses; *see* also **merosin**.

lampbrush chromosomes: large, actively transcribing chromosomes in the oocytes of some vertebrates, named for their characteristic appearance under low magnification. They contain hundreds of paired DNA loops covered with newly synthesized RNAs that extend outward from the main axis.

Langerhans cells: LC cells: epidermal stellate cells with long cytoplasmic extenions that take up antigens, process them, present the derivatives to T lymphocytes, and are implicated as mediators of delayed hypersensitivity reactions. The typical cell has a characteristic round or square inclusion (Birbeck granule), and cell surface markers that include CD1, class II (HLA-DR), and "nonclassical" MHC class I (T6) antigens. Many LC cells additionally express Fcγ receptors and receptors for complement factors 1 and 3; and some make interleukin-2-like growth factors and display cytotoxicity that is not MHC restricted. It has been proposed that one subpopulation originates in the bone marrow, and another in the thymus gland, and that interleukin-2-dependent subtypes are post-thymocytes. (Thymus gland interdigitating cells have similar properties.) The cells in skin migrate, carry antigens to the lymph nodes and spleen, and elsewhere, and can convert to lymph node dendritic cells identical with or related to lymph node interdigitating and/or veiled types. They differ from dendritic epidermal cells (which possess γδ chain type T lymphocyte receptors, and do not express MHC antigens).

Langerhans islets: *see* **islets of Langerhans**.

Langhans cells: L cells; cuboidal chorionic villi cytotrophoblast cells, used to study the synthesis of placental proteins.

Langhans giant cells: multinucleated cells in granulomatous lesions of individuals with leprosy, tularemia, and tuberculosis.

lanosterol: lanosta-8,24-dien-3-ol; an intermediate in pathways for biosynthesis of cholesterol, ergosterol, and related lipids, formed from squalene.

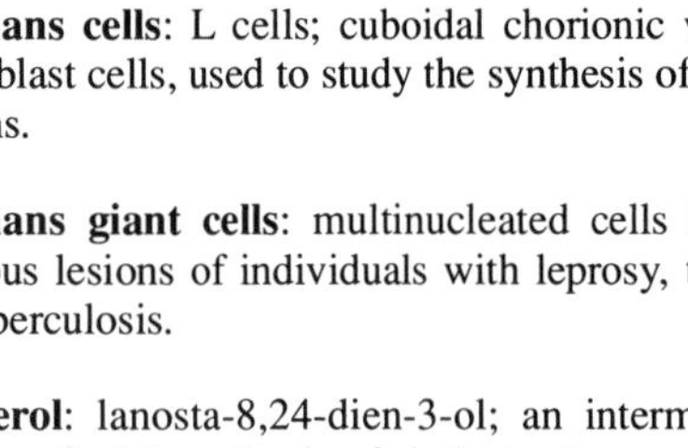

CH₃

HO

lanthanum: La; an element of the rare earth group (atomic number 57, atomic weight 138.906.) Although trivalent, the cations are similar in size to Ca^{2+} ions. They inhibit transport through receptor activated (but not voltage gated) calcium channels, and block mitochondrial Ca^{2+} uptake without affecting electron transport. Although they influence certain responses to Mg^{2+}, lanthanum salts are used to investigate some aspects of calcium metabolism, and also as negative stains in electron microscopy.

laparotomy: surgical incision through the abdomen, usually to gain access to the peritoneal cavity and its components.

lapine: derived from, or characteristic of rabbits and related species.

lap joints: intermediate structures formed during genetic recombination, in which gaps separate the ends of the broken DNA strands of two homologous chromosomes:

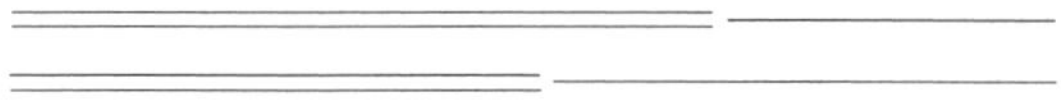

The two components of each strand later join:

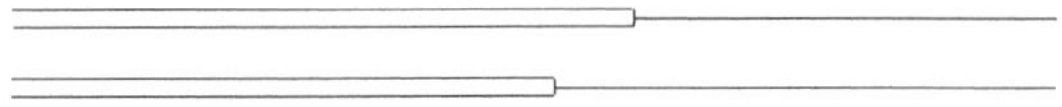

large external transformation protein: LETS; a high molecular weight cell surface protein that mediates cell:cell adhesions and interactions.

large granular lymphocytes: LGL: a morphologically defined subset of lymphocytes that accounts for approximately 5% of the population in human blood. Most have Fcγ, interleukin-2 and CR3 type complement receptors, display killer (K) and/or natural killer (NK) activity, and contribute to natural resistance against cancer and some infections. LGLs are also called null cells, since they do not have complete sets of characteristics for either B or T lymphocyte types. Immature precursors initially express some lymphocytes surface markers, but later acquire macrophage types; and some additionally make asialo-GM1 (a marker for monocytes and granulocytes); but they are neither phagocytic nor adherent.

large intestine: the distal portion of the gastrointestinal tract, named for its large diameter. It extends from the end of the ileum to the anus, and includes the **cecum** and **colon** (*q.v.*), and rectum (and also the vermiform appendix, which is not a digestive system organ).

large T antigen: *see* **Simian virus S40**.

lariat: a loop. A lariat forms during premessenger RNA processing when an endonuclease cleaves the bond between an exon and upstream intron, and a phoshodiesterase bond joins the cleaved region of the intron with its other end (which is adjacent to a different exon). The lariat is released when the link with the second exon is broken, and the two exons are joined.

Laron dwarfism: a form of growth retardation in which growth hormone levels are high, and somatotrope responses to growth hormone releasing hormone (GRH) are exaggerated, but little or no insulin-like growth factor-I (IGF-I) is made (and production cannot be stimulated with exogenous GH). Some individuals have abnormal GH receptors, and can respond to exogenous IGF-I. Others have postreceptor defects.

larvae: immature individuals of some species that hatch from eggs. The term applies to fish embryos, tadpoles, endoparasites, caterpillars, maggots, and other animal types.

larviparous: describes species in which zygotes develop to larval stages within the female reproductive tracts.

laser: (1) an acronym for light amplification by stimulated emission of radiation; (2) devices that generate and amplify electromagnetic radiation coherent in phase and frequency in the ultraviolet, visible, or infrared region of the spectrum, and produce narrow, intense, nondiverging beams. They are used in investigative and diagnostic procedures, to destroy pathological tissue in discrete regions, and to control bleeding during surgery.

Lasix: a trade name for furosemide.

late genes: DNA segments transcribed after **immediate early genes** (*q.v.*) are activated.

latent: existing, but not detected; describes, for example infections whose effects have not as yet been manifested, or responses to a hormone that require time to develop. *See* also **latent period**.

latent period: the time interval between presentation of an exogenous factor and the first manifestation of a response. Its duration depends on the parameter measured. In endocrinology, the *absolute* latent period is the time during which no response to a hormone that contacts its target cells can be detected. The *relative* latent period extends from the earliest manifestation to when the maximum response for that dose is attained. Latent periods provide some information on the mechanisms of action. They are measured in seconds for effects mediated via plasma membrane transport or activation of preexisting enzymes, and in minutes if new proteins must be made with pre-existing messenger RNAs. Successively longer ones are required for synthesizing new RNAs, replicating DNAs, and passage through cell cycles. Triiodothyronine invokes a few responses rapidly, but maximum elevation of metabolic rates requires weeks to develop.

latent virus: a virus that does not invoke signs of infection in host cells until it is activated (for example by toxins, radiation, other viruses, responses to stress, or substantial changes in the concentrations of naturally occurring cell components).

lateral: side; away from the midline; *cf* **medial**.

lateral geniculate nuclei: bilateral clusters of thalamic neurons that receive inputs from the optic nerves, and mediate both visual perception and synchronization of body rhythms with photoperiods.

lateral hypothalamic area: LHA: hypothalamic regions that include the lateral hypothalamic, lateral preoptic, and tuberomammillary nuclei. They communicate with the limbic system and pineal gland via the medial forebrain bundles, and have been said to contain "feeding centers" and "pleasure-reward centers".

lateralization: functional and/or morphological differences between similar structures on the two sides of a bilaterally symmetric organism. The term is most commonly applied to the brain, in which the left side controls most motor functions on the right side of the body, receives sensory inputs from that side, and in most humans contains regions not represented on the right side that control speech. The "right brain" controls left side motor functions and sensations, and is said to be more prominently involved in three-dimensional sense, creativity, and abstract thought. The amount of lateralization varies from one individual to another. There are controversies concerning the separation of some functions (such as logical reasoning). *See* also **corpus callosum**.

late replicating X chromosome: in cell cycle S phases of proliferating mammalian somatic cells that contain two or more X chromosomes (including those of normal females), the X chromosome that persists in condensed states for longer time periods than its counterpart, and replicates later than the non-condensed chromosome. *See* also **X inactivation**.

Lathrus odoratus: the common sweet pea. LOA, an agglutinin extracted from it, binds to D-glucose and D-mannose, and to glycosides that contain those sugars.

lathyrism: a condition in which spastic paresis and sensory impairment of the lower limbs follows ingestion of peas of the *Lathyrus* genus. Laboratory animals fed large amounts also develop aortic aneurysms which can rupture. The active component is β-aminopropionitrile (shown below), an inhibitor of lysyl oxidase and some other enzymes.

$$H_2N - CH_2 - CH_2 - C \equiv N$$

Latin squares: diagrams used to design experiments that avoid errors related to improper assignments of treatments to experimental groups, and to assess the effects of a set of treatments when the responses are influenced by two or mote independent variables. In the example shown, the variables are the ages of the subjects, the kinds of agents administered (A, B, C, and D, which can be four chemically related steroids, or four different dosages of the same kind), and the hours (times of day) for administration. Subjects of each age group receive each of the treatment types, at each of the times. No letter appears more than once in any column or row, and no letter is omitted from any of them. The squares can be used in conjunction with analyses of variance to separate differences related to the treatment types from the effects of the other factors.

Hour:	6	12	18	24
age 15	A	B	C	D
age 30	B	D	A	C
age 45	C	A	D	B
age 60	D	C	B	A

α-latrotoxin: α-LT; a major protein in the venom of the black widow spider, *Latrodectus matans tredecimguttatus* that strongly stimulates and then paralyzes vertebrate myoneural junctions, and promotes exocytosis from small synaptic vesicles. It is an approximately 130K acidic, single chain molecule devoid of proteolytic and lipolytic activity that invokes massive release of acetylcholine, norepinephrine, gamma aminobutyric acid (GABA), and other small molecules, but does not act on large, dense core vesicles that contain peptide type neurotransmitters. It binds to a neurexin on presynaptic membranes and also opens divalent ion channels.

LATS: long-acting thyroid stimulator.

LATS-P: long-acting thyroid stimulator protector.

Laurence-Moon-Biedl syndrome: a rare autosomal recessive disease in which early manifestations include retinitis pigmentosa, mental retardation, obesity, and commonly also renal abnormalities and polydactylism. The levels of both luteinizing and follicle stimulating hormones (LH and FSH) are subnormal, but the testes can respond to human chorionic gonadotropin (hCG). At least half the victims have hypogonadotropic hypogonadism; and delayed puberty is common in others.

LAV: lymphadenopathy associated virus; *see* **human immunodeficiency viruses**.

LBP: lipopolysaccharide binding protein; *see* **CD14**.

L-cadherin: *see* L-**cadherin**.

l. caeruleus: l. ceruleus; l. coeruleus; *see* **locus ceruleus**.

L calcium channels: *see* **calcium channels**.

L-CAM: *see* **liver cell-adhesion molecule**.

LCAT: lecithin:cholesterol acyltransferase.

LC cells: Langerhans cells of the epidermis.

L cells: (1) intestinal cells that secrete glicentin and related peptides, including oxytomodulin and glucagon-like peptides I and II; (2) Langerhans cells; (3) Langhans cells; (4) a fibroblast line derived from C3H mice, used to support virus growth; *see* also **L cell conditioned media**; (5) null cells with killer (K) and/or natural killer (NK) properties.

L cell conditioned media: fluid collected from cultures of L cells (definition 4). It contains mast cell colony stimulating factor (M-CSF), and is used to support the growth of some hemopoietic cell types.

l. ceruleus: locus ceruleus.

L chain: *see* **light chain**.

lck: a proto-oncogene of the *src* family that codes for pp56^{lck}, a protein kinase expressed at high levels by T lymphocytes that associates with the cytoplasmic faces of CD4 and CD8, and is implicated in T cell development and functions. Soon after cell stimulation, CD45 promotes dephosphorylation of tyrosyl moieties on the enzyme, and thereby rapidly increases its activity. Insertion of a promoter from a Moloney murine leukemia virus leads to overexpression of the gene in lymphoma cells.

LD$_{50}$: the dose that kills one-half of a population exposed to a potentially lethal factor (such as ionizing radiation or a pharmacological agent) within a specified time period.

LDH: lactic dehydrogenase.

LDL[s]: *see* **low density lipoproteins, lipoproteins**, and **apolipoproteins**.

LDL receptor[s]: 115K transmembrane proteins that recognize apoprotein B-100, bind low density lipoproteins with high affinity, and promote endocytosis. They provide cells with cholesterol and other LDL components, and regulate plasma cholesterol levels. In fibroblasts, steroid hormone secreting, and some other cell types, the receptors reside in coated pits. After internalization, the vesicles fuse with endosomes, shed their coats, and deliver their contents. The lipids are retained within the cells, as transport vesicles that bud from the endoplasmic reticulum recycle the receptors to the plasma membranes. The human type has 840 amino acid moieties. Receptor defects, or inability to make sufficient numbers of normal types, leads to hypercholesterolemia.

LDL receptor related protein: LRP; a protein that mediates clearance of chylomicron remnants, and internalization of plasminogen activator-inhibitor, α_2-microglobulin-protease, and other protease inhibitor complexes. It is present on blastocyst surfaces, where it mediates internalization of receptor-protease inhibitor complexes, and is essential for completion (but not initiation) of implantation.

L-DOPA: levodopa.

LE: (1); lupus erythematosus; (2) leu-enkephalin.

lead: Pb; a heavy metal element (atomic number 82, atomic weight 207.2). When ingested or inhaled in vapor form, it is absorbed, taken up by erythrocytes, and rapidly distributed to soft tissues (especially liver and kidneys). Pb later deposits in bones, teeth, hair, and fingernails. Small amounts also accumulate in the neurons of basal ganglia and some other brain regions. The toxic effects result from binding to sulfur, oxygen, and nitrogen containing groups of a wide variety of biological molecules, and most obviously affect neuromuscular, gastrointestinal, renal, hemopoietic, and nervous system functions. Lead sheets are used as shields to protect against X-ray penetration.

leader sequences: signal sequences: 13-36 amino acid segments with at least one negatively charged and 10-15 hydrophobic moieties, at the *N*-termini of certain peptides undergoing elongation on ribosomes. Proteins whose synthesis begins in this way are destined for secretion, incorporation into lysosomes, or insertion into plasma membranes. Soon after the leader sequence is formed, a cytoplasmic signal recognition particle (SRP, composed of ribonucleic acids and proteins) binds to the ribosome and transiently slows or arrests peptide chain elongation. The SRP-ribosome-peptide complex then moves to the endoplasmic reticulum membrane and binds to an SRP-receptor (docking protein). The nascent polypeptide chain is then directed across the membrane to the endoplasmic reticulum lumen, in which translation is completed. Most leader sequences are cleaved by signal peptidases before chain elongation resumes; but a few secreted proteins contain segments that with comparable translocation functions that are retained in the finished molecules.

leading strand: the DNA strand that directly engages in replication without fragmentation; *cf* **lagging strand**.

leaky junctions: association sites for adjacent epithelial cells with low electrical resistances that permit intercellular exchanges of water and small ions. *Cf* **tight junctions**.

least squares method: a statistical procedure for calculating the line of best fit for a linear regression curve of a normally distributed parameter. The independent variable is plotted along the X axis. The theoretical value for $\overline{Y}$ (the average value of the dependent variable that corresponds to $\overline{X}$, the average value for the measured Xs) is then estimated. A line then drawn through points $\overline{X}, \overline{Y}$

shows Y values that yield the lowest numbers when the sum of $(Y - \overline{Y})^2$ is calculated. The slope of the line, b, = $\Sigma xy / \Sigma x^2$, where $x = X - \overline{X}$, and $y = Y - \overline{Y}$.

Lebistes reticularis: the guppy, a species of small fishes with short life-cycles, used for studies of development and factors that affect it, and to investigate sex chromosome inheritance and functions, and other genetic processes.

LE-CAMs: lectin binding cell adhesion molecules; selectins; endothelial cell leukocyte adhesion molecule-1 (ELAM-1), GMP-140/PADGEM, a protein known as Leu 8 in the mouse and TQ1 in humans, homing receptor LE-CAM-1 (Mel-14), and other molecules with carbohydrate recognition domains that display calcium-dependent binding to lectins. Specific types mediate adhesive interactions between certain cell types, for example circulating leukocytes and vascular endothelium, or leukocytes and activated blood platelets. They contribute to the accumulation of neutrophilic leukocytes and monocytes at sites of inflammation, and play roles in leukocyte migration into and out of the lymphoid organs. Participation in hematogenous dissemination of lymphoid malignancies has been suggested.

LE-CAM-1: *see* **LE-CAMs** and **Mel-14**.

LE cells: (1) neutrophilic leukocytes in the blood and spleen of individuals with lupus erythematosus that contain phagocytosed nuclei from other cells; (2) initially normal leukocytes that have been converted to LE types by exposure to antinuclear globulins in sera of individuals with the disease.

lecithin: (1) vitellin; (2) any 1,2-diacylglycerophosphoryl choline; *see* **phosphatidylcholine**.

lecithin: cholesterol acyltransferase: LCAT; an enzyme made mostly in the liver and delivered to the bloodstream (but also present in lymph and cerebrospinal fluid) that catalyzes: lecithin + cholesterol → lysolecithin + cholesterol ester. It acts mostly on high density lipoprotein particles (HDLs), and is activated by apoprotein A-1. The cholesterol esters are taken up by intermediate and very low density lipoproteins (IDLs and VLDLs). In a rare, inherited disorder manifested by development of corneal opacity early in life and atherosclerosis and renal dysfunction during the third and fourth decades, impaired ability to make the enzyme causes elevation of blood free cholesterol levels (with low cholesterol ester concentrations).

lectins: proteins or glycoproteins that bind with high affinity to specific kinds of oligosaccharide moieties of glycoproteins and glycolipids (*see* also **LE-CAMs**). Most animal types are integral membrane proteins with binding sites oriented to cell exteriors. Several kinds made by hepatocytes and Kupffer cells function as glycoprotein receptors. Different ones contribute to morphogenesis and cell differentiation, cell migration (including guided migration of postmitotic neurons along astrocyte processes, and of lymphocytes to and from homing sites), phagocytosis, endocytosis, agglutination, fertilization, oocyte activation, and other processes; and a few are binding sites for microorganisms. Plants use lectins for symbiosis and protection against pathogens. Some bacterial lectins bind to and agglutinate erythrocytes and other animal cell types. Preparations of plant seeds, bacteria, molds, hemolymph, hemocytes, sexual organs, albumin glands, and egg cells are used to study cell surface components. Their specificities permit identification of cell types and states of maturation. Some activate by promoting receptor clustering; and several kinds that bind to asparagine-linked oligosaccharides are mitogenic for receptive targets. Lectins immobilized on activated agarose are used to separate morphologically similar cell types with different immunological properties, and to collect glycoconjugates for analytical procedures. Concanavalin A, pokeweed mitogen, soybean and wheat-germ agglutinins, phytohemagglutinin, ricins, and the fava, lima bean, lotus seed, and peanut lectins, all obtained from plants, and several from invertebrates, such as *Helix pomatia* (a snail), *Limulus polyphemus* (a crab), *Homerus americanus* (a lobster), and *Limax flavus* (a slug), are among the more widely used types.

Lee-Boot effect: suppression or prolongation of ovarian cycles of mice and some other rodent species, when females are housed in groups and isolated from males. It is attributed to the effects of an estrogen-dependent pheromone released to urine that acts on vomeronasal organs of recipients, lowers luteinizing hormone (LH), and elevates prolactin levels. Urine-soaked bedding from the cages of other normal females, or from estrogen-injected ovariectomized animals can invoke the same responses in isolated female recipients (but urine from untreated ovariectomized animals is ineffective). The responses are abolished if the vomeronasal organs of the recipients are destroyed, or if dopamine (which lowers prolactin levels) is administered.

leeches: annelid worms of the genus *Hirudo*. Some species are used to remove blood from necrotic areas, as a source of anticoagulants (*see* **hirudin**), and in morphogenesis studies.

legal sex: the gender officially assigned to an individual, usually at the time of birth, and usually on the basis of phenotype; *cf* **chromosomal sex**.

leghemoglobin: myoglobin-like pigments in leguminous plant root nodules that bind oxygen, and thereby protect nitrogenase against degradation. Soy beans are a major source for investigative use.

legume: the pod or fruit of a pea, bean, lentil, or related plant that engages in symbiosis with microorganisms to accomplish nitrogen-fixation.

leiomyomas: benign neoplasms derived from smooth muscle cells. Uterine fibroid tumors are the most common types.

Leishmania: a genus of flagellate protozoa of the Trypanosome family. Various species undergo early development in sandflies, and then infect vertebrate hosts and cause ulceration and other mucocutaneous diseases.

They are disseminated via lymphatic vessels, and are ingested by, and live within macrophages.

Leishman stain: a mixture that contains methylene blue and eosin in absolute alcohol, used for differential staining of leukocytes on blood smears.

lek: a site where males of a species congregate for courtship displays to females. The term is usually applied to bird, reptile, and other animal types in which females select their mates.

lemma: an outer membrane or sheath; *see*, for example **oolemma** and **neurilemma**.

lentiviruses: transmissible retroviruses that invoke slow, progressive effects after long, usually asymptomatic latent periods.

leprosy: chronic, progressive diseases that destroy body tissues caused by *Microbacterium leprae*, in which cellular (but not humoral) immunity is severely impaired. The organisms have waxy coats that protect them against attack by lysosomal enzymes, and can survive in Schwann cells and macrophages.

leptotene: the first of five stages of meiotic prophase, during which replicated chromosomes appear as thin threads with clearly defined chromomeres. It is followed by zygotene.

lergotrile: 2-chloro-6-methyl-8β-cyanomethyl-ergoline; a semi-synthetic ergot alkaloid derivative that exerts dopamine-like inhibition of prolactin secretion. It was initially developed to treat Parkinson's disease, but hepatotoxicity precludes its use for this purpose.

Lesh-Nyhan Syndrome: an X-linked recessive disease in which synthesis of hypoxanthine guanine phosphoribosyltransferase (HPRT) is impaired. The manifestations include uric acid accumulation, as well as mental retardation and other developmental defects, and self-destructive behavior. Afflicted males do not usually survive beyond childhood. Because of random X chromosome inactivation, only some cells of female heterozygotes lack the enzyme.

lethal mutations: DNA defects that cause premature death.

let-down factor: milk let-down factor; *see* **oxytocin**.

Leu: L; leucine.

Leu antigens: glycoproteins that bind antibodies directed against murine immune system cells. Most are similar to or identical with antigens known by other names (see

table). Distinctions are made between B and T lymphocyte types (*see* **Lyb** and **Lyt**).

Leu 1: CD5, T1, Ly1	Leu 6: CD1, T6
Leu 2: CD8, T8, Lyt2,3, OKT8	Leu 7: natural killer cell antigen
Leu 3: CD4, T4, L3T4, OKT4	Leu 11: Fcγ receptor
Leu 4: CD3, T3, OKT3	Leu 15: CR3, Mac-1, OKM1
Leu 5: CD2, T11	

leucine: L; Leu; 2-amino-4-methyl valeric acid; α-amino isocaproic acid; a hydrophobic, ketogenic, essential amino acid. It is a component of the active sites of some enzymes and of many other proteins, an energy source, and a stimulant for insulin and growth hormone secretion. Insulin accelerates its uptake by skeletal muscle and some other cell types. The degradation begins with deamination to yield α-keto isocaproic acid. Skeletal muscle uses the amino groups released to synthesize alanine from pyruvate. *See* also **leucine zipper**.

leucine aminopeptidase: a zinc regulated exopeptidase that catalyzes removal of *N*-terminal amino acids from many peptides and proteins (but not ones with terminal arginine or lysine moieties). Preparations are used to analyze amino acid sequences.

leucine zipper: an α-helix configuration within a protein molecule, with leucyl moieties at every seventh position, located adjacent to a region rich in basic amino acids. The helix can interdigitate with similar configurations on other proteins to form noncovalently associated homodimers or heterodimers, in which the basic amino acids contribute to the binding. Leucine zippers within receptors for steroid and some other hormones, and within Jun, Fos, and other transcription factors, mediate dimerizations essential for functional binding to DNA segments, and, in some cases, for interactions with other regulatory factors.

leuco-: leuko-; a prefix meaning white.

leucocyte: leukocyte.

leucovorin: folinic acid; 5-formyltetrahydrofolate; CF; **citrovorum factor** (*q.v.*); a ubiquitous compound made from 5,10-methenyltetrahydrofolate via an irreversible reaction catalyzed by serine hydroxymethyltransferase (SMHT). The precursor can be restored by methenyltetrahydrofolate synthetase. Several derivatives of stored CF are essential cofactors for the biosynthesis of purines, pyrimidines, thymidylate, and methionine, and for other reactions that require transfers of one-carbon moieties. Regulatory functions are suggested by observations that it exerts slowly developing, but highly potent inhibition of SMHT, and of other folate-dependent enzymes involved in nucleic acid and amino acid synthesis. CF accounts for 10-15% of folates in vertebrate cells, with highest levels in the liver. Soy beans, rice kernels, some other plant seeds, and yeast cells store large amounts. It is an effective agent for ameliorating hematological and some other toxic effects of chemotherapeutic agents such as methotrexate in cancer patients, and an essential growth factor for *Pediococcus acidlactici* (formerly known as *Leuconostoc citrovorum*), *Lactobacillus casei*, and other microorganisms.

leu-enkephalin: LE; H$_2$N-Tyr-Gly-Gly-Phe-Leu; a pentapeptide cleaved from proenkephalin and prodynorphin that interacts mostly with δ-type opioid receptors, and to a lesser extent with μ types. It is made in the central nervous system, neurohypophysis, adrenal medulla, and gastrointestinal and reproductive system organs, by mast, helper T lymphocyte, macrophage, and other normal cell types, and by T cell lymphoma and mastocytoma cells; and it functions as a neurotransmitter, neuromodulator, and immune system regulator. Most effects (including some on the immune system) are mediated via influences on neurons, and many involve interactions with other regulators. In common with metenkephalin (ME), most of the roles in body defenses (including modulation of phagocytosis, cell-mediated toxicity, and leukocyte chemotaxis) are biphasic (stimulatory in low concentrations, but inhibitory at higher ones). They are also short-lived, because of rapid degradation by enkephalinases and aminopeptidases. LE is less potent than ME in many systems, but may interact with common receptors in the brain. The presence of peripheral receptors that do not bind ME, and developmental changes in the relative amounts of the receptor types synthesized, suggest specific functions.

leukemia: several malignant diseases of the hematopoietic system, in most of which leukocytes precursor cells proliferate excessively and fail to undergo terminal differentiation. Classification systems are based on both timing patterns and the cell type(s) involved. *Acute lymphoblastic* forms occur most commonly in young individuals, and the major circulating cell types are very immature lymphocyte precursors. Granulocyte and monocyte precursors proliferate in *acute myeloblastic* leukemia, which is more common in adults. Other terms applied to various acute forms include promyelocytic, myelomonocytic, monocytic, and lymphocytic leukemias, and erythroleukemia. *Chronic lymphocytic* and *chronic myelocytic* types develop slowly, and are also more common in older persons. In the former, most circulating cells resemble normal lymphocytes, whereas in the latter they are usually neutrophils and their precursors, but can include eosinophils or basophils. The major problems are leukocytosis, which impairs circulatory functions, and bone marrow invasion by leukocyte precursors that severely limits erythroid precursor proliferation and differentiation. *Leukopenic* leukemia is a rare type, diagnosed on the basis of neoplastic changes in the bone marrow, in which the numbers of circulating leukocytes can be subnormal, and susceptibility to infection is increased. Various forms of leukemia have been linked with gene mutations or chromosomal translocations that invoke excessive production of growth factors. The genes implicated include *myc*, *abl*, and *hox-2*. Human chromosome 11 is a major site for chromosome breakage that leads to dysregulation; *see* also **Philadelphia chromosome**. Several kinds of viruses invoke leukemias in laboratory animals and domestic cats. Environmental toxins and some pharmacological agents induce other forms of the disease. Calcitriols are among the physiological stimulants for cell differentiation; and analogs, such as 1,25-dihydroxy-16-23-yne-cholecalciferol, that are far less potent than the naturally occurring hormone for effects on calcium metabolism, can confer beneficial effects. Many kinds of leukemia cells express glucocorticoid receptors, and the steroids are used in high concentrations (usually in conjunction with other agents) to treat certain forms. Steroids do, however, exert undesirable side-effects (*see* **Cushing's syndrome**).

leukemia growth factor: one of the names applied to a member of the basic fibroblast growth factor family.

leukemia inhibitory factor: LIF; embryonal cell differentiation inhibiting activity, DIA; human interleukin for DA cells, HILDA; differentiation retarding factor, DRF, D-factor; hepatocyte stimulating factor III, HSFIII; melanoma derived lipoprotein lipase inhibitor I, MLPI; cholinergic neuron differentiation factor; a pleiotropic 60K glycoprotein cytokine known under many names because several investigators obtained it from various sources (including fibroblast feeder, ascites, testicular teratoma, hepatoma, and melanoma cells), and studied it under diverse conditions. Forms that diffuse freely, and others that anchor to extracellular matrices have been identified. The A type differs from the B in glycosylation but not amino acid composition. LIF is believed to function physiologically as a factor that maintains self-renewal of hematopoietic cell precursors. Its effects on more mature precursors vary with the cell types (stimulation of differentiation and inhibition of proliferation in some, and the opposite effects on others). The net influences lead to increases in erythroid and megakaryocyte components, and decreases in lymphocyte numbers. In cell cultures, LIF promotes proliferation of a murine interleukin-3-dependent (DA) cell line, and it additionally induces some mouse leukemia cells to differentiate to macrophages. A burst of LIF synthesis that occurs in endometrial glands around the time when blastocysts arrive in the uterus, and subsides soon afterward, suggests roles in implantation. The surge does not require the presence of viable fetuses, and does not occur at the usual time after conception if implantation is artificially or physiologically delayed; but it can be induced by estrogens during diapause. Although embryos are not known to make it, LIF maintains embryonal stem cells in a totipotent proliferative state by inhibiting differentiation (but is not directly mitogenic). In certain neuron precursors, it determines the kinds of neurotransmitters synthesized. Postnatally, LIF levels are low in most tissues, but are high in neonatal skin and in adult intestinal cells; and in mature individuals, the peptide stimulates bone remodeling and hepatic synthesis of acute phase proteins. The ability of injected LIF to induce cachexia and triglyceridemia in laboratory animals is attributed to inhibition of lipoprotein lipase.

leuko-, **leuco-**: a prefix meaning white.

leukocytes: leucocytes; white blood cells. Neutrophils (polymorphonuclear leukocytes), eosinophils, and basophils are named for the staining properties of their granules. Monocytes and lymphocytes are said to be agranular, but *see* **large granular lymphocytes**. *See* also individual leukocyte types.

leukocyte adhesion deficiency: LAD; an autosomal recessive disease that affects the synthesis of LFA-1 (lymphocyte function associated antigen-1), complement receptor 3 (CR3), and p150,95, and thereby increases susceptibility to recurring pyogenic infections. Leukocyte and phagocyte adhesion and mobility, interferon γ production, and natural killer cell activity are all impaired; but T cell functions are retained.

leukocyte adhesion inhibitor: LAI; *see* **interleukin-8**.

leukocyte adhesion proteins: members of the integrin superfamily of cell surface glycoproteins expressed on leukocyte cell surfaces with a common 95K subunit (CD18). They mediate cell-to-cell adhesion and contribute to immune system and inflammatory responses. The α subunits for LFA-1 (lymphocyte function associated antigen-1), Mac-1, and p150,95 are, respectively, CD11a (180K), CD11b (170K), and CD11c (150K).

leukocyte common antigen: L-CA; T200; CD45; carbohydrate-rich 180-200K cell surface glycoproteins with transmembrane and cytoplasmic domains, expressed on most leukocytes (but not on other cell types). In mice, they are identified with antibodies directed against Ly5. Their synthesis is directed by a single gene whose premessenger RNA undergoes differential splicing. Microheterogeneities result from differences in glycosylation, and to some extent phosphorylation. All L-CAs share certain antigen determinants, but some are specific for either B or T lymphocytes. They are believed to couple environmental signal perception with cytoskeletal responses.

leukocyte inhibitory factor: a 68K lymphokine that inhibits migration of neutrophilic leukocytes. It differs from migration inhibitory factor (whose activity cannot be inhibited by serine esterase inhibitors), and from leukemia inhibitory factor (although the acronym LIF has been applied to both).

leukocyte interferon: leukocyte IFN; IFNα; *see* **interferon α**.

leukocytosis: increased numbers of circulating leukocytes. Usually, only specific types are involved. The term *granulocytosis* is often applied to the increased numbers of neutrophilic leukocytes released when combatting bacterial infections. Eosinophilia occurs in allergic reactions and responses to some parasitic organisms. Certain kinds of infections invoke lymphocytosis or monocytosis. Basophilia is less common, but can be invoked by a few allergens. In most forms of leukemia, immature or abnormal cell types account for much of the leukocytosis.

leukocytotaxis: migration of leukocytes to sites of inflammation or injury.

leukodystrophy: several inherited nervous system diseases that lead to progressive loss of myelin. The manifestations include dementia, spasticity, cerebellar dysfunction, and both visual and somatosensory perception impairment. The most common forms are *metachromatic leukodystrophies*, in which autosomal recessive defects affect arylsulfatase A (an enzyme that catalyzes conversion of sulfatides to cerebrosides). Sulfatide accumulation destabilizes myelins, destroys oligodendroglia, and may directly damage neurons. *Globoid cell* types (Krabbe's disease) invoke similar effects, but are attributed to galactosylceramide β-galactoside deficiency, which leads to accumulation of galactosyl sphingosine (a metabolite that inhibits mitochondrial function). *Adrenoleukodystrophies* are peroxisomal disorders that block the ability to degrade very long-chain fatty acids. Both sex-linked and autosomal forms are known; and both can destroy adrenocortical cells before neurological symptoms develop.

leukoencephalitis: inflammatory disorders that affect mostly white matter components of the brain.

leukokines: lymphokines, monokines, and other peptides released by activated leukocytes.

leukokinin: an α-globulin precursor of tuftsin that is made in the spleen.

leukopenia: excessively low numbers of circulating leukocytes; *cf* **leukocytosis**. The causes include autoimmune disorders that destroy bone marrow tissue, exposure to radiation, some poisons, some therapeutic agents, and severe nutritional deficiencies.

leukophores: iridophores.

leukopoiesis: leukocyte formation and release.

leukopoietin: an uncharacterized stimulant for leukopoiesis. Regulators that may contribute to its effects on leukocyte precursor proliferation and differentiation include colony stimulating factors and some interleukins.

leukosialin: a major cell surface glycoprotein expressed on monocytes, granulocytes, T lymphocytes, and some B lymphocytes, that markedly affects cell surface charge, and is believed to play roles in cell activation and immune system responses. It may be identical with sialophorin (CD43). The distribution of isoforms that differ in *O*-linked oligosaccharide composition is cell type-specific.

leukosis: abnormal proliferation of any white blood cell type. The term applies to the manifestations of leukemias and some other malignant diseases, but not to the transient forms of leukocytosis that occur in response to allergens and infectious organisms.

leukotaxins: agents that promote directed movements of leukocytes.

leukotrienes: LTs; highly potent polyunsaturated carboxylic acids made by granular leukocytes, macrophages, basophils, mast cells, non-phagocytic lung cells, brain, and microvascular endothelium. Most are synthesized from arachidonate (AA), and have four double bonds (indicated by the subscript); but dihomogamma-linoleic, linoleic, and eicosapentaenoic acids are precursors of a few with three or five. The rate-limiting factor for biosynthesis is the availability of free substrates, which are liberated by platelet activating factor (PAF) and other phospholipase activators. 5-lipoxygenase catalyzes: AA + O_2 → 5-hydroperoxyeicosanoic acid (5-HPETE), and leukotriene A synthetase dehydrates the product to leukotriene A_4 (LTA$_4$), which is 3-(1,3,5,8-tetradecatetraenyl)-oxyrane-butanoic acid. Although LTA$_4$ is unstable, and can revert nonenzymatically to hydroxy-fatty acid metabolites, it is the precursor of other LTs. Leukotriene B synthetase catalyzes its conversion to leukotriene B_4 (LTB$_4$), 5,12-dihydroxy-6,8,10,14-eicosatetraenoic acid. Glutathione-S-transferase promotes LTA$_4$ combination with glutathione to yield LTC$_4$, N-[S-[1-(4-carboxy-1-hydroxybutyl)-2,4,6,9-pentadecatetraenyl]-N-L-γ-glutamyl-L-cysteinyl]-glycine; and gamma glutamyltranspeptidase catalyzes conversion of LTC$_4$ to LTD$_4$, N-[S-[1-(4-carboxy-1-hydroxybutyl)-2,4,6,9-pentadecatetraenyl]-L-cysteinyl] glycine. An amino peptidase acts on the product to yield LTE$_4$ (6-[2-amino-2-carboxyethyl)-thio]-5-hydroxy-

7,9,11-14-eicosatetraenoic acid. Addition of a γ-glutamyl group to LTE$_4$ yields LTF$_4$:

arachidonic acid → 5-HPETE + O_2	[lipoxygenase]
5-HPETE + O_2 → LTA$_4$	[leukotriene A synthetase]
LTA$_4$ + O → LTB$_4$	[leukotriene B synthetase]
LTA$_4$ + glutathione → LTC$_4$	[glutathione S-transferase]
LTC$_4$ → LTD$_4$ + glutamate	[gamma glutamyl transpeptidase]
LTD$_4$ → LTE$_4$ + glycine	[aminopeptidase]
LTE$_4$ + glutamate → LTF$_4$	[transpeptidase]

Various members of the group are extremely potent stimulants for vascular and bronchiolar smooth muscle, and for leukocyte activation, migration, and adhesion. They mediate some endotoxin effects (including restriction of renal blood flow and glomerular filtration that can in extreme cases lead to renal failure). They also depress myocardial contractility and decrease coronary blood flow, invoke asthma and other allergic responses, and contribute to injury associated with inflammation; and they are implicated in the etiology of arthritis, psoriasis, and other diseases. The slow reactive substance of anaphylaxis (SLR-A), a mixture of LTC$_4$, LTD$_4$, and LTE$_4$. LTB$_4$, is especially potent for stimulating polymor-

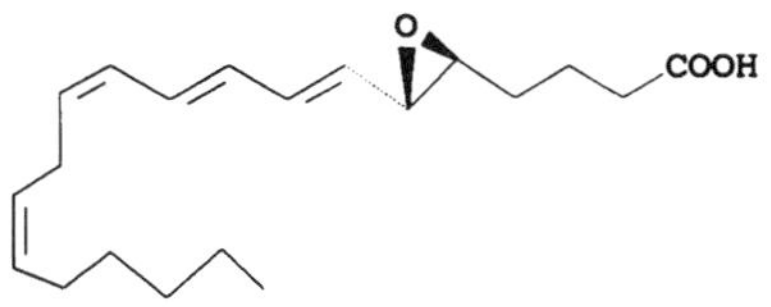

LTA$_4$

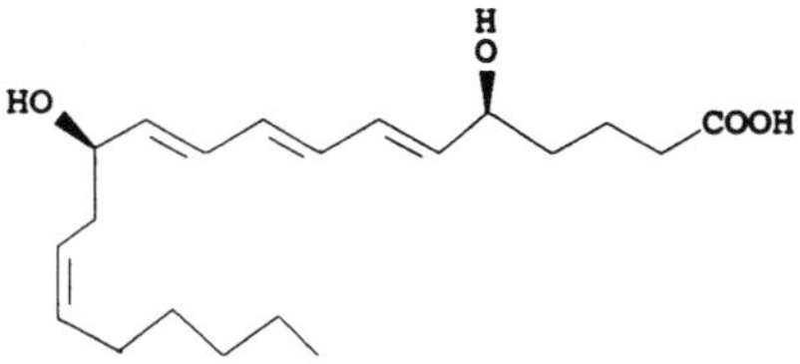

LTB$_4$

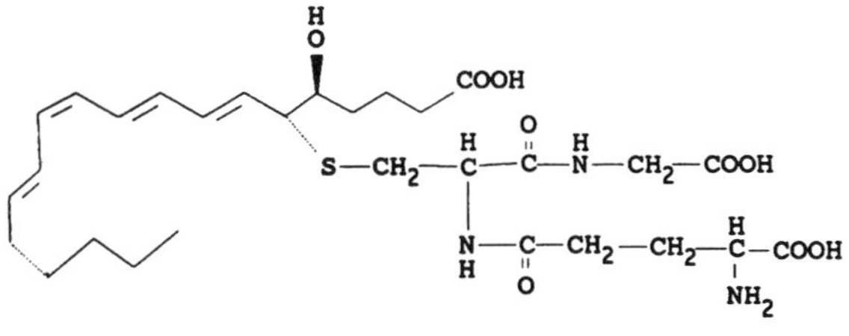

LTC$_4$

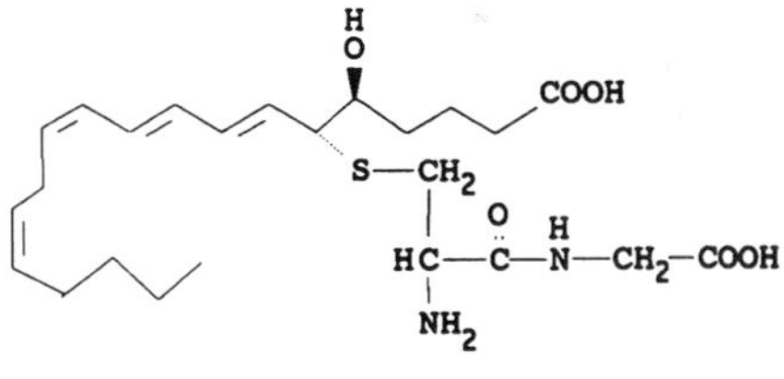

LTD$_4$

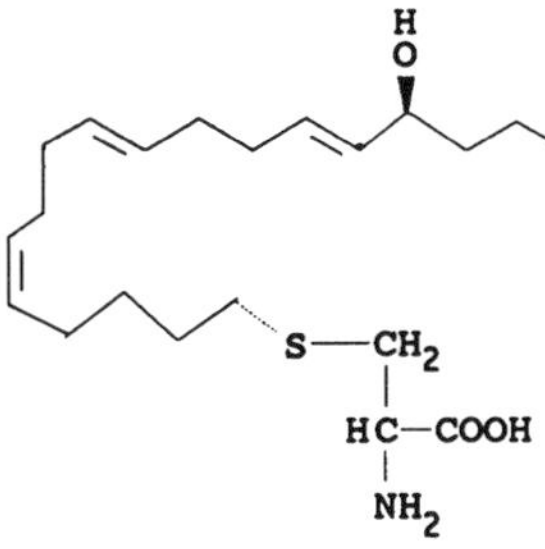

LTE$_4$

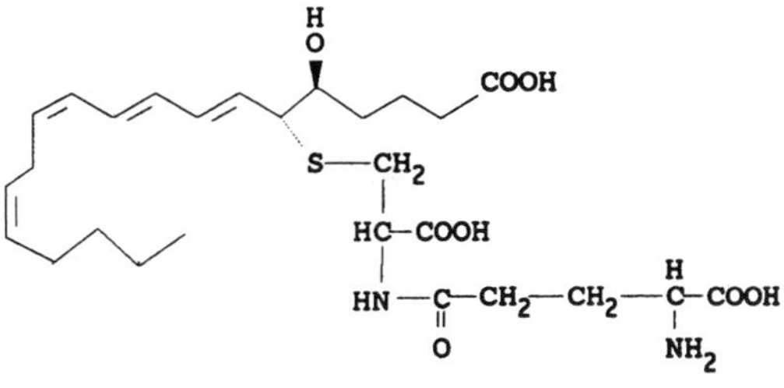

LTF$_4$

leukotrienes

phonuclear leukocyte chemotaxis, aggregation and adherence, and the release of oxygen radicals and proteolytic enzymes. In the hypothalamus, LTC$_4$ promotes the release of gonadotropin releasing hormone (GnRH), and also augments luteinizing hormone (LH) release via direct effects on the adenohypophysis. In the cerebellum, it activates Purkinje cells. C$_4$, D$_4$, and E$_4$ types all stimulate intestinal, uterine, and urinary tract (as well as bronchiolar) smooth muscle contraction, promote mucus secretion, and augment the permeabilities of postcapillary venules.

leukotriene synthetases: *see* **leukotrienes**.

leukoviruses: Rous sarcoma, Maloney, feline leukemia, and several other RNA retroviruses that invoke leukemia and tumor formation.

leupeptins: tripeptide serine-cysteine protease inhibitors derived from *Actinomyces* species. The term is most commonly applied to *acetyl*-Leu-Leu-Arg-hemisulfate. It can enter cells, is effective against plasmin, trypsin, papain, and some other enzymes, and exerts anti-inflammatory effects *in vivo*. When added to assay systems, it protects biological molecules against degradation by endogenous enzymes.

leuprolide: leuprorelin; 5-oxo-Pro-His-Trp-Ser-Tyr-D-Leu-Leu-Arg-Pro-ethylamide; a highly potent, long-acting gonadotropin releasing hormone (GnRH) receptor agonist. By desensitizing gonadotropes, it suppresses gonadotropin (and thereby gonadal steroid hormone) secretion. It is used (usually in acetylated form) to treat prostatic cancer, metastatic breast cancer, endometriosis, and idiopathic precocious puberty, and as a laboratory tool.

levallorphan: 17-(2-propenyl)morphinan-3-ol; a levorphanol analog and opioid receptor antagonist that alleviates respiratory depression and other effects of narcotic overdosage.

levamisole: tetramisole; (*S*)-2,3,5,6-tetrahydro-6-phenylimidazo[2,1-*b*]thiazole; a ganglionic stimulant that invokes paralysis in small animals, used to treat helminth infections and as a laboratory tool. It is also an immunostimulant that promotes T cell differentiation. High concentrations additionally inhibit fumarate reductase, and hepatic, placental, bone, and some tumor (but not intes-

tinal) alkaline phosphatases. In combination with 5-fluorouracil, it controls the growth of neoplasms.

levarterenol: the levorotary isomer of norepinephrine. Its effects are qualitatively similar to those of the naturally occurring dextrorotary form, but more potent.

levator ani muscles: striated muscles that support the prostate gland and draw the anus upward during defecation and copulation. A bioassay system formerly used for anabolic steroids is based on their abilities to promote dose-dependent growth in rodents.

levo-: a prefix meaning left, as in levorotary.

levodopa: L-DOPA; 3-hydroxy-L-tyrosine; dihydroxyphenylalanine; an intermediate in the pathway for biosynthesis of dopamine from tyrosine, via a reaction catalyzed by tyrosine hydroxylase. Unlike dopamine, it is orally effective, and can cross blood-brain barriers. Since it is converted to dopamine in the brain, it used (often in conjunction with agents that inhibit the systemic conversion) to treat Parkinson's disease; but *see* also **selegiline**.

levonorgestrel: the levo form of **norgestrel** (*q.v.*). It slows gonadotropin releasing hormone (GnRH) pulse frequency, and is incorporated into intrauterine devices to decrease menstrual bleeding.

levorotary: l; describes substances that rotate the plane of polarized light to the left; *cf* **dextrorotary**. L-isomers are not necessarily levorotary.

levorphanol: 17-methylmorphinan-3; the tartrate ester is an orally and subcutaneously effective synthetic narcotic analgesic.

levothyroxine sodium: L-thyroxine sodium: the sodium salt of the L isomer of **thyroxine** (*q.v.*), used to treat hypothyroidism and maintain hormone functions after thyroidectomy, In laboratory animals, it is used to study hyperthyroidism, suppress thyrotropin (TSH) secretion, and

levothyroxine sodium

maintain animals in euthyroid states when thyroidectomy is performed to investigate the effects of calcitonin deprivation.

levulinic acid: 4-oxopentanoic acid; an intermediate in the pathway for porphyrin biosynthesis; *see* δ-**amino-levulinic acid**.

levulose: an obsolete term for fructose (which, in its naturally occurring form, is levorotary).

Lewis acid: a substance that can accept electron pairs that are not necessarily associated with hydrogen ions; *see* **Lewis base**.

Lewis base: a substance that can donate electron pairs that are not necessarily associated with hydrogen ions. It can combine with a Lewis acid. The actions of several enzymes depend on such groups. *See* also **CD15**.

Lewis blood group: soluble blood plasma antigens that are adsorbed by erythrocytes.

Lewis reaction: localized formation of a red flare and elevated wheal in response to histamine.

Leydig cells: *see* **interstitial cells of the testis**.

LFA, LFA-1, LFA-2, LFA-3, LFA-4: *see* **lymphocyte function-associated antigens**.

LFD: least fatal dose; the smallest amount of a pharmacological or other agent that kills significant numbers of test cells or animals.

LGLs: large granular lymphocytes.

L-I glycoprotein: *see* **neural-glial cell adhesion factor**

LH: luteinizing hormone.

LH-RF: luteinizing hormone release factor; *see* **luteinizing hormone releasing hormone**.

LH-RH: luteinizing hormone releasing hormone.

LH surge: the rapid, massive release of luteinizing hormone (LH) that precedes, and is essential for ovulation, mediated primarily by a rapid rise in luteinizing hormone releasing hormone (GnRH) levels in most species with estrous cycles. In humans and many other primates, sustained high estrogen levels during the follicular phases of ovarian cycles promote LH synthesis and and storage in gonadotropes. Small amounts of progesterone released shortly before ovulation facilitate LH discharge.

Li: lithium.

libido: sexual interest, desire, or drive.

library: *see* **gene library**.

Librium: a trade name for chlordiazepoxide hydrochloride.

licorice: *see* **glycyrrhiza** and **carbenoxolone**.

lidocaine: 2-(diethylamino)-*N*-(2,6-dimethylphenyl)acetamide; an agent that elevates depolarization thresholds, especially in sensory neurons and cardiac Purkinje cells. It is used as a local anesthetic, and for long-term control of dysrhythmias.

lidocaine

Lieberkühn, crypts of: small intestinal mucosa pits that contain **Lieberkühn glands** (*q.v.*).

Lieberkühn glands: small, simple tubular glands, most abundant near the bases of villi in the small intestine mucosa, but also present in the large intestine. They produce a watery secretion that dilutes the luminal contents and provides a vehicle for absorption of small, soluble molecules. The stimuli for secretion include cholecystokinin (CCK), vasoactive intestinal peptide (VIP), and a 27-amino acid VIP-like peptide (PHM in humans, and PHI in several other mammalian species).

Lieberman-Burchard reaction: a colorimetric procedure for measuring cholesterol and related unsaturated sterols, based on generation of a blue-green compound with maximum absorption at 620nm when the test solution is mixed with concentrated sulfuric acid and acetic anhydride.

LIF: an acronym used for both leukocyte inhibitory factor and leukemia inhibitor factor.

Li-Fraumeni syndrome: high tendency to develop multiple malignant tumors in brain, bone marrow, mammary glands, adrenal cortex, colon, and other soft tissues, and in bone, attributed to a germline mutation that impairs synthesis of p53. The manifestations can begin during childhood, and can affect more than one organ. (When one cancer is removed, it is common for another to appear, especially after radiation therapy.)

ligaments: fibrous bands that strengthen joints.

ligand: a substance that binds with high affinity to another (usually larger) molecule. Hormones and neurotransmitters are ligands for receptors, metals for porphyrins, oxygen for hemoglobin, and oligosaccharides for lectins.

ligand gated channels: ion channels in membranes whose functions are regulated by organic signalling molecules such as hormones, neurotransmitters, or cyclic nucleotides. *Cf* **voltage gated channels**.

ligase: an enzyme that joins two molecules, usually in a reaction coupled to hydrolysis of a high energy phosphate compound and the formation of a diester bond; *see* for example **DNA** and **RNA ligases** and **synthetases**.

ligation: binding; in molecular biology, formation of phosphodiester bonds that link linear nucleic acid molecules.

light: (1) electromagnetic radiation with wavelengths of 180-1000 nm. Human retinal photoreceptors are activated by "visible" (400-700 nm) light. *See* also **pineal gland**. Ultraviolet radiation (180-400 nm) is required for photosynthesis and for vitamin D formation in the skin. Excessive amounts can damage DNAs and other large molecules and invoke mutations. Infrared radiation (700-1000 nm) is perceived as heat. Many analytical proce-

lignoceric acid

dures are based on absorptions at specific wavelengths. In *polarized* light, all vibrations are confined to a single plane. *See also* **bioluminescence, fluorescence, photosynthesis.** and **microscopy.**

light chain: L chain; usually (1) the shorter (kappa or lambda) polypeptide component of an immunoglobulin or related molecule; (2) the shorter chain of a dimeric polypeptide, glycopeptide, protein, or glycoprotein (for example of myosin).

light meromyosin: LMM; *see* **meromyosin.**

light microscopy: *see* **microscopy.**

light reaction: *see* **photosynthesis.**

lignoceric acid: $CH_3(CH_2)_{22}COOH$; tetracosanoic acid; a component of some cerebrosides.

LIM: a cysteine-rich, metal binding domain common to several proteins that acts on oxidation-reduction sensitive mechanisms for transcription control. The name derives from the products of three genes, *lin-11* (a regulator of cell division during vulval development in *C. habditus*), *Isl-I* (*islet-1*, initially identified as an insulin gene enhancer, but now known to be expressed, along with *SCI*, by motor neuron precursors during the earliest stages of differentiation), and *mec-3* (essential for neuron development in *C. habditis*).

limbic system: the brain region that apposes the medial walls of the cerebral hemispheres, and includes the cingulate gyrus, hippocampus, amygdala, fornix, and parts of the hypothalamus and midbrain. It is implicated as the site for regulation of mood, motivation, overt expression of emotions, and some autonomic and endocrine system functions.

limb bud: a vertebrate embryo structure composed mostly of mesenchyme surrounded by epithelium that gives rise to an appendage.

lime sacs: amphibian paravertebral organs that store calcium. Their functions are regulated by calcitonin, prolactin, and other hormones.

liminal stimulus: threshold stimulus; minimal stimulus; a stimulus with just sufficient intensity and duration to invoke a response; *cf* **maximal** and **supramaximal stimulus.**

limonene: 1-methyl-4-(1-methylethenyl)cyclohexene; an aromatic, irritating terpene component of citrus fruit skin and other plant oils.

limpets: marine gastropods with open conical shells. *Megathura crenulata* (the keyhole limpet) makes hemocyanin (a copper-containing respiratory pigment used as

an antigen to study immune system functions). *Patella vulgata* and other molluscs are good sources of β-glucuronidase and sulfatase.

Limulus polyphemus: the horseshoe crab. Its compound eyes are used to study visual system functions. Components used for other studies include hemocyanin and actin (which is not associated with myosin in the sperm). Its amebocytes contain a lysin that is activated by endotoxin.

lincomycin: methyl-6,8-dideoxy-6[[(1-methyl-4-propyl-2-pyrrolidinyl)carbonyl]amino]-1-thio-D-erythro-α-D-galacto-octopyranoside; an antibiotic made by *Streptomyces lincolnnensis* that blocks protein synthesis by binding to 50S ribosomal subunits and inhibiting peptidyltransferase reactions. It has been replaced for clinical use by clindamycin.

line: (1) a subpopulation of homozygous individuals phenotypically distinct from other members of the species; (2) a genetically distinct set of cells derived from a single parent cell; (3) a connection between two points; (4) a boundary between two areas.

LINE: long interspersed element; long interspersed DNA segment; *see* **LINE-1.**

LINE-1, L1: highly repetitive, adenine and thymine rich 5-7Kb DNA segments dispersed throughout mammalian genomes, located mostly in Giemsa positive bands. Since many are close to transcribed genes, roles in regulation of polyadenylation have been proposed. LINE-1 segments contain open reading frames, with reverse transcriptases and other sequences similar to ones made by viruses. Transposable types are believed to be made from RNA templates and then inserted. In humans, 10^4 - 10^5 copies account for 4% of the total DNA. A 38K protein product has been identified in teratocarcinoma and choriocarcinoma cells. Comparable DNA components in other species include *Drosophila* F elements, and a cin4 element in plants. *Cf* ***Alu*** **sequences.**

lineage: (1) direct descendants of a cell or a subpopulation of individuals; (2) a population with a set of genetic traits derived from an ancestral species; (3) a precursor cell type that differentiates along a defined pathway.

linear regression: statistical analysis of the dependence of measured values of Y (a dependant variable, such as rat prostate gland weights) on those of a chosen independent variable, X (e.g. log dose of testosterone administered), when both X and Y are continuous, and a straight line can join X,Y points. If X can be accurately measured, $Y = \alpha + \beta X + \varepsilon$, where α is a constant related to the parameters, β is the slope of the line, and ε is the random error for measuring Y. The positive value of β thus obtained lends support to the hypothesis that the weights relate directly to the hormone dosages. Over a limited dosage range, the slope can be used to predict Y values that were not measured.

Lineweaver-Burk plot: a graph in which the reciprocal of the reaction velocity (1/V) is plotted on the Y axis, and the reciprocal of the substrate concentration (1/S) on the X. This double transformation of the Michaelis-Menton equation yields a straight line whose slope = K_M/V_{max}. The Y intercept = $1/V_{max}$, and the X intercept = $1/K_m$. Graphs for competitive inhibitors of the same enzyme have common Y intercepts; those for noncompetitive inhibitors have common X intercepts. The effects of uncompetitive inhibitors show up as parallel lines.

lingual: relating to the tongue.

linkage: in genetics, the tendency to co-inherit two or more nonallelic genes that reside on the same chromosome. It occurs most often when the genes are close to each other. *See* also **crossing over** and **linkage disequilibrium**.

linkage disequilibrium: the preferential association of one allele with another on the same chromosome that leads to co-inheritance with greater frequency than would be predicted on the basis of random assortment. The tendency to inherit certain pairs of major histocompatibility alleles can contribute to familial patterns of susceptibility (or resistance) to some diseases. A normal gene linked to a mutated one can be used as a marker.

linkage equilibrium: the appearance (and random inheritance) of all possible combinations of linked genes in a population undisturbed by extraneous factors such as migration or selective mating.

linkage map: a diagram showing the relative positions of genes on chromosomes.

linkers: synthetic oligodeoxyribonucleotides with specific restriction endonuclease sensitive sites. They are used to clone DNA fragments and construct vectors.

linker DNA: a linear DNA segment that joins adjacent nucleosomes. It is less condensed than nucleosomal DNA, and provides recognition sites for restriction endonucleases. Although it does not bind most nucleosome histones, it associates loosely with histone H1.

link protein: a small, globular protein that noncovalently attaches the core protein (and its associated keratan sulfate or chondroitin sulfate groups) to hyaluronic acid in some proteoglycans.

linoleic acid: 9,12-octadecadienoic acid (18:Δ9,12); an essential fatty acid, ingested as a triacylglycerol component of corn, peanut, cottonseed and other vegetable oils. It (and several of its metabolites) are incorporated into animal triacylglycerols, phospholipids, and other lipids, from which they can be liberated by lipolytic enzymes. Liver cell enzymes catalyze its conversion to some longer chain fatty acid components of nervous tissue, and (via intermediates) to arachidonic acid and other eicosanoid precursors; *see* also **linolenic acid**. Some steps in the pathways (which involve dehydrogenation, rearrangements of double bonds, and chain elongation) are shown.

---

linoleic - 2H $\rightarrow$ linolenic   linolenic - 2H $\rightarrow$ γ-linolenic acid

γ-linolenic + 2C $\rightarrow$ dihomo-γ-linolenic

dihomo-γ-linolenic + 2H $\rightarrow$ arachidonic

arachidonic - 2H $\rightarrow$ eicosapentaenoic

---

linolenic acid: 9,12,15-octadecatrienoic acid; 18:Δ6, 9,12; an essential fatty acid, present in some plant oils, but derived mostly from **linoleic acid** (*q.v.*). It is incorporated into animal lipids, from which it can be liberated by lipases and esterases, converted to other unsaturated fatty acids, and serve as an intermediate for eicosanoid biosynthesis.

di-homo-γ-linolenic acid: 8,11,14-eicoastrienoic acid; 20:Δ8,11,14; an intermediate in the pathway for biosynthesis of eicosanoids; *see* also **linoleic acid**.

Lioresal: a trade name for baclofen.

linoleic acid

linolenic acid

di-homo-γ-linolenic acid

liothyronine: L-triiodothyronine.

lipases: enzymes that catalyze hydrolysis of ester bonds between fatty acids and other moieties. Triacylglycerol lipases (triglyceride lipases) degrade fats to fatty acids and diacylglycerols. Diacylglycerol lipases act on the products to form monoacylglycerols and fatty acids, and monoacylglycerol lipases degrade monoglycerides to glycerol and fatty acids. Lipases in pancreatic juice digest dietary fats. Adipose tissue types release fuels used by other cells. Hepatic enzymes provide fatty acid fuels to the liver, and release some molecules to the bloodstream. Commercial preparations are obtained from porcine pancreas, wheat germ, and some microorganisms. *See* also **lipoprotein lipases** and **phospholipases**.

lipemia: high blood lipid content. A transient condition that imparts an opalescent ("milky", lactescent) appearance to blood develops when lipid-rich meals are absorbed from the small intestine. More specific terms (such as triglyceridemia) are applied when the high levels persist. The causes include insulin deficiency (which lowers lipoprotein lipase activity) and inherited defects that impair formation of lipoprotein particles and/or removal of their associated lipids.

lipids: fats, phospholipids, glycolipids, steroids, lipoproteins, waxes, terpenes, and other organic compounds that are soluble in lipid solvents and insoluble in water.

lipid A: the active, membrane-associated component of endotoxin (lipopolysaccharide, LPS), released when infecting gram negative bacteria die. It attaches to macrophages via LPS binding proteins (LPS receptors), activates CD14, and thereby promotes the release of tumor necrosis factor-α (TNFα), interleukins 1, 6, and 8, prostaglandin E_2, thromboxanes, and platelet activating factor (PAF); and it also stimulates formation of hydrogen peroxide, nitric oxide, and oxygen free radicals. The resulting elevation of body temperature and immune system stimulation, in conjunction with macrophage products, contributes to defenses against the organisms; but excessive amounts of the cytokines can cause hyperthermia, hypotension, clot formation, and, in extreme cases, circulatory shock. Lipid A is a β-1,6-D-glucosamine disaccharide with two *N*-linked hydroxymyristic acid moieties, two *O*-linked phosphates, and three *O*-linked long-chain fatty acids, joined to the endotoxin O antigen by a deoxyketooctanoate trisaccharide. Gram negative bacteria incorporate it into highly ordered phospholipid membranes, in which LPS increases fluidity and decreases permeability. Mutants that do not synthesize lipid A are easily damaged by environmental chemicals, and cannot reproduce. Commercial prepara-

tions are used as immune system stimulants, to study the effects of the cytokines, and to elevate body temperature in laboratory animals. The various types from *E. coli*, *Salmonella*, and other microorganisms differ somewhat in fatty acid content. Newer synthetic ones have facilitated investigations, and hold promise for the design of therapeutic agents.

lipid bilayer: *see* **phospholipid bilayer**.

lipid droplets: cell inclusions composed predominantly or entirely of lipids. Most cells that synthesize steroid hormones store cholesterol esters in this way.

lipidosis: any condition in which excessive lipid is stored in reticuloendothelial cells; *see*, for example **Niemann-Pick disease** and **leukodystrophy**.

lipid vesicles: *see* **liposomes**.

lipoamide: 6,8-thioctic acid amide; a cofactor, synthesized from lipoic acid + lysine, for pyruvate dehydrogenase, α-ketoglutarate dehydrogenase, and related enzyme complexes that catalyze oxidative decarboxylation reactions. It accepts acetyl groups from thiamine pyrophosphate (TPP) and transfers them (via an acetyllipoamide intermediate) to coenzyme A.

lipoblasts: connective tissue cells that differentiate to adipocytes.

lipocaic: an uncharacterized substance in exocrine pancreas extracts that protects pancreatectomized dogs against developing fatty livers.

lipochromes: carotene, lipofuscin, and other lipid-soluble yellow, orange and red pigments.

lipocortins: calcium and phospholipid binding proteins that contribute to the anti-inflammatory effects of glucocorticoids. They decrease the availability of arachidonic acid for eicosanoid synthesis by binding to phospholipase A_2 substrates. (An earlier concept that lipocortins directly inhibit phospholipase A_2 has been discarded.) They are also substrates for several kinases; and they exert autocrine and/or paracrine effects, some of which are unrelated to the influences on the phospholipases. Other names introduced by investigators who isolated them from various sources include lipomodulin (from neutrophilic leukocytes), macromodulin (from macrophages), renomodulin (from kidneys), and endocortin (from epithelium). Additional sites of synthesis include thymus gland, spleen, skin, intestine, brain, and fibroblasts. Glucocorticoids induce the messenger RNAs, but other factors are needed to augment production of the proteins. Lipocortin I, which is identical to calpactin-II (p35), inhibits leukotriene C$_4$-induced release of thromboxane A$_2$, and also prolactin synthesis and release in the placenta; and it is believed to play roles in parturition. Lipocortin II is identical to the heavy chain (p36) of calpactin-I. There is approximately 50% homology between p35 and p36. A lipocortin-III has also been identified. Most cell types make at least two other members of the protein family, which includes protein II/endonexin, placental IBC (inhibitor of blood coagulation), human placental endonexin, and calectrin (p68/67); *see* also **annexins**.

lipodystrophy: lipid metabolism disorders in which fat stores are depleted in one or more parts of the body (and in some cases accumulate excessively at other sites). Generalized, severe conditions are often associated with lipemia, insulin resistance and other endocrine system dysfunctions, hepatomegaly, and/or nephrotic syndrome. Localized lipodystrophy commonly develops at sites of repeated insulin injection in individuals with diabetes mellitus.

lipofuscins: yellowish to brownish lipid-containing pigments, believed to be oxidation and polymerization products of lipids processed in lysosomes. They accumulate in granules of the cells of the testes, adrenal cortex, adipose tissue, liver, and pineal gland, in cardiac and smooth muscle, and in neurons, macrophages, and arteriosclerotic plaques. In some species, including humans, they impart the characteristic coloration of corpora lutea. The amounts increase with advancing age at some sites.

lipogenesis: fat synthesis. *See* **triacylglycerols** and **fatty acid synthetase.**

α-**lipoic acid**: thioctic acid; 1,2-dithiolane-3-pentanoic acid; pyruvate oxidation factor; protogen A; acetate replacing factor; a lipid initially identified as a growth factor for microorganisms, and once classified as a member of the vitamin B complex (but now called a pseudovitamin since animals can make small amounts). Lipoic acid is formed via oxidation of the thiol groups of 6,8-

dimercaptooctanoic acid, and it serves as the lipoamide precursor.

lipolysis: hydrolytic degradation of triacylglycerols. It is inhibited by insulin, and augmented by norepinephrine, glucagon, and other hormones. *See* also **lipases**.

lipomas: benign tumors composed of mature adipocytes that are normal in appearance.

lipomodulin: a name given to the **lipocortin** (*q.v.*) identified in neutrophilic leukocytes.

lipophilic: soluble in nonpolar solvents; hydrophobic; *cf* **hydrophilic**.

lipophores: erythrophores and other chromatophores that contain lipid-soluble pigments.

lipophorins: high-density lipoproteins in insect hemolymph.

lipopolysaccharide: usually (1) endotoxin (LPS); (2) any molecule composed of lipid and polysaccharide moieties.

lipoprotein[s]: although it can designate any compound composed of protein and lipid moieties (such as lipovitellin), the term is most commonly applied to particles with hydrophobic cholesterol ester and triacylglycerol cores surrounded by amphipathic layers of phospholipids, proteins, and free cholesterol. The particles can be separated by ultracentrifugation, and are classified on the basis of density. *Chylomicrons*, made mostly in the small intestine, transported to lymph, and released to the bloodstream, are the lightest, largest, and lowest in protein and phospholipid content, and the only ones that lack surface charges. They carry dietary lipids, mostly triacylglycerols (but also vitamin A, which is used as a marker), and absorb apo-E from other particles. Lipoprotein lipases hydrolyze the triacylglycerols, release fatty acids for use by all cell types, and convert them to chylomicron remnants which are taken up by the liver. (Some di- and monoacylglycerols are also released and further degraded by endothelium.). Electrophoresis terms applied to the others are pre-β (mostly very low density lipoproteins, VLDLs), "broad β" or slow β (inter-

Type	Density	Apoprotein [Types]	Cholesterol	Triacylglycerols	Phosolipids
Chylo-micron	<.95	1.7-2 [B-48; some C, E]	7-8	83-98 (5-6 ester)	7
VLDL	.95-1.006	8-9 [B-100; some C, E]	0-22 (13-15 ester)	50-51	18-19
IDL	1.006-1.019	9-19 [B-100; some C, E]	23-44	12-49	20-21
LDL	1.019-1.063	20-25: [B-100; some C, E]	45-46 (37-38 ester)	8-11	22
HDL	1.063-1.21	33-50 [A-I, A-II, C, E]	22-30 (18-23 ester)	4-8	23-29

lipoproteins

417

mediate density lipoproteins, IDLs), β (low density lipo-proteins, LDLs), and α (high density lipoproteins, HDLs). Apoprotein families are identified by letters, and subtypes within them by numbers (*see* **apolipoproteins** and specific types). Typical percentages of lipoprotein components are shown in the table, but the values fluctuate under physiological conditions, vary with age, and are affected by diet, several hormones, and genetic factors. Lipoprotein lipases are activated by Apo-CII (enzymes secreted by many cell types that reside on endothelial cell surfaces). Local controls over their synthesis affect fatty acid uptake. Carbohydrates and insulin promote enzyme synthesis in adipocytes, but fasting accelerates it in the heart, and factors associated with parturition increase it in mammary glands. Most VLDLs are made by the liver, and contain Apo-B100 (which is essential for their formation); but small numbers with Apo-B48 originate in the intestine. Their cholesterol content is affected by hormones and by saturated fatty acids. Lipases convert VLDLs to IDLs (VLDL remnants). During infections, tumor necrosis factor-α (TFNα) rapidly increases VLDL synthesis and processing by stimulating hepatic synthesis of fatty acids and inhibiting lipoprotein lipases. IDLs give up Apo B, C, and E and are converted to LDLs. The LDLs deliver cholesterol to cells via receptor-mediated endocytosis. They can increase prostaglandin and prostacyclin synthesis by providing substrate (but arachidonic acid and LDL receptors exert negative feedback control over PGH synthetase). The receptors reside in clathrin-coated pits. Adrenocorticotropic hormone (ACTH) and luteinizing hormone (LH) increase receptor numbers in adrenal cortices and gonads, respectively; and high cholesterol levels decrease them in fibroblasts and some other cell types. When LDL

receptors are saturated, and the lipid components undergo peroxidation or acetylation, macrophages also take up LDL cholesterol (and this contributes to atherosclerosis). Discoid, nascent HDLs are made mostly in the liver, but also in the small intestine. They take up free cholesterol from other lipoproteins, and contain a lecithin:cholesterol acyltransferase (LCAT) which is activated by Apo-AI, and catalyzes cholesterol esterification. The stored esters change the discoid particles to spherical HDLs. Three subtypes are known, HDLc, HDL₂, and HDL₃, but only the 2 and 3 types achieve high concentrations in blood plasma. They transport excess cholesterol to the liver, and thereby accelerate bile salt formation and lower circulating levels. Estrogens and polyunsaturated fatty acids elevate, and testosterone lowers HDL₂ levels, which are large (density 1.063-1.0125) and lipid-rich. The concentrations of HDL₃ (density 1.0125-1.21) are not affected by hormones or diet. They inhibit LDL interactions with platelets. In rats and some other species, HDLs are important sources of cholesterol for steroid hormone synthesis.

lipoprotein lipases: LPL; diacylglycerol lipases: enzymes that catalyze hydrolytic degradation of circulating lipoprotein triacylglycerols. They are made by adipocytes and some other cell types, and are present on endothelial surfaces of blood capillaries. Insulin promotes their synthesis, and heparin activates preexisting enzymes.

lipoprotein(a): 450K-750K lipoproteins that contain **apoprotein(a)** (*q.v.*).

lipoprotein-associated coagulation inhibitor: LACI; a glycoprotein that binds coagulation factors Xa and VII A, and inhibits the extrinsic pathway for blood clotting. It is made by endothelial cells and megakaryocytes, and is present in blood platelets.

liposomes: (1) lipid-storing organelles, for example ones that hold reserve supplies of cholesterol esters in adreno-cortical and other steroid synthesizing cells; (2) spherical particles formed by lipid bilayers that enclose aqueous compartments, used to study transport mechanisms. Artificially constructed liposomes can deliver specific kinds of molecules (such as nucleic acids and toxins) for therapeutic or investigative purposes. Most are rapidly taken up by reticuloendothelial cells.

lipoteichoic acids: compounds composed of **teichoic acid** (*q.v.*) and glycolipids in the cell walls of most gram positive bacteria. They mediate binding to host cells.

lipotropes: lipotrophs; adenohypophysial cells that synthesizes β-lipotropin; *see* also **corticolipotropes** and **corticotropes**.

lipotropic: fat mobilizing.

β-**lipotropin**: β-lipotrophin; β-LPH; lipotropic hormone; lipolytic hormone; adipokinetic hormone; 91-amino acid, single chain polypeptides cleaved from proopiomelanocortin (POMC), and secreted in equimolecular quantities with adrenocorticotropic hormone (ACTH) by corticotropes in response to stress and some other stimuli. Although β-lipotropins can release fatty acids from adipose tissue triacylglycerols, they are less potent than other regulators, and no physiological function has been established. The cleavage products in corticotropes and melanotropes include β-endorphin (amino acids 61-91) and related molecules, as well as γ-lipotropin (amino acids 1-58). The sequences for metenkephalin (amino acids 61-65) and some other opioid peptides are contained within the molecules, but those peptides are derived from other precursors (*see* **prodynorphin**). "β-melanocyte stimulating hormone" (amino acids 41-58) is not known to be cleaved under physiological conditions. Since β-LPHs have long plasma half-lives, they are used as markers for corticotrope secretory functions.

γ-**lipotropin**: γ-**LPH**: 58-amino acid peptides cleaved from proopiomelanocortin (POMC) that can be further cleaved to β-endorphin and other peptides.

lipovitellin: a 400K egg yolk lipoprotein cleaved from vitellogenin. Yolk platelets of many oviparous species contain complexes composed of one molecule of lipovitellin and two of phosphvitin.

lipoxins: tetrahydroxy polyunsaturated fatty acid oxidation products made by neutrophilic leukocytes, eosinophils, and other cell types, formed from 5,12-di-HETE (*see* **hydroxyeicosatetraenoic acids** and **lipoxygenases**) via a 5,6-epoxy intermediate. They modulate inflammatory reactions, exert other effects, and are implicated in the etiology of some pathological processes. Lipoxin A₄ blocks the actions of natural killer cells on some targets, promotes slowly-developing bronchoconstriction, augments capillary permeability, and facilitates the

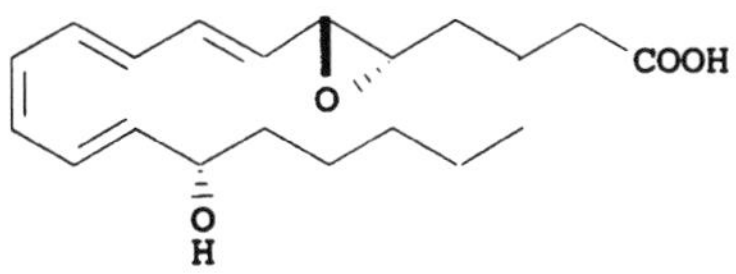

5,6-epoxy intermediate

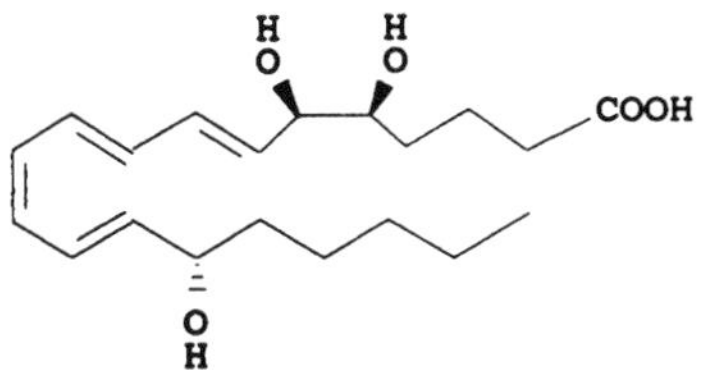

lipoxin A

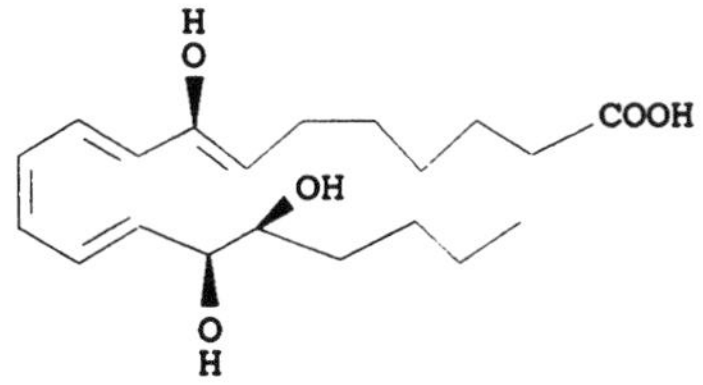

lipoxin B

release of hydrolases and superoxide free radicals by destabilizing lysosomal membranes. Lipoxin B shares the first two properties.

lipoxygenases: LOs; enzymes in leukocytes, macrophages, endothelium, and other cell types that convert polyunsaturated fatty acids to hydroperoxides and other reactive products. They are named for the carbon positions on which they act (*see* **hydroxyeicosatetraenoic acids**). 5-lipoxygenases are dual-function complexes that promote Ca^{2+} and ATP-dependent oxidation and dehydration. The leukocyte form comprises a 75-80K polypeptide chain plus one membrane-bound and two cytosolic cofactors. (Enzymes in other cell types may not require the same cofactors.) It converts arachidonic acid to an intermediate which rapidly forms 5-hydroperoxyeicosatetraenoic acid (5-HPETE). The latter is a direct precursor of both 5-hydroxyeicosatetraenoic acid (5-HETE) and leukotriene A_4. The same enzyme converts 15-HPETE (formed in a 15-lipoxygenase reaction) to 5,6- and 14,15- epoxytetraenes. Opening of the epoxide rings then yields lipoxins A and B, and their isomers. 15-HETE is chemotactic for circulating monocytes, and it acts on endothelial cells to promote the release of several derivatives with similar properties. It additionally stimulates endothelial cell mitosis, and can damage those cells. The likelihood that it contributes to atherosclerosis is supported by observations that it accelerates vascular smooth muscle migration and oxidizes low density lipoproteins. 12-lipoxygenase generates 12-HPETE (and 12-HETE), and also acts on 5-HPETE to yield 5,12-di-HPETE and 5,12-di-HETE. Related enzymes promote formation of 8,15-di-HETE and other hydroxy acids. Plants make lipoxygenases; and soybean preparations are used in some studies.

liquid scintillation counters: devices for measuring radioactivity, in which light flashes emitted when ionizing particles or electromagnetic photons strike dissolved fluorescent chemicals are captured by photomultiplier tubes, transformed into electric pulses, amplified, and routed through scalers for counting.

lisinopril: Zestril; Novatec; Vivatec; (*S*)-1-[N^2-(1-carboxy-3-phenylpropyl)-L-proline dihydrate; a long-acting, orally effective angiotensin converting enzyme inhibitor (which also slows kallidin degradation). It is used to treat some forms of hypertension.

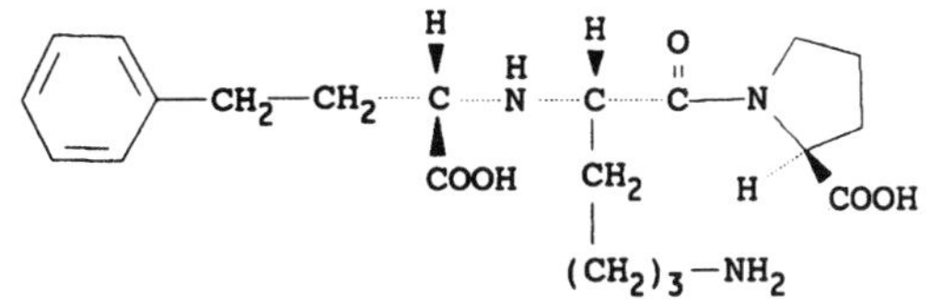

Lissamine: rhodamine B.

Lissauer, tract of: tractus dorsolateralis; a small fascicle of myelinated and unmyelinated fibers near the surface of the spinal cord on each side, between the dorsal and lateral funiculi. It transmits messages from receptors for pain, touch, proprioception, and heat.

lisuride: 3-(9,10-didehydro-6-methyl-ergolin-8α-yl)-1, 1-diethylurea; a D_2-type dopamine receptor agonist, D_1-type antagonist, and partial serotonin agonist. It is used (outside the United States) to treat Parkinson's disease, suppress prolactin secretion, and relieve migraine headaches, but can invoke hallucinations and other psychic dysfunctions.

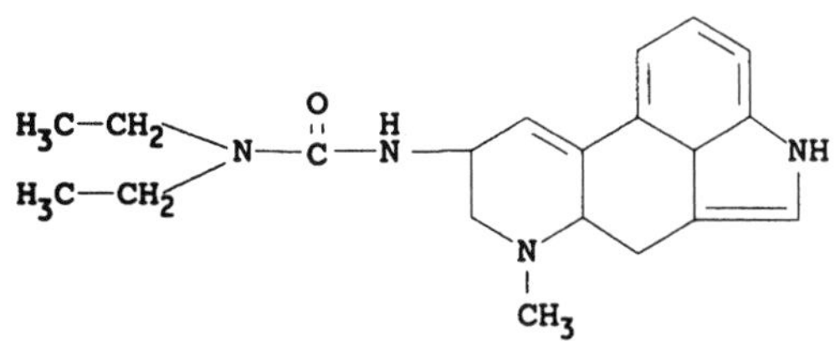

lith-: a prefix meaning stone, as in lithiasis.

lithiasis: the presence of calculi, usually in the kidneys or gallbladder.

lithium: Li; an element (atomic number 3, atomic weight 6.941). Li^+ blunts the responses of many cell types to their natural stimulants, in part by inhibiting several phosphatases. By slowing inositol-1-phosphate hydrolysis, it depletes the supply of free inositol for phosphatidylinositol (PI) synthesis, and thereby diminishes production of inositol-1,4,5-triphosphate ($IP_{1,4,5}$). This dampens neuron reactivity to muscarinic, α-adrenergic, and other stimuli, and is believed to mediate some of the mood-stabilizing influences in manic-depressive illness. It may act preferentially on hyperresponsive neurons, since psychotropic changes are not observed when moderate amounts are taken by healthy subjects. Although it does not seem to directly affect adenylate cyclases in the brain, it attenuates the cAMP-mediated actions of several hormones. It can invoke dehydration and thirst by affecting vasopressin-mediated water conservation in the kidneys, and decrease gastrin-mediated hydrochloric acid production in the stomach. Depression of thyroid gland responses to thyroid stimulating hormone can elevate thyrotropin (TSH) levels sufficiently to inovke goiter formation; but influences on parathyroid hormone targets can cause hypercalcemia and osteopenia. Li^+ also blunts responses to adrenocorticotropic hormone (ACTH); and diminished pancreatic β cell sensitivity to glucose can lead to hyperglycemia. Although Li^+ can replace Na^+ at some sites, it is not an effective substrate for Na^+/K^+-ATPases. It elicits single depolarizations in adrenomedullary cells, but then inhibits depolarization and Ca^{2+}-dependent release of catecholamines. The toxic effects of high concentrations include vomiting, diarrhea, ataxia, tremors, convulsions, and coma.

lithocholic acid: 3α-hydroxycholanic acid; one of the bile acids.

litorin: pGlu-Gln-Trp-Ala-Val-Gly-His-Phe-Met-NH$_2$; an amphibian peptide chemically and biologically related to ranatensin, neuromedin B, bombesin, and the *C*-terminal decapeptide of gastrin releasing peptide (GRP).

"little" hormones: low molecular weight forms of hormones that also exist as larger entities, for example little gastrins, and little ACTHs. They can have fewer amino acids, and/or carbohydrate moieties than their "big" counterparts. Some truncated forms exert the same short-range actions, but (since they are more rapidly degraded and/or excreted) are ineffective for long-range effects. (Whereas both big and little gastrins stimulate hydrochloric acid secretion, only the big types are trophic for gastric mucosa.) A few small types act preferentially on specific receptor isoforms.

littoral: usually describes organisms that live at seashores.

littoral cells: flattened cells that line the walls of blood and lymph sinuses.

liver: the largest encapsulated gland of the body. Its many functions, which are critical for survival, include control of blood glucose levels (via direct uptake from hepatic portal vessels, glycogenesis, glycogenolysis, and gluco-

neogenesis), regulation of lipid metabolism (via synthesis of fatty acids, triacylglycerols, phospholipids, cholesterol, and other molecules, fatty acid oxidation, ketogenesis, formation of very low density lipoproteins, uptake of lipoprotein remnants, and production and secretion of bile acids), synthesis of most plasma proteins (including albumin, coagulation factors, hormone-binding globulins, and acute-phase types), conjugation and degradation of hormones, synthesis of insulin-like growth factor-I and some other hormones, conversion of vitamin D to 25-dihydroxycholecalciferol, destruction of worn out erythrocytes, conversion of hemoglobin to bile pigments, excretion of numerous waste products (including bile pigments) to the intestine, ureagenesis, storage of vitamins and other nutrients, and uptake and metabolism (including detoxification) of many drugs and environmental chemicals. Insulin and glucagon are among the major regulators of the metabolic activities.

liver cell adhesion molecule: L-CAM; a 124K glycoprotein initially identified in the livers of chick embryos, but present on most non-neuronal cells. It is similar to but not identical with uvomorulin. L-CAM mediates calcium-dependent homophilic adhesion, and is implicated as a regulator of morphogenesis, wound healing, and other functions.

liver lactogenic factor: a hepatic peptide, distinct from prolactin and synlactin, that affects milk production.

LL: continuous bright light (a condition used to study pineal gland functions and circadian rhythms).

LLC-PK: a porcine kidney cell line.

LMM: light meromyosin; *see* **myosin**.

lobeline: 1-methyl-α,α-diphenyl-2,6-piperidinediethanol; an alkaloid derived from *Lobelia inflata* herb that exerts nicotine-like effects on acetylcholine receptors (initial stimulation followed by depression). The targets for acute effects include the respiratory center of the medulla oblongata, chemoreceptors involved in breathing and cardiovascular reflexes, the gastrointestinal tract, and the adrenal medulla. It has been used as a respiratory stimulant, but has not proven effective for treating addiction to tobacco.

Locke-Ringer solution: a solution isotonic to mammalian cells, used to sustain the viability of excised organs. One liter contains 9.0g NaCl, 0.42g KCl, 0.24g CaCl$_2$, 0.20g MgCl$_2$, 0.5g NaHCO$_3$, and 0.5g glucose.

locus: location; in genetics, the position of a gene on a chromosome.

locus ceruleus: locus caeruleus; locus coeruleus: a melanin-rich region of the brain near the cerebral aqueduct, named for its blue color. It contains noradrenergic neurons whose axons project to the neurohypophysis, hypothalamus, cerebellum and cerebral cortex, and it receives inputs from the paraventricular nuclei of the hypothalamus.

LOD score: the logarithmic ratio of the observed frequency for co-inheritance of two traits to the frequency that would be expected if there were no genetic linkage. A score of 3 (1000:1 odds in favor) is accepted as an indication of linkage, whereas a score of -2 (100:1 against) suggests independent inheritance.

Loestrin 1/20, **Loestrin 1.5/30**; trade names for oral contraceptives that contain, respectively, 0.02 mg ethinyl estradiol plus 1.0 mg norethindrone acetate, and .03 mg ethinyl estradiol plus 1.5 mg norethindrone acetate, per pill.

logarithmic growth phase: the stage during which organisms double their numbers in a specified time period.

Loligo paelei: the giant squid, a cephalopod of the phylum Mollusca. Its large axons are used to study neurotransmission, learning, and behavior.

Lomotil: a trade name for a mixture of atropine and diphenoxylate hydrochloride used to control diarrhea. The latter (shown below), is a μ-type opioid receptor antagonist with properties similar to those of meperidine,

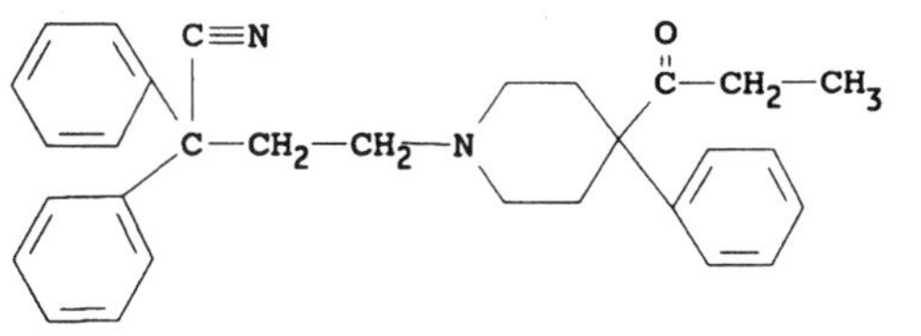

long acting thyroid stimulator: LATS; an IgG immunoglobulin in the sera of approximately 50% of individuals with Graves' disease, made by a subset of lymphocytes, but not negatively regulated by T_3. It binds thyroid stimulating hormone (TSH) receptors, exerts delayed, sustained TSH-like actions on mouse thyroid glands, and may contribute to disease symptoms in some cases. There is no direct relationship between its levels (or presence) and the severity of hyperthyroidism or exophthalmos. *See* also **thyroid stimulating antibodies** and **long acting thyroid stimulator-protector**.

long acting thyroid stimulator-protector: LATS-P; an IgG immunoglobulin in the sera of approximately 90% of individuals with Graves' disease (including some who are LATS-negative) that blocks LATS binding to human thyroid gland plasma membrane preparations. It stimulates human, but not mouse thyroid glands. *See* also **long acting thyroid stimulator**.

long feedback loops: pathways for controlling hormone secretion and other processes that involve transport of two or more regulators through the systemic bloodstream. For example, adrenocorticotropic hormone (ACTH) made by adenohypophysial corticotropes stimulates glucocorticoid secretion in adrenocortical cells, and circulating glucocorticoids inhibit ACTH secretion. *Cf* **short** and **ultrashort feedback loops**.

long interspersed DNA segments: long repetitive DNA base sequences formed via reactions that use RNA templates and reverse transcriptases; *see* also **LINE-1**.

long terminal repeats: LTRs; identical sequences with hundreds of base pairs, located at both ends of double-stranded DNA molecules, that are synthesized from retroviral RNAs via reactions catalyzed by reverse transcriptases. They contain inverted repeats, and are essential for provirus integration into host DNA. The upstream component performs promoter and enhancer functions, and the downstream one is a polyadenylation site. Similar sequences in eukaryotes mediate integration of transposons.

long term potentiation: LTP; a form of synaptic plasticity, characterized by heightened postsynaptic neuron responsivity. It is invoked by high-frequency, repetitive stimulation (usually by a presynaptic neuron), or by providing additional stimuli to already depolarized neurons. Once established, it can persist for days or weeks. The prolonged responses involve activation of NMDA (*N*-methyl-D-aspartate), and possibly also AMPA (3α-aminomethyl isoxazole propionic acid) sensitive receptors, elevation of intracellular Ca^{2+} levels, and changes in synaptic structure. LTP in the hippocampus is believed to mediate learning and long-term memory.

Lonitin: a trade name for minoxidil.

loop diuretics: furosemide, ethacrynic acid, and other agents that increase urine volume by inhibiting Cl⁻ and Na⁺ transport across kidney ascending Henle loops. Most additionally affect proximal tubule ion transport; and some act on more distal nephron segments. Since they invoke very large peak responses, they are called high-ceiling diuretics.

loop of Henle: a nephron component, comprising a descending limb that receives processed filtrate from the proximal convoluted tubule and is permeable to both sodium chloride and water, a thin hairpin turn, and an ascending limb that delivers filtrate to the distal convoluted tubule and is impermeable to sodium ions. The loops run parallel to vasa recta, which carry blood in a direction opposite to the flow of tubular fluid. Long Henle loops that descend into the renal medulla have thick ascending limb segments that extrude chloride (and sodium) ions to the surrounding interstitial fluid, and function as countercurrent multipliers that establish osmotic gradients essential for vasopressin actions on collecting ducts. Vasopressin may contribute to formation and maintenance of the gradients by regulating divalent cation transport across the loops.

loperamide: 4-(4-chlorphenyl)-4-hydroxy-*N*,*N*-dimethyl-α,α-diphenyl-1-piperidinebutanamide; a μ-type opioid receptor agonist that exerts morphine-like effects on the nervous and cardiovascular systems, and on the pituitary gland and smooth muscle. It is used as an analgesic, and to arrest diarrhea. Only minute amounts of therapeutic dosages cross blood-brain barriers. Imodium is a trade name for loperamide hydrochloride.

Lopid: a trade name for gemfibrozil.

loperamide

Lopressor: a trade name for metoprolol.

lorazepam: Ativan; 7-chloro-5-(2-chlorphenyl)-1,3-dihydro-3-hydroxy-2*H*-1,4-benzodiazepin-2-one; a benzodiazepine type depressant used for preanesthetic medication, to induce or maintain general anesthesia (often in combination with other agents), and to treat some forms of anxiety and insomnia. Its duration of action is much shorter than that of diazepam.

lordosis: (1) the characteristic posture assumed by females in response to vulval stimulation during receptive phases of estrous cycles: dorsiflexion of the spine, elevation of the head and rump, and movement of the tail away from the vaginal orifice. Receptivity is conferred by high estrogen levels in the supraoptic region of the brain. Although usually initiated by a male during mating, it can be elicited artificially with a glass rod. *See also* **lordosis quotient**; (2) a skeletal deformity that affects the curvature of the lumbar and cervical spine.

lordosis quotient: lordosis:mount ratio; within a specified time period, the number of lordosis responses to stimulation, divided by the number of mounts by a conspecific male. The value is related to the estrogen levels in the female brain, but other factors account for the considerable variation among normal females.

Lorelco: a trade name for probucol.

lorglumide: 4-[(3,4-dichlorobenzoyl)amino]-5-(dipentylamino)-5-oxopentanoic acid; an orally effective cholecystokinin (CCK) receptor antagonist.

Losec: a former trade name for omeprazole. To avoid confusion with Lasix, it has been replaced by Prilosec.

lotus seed lectin: an agglutinin that binds to oligosaccharide α-fucose moieties. It promotes erythrocyte clumping, but is not blood type specific.

lovastatin: *see* **mevinolin**.

low density lipoproteins: LDLs; β-lipoproteins with densities of 1.006-1.063, and diameters of 300-850 Å, derived from very low density lipoproteins (VLDLs); *see* **lipoproteins**. Most contain 20-25% by weight of apoprotein B-100, and small quantities of fatty acids. Typical levels of other constituents are cholesterol (45-46%), phospholipids (20-25%), and triacylglycerides (8-11%). Hepatic, adrenocortical, gonadal, and some other cell types take up LDLs via receptor-mediated endocytosis. The cholesterol is used directly, or is esterified and stored, and the receptors are recycled to the plasma membranes. High intracellular cholesterol levels inhibit local cholesterol biosynthesis, and they lower LDL receptor numbers. Acetylation and oxidation of LDLs by macrophage enzymes is believed to contribute to atherosclerosos. Observed effects of LDLs on immune system functions include inhibition of T lymphocyte proliferation.

Lowry reagent: a reagent for colorimetric determination of total protein content. When the cupric ions in alkaline tartrate react with peptide bonds, the phenol component generates a blue-purple complex that absorbs light at 550-750 nm.

LPAM-1: murine lymphocyte Peyer's patch adhesion molecule-1; a heterodimeric protein that mediates lymphocyte homing to high endothelial venules of Peyer's patches (but not to peripheral lymph nodes). The 160K α subunit, similar to VLA-4 (very late antigen-4) is linked to a 130K β type.

β-LPH: β-lipotropin.

γ-LPH: γ-lipotropin.

LPL: lipoprotein lipase.

LPS: lipopolysaccharide.

LRF: luteinizing hormone release factor; *see* **luteinizing hormone releasing hormone**.

LRH: luteinizing hormone releasing hormone.

LRH analogs: GnRH analogs; synthetic peptides that act on receptors for luteinizing hormone releasing hormone. Most are potent, long-acting agonists that stimulate gonadotropin secretion when administered intermittently, and are used to diagnose and treat some forms of hypogonadism. Continuous presentation desensitizes the gonadotropes, downregulates LRH receptor numbers, and secondarily shuts down gonadal steroid secretion. Other analogs are direct antagonists. Both forms of inhibition can be used to arrest precocious puberty, alleviate endometriosis, and slow the growth of some cancers. The resulting estrogen (or androgen) deficiency precludes direct application to contraception, but methods which involve administration during specific phases of the menstrual cycle, and use in combination with steroids are under investigation.

LRH-like peptides: (1) gonadocrinins; (2) LRH analogs.

LSD: lysergic acid diethylamine.

LT: (1) lymphotoxin; *see* **tumor necrosis factor-β**; (2) leukotriene.

α-LT: α-latrotoxin.

L3T4: the mouse equivalent of human T4 (CD4), an antigen on the surfaces of helper type (T_H) T lymphocytes that contributes to recognition of class 2 type major histocompatibility complex molecules and cell activation.

LTA$_4$, LTB$_4$, LTC$_4$, LTD$_4$, LTE$_4$: *see* **leukotrienes**.

LTH: *see* **luteotropic hormone**.

LTP: long-term potentiation.

L1 transposable elements: *see* **LINE-1**.

Lubrol PX: a trade name for an approximately 600K polyethylene glycol monododecyl ether polymer. It is a nonanionic detergent, used to dissolve membrane-bound adenylate cyclases, and applied topically as local anesthetic, antipruritic, and sclerosing agent.

$$CH_3(CH_2)_9(CH_2CH_2O)_nH_n$$

luciferases: enzymes obtained from the tails of the firefly, *Photinus pyralis*, and from *Vibrio* species that are used for ATP assays; *see* **luciferins**.

luciferins: luciferase substrates obtained from fireflies, sea pansies (*Renilla reniformis*), limpets (*Latina neritoides*), and other sources, used to measure ATP levels in the picomole range. They form luciferin-adenylates that are oxidized by luciferinases to oxyluciferins + CO_2. The amount of light emitted by the reactions is directly related to the ATP level. The color depends on the luciferin structure. Animals use the reactions to signal other members of the species. Firefly luciferin (D-luciferin, shown below) is 4,5-dihydro-2-[6-hydroxy-2-benzothiazolyl]-4-thiazolecarboxylic acid. Luciferin 6′-ethyl ether, 4,5-dihydro-2-[6-ethoxy-2-benzothiazolyl]-4-thiazolyl-]-4-thiazonline carboxylic acid, a luciferin analog, is used to inhibit luciferin-luciferase light emission reactions.

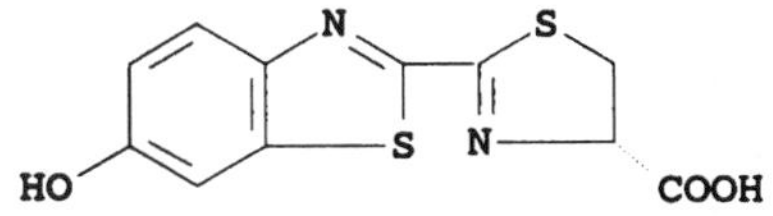

Lucifer yellow CH: 6-amino-2-[(hydrazinocarbonyl)-amino]-2,3-dihydro-1,3-dioxo-1*H*-benz-[de]isoquinoline-5,8-disulfonic acid dilithium salt; a fluorescent dye avidly taken up by retinal cells. Since it is also taken up by neurons, and transferred from one to another, it can identify functional connections.

Lugol's solution: a concentrated solution of potassium iodide and iodine. The iodide, which is avidly taken up by thyroid gland follicular cells, can protect against damage to the glands in individuals accidently exposed to I^{131}, by displacing the radioactive isotope. Although widely used in the past to treat some forms of hyper-

Lucifer yellow

thyroidism (*see* **Wolf-Chaikoff effect**), it is now prescribed only in special cases.

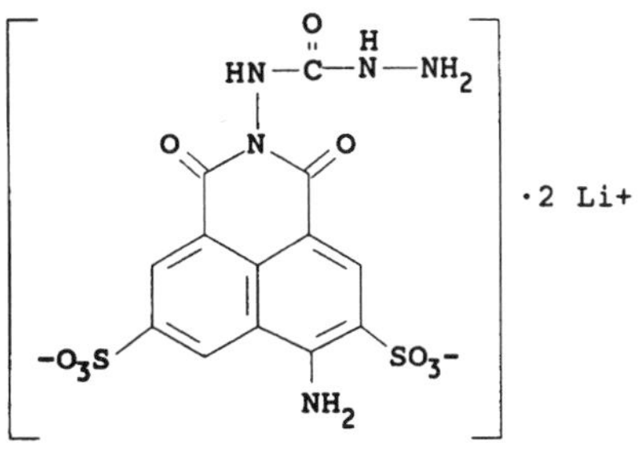

lumazine: 2,4(1*H*,3*H*)-pteridinedione; an indicator dye that emits green fluorescence in alkaline solutions, and blue in acids.

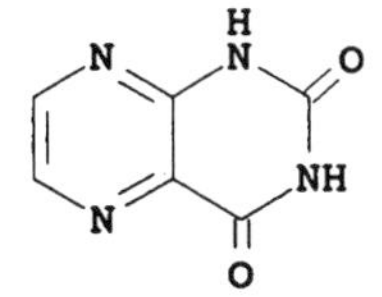

lumen: a cavity or channel.

lumicolchicines: two or more substances obtained by exposing colchicine to ultraviolet radiation. They do not inhibit tubulin polymerization, but exert *nonspecific* colchicine-like effects, and are used as control agents for studies of microtubule functions.

lumichrome: 6,7-dimethylalloxazine; a fluorescent dye formed by exposing riboflavin to ultraviolet radiation. It is used for riboflavin assays.

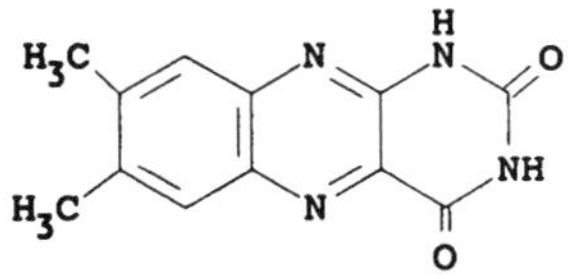

Luminal: a trade name for phenobarbital.

luminol: 5-amino-2,3-dihydro-1,4-phthalazinedione; a reagent for detecting copper, iron, cyanides, and peroxides. It emits light when oxidized by hydrogen peroxide in the presence of myeloperoxidase, and is used to assess the activities of granular leukocytes.

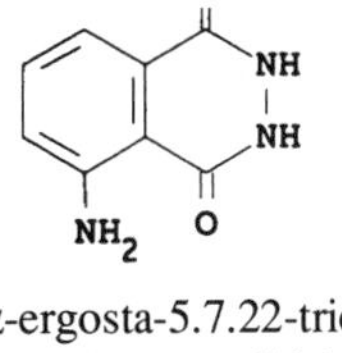

lumisterol: 9β,10α-ergosta-5.7.22-triene-3β-ol; a steroid chemically related (and convertible) to cholecalciferol, formed when provitamin D_3 is exposed to ultraviolet radiation.

lumones: chemical messengers released to the gastrointestinal tract lumen.

lumisterol

lungs: in addition to respiratory epithelium (essential for O_2 and CO_2 exchange), the lungs contain numerous cell types that synthesize surfactant, prostaglandins, histamine, vasoactive intestinal peptide (VIP), substance P, opioid peptides, somatostatin, and other hormones. Transformed tumor types can release large quantities of growth hormone (GH), adrenocorticotropic hormone (ACTH), vasopressin, bradykinin, and other regulators. Since all blood delivered to arteries must traverse them, the lungs provide a unique site for processing plasma components. An angiotensin converting enzyme on endothelial cell surfaces converts circulating angiotensin I to angiotensin II in a single passage. Different ectoenzymes cleave kallikreins. Regulators rapidly inactivated by lung enzymes include eicosanoids, bradykinin, serotonin, norepinephrine, acetylcholine, and adenine nucleotides. (Epinephrine, dopamine, oxytocin, vasopressin, and angiotensin II are among the ones not affected).

Lupron: a trade name for leuprolide acetate.

luprostiol: $9\alpha,11\alpha,15$-trihydroxy-16-*m*-chlorophenoxy-13-thia-17,18,19,20-tetranor-5-prostenoic acid; a luteolytic prostaglandin analog used in veterinary medicine to regulate estrus cycles.

lupus: a term initially applied to localized skin destruction, but now used only in conjunction with other terms; *see*, for example **lupus erythematosus** and **lupus vulgaris**.

lupus erythematosus: chronic inflammatory connective tissue system disorders whose manifestations include cutaneous lesions. The *discoid* type is limited to the skin (usually of the face and scalp), often with effects on the cheek regions that impart a "wolf-like mask". *Systemic lupus erythematosus* (SLE) is a chronic, remitting and relapsing disease that can affect the joints, kidneys, lungs, heart, and other structures. It is usually caused by immune system dysfunction, in which antibodies directed against cell constituents (including small ribonucleoproteins) are produced and released to the bloodstream. Reversible forms are invoked in susceptible individuals by hydralazine, chlorpromazine, and some other drugs.

lupus erythematosus cells: cells obtained from individuals with systemic lupus erythematosus; but *see* **LE cells**.

lupus vulgaris: a severe, rare form of skin tuberculosis.

luteal cells: *see* **corpus luteum**.

luteal phase: the stage of the ovarian cycle that begins with formation of one or more corpora lutea, during which progesterone is the major gonadal steroid hormone secreted. The durations and control factors vary widely with the species. *See* **corpus luteum** and **progesterone**.

luteectomy: removal of one or more corpora lutea. Both unilateral and bilateral luteectomy are performed to study ovarian factors involved in reproductive cycle controls.

lutein: a yellow to brown lipochrome chemically related to xanthophyll, in egg yolk, adipocytes, and the corpora lutea of some species (including humans).

luteinization: morphological changes associated with conversion of an emptied Graafian follicle to a corpus luteum, and/or the biochemical changes associated with acquisition of the ability to secrete large amounts of progesterone.

luteinization stimulants, luteinization inhibitors: physiological regulators other than luteinizing hormone (LH) that affect corpus luteum formation, survival, and functions.

luteinizing hormone: LH; lutropin; interstitial cell stimulating hormone, ICSH; approximately 30K species specific glycoprotein hormones secreted by gonadotropes that stimulate testosterone secretion in testes and ovaries. The α subunits are similar to or identical with those of follicle and thyroid stimulating hormones (FSH and TSH), and human chorionic gonadotropin (hCG). The β subunits are biologically and chemically related to those of hCG, but lack the *C*-terminal extensions, are less heavily glycosylated, and have shorter half-lives. LH surges are essential for ovulation and subsequent formation of corpora lutea. They initially stimulate the secretion of large quantities of progesterone; but progesterone secretion continues when the steroid levels rise sufficiently to inhibit LH release. LH also promotes formation of receptors for low density lipoproteins (LDLs), activates cholesterol esterase, augments cholesterol side-chain cleavage, and affects other enzymes involved in androgen biosynthesis. Most effects are mediated via cAMP. The testicular receptors are on Leydig cells (but the testosterone released affects Sertoli, peritubular, and germinal types). In immature ovarian follicles, LH receptors are expressed only by theca cells, but FSH and estrogen promote their appearance on granulosa cells of more mature follicles. Chronically elevated LH levels down-regulate the receptor numbers. LRH (GnRH) stimulates LH synthesis and release by gonadotropes, and testosterone inhibits both processes. Estrogens acutely and directly inhibit LH release, but they act over longer time periods to invoke LH surges by increasing gonadotrope sensitivities to GnRH, and thereby promoting gonadotropin synthesis and storage. LH and related peptides made in the brain affect behavior and other functions that are not mediated via testosterone.

luteinizing hormone releasing hormone: LH-RH; LRH; a term used synonymously with gonadotropin releasing hormone (GnRH) by many authors, since it is a hypothalamic hormone that stimulates the secretion of both follicle stimulating and luteinizing hormones (FSH and LH). However, other regulators exert important controls over FSH. The major form, made by several species, has the amino acid sequence p-Glu-His-Trp-Ser-Tyr-Gly-Leu-Arg-Pro-Gly-NH_2. It initially promotes release of preformed hormones, later stimulates gonadotropin synthesis, and also acutely accelerates formation of LRH receptors. When administered to gonadotropes previously deprived of the regulator, its "priming" effects sensitize the cells to subsequent presentation. However, although pulsatile release maintains gonadotrope structure and function and LH-RH receptor numbers, continuous presentation invokes desensitization and receptor down-regulation. LRH secretion is regulated by several neurotransmitters (including catecholamines which stimulate and opioid peptides which inhibit). Testosterone exerts negative feedback control, but the effects of estrogens vary with the levels and duration of presentation (see **ovarian cycles**). *See* also **inhibins**, **activins**, **folliculostatin**, and **gonadocrinin**.

luteolysins: physiological or pharmacological agents that promote corpus luteum degeneration (luteolysis). Prostaglandin $F_{2\alpha}$ is a major type.

luteolysis: corpus luteum demise. During normal ovarian cycles in which conception does not occur, corpora lutea (CL) deteriorate at times characteristic for the species, and are replaced by corpora albicantia. In women, usually just one CL forms, and survives for 10-12 days. In some species, several form and deteriorate; but in rats, mice, and many others with short cycles, ones that partially mature during a cycle persist and complete development in subsequent ones. Prostaglandin $F_{2\alpha}$, which is believed to be the major luteolysin, is released by uterine cells, at least in some species. However "programmed death" can progress without it. If conception occurs in women, **human chorionic gonadotropin** (*q.v.*) transforms the structures into corpora lutea of pregnancy (which survive for around three months). Related trophoblast hormones perform comparable functions in many other species; but some require the support of adenohypophysial regulators.

luteomas: (1) tumors comprising mostly hyperplastic luteal cells. Androgen-secreting nodules can form during the third trimester of pregnancy, but usually regress after parturition; (2) granulosa-theca cell tumors that have undergone luteinization.

luteostatic agents: physiological or pharmacological agents that prolong the lives of corpora lutea. Estrogens, progestins, and relaxin are among the regulators that exert such activity during ovarian cycles and pregnancy in various species; but chorionic gonadotropins and other placental and uterine hormones (and adenohypophysial ones in some species) assume major importance during pregnancy.

luteotropes: luteotrophs; a term formerly applied to adenohypophysial lactotropes, since prolactin maintains corpora lutea in some species. However, since prolactin is not a physiological stimulant for many other animal types, the term is no longer used.

luteotropic hormone: luteotrophic hormone; LTH; a term initially applied to the hormone secreted by **luteotropes** (*q.v.*), but now used more generally for factors that contribute to corpus luteum survival and functions.

lutropin: luteinizing hormone.

luzindole: N-0774; 2-benzyl-*N*-acetyltryptamine; a competitive inhibitor for some melatonin receptor subtypes, and a partial agonist for others.

LVP: lysine vasopressin; *see* **vasopressins**.

LXA₄, LXB₄: *see* **lipoxins**.

LY 141B: pergolide.

LY 1140: fluoxetine.

LY 53,587 maleate: 6-methyl-1-(1-methylethyl)-ergoline-8β-carboxylic acid 2-hydroxy-1-methylpropyl ester maleate salt; a selective vascular and brain 5-HT_2 type serotonin antagonist, with very low affinity for α_2-adrenergic types.

LY 83,583: 6-aniloquinoline-5,8-quinone; a potent inhibitor of soluble cyclic guanylate cyclases that does not act on adenylate cyclases. It blocks nitric oxide generation by endothelial cells, atrial natriuretic factor influences on ion channels, cGMP-mediated relaxation of aortic smooth muscle, and both antigen and interleukin-1 stimulated generation of leukotriene release.

LY 134,046: 8,9-dichloro-2,3,4,5-tetrahydro-1*H*-2-benz-azepine hydrochloride; a selective inhibitor of phenyl-ethanolamine-*N*-methyltransferase (PNMT).

LY 278,584: 1-methyl-*N*-(8-methyl-8-azabicyclo[3,2,1]-oct-3-yl)-1-*H*-indazole-3-carboxamide maleate; a selective 5HT$_3$ type serotonin receptor antagonist.

Ly antigens: several antigens expressed on the surfaces of mouse lymphocyte subsets that contribute to immune system functions, and are used as differentiation markers. Most are analogous to human CD or T types. Ly1 and some others are on both B and helper type T cells. Thymocytes and more mature lymphocyte precursor cells that are Ly^{1,2,3} positive are the precursors of both Ly^{1+} (CD^{4+} related) and Ly$^{2,3+}$ (CD8$^+$ related) cells. The term *Lyt* is used for some subtypes limited to mouse T lymphocytes, and *Lyb* for ones on B cells.

lyases: aldolases, deaminases, decarboxylases, dehydratases, and other enzymes that catalyze non-hydrolytic cleavage of C—C, C—O, or C—N bonds, with no oxidation or reduction.

17,20-lyase: C17,C20-lyase: enzymes essential for androgen and estrogen synthesis that use the P450 for 17-α-hydroxylase to cleave steroid side-chains.

Lyb antigens: glycoproteins on mouse B lymphocytes. Lyb1 is the mouse equivalent of CD5. Lyb3 and Lyb7 appear during early B cell development, and affect interactions with complement receptors. Lyb5, expressed by mature B cells, affects responses to T lymphocyte-independent antigens.

lymph: extracellular fluid, initially formed as a blood filtrate that is taken up by lymph capillaries near the venous ends of blood capillaries. Lymph capillaries (with valves that permit flow in just one direction) transport it to larger lymphatic vessels. It passes through lymph nodes and other lymphatic organs, where it picks up lymphocytes, and is ultimately delivered to the systemic bloodstream via the right lymphatic and thoracic ducts which drain, respectively, to the right and left subclavian veins. The functions include lymphocyte transport, and return of albumin leaked from blood capillaries. Edema develops when lymphatic vessels are obstructed. Normal lymph has a lower protein content than blood and does not contain erythrocytes. *See* also **lacteals**.

lymphadenitis: inflammation of one or more lymph nodes.

lymphadenoma: (1) lymphoma; (2) Hodgkin's disease.

lymphangiectasis: dilation of lymphatic vessels.

lymphangiomas: benign tumors composed of lymph vessels lined with endothelium.

lymphatic organs: all lymphatic system structures, including the lymph nodes, tonsils, thymus gland, spleen, Peyer's patches, and bone marrow.

lymphedema: accumulation of interstitial fluid, caused by obstruction of lymphatic vessels.

lymph nodes: small, bean-shaped, encapsulated lymphatic organs. Each contains a loose network of reticular tissue (stroma) that holds large numbers of lymphocytes, macrophages, and accessory cells. The superficial cortex has densely packed nodules (follicles), with germinal centers in which B lymphocytes proliferate. The deeper paracortex contains loosely arranged T lymphocytes. Cells formed in the nodes (and recirculating ones) pass through a medullary sinus, and leave via specialized high endothelial venules. Flow is slow, because there are more afferent than efferent vessels. As it traverses the sinuses, lymph is filtered, and both macrophages and dendritic cells take up foreign antigens. Macrophages also remove damaged cells, microorganisms, and debris. In a typical response to a T cell-dependent antigen, lymph flow transiently accelerates, but cell adhesion molecules, such as lymphocyte function associated antigen-1 (LFA-1) soon promote lymphocyte retention, and T cells proliferate. Later, antigen-specific B cells proliferate and are released to the bloodstream.

lymphoblasts: (1) immature lymphocyte precursor cells; (2) B or T lymphocytes that have enlarged in response to an antigen and entered proliferative phases.

lymphocytes: leukocytes that differentiate from lymphoblasts (definition 1). They produce interleukins, interferons, and other cytokines, as well as several hormones usually associated with "typical" endocrine glands, and are the major mediators of immune system functions. *See* **B** and **T lymphocytes, large granular lymphocytes,** and **memory cells.**

lymphocyte activating factor: LAF; *see* **interleukin-1**.

lymphocyte function-associated antigens: LFAs: proteins on T lymphocyte surfaces that mediate non-immunological adhesion to antigen-presenting and other cell types. The adhesion precedes, and is essential for T cell activation by specific antigens. *See* specific types.

lymphocyte function associated antigen-1: LFA-1; an integrin on all leukocyte plasma membranes, composed of CD11a (the 180K α subunit) noncovalently linked to CD18 (a 95K β type common to all members of the family). Its major ligand is intercellular adhesion molecule-1 (ICAM-1), but it also binds ICAM-2, umbilical cord venule components, and some other molecules.

When activated by kinase C, LFA-1 strengthens T cell and monocyte homotypic adhesion, and also T cell: monocyte, T lymphocyte:endothelial, and monocyte: epithelial cell interactions. It contributes to lymphocyte retention in lymph nodes during early responses to T cell-dependent antigens, and may be required for antigen presentation. CD2 persistently activates, whereas CD3 inactivates. LFA-1 also plays roles in chemotaxis, opsonization, and superoxide generation.

lymphocyte function-associated antigen-2: LFA-2; CD2; T11; Leu 5; sheep erythrocyte receptor; 50K proteins on T lymphocytes, thymocytes, and some natural killer cells that mediate adhesion to human and sheep erythrocytes, and contribute to T cell activation and proliferation. Binding to LFA-3 is independent of, but complementary to LFA-1:ICAM-1 interactions.

lymphocyte function-associated antigen-3: LFA-3; 55-70K proteins on all B and T lymphocytes (but not thymocytes), and on monocytes, granulocytes, platelets, fibroblasts, and endothelial cells. They bind LFA-2, and mediate T cell adhesion and T cell activation, but inhibit the cytolytic effects of T_C cells.

lymphokines: peptides and glycoproteins secreted by lymphocytes that mediate immune system functions (but differ from antibodies and complement components). Examples include interleukins, interferons, and tumor necrosis factor-β (TNFβ). *See* also **monokines** and **cytokines**.

lymphokine activated killer cells: LAK cells; cytotoxic T lymphocytes that have been activated *in vitro* by high concentrations of interleukin-2. When re-infused into donors, they promote regression of some kinds of tumors. T_C cells can also be activated by interferons.

lymphomas: malignant tumors, usually in lymphatic organs, derived from lymphoreticular tissue. *See*, for example **Hodgkin's disease** and **Burkitt's lymphoma**.

lymphomatosis: the presence of numerous lymphomas.

lymphotoxin: LT; usually, (1) tumor necrosis factor-β; (2) any cytotoxic lymphokine.

lynestrenol: ethinylestrenol; 19-nor-17α-preg-4-en-20-yn-17-ol; a synthetic progestin component of Ovanon and some other oral contraceptive preparations.

Lynoral: a trade name for ethinyl estradiol.

Lyon hypothesis: the concept that one X chromosome in normal (XX) females (and all but one in individuals with more than two X chromosomes) undergoes random inactivation in somatic cells. In heterozygotes, this leads to expression of certain alleles in some somatic cells, and different ones in other cells. The inactivation is incomplete; both alleles in pseudoautosomal regions (which include genes for sulfatases and some other enzymes) continue to function; and, although two functioning X chromosomes are required for oogenesis, three or more impair fertility. Activation is non-random at certain developmental stages; *see* **trophoblast**.

Lyonization: *see* **Lyon hypothesis**.

lyophilic: describes substances that are easily dispersed because of high affinities for solvents; *cf* **lyophobic**.

lyophilization: rapid freezing and dehydration under a high vacuum. Many otherwise unstable compounds can be preserved by the processes, in most cases without refrigeration.

lyophobic: describes substances that are not easily dispersed because of low affinities for the solvents; *cf* **lyophilic**.

lypressin: lysine vasopressin.

lysenkoism: the concepts that acquired characteristics are inherited, and that genes are not the major determinants of inheritance.

lysergic acid: 9,10-didehydro-6-methylergoline-8-carboxylic acid; an ergot alkaloid; *see* lysergic acid diethylamide.

lysergic acid diethylamide: lysergide; LSD' 9,10-didehydro-N,N-diethyl-6-methylergoline-8β-carboxamide; a lysergic acid preparation that is more potent than the parent compound. It is a partial serotonin receptor agonist that acts preferentially on presynaptic $5H_2$ subtypes. Although it directly inhibits locus ceruleus neurons, LSD augments sensitivities to catecholamines, and thereby exerts effects that include pupil dilation, piloerection, vasoconstriction, tachycardia, body temperature elevation, and hyperreflexia. It affects all levels of the central nervous system, and can invoke hallucinations, mood changes, sensory distortions, paresthesias, dizziness, nausea, delusions, panic reactions, and persistent psychotic reactions with flashbacks. Tolerance often develops, and is attributed to down-regulation of receptor numbers.

lysin: (1) a specific kind of complement-fixing antibody; (2) any agent that destroys cells by enhancing plasma membrane permeability (which permits entry of substances normally excluded and leakage of cytoplasmic components). Examples include bacteriolysins, and some agents released by cytotoxic immune system cells. The term is also applied to sperm lysins and some other proteolytic enzymes.

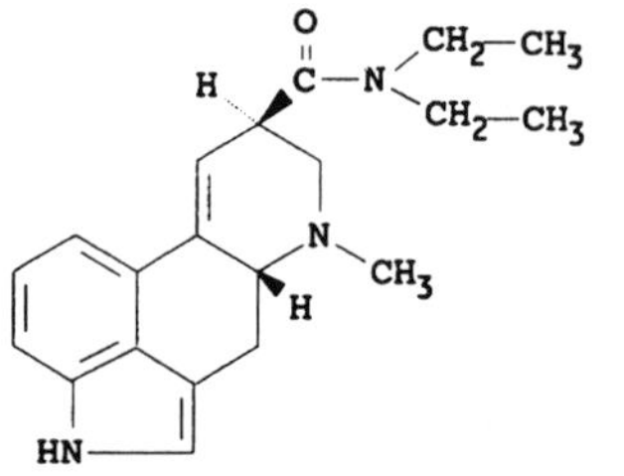

lysergic acid diethylamide

lysine: Lys; L; 2-6-diaminohexanoic acid; a basic essential amino acid, and a component of many proteins. Severe deficiencies cause anemia, and can be fatal. Lysine is a precursor of the **hydroxylysine** (*q.v.*), allysine, and other derivatives that form collagen chain cross-links, and it combines with allysine moieties to form the desmosine and isodesmosine components of elastin cross-links. Many prohormones have Lys-Lys and/or Lys-Arg bonds that are cleaved to yield the active regulators.

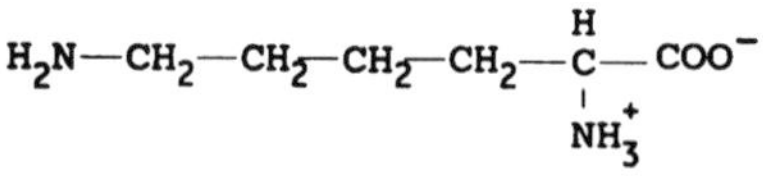

$$H_2N-CH_2-CH_2-CH_2-CH_2-\overset{\overset{H}{|}}{\underset{\underset{NH_3^+}{|}}{C}}-COO^-$$

lysine bradykinin: kallidin.

lysine vasopressin: LVP; 8-α-lysine vasopressin; a hypothalamic hormone made by pigs and some other species. Although slightly less potent than its arginine counterpart, its effects are qualitatively similar; *see* **vasopressins**. Synthetic LVP is used in nasal sprays to treat diabetes insipidus. The cysteine moieties in the structure shown join to form a ring.

Cys-Tyr-Phe-Gln-Asn-Cys-Pro-Gly-NH$_2$

lysis: (1) cell destruction by a lysin; (2) the process by which a bacteriophage lyses, and thereby destroys its host cell; *cf* **lysogeny**.

lysogeny: a stage in the life cycle of some bacteriophages, during which its DNA covalently inserts into bacterial host genomes at specific sites, and is replicated with host DNA. A repressor protein blocks entry into the lytic phase of the cycle (*see* **lysis**, definition 2).

lysokinase: tissue plasminogen activator.

lysolecithin: the product obtained when the fatty acid moiety at the 2-position of a lecithin is removed, for example by the action of a phospholipase A$_2$ or LCAT (lecithin:cholesterol acyltransferase). It labilizes membranes and lyses erythrocytes and other cell types.

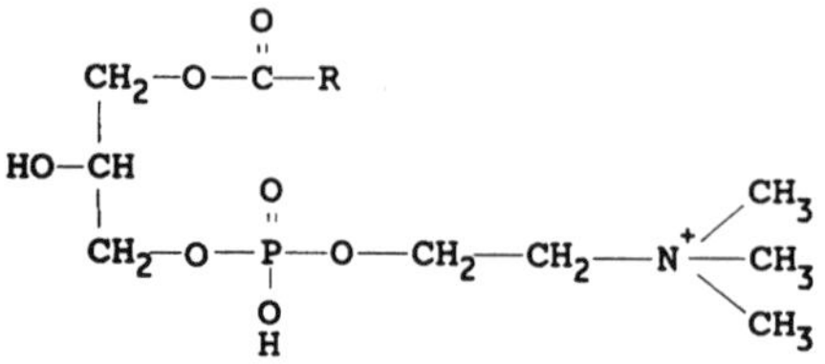

lysophosphatidic acids: 1-acylglycerol-3-phosphates; glycerophosphates esterified with fatty acids on carbon-1 and phosphate on carbon-2. They are synthesized in reactions of the general type: glycerol-3-phosphate + R—CO—CoA → lysophosphatidic acid + CoA (in which R—CO—CoA is a fatty-acyl-coenzyme A), and can react with additional fatty acyl—CoAs to form phosphatidic acids (precursors of triacylglycerols and phospholipids). An alternate pathway for synthesis (from a glycolysis intermediate) is: dihydroxyacetone-phosphate + R—CO—CoA → acyl—dihydroxyacetone phosphate + CoA, followed by reaction of the phosphate with NADPH + H$^+$ to yield the lysophosphatidic acid + NADP$^+$.

lysosomal enzymes: approximately 40 hydrolases (glycosidases, proteases, lipases, phospholipases, phosphatases, esterases, nucleases, and sulfatases) with low pH optima that are incorporated into **lysosomes**, (*q.v.*). Most are soluble glycoproteins, synthesized on rough endoplasmic reticulum (RER), co-translationally glycosylated on asparagine moieties, and directed to the RER lumen. Vesicular carriers transport them to the *cis* Golgi compartment, in which two enzymes catalyze acquisition of phosphomannosyl residues. They then cross the *medial* and *trans* Golgi compartments and emerge in clathrin coated vesicles that bud from the *trans* region. **Mannose-6-phosphate receptors** (*q.v.*) on the vesicles bind the enzymes and separate them from other proteins. The vesicles then lose their clathrin coats, and fuse with prelysosomes, in which high acidity facilitates dissociation of enzyme-receptor complexes. The receptors are recycled to the Golgi membranes in clathrin coated vesicles that bud from the endoplasmic reticulum. The enzymes are retained and phosphorylated, as the remaining components mature to lysosomes. Extracellular acidic hydrolases recognized by plasma membrane mannose-6-phosphate receptors are also incorporated into lysosomes.

lysosomes: organelles that enclose **lysosomal enzymes** (*q.v.*), with membranes that use ATP-driven proton pumps to maintain internal pHs of approximately 5. Under most conditions, the enzymes do not leave the organelles; and their activities are minimal at normal cytoplasmic pH levels (which are closer to 7.2). One function is regulation of hormone receptor numbers. Hormone-receptor complexes taken up by endocytosis are transferred to endolysosomes and dissociated into component parts in much the same way as lysosomal enzymes. Most hormones and some receptors are degraded; but other receptor types are recycled to plasma membranes. Similarly, low density lipoprotein (LDL) receptors are recycled, as lysosomal esterases provide cells with free cholesterol. Phagocytic cells incorporate microorganisms and debris into phagosomes, which fuse with endolysosomes and deliver their contents for degradation. Autophagosomes that contribute to the destruction of intracellular components such as degenerating organelles and excessive amounts of some lipids, are formed when membranes enclose the substances. They fuse with lysosomes to form phagolysosomes (autophagolysosomes) in which the substances are degraded. **Tay-Sachs** and **Gaucher's diseases** (*q.v.*) are disorders caused by inability to adequately degrade certain molecular species. Phagolysosomes are additionally involved in bone resorption, remodeling during morphogenesis, and involution of structures such as uteri following parturition and mammary glands when lactation is terminated. In thyroid glands, they take up thyroglobulins and release thyroxine and triiodothyronine. Nutrient deprivation lowers cytoplasmic pH and labilizes lysosomal membranes. The released enzymes then provide fuel, amino acids, and other substances by acting on glycogen, triacylglycerols, proteins, and other large molecules. When hypoxia and other conditions that lower cytoplasmic pH lead to their release, the enzymes can damage cells and/or enter the bloodstream, cleave plasma proteins, and generate biologically active peptides. The protective effects of glucocorticoids during inflammatory response are attributed in part to stabilization of membranes that would otherwise release mediators. *See* also **mannose-6-phosphate receptors**.

lysosphingolipids: products released when phospholipases catalyze removal of fatty acid components of sphingolipids. They are potent inhibitors of some kinase C isozymes.

lysozyme: muramidase; a 14.6K cationic protein in tears, saliva, milk, blood, nasal mucus, and other fetal and adult animal fluids, and also in egg-white, some molds, and some plant fluids. It catalyzes hydrolysis of linkages between *N*-acetylmuramic acid and *N*-acetylglucosamine, and thereby destroys bacterial cell walls. It additionally acts against some viruses, and may also function as a lubricant.

lysyl hydroxylase: an enzyme that catalyzes conversion of lysine to 5-**hydroxylysine** (*q.v.*) and is essential for normal formation of collagen cross-linkages.

lysyl oxidase: an enzyme essential for cross-linking collagen and elastin peptide chains. It catalyzes copper and pyridoxal phosphate-dependent reactions that convert lysine to allysine, and hydroxylysine to hydoxyallysine. *See* **hydroxylysine**.

Lyt antigens: glycoproteins expressed on the surfaces of mouse T lymphocytes. Lyt1 and Lyt2 are also known, respectively, as Ly1 and Ly2; *see* also **Ly antigens**.

lytic complex: an approximately 2000K complex of complement factors C5b, 6, 7, 8, and 9, that mediates cell lysis.

M

M: (1) methionine; (2) moles per liter; (3) mega; (4) morgan.

m: (1) meter; (2) milli-; (3) median; (4) murine, as in mPRL.

m: meta.

μ: micro-; (2) micron (μ is preferred); *see also* **IgM** and μ-type **opioid receptor**.

M1, M2, etc.: *see* **muscarinic** and **melatonin receptors**.

4-MA: DMAA; *N,N*-diethyl-4-methyl-3-oxo-4-aza-5α-androstane-17ß-carboxamide; an agent used to inhibit 5α-reductase.

Mab: monoclonal antibody.

MAC: membrane attack complex.

M.A.C.: maximal allowable concentration; a unit used for toxins.

Mac-1: CR3; Leu-15; OKMI; an integrin composed of a 95K integrin β subunit (CD18) noncovalently linked to 170K α subunit (CD11b), expressed on the surfaces of macrophages, monocytes, granulocytes, natural killer cells, and some T lymphocytes that facilitates neutrophilic leukocyte accumulation at sites of inflammation, enhances phagocytosis by binding to the complement component iC3b, and contributes to blood coagulation by binding coagulation factor X.

Mac-2: two or more closely related glycoproteins expressed on the surfaces of monocytes and macrophages that bind IgE and laminin, mediate cell-to-cell and cell-to-extracellular matrix adhesion, and are believed to contribute to tumor metastasis.

MAC 117: *see* c-**erbB**.

Macaca mulatta: the Rhesus monkey.

macrocortin: *see* **lipocortins**.

macrocytes: abnormally large erythrocytes, for example of the kinds that circulate in individuals with pernicious anemia.

macroglia: astrocytes and oligodendrocytes; *cf* **microglia**.

macroglobulins: 400K and larger globular plasma proteins, and related proteins made at other sites. Most affect the activities of proteases.

α$_1$-**macroglobulin**; α$_1$; a protein fraction, separable by electrophoresis from α$_2$-macroglobulin, composed mostly of immunoglobulin M (IgM).

α$_2$-**macroglobulin**: α2-M; a 680-725K tetrameric acute phase plasma protein, with 170K subunits homologous to complement proteins C3 and C4. It binds to serine-, thiol-, carboxy-, and metalloproteinases, and inhibits trypsin, chymotrypsin, kallikreins, plasmin, thrombin, thermolysin, and some other proteolytic enzymes; but the binding activates enzymes that degrade fibrin, angiotensin, and vasopressin, and other substrates. It also contributes to the clearance of proteases, and is used as a probe for receptor-mediated endocytosis. Glucocorticoids synergize with interleukin-6 to induce it in the liver. Hepatic cirrhosis, nephrotic syndromes, and severe burns are among the conditions that elevate the levels. α$_2$-M also binds transforming growth factor-β (TGFβ), basic fibroblast growth factor (bFGF), platelet derived growth factor (PDGF), interleukins 1 and 6, and some other mitotic stimulants, promotes lymphocyte regeneration in irradiated animals, and stimulates the growth of cultured cells. Receptors have been identified on fibroblasts, macrophages, and tumor cells. Some of the protein in ovarian follicular fluid is derived from the blood, but small amounts are synthesized by luteal cells. The protein made in Sertoli cells is believed to protect developing spermatozoa against the effects of proteolytic enzymes released by degenerating ones (which are phagocytosed), and by different enzymes that mediate seminiferous tubule remodeling. The concentrations in the testis are controlled locally, and can be elevated by glucocorticoids. They are unrelated to blood levels, and are not affected by IL-6, follicle stimulating hormone (FSH), testosterone, or P-Mod-S.

macrolecithal: describes egg cells that contain large quantities of yolk; *cf* **microlecithal**.

macrolides: several antibiotics made by *Streptomyces* that inhibit protein synthesis by binding to 50S ribosomal subunits; *see*, for example **erythromycin**.

macromeres: large blastomeres. In oviparous vertebrates, they occur predominantly in vegetal hemispheres, and divide more slowly than animal hemisphere cells.

macromolecules: large, high molecular weight molecules, such as proteins, nucleic acids, and polysaccharides.

macronutrients: foods required in relatively large amounts as fuels and/or protoplasmic building blocks; *cf* **micronutrients**.

macrophages: large, long-lived, noncirculating phagocytes derived from bone marrow stem cells via the monoblast → promonocyte → monocyte pathway. They are widely distributed, mostly as reticuloendothelial system components. Their properties vary with the locations. Names applied to special kinds include peritoneal and spleen macrophages, histiocytes (in fibrous connective tissues), alveolar macrophages (in lungs), Kupffer cells (in liver), and astrocytes (in nervous tissue). The cells ingest and destroy microorganisms, cell debris, and some tumor cells, via mechanisms that involve FcR1 and complement receptors, and take up acetylated low density lipoproteins via "scavenger" types. Some fuse and develop into osteoclasts, Langerhans giant cells, and other specialized types; *see* also **foam cells**. Others ingest, process, and present antigens to lymphocytes. When stimulated, they secrete more than 100 substances, including interleukin-1, interferons, prostaglandins, leukotrienes, macrophage inflammatory proteins 1 and 2 (MIP-1 and MIP-2), tumor necrosis factor-α (TNFα), neutrophil activating protein, collagenase, elastase, acid proteases, properdin, sulfatases, phosphatases, free radicals, complement components, plasmin inhibitors and α_2-macroglobulins, many of which mediate inflammation and immune system responses. Basic fibroblast and platelet-derived growth factors (bFGF and PDGF), transforming growth factors α and β (TGFα and TGFβ), and amphiregulin-like glycoprotein promote proliferation of fibroblasts, epithelial cells and keratinocytes, and contribute to tissue repair and wound healing. Roles in blood coagulation involve binding to Mac-1 receptors and release of platelet activating factor (PAF).

macrophage activating factor: MAF: a cytokine released during inflammatory reactions that may be identical with macrophage inhibitory factor (MIF). It promotes retention of macrophages at sites of inflammation, and enhances their phagocytic, tumoricidal, and bactericidal activities. Interferons α and β (IFNα and IFNβ), and tumor necrosis factor-α (TNFα) are among the stimulants for its release. IFNγ augments its effects.

macrophage colony stimulating factor: M-CSF; macrophage stimulating factor; colony stimulating factor-1, CSF-1; 45-90K acidic glycoproteins in blood, urine, lungs, bone marrow and spleen stroma, and in conditioned media from pancreatic, some cancer, and some embryonic cells. It is made by fibroblasts, macrophages, endothelial cells, activated lymphocytes, and other cell types. Human M-CSF is composed of two identical 26K plus two identical 16K polypeptide chains. A mouse form is a 70K dimer. Low concentrations promote survival, proliferation, and maturation of monocyte precursor (but not stem) cells, and formation of macrophage colonies in bone marrow. Higher ones enhance granulocyte precursor survival, proliferation, and maturation (but do not

directly activate those cells). They contribute to inflammatory reactions, augment antigen-dependent killing of tumor cells, and induce granulocyte-macrophage colony stimulating factor (GM-CSF), interleukin-1, prostaglandins, plasminogen activator, and other mediators. Endotoxin promotes M-CSF synthesis, whereas lactoferrin (released by granulocytes) inhibits.

macrophage colony stimulating factor receptors: 165K glycoproteins on the surfaces of bone marrow stem cells, promonocytes and monocytes. They are chemically related to a protein whose synthesis is directed by the *fms* oncogene.

macrophage fusion factor: Mff; *see* **interleukin-4**.

macrophage inflammatory proteins: MIPs; heparin-binding peptides released by activated macrophages that participate in inflammation by recruiting and activating granulocytes. Their production is stimulated by endotoxin. Macrophage inflammatory protein-1 (MIP-1) is an 8K doublet that promotes oxidative bursts and is weakly chemotactic. Macrophage inflammatory protein-2 (MIP-2) is a 6K cationic protein chemically related to the platelet factor 4, and to the products of murine *gro* and *KC* genes. It is strongly chemotactic, and can invoke lysozyme release, but does not promote oxidative bursts. An earlier concept that MIPs are identical to neutrophil activating protein has been discarded.

macrophage inhibiting factor: MIF; peptides and/or glycoproteins released by activated lymphocytes, named for their ability to retain macrophages and monocytes at inflammatory sites by inhibiting their mobility. They promote adhesion of macrophages to other cells, and enhance phagocytosis. Some components may be identical with macrophage activating factor.

macrophage stimulating factor: *see* **macrophage colony stimulating factor**.

macula adherens: spot desmosome.

macula densa: a component of the juxtaglomerular apparatus in the distal convoluted tubule of the nephron. It senses the rates at which ions in distal tubular fluid travel to the collecting ducts, contributes to the regulation of renin secretion, and is a major participant in tubuloglomerular feedback.

macule: a spot.

MAF: macrophage activating factor.

MAG: myelin-associated glycoprotein.

magainins: two peptides in the skin of the *Xenopus levis* toads, biologically related to mammalian defensins, insect cecropins (sarcotoxins), and melittin. Magainin I is H_2N-Gly-Ile-Gly-Lys-Phe-Leu-His-Ser-Ala-Gly-Lys-Phe-Gly-Lys-Ala-Phe-Val-Gly-Glu-Ile-Met-Lys-Ser-OH. In magainin II, a Lys- replaces the Gly at position 10, and an Asn- replaces the Lys at position 22. The peptides are broad-spectrum antibiotics, effective against gram positive and gram negative bacteria, many protozoa, and some fungi. They interfere with the build-up of proton gradients essential for ATP synthesis by opening membrane channels, and may also play roles in wound healing.

magnesium : Mg; an element (atom number 12, atomic weight 24.312). It is a component of chlorophyll porphyrin complexes, and a cofactor for mitochondrial phosphotransferases involved in ATP generation, ATPases, adenylate cyclase, guanylate cyclase, and other enzymes. (The substrate for most ATP-hydrolyzing enzymes is Mg-ATP.) Mg facilitates amino acid activation and attachment to ribosomes, and is needed for DNA synthesis and transcription. It is also an important regulator of cardiac structure and function. Deficiencies lead to degenerative changes, whereas sudden high elevations invoke diastolic arrest. Additionally, it participates in control of parathyroid hormone (PTH) secretion, and modifies the calcium-mobilizing effects. (Deficiency is associated with low PTH levels, phosphate retention, and low cholecalciferol 1α-hydroxylase activity). Calciferols, in turn, accelerate intestinal absorption of dietary magnesium. Small amounts in bone mineral may directly affect bone formation. Mg also modifies the caloric actions of thyroid hormones; and triiodothyronine (T_3) affects Mg levels in blood. In the central nervous system, the ability of Mg to attenuate glutamate toxicity is attributed to influences on NMDA (N-methyl-D-aspartate) sensitive receptor channels. Pharmacological levels of Mg^{2+} interfere with Ca^{2+} effects on skeletal muscle, neurons, and secretory cells, in part by blocking voltage-dependent calcium channels. Very high concentrations are anesthetics. Regulators of Mg excretion to the urine include parathyroid hormone, calciferols, calcitonin, glucagon, aldosterone, and urotensins. $MgSO_4$ is a cathartic that acts via both osmotic mechanisms and stimulation of cholecystokinin release. Mag-FURA and Mag-QUIN are Mg-specific agents analogous to the ones used as calcium indicators.

magnetic resonance imaging: MRI; nuclear magnetic resonance; NMR; noninvasive diagnostic procedures for high resolution visualization of organs and tissues that also provide information on chemical composition (for example on glycogen stores in liver and muscle). In the most commonly used method, hydrogen ion nuclei are lined up by a magnetic field and then briefly exposed to a second magnetic field at right angles to the first. The voltage created when the second field is cut off is detected and relayed to a computer for analysis.

magnocellular nuclei: clusters of large neuron cell bodies in the hypothalamus, a term usually applied to cells of the supraoptic and paraventricular nuclei and adjacent regions that secrete vasopressin, oxytocin, the associated neurophysins, and other regulators. The neurons send out long axons, most of which form the hypothalamo-hypophysial nerve tracts that terminate in the neural lobe. (Some axons travel directly to the median eminence and elsewhere). The neurons are functionally associated with other brain regions; and some communicate with the pineal gland.

main olfactory bulbs: MOB; paired masses of gray matter on the ventral surface of the cerebral cortex, beneath the frontal lobes, in which nerve bundles that originate in the olfactory mucosa synapse with those of the olfactory tracts. The olfactory (first cranial) nerve on each side includes the bulb and the tract. The MOB are essential for conscious perception of odors, and processing of the information; *cf* **accessory olfactory bulbs**.

maitotoxin: a polyether made by the tropical dinoflagellate, *Gambierdiscus toxicus* and related species, and by some tropical fish, that indirectly activates L type voltage-dependent calcium channels, and is more selective for promoting Ca^{2+} uptake than A23187. (It does not bind to the dihydropyridine site.) By elevating cytoplasmic Ca^{2+}, it promotes the release of many hormones and neurotransmitters.

major basic protein: MBP; a protein stored in and released from the granules of **eosinophils** *(q.v.)* that contributes to parasite killing.

major histocompatibility complex: MHC; a large set of genes on human chromosome 6 (and on mouse chromosome 17) that codes for proteins essential for immune system functions (*see* **class 1, 2,** and **3 proteins** and **tumor necrosis factors**), and also for steroid 21-hydroxylase cytochrome P450, and some other molecules. Terms applied to the gene sets of specific species include HLA (human), H-2 (mouse), GPLA (guinea pig), Rt-1 (rat), and DLA (dog). Humans inherit 4 of 100 possible sets of alleles. Certain combinations affect the tendencies to develop autoimmune diseases. Class II genes (DP, DQ, and DR) are separated from class I types (B, C, and A) by class III types, C2, Bf (for properdin), C4A, C4B, and ones that code for 21-hydroxylase.

Malachite green: N,N,N′,N′-tetramethyl-4,4-diaminotriphenylcarbenium oxalate; a biological stain and acid-base indicator, and a reagent for chemical determinations of inorganic phosphate and sulfurous acid. It is used to kill parasites that attack fish.

malacia: morbid softening of tissue. The term is also used as a suffix, as in osteomalacia.

malate: *see* **malic acid**.

malate-aspartate shuttle; a set of reactions in heart and liver that mediates net transfers of electrons across mitochondrial membranes, via the overall, reversible effect: cytosolic NADH + H⁺ + mitochondrial NAD⁺ ⇄ cytosolic NAD⁺ + mitochondrial NADH + H⁺. It is needed to generate mitochondrial NADH from cytoplasmic fuels that yield the reduced coenzyme, because neither pyridine nucleotides nor oxaloacetate diffuses across mitochondrial membranes. Cytoplasmic oxaloacetate gains hydrogen atoms and electrons when it reacts with cytosolic NADH + H⁺ to yield malate + NAD⁺. Malate then enters the mitochondrion, engages in the reverse reaction, and thereby forms oxaloacetate and reduces mitochondrial NAD⁺ to NADPH + H⁺. Intramitochondrial oxaloacetate then reacts with α-ketoglutarate to yield aspartate. After entering the cytoplasm, aspartate reacts with α-ketoglutarate to regenerate oxaloacetate. (Intramitochondrial oxaloacetate can also enter the tricarboxylic acid cycle.) *See* also **malate-oxaloacetate** and **glycerophosphate shuttles**.

malate dehydrogenase: (1) an NAD⁺ dependent enzyme that converts malate to oxaloacetate; (2) the NADP⁺ dependent malic enzyme that catalyzes malate dehydrogenation.

malate-oxaloacetate shuttle: during gluconeogenesis, pyruvate is converted in mitochondria to oxaloacetate, which does not diffuse across mitochondrial membranes (*see* also **malate-aspartate-shuttle**). It is reduced to malate (which does cross). In the cytoplasm, malate is re-oxidized to oxaloacetate and is then used to generate phosphoenolpyruvate.

malate synthetase: *see* **glyoxylate cycle**.

male: (1) describes the chromosome makeup, phenotype, and/or behavior of the members of a species who produce spermatozoa or related types of gametes (and also of immature individuals and reproductively incompetent ones with similar characteristics); (2) an individual with the described characteristics.

male pseudohermaphroditism: *see* **pseudohermaphroditism**.

maleic acid: *cis*-butanedioic acid; toxilic acid; a fumaric acid isomer, used as a competitive inhibitor of malate dehydrogenase, an antioxidant, and a component of some buffers.

maleic hydrazide: 1,2-dihydro-3,6-pyridazine dione; an agent that damages mitochondria and inhibits the growth of plants.

malic acid {malate ion}: hyrdroxysuccinic acid; a tricarboxylic acid cycle intermediate made from fumarate and oxidized to oxaloacetate. It is a component of some fruits, and is used as a food additive. *See* also **malate-aspartate shuttle**.

malic enzyme: an enzyme induced by triiodothyronine (T₃) that catalyzes: malate + NADP⁺ → oxaloacetate +

NADPH + H⁺. It generates NADPH for synthetic reactions.

malignancy: (1) a cancerous growth; (2) the tendency to progress to transformation and metastasis, or to virulence.

malignant: (1) tending to become progressively worse, or to increase in virulence; (2) describes tumors that metastasize; *cf* **benign**.

Mallory's phosphotungstic acid-hematoxylin: a dye mixture used to stain muscle fibrils, glial fibrils, cilia, and fibrin. *See* **hematoxylin**.

malonyl-ACP: an intermediate in the pathway for biosynthesis of fatty acids from acetyl-coenzyme A. It is made in the reaction catalyzed by malonyl transacylase: malonyl-coenzyme A + acyl carrier protein → malonyl-ACP + coenzyme A. It then reacts with acetyl-ACP to yield acetoacetyl-ACP + ACP + CO₂ in a reaction catalyzed by acyl-malonyl-ACP condensing enzyme.

malonyl-coenzyme A: an intermediate in the pathway for biosynthesis of fatty acids from acetyl-coenzyme A, formed in a rate-limiting reaction catalyzed by acetyl-coenzyme A carboxylase: acetyl-CoA + ATP + H₂O → malonyl-CoA + ADP + Pi + H⁺. *See* **malonyl-ACP**.

malonyldialdehyde: MDA; a by-product of reactions in which prostaglandin PHG₂ is converted to hydroxy-eicosanoids. It cross links some proteins, contributes to the formation of atherosclerotic lesions by binding to apoprotein B lysyl moieties to form low density lipoprotein (LDL) conjugates that are taken up by macrophages, and is also believed to participate in some physiological processes. The levels are used as measures of lipid peroxidation.

MALT: mucosa associated lymphoid tissue; a network of cells in gastrointestinal tract and other mucous membranes that contributes to immune system functions, and especially to protection against bacterial invasion.

maltose: 4-*O*-α-D-glucopyranosyl-D-glucose; a disaccharide component of several plant foods, and formed in animals during starch and glycogen digestion. Maltase catalyzes the reaction: maltose + H₂O → 2 glucose.

mammary glands: epithelium-derived glands of Eutherian and Metatherian mammals that produce milk when prepared by sufficient amounts of hormones presented in the right sequences, and others that sustain the function. In most species, estrogens are essential for duct, and progesterone for alveolar maturation; and prolactin is one of the regulators universally required for lactation. High levels of progesterone during pregnancy inhibit lactose synthesis (*see* **lactose synthetase**). Oxytocin promotes milk release by stimulating myoepithelial cell contraction. Platelet derived growth factor-like peptides, epidermal growth factor (EGF), insulin-like growth factor-I (IGF-I), and transforming growth factors α and β (TGFα and TGFβ) are among the regulators identified in normal tissues; and some tumors make large amounts. In women who are not pregnant or lactating, the glands contain substantial quantities of adipose tissue. When the high levels of gonadal and other hormones during pregnancy complete the preparations for lactation, much of the adipose tissue is replaced by cells that produce milk and transport it to the nipples. (Although some adipose tissue is required for maturation, most other species accumulate only small amounts.) There is less extensive development of the glands in non-pregnant mammals of most other species; and in rodents, androgens inhibit maturation in males. Simple structures that more closely resemble sweat glands develop in female Prototheria. *See* also **milk**, **mouse mammary tumor virus**, and *int-2*.

mammary tumor virus: *see* **mouse mammary tumor virus**.

mammillary region of the hypothalamus: a component of the limbic system in the posterior region of the hypothalamus that contributes to olfaction, taste perception, and some forms of behavior.

mammogenesis: mammary gland development.

mammosomatotropes: somatomammotropes; adenohypophysial cells that secrete both prolactin and growth hormone. Some may be somatotrope or lactotrope precursors.

mammotropes: mammotrophs; lactotropes; acidophilic adenohypophysial cells that synthesize and secrete prolactin; *see* also **mammosomatotropes**. Estrogens are major stimulants of cell proliferation and secretory activity, and dopamine is a major inhibitor. *See* also **prolactin inhibitory factor**, **prolactin release factor**, and **gonadotropin associated peptide**.

mammotropin: mammotrophin; *see* **prolactin**.

3,4-dihydroxy-mandelic acid: a metabolite formed mostly outside the central nervous system when monoamine oxidases catalyze oxidative deamination of epinephrine and norepinephrine. The intermediate, 3,4-dihydroxyglycoaldehyde, is converted mostly to 3,4, dihydroxyphenylethylglycol in nervous tissue.

manganese: Mn; an element (atomic number 25, atomic weight 54.93). It is an essential trace metal that forms ions with valences of 2^+, 3^+, 4^+, 6^+, or 7^+. Since it is a cofactor for arginase, succinic dehydrogenase, prolidase, and some peptidases, it is needed for normal lipid metabolism, glycosaminoglycan synthesis, and development of the nervous, skeletal, and reproductive systems, and for maintaining reproductive system functions and lactation. Deficiencies impair controls over insulin secretion and degradation.

mannitol: cordycepic acid; a naturally occurring alcohol formed from mannose. It is used as an osmotic type diuretic, to lower cerebrospinal fluid and intraocular pressures, and as a flavoring agent. The hexanitrate is a vasodilator.

mannoheptulose: a 7-carbon sugar in avocado and some other foods. Cells metabolize small amounts, but most of the ingested sugar is excreted to urine. It blocks glucose phosphorylation by competing with it for hexokinase, and inhibits insulin secretion.

mannose: an aldohexose that differs from glucose in the arrangement of atoms around the second carbon. It binds to glucose carriers, is phosphorylated by hexokinase, and is used as a fuel (*see* **mannose-6-phosphate**). It is also directly incorporated into some oligosaccharides and glycoproteins. *See* also **mannose-6-phosphate receptors**.

mannose-6-phosphate: a compound formed from mannose + ATP that attaches to molecules targeted for transport to lysosomes, and binds to receptors on lysosomal membranes. Mannose-6-phosphate isomerase (phosphomannose isomerase) catalyzes its conversion to fructose-phosphate (which is used in glycolysis). *See* also **mannose-6-phosphate receptors**.

mannose-6-phosphate

mannose-6-phosphate receptors: integral membrane proteins that recognize mannose-6-phosphate moieties on glycoproteins and glycosaminoglycans. Low affinity, divalent cation-dependent Golgi types transport the molecules to phosphatase-containing acidic vesicles (prelysosomes) that fuse with, and deliver their contents to preexisting lysosomes. *See* **lysosomal enzymes** and **lysosomes**. Higher affinity, cation independent forms contribute to the redistribution and secretion of many substances. The ones on lymphoid organ postcapillary venules recognize lymphocyte homing receptors. In mammals, **insulin-like growth factor-II (IGF-II) receptors** (*q.v.*) bind mannose-6-phosphate at sites different from ones that bind the hormone, and function as cation-independent types that mediate internalization of hormone-receptor complexes and extracellular enzymes, and are needed for processing of transforming growth factor-β (TGFβ) precursors to active forms. Estrogens down-regulate high affinity receptors in mammary glands and some other organs. Their ability to promote the secretion of certain enzymes and growth factors is attributed in part to this activity, since the limited numbers of binding sites are rapidly saturated by cytoplasmic compounds. (Estrogens also induce several enzymes and growth factors via different mechanisms.)

mannosidases: enzymes that hydrolyze bonds between mannose moieties and alcoholic groups. Endoplasmic reticulum and Golgi enzymes excise mannose groups during *N*-linked oligosaccharide processing, and lysosomal types degrade gangliosides.

α-mannosidosis: accumulation of GM2 gangliosides in a subpopulation of cerebral cortex pyramidal neurons, which then extend ectopic dendrites. The conditions are caused by metabolic defects in which excessive amounts of GM3 are converted to GM2, or conversion of GM2 to GM1 is impaired, and lysosome degradative capacity is overwhelmed. Swainsonine invokes similar defects in laboratory animals.

manoalide: 4-[3,6-dihydro-6-hydroxy-5-[4-methyl-6-(2,6,6-trimethyl-1-cyclohexen-1-yl)-3-hexenyl]-2*H*-pyran-2-yl]-5-hdyrdoxy-2-(5*H*)-furanose; a compound made by *Luffanella variabilis* that inhibits phospholipase A$_2$ and C isozymes.

MAO, MAO-A, MAO-B: *see* **monoamine oxidases**.

MAP[s]: (1) microtubule-associated proteins; (2) mitogen activated serine-threonine protein kinases.

MAP-2: microtubule-associated protein-2.

manoalide

MAP kinases: *see* **mitogen activated kinases**.

maple syrup disease: autosomal recessive disorders named for the characteristic odor of the urine, in which the metabolism of branched chain amino acids (isoleucine, leucine, and valine) is impaired. The manifestations include ketoacidosis, seizures, and coma. Some infants die soon after birth. Ones that survive for a time suffer mental and physical retardation. Effective treatments include diets restricted in those amino acids, and administration of thiamine (which accelerates degradation).

maprotiline: *N*-methyl-9,10-ethanoanthracene-9(10*H*)-propanamine; an antidepressant that blocks sodium-dependent neuronal uptake of catecholamines.

marasmus: a condition in children caused by nutritional deprivation (often complicated by diarrhea) in which growth is severely retarded; *cf* **kwashiorkor**.

MARCKS: myristoylated alanine-rich C kinase substrate.

Marezine: a trade name for cyclizine hydrochloride.

Marfan syndrome: an autosomal dominant disorder in which formation of connective tissue (especially collagen components) is impaired. Its usually affects the eyes, cardiovascular system, and skeleton. Ruptured aneurysms are major causes of death.

marginal bands: cytoskeletal structures that associate with plasma membranes and maintain cell shape. They have been studied most intensively in erythrocytes.

margination: (1) leukocyte accumulation along the walls of small blood vessels at sites of injury during early stages of inflammation (when cell surface adhesive properties are altered); (2) migration of granules to cell peripheries. It is preceded by redistribution of Ca^{2+} and changes in the cytoskeleton, and can be inhibited by trifluoperazine.

marihuana, marijuana: the dried leaves, stems and flowers of *Cannabis sativa*; *see* **cannabis**.

marker: (1) a radioactive element, fluorescent dye, enzyme, or other label used to identify or track a specific kind of molecule, organelle, or cell; (2) a component expressed on a single cell type, a set of closely related cell types, or at a specific stage of differentiation that can be used for identification (usually with a specific antibody); (3) a gene associated with specific phenotypic characteristics whose locus is known, and can be used to investigate the location of a mutation.

marker enzymes: enzymes restricted to certain cell components that are used for identification. Examples include cytochrome c (in mitochondria), acid phosphatase (in lysosomes), and catalase (in peroxisomes). The purity of cell fraction preparations is assessed by testing for contaminating enzymes.

marsupials: Metatheria; a subclass of mammals that includes kangaroos, opossums, koala bears, wombats, and wallabies. The young are born in a very immature state, and (in most species) are carried in pouches during early developmental stages.

marsupium: usually, (1) the pouch of a marsupial in which the young undergo early development; (2) the scrotum.

mas: a proto-oncogene that codes for transmembrane AT_2-type angiotensin II receptors in the cerebral cortex and hippocampus, and is believed to regulate the development and functions of some neurons by activating a G protein. Transfection transforms NIH 3T3 cells.

masculinization: (1) acquisition of male type structures and/or the central nervous system characteristics associated with male-type behavior patterns; *cf* **defeminization**; (2) virilization of a female.

masked RNA: messenger RNA that is protected against nuclease degradation. Large quantities are stored in the oocytes of many species.

masking protein: a nuclear protein that affects gene transcription by blocking binding sites for enhancers or other regulatory proteins.

mass action, **law of**: the principle that the rate of a reaction is proportional to the concentrations of the reactants (when the enzyme level is not rate-limiting).

mass number: the number of protons plus neutrons in the nucleus of an element.

Masson's trichrome stain: a dye mixture that contains ponceau R, acid fuchsin, and aniline blue or light green. It is used to stain connective tissue fibers.

mass spectrometers: mass spectrographs: instruments used to measure the concentrations of trace metals and other atomic components, in which patterns generated by deflecting the paths of streaming charged particles are recorded on photographic plates.

mast cell[s]: noncirculating cells in connective tissues, serosal cavities, mucous membranes, skin, nervous tissue, and some other sites. They have large granules with negatively charged proteoglycans that complex with positively charged proteases and histamine, and can be identified with dyes such as toluidine blue and Alcian blue. When antigens bind to their high affinity IgE receptors, they release proteases similar to chymotrypsin and trypsin, hexosaminidase, glucuronidase, aryl sulfatase,

and other enzymes, and also platelet activating factor (PAF), eicosanoids, and chemotaxins for eosinophils and neutrophils. At many sites, they additionally release heparin, histamine, and other amines (including serotonin in some species). Mast cells mediate allergic reactions, and contribute to inflammation, ovulation, bone resorption, some central nervous system functions, and other processes. They share morphological and functional characteristics with basophilic leukocytes, and derive from the same precursors; but most proliferate and complete differentiation after leaving the bone marrow. Interleukin-3 is a major regulator of precursor cell differentiation. IL-4 and factors acquired when fibroblasts interact with a *c-kit* gene product expressed on mast cell surfaces contribute.

mast cell growth enhancing activity: MEA; *see* **interleukin-9**.

mast cell growth factor: steel factor; *see* **stem factor**.

mast cell growth factor-1: MCGF-1; *see* **interleukin-3**.

mast cell growth factor-2: MCGF-2; *see* **interleukin-4**.

masto-: a prefix (1) meaning mammary gland or breast; (2) that refers to the mastoid process of the temporal bone.

mastocytomas: mast cell tumors.

mastoparan: Ile-Asn-Leu-Lys-Ala-Leu-Ala-Ala-Leu-Ala-Lys-Lys-Ile-Leu-NH$_2$; a neurotoxic peptide that promotes mast cell degranulation.

MAT: mating type locus; the yeast gene region that controls mating factor expression.

maternal antibodies: antibodies transferred from mothers to fetuses. Some confer resistance to infections that persists perinatally.

maternal immunity: the form of passive immunity acquired by a fetus or infant via antibodies taken up from the placenta or ingested with colostrum.

maternal inheritance: cytoplasmic inheritance; extranuclear inheritance; transmission of mitochondria, messenger RNAs, viruses, or other nongenomic cell components from parent cells or female organisms to progeny. Oocytes transmit many factors this way.

maternal mRNAs: messenger RNAs in oocytes, most of which are activated soon after fertilization, and mRNAs in young embryos derived from them.

mating: (2) in complex animals, association of individuals for sexual reproduction; (2) in unicellular organs, conjugation.

mating factors: usually, oligopeptide pheromones released by yeasts, bacteria, and other small organisms that promote expression of factors essential for fusion of haploid cells to form spore generating diploid types. Enzymes encoded by yeast *kex2* genes catalyze their formation from precursor proteins. The *S.cerevisiae* α_1 mating factor is H$_2$N-Trp-His-Trp-Leu-Gln-Leu-Lys-Pro-Gly-Gly-Pro-Met-Tyr. Organisms that express α pheromone fuse with others that make *a* factor (a 12-amino acid peptide similar to the α type), and form α/*a* diploids. Each cell makes just one kind, which arrest cells that make the other in the G_1 phases of their cell cycles. However, switching can occur via processes that involve endonuclease catalyzed excision of *MAT* locus base sequences and insertion of previously "silent" DNA. *See* also **mating types**.

mating types: inherited differences in cell surface characteristics that affect mating in many species whose life cycles involve a haploid phase. Most molds and yeasts have two types, A and *a*, or *a* and α. The receptors are integral membrane proteins of the rhodopsin/adrenergic β receptor family that couple to G proteins. Bacteria types are + and −. Only unlike cells fuse to form diploid organisms.

matrilinear inheritance: cytoplasmic inheritance of factors derived from the female parent.

matrins: *see* **nuclear matrix**.

matrix [matrices]: (1) extracellular matrix; (2) a ground substance into which other materials can be embedded.

matrix gla protein: MGP; a vitamin K-dependent 79-amino acid protein in dentin, bone and cartilage. In cartilage, it appears to protect against premature mineralization. In osteoblasts, its production is regulated by 1,25-dihydroxycholecalciferol (1,25-dihydroxyvitamin D).

matrocliny: inheritance in which the progeny more closely resemble the female than the male parent.

maturases: proteins required for intron excision from premessenger RNAs. They are believed to hold the precursor RNA molecules in configurations that render them susceptible to the actions of endonucleases.

maturation promoting factor; *see* **MPF**.

maturity onset diabetes mellitus: MOD; *see* **diabetes mellitus**.

maturity onset diabetes mellitus in the young: MODY; *see* **diabetes mellitus**.

Mauthner cells: M cells; large neurons in the mesencephalons of teleost fish brains that control escape reflexes.

maximum permissible dose: the greatest amount of ionizing radiation that meets safety standards for individual exposure.

May-Grunwald stain: a dye mixture very similar to Wright's stain, but prepared with oxidized methylene blue. It is used to stain blood smears for leukocyte counting.

mazindol: 5-(4-chlorophenyl)-2,5-dihydro-3H-imidazo-[2,1-a]isoindol-5-ol; an agent that blocks norepinephrine uptake. It is a central nervous system stimulant and appetite depressant, used to treat some forms of obesity because it is less addictive and invokes fewer other undesirable effects than amphetamines.

MBH: medial basal hypothalamic region.

6-MBOA: 6-methoxybenzoxazolinone; a component of fresh grass and some other plants that triggers springtime reproductive system recrudescence in *Microtus montanus* (mountain voles). When added to the diet during winter months, it promotes testicular growth in males, and prepares females for conception. The precursor, 2,4-dihydroxy-7-methoxy-2*H*-1,4-benzoxazin-3-(4*H*)-one (DIMBOA) is stored in young, growing seedlings, and is rapidly converted to 6-MBOA by an enzyme released in response to injury when animals feed.

MBP: (1) myelin basic protein; *see* also **MAP kinases**; (2) major basic protein, *see* **eosinophils**.

mc: millicurie.

MCD peptide: a neurotoxic peptide in the venom of the European honey bee, *Apis mellifera* that stimulates histamine release from mast cells, blocks voltage gated K^+ channels, affects long-term potentiation, and invokes convulsion at high concentrations.

M cells: (1) epithelial cells of Peyer's patches that transport antigens and other molecules, and some microorganisms from the intestinal lumen to lymphocytes within the patches; (2) Mauthner cells.

MCGF-1: mast cell growth factor-1: *see* **interleukin-3**.

MCGF-2: mast cell growth factor-2: *see* **interleukin 4**.

MGF: mast cell growth factor; *see* **steel factor**.

MCH: melanin concentrating hormones.

McN-A-343: 4-(*N*-[3-chlorophenyl]carbamoyloxy)-2-butynyltrimethammonium chloride; an M_1 type muscarinic receptor agonist that acts on myenteric plexus inhibitory neurons. It also stimulates sympathetic ganglia

DIMBOA

6-MBOA

McN-A-343

neurons, but does not affect cardiac or vascular muscle postganglionic receptors.

MCP: membrane cofactor protein; *see* **CD46**.

MCR: metabolic clearance rate.

M-CSF: macrophage colony stimulating factor.

McCune-Albright syndrome: a form of precocious puberty associated with hypothyroidism, hirsutism, acne, cafe-au-lait pigmentation, facial deformities, phako-matosis, and often also multiple neurological lesions, at-tributed to genetic mosaicism and formation of excessive quantities of growth factors that stimulate somatotropes, melanocytes, osteoblasts, and steroid hormone synthesiz-ing cells.

M currents: K^+ ion currents that slowly invoke depolar-ization. The channel type in hippocampus pyramidal cells is blocked by muscarinic agents and inositol-1,4,5-triphosphate ($IP_{1,4,5}$), but not by phorbol ester invoked kinase C activation or diacylglycerols. In sympathetic ganglia, phorbol esters partially block, but $IP_{1,4,5}$ does not.

MD: macula densa.

MDA: (1) malonyldialdehyde; (2) 3,4-methylenedioxy-amphetamine.

MDC: monodansylcadaverine.

MDCK: Madin-Darby canine kidney cells. They are used to study transport and other epithelial cell functions.

MDCNF: monocyte derived neutrophil chemotactic fac-tor; *see* **neutrophil activating protein-1**.

MDI: Müllerian duct inhibitor.

MDL-26630 trihydrochloride: 1,5-(dimethylamino)-piperidine hydrochloride; a spermidine analog that ac-tivates NMDA receptor polyamine sites.

MDMA: ecstasy; *see* 3,4-**methylene-dioxymetham-phetamine**.

MDNCF: monocyte-derived neutrophil chemotactic fac-tor; *see* **interleukin-8**.

MDP: *see* **muramyl peptides**.

MDR: multidrug resistance.

mdr1: *see* **multidrug resistance**.

2-ME: 2-mercaptoethanol.

MeAIB: N-methyl-α-aminoisobutyric acid; a nonmeta-bolizable amino acid analog used to study amino acid transport.

mean: average; a statistical measure obtained by dividing the sum of all values by the numbers of measurements. It is usually represented as X and used in conjunction with other calculations (*see*, **standard deviation** and **stand-ard error**). For large, normally distributed populations, it is a good indicator of the central value around which others are distributed; but a single extraordinarily large or small value can markedly affect it and convey a wrong impression when the numbers are small; *cf* **median**.

MEA-peptic ulcer syndrome,: multiple endocrine adenomatosis: *see* **multiple endocrine neoplasia**.

MECA: 5′-N-methylcarboxamidoadenosine; an A_2 type adenosine receptor agonist.

mecamylamine: N-2,3,3,-tetramethyl-2-norbornan-amine; a ganglionic blocking agent used to treat some forms of hypertension.

meclizine: Antivert; 1-(p-chlorobenzhydryl)-4-(m-meth-ylbenzyl)piperazine; a long-acting H_1 type histamine receptor antagonist used to control motion sickness, and also vomiting from other causes such as chemotherapy and vestibular apparatus disease.

meclizine

meclofenamic acid: 2-[2,6-dichloro-3-methylphenyl)-amino]benzoic acid; a nonsteroidal anti-inflammatory, analgesic, antipyretic agent that inhibits prostaglandin synthesis.

meconium: (1) the black or greenish black matter in the lower intestine of a newborn infant, and the fecal matter discharged during the first few days after birth; (2) the juice of the opium poppy.

M.E.D.: minimum effective dose.

media: (1) middle layer, as in tunica media; (2) preparations in which cells are cultured; *conditioned* media contain cell secretions, and are sources of locally produced growth factors; (3) agents used to hold or transport substances, or in which interactions occur; (4) in radiology, components more (or less) opaque than the tissues investigated, used for contrast; (5) resins, polymers, or other materials used to mount objects for microscopy.

medial: toward the midline of the body; *cf* **lateral**.

medial basal hypothalamic region: MBH; the inferior region of the hypothalamus that includes the arcuate (infundibular) and ventromedial nuclei. It contains neurons that secrete gonadotropin releasing hormone (GnRH), growth hormone releasing hormone (GRH), somatostatin, and other regulators.

medial forebrain bundles: MFB; nerve fiber tracts that course through the lateral hypothalamus and communicate with the forebrain, limbic system, and pineal gland.

median: the middle number of a distribution when all values are arranged in ascending or descending order; *cf* **mean**.

mediastinum: (1) a midline septum; (2) a mass of tissue between the lungs that extends from the sternum to the vertebral column and includes the heart, large blood vessels, thymus gland, esophagus, trachea, bronchi, and parts of the vagus nerves.

medium: singular of media, definitions 2 through 5.

MEDLARS: medical literature retrieval system; a computerized system compiled by the National Library of Medicine.

MEDLINE: an international database of biomedical literature; a component of MEDLARS.

medroxyprogesterone: 6α-methyl-17α-hydroxy-progesterone; a synthetic progestin used to treat endometriosis and polycystic ovary disease. The 17-acetate is combined with ethinyl estradiol in several oral contraceptive preparations. A depot form is used for long-term effects.

medulla: an inner region or layer, as in adrenal or renal medulla.

medulla oblongata: the caudal part of the brain that joins the pons with the cervical spinal cord, and forms the floor of the lower half of the fourth ventricle. It contains nuclei for the glossopharyngeal, vagus, spinal accessory, and hypoglossal cranial nerves, and axons that communicate with the cerebellum, thalamus, and cerebral cortex. Some of the neurons are components of "vital centers" (e.g. for breathing and swallowing), and others are essential for many cardiovascular, pulmonary, digestive system, and other reflexes. The pyramidal and extrapyramidal nerve tracts, and fibers that ascend from the spinal cord pass through this region.

medullarin; medullarine; a hypothetical substance made in the central part of an indifferent gonad that promotes differentiation of the testis; but *see* **testis determining genes**.

medullary carcinomas: usually, calcitonin-secreting thyroid gland tumors.

mefenamic acid: 2-[(2,3-dimethylphenyl)amino]-benzoic acid: a nonsteroidal anti-inflammatory, antipyretic analgesic that inhibits prostaglandin synthesis.

mega-: a prefix meaning million or very large.

Megace: a trade name for megestrol acetate.

megakaryocytes: very large cells that differentiate in the livers of embryos and young fetuses, and in the bone marrow at later stages of development. When mature, they undergo fragmentation, and each cell yields 1000-1500 thrombocytes. *See* also **thrombopoietin**.

megakaryocytopoiesis: formation of blood platelets; *see* **megakaryocytes**.

megestrol acetate: Megace; 6-dehydro-6-methyl-17α-acetoxy-progesterone; a synthetic progestin, used alone for its progesterone-like actions and to treat some cancers, and in combination with ethinyl estradiol in several oral contraceptive preparations.

melanins

meiosis: reduction divison; nuclear division that (when associated with cytokinesis) leads to the formation of haploid gametes (and plant spores). The prophase of meiosis I is long, preceded by chromosome replication, and divided into leptotene, zygotene, pachytene, diplotene, and diakinesis stages. Homologous chromosomes pair during zygotene Since crossing over occurs during pachytene, the division produces two genetically dissimilar cells, each containing two copies of a single set of alleles. Meiosis II immediately follows (without chromosome replication) to form the haploid cells. *See* also specific stages, **spermatogenesis**, and **oogenesis**.

MEL-14: Mel-14; a monoclonal antibody directed against murine glycoprotein gp100^{MEL-14}, a cell adhesion molecule expressed on bone marrow and peripheral blood granulocytes that contains a lectin domain and mediates the initial adhesion of granulocytes to endothelial cell walls and to sites of inflammation. The protein is shed after the cells are activated. This releases them from the endothelium, and protects against adherence to nonspecific sites. Leukotriene B$_4$ (LTB$_4$), tumor necrosis factor-α (TNFα), complement fragment C5a, and some phorbol esters are among the agents that lower cellular levels of the glycoprotein and induce expression of Mac-1. MEL-14 also recognizes gp90^{MEL-14} on lymphocyte surfaces that mediates adhesion to homing receptors on high endothelial venules of peripheral lymph nodes (but not on Peyer's patches).

melanins: widely distributed pigments synthesized from tyrosine and dihydroxyphenyl compounds, via processes that include oxidation and polymerization (*see* **tyrosinase**), in skin, hair, feathers, nipples, and connective tissues, substantia nigra and other nervous tissue, pineal gland, eye choroid coat, and elsewhere. Dark brown and black animal pigments ("true" melanins, sepiomelanins) are mostly polymers of indole 5,6-quinone and 5,6-dihydroxyindole-2-carboxylic acid. Phaeomelanins contain sulfur, and are yellow, orange-colored, red, or light brown. Some dark plant pigments (allomelanins) are polymers of different composition that do not contain nitrogen.

melanin concentrating hormones: MCH: small pituitary gland and brain peptides that regulate skin pigmentation. Asp-Thr-Met-Arg-Cys-Met-Val-Gly-Arg-Val-Tyr-Arg-Pro-Cys-Trp-Glu-Val, a peptide in teleost neurointermediate lobes (with bonds connecting the cysteine moieties), lightens skin color in bony fishes by promoting melanosome consperson (aggregation), antagonizes some other effects of α-melanocyte stimulating hormone (α-MSH), and suppresses α-MSH release. Its receptors differ from the ones that mediate norepinephrine (α-adrenergic) consperson; but α-MSH opposes the effects of both regulators. Some shorter fragments, such as MCH 1-14, display similar potency; but they promote dispersion in tetrapods. A related cyclic peptide, Asp-Phe-Asp-Met-Thr-Arg-Cys-Met-Leu-Gly-Arg-Val-Tyr-Arg-Pro-Cys-Trp-Gln-Val is made in rat intermediate lobes, possibly by cell types other than melanotropes. Two 132-amino acid prepro-MCHs and their messenger RNAs are expressed in hypothalamic neurons that project to the cerebral cortex, brainstem, and neurohypophysis in fishes, amphibians, and mammals. Their cleavage products appear to be neurotransmitters and/or neuromodulators that decrease stress associated, corticotropin release hormone (CRH)-mediated release of adrenocorticotropic hormone (ACTH). Possible relationships to a previously described W substance of pituitary extracts have not been elucidated.

melanoblasts: melanocyte precursor cells that originate in the neural crests.

melanoblastomas: malignant tumors that contain melanoblasts.

melanocyte: (1) any melanin producing cell; (2) a cell type that synthesizes melanin, but does not contain moveable pigment organelles; *cf* **melanophore**. *Amelanocytic melanocytes* are related types that have not accumulated the pigments, but are capable of making them. *Dendritic* melanocytes extend long cytoplasmic processes that transfer pigment to keratinocytes and other cell types.

melanocyte concentrating hormones: *see* **melanin concentrating hormones**.

melanocyte growth stimulating activity: MSGA; an uncharacterized factor, different from other known regulators, implicated as an autocrine growth stimulant for melanoma, lung cancer, and skin cancer cells.

melanocyte inhibiting hormones: α-melanocyte-stimulating hormone (α-MSH) release is controlled mostly by neural factors, including gamma-aminobutyric acid (GABA), and others that inhibit. The term *MIF* has been applied to specific peptides initially said to be physiological inhibitors of α-MSH release and/or its actions on pigment cells, but whose functions have not been elucidated. Pro-Leu-Gly-NH$_2$, the side-chain of oxytocin, has been given the names melanostatin-1, MSH-release inhibiting factor, and MIF-1. Tocinoic acid (the cyclic 6-amino acid peptide equivalent to oxytocin minus the Pro-Leu-Gly-NH$_2$ side-chain) is MIF-2. The hypothalamus contains enzymes that cleave oxytocin, the peptides have been extracted from rodent hypothalami and pituitary glands, and high affinity binding sites for MIF-1 have been identified. Under some conditions, MIF-1 does, in fact, promote melanophore consperion, mostly by opposing dopamine and opioid peptide actions. It also antagonizes other effects of those regulators, including analgesia, and influences on behavior and skeletal muscle functions. A tetrapeptide, Tyr-Leu-Pro-Gly-NH$_2$, that also binds with high-affinity to hypothalamic sites, exerts similar effects on the central nervous system, but not on pigment cells.

melanocyte stimulating hormones: MSHs; melanotropins; hormones that stimulate any of the following in cells of melanocyte lineage: proliferation, differentiation, melanin synthesis, and/or melanin dispersion. The ones made by pars intermedia cells are also known as intermedins. *See* **α-, β-**, and **γ-melanocyte stimulating hormones, morphological color changes,** and **physiological color changes.**

α-melanocyte stimulating hormone: α-MSH; α-melanotropin; a peptide cleaved from proopiomelanocortin (POMC) that contains the first 13 amino acids of adrenocorticotropic hormone (ACTH), and is usually acetylated and amidated as in *acetyl*-Ser-Tyr-Ser-Met-Glu-His-Phe-Arg-Trp-Gly-Lys-Pro-Val-NH$_2$. It is made in the pars intermedia of animals that possess that pituitary gland component, in neurointermediate lobes of some other vertebrates, and in scattered cells within the human hypophysis. Although best known as the most potent melanocyte stimulating hormone thus far identified, it exerts other effects, including stimulation of fetal growth. Correlations between pars intermedia size and the ability to withstand water deprivation, morphological changes in response to hypertonic saline, and influences of the peptide on sodium transport, natriuresis, vasopressin, and aldosterone secretion, are all consistent with roles in water and electrolyte balance. α-MSH secretion by pituitary glands is mostly under inhibitory control. Dopamine appears to be the major regulator, and it also slows acetylation. Other inhibitors include melatonin and arginine vasotocin; *see* also **melanocyte release inhibitory factors.** Chemically related α-MSHs that affect pigmentation are made by fishes. In humans, the pars intermedia disintegrates as the pituitary gland matures, and adenohypophysial cells may not make sufficient modified peptide after birth to control pigmentation; but *see* **γ-melanocyte stimulating hormone**. A non-acetylated α-MSH is made in the hypothalamus and other

brain regions of humans and other vertebrates, in which it functions as a neurotransmitter and neuromodulator (but is inactive on melanophores and melanocytes). Brain α-MSH, affects learning, memory, some forms of behavior, body temperature, and other functions, and can inhibit the release of thyrotropin releasing hormone (TRH). It also antagonizes many effects of β-endorphin. For example, it is hyperalgesic, promotes arousal, and blocks β-endorphin inhibition of sexual behavior and luteinizing hormone (LH) secretion, as well as β-endorphin mediated stimulation of prolactin release. Acetylcholine acts on both M$_1$ type muscarinic and nicotinic acid receptors to promote brain MSH release. Other stimulants include TRH and corticotropin releasing hormone (CRH), whereas gamma aminobutyric acid (GABA) and neuropeptide Y inhibit. Some non-acetylated α-MSH may be released to the systemic bloodstream. High affinity receptors have been identified in Harderian and lacrimal glands and at many other sites, including duodenum, pancreas, salivary glands, urinary bladder, spleen, and some accessory reproductive glands. Some actions seem to involve synergisms with androgens. α-MSH stimulates lipogenesis in brown adipose tissue and in sebaceous glands, but is lipolytic in white adipose tissue. It can also increase the secretion of glucagon and insulin. When the first 13 amino acids are cleaved from the ACTH component of POMC, corticotropin-like intermediate peptide (CLIP, amino acid moieties 18-39) is also made. Since CLIP regulates fetal pituitary glands, it has been suggested that some α-MSH is a byproduct.

β-melanocyte stimulating hormones: β-MSHs; 16-18 amino acid peptides that exert weak α-MSH-like actions. The sequences are contained with the β-lipoprotein component of proopiomelanocortin, and have been found in pituitary gland extracts, but it is not known if they are cleaved from proopiomelanocortin (POMC) under physiological conditions. The amino acids shared with α-MSH are underlined in the structure shown: Asp-Glu-Gly-Pro-Tyr-Arg-Met-Glu-His-Phe-Arg-Trp-Gly-Ser-Pro-Pro-Lys-Asp.

γ-melanocyte stimulating hormone, γ-MSH: a peptide contained within the 16K *N*-terminal region of proopiomelanocortin (POMC), believed to be secreted by corticotropes, and to accelerate steroidogenesis in the adrenal cortex and gonads by augmenting cholesterol esterase activity. It is not known if the weak melanocyte stimulating activity is physiologically significant; *cf* **α-melanocyte stimulating hormone**. The amino acids shared with α-melanocyte stimulating hormone are underlined: Tyr-Val-Met-Gly-His-Phe-Arg-Trp-Asp-Arg-Phe-Gly.

melanocyte stimulating hormone release factor: MRF; Cys-Tyr-Ile-Gln-Asn-OH; a linear peptide composed of the five amino acid moieties of tocinoic acid, which may be cleaved from oxytocin. It is a proposed stimulant for MSH secretion, but a physiological function has not been established.

melanocytomas: moles and other benign tumors that contain cells derived from dermal melanocytes.

melanogenesis: melanin synthesis.

melanomas: malignant tumors derived from cells of melanocyte lineage.

melanophore[s]: chromatophores; cells that contain melanosomes (moveable melanin-containing organelles), in the skins of amphibians and some other poikilotherms. *See* also **physiological color changes** and **melanocytes**.

melanophore index: MI; a morphological measure of melanosome dispersion, used in melatonin bioassays. Cells that display maximal aggregation are said to be punctate, and those with maximal dispersion, reticulate. The three intermediate stages are punctate-stellate, stellate, and punctate-reticulate. The assay has limited precision, in part because it is subjective; but it does provide a rough estimate of the hormone concentration. Attempts to improve it with photometric measurements of the amounts of light blocked by melanosomes have not been successful.

melanosis: deposition of brown and/or black pigments that contain melanins (often in combination with lipofuscins) in tissues that do not normally have detectable amounts.

melanosomes: melanin-containing pigment organelles; *see* **melanophores**.

melanostatin: a general term for regulators that inhibit the secretion and/or actions of melanocyte stimulating hormones; *see* **melanin concentrating hormones**, **melanocyte inhibiting hormones**, **melatonin**, and α-**melanocyte stimulating hormone**.

melanotropes: adenohypophysial cells that secrete α-melanocyte stimulating hormone (α-MSH), in the pars intermedias or neurointermediate lobes of many species, and in other parts of the mature human hypophysis. At least some also secrete corticotropin-like intermediate peptide (CLIP).

melanotropins: *see* **melanocyte stimulating hormones**.

melatonin: MLT; *N*-acetyl-5-hydroxytryptamine; a hormone synthesized from serotonin in pineal glands, retinas and Harderian glands, and also in the gastrointestinal tract. In some species, the rate-limiting step is formation of the *N*-acetylserotonin precursor; in others it is the reaction catalyzed by hydroxyindole-*N*-methyltransferase. Norepinephrine (acting mostly on β-type receptors), vasoactive intestinal peptide (VIP), and acetylcholine acting on both M_1-type muscarinic and nicotinic receptors, all stimulate MLT synthesis in the pineal. Norepinephrine actions on $α_2$ type adrenergic receptors, and the effects of environmental light on the suprachiasmatic nuclei (SCN) of the hypothalamus inhibit. In both diurnal and nocturnal species, larger amounts are made during darkness (more at night than during the day, and more in winter than in summer); and there are circadian variations in the numbers of MLT receptors. The hormone transduces photoperiod signals that regulate several circadian and seasonal rhythms. It directly affects locomotor activity patterns in birds, and influences grooming and sexual behavior in laboratory rodents. In humans, it affects mood and invokes drowsiness and sleep. Excessive secretion or deranged circadian patterns are implicated as causes of seasonal affective disorder (SAD); and afflicted individuals improve when exposed every morning to very bright light. Similar treatment (and artificial changes in light-dark cycles) have been used to reset sleep-wake rhythms in individuals with insomnia, and in ones experiencing jet-lag. The ability of MLT to augment growth hormone secretion may be related to its effects on sleep. Other central nervous system effects include modulation of cerebellar GABAergic neuron activity, and changes in cerebrocortical GABA receptor numbers. The effects on body temperature and metabolic rate have been linked with influences on the secretion of triiodothyronine (T_3) and other hormones, stimulation of cerebral vessel smooth muscle, and acceleration of brown adipose tissue formation in rodents. The numerous influences on reproductive system functions include inhibition of follicle stimulating and luteinizing hormone (FSH and LH) release under certain conditions, and interactions with anterior hypothalamic neurons that mediate seasonal changes in prolactin secretion. Roles in regulation of the timing of puberty onset have been suggested. In juvenile laboratory animals, MLT acts on the anterior hypothalamic area to increase the numbers of androgen receptors involved in negative feedback control of LH, changes receptor affinities, and thereby retards testicular growth and androgen secretion. A decline in MLT production around the time of puberty onset in humans and other animals has been described by some investigators; and, in Northern hemisphere locales with large seasonal differences in photoperiods, the first menstrual period occurs most frequently in June (a time when MLT levels are low). In older animals of some species, it mediates seasonal regression of the gonads, and appears to be a major mediator of seasonal implantation delay (diapause). In women, it contributes to the regulation of estrous and menstrual cycles (and bright light alleviates irregularities in some). It may also be directly involved in seasonal differences in fertility. (More non-identical twins are conceived during the summer than during the winter in some countries.) Other seasonal changes affected in some species include fur thickness, coat color, and antler growth. MLT is additionally reported to exert stimulatory influences over some immune system functions, and inhibitory ones on tumor growth and on some aging processes. Caloric restriction in laboratory animals can attenuate age-related declines in MLT production and elongate life spans. In poikilotherms, MLT promotes melanophore conspersion and can decrease melanin synthesis. Some metabolites, including 6-hydroxymelatonin (made in the liver), *N*-acetyl-5-methoxykinurenine (which accumulates in the central nervous system), *N*-methylated methoxytryptamines, and 5-methoxytryptamine are mediators or inhibitors of certain MLT actions. *See* also 5-**methoxytryptophol** and 5-**hydroxytryptophophol**.

melatonin receptors: cell components that mediate melatonin actions. An M1 type in retinas binds inhibitory G proteins, decreases dopamine release in the retina, and affects photoreceptor disk shedding. An M2 type at other

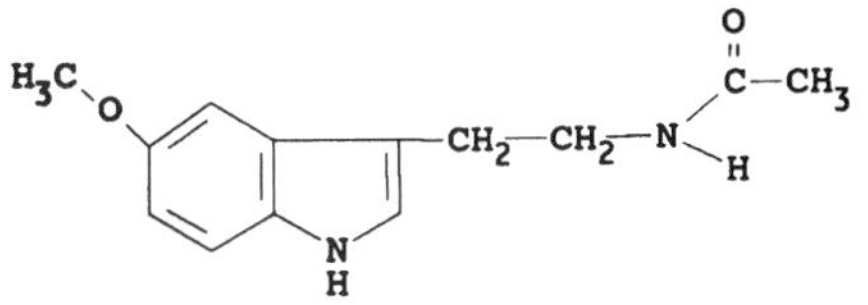

melatonin

melphalan

sites binds stimulatory G proteins. Receptors have been identified in the anterior hypothalamic area, the paraventricular nuclei of the hypothalamus, the median eminence, the pars tuberalis of the adenohypophysis, the choroid plexus, and Harderian glands.

6-hydroxy-**melatonin**: a melatonin metabolite formed in the liver. Some is directly excreted to urine, but most is first converted to a sulfate or glucuronide conjugate.

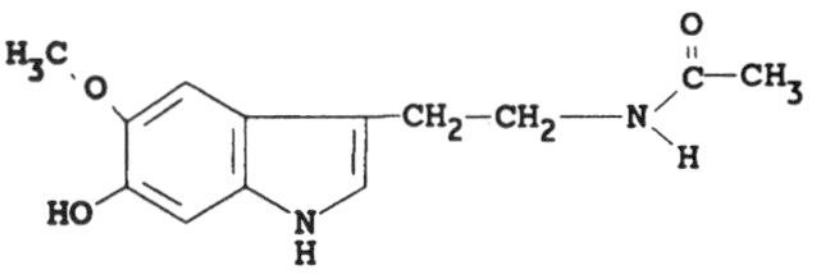

6-OH melatonin

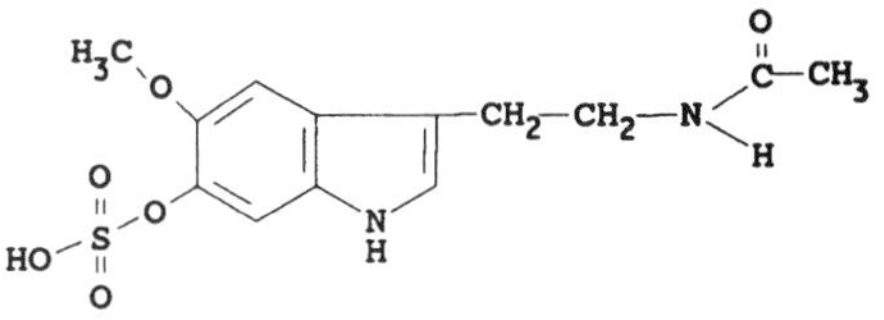

melatonin sulfate

melittin, mellitin: an alkaline mixture from the venom of the honey bee (*Apis mellifera*) that kills gram positive bacteria. Its major component, Gly-Ile-Gly-Ala-Val-Leu-Lys-Val-Leu-Thr-Thr-Gly-Leu-Pro-Ala-Leu-Ile-Ser-Trp-Ile-Lys-Arg-Lys-Arg-Gln-Gln-NH$_2$, is cleaved to a form that activates phospholipase A_2, and thereby generates lysophosphatides and releases arachidonic acid. Lysophosphatides lyse erythrocytes and some other cell types. Arachidonic acid acts directly at some sites, and via conversion to eicosanoids at others. Mellitin also binds calmodulin in a calcium-dependent manner, and inhibits several calmodulin-regulated enzymes. The hydrophobic nature of the molecule probably accounts for its ability to form ion pores in membranes (since an all-D isomer is equally effective for this, but not the other actions).

Mellaril: a trade name for thioridazine hydrochloride.

melphalan: L-phenylalanine mustard; L-sarcolysine; an orally effective alkylating agent with actions similar to those of other nitrogen mustards, used to treat multiple myeloma and some ovarian, breast, and other neoplasms. It does not cause hair loss and some other undesirable effects of different chemotherapeutic agents; and normal cells repair the DNA damage inflicted more rapidly than some malignant types. However, melphalan can depress hematopoiesis, and is carcinogenic.

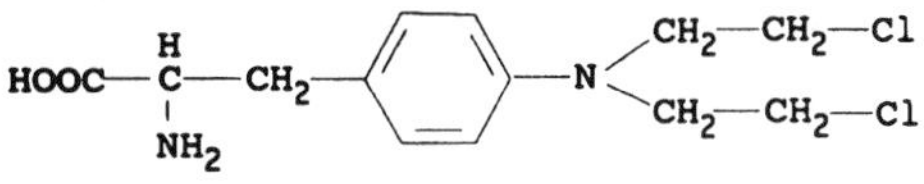

membrane attack complex: MAC; a complex formed when **complement** (*q.v.*) is activated by either classical or alternate pathways. It rearranges plasma membrane lipid bilayers, and promotes formation of pores that coalesce and lyse cells by permitting loss of cytosolic K^+ and entry of Na^+ and water.

membrane fluidity: a property of plasma membranes that facilitates lateral mobility of integral membrane proteins and other molecules, and affects permeability, cell surface receptor aggregation, enzyme activation, and other processes. High temperatures and large quantities phospholipids rich in unsaturated fatty acids augment it, whereas cholesterol is a major opposing factor.

memory cells: lymphocytes "sensitized" by specific antigens that are retained in lymphatic organs during primary immune responses. They do not contribute to early reactions, but are rapidly released to the bloodstream and activated if the same antigen is presented at a later time, and are major participants in secondary responses. The term is often applied to long-lived B cells that produce IgD type immunoglobulins and express CR1 and CR2 receptors; but shorter-lived T type memory cells are also made.

MEN: multiple endocrine neoplasia.

menadione: 2-methyl-1,4-naphthoquinone; vitamin K_3; a synthetic preparation with vitamin K properties, used to treat prothrombin deficiencies and dicumarol poisoning.

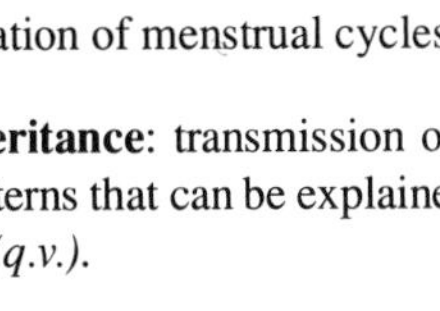

menalgia menorrhalgia: painful menstruation; dysmenorrhea.

menarche: initiation of menstrual cycles.

Mendelian inheritance: transmission of genetic factors according to patterns that can be explained on the basis of **Mendel's laws** (*q.v.*).

Mendel's laws of inheritance: two basic concepts, and some events that logically follow. The *law of segregation* states that alleles (on different chromosomes) separate during meiosis in a manner that leads to transmission of a single type to each of the gametes, and the *law of independent assortment* that unlinked genes are transmitted in a random manner, so that inheritance of one allele is unrelated to inheritance of the others. *See* also **sex linked inheritance**, **homozygotes**, and **heterozygotes**.

meninges: three membranes that cover the brain and spinal cord: the dense fibrous outer *dura mater*, the underlying, wispy, trabecular *arachnoid*, and the fine inner *pia mater* that adheres to neural tissue.

menopausal gonadotropins; menotropins; gonadotropins extracted from the urine of postmenopausal women, used mostly for their high follicle stimulating hormone (FSH)-like activity, to treat gonadotropin deficiencies, and to promote the maturation of large numbers of ovarian follicles for *in vitro fertilization*. **Clomiphene** (*q.v.*) is now preferred for enhancing fertility in women capable of ovulation, since it is difficult to assess the gonadotropin dosages required, and excessive amounts increase the probability that too many zygotes will form. (The urine contains high gonadotropin concentrations because cessation of ovarian cycles decreases the negative feedback control over gonadotropin production otherwise exerted by ovarian steroids.)

menopause: (1) cessation of ovarian and menstrual cycles. The term usually refers to normal events that occur in most women between the ages 45 and 60 (earlier in some), but is also applied when the cycles stop because of premature ovarian failure or ovariectomy; (2) the time period during which ovarian function declines and cycles cease, and the associated physiological and psychological manifestations; *see* **climacteric**.

menorrhagia: excessive blood loss during menstruation.

menorrhalgia: menalgia; dysmenorrhea.

menorrhea: the blood loss associated with normal menstrual cycles; *cf* **amenorrhea** and **menorrhagia**.

menses: (1) menstruation; (2) the phase of the female primate reproductive cycle during which menstruation occurs.

menstrual cycles: recurring primate endometrial cycles that begin at menarche and continue to menopause (but are arrested during pregnancies); *see* also **menstrual phase**.

menstrual phase: the stage of the primate ovarian cycle initiated by demise of the corpus luteum, during which blood and the debris formed by degenerative changes in the endometrium are discharged to the vagina.

menstruation: the discharge of blood and cell debris during the menstrual phase of the primate endometrial cycle.

mensual: monthly.

mepacrine: quinacrine; N^4-(6-chloro-2-methoxy-9-acridinyl)-N^1, N^2-diethyl-1,4-pentanediamine; an agent that inhibits phospholipase A_2. The hydrochloride (Atabrine hydrochloride) has been used to treat malaria, other protozoal, and tapeworm infections; but the toxic effects can include blood dyscrasias, optic neuropathy, vomiting, dizziness, and dermatitis.

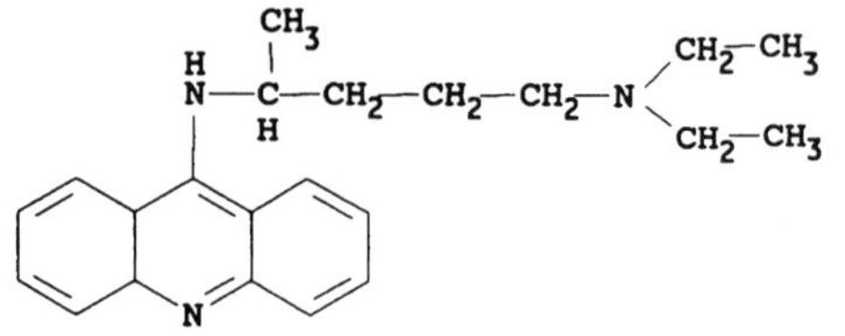

mepacrine

mepartricin: the methyl ester of **partricin** (*q.v.*). It is a polyene antibiotic with therapeutic properties similar to those of amphotericin, but is less nephrotoxic.

meperidine: 1-methyl-4-phenyl-4-piperidinecarboxyl acid ethyl ester; a synthetic agent used for its analgesic and anti-spasmolytic properties. It acts on µ-type opioid receptors and exerts morphine-like effects, such as respiratory depression, pupillary constriction, and dysphoria. Repeated use can lead to addiction.

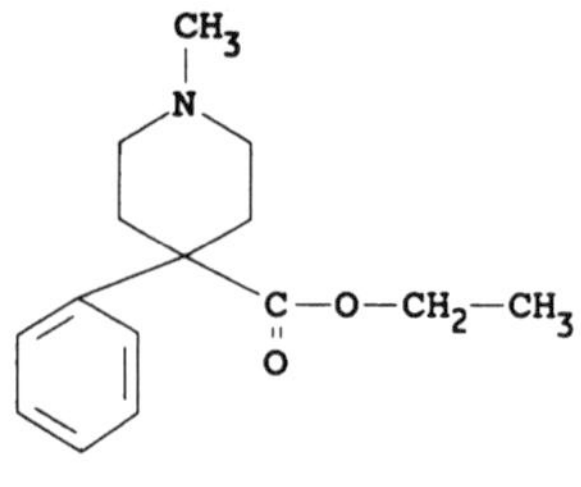

mephenesin: 3-(2-methylphenoxy)-1,2-propanediol; Atensin; a centrally acting skeletal muscle relaxant that slows transmission through spinal and supraspinal pathways, but invokes little or no sedation.

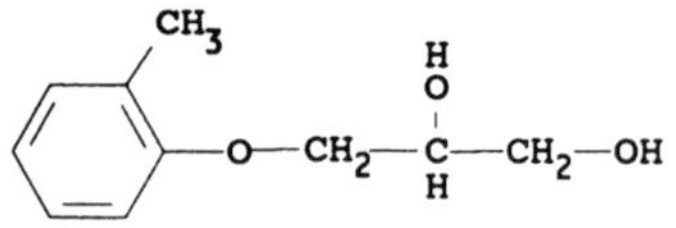

mephenhydramine: 2-(1,1-diphenylethoxy)-*N,N*-dimethylethanamine; an H_1 type histamine receptor antagonist used to alleviate allergic reactions.

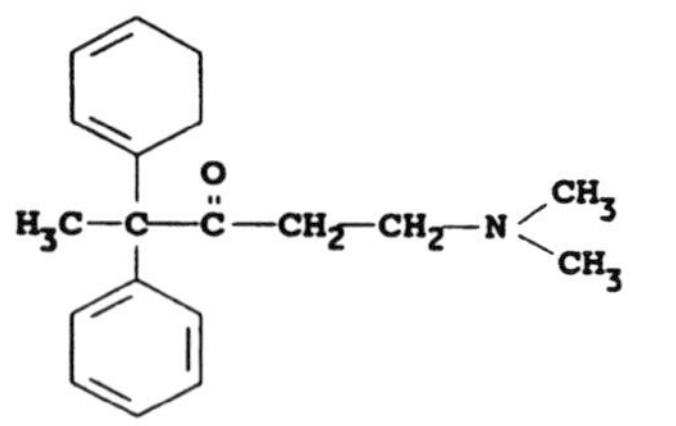

mephentermine: trimethylbenzene ethanamine; an orally effective agent with properties similar to those of ephedrine. It is used as a nasal decongestant, and to treat some forms of hypotension. In addition to its α_1 type adrenergic receptor agonist activity, it promotes norepinephrine release from sympathetic nerve endings.

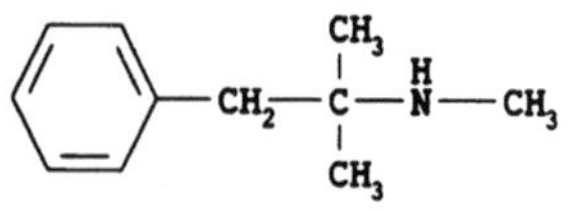

444

mephenytoin: 5-ethyl-3-methyl-5-phenyl-2.4-imidazol-idenedione; an orally effective anti-convulsant, used to treat of some forms of epilepsy. It invokes sedation, and is more toxic than some other phenytoins.

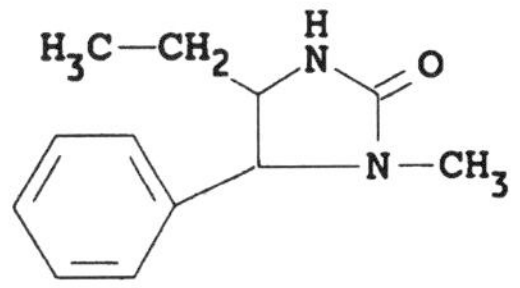

meprednisone: 16-β-methyl-prednisone; an orally effective cortisol analog, used to treat inflammatory, allergic and rheumatic conditions, and effective against some neoplasms.

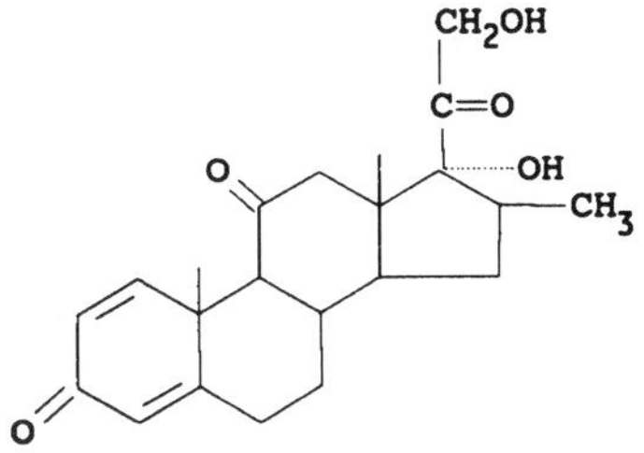

meprin: a plasma membrane metalloendopeptidase that degrades insulin B chains and some other peptides.

meprobamate: 2-methyl-2-propyl-1,3,-propanediol; a central nervous system depressant, used as an anxiolytic and sedative, and to alleviate insomnia. Large doses relax skeletal muscle.

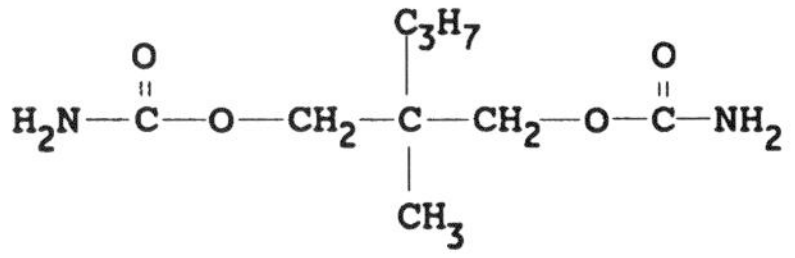

mepyrapone: metyrapone.

meq: milliequivalent.

MER-25: ethamoxytriphetol; 1-[p-(2-diethylamino-ethoxy)phenyl]-2-(p-anisyl)ethanol; a nonsteroidal estrogen receptor antagonist, used as an investigative tool, and to arrest the growth of some neoplasms.

MER-29: triparanol; 2-(p-chlorophenyl)-1-[p-diethyl-aminoethoxyphenyl]-1-(p-tolyl)ethanol; an agent that inhibits cholesterol synthesis. It is too toxic for clinical use.

mercaptans: reducing agents that contain —C—SH groups.

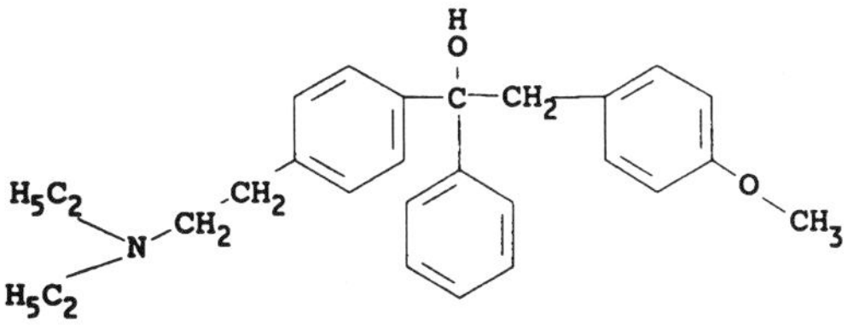

MER-25

mercaptoacetate: thioglycolic acid; an agent that binds to proteins, reduces disulfide bonds, and affects other properties. It is used to protect tryptophan in amino acid analyses, as a reagent for determination of iron, tin, molybdenum, and silver, and in bacteriological media. It also blocks fatty acid oxidation by inhibiting acyl-coenzyme A dehydrogenase, accelerates fatty acid mobilization, and promotes ATP conversion to ADP. The calcium salt is a depilatory; and ammonium salts are components of permanent wave lotions.

$$HS—CH_2—COOH$$

mercaptoethanol; thioglycol; 2-hydroxyethyl mercaptan; a reducing agent that converts disulfide bonds to sulfhydryl groups. It is used as a laboratory tool to arrest mitosis, inhibit dopamine β-hydroxylase, prepare proteins for electrophoresis, and protect catalysts against oxidative polymerization.

$$HS—CH_2—OH$$

3-**mercaptopicolinic acid**: 3-MPA: a phosphoenol-pyruvate carboxykinase inhibitor.

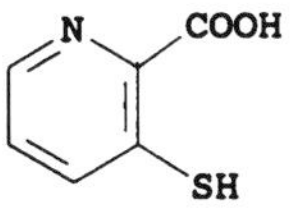

6-**mercaptopurine**: 6-MP: 6-purinethiol; a hypoxanthine analog used as an immunosuppressant and antineoplastic agent, effective against acute granulocytic, acute lymphocytic, and chronic granulocytic leukemias. Hypoxanthine-guanine phosphoribosyltransferase (HGPRT) catalyzes its conversion to 6-thio-inosine-phosphate, which accumulates and inhibits several enzymes essential for nucleic acid synthesis. It is also slowly converted to thioguanine deoxyribonucleotide, which incorporates into DNA.

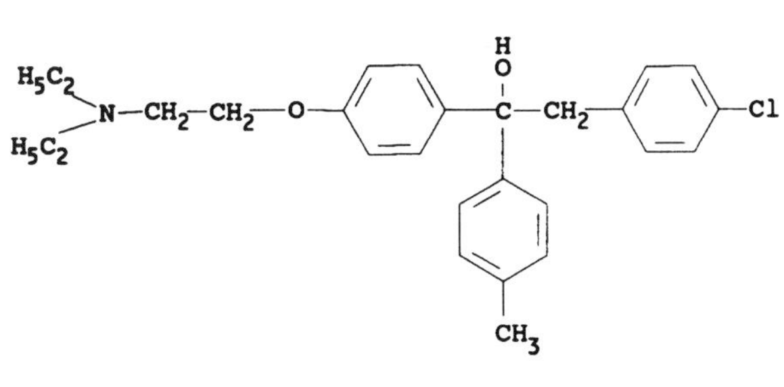

MER-29

445

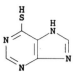

6-mercaptopurine

mercury: Hg; a metallic element (atomic number 80, atomic weight 200.59). It forms covalent bonds with sulfur atoms of enzymes whose active sites contain —SH groups, and displays weaker affinities for phosphoryl, carboxyl, amide, and amine groups. Monovalent salts, such as mercurous chloride (calomel) have been used as antiseptics, cathartics, and diuretics; and some organic mercurials (for example mersalyl) are still employed as diuretics. Divalent salts, are highly toxic and strong irritants, but were once used to treat syphilis.

Merkel's cells: Merkel-Ranvier cells; clear cells in epidermis basal layers that contain catecholamines, and are morphologically similar to melanocytes.

Merkel's discs: Merkel corpuscles; epidermal touch receptors. They are small and cup-shaped, each composed of the endings of a single nerve fiber in contact with an epithelial cell.

mero-: a prefix used for fragments of larger compounds, as in meromyosin and meroreceptor.

meroblastic cleavage: incomplete or partial cleavage; division of a blastomere, with no concomitant separation of yolk.

merocrine: describes glands that produce watery secretions; *cf* **holocrine** and **apocrine**.

merocyte: a cell type in the yolk region of a fertilized macrolecithal ovum, derived from a nonfertilizing spermatozoan.

meromyosins: fragments formed when myosin is digested with trypsin. The heavy meromyosin component (HMM) is a short rod with two globular domains that contains the hinge region, the ATPase, and the actin binding sites. Light meromyosin is the helical component that interacts with other light meromyosin molecules, and forms most of the thick filament.

merosins: tissue-specific 300K basement membrane-associated glycoproteins structurally similar to laminin, with 40% amino acid identity. They occur in human placenta trophoblastic tissue, and in striated muscle and peripheral nerves, and are implicated as regulators of tissue differentiation and maturation.

merospermy: a form of gynogenesis, in which the sperm nucleus makes contact with the oocyte nucleus and stimulates, but then degenerates without imparting its DNA.

merozoite: the motile sporozoan formed during the life-cycle of the malaria parasite that arises from asexual division in the liver and is released to the bloodstream.

mesangial cells: stellate cells of the renal glomerular tuft microvasculature that extend processes between epithelial cells and the basal lamina. They derive from smooth muscle, and are believed to contribute to the control of blood flow. Regulators that stimulate their contraction include angiotensin II, vasopressin, norepinephrine, platelet activating factor (PAF), platelet derived growth factor (PDGF), histamine, prostaglandin $F_{2\alpha}$, leukotrienes C and D, and thromboxane A_2. Dopamine, atrial natriuretic peptides, and PGE_2 are among the factors that promote relaxation. Mesangial cells are also phagocytic, and may function as accessory cells that participate in immune responses by presenting antigens.

mesangium: the thin membrane that supports the capillary loops of renal glomeruli; *see* also **mesangial cells**.

mescaline: 3,4,5-trimethyoxyphenylethylamine; an alkaloid from the flowering heads of the peyote cactus, *Lophophora williamsii*. It alters perception, affects mood, invokes hallucinations, and is used in tribal rites. At least some of the effects involve interactions with serotonin receptors.

mesectoderm: embryonic tissue derived from the neural crest of the head region that contributes to the formation of meninges.

mesencephalon: midbrain; (1) the second of the three primary embryonic cerebral vesicles; (2) the part of the brain stem that develops from the middle primary vesicle and lies between the diencephalon and the pons. It surrounds the cerebral aqueduct, and includes the corpora quadrigemina (required for eye and ear reflexes), the nuclei for the oculomotor and trochlear nerves, the cerebral peduncles (crus cerebri) traversed by the corticospinal tracts, the substantia nigra, and the red nucleus. Axons that communicate with the thalamus and pineal gland pass through this region. Regulators identified there include cholecystokinin (CCK) and dopamine.

mesenchymal cells: cells that originate in the embryonic mesenchyme. Some persist as precursors of fibroblasts, chondroblasts, osteoblasts, adipocytes, and other connective tissue cell types.

mesenchyme: tissue derived mostly from mesoderm that forms loose networks in embryos and gives rise to more mature connective tissues. It transports chemical messengers to neighboring epithelium that affect growth and differentiation.

mesenteric: (1) pertaining to the mesentery; (2) a term applied to the liver, pancreas, intestine, and spleen, and to the blood vessels and nerves that supply them.

mesentery: a membranous fold that attaches visceral organs to the body wall.

meso-: a prefix denoting (1) middle; (2) connecting; (3) in chemistry, an atom that forms a bridge, or an isomer that contains asymmetric components but is not asymmetric when assembled; *see* for example **tartaric acid**.

mesoderm: (1) the middle of the three primary embryonic germ layers. It divides into outer somatic and inner splanchnic components, and gives rise to connective, musculoskeletal, and blood vascular tissues, and to parts of the kidneys, gonads, and adrenal glands; (2) a term that additionally includes the extraembryonic mesoderm (which contributes to the formation of fetal membranes).

mesolecithal: describes oocytes or ova that contain moderate amounts of yolk; *cf* **macrolecithal** and **microlecithal**.

mesomorph: an individual of medium stature, with a well-proportioned, usually muscular body; *cf* **ectomorph** and **endomorph**.

mesonephros: Wolffian body; the second of the three kidney types formed prenatally in mammals. It replaces the pronephros, contributes to development of the urinary and reproductive systems, and is replaced by the metanephros. It persists as the permanent kidney in reptiles.

mesothelial cells: flat epithelial cells derived from mesoderm that line the peritoneal, pleural, pericardial, and other serous cavities, and form the secretory epithelium of the kidneys.

mesotocin: MT; a neurohypophysial peptide made by birds, reptiles, amphibians, and lungfishes that is chemically and biologically related to oxytocin and vasopressin. It is a vasodilator that lowers blood pressure in most species, but a stimulant for nonvascular smooth muscle. In mammals, it promotes contraction of uterine and myoepithelial cells, but does not mediate water retention. The amino acid sequence is: Cys-Tyr-Ile-Gln-Asn-Cys-Pro-Ile-Gly-NH$_2$, with a bridge between the two cysteine moieties.

Mesozoic: the era, preceded by the Paleozoic, and followed by the Cenozoic, believed to have extended from 180 to 125 million years ago, divided into three periods: *Triassic*, dominated by reptiles and conifers, during which the first primitive mammals appeared; *Jurassic*, the age of dinosaurs, during which bony fish and the first flowering plants evolved; and *Cretaceous*, when reptiles assumed dominance but dinosaurs became extinct, marsupial mammals appeared, and the numbers of flowering plants and insects increased.

messenger RNAs: mRNAs; **ribonucleic acids** (*q.v.*) that direct translation of specific proteins, formed from primary transcripts (premessenger RNAs) whose synthesis is catalyzed by RNA polymerase II. Processing of eukaryote primary transcripts usually involves capping, polyadenylation, and excision of one or more introns.

mestranol: 17α-ethinylestradiol 3-methyl ether; an orally effective estrogen receptor agonist. It is a component of Enovid, Ortho-Novum, C-Quens, Metrulen, and other oral contraceptive preparations.

mesylate: methane sulfonate.

Met: M; methionine.

met: a proto-oncogene that codes for an approximately 190K transmembrane protein which undergoes autophosphorylation when activated by its ligand. The product is a receptor for both hepatocyte growth factor (which appears to be identical with scatter factor and human lung fibroblast derived mitogen) and for a hepatocyte growth factor antagonist. Amplification and overexpression, invoked by fusion with a segment from chromosome 1, has been detected in human gastric cancer cells and some of their precancerous precursors, and also in a chemically transformed human osteosarcoma cell line.

***f*Met:** formyl methionine; *see* **methionine**.

meta-: *m*-: a prefix for benzene compounds with substitutions at positions 1 and 3 (*cf* **ortho** and **para**), and for polymeric acid anhydrides such as metaphosphoric acid.

metabolic acidosis: nonrespiratory disorders in which accumulation of acidic metabolites or loss of alkali leads to lowering of the blood plasma pH and NaHCO$_3$:HHCO$_3$ ratio. The causes include starvation, insulin deficiency, and other conditions that accelerate lipolysis and/or inhibit lipogenesis, ingestion of high-fat, low-carbohydrate, or sodium deficient diets, and conditions such as aldosterone deficiency that impair renal reabsorption of sodium and bicarbonate. In *compensated* metabolic acidosis, accelerated carbon dioxide loss via the lungs decreases the HHCO$_3$ content and thereby raises the NaHCO$_3$:HHCO$_3$ ratio. However, the total bicarbonate concentration is subnormal. *Cf* **metabolic alkalosis** and **respiratory acidosis**.

metabolic alkalosis: nonrespiratory disorders in which accumulation of alkaline metabolites or loss of acidic ones leads to elevation of the blood pH and NaHCO$_3$:HHCO$_3$ ratio. It is often associated with hypokalemia. The causes include mineralocorticoid excess and ingestion of very alkaline diets. In *compensated* metabolic alkalosis, decreased carbon dioxide excretion by the lungs leads to retention of HHCO$_3$ and lowering of the NaHCO$_3$:HHCO$_3$ ratio. (The total bicarbonate concentration is elevated). *Cf* **metabolic acidosis** and **respiratory alkalosis**.

metabolic burst: *see* **respiratory burst**.

metabolic clearance rate: MCR: a measure of how rapidly a substance is removed from a compartment via sequestration, chemical modification, and/or excretion.

Plasma clearance rates do not necessarily reflect time courses for hormone actions, since some regulators bind avidly to target cells and/or initiate persistent secondary events.

metabolic pathway: a coordinated series of chemical reactions that leads to the formation of specific end products.

metabolic rate: heat production rate, usually expressed in Calories per hour per square meter of body surface for humans and other large animals (*see* also **basal metabolic rate**). For tissues, units such as calories per hour per milligram are more commonly used. Although they can be determined directly, the values are usually obtained by measuring oxygen consumption rates and calculating the heat equivalents.

Metabolin: a trade name for thiamine hydrochloride.

metabolism: all chemical processes used by living organisms to synthesize body components and/or obtain energy (including anabolism and catabolism). *See* also **intermediary metabolism**.

metabolite: any substance produced by a chemical reaction within a living organism.

metacentric: describes chromosomes with centrally located centromeres.

metachromasia: describes substances in which a component assumes a color different from surrounding ones, or a color different from that of the applied biological stain. In the second case, it usually involves polymerization of the dye.

metafemale; superfemale: (1) a vertebrate with a female phenotype and more than the usual numbers of female-type sex chromosomes. Humans with XXX and XXXX patterns usually have low fertility and suffer other dysfunctions; (2) an insect with an X chromosome: autosome ratio greater than one, a condition associated with diminished viability.

metagenesis: alternation of generations. The life cycles of some invertebrates involve two diploid stages. In higher plants, one stage is haploid.

metal: any element that can form cations in solution.

metalloenzymes: enzymes that contain or bind metallic elements essential for their functions. In some cases, the element participates directly in the reactions; in others, it stabilizes active configurations.

metallothioneins: 10K cysteine-rich proteins (metallothioneins I, II, and their subtypes), made in liver, kidney, intestine, lung, spleen, brain, skin, placenta, yolk sac, and elsewhere. They avidly bind heavy metals, promote tissue-specific redistribution of zinc (for example from blood plasma to liver, bone marrow, and thymus glands), and of copper, and thereby contribute to regulation of growth processes and membrane stabilization. They are also oxygen radical scavengers, and can protect against heavy metal poisoning. The levels rise in response to heat, cold, food deprivation, and other forms of stress. Inducers include heavy metals, glucocorticoids,

epinephrine, and glucagon. Interleukins 1α and 6 probably act indirectly, by affecting glucocorticoid release. Since metallothionein promoters attached to the coding regions of other genes and promote transcription when activated by cadmium, zinc, and other factors, they are incorporated into plasmids, and used to stimulate the production of growth hormone and other proteins.

metamale: in *Drosophila* and some other insects, an animal with one X chromosome and three sets of autosomes; *cf* **metafemale**.

metamerism: serial repetition of similar structures, for example of earthworm segments. Vertebrate embryos form several kinds of metameres, most of which fuse during organogenesis. Rib cages and vertebral columns are examples of structures that retain the patterns.

metamorphosis: a substantial change in form. Most commonly (1) body changes associated with maturation, such as transformation from a larva to a reproductively competent adult (as in insects and amphibians); *cf* **neoteny**. Triiodothyronine is the major stimulant for many species, whereas prolactin inhibits in some; (2) changes in tissue structure, such as fatty degeneration.

metamyelocytes: bone marrow cells that differentiate from myelocytes and mature to neutrophilic leukocytes.

Metandren: a trade name for methyltestosterone.

metanephrine: 3-methyl-epinephrine: a metabolite formed when epinephrine is inactivated by catecholamine-*O*-methyltransferase (COMT.) Some metanephrine is excreted to urine, but most is further metabolized to vanillyl mandelic acid outside the nervous system, or to 3-methoxy,4-hydroxyphenylethylglycol (MOPEG) in neurons.

metanephros: the permanent kidney that develops in mammalian embryos; *cf* **mesonephros**.

metaphase: the stage of mitosis or meiosis that follows prophase, in which condensed chromosomes arrange along the equatorial plane. It is followed by anaphase.

metaphase plate: equatorial plate; the plane of the spindle along which chromosomes align during meiosis and mitosis.

metaphit methanesulfonate: 1-(1,3-isothiocyananto)-phenyl)-cyclohexylpiperidine methylsulfonate; a phencyclidine (PCP) derivative that promotes irreversible acylation of compounds believed to be specific phencyclidine (PCP) receptors in rat brains, and sigma (σ) receptors in guinea pig brains. It is a noncompetitive inhibitor that blocks PCP influences on cerebral glucose utilization and behavior, and may additionally act on NMDA (*N*-methyl-D-aspartate) receptors.

metaphysis: (1) the growing end of the diaphysis of an immature long bone, adjacent to the epiphysial cartilage;

metaphit methanesulfonate

(2) the bony region in an adult that forms from the preceding, and fuses with the epiphysis.

metaplasia: abnormal transformation of one kind of differentiated adult tissue into another within an organ. It can occur in response to injury or a pathological condition. *Cf* **neoplasia**.

metapramine: 10,11-dihdyro-*N*,5-dimethyl-5*H*-dibenz-[*b*,*f*]azepin-10-amine; a tricyclic antidepressant with properties similar to those of imipramine.

metaproterenol: 5-[1-hydroxy-2-[1-methylethyl)amino]ethyl]-1.3-benzenediol; a sympathomimetic agent, fairly selective for β₂-type adrenergic receptors that resists methylation by catecholamine-*O*-methyltransferase, used orally and as an inhalant for long-term treatment of obstructive airway diseases, and to alleviate acute bronchospasm.

metaraminol: *m*-hydroxyphenylpropanolamine; an agent that blocks neuronal uptake of catecholamines, and thereby enhances and prolongs their effects. It is used to treat some forms of hypotension.

metastasis: transfer of disease from one body site to another. The term usually refers to the migration of tumor cells and the establishment of secondary tumors, but is applied in other ways, for example to the spread of an infection or its secondary effects.

metastatic calcification: deposition of calcium salts in soft tissues. Vascular smooth muscle, kidney tubules, and myocardium are common sites; but it can occur in skin and elsewhere. The most severe generalized conditions are initiated by high calcitriol levels, (which elevate both calcium and phosphate concentrations in extracellular fluids). Other causes include chronic hypercalcemia (invoked by hyperparathyroidism, or by tumors that secrete parathyroid-like peptides), and chronic hyperphosphatemia secondary to renal dysfunction. Localized deposition, for example in bursae, can occur at sites of injury when blood mineral levels are in the normal range.

metapyrone: metyrapone.

metaxalone: 5-(3,5-dimethylphenoxymethyl)-2-oxazolidone; a central nervous system depressant that acts preferentially on interneurons. It is used to alleviate skeletal muscle spasms.

metazoan: (1) any multicellular animal; (2) an animal with more than one kind of tissue.

metazocine: 2'-hydroxy-2,5,9-trimethyl-6,7-benzomorphan; a synthetic narcotic, equipotent with morphine, that acts on the same receptors.

metecdysis: the stage of a molting cycle that immediately follows shell shedding.

metencephalon: (1) the embryonic brain component that develops from the rhombencephalon and gives rise to the pons and cerebellum; (2) the pons.

metenkephalin: methionine enkephalin; ME; Tyr-Gly-Gly-Phe-Met; a peptide cleaved from proenkephalin A in brain, spinal cord, sympathetic nerves, adrenal medulla, pituitary gland, heart, gut, reproductive system organs, and elsewhere. The amino acid sequence is identical with moieties 61-65 of β-lipotropin, but ME is not derived from that peptide. Although many of the effects are mediated via δ-type opioid receptors, ME also interacts to some extent with μ types. However, it is a weaker analgesic than morphine, β-endorphin, and leu-enkephalin. ME functions as a neurotransmitter and neuromodulator that affects behavior, and is implicated as a mediator of olfaction and other forms of sensory perception. It co-localizes with catecholamines in sympathetic system neurons and adrenal medulla cells, and is co-secreted in response to many forms of stress. In the digestive system, it antagonizes motilin-stimulated phasic stomach contractions, and exerts complex effects on the small intestine (activation of quiescent muscle via both acetylcholine release, and direct stimulation of the deep muscular plexus, but inhibition of active muscle via effects on the myenteric plexus). ME is also made by germinal, Sertoli, and Leydig cells of the testis, concentrates in acrosomes, and is implicated as a mediator of sperm motility and fertilization. Roles in female reproductive system functions are suggested by cyclic changes in ovarian follicular fluid levels (highest during metestrus and diestrus in rodents, and further elevated if progesterone is administered after estrogen priming). Progesterone directly raises the levels in uterine fluid. In common with other opioids, it can augment prolactin and growth hormone secretion; and it also affects gamma aminobutyric acid (GABA) and neurohypophysial peptide levels (but is less effective for inhibition of luteinizing hormone release than β-endorphin). Additionally, it participates in baroreceptor reflexes, stimulates lymphocyte proliferation, and affects chromatophore movements in poikilotherms.

metenkephalin-RF: Tyr-Gly-Gly-Phe-Met-Arg-Phe; one of several biologically active opioid peptides cleaved from proenkephalin A, in adrenal glands and at some other sites. It exerts metenkephalin-like effects by acting on δ type opioid receptors, but is a more potent ligand for μ type receptors.

metenkephalin-RGL: Tyr-Gly-Gly-Phe-Met-Arg-Gly-Leu; a biologically active opioid peptide cleaved from proenkephalin A that acts mostly on κ and δ type opioid receptors; *cf* **metenkephalin** and **metenkephalin-RF**.

metergoline: methergoline: D-N-carbobenzoxydihydro-1-methyllysergamine; a serotonin receptor antagonist chemically related to ergot alkaloids. It is also a dopamine receptor agonist, used to inhibit prolactin secretion.

metestrus: the phase of the estrous cycle that follows ovulation, during which some progesterone is secreted and the endometrium is prepared for implantation. It is followed by diestrus. *Cf* **estrus**.

metformin: N-N-dimethylimidodicarbonimidic diamide: a "second generation" biguanide type oral hypoglycemic agent. It has replaced phenformin (which often invokes lactacidosis), but is contraindicated in individuals with renal dysfunction.

methacholine: mecholyl; 2-(acetyloxy)-N,N,N-trimethyl-1-propanaminium; a broad-spectrum muscarinic type acetylcholine receptor agonist that is slowly degraded by cholinesterases. The bromide, chloride, and iodide salts are used in the diagnosis of bronchial asthma, and to treat paroxysmal tachycardia.

methadone hydrochloride: 6-dimethylamino-4,4-diphenyl-3-heptanone hydrochloride; an orally effective agent that acts on μ type opioid receptors. It is used mostly to treat morphine and heroine withdrawal symptoms, and to maintain morphine and heroine addicts, but also to some extent as an analgesic and, in low doses, as an antitussive. Many effects (including euphoria) closely resemble those of morphine; but tolerance develops more slowly. The (+) isomer is less addictive than the (−), and does not cause respiratory depression. Methadone also inhibits the growth of some lung cancer cells, probably by acting on κ receptors. This activity can be blocked with naltrexone, cycloheximide, or actinomycin D, but not with nicotine, pertussis toxin, or some other agents that affect the growth inhibiting effects of morphine.

methallibure: N-methyl-N′-(1-methyl-2-propenyl)-1,2,-hydrazinecarbothioamide; an agent used to stimulate production of some pituitary gland hormones in swine. It inhibits gonadotropin secretion, and can block implantation.

methamphetamine: d-deoxyephedrine; a sympathomimetic agent with actions similar to those of amphetamine, but a more potent central nervous system stimulant. It suppresses appetite, but exerts toxic effects. Its value in the treatment of obesity has been questioned.

methandriol: 17α-methyl-androstenediol; 5,6-dehydro-androsterone; a synthetic androgen used for its anabolic effects; *see* **anabolic steroids**. The trade names include Protandren, Neosteron, and Stenediol. Probolin is the dipropionate conjugate.

methandrostenolone: 17-hydroxy-17α-methyl-androsta-1,4-diene-3-one; a synthetic androgen used for its

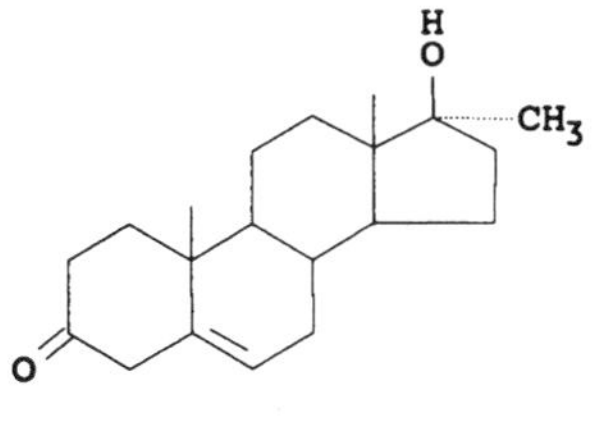

methandriol

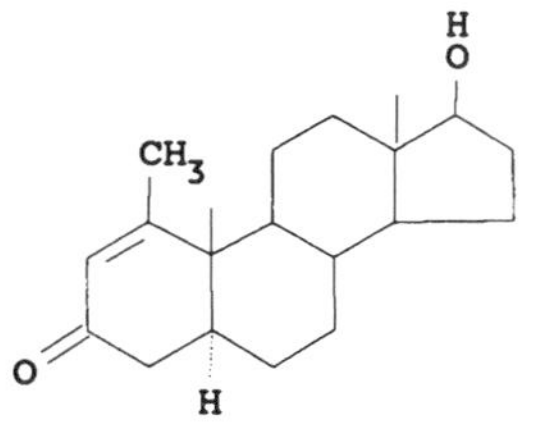

methenolone

anabolic effects; *see* **anabolic steroids**. The trade names include Dianobol, Nabolin, and Stenolon.

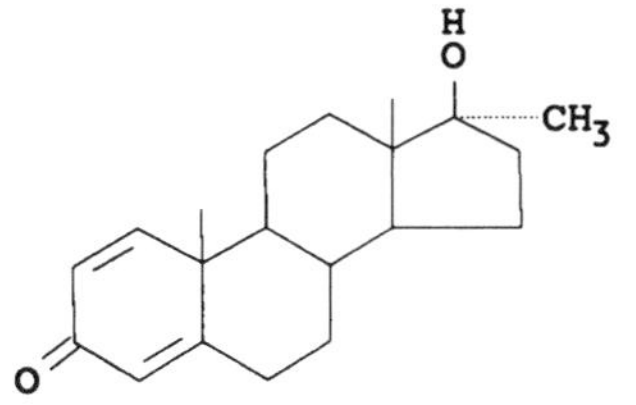

methanol: wood alcohol; CH_3—OH; a solvent used in numerous industrial, pharmaceutical, and laboratory procedures. It is highly toxic if ingested, and can cause acidosis, dizziness, convulsions, blindness, pancreatic necrosis, and respiratory failure. Some of the effects are attributed to formation of formic acid and other metabolites.

methazolamide: 5-acetylamino-4-methyl-Δ^2-1,3,4-thiadiazoline-2-sulfonamide; a carbonic anhydrase inhibitor used to treat glaucoma.

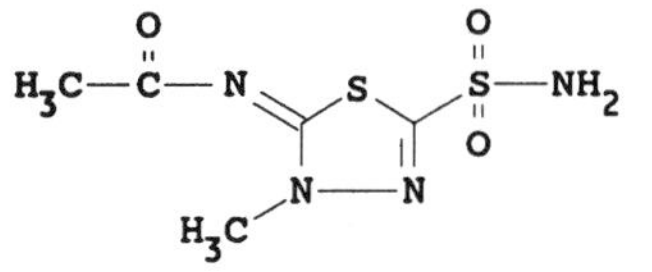

methemoglobin: ferrihemoglobin; hemoglobin in which the iron atom has been oxidized to Fe^{3+}. Very small amounts form under normal conditions. Nitrites and high doses of phenacetin, sulfonamides, and several other agents markedly increase the levels. Cyanide kills by poisoning the cytochrome system. If nitrites are administered very soon after exposure, they promote methemoglobin formation, and the Fe^{3+} component binds tightly to the cyanide. The treatment does not seriously compromise respiratory gas exchange, since only limited amounts of methemoglobin (which does not transport oxygen) are formed.

methemoglobin reductase: NADH diaphorase; an erythrocyte enzyme that protects against methemoglobin accumulation by catalyzing transfer of electrons from methemoglobin to NAD^+.

methenolone: 17β-hydroxy-1β-methyl-5α-androst-1-en-3-one; a synthetic androgen used for its anabolic effects; *see* **anabolic steroids**. Primobolan is one of the trade names.

methimidazole: methimazole; MMI; mercaptothiazole; methylmercaptimidazole; Tapazole; 1-methyl-2-mercap-

toimidazole; 1,3-dihydro-1-methyl-2*H*-imidazole-2-thione; an agent that inhibits thyroxine synthesis by acting on the peroxidase that catalyzes iodine oxidation and incorporation into thyroglobulin. It has little effect on peripheral conversion of thyroxine (T_4) to triiodothyronine (T_3); *cf* **propylthiouracil**. However, it indirectly lowers T_3 levels, and is used in conjunction with other agents for this purpose. The therapeutic effects in some forms of hyperthyroidism are attributed in part to additional suppression of autoimmune processes. The most common side effects are allergic reactions. Toxicity is rare, but MMI has been known to invoke hepatitis, arthritis, and bone marrow depression.

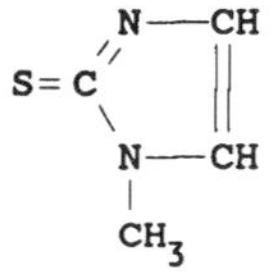

methionine: an essential amino acid, and a component of most proteins (including many enzymes), and of numerous biologically active peptides. It reacts with ATP to form *S*-adenosylmethionine, a donor of methyl groups for the biosynthesis of acetylcholine, epinephrine, melatonin, spermine, and other compounds. Homocysteine made in those reactions is a substrate for homocysteine methyltransferase, which regenerates methionine by transferring methyl groups from N^5-methyltetrahydrofolate. Oxidants can abolish the functions of methionine-containing molecules by converting them to methionine sulfoxides. (The emphysema that develops in susceptible individuals who smoke is attributed to such destruction of an elastase inhibitor.) Methionine is also the first amino acid attached to ribosomes during translation in eukaryotes. (In prokaryotes, it is *formyl*-methionine, *f*-Met). Methionine deficiency effects include anemia, hypoproteinemia, hair loss, accumulation of fat in and necrosis of the liver, and kidney damage. Methionine affinity for cyanogen bromide is used in protein analysis.

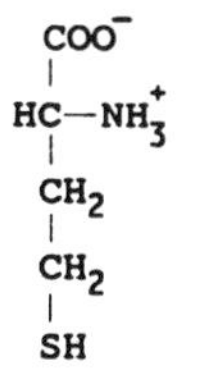

homocysteine

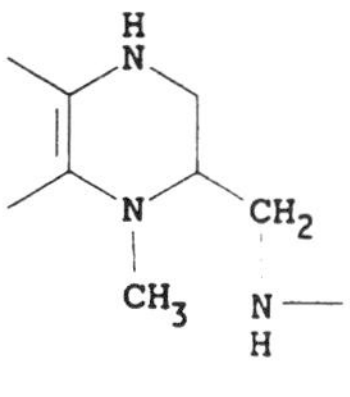

N^5-methyltetrahydro-folate

451

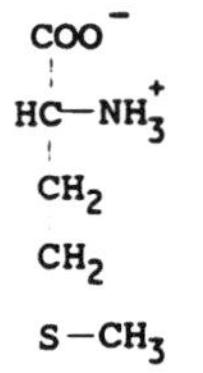

methionine 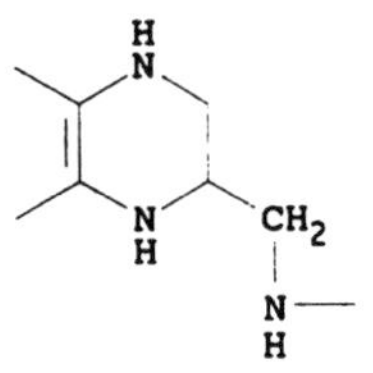   tetrahydrofolate 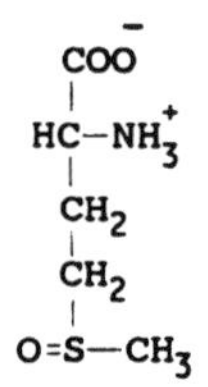   methionine sulfoxide

methionine adenosyltransferase: *see* **S-adenosylmethionine**.

methionine-enkephalin: *see* **metenkephalin**.

methionine sulfoxide: a toxic metabolite formed when oxidants act on **methionine** (*q.v.*).

methionine sulfoximine: an agent used to inhibit glutamine transferase, and to measure methionine production by microorganisms.

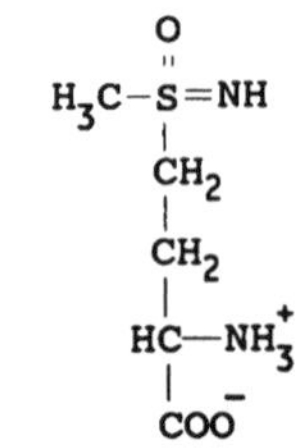

methiothepin mesylate: 1-[10,11-dihydro-8-(methylthio)-dibenzo[*b,f*]thiepin-10-yl]-4-methylpiperazine mesylate; a 5HT$_1$ type serotonin receptor antagonist that acts on autoreceptors.

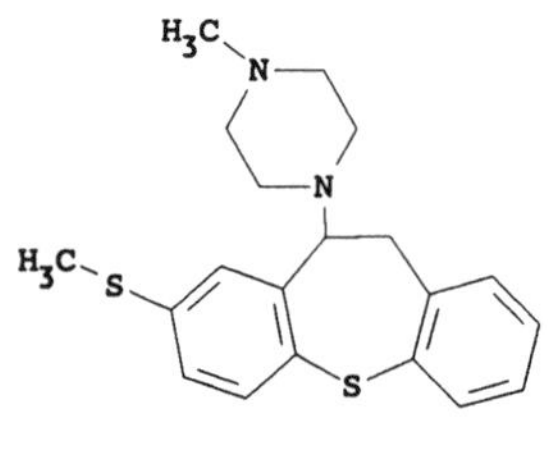

methoctramine tetrachloride: *N,N'*-bis[6-[[(2-methoxyphenyl)methyl]amino]hexyl]-1,8-octane diamine tetrahydrochloride; a highly selective M$_2$ type muscarinic receptor antagonist.

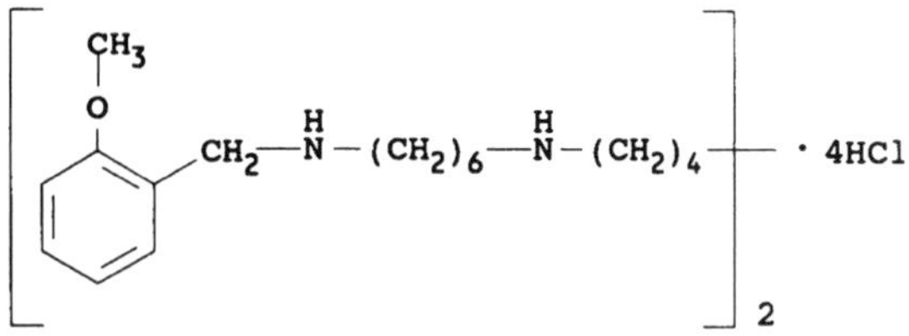

methoctramine tetrachloride

methohexital sodium: 5-allyl-1-methyl-5-1-(1-methyl-2-pentynyl)barbituric acid sodium salt; an ultrashort acting barbiturate, used for anesthesia.

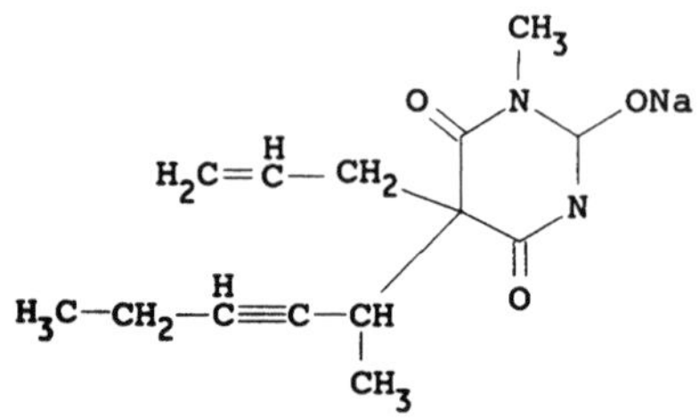

methotrexate: amethopterin; 4-amino-N^{10}-methylpteroylglutamic acid; a very potent antimetabolite that blocks folic acid functions by binding to and inhibiting dihydrofolate reductase. It is used as an immunosuppressant to treat psoriasis, granulomatosis, and severe cases of rheumatoid arthritis, and to protect against transplant rejection. It is also effective against choriocarcinomas and osteosarcomas, and can accomplish temporary remission in some forms of leukemia. Some of the toxic effects are minimized by simultaneous administration of leucovorin. Certain microorganisms resist the effects via gene amplification that leads to the production of large quantities of the enzyme. Cloning vectors containing the gene are used to identify methotrexate transformants.

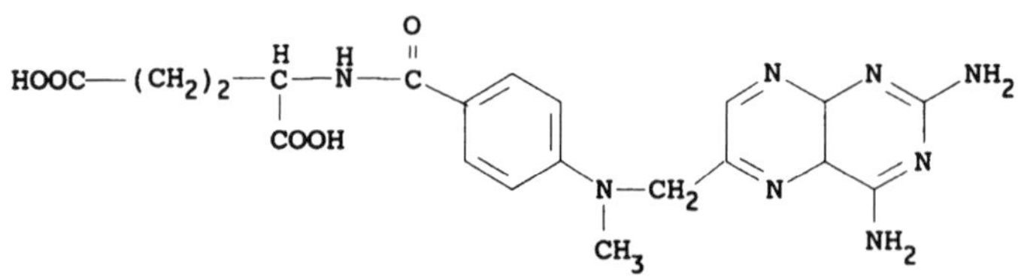

methotrexate

methoxamine: Vasoxyl; α-1-(aminoethyl)-2,5-dimethoxy-benzene methanol; a highly selective α_1-type adrenergic receptor agonist. The hydrochloride is administered intravenously to arrest paroxysmal tachycardia, and to treat some forms of hypotension.

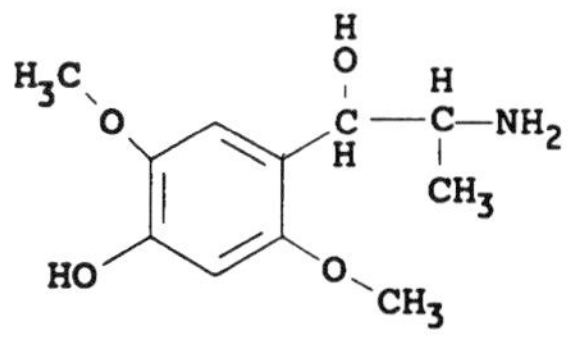

6-methoxybenzoxazolinone: *see* 6-**MBOA**.

methoxyestrogens: two of the compounds are shown; *see* **catechol estrogens**.

3-methoxy,4-hydroxyphenylethylglycoaldehyde; a metabolite formed when norepinephrine and epinephrine are degraded by both catecholamine-*O*-methyltransferase (COMT) and monoamine oxidase (MAO). Centrally, most is reduced to 3-methoxy,4-hydroxy-phenylethylglycol, conjugated with sulfate, and released for excretion to the urine. Peripherally, most is oxidized to vanillylmandelic acid (VMA). *See* also **MOPEG**

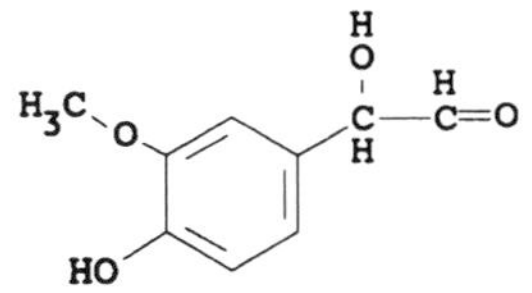

3-methoxy,4-hydrdroxyphenylethylglycol: MOPEG, MPG; an epinephrine and norepinephrine metabolite made mostly in the central nervous system; *see* 3-**methoxy,4-hydroxyphenylethylglycoaldehyde**.

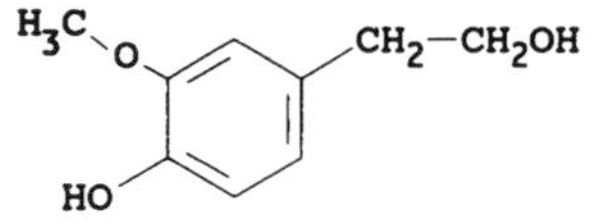

5-methoxyindole acetic acid: 5-MIAA; a serotonin metabolite, formed from 5-hydroxyindole acetic acid (5-HIAA) via a reaction catalyzed by hydroxyindole-*O*-methyltransferase (HIOMT).

2-methoxy-3,4-methylenedioxyamphetamine: ecstasy; *see* **MMDA**.

1-(2-methoxyphenyl)piperazine hydrochloride: 2-MPP hydrochloride; a selective $5HT_1$ type serotonin receptor agonist.

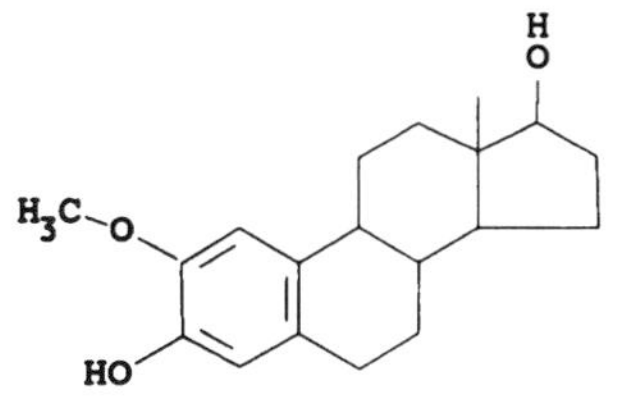

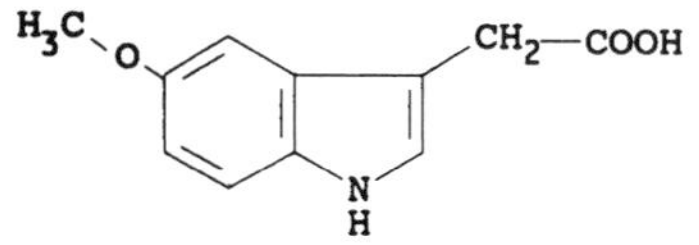

5-methoxyindole acetic acid

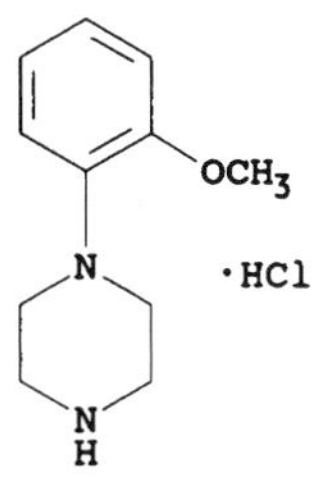

1-(2-methoxyphenyl)piperazine hydrochloride

6-methoxypurine: a guanine analog. It is a potent inhibitor of phosphoribosyltransferases. The enzymes catalyze nucleic acid base reactions with 5-phosphoribosyl-1-pyrophosphate (PRPP) to yield the corresponding ribonucleotides + P-P.

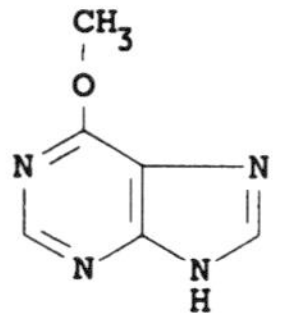

5-methoxytryptamine: 3-(2-aminoethyl)-5-methoxyindole: a tryptophan metabolite, formed via reactions catalyzed by tryptophan decarboxylase and catecholamine-*O*-methyltransferase (COMT). It exerts potent serotonin-like effects, and can potentiate the actions of some sedatives and hypnotics.

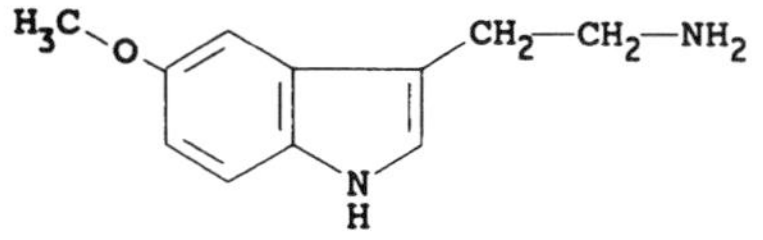

5-methoxytrytophol: a serotonin metabolite made in pineal glands that may function as a physiological inhibitor of gonadotropin secretion.

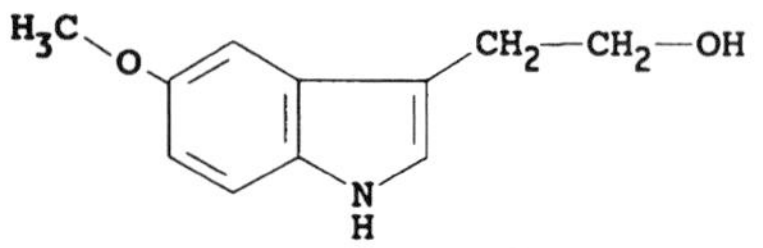

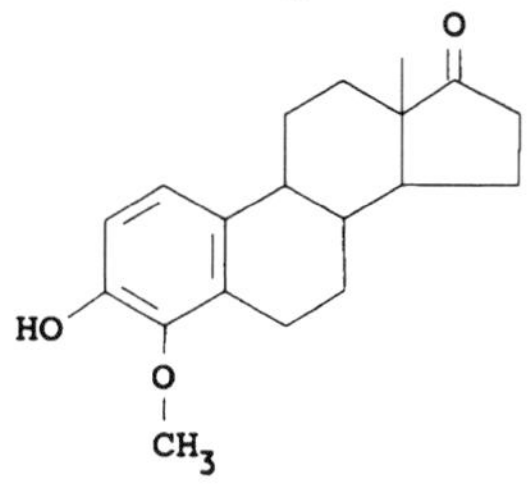

2-methoxy estradiol

4-methoxy estrone

453

1-methyl adenine: a hormone that stimulates germinal vesicle breakdown in invertebrate oocytes. 1-methyl adenosine exerts similar effects in some species.

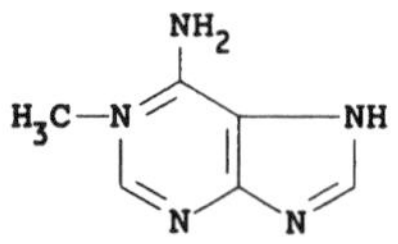

methyl alcohol: methanol.

methylamine: a flammable corrosive gas used to manufacture organic compounds. It promotes ligand-receptor dissociation and accelerates receptor recycling by accumulating in lysosomes and elevating the internal pH.

N^G-**methylarginine**: an arginine analog used to inhibit nitric oxide synthetase.

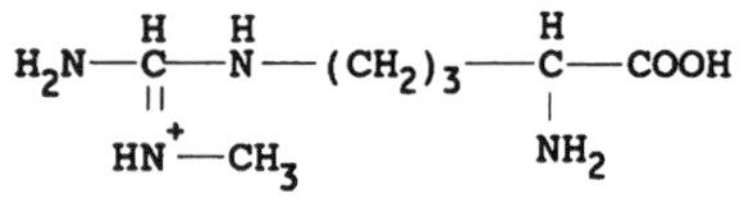

N-**methyl**-D-**aspartate**: *see* **NMDA**.

methylation: addition of methyl groups; *see* **methionine**. Selective methylation of DNA bases inactivates some genes, and mediates cell type specific effects on transcription.

methylcarbaminocholine: methylcarbachol; a nicotinic type acetylcholine receptor agonist that acts preferentially on autoreceptor types.

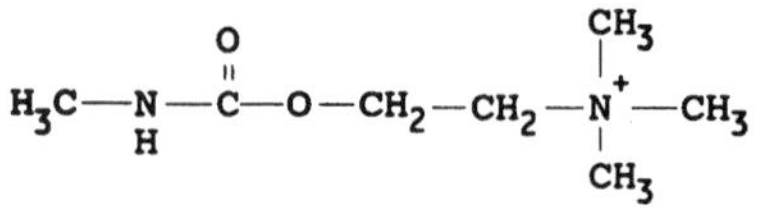

methylcholanthrene: 3-MECA; a carcinogenic hydrocarbon.

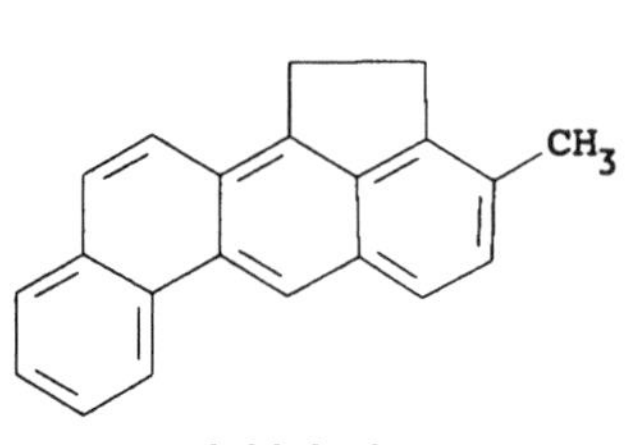

α-**methyldopa**: Aldomet; 3-hydroxy-α-methyl tyrosine; an agent that crosses blood-brain barriers and is rapidly converted α-methyldopamine, α-methylnorepinephrine, and α-methylepinephrine. The norepinephrine derivative is a potent α₂ type adrenergic receptor agonist that decreases norepinephrine secretion, promotes vasodila-

methylcholanthrene

tion, and is used (usually in conjunction with diuretics) for its antihypertensive effects. Aldomet also depletes brain epinephrine stores. The side effects can include sedation, headache, blurred vision, parkinson-like symptoms and (in rare cases) liver injury. Although it also inhibits DOPA decarboxylase, its major effects are no longer attributed to this property.

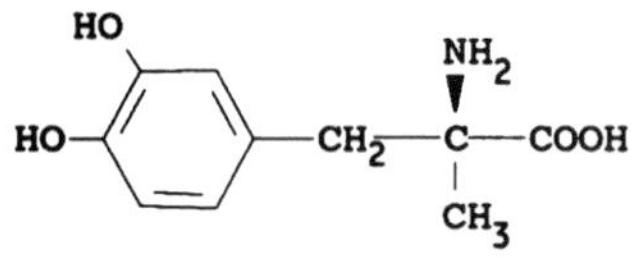

3-*O*-**methyldopa**: 3-methoxy-tyrosine: a tyrosine degradation product, formed in a reaction catalyzed by catecholamine-*O*-methyltransferase (COMT). It crosses bloodbrain barriers and is slowly converted to dopamine.

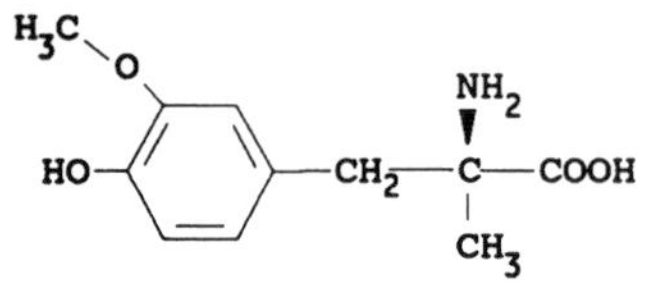

methylene adenosine triphosphates: both αβ (AMP-CPP) and βγ (AMP-PCP) forms are potent P₂ type purinergic receptor agonists.

methylene blue: methylthionium chloride; a hydrogen and electron acceptor, used as an indicator in oxidation-reduction reactions, a bacteriological stain, an antiseptic, an antidote for cyanide and nitrate poisoning, and to inhibit soluble guanylate cyclases.

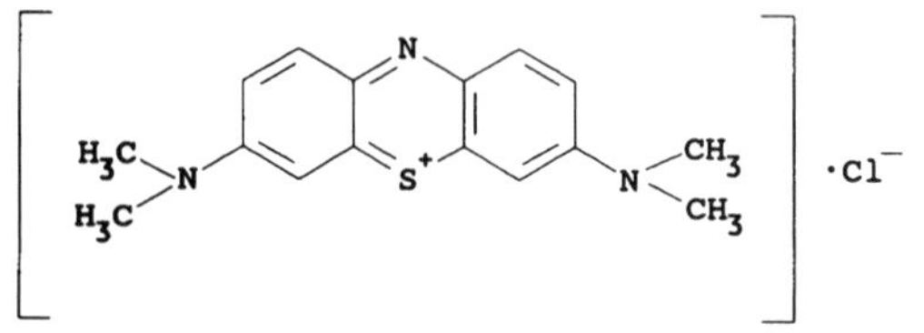

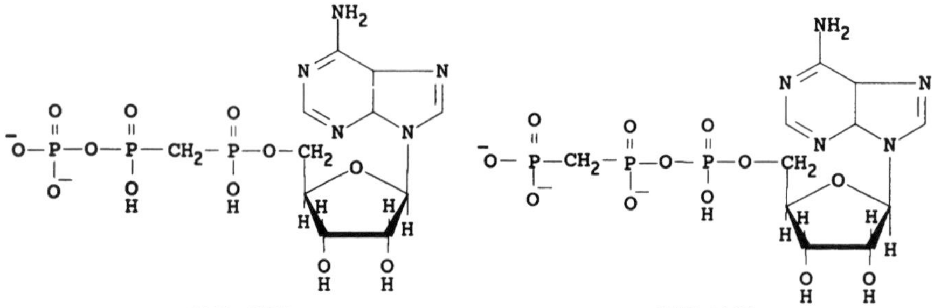

AMP−CPP

AMP−PCP

methylene adenosine triphosphates

3,4-methylenedioxyamphetamine: MDA; a mescaline-like psychedelic agent taken directly, and formed when **MMDA** (ecstasy, *q.v.*) is ingested. The effects are similar to those of lysergic acid diethylamide (LSD); but at high dosages amphetamine-like actions are more pronounced.

3-methyl-GABA *bis*-naphthalene sulfonate: an activator of GABA aminotransferase that can suppress convulsions.

methyl green: 4-[[4-(dimethylamino)phenyl][4-(dimethylimino)-2,5-cyclohexadien-1-ylidene]-methyl]-*N*-ethyl-*N*,*N*-dimethylbenzenaminium bromide chloride; a biological stain for undegraded DNA in cells and electrophoresis studies.

2-methylhistamine: an H_1 type histamine receptor agonist.

4(5)-methylhistamine: an H_2-type histamine receptor antagonist.

(*R*)α-methylhistamine: an H_3 type histamine receptor agonist.

α-methylhistidine: a histidine analog used to inhibit histidine decarboxylase.

methylmalonyl coenzyme A: a metabolite formed during degradation of methionine, isoleucine, and valine, and of fatty acids with odd numbers of carbon atoms. It is converted to succinyl-coenzyme A via a reaction catalyzed by methylmalonyl coenzyme A mutase (one of the few enzymes that requires a coenzyme derived from vitamin B_{12}). Vitamin B_{12} deficiency, and inherited defects that impair the reactions invoke severe metabolic acidosis.

methylmelamines: several alkylating agents effective against advanced ovarian cancers and some other neoplasms, but strongly cytotoxic and mutagenic. *See*, for example **tetraethylmelamine.**

methylmercaptoimidazole: *see* **methimazole.**

methyl methanesulfonate: an agent that binds to, and alters the functions of sulfhydryl groups on enzymes, and is mutagenic.

2′-methyl MPTP hydrochloride: 1-methyl-4-(2-methylphenyl)-1,2,3,6-tetrahydropyridine hydrochloride; a highly potent dopaminergic neurotoxin, used as a substrate for assaying B type monoamine oxidases.

N′-**methyl-*N″*-nitro-*N*-nitrosoguanidine**: MNNG; a laboratory tool used to invoke mutagenesis and carcinogenesis.

methylnitrosoureas: MNUs; highly toxic alkylating agents, used to treat myeloid leukemias and some other neoplastic diseases. Streptozotocin-MNU (in which the R group is obtained from glucose) binds with high affinity to pancreatic beta cells, and arrests the growth of islet cell carcinomas. When administered to laboratory animals, the kinds of mutations invoked vary with the ages of the subjects.

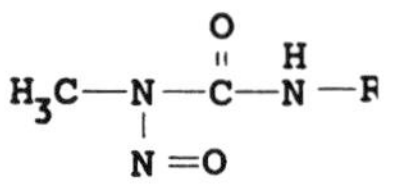

α-methylnorepinephrine: a "false neurotransmitter" (*q.v.*), formed from α-methyldopa.

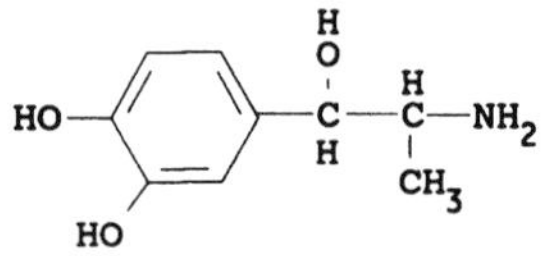

methylphenyltetrahydropyridine: *see* **MPTP**.

methyl red: 2-[[4-(dimethylamino)phenyl]azo]-benzoic acid; an indicator used to assess the pH of culture media, and for titrating weak bases. It exerts weak estrogen-like effects.

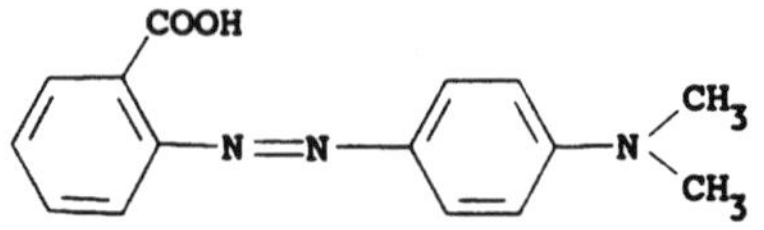

17α-methyltestosterone: a testosterone derivative used for its androgenic and anabolic effects.

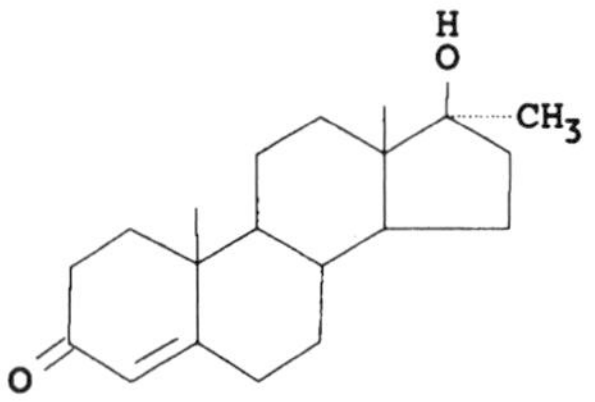

2-methylthioadenosine triphosphate: a P_2 type purinergic agonist. The trisodium salt labeled with ^{32}P is used to identify the receptors. The tetrasodium salt is resistant to hydrolysis.

methylthiouracil: 6-methyl-2-thiouracil; an inhibitor of iodine oxidation and incorporation into thyroglobulin,

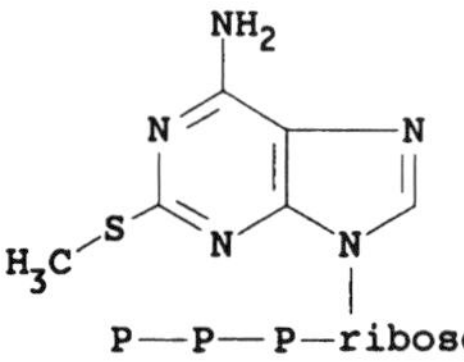

α-methyl-*p*-tyrosine

2-methylthioadenosine triphosphate

used to treat some forms of hyperthyroidism; *see* also **thiouracils**.

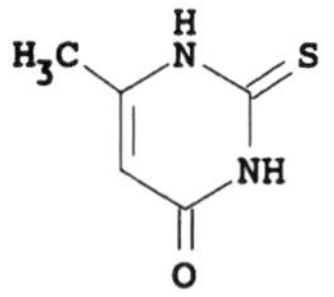

methyltransferases: enzymes that transfer methyl groups to acceptor molecules; *see*, for example **catechol-*O*-methyltransferase** (COMT), **hydroxyindole-*O*-methyltransferase** (HIOMT), and **histamine-*N*-methyltransferase**. Most act on two or more chemically related substrates.

methyltrienolone: 17-β-hydroxy-methylestra-4,9,11-trien-3-one; a photoreactive synthetic androgen receptor agonist, used as a ligand for receptor studies.

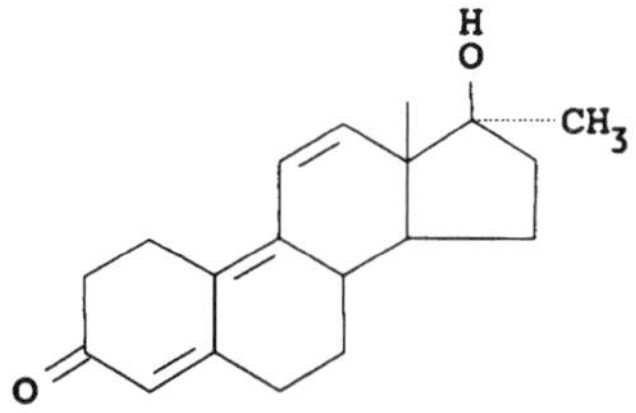

methyltrienolone binding protein: MTBP; 67K species-specific proteins in human placenta and chorion (but not umbilical cord, amnion, or other androgen responsive tissues), believed to contribute to sequestration of androgens and/or transport of related steroids that can be converted to estrogens. In the presence of NAD^+, it binds methyltrienolone with high affinity, and both testosterone and androstenedione with moderate affinity (but does not bind dihydrotestosterone). It differs from classical androgen receptors, rodent androgen binding protein, and testosterone-estrogen binding protein (SHBG).

α-methyltyrosines: agents used to study catecholamine localization and functions. Both *para*- (αMPT) and *meta*- (αMMT) forms inhibit tyrosine hydroxylase.

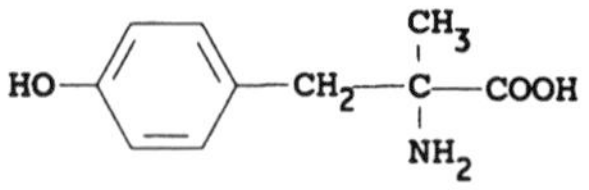

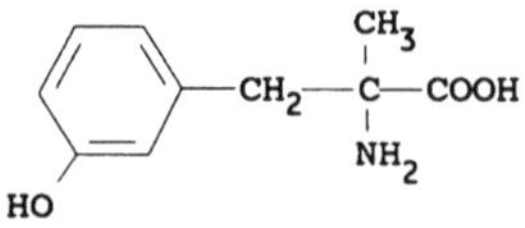

α-methyl-*m*-tyrosine

methylxanthines: caffeine, theophylline, theobromine and other naturally occurring xanthine alkaloids, and related compounds such as isobutylmethylxanthine. In addition to varying degrees of inhibition of cyclic AMP phosphodiesterases, they exert other biological actions. *See* specific types.

methysergide: 1-methyl-*d*-lysergic acid butanolamide; a compound chemically related to lysergic acid and its diethylamide (LSD) that inhibits serotonin stimulation of smooth muscle contraction, but has little effect on the central nervous system. It is used to prevent (but not treat) migraine and other vascular headaches.

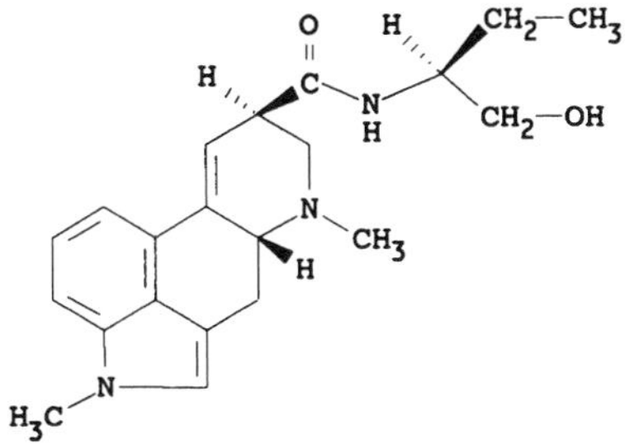

metiamide: *N*-methyl, *N'*-[2--[[(5-methyl-1-*H*-imidazole-4-yl)methyl]thio]-ethyl]thiourea; an H_2-type histamine receptor antagonist.

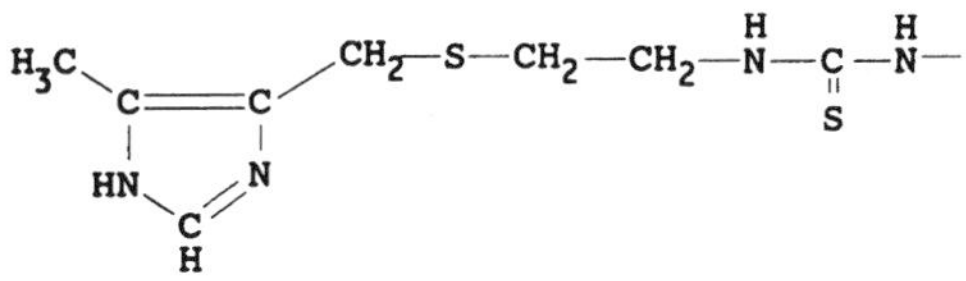

*f***Met-Leu-Phe**: FMLP; an amino acid sequence contained within, and believed to be the active component of several chemotactic agents that elevate cytosolic Ca^{2+} and recruit leukocytes and macrophages to sites of inflammation.

metoclopramide: 4-amino-5-chloro-*N*-[(2-diethylamino) ethyl]-2-methoxybenzamide; a dopamine receptor antagonist that crosses blood-brain barriers, and is used to alleviate vomiting. It exerts some effects on serotonin receptors.

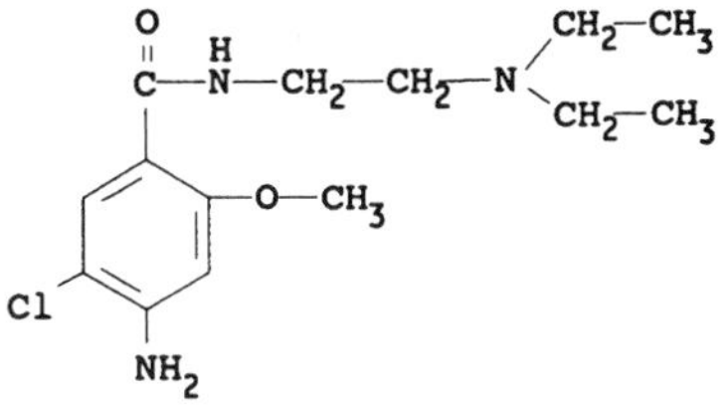

metorphamide: *see* **adrenorphin**.

metrial glands: structures that develop in the uteri of pregnant rats, rabbits, mice, hamsters, and guinea pigs. They contain natural killer (NK)-like cells that are believed to destroy aberrant trophoblastic and fetal cells, and to suppress immune responses that could lead to fetal rejection. The may also block fetal cell migration to the maternal system.

metropolol: 1-[4-(2-methoxyethyl)phenoxy]-3-[(1-methylethyl)amino]-2-propanol; a selective β_1-type adrenergic receptor antagonist, used to treat some forms of hypertension.

metyrapone: metapyrone; mepyrapone; 2-methyl-1,2-di-3-pyridyl-1-propanone; SU-4885; an inhibitor of the 11β-hydroxylase enzyme required for glucocorticoid biosynthesis. High concentrations also inhibit 18-hydroxylase and 18-hydroxysteroid dehydrogenase (needed for aldosterone synthesis) and cholecalciferol 25-hydroxylase. It is used to assess the ability to secrete adrenocorticotropic hormone (ACTH) and some other hormones, to treat Cushing's syndrome, to inhibit the growth of some tumors, and as an investigative tool.

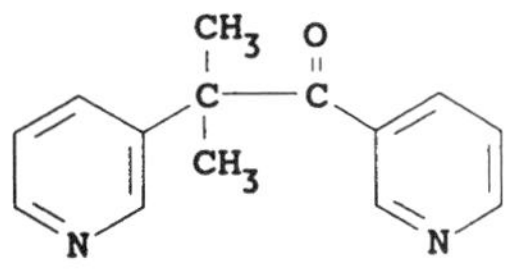

mevalonate: 3,5-dihydroxy-3-methylvalerate; a metabolite formed from 3-hydroxy-3-methyl-glutaryl coenzyme A via a reaction catalyzed by hydroxymethyl-glutaryl-coenzyme A reductase (HMG-CoA reductase), the rate-limiting enzyme for cholesterol biosynthesis.

mevastatin: compactin; 6-demethylmevinolin; an agent isolated from *Penicillium citrinum*. It is a potent inhibitor of hydroxymethyl-glutaryl-coenzyme A reductase (HMG-CoA reductase), with properties similar to those of **mevinolin** *(q.v.)*.

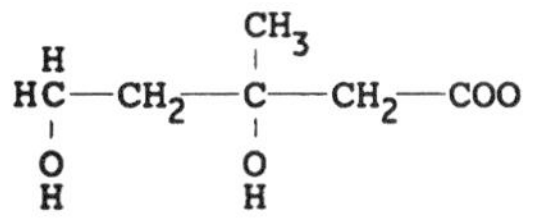

mevinolin: MK803; lovastatin; Mevacor; 2-methylbutanoic acid 1,2,3,7,8,8a-hexahydro-3,7,-dimethyl-8-[2-(teterahydro-4-hydroxy-6-oxo-2*H*-pyran-2-yl)ethyl]-1-naphthalenyl ester; 6α-methylcompactin; a potent inhibitor of hydroxymethyl-glutaryl-coenzyme A reductase

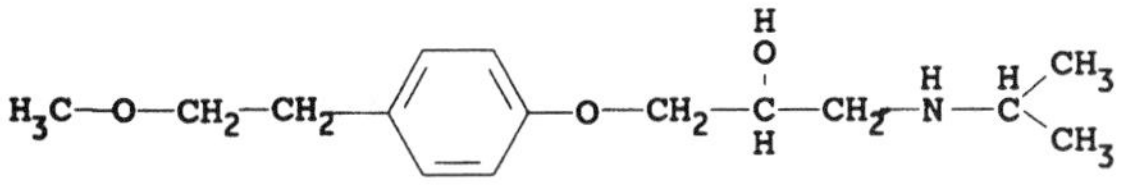

metropolol

457

(HMG-CoA reductase) that also lowers circulating tri-acylglycerol levels, obtained from *Aspergillus terreus* and other fungi. It is used to lower LDL-cholesterol levels in individuals at high risk for myocardial infarction, with primary hypercholesterolemia, and with secondary hypercholesterolemia associated with diabetes mellitus and nephrotic syndrome. The side-effects include gastrointestinal upsets, headaches, and skin rashes. In some individuals, it adversely affects the activities of several hepatic enzymes, can cause jaundice, and (in combination with other agents) invokes myopathies. High doses are teratogenic and can cause cataracts in laboratory animals.

MFB: medial forebrain bundles.

Mg: magnesium.

MGB6: mitoguazone.

MGF: mast cell growth factor; *see* **steel factor**.

MGP: matrix gla protein.

MGSA **genes**: melanoma growth stimulating genes; *see* *GRO*.

MHC: major histocompatibility complex.

MHC restriction: the requirement that T lymphocytes bind to MHC glycoproteins (class I for cytotoxic, and class II proteins for helper types) to perform antigen-stimulated immune system functions.

MHPG: 3-methoxy-4-hydroxy-phenylethyl-glycol; *see* 3-**methoxy-4-hydroxyphenylethylglycol**.

MI: melanocyte index.

MIAA: 5-methoxyindole acetic acid.

mianserin: 1,2,3,4,10,14*b*-hexahydro-2-methyldibenzo-[*c,f*]pyrazino[1,2-a]-azepine; a 5-HT$_2$ serotonin receptor antagonist with some inhibitory effects on histamine and α_2 adrenergic types.

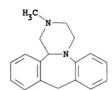

micelles: colloidal clusters of amphipathic molecules. Bile salt micelles with polar ends oriented towards the aqueous environment of the intestinal lumen break up large lipid globules, adsorb dietary lipids and transport the lipids to intestinal epithelial cells.

Michaelis constant: K$_m$; the substrate concentration for a reaction at which half-maximal velocity is achieved when the enzyme concentration is fixed and is not rate-limiting. It is a measure of the affinity of the enzyme for the substrate (but cannot be used when other substances bind to and affect substrate configurations).

Michaelis-Menten equation: an equation for the hyperbolic curve obtained for reactions of the kinds cited above (*see* **Michaelis constant**), when the substrate concentration [S] is plotted on the X axis, and the velocity on the Y. The Michaelis constant is calculated from: v = V$_{max}$ [S] / [S] + Km, where v and V$_{max}$ are, respectively, the initial and maximum velocities. V$_{max}$ is related to the amount of active enzyme.

micro-: a prefix meaning (1) small; (1) μ or 10^{-6}, as in microliter (μL), microgram (μgram), or micromolar (μM).

microangiopathy: basement membrane thickening and other pathological changes in small blood vessels. It occurs commonly in individuals with diabetes mellitus, even when blood glucose concentrations are moderately well controlled.

microbodies: small, dense, membrane-enclosed particles with granular matrices that hold oxidase enzymes, located near the endoplasmic reticulum. Most are spherical, with diameters of approximately 0.5 nm, but some have other shapes; and sizes can range from 0.2-1.7 nm. Peroxisomes are the major types in higher animals. In plants, fungi and protozoa, most are glyoxysomes.

microcytes: abnormally small erythrocytes, usually caused by protein deficiency.

microfilaments: fine unbranched strands, with diameters of 6-7 nm, in all eukaryotic cells. They strengthen cell membranes, participate in cell motility and intracellular translocations, contribute to the establishment and maintenance of cell shape, are components of desmosomes and microvilli, and can transmit signals from cell environments to cell interiors. Some anchor organelles to microtubules, cell proteins to plasma membranes, or cells to extracellular matrices. Most comprise two actin strands twisted around each other. Contraction involves interactions with myosin. Skeletal muscle types additionally contain tropomyosin and troponins; and erythrocyte types have spectrin. Loose microfilament networks form when α-actinin or filamen binds to form cross-links. More orderly bundles are held together by fimbrin. Vinculin links actin to cell membranes, and ankyrin binds to spectrins. Fragmin, gelsolin, and villin at microfilament ends are implicated as regulators of length, whereas profilin blocks actin polymerization by binding to its monomers. Cytochalasin B disrupts the functions.

microcurie: μC; a unit of atomic radioactivity, equivalent to 3.7 x 10^4 becquerels (disintegrations per second).

microenvironment: the fluid and other substances that immediately surround a cell, cell component, or tissue.

microglia: small, motile, non-neural phagocytic cells in nervous tissues, derived from mesoderm. They protect against infections and remove cell debris.

microglobulins: small globular proteins or their fragments; *see* β_2-**microglobulins**.

β_2-**microglobulins**: β_2m: highly conserved, nonglycosylated 11.6K proteins (96 amino acids in humans) on most cell types, and also released to extracellular fluids. They have immunoglobulin-like domains, but their synthesis is not directed by major histocompatibility complex genes. The proteins are expressed in very young embryos, in which the term *thymotaxin* has been applied (since they perform chemotactic functions in fetal thymus glands). β_2-Microglobulins associate noncovalently with CD1 and the heavy chains of most other class 1 proteins, and are essential for transporting immunoglobulins from endoplasmic reticula to cell surfaces, and for the development and functions of $\alpha\beta$ and some $\delta\gamma$ type CD4$^-$8$^+$ (cytotoxic) T cells (but not for all $\delta\gamma$ subsets). They associate with Fc receptors in fetal and neonatal gut cells, and mediate IgG uptake from milk in neonatal animals. Additionally, they augment collagenase activity in fibroblasts, and a soluble form is made by synovial types. Roles in other functions (including fertility and olfaction) are controversial; but some mutants unable to make the protein are sterile.

microheterogeneity: small differences among closely related molecules that can affect the weights, surface charges, metabolic clearance rates, activities, and other properties. For most proteins and peptides, they are related to differences in the amounts and/or kinds of glycosylation; but many undergo other covalent changes (such as phosphorylation, methylation, amidation, acetylation, or sulfation), and a few differ slightly in amino acid make-up. Usually, all members of a group perform qualitatively similar functions.

microinjection: usually, injection of substances into individual cells or cell nuclei.

microlecithal: describes egg cells that contain small quantities of yolk; *cf* **macrolecithal** and **mesolecithal**.

micromanipulators: devices attached to light microscopes that are used to move or dissect minute objects.

micromanometers: devices for measuring gases emitted by cells, or by small amounts of tissue and/or tissue fluids.

micromeres: small blastomeres formed during uneven cleavage. They accumulate in animal poles of amphibian and other embryos, give rise to nervous system and other structures, and divide more rapidly than macromeres.

micrometers: devices for measuring objects viewed under microscopes.

micron: μ; a unit of length equivalent to 10^{-6} meters.

micronucleus: the smaller of two nuclei in some protozoa. It is diploid and transcriptionally active, and participates in meiosis and autogamy.

micronutrients: dietary components required in very small amounts, such as vitamins and trace minerals; *cf* **macronutrients**.

microphages: small phagocytic cells, usually neutrophilic leukocytes; *cf* **macrophages**.

microphallus: an undersized, poorly developed penis, usually caused by an androgen receptor defect or impaired ability to synthesize testosterone 5-α-reductase.

micropinocytosis: cell uptake of liquids or very small vesicles; *see* **pinocytosis**.

micropore filters: meshworks of cellulose acetate or nitrate with defined pore sizes, used to remove microorganisms and macromolecules. Millipore is a trade name.

microprolactinomas: small pituitary adenomas that secrete minute quantities of prolactin.

micropuncture: insertion of a small probe or cannula into a cell. Micropipettes are inserted into renal tubule lumens, to collect and analyze the fluid.

microscopes: instruments with magnifying devices that are used to observe the fine structures of tissues, cells, cell components, and other objects, and/or obtain information on surface properties. In *optical* types, light in the visible range transmitted through objects is manually focused by glass lenses, and specimens are viewed directly with the eyes. The highest magnifications (up to 1000-1200X) are achieved when light refraction by air is minimized by immersing objective lenses in oil films that cover the specimens. In *darkfield* microscopy, specimens are also directly observed, but illumination from the sides causes tiny objects not otherwise easily defined to appear light against dark backgrounds. *Fluorescence* microscopy uses ultraviolet light to detect light-emitting substances. *Transmission electron* m. (TEM) permits observation of much smaller entities, since electrons (rather than light beams) are sent through the objects, and grids focus them on fluorescent screens or photographic plates. Although useful for many purposes, the disadvantages include the need to prepare ultrathin sections (which limits the amount of material that can be examined), and for maintaining a vacuum (which distorts some structures). Various techniques, such as shadowing with heavy metals, enhance the versatility. Since electrons are bounced off specimen surfaces in *scanning electron* m. (SEM), larger objects can be studied. Several devices with special purposes have recently been developed, but most require modifications for application to cells and other biological materials. *Scanning tunneling* m. (STM), with probes that move a few nanometers above the surfaces (and do not damage specimens) can differenitate individual atoms. Low voltages applied between the probes and the specimens create small tunneling currents (electron flows) whose magnitudes depend on the sizes of the gaps. Computer-assisted recording of the up and down movements required to maintain constant voltage can provide topological maps of specimen surfaces; but applications to nonconducting materials (most biological types) are limited. *Atomic force* m. probes directly contact specimen surfaces and measure irregularities. Since they do not use currents, the techniques can be applied to nonconducting specimens; and some success has been achieved in defining protein structures. They do, however, distort surfaces, and this limits resolution with soft materials. *Scanning thermal* m. have tiny thermocouples that monitor the temperatures of living cells.

microsomal fractions: centrifuged cell homogenate fractions that contain ribosomes and other membranous components; *see* **microsomes**.

microsomes: vesicles formed when cell homogenates are subjected to high speed centrifugation. The heavier ones, derived from rough endoplasmic reticulum, have ribosomes and can be separated from lighter ones, derived from smooth endoplasmic reticulum.

microtomes: devices for cutting thin sections of embedded materials for microscopy. *Ultra-microtomes* are used for electron microscopy.

microtrabecular lattices: cytoskeletal structures dispersed throughout the cytoplasm of most cell types, composed mostly of cross-linked microfilament and intermediate filament networks, microtubules, and associated ribosomes. They are visible in electron micrographs.

microtubule[s]: MTs; rigid, hollow, rodlike cytoskeleton components with outer and inner diameters of approximately 24 nm and 14 nm, respectively. In higher eukaryotes, assembly begins with the formation of dimers composed of globular, 450-amino acid α-tubulin and β-tubulin subunits. The dimers join head to tail ($\alpha\beta \rightarrow \alpha\beta \rightarrow \alpha\beta \rightarrow$) to form polarized, helical protofilaments that assemble, side-by side, into protomers (single microtubules), each with 13 longitudinally arranged protofilaments surrounding a central core that appears hollow in electron micrographs. In most cell types, pre-assembled protomers undergo regulated polymerization, via processes that involve GTP binding, with plus ends growing more rapidly than minus ones. Proteins can move along assembled microtubules in specific directions (neuronal kinesin from minus to plus ends, and dynein from plus to minus). Some microtubules are attached to microtubule organizing centers, and small amounts of a different protein, γ-tubulin mediate attachments to pericentriolar organizing regions. γ-Tubulin is present in small amounts during cell cycle interphases. The levels rise during late G_2, are high during prophase and metaphase, and fall again during anaphase and telophase. Centrioles are pairs of centrosomes, each composed of microtubules arranged in nine triplets, surrounded by centriolar matter. (Each triplet has one complete, A type protofilament, linked to two incomplete B types.) Microtubules that separate from organizing centers can form axonemes, each composed of two associated microtubules (A and B subfiber doublets) plus microtubule-associated proteins. Depolymerization seems to require a tubulin activated GTPase. Several genes code for tubulins. The various products are approximately 40% homologous. They undergo reversible posttranslational modifications that include phosphorylation, acetylation, glutamylation, and removal of terminal tyrosyl moieties. The composition varies with the cell type, state of differentiation, and microenvironment, and affects polymer stability as well as interactions with microtubule associated proteins and other cell components. Physiological regulators include Ca^{2+} ions and hormones (some of which act via Ca^{2+}). Other factors that affect the properties include temperature changes, deuterium, and pharmacological agents (*see* **colchicine, colcemid, nocodazole, vinblastine, vincristine,** and **taxol**.) Microtubules bind to membranes and other cell components, and play essential roles in morphogenesis and axon growth. They contribute to the establishment and maintenance of cell shape, and are components of cilia, flagella, and mitotic spindles. They also form "tracks" for intracellular transport of organelles and cell inclusions, and mediate axonal movements of neurotransmitters, hormone secretion, melanosome dispersion, and other processes.

microtubule-associated proteins: MAPs; several proteins that bind to and affect the functions of microtubules. The fibrous group includes high molecular weight (200-300K) and tau (40-60K) types, which stabilize polymerized units, facilitate bundling and binding to other cell components, and may modify the motor activities. Tau proteins appear to be essential for axon formation and growth. The "motor" types, with tubulin-activated ATPases, include kinesin (which mediates transport of organelles towards the plus [growing] ends of microtubules, and is a component of mitotic spindles in many cell types), dyneins (which promote transport to the minus ends), and dynamin (which drives sliding of one tubule along another). *See* also **microtubule associated protein-2**.

microtubule associated protein 1B: MAP-1B; a filamentous protein in cross-links between microtubules, and between the tubules and other cytoskeletal components. It contributes to neuron morphogenesis. The gene that directs its production in humans is adjacent to the spinal muscular atrophy locus; and it has been suggested that MAB-1 gene mutations contribute to anterior horn motor neuron degeneration.

microtubule associated protein-2: MAP-2; abundant neuronal proteins that inhibit microtubule functions when they undergo an MAP-2 kinase catalyzed phosphorylation. (*See* also **mitogen activated kinases**.) They accumulate in larger amounts in dendrites than in axons, possibly because of differences in metabolism or microenvironments.

microtubule organizing centers: MTOC; sites for microtubule assembly and disassembly. The pericentriolar matter directs formation of asters and spindles during mitosis and meiosis.

Microtus: a genus of Arctic rodents that includes voles and meadow mice. The animals are used for studies of reproduction, inheritance, and biological rhythms.

microvilli: (1) tiny cylindrical projections on the surfaces of cells that augment surface areas and thereby facilitate absorption and endocytosis. Because of their appearance in electron micrographs, surfaces that contain large numbers are called brush borders; (2) minute cytoplasmic extensions of trophoblast cells.

micturition: urination.

midbrain: *see* **mesencephalon**.

MIF: (1) macrophage inhibitory factor; (2) melanocyte inhibiting hormones.

MIF-1, **MIF-2**: *see* **melanocyte inhibiting hormones**.

mifentidine: *N*-(*p*-imidazol-4-ylphenyl)-*N'*-isopropyl-formamidine; an H_2 type histamine receptor antagonist used to decrease the activities of gastric glands.

mifepristone: RU 486; RU 38486; 11β, 17β-11-[4-(dimethylamino)-phenyl]-17-hydroxy-17-(1-propynyl)-estra-4,9-diene-3-one; a progesterone receptor antagonist that blocks progesterone binding to its receptor by stabilizing the receptor association with heat shock protein 90. It may also interfere with receptor-DNA interactions. Moderate amounts prevent implantation and interrupt established pregnancies at early stages. In France, Great Britain, and some other countries, it is used in conjunction with prostaglandin analogs to induce abortion at any time during the first eight weeks after conception. The PGE_1 analogs (sulprostone and gemeprost) are not available in the United States, but studies with misoprostol have been performed. Pregnancy termination was achieved in 99% of women tested, with no adverse effects on conceptuses in the others. The procedure is not been advocated for women who have experienced amenorrhea for more than 50 days, are older than 35 years, or are heavy smokers. Fertility control by use of mifepristone once monthly to block formation of a receptive endometrium is under investigation. The anti-progesterone actions are also useful for treating endometriosis and some kinds of neoplasms. Larger amounts are glucocorticoid receptor antagonists that alleviate many of the manifestations of Cushing's syndrome, and inhibit the growth of some cell types. In the United States, RU-486 has been approved for treating some inoperable brain tumors.

migration inhibiting factor: MIF; *see* **macrophage inhibiting factor**.

MIH: molt inhibiting hormone.

mil: a chicken sarcoma oncogene that codes for a protein with tyrosine kinase activity.

milk: (1) the secretory product of fully differentiated mammary glands. In addition to casein, lactalbumin, lactose, lipids, vitamins, minerals, and other nutrients, it contains prolactin, calcitonin, opioid peptides, several growth factors. and other regulators. Its immunoglobulin content is lower than that of colostrum. The composition varies with the species, changes within an individual in a manner complimentary to the needs of growing infants, and differs from one part of the day to another. The approximate composition of human milk after lactation is established is water 88%, protein 0.9%, fat 4%, and lactose 7%. It supplies 70 Calories per 100 ml. The volume is augmented by stimuli from nerve endings in the nipples (*see* **suckling reflex** and **oxytocin**), and is also affected by maternal nutrition, stress, and other factors. The hormonal requirements for maintaining lactation vary with the species, but universal ones include prolactin, glucocorticoids, and insulin (whereas progesterone and some other gonadal steroids inhibit); *see* also α-**lactalbumin** and **galactorrhea**; (2) related nutrients made by the simpler glands of monotremes; (3) the products elaborated by bird crop sacs; (4) other substances that physically resemble milk, for example uterine secretions made by some pregnant mammals.

milk letdown factor: *see* **oxytocin**.

milliequivalent: Meq; milligram equivalent weight; the atomic weight in milligrams, divided by the valence number. *See* also **gram equivalent weight**.

millimicron: mμ; 10^{-9} meter; the term nanometer is now preferred.

mimicry: imitation by one species of characteristics of another, usually of a type that improves the chances of survival. *Antigenic* mimicry is production by one species of antigens chemically unrelated to those of another, but capable of cross-reacting with the same antibodies. It can contribute to the development of autoimmune diseases and abnormal immunological tolerance.

mineralocorticoids: steroid hormones secreted by the adrenal cortex that act on kidney cells to promote Na^+, HCO_3^- and water retention, H^+ and K^+ excretion, and exert other effects; *see* **aldosterone**, the major type in mammals. Small amounts of 11-deoxycorticosterone and some others are made under normal conditions. Excessive amounts of certain types cause some forms of hypertension.

minigenes: chromosome segments that code for variable regions of immunoglobulin light and heavy chains.

mini hormones: low molecular weight peptide hormone isoforms; *see*, for example **gastrins**.

minipills: oral contraceptive preparations that contain progestins but no estrogens, developed when it was believed that estrogens caused most of the toxic effects of combined steroid preparations. They act on uterine cervical and endometrial glands, without necessarily blocking ovulation, and are therefore less dependable than estrogen-progestin combinations. They can, however, potentiate lactation-associated infertility, and (since estrogens enter milk) have been recommended for use by women who are nursing infants. (Some depot preparations of progestins are, however, effective contraceptives.)

minor histocompatibility antigens: cell surface antigens whose synthesis is directed by genes outside the major histocompatibility complex. They usually invoke only weak immunological responses, possibly because few cytotoxic lymphocytes recognize them, and the recognition processes require the presence of MHC antigens. Most commonly used serological methods do not detect them, and it is difficult to obtain antibodies directed against them. Under special conditions, a single type can mediate transplant rejection (*see*, for example **H-Y antigen**); but usually the collective effects of several are needed.

minoxidil: Rogaine; 2,4-diamino-6-piperidinopyrimidine; an agent initially used to treat some resistant forms of hypertension. After conversion to its active form (minoxidil-*O*-sulfate) via a reaction catalyzed by a hepatic sulfotransferase, it dilates arterioles and venules by increasing plasma membrane permeability to K^+ and promoting hyperpolarization (and to some extent by inhibiting α_1 adrenergic receptors). When applied topically on a regular basis, it promotes growth of scalp hair in some individuals with male pattern baldness, probably by accelerating cutaneous blood flow. However, the effects are limited, and are maintained only when the preparation is used. Hair growth on the face, back, and legs is an undesirable side-effect of use for hypertension in women. Minoxidil also enhances renin release, and the angiotensin generated stimulates aldosterone secretion. The resulting sodium and water retention are augmented by reflex inhibition of α_1 type adrenergic receptors that affect proximal tubule reabsorption. (Adrenergic receptor inhibition leading to vasodilation is not opposed by angiotensin.)

miosis: constriction of the pupils of the eyes; *cf* **mydriasis**. The major physiological stimulant is acetylcholine released from oculomotor nerves. Since miosis facilitates aqueous fluid drainage, cholinergic agents are used to treat glaucoma.

MIP-1, MIP-2: *see* **macrophage inflammatory proteins**.

MI proteins: *see* **superantigens**.

MIS: Müllerian inhibitory substance; *see* **Müllerian duct inhibitor**.

mismatch repair: a process for repairing newly synthesized DNA segments with improperly placed nitrogenous bases, accomplished by replacing a single base or nucleotide. The aberrant component is recognized by its effects on the three-dimensional structure, and is excised by an endonuclease. After it is replaced by a correct type, a DNA polymerase links the DNA segment.

misoprostol: Cytotec; a mixture of four isomers of 15-deoxy-16-hydroxy-16-methyl-PGE_1 methyl ester. They are PGE_1 analogs, prescribed to protect against development of, and to facilitate healing of gastric ulcers in individuals taking large doses of **nonsteroidal anti-inflammatory drugs** (NSAIDs, *q.v.*). They augment mucosal blood flow, and mucus and bicarbonate production, but can cause diarrhea, cramps, and other undesirable effects. They do not counteract the kinds of toxicity invoked by drug actions unrelated to inhibition of prostaglandin synthesis, and are reported to be no more effective than placebos in some individuals who experience gastric upsets. The (+)-*S* form is shown. *See* also **mifepristone**.

mispairing: bases on one DNA strand that are not complementary to bases at the same positions on the other strand.

missense mutation: a change in a DNA molecule that leads (via transcription and translation) to formation of an abnormal protein.

mistranslation: insertion of a wrong amino acid into a growing peptide chain, caused by a defect in the transfer RNA, the ribosome, or the enzyme that attaches the amino acid to the tRNA.

MITs: monoiodotyrosines.

mithramycin: mitramycin; plicamycin; aurelic acid; an antibiotic made by *Streptomyces tanashiensis* that inhibits RNA synthesis in many cell types, and is used to treat testicular tumors. Since it also lowers plasma calcium and alkaline phosphatase levels, and is believed to exert direct inhibitory influences on osteoclasts, it can alleviate the hypercalcemia associated with some cancers, and the excessive bone remodeling of Paget's disease.

mitochondria: self-replicating organelles of all cells that engage in oxidative phosphorylation. Most are rods, but the shapes, sizes, and numbers vary with cell type and the physiological status. A thin, smooth outer membrane faces the cytoplasm, maintains organelle structure, holds phospholipase A_2, monoamine oxidase, and some other enzymes, and permits diffusion of small molecules and ions. Cardiolipins are among the factors that limit the permeability, whereas porins form aqueous channels. The outer membrane is separated from an inner one with many folds (cristae) that confer a large surface. The inner membrane holds adenylate kinase, creatine kinase, deoxyribonuclease, electron transport chain components, and iron sulfur proteins that are used for cholesterol side-

mithramycin

chain cleavage, some hydroxylation reactions involved in steroid and secosteroid hormone synthesis, and drug metabolism. It encloses a fluid filled central cavity (matrix). Enzymes on the surface facing the matrix include ATP synthetase/ATPase, carnitine palmitoyltransferase, and some dehydrogenases. The matrix holds approximately 2/3 of the organelle protein, including soluble enzymes for the tricarboxylic acid cycle, gluconeogenesis, fatty acid oxidation, and the urea cycle. Mitochondria also have transport systems for calcium uptake, and different ones for calcium release; and the small amounts of free Ca^{2+} ion within the matrix affect the activities of several enzymes. When cytoplasm contains more calcium than can be controlled by other cell components (*see* **endoplasmic reticulum**), the reaction: $3\ Ca^{2+} + 2\ HPO_4^{2-} \rightleftharpoons Ca_3(PO_4)_2 + 2\ H^+$ facilitates sequestration of the excess in an inactive, but recruitable form. Since phosphate is taken up from the cytoplasm, and H^+ is released to it, the reaction affects cytoplasmic pH and inorganic phosphate levels. Most mitochondrial proteins are made on cytoplasmic ribosomes and imported, but bacteria-like mitochondrial genes and mitochondrial ribosomes direct formation of a few.

mitochondrial genes: DNA within mitochondria that directs the synthesis of some mitochondrial proteins. It replicates, and is transmitted to daughter cells during meiosis and mitosis (*see* **maternal inheritance**). The human mitochondrial genome contains approximately 16,500 nucleotides, and controls formation of two ribosomal RNAs, 22 transfer RNAs, and 22 proteins.

mitogen[s]: agents that promote cell proliferation.

mitogen activated protein kinases: MAP kinases; extracellular signal regulated protein kinases; ERKs; serine-threonine protein kinases that regulate cell cycle progression and cell proliferation, lymphocyte functions, germinal vesicle breakdown, and other processes, and can contribute to cell transformation. They require phosphorylation on both tyrosyl and serine and/or threonine moieties by MAP kinase kinases to achieve full activity, and can be inactivated, not only by both protein phosphatase 1B and more specific phosphotyrosine phosphatases, but also by protein phosphatase 2 and other phosphoserine phosphatases. The MAP kinases kinases (MPKKs) undergo autophosphorylation and can be inac-

tivated by 2A phosphatases. MAP kinases are ubiquitously expressed in eukaryote cells, but are inactive until affected by stimulants. Some types are distinguished by superscripts related to their molecular weights (as in p42^{mpk}, p43^{erk1}, and p44^{mpk}), but a few are known under two or more names. For example, p42^{mpk} is also called ERK-2. Most promote phosphorylation of microtubule associated protein-2 (MAP-2) and of myelin basic protein (MBP), and at least some act on ribosomal S6 kinases, phospholipase Cγ and other second messenger generators, as well as on cytoskeletal components and membrane bound molecules that mediate Na^+/H^+ and other ion exchanges. The MAP kinases are components of complex cascades, initiated in various cell types when receptors for insulin, insulin-like growth factor-I (IGF-I), epidermal growth factor (EGF), nerve growth factor (NGF), colony-stimulating factor-1 (CSF-1, M-CSF), platelet-derived growth factor (PDGF), and some other mitogens that undergo ligand activation of their tyrosine kinase components and autophosphorylation. The enzymes contain SH2 and related domains that directly recognize components of tyrosine-phosphorylated receptors, and are thereby affected by mechanisms that do not require soluble second messengers. MAP kinases are also activated when G-coupled receptors for thrombin, serotonin, acetylcholine and some other regulators bind their ligands, and by some oncogene products. Phosphatidylinositol-3-kinase is a component of cascades initiated by the binding of p21^{ras} and other small G proteins to guanosine triphosphate (GTP), and it has been suggested that its effects include generation of receptors for as yet unidentified intracellular ligands. A pathway initiated by RAS, with Raf-1 as an intermediate has been described. Since the kinases provide sites for convergence of diverse signaling pathways, and profoundly affect cell functions, they have also been called "switch" kinases.

mitoguazone: MBG6; methylglyoxal-*bis*(guanyl)hydrazone; an antineoplastic agent used to treat myelogenous leukemia, and an inhibitor of *S*-adenosyl methionine transferase.

mitomycins: antibiotics derived from *Streptomyces caespitosus*, that inhibit DNA synthesis, cross-link DNA molecules, are weakly immunosuppressive, and can be

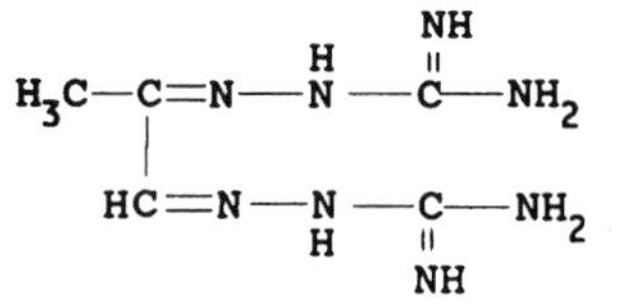

mitoguazone

teratogenic in rodents. They are used to treat several kinds of cancers. Mitomycin C (shown below) is [1αR]-6-amino-8-[[(aminocarbonyl)oxy]methyl]-1,1a,2,8, 8a, 9b-hexahydro-8a-methoxy-5-methylazirino[2′3′:3,4]pyrrolo[1,2-a]indole-4,7-dione.

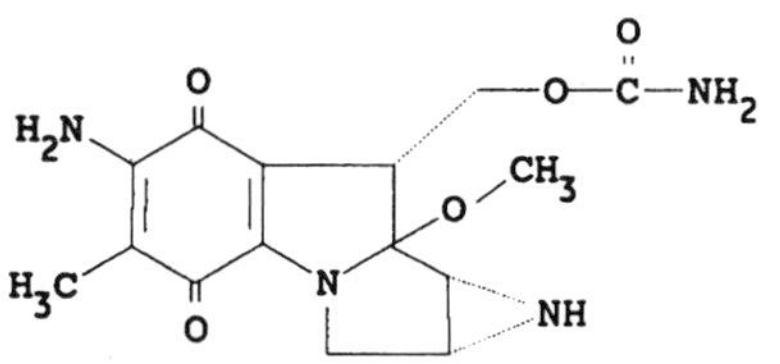

mitosis: the usual process of nuclear division in eukaryote somatic cells, in which segregation and separation of chromosomes leads to the formation of two daughter nuclei that are genetically identical to each other and to the parent cell nucleus; *cf* **meiosis**. Although one phase merges into the next, the events are divided (for discussion) into **prophase**, **metaphase**, **anaphase**, and **telophase** *(q.v.)*. Mitosis is preceded by interphase, during which the chromosomes replicate. In most (but not all) cases, cytokinesis begins during telophase. When no qualifying terms are used, open mitosis, in which the nuclear membrane breaks down, is implied. *See* also **closed mitosis** and **cell cycles**.

mitotane: 1-chlor-2-[2.2-dichloro-1-(-4-chlorophenyl)-ethyl]benzene; *o′p′*-DDD; an anti-neoplastic agent chemically related to the insecticide DDT that kills adrenocortical cells. It is used to destroy some adrenocortical cancers, and to invoke hormone deficiency in laboratory animals.

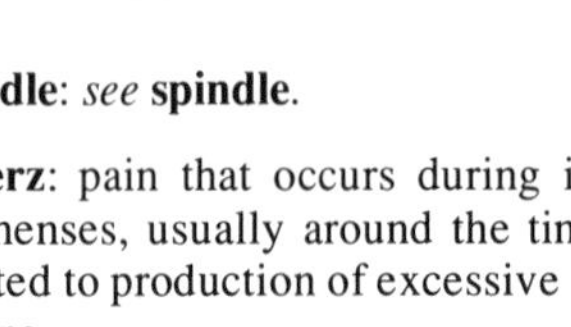

mitotic index: the ratio of the numbers of cells engaged in mitosis at a specific time to the total numbers in the sample.

mitotic spindle: *see* **spindle**.

mittelschmerz: pain that occurs during intervals between the menses, usually around the time of ovulation, attributed to production of excessive quantities of prostaglandins.

MIX: methyl isobutyl xanthine; *see* **isobutyl methylxanthine**.

mixed function oxidases: mixed function oxygenases; monooxygenases; enzymes that catalyze reactions in which one atom of an oxygen molecule incorporates into

the substrate and the other joins with hydrogen atoms (usually donated by NADH or NADPH) to form water; *cf* **dioxygenases**. The enzymes are components of pathways for the biosynthesis of steroid and secosteroid hormones, catecholamines, collagens, and other compounds, and for tyrosine and phenylalanine degradation.

mixed lymphocyte reactions: MLRs; proliferative responses, usually measured as functions of tritiated thymidine incorporation into the DNA, that occur when lymphocytes from two genetically different individuals are mixed *in vitro*. A *one way* MLR is achieved by irradiating one of the cell populations (or by treating it with a DNA synthesis inhibitor) prior to the test.

MK-421: enalapril.

MK-486: carbidopa.

MK 801: dizocilpine; 10,11-dihydro-5-methyl-5*H*-dibenzo[a,d]cyclohepten-5,10-imine; a noncompetitive antagonist for *N*-methyl-D-aspartate (NMDA) and phencyclidine (PCP) receptors, used to identify those receptors, as anticonvulsants for treating some forms of epilepsy, and to protect against damage by some neurotoxins.

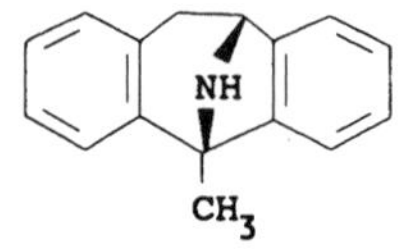

MK 803: mevinolin.

MLCK: myosin light-chain kinase.

MLD: (1) median lethal dose; (2) minimum lethal dose.

M line: the central part of the A band of a striated muscle sarcomere. It contains myomesin, creatine kinase, and glycogen phosphorylase, and controls the spacings between thick filaments.

f-**MLP**: *f*-Met-Leu-Phe-OH: formyl-methionyl-leucyl-phenylalanine; a receptor binding component of larger molecules made by macrophages that contribute to inflammatory reactions. The isolated peptide is directly chemotactic for neutrophilic leukocytes, and is used to study the functions. The effects have been linked with phospholipase activation and arachidonic acid release.

MLR: mixed lymphocyte reaction.

MLT: melatonin.

N^5-**MMA**: monomethyl arginine acetate; the L form (L-NMMA) is a potent inhibitor of nitric oxide synthetase; the D isomer (D-NMMA) is less active.

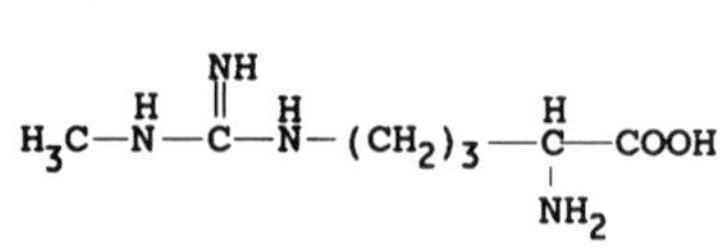

MMDA: ecstasy; 3,4-methylenedioxymethamphetamine; a psychedelic drug that exerts effects similar to those invoked by mescaline, LSD (lysergic acid diethyla-

464

mide), and methamphetamine, including hallucinations and influences on the cardiovascular system. Tolerance to the psychic effects develops rapidly, but sensitivity is regained if the drug is not used for several days. Objections to use of MMDA as an adjunct in some forms of psychotherapy include serotoninergic neuron damage after repeated administration.

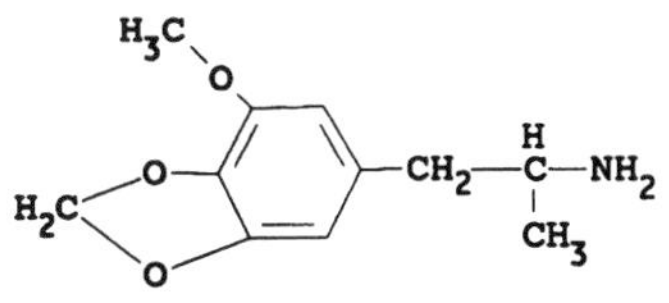

MMDA

MMI: methimazole.

MMTV: mouse mammary tumor virus.

MMT: metallothionein.

Mn: manganese.

MNS blood group: human blood in which certain antigens are expressed on erythrocytes. The genes that code for MM, MN, and NN phenotypes segregate independently of those for ABO types. Alloimmunization reactions can invoke a neonatal hemolytic disease.

MNU: methylnitrosourea.

Mo: molybdenum.

MOB: main olfactory bulbs.

mobile genetic elements: *see* **transposable genetic elements**.

Mo cells: gastrointestinal tract cells that synthesize motilin.

MOD: maturity onset type **diabetes mellitus** (*q.v.*).

modulation: change from one kind of differentiated cell to another, as from osteoblast to osteocyte; *cf* **differentiation**. *See also* **neuromodulators**.

MODY: maturity onset type diabetes in the young; *see* **diabetes mellitus**.

moiety: a chemical group within a larger molecule, such as an amino acid or sugar component of a glycoprotein.

molal solution: an aqueous solution prepared by dissolving one gram molecular weight of solute in each 1000 ml of water. The volume that contains 1 GMW can be smaller or greater than one liter; *cf* **molar solution**.

molar solution: an aqueous solution that contains one gram molecular weight of solute per liter; *cf* **molal solution**.

mole: gram molecular weight; GMW; a quantity of a pure compound equal in grams to the number for its molecular weight.

mollusks: animals of the phylum Mollusca, which includes snails, slugs, mussels, oysters, clams, squid, octopuses, cuttlefish, and nautiluses.

Moloney murine leukemia virus: MoMuLV; a replication-competent retrovirus that causes leukemias and lymphomas in mice and rats when it integrates into the host DNA and promotes overexpression of proto-oncogenes such as *lck*, *evi-1*, and *pim-1*. The effects, which become apparent after latent periods of 2-6 months, depend on the location. The virus is not known to code for an oncogene, and is not transmitted via the germ line to progeny. It is used with some replication-defective types to induce neoplasms in laboratory animals.

Molony murine sarcoma virus: a replication-defective retrovirus that induces fibrosarcomas in rodents; *see* also *mos*.

molting hormone: MH: *see* **ecdysone**.

molybdenum: Mo; a metallic element (atomic number 42, atomic weight 95.94), supplied by the diet and needed in trace amounts. It is a cofactor for xanthine, sulfite, and aldehyde oxidases in animals, and for nitrate reductase in nitrogen-fixing microorganisms. High concentrations are used to stabilize unoccupied steroid hormone receptors. Some of its effects are related to inhibition of phosphatase enzymes.

monactin: *see* **nonactin**.

monensin: 2-[5-ethyltetrahydro-5-[tetrahydro-3-methyl-5-[tetrahydro-6-hydroxy-6-(hydroxy-methyl)-3,5-dimethyl-2*H*-pyran-2-yl-]-2-furyl]-2-furyl]-9-hydroxy-β-methoxy-α-γ,2,8-tetramethyl-1,6-dioxaspiro[4,5]-decane-7-butyric acid; an antiprotozoal, antifungal, and antibacterial agent made by *Streptomyces cinnamonensis*. It is a polyether carboxylic acid, used as monovalent cation ionophore with high selectivity for Na$^+$. It also transports small amounts of K$^+$, and affects Na$^+$/H$^+$ antiport. After entering cells, it raises the pH of endocytic vesicles, blocks vesicle transit from the Golgi apparatus to the

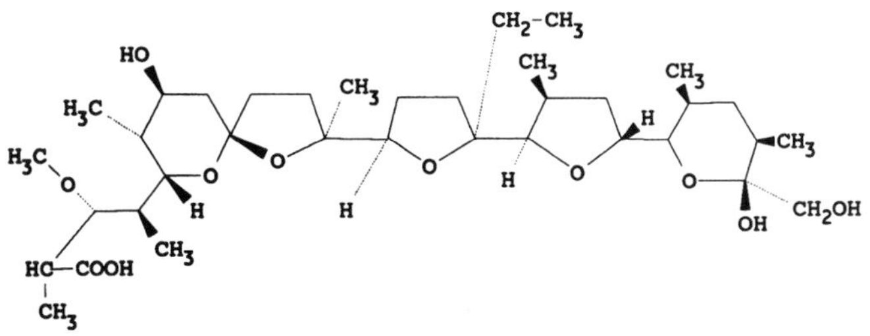

monensin

465

plasma membrane, and inhibits terminal glycosylation of proteins.

Monera: a kingdom of living organisms that includes bacteria and blue-green algae.

monoamine oxidases: MAOs; enzymes that catalzye oxidative deamination of catecholamines, serotonin, histamine, tyramine, and several other amines. Most of the aldehydes formed are further oxidized to acids in the periphery, but reduced to alcohols in the central nervous system. The A type (MAO-A), which acts preferentially on epinephrine, norepinephrine, and serotonin, predominates in sympathetic nerves; and high levels are found in the spleen, superior cervical ganglia and intestine. Blood platelets, pineal gland parenchymal cells, and corpus striatum neurons contain MAO-B, which preferentially degrades tryptamine and some related molecules. Brain and liver have equal amounts of A and B, and dopamine and tyramine are substrates for both. MAOs differ from histaminase, spermine oxidase, and several other enzymes that catalyze oxidative deaminations.

monoamine oxidase inhibitors: agents with high specificities for monoamine oxidases. Clorgyline, which is selective for MAO-A, is used as an antidepressant. Deprenyl preferentially inhibits MAO-B, and is used to treat Parkinson's disease. Pargyline acts on both isozymes.

monoecious: possessing both male and female type gonads, a term usually applied to plants, but also to a few animal types (such as tapeworms) in which the condition is regarded as normal for the species. *See* also **hermaphrodites**.

monestrous: having just one estrus cycle per season, or per year.

monoblasts: immature bone marrow cells that differentiate from hemopoietic stem cells, and mature (via a promonocyte stage) to circulating monocytic leukocytes.

monocentric: describes a chromosome with a single centromere. (Most chromosomes of higher animals are monocentric.)

monocistronic RNA: a messenger RNA that directs translation of just one kind of protein.

monoclonal: describes (1) a set of identical cells derived, via mitosis, from a single parent cell; (2) an antibody that reacts with just one kind of antigen.

monoclonal antibody: Mab; an immunoglobulin raised against a single, purified antigen; *cf* **polyclonal antibody**. Some Mabs bind with high affinity to two or more different proteins, but they are much more selective than polyclonal types.

monocytes: ameboid, phagocytic leukocytes that differentiate from monoblast precursors, and are released to the bloodstream. They are attracted to, and accumulate at sites of inflammation, and can develop into macrophages in the liver, lungs, and other organs. Under normal conditions, approximately 4-6% of human circulating leukocytes are monocytes. *See* also **infectious mononucleosis**.

monocyte derived neutrophil chemotactic factor: a 6K protein (different from *f*-MLP), made by monocytes, that is chemotactic for neutrophilic leukocytes.

monodansylcadaverine: MDC; dansylcadaverine; an agent used to inhibit transglutaminase.

monogamy: the reproduction pattern in which one male and one female form an exclusive, stable mating pair.

monogenic: directed by a single gene.

mongolism: an obsolete term for Down's syndrome.

monohybrids: describes the heterozygous progeny of homozygous parents who are genetically identical except for alleles at one specific locus.

monoiodothyronines: T_1; biologically inactive triiodothyronine (T_3) and thyroxine (T_4) degradation products. Small amounts are formed in thyroid glands; but most arise in peripheral tissues, and especially in the liver. The iodine substitution can be on any of the positions shown: 3, 3′, 5, or 5′. Monoiodothyronines can be directly excreted, further deiodinated to thyronine (T_o), or conjugated at the 4′ position with sulfate or other groups before or after deiodination.

monoiodotyrosine: MIT; 3-iodotyrosine; a by-product formed when iodothyroglobulin is digested in thyroid glands to yield thyroxine and triiodothyronine. It is usually degraded within the glands, but small amounts are released to the bloodstream. Although generally regarded as biologically inactive, high levels can inhibit tyrosine hydroxylase.

monokines: interleukin-1, interferons, tumor necrosis factor-α, and other low molecular weight mediators of immune responses, released by monocytes and/or macrophages. *See* also **lymphokines**.

monolayer: a single, flat layer, for example of cultured cells growing on a support.

monomer: a molecule that contains a single unit, such as one peptide chain; *cf* **dimers** and **polymers**.

mononuclear leukocytes: usually, monocytes.

mononucleosis: conditions in which the blood contains excessive numbers of monocytes; *see* **infectious mononucleosis**.

monooxygenases: *see* **mixed function oxygenases**.

monovular species: species in which a female characteristically releases a single mature oocyte during each ovarian cycle; *cf* **polyovular**.

monosodium glutamate: MSG: a neurostimulant at very low dosages, and a neurotoxin at higher ones. Small amounts are used to enhance food flavors and the palatability of some bitter drugs; but even these invoke "Chinese restaurant syndrome" (headache, muscle spasms, and other forms of discomfort) in susceptible individuals by acting on glutamate receptors. Somewhat larger amounts are used to treat hepatic coma. Repeated administration severely impairs nervous system development in young rodents, and is especially toxic for the arcuate nuclei of the hypothalamus, the median eminence, the optic nerves, and in some cases also the circumventricular organs. Direct effects on the firing of spinal cord neurons have also been described; and at least some actions involve inhibition of opioid peptide functions. MSG can impair somatic growth by affecting neurons that make growth hormone releasing hormone (GRH), invoke gonadal dysfunction by destroying neurons that secrete gonadotropin releasing hormone (GnRH), and cause excessive production of proopiomelanocortin (POMC) peptides. The obesity that develops in laboratory animals is attributed to combined influences on several kinds of central nervous system components.

$$HOOC-CH_2-CH_2-\overset{\overset{\displaystyle NH_2}{|}}{\underset{\underset{\displaystyle H}{|}}{C}}-COONa$$

monosome: a single messenger RNA-ribosome complex; *cf* **polysome**.

monosomy: absence of one member of an allele pair, a term usually used in conjunction with the chromosome number, as in monosomy 22.

monospermy: fertilization by a single spermatozoan; *cf* **polyspermy**.

monotocous: giving birth to a single offspring per pregnancy.

monotremes: members of the mammalian subphylum Prototheria (order Monotremata). They lay eggs, and have rudimentary mammary glands that lack nipples and somewhat resemble sweat glands. The duck-billed platypus and the spiny anteater (echidna) are the only known living representatives.

monozygotic: describes genetically identical twins, triplets, and larger numbers of siblings that develop from a single zygote; *cf* **dizygotic**.

moon face: excessive fat deposition on the cheeks, a condition that occurs in response to excessive amounts of glucocorticoids (for example in individuals with Cushing's syndrome, and in ones given repeated large doses to alleviate inflammatory disease symptoms, treat some leukemias, or facilitate transplant acceptance). It is usually associated with fat deposition on the back of the neck and on the trunk, and depletion of adipose tissue in the limbs.

MOPEG: usually, 3-**methoxy,4-hydroxyphenylethylglycol** (*q.v.*); *see* also 3-**methoxy,4-hydroxyphenyllethylglocaldehyde**.

MOPP: the combination of nitrogen mustard (mechlorethanamine), vincristine (Oncovin), procarbazine, and prednisone, used to treat Hodgkin's disease.

MOPS: 4-morpholinopropane sulfonic acid; a phosphate-free buffer used to maintain a pH of approximately 7.2 in biological preparations. (Activity is retained over pH 6.5-8.0.)

$$O \diagdown \underset{\diagdown}{\diagup} N - (CH_2)_3 - SO_3H$$

morbidity: (1) a diseased condition; (2) the tendency of a factor to cause disease; (3) the numbers of sick persons, or the numbers of new cases of an illness observed in a population during a specified time period.

morgan: a unit for distances between two genes on a chromosome. The probabilities that crossing over will occur during meiosis are 100%, 10% and 1%, respectively, for distances of one morgan, one decimorgan, and one centimorgan.

morning after contraceptives: agents taken postcoitally to avoid pregnancy. Large doses of synthetic estrogens promote expulsion of oocytes and very young conceptuses by stimulating the contraction of reproductive tract smooth muscle, but usually also invoke cramping pain; and repeated use may damage hypothalamic mechanisms that control ovarian cycles. Prostaglandin $F_{2\alpha}$ (PGF$_{2\alpha}$) can exert similar effects, but must be infused (since it is rapidly destroyed). Longer acting prostaglandin analogs can avert this problem, but, in addition to the undesirable effects that include severe cramps, diarrhea, and vasoconstriction, they can cause fetal defects if abortion is not achieved. RU-486 is a safer, less toxic alternative that is not currently available for this purpose in the United States.

morphinan: (4aR)-1,3,4,9,10,10aα-hexahydro-2H-10α, 4aα-(iminoethano)phenanthrene; a compound used for the nomenclature of morphine and related alkaloids (such as codeine and thebaine).

morphine: 7,8-didehydro-4,5-epoxy-17-methylmorphinan; the major opioid alkaloid obtained from the *Papaver somniferum* poppy (which contains at least 20 others). It is used directly, and to prepare chemically related agents such as apomorphine, naloxone, nalorphine, heroine, methadone, meperidine (Demerol), and paregoric (which contains other substances). Morphine is a central nervous

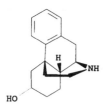

morphinan

system depressant that affects mood, inhibits cough reflexes, and can cause respiratory arrest, but stimulates gastrointestinal and urogenital tract smooth muscle, and invokes miosis. It is used to diminish the kinds of pain not affected by aspirin-type analgesics (especially continuous dull types that originate in visceral organs, and the severe pain associated with biliary and renal colic and myocardial infarction). It also alleviates the associated anxiety and other unpleasant psychological effects. (Some individuals state that they continue to sense pain but are not disturbed by it.) It is usually not addictive when taken for short time periods. Although problems arise with chronic use, especially when administration is on a regular schedule, there is a growing tendency to provide it for patients with advanced cancers. Morphine acts mostly on μ-type opioid receptors, but also binds to other types. Some of its actions are mediated via changes in Ca^{2+} uptake and inhibition of adenylate cyclase. "Addicted cells" make more of the enzyme, and display excessive activity when the drug is withdrawn.

morphogen: (1) any agent that promotes differentiation of tissues and organs; (2) a regulator whose concentration gradient serves as a position indicator during development. The concept that **retinoic acid** (*q.v.*) acts in this way has been questioned.

morphogenesis: developmental processes that lead to acquisition of structures characteristic of more mature members of the species. It involves the actions of morphogens, and interactions between cell surface and extracellular matrix components.

morphogenetic movements: invagination, evagination, dorsal convergence, and other forms of cell and cell group migrations that change the positions and shapes of, and affect the ultimate fates of embryonic precursor cells.

morphological color change: slowly-developing color changes that result from changes in the sizes, numbers, locations, and pigment producing capacities of melanocytes; *cf* **physiological color change**.

morphology: the study of structure and form.

morula: a mulberry-like cell ball, formed during early cleavage stages, that rapidly develops into a blastocyst. The cells are similar in appearance, and small (since all of the cytoplasm is derived from the zygote).

mos: a proto-oncogene that directs formation pp39*mos*, a phosphoprotein with serine-threonine kinase activity that is also known as **cytostatic factor** (*q.v.*), since high levels arrest cleavage of two-cell embryos in metaphase. pp39*mos* binds to and phosphorylates tubulins (type β more than type α), stabilizes spindles during cell division, and contributes to the control of intracellular organelle transport. It also phosphorylates, and thereby inactivates a protease that degrades cyclin B (a component of **MPF**, *q.v.*). It is expressed in both male and female germinal cells, in which it regulates meiosis. (In *Xenopus* oocytes, synthesis of the protein is essential for initial activation of MPF, and anti-sense RNAs that impede its formation block hormone-stimulated germinal vesicle breakdown; but in mouse oocytes, MPF is activated prior to initiation of meiosis I. The cells can therefore complete the first division in the presence of the anti-sense RNA; but they cannot enter meiosis II.) The high levels of pp39*mos* in very young embryos affect mitosis and contribute to cell differentiation. Most mature cell types, including neurons, make small amounts, and the production is tightly regulated. Over-expresssion invokes behavioral abnormalities and degenerative changes in neurons, neuroglia, and blood-brain barrier cells, and can invoke plasmacytomas in rodents. It is not known if the transforming potential is directly related to dysregulation of cell cycle control via influences on MPF, or involves phosphorylation of other proteins. *V-mos* is a Moloney sarcoma retrovirus oncogene that inserts into host DNA, and codes for a related, but truncated, 37K phosphoprotein, p37*env-mos*.

mosact: Asp-Ser-Asp-Ser-Ala-Glu-Asn-Leu-Iso-Gly; a peptide made by sand dollar oocytes that binds to and activates the guanylate cyclase of spermatozoa of the same species. *See* also **resact** and **speract**.

mosaic: (1) an individual with cells of two or more genetic types. A zygote can acquire an abnormal chromosome number if segregation and separation do not proceed in the usual manner during gametogenesis. One or more chromosomes can then be deleted from (or duplicated in) some cells during cleavage, and the changes passsed on to the progeny. Chimeras have cells from two or more different genetic sources. The condition can arise from polyspermy, fertilization of a secondary oocyte, or incorporation of a polar body (which may also have been fertilized) into the conceptus. Nonidentical twins that share placental blood vessels can also exchange cells. XX/XO, XX/XY, XXX/XX and XXY/XO are among the sex chromosome patterns compatible with survival; *see* also **hermaphroditism**; (2) expression of some alleles in certain cells and different alleles in others, because of random X chromosome inactivation.

mosaic receptors: receptors with two or more domains, each of which binds its own kind of ligand.

468

motilin: 22K species specific peptides, chemically related to pancreatic polypeptide, peptide YY, and neuropeptide Y, made in intestinal Mo cells, some specialized intestinal argentaffin cells, and in the brain. The porcine type has the sequence: H$_2$N-Ala-Pro-Leu-Glu-Pro-Val-Tyr-Pro-Gly-Asp-Asn-Ala-Thr-Pro-Glu-Gln-Met-Ala-Gly. Motilins stimulate stomach and intestinal motility and pepsin secretion, and can initiate myoelectrical discharges in the duodenum that are propagated to more distal regions of the small intestine. Factors promoting their release include acids, fats, pancreatic juice components, bile in the duodenum, cholinergic and non-cholinergic vagal discharges, and circulating bombesin and bombesin-related peptides (*see* **gastrin releasing peptide**). Somatostatin is an inhibitor. Larger peptides that react with the same antibodies may be precursors.

motility factor: *see* **scatter factor**.

motor end plate: myoneural junction; *see* **neuromuscular junction**.

Motrin: a trade name for ibuprofen.

mouse: the common domesticated laboratory mouse is *Mus musculus*. The strains bred for specific purposes include *Balb*, *db*, *ob*, *NZB*, *nude*, *Snell-Bagg*, and *SCID*, as well as agouti (CBA, C3H), and black (C$_{57}$, C$_{58}$) types. *Mus caroli* is a wild mouse of southeastern Asia that has the same chromosome number but does not hybridize with domestic species. Animals of different genera used in some studies include the deer mouse (*Peromyscus maniculatas*), the white footed mouse (*Peromyscus lucopus*), and field mice (meadow mice, voles, *Arvicola* or *Microtus*). Their small sizes and short gestation periods provide special advantages for studies of reproductive and immune system functions, and of inheritance. Transgenic animals are prepared by inserting fertilized oocytes injected with foreign DNAs into pseudopregnant females.

mouse anti-alopecia factor: myoinositol.

mousebane: aconite.

mouse mammary tumor virus: MMTV; a retrovirus that integrates into host DNA and augments the expression of proto-oncogenes (especially *int-1* and *int-2*) that cooperate with other oncogenes to promote development of mammary gland tumors in mice. The virus is transmitted in milk, and has therefore also been called *milk factor*. Since the activity of the promoter is enhanced by glucocorticoids, MMTVs are used in transfection studies.

mouse test for pregnancy: *see* **Aschheim-Zondek test**.

mouse urinary protein: MUP; a complex of at least seven similar, hormonally controlled, negatively charged 17-22K proteins in the urine of adult female mice. They are believed to function as transporters that facilitate penetration of a female urinary pheromone into the nasal mucosae of conspecific males. The pheromone acts on the vomeronasal organs of the recipients and augments the release of luteinizing hormone (LH).

moxestrol: RU 2858; 11β-methoxy-ethynylestradiol; a synthetic estrogen.

M-6-P: mannose-6-phosphate.

6-MP: (1) 6-mercaptopurine; (2) 6-methylene-4-pregnene-3,20-dione, a steroid 5α-reductase inhibitor, used to block conversion of testosterone to 5α-dihydrotestosterone.

3-MPA: 3-mercaptopicolinic acid.

MPF: a cell component initially named maturation promoting factor because it terminates metaphase arrest in *Xenopus* oocytes. Other terms, based on different observations, include *mitosis promoting factor*, *meiosis promoting factor*, *M-Phase H1 kinase*, and *growth associated kinase*. Since it is essential for entry into M phases of both mitosis and meiosis, *M phase promoting factor* is now preferred. MPF is a dimer composed of a 34K subunit (p34^{cdc2}) with serine-threonine kinase activity, and a B cyclin regulatory subunit (45K in some species, but a 56K product of the *cdc13* gene in fission yeast). The 34K component is similar to a protein of the same size with comparable functions whose synthesis is directed by the *cdc2* gene of fission yeast (*Schizosaccharomyces pombe*) and to the *CDC28* product of budding yeast (*Saccharomyces cerevisiae*). The human counterpart is *CDC2Hs*, in which *Hs* stands for *Homo Sapiens*. MPF is always present, but is maintained in an inactive state during interphase by phosphorylation of a

6-mercaptopurine

6-methylene-4-pregnene-
3,20-dione

469

tyrosyl moiety of its ATP-binding domain. In fission yeast, genes *wee1* and *mlk* contribute to inactivation. p107*wee1* prevents dephosphorylation, and thereby premature division of cells that have not attained adequate size. Incompletely replicated DNA also blocks, but its relationship to the other factors has not been defined. A different gene codes for p80*cdc25*, a phosphatase that activates. The *CDC14* gene of budding yeasts codes for a similar phosphatase; and other eukaryote cells are believed to make analogous factors. In contrast to p34*cdc2*, cyclins that accumulate during G phases attain peak levels at M onset, and then undergo ubiquitin-mediated degradation. Among other functions, they affect p34*cdc2* subcellular location and substrate specificities. After association with the cyclin and other cell components, p34*cdc2* undergoes phosphorylation at specific serine and threonine sites, and this leads to stabilization of the dimer as well as kinase activation. Activated MPF participates (directly, and/or via influences on other enzymes) in all events required to achieve metaphase (chromatin condensation, nuclear envelope breakdown, and the cytoskeletal reorganization involved in spindle formation). It may additionally act autocatalytically as a kinase for other p34*cdc2* molecules and participate in complex cascades. The affected substrates, and the consequences (shown in brackets) include nuclear lamins [depolymerization], nucleolin [nuclear reorganization], vimentin [intermediate filament disassembly], caldesmon [inhibition of the actomyosin ATPase activity that mediates microfilament contraction], histone H1 [chromatin condensation], and p53 [possibly for protection against transformation]. Other substrates demonstrated *in vitro* include RNA polymerase [transcription inhibition], elongation factor EF-1γ [translation inhibition], myosin light chain kinase [contractile ring activation], microtubule associated protein kinase [microtubule reorganization], and p105*Rb* [an anti-oncogene]. It is also believed to contribute to ubiquitin-mediated proteolysis of cyclin B (an event essential for exit from metaphase). Its activity is measured *in vitro* with casein kinase II, but no physiological function has been linked to effects on that enzyme. Cytostatic factor, p39*mos*, a serine-threonine kinase, prevents the degradation, possibly by promoting phosphorylation (and thereby inactivation) of a protease. Excessive amounts invoke metaphase arrest. Cyclins may contribute to p39*mos* degradation. Although metaphase controls appear to be similar in all eukaryote cell types, numerous cell-type and species differences in the regulation of events that lead to G1 → S transition have been observed. A cyclins accumulate earlier than B types, and it has been proposed that the controls involve association of an A cyclin with a 32-33K protein that closely resembles p34*cdc2*. A gene that directs its synthesis (*cdc2B*, *cdck2*) has been described. *See also* **S phase promoting factor** and **cyclins**.

M phase: the stage of **cell cycle** (*q.v.*) during which mitosis occurs.

M phase promoting factor: *see* **MPF**.

MPD: maximal permissible dose.

M peptide: H$_2$N-Tyr-Gly-Lys-Val-Glu-Gln-Leu-Ser-Pro-Glu-Glu-Glu-Glu-Lys-Arg-Ile-Arg-Arg-Glu-Arg-Asn-Lys-Met-Ala-Ala-Ala-OH; a biologically active c-fos fragment.

MPO: myeloperoxidase.

MPP: *see* **MPTP**.

2-MPP: *see* 1-(2-**methoxyphenyl**)**piperazine hydrochloride**.

M protein: a component of skeletal muscle myofibrils, located at sites where myosin molecules join tail to tail.

MPTP: 1-methyl-4-phenyl-1,2,3,6-tetrahydropyridine; a contaminant of some heroine preparations that is converted, via a reaction catalyzed by monoamine oxidases, to 1-methyl-4-phenylpyrimidinium ions (MPP$^+$). The ions inhibit mitochondrial oxidation of NAD-linked substrates, and aerobic oxidation of NADH. After uptake by dopaminergic neurons, and accumulation in the substantia nigra, they destroy neurons that regulate extrapyramidal system functions and invoke an irreversible Parkinson-like disorder.

MR: methyl red.

MR2266: a selective antagonist for κ type opioid receptors.

MRF, MRH: *see* **melanocyte stimulating hormone release factors**.

*f***MRFa**: *formyl*-Phe-Met-Arg-Phe-NH$_2$; a neuropeptide that rapidly decreases leukotriene-mediated rapid neuromuscular transmission in invertebrates, and is implicated as a major mediator of long-term synaptic plasticity. By decreasing the magnitude of voltage-dependent currents that promote Ca^{2+} uptake across plasma membranes during stimulus-invoked depolarization, and diminishing cell sensitivity to high Ca^{2+} levels (with consequent effects on exocytosis), it sustains presynaptic inhibition of acetylcholine release. The effects are specific, and can be reversed with tubocurarine.

MRI: magnetic resonance imaging.

mRNAs: messenger ribonucleic acids.

MRP8, MRP14: *see* **S-100**.

MPTP

MPP$^+$

MS: multiple sclerosis.

ms: millisecond.

MSA: multiplication stimulating activity; *see* **insulin-like growth factor-II**.

MSG: monosodium glutamate.

MSGA: melanoma growth stimulating activity.

MSH, α-, β-, γ-MSHs: *see* **melanocyte stimulating hormones**.

M subunits: *see* **lactic dehydrogenase**.

MT: (1) mesotocin; (2) methyltyrosine.

MTBP: methyltrienolone binding protein.

mtDNA: mitochondrial DNA.

MTOC: microtubule organizing center.

MTol: 5-methoxytryptophol.

MTT: 3-(4,5-dimethyl-2-thiazolyl)-2,5-diphenyl-2H-tetrazolium bromide; a biological stain that changes from yellow to blue when taken up by cells, and a reagent for xanthine oxidase determinations.

mucic acid: galactaric acid.

mucins: major constituents of nasal, salivary, gastric, intestinal, and other mucous gland secretions that lubricate, perform buffer functions, protect underlying cells against mechanical and chemical injury, and trap microorganisms and other foreign matter for movement by cilia by forming viscoelastic gels (in which Ca^{2+} and other cations attach to the negative charges). They are high molecular weight polyanionic glycoproteins with large numbers of sialic acid groups, and mostly sulfated polysaccharides. The composition (and especially the carbohydrate content) varies with both location and species.

mucopolysaccharides: glycosaminoglycans.

mucopolysaccharidoses: inherited disorders, such as Hunter syndrome and Hurler's disease, in which excessive amounts of glycosaminoglycans accumulate because of lysosomal enzyme deficiencies.

mucoproteins: glycosaminoglycans covalently linked to proteins; *see* **proteoglycans**.

mucosa, mucous membrane: membranes that line the mouth, the nose, and the internal surfaces of the respiratory, gastrointestinal, urinary, and reproductive tracts, composed of stratified epithelium with merocrine, mucus-secreting goblet cells.

mucus: the viscous secretions made by mucous membrane goblet cells. Mucins are major components.

mule: a sterile hybrid female offspring of a female horse (with 64 chromosomes) and a male donkey (with 62). It has 63 chromosomes.

Müller cell: (1) a retinal gliocyte (elongated neuroglial supporting cell); (2) any supporting cell for epithelium, such as a Sertoli cell.

Müllerian ducts: paramesonephric ducts; paired embryonic structures that give rise to the uterus, Fallopian tubes, and upper vagina in females, but undergo atrophy in normal males. *See* also **Müllerian duct inhibitor**.

Müllerian duct inhibitor: MDI; Müllerian inhibitory substance, MIS; anti-Müllerian hormone, AMH; Müllerian regression factor: a 72K peptide chemically related to inhibins and transforming growth factor-β (TGFβ), initially identified as the factor synthesized by embryonic and fetal Sertoli cells that acts during a critical stage of development to promote Müllerian duct regression in male mammals. It is also made by older male fetuses, in which it contributes to descent of the testes. It can be detected in boys until the end of the second year; but the form produced after birth may differ from the fetal type. (A messenger RNA detected during late gestation in rats is smaller than the one made earlier.) MDI synthesis is constitutive in embryos, but testosterone may later exert some synergistic influences. Estrogens antagonize some actions. MDI displays phosphatase activity that is opposed by protein kinase A. Some effects have been linked with interference with phosphorylation of epidermal growth factor (EGF) receptors and dephosphorylation of nucleotides. Little or nor MDI is made in fetal ovaries; but the peptide is present in juveniles, and in follicular fluids of more mature organs. It may inhibit oocyte meiosis and aromatase activity, but stimulate follicular cell maturation and contribute to controls for follicle selection. There is some evidence that it protects against development of ovarian cancers. It has also been observed to suppress fetal lung surfactant synthesis.

multi-CSF: multi-colony stimulating factor; *see* **interleukin-3**.

multidrug resistance: MDR; ability to resist the damaging effects of several lipophilic cytotoxic agents (including ones that vary widely in chemical makeup and act via diverse mechanisms). A multidrug resistance gene (*mdr1*) that codes for a plasma membrane-associated transport ATPase has been identified in several kinds of cancer cells refractory to chemotherapeutic agents; *see* **P-glycoprotein**. It undergoes amplification in response to many cytotoxic agents, and is believed to promote extrusion of numerous lipophilic compounds. Agents that inhibit the pump, and substrates that compete with the drugs, counteract the effects. Some mutations that alter P-glycoprotein composition affect the drug specificities. Multidrug resistance is often associated with enhanced sensitivities to steroid hormones, local anesthetics, and Ca channel blocking agents.

multidrug resistance gene: *mdr-1*; *see* **multidrug resistance**.

multienzyme complex: a set of physically associated enzymes that catalyzes successive steps in a metabolic pathway, but does not release the intermediates; *see*, for example **pyruvate dehydrogenase**, and **fatty acid synthase**. The association augments synthetic efficiency by shuttling intermediates from one enzyme to the next. Steroid hormone synthesis may be accomplished in this way.

multifactorial inheritance: genetic transmission that requires participation of two or more genes.

multifunctional enzyme: an enzyme that catalyzes two or more reactions, usually because it possesses two or more active (substrate binding) sites. The C17,C20-lyase/17α-hydroxylase used for androgen biosynthesis is one example.

multigene family: a set of genes derived from a single ancestral precursor via duplications and mutations. The components usually direct production of chemically related proteins, with some species differences in composition. Examples include prolactin/growth hormone, histocompatibility antigen, immunoglobulin, actin, hemoglobin, tubulin, keratin, heat shock protein, integrin, and histone protein family gene sets.

multigravida: a women who has been pregnant several times; *cf* **primigravida**.

multimers: molecules with several subunits; *cf* **monomer** and **dimers**.

multinucleate: describes cells with several nuclei. Examples include skeletal muscle fibers, osteoclasts and other macrophage-derived types, and some liver cell types.

multiparous: (1) having had two or more pregnancies that culminated in the birth of viable offspring; (2) producing several offspring at one time.

multiple allelism: the presence of various forms of a gene type within a population.

multiple endocrine adenomatosis: *see* **multiple endocrine neoplasia**.

multiple endocrine neoplasia: MEN; familial multiple endocrine neoplasia; inherited defects that lead to the formation of tumors derived neuroendocrine cells, and to ectopic hormone secretion. The most prevalent type is MEN 1 (multiple endocrine adenomatosis, MEA-peptic ulcer syndrome, Werner's syndrome), an autosomal dominant form. Parathyroid hyperplasia is the most common manifestation; but afflicted individuals often have additional tumors that originate in pancreatic islet cells (gastrinomas that invoke Zollinger-Ellison syndrome, glucagonomas, or insulinomas). Alternatively, or in addition, they can have pituitary gland tumors (some of which secrete growth hormone, prolactin, and/or adrenocorticotropic hormone). A few also have VIPomas (*see* **Verner-Morrison syndrome**); and there are cases in which adrenocortical, thyroid, and other cell types are additionally affected. A normal *MEN-1* gene on human chromosome 11 (11q13) is believed to protect against uncontrolled proliferation of the cell types. In some individuals with MEN-1, one allele has been deleted from the genome, and the other has undergone mutation. In MEN-2a (Sipple's syndrome) the characteristic findings are thyroid gland medullary carcinomas that secrete calcitonin and/or calcitonin gene related peptide (CGRP), often in conjunction with parathyroid gland hyperplasia. The terms *MEN-2b* and *Schmidt's syndrome* have been applied, respectively when medullary carcinomas are associated with pheochromocytomas or Addison's disease. Other products produced by some MEN-2 medullary carcinomas include katacalcin, substance P, serotonin, prostaglandins, adrenocorticotropic hormone, and carcinoembryonic antigen (CEA). In MEN-3, parathyroid and adrenomedullary tumors are associated with mucosal neuromas.

multiple myelomas: plasma cell cancers derived from a single aberrant cell that undergoes uncontrolled proliferation. They usually originate in bone marrow and destroy osseous tissue, but can infiltrate into visceral organs. The cells release monoclonal antibodies and Bence-Jones protein (myeloma protein light chain monomers and/or dimers) that are excreted to urine.

multiple sclerosis: MS; diseases in which destruction of brain and spinal cord myelin slows conduction of action potentials and alters the distribution of Na^+ channels. The suggested causes include T lymphocyte mediated production of autoantibodies directed against myelin basic protein, release of proteases, and processes initiated by a slow virus. The manifestations include recurring episodes of neurological dysfunction (such as disturbances in proprioception, muscle weakness and spasticity, and vertigo), interspersed with periods of remission during the early stages, but ultimately continuous and progressive.

multiplication stimulating activity: MSA; *see* **insulin-like growth factor-II**.

multipotent colony stimulating factor: multi-CSF; *see* **interleukin-3**.

multivesicular bodies: secondary lysosomes.

MUP: mouse urinary protein.

muramic acid: 2-amino-3-*O*-(1-carboxymethyl)-2-deoxyglucose. A repeating unit of a bacterial cell wall peptidoglycans, in which *N*-acetylmuramic acid links at one end to *N*-acetylglucosamine, and at the other to a peptide chain.

muramidase: **lysozyme** (*q.v.*); a hydrolytic enzyme that degrades muramic acid. It is secreted by tear glands, and provides some protection against bacterial infections.

murarmyl peptides: muramic acid-containing peptidoglycans. Mammalian types are believed to derive from bacterial cell wall components that serve as vitamin-like precursors, taken up and processed to peptides by macrophages. (Germ-free animals can get precursors from dead bacteria in foods.) A synthetic peptide, muramyl dipeptide (MDP), *N*-acetylmuramyl-L-alanyl-D-isoglutamine, is an immune system stimulant believed to act on specific receptors, that can replace mycobacteria in Freund's complete adjuvant. The effects elicited include augmentation of natural killer (NK) cell activity, activation of granular leukocytes and of the complement cascade, induction of cell-mediated immune responses, modulation of humoral immunity, and stimulation of leukocytosis and lymphocyte proliferation. It is pyrogenic, and it increases vascular permeability, promotes blood platelet lysis, enhances fibroblast proliferation, accelerates osteoclastic bone resorption, and provides resistance to tumor growth. Most effects are attributed to stimulation of interleukin-1, prostaglandin E_2 (PGE$_2$), and serotonin release. Its ability to invoke slow-wave sleep and fever may result from direct actions on the brain, as well as influences mediated by second messengers. A sleep factor (SF) in mammalian urine and peritoneal fluid with a muramyl peptide component is an immunostimulant.

murein: a cross-linked peptidoglycan in bacterial inner cell walls that contains glucosamine and *N*-acetyl-muramic acid.

murexine: β-(4-imidazolyl)acrylcholine; urocanylcholine; a muscle relaxant made by *Murex trunculus* and related molluscs that exerts both nicotinic and curariform effects.

murine: usually, (1) derived from or characteristic of mice; (2) derived from or characteristic of mice, rats, and related rodents.

murine leukemia viruses: retroviruses that cause leukemia in rodents. Abelson, Friend, Moloney, Rauscher, and some other types (named for investigators who described them) invoke mutations and/or overexpression of specific proto-oncogene types.

murine sarcoma viruses: Harvey, Kirsten, Moloney, and related retroviruses that promote the development of sarcomas and other tumors in rodents by causing mutations and/or overexpression of specific proto-oncogene types.

muscarine: tetrahydro-4-hydroxy-*N,N,N*,5-tetramethyl-2-furanmethanaminium; an alkaloid made by the poisonous mushroom, *Amanita muscaria* and some other fungi. It is a potent, nonselective agonist for muscarinic type acetylcholine receptors.

muscarinic: describes (1) a set of acetylcholine receptor types; *cf* **nicotinic**; (2) effects elicited when those receptors bind their ligands, such as decreased cardiac rate and contractile force, bronchoconstriction, increased gastrointestinal tract secretion and motility, vasodilation, salivation, and miosis.

muscarinic receptors: a major class of acetylcholine receptors on all parasympathetic effector cells, some brain neurons, and many endocrine glands. Five different genes direct the synthesis of subclasses M1 through M5, and there is evidence for subtypes within each of the subclasses; *see* also **muscatinic receptors**. All known types are approximately 70K glycoproteins, 27% carbohydrate by weight, with seven plasma membrane spanning regions. They display homologies with adrenergic and some other G protein coupled types, and undergo homologous desensitization when continuously activated. The effects of ligand binding include vasodilation, slowing of conduction and weakening of contractile force in the heart, and activation of many exocrine and endocrine glands. Strong stimulation can additionally stimulate mitogenesis in immature nerve cells that retain the ability to divide. Broad spectrum muscarinic agonists that act on all types include muscarine, pilocarpine, and bethanechol. The presence of more than one kind of receptor on a single cell, and the ability of a single type to mediate its effects by more than one mechanism complicate attempts to identify the locations and functions of subtypes with more selective ligands. Pyrenzepine studies suggest that M1 receptors activate a guanylate cyclase and mediate memory processes in the cerebral cortex. Binding to hippocampus neurons declines with age in normal individuals; and some aspects of Alzheimer's disease have been linked with defects. M3 and M5 types, which couple to pertussis toxin insensitive G proteins, resemble M1 in several ways. Activation augments phospholipase Cγ activity, generates diacylglycerols and inositol phosphates, elevates cytosolic Ca^{2+} levels, and opens Ca^{2+}-dependent K^+ channels. The effects of ATP (which is stored in secretory granules of many cholinergic neurons, and is co-released with that neurotransmitter) on phospholipase A_2 activation and arachidonic acid release are also enhanced. Some subtypes additionally activate adenylate cyclases. In contrast, M2 and M4 receptors interact with pertussis toxin *sensitive* G proteins, and can mediate adenylate cyclase inhibition and augment chloride conductance. Differences between M2 "glandular" vs "cardiac" types have been described by some investigators; but others suggest that M4 is similar to or identical with what has been called the glandular form. Mixed agonists that additionally act on nicotinic type acetylcholine receptors include carbachol and arecoline. Moderate levels of atropine and scopolamine antagonize only muscarinic effects, but very high atropine dosages additionally affect sympathetic ganglia nicotinic receptors.

muscatinic: describes acetylcholine receptors with binding sites for both muscarinic and nicotinic agonists, that mediate both kinds of effects. A receptor of this type mediates catecholamine release in the bovine adrenal medulla.

muscimol: 5-aminoethyl-3-hydroxyisoxazole; a GABA$_A$ type gamma aminobutyric acid receptor agonist.

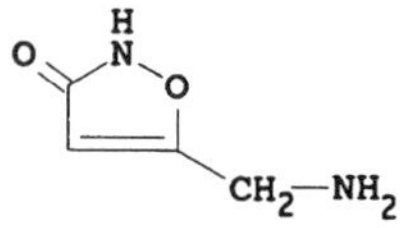

muscles: organs specialized for contraction. The term *striated* is usually applied to skeletal types, because of the appearance under high magnification. It has orderly arrangements of thick myosin filaments and thin filaments (which contain actin, tropomyosin, and troponins, and slide along the thick ones during contraction). In addition to moving the diaphragm and bones, it contributes to glucose homeostasis and is a major source of body heat. It is under voluntary control, and usually contracts only when acetylcholine is released from motor nerve terminals. The cells are long, multinucleated syncytia, well supplied with mitochondria. *Cardiac* muscle is also striated, but the cells are small, with single nuclei. They display intrinsic rhythmicity, and communicate via intercalated discs to achieve coordinated contraction. The activities are directed by the sino-atrial and atrioventricular nodes and associated structures; but stretch, parasympathetic and sympathetic innervations, and humoral factors (including circulating hormones, carbon dioxide and inorganic ions) affect the rate and force of contraction. Cardiac muscle is not under direct voluntary control (but *see* **biofeedback**). The myocytes are major sources of circulating natriuretic hormones. *Smooth* muscle is involuntary. At most sites, it contracts and relaxes more slowly than striated types; but small muscles in the eyes function quite differently from larger ones in the digestive tract, reproductive system, and at some other sites. Much of the activity is intrinsically regulated; but neurotransmitters, stretch, and other factors contribute to the controls. *See* specific muscle types, and *see* also **myoid** and **myoepithelial cells**.

muscle spindles: sensory organs within skeletal muscles that contribute to adjustment of tone, and to the ability to sustain the strong contractions required for holding weights and maintaining posture. Each comprises 3-10 small intrafusal fibers that run parallel to the large extrafusal fibers (the major muscle components). Both ends contain actin and myosin, are innervated by small, afferent gamma motor neurons, and are anchored to perimysium and epimysium. When they contract, they stretch the central region, and thereby activate a noncontractile mechanoreceptor which communicates with the large afferent motor nerve that innervates the extrafusal fibers. Stimulation of the motor nerve is accompanied by simultaneous activation of a gamma nerve that acts on the spindle fiber ends. If contraction of the extrafusal fibers is of sufficient magnitude, the muscle shortens, and the spindle sensor is inactivated. However, if extrafusal fiber contraction is too weak for its purpose, the spindle sensor is stretched, and it sends messages to the large motor neuron that augment extrafusal fiber contraction. Spindle fibers are the major mediators of stretch reflexes, since they are activated when a tendon is tapped. Diabetes mellitus is one of the conditions in which neuron damage can weaken or abolish stretch reflexes.

muscone: *see* **musks**.

Mus musculus: the laboratory mouse.

musks: aromatic substances obtained from the musk glands of several male mammals and some plants, and synthetic agents with similar properties. The naturally occurring types contain pheromones that affect the reproductive behavior of members of the opposite sex of the species. A major aromatic component is muscone, 3-methylcyclopentadecanone (shown below). Most others are chemically related macrocyclic ketones or lactones with approximately 15 carbon atoms. Both natural and synthetic types are used as fixatives in the perfume industry.

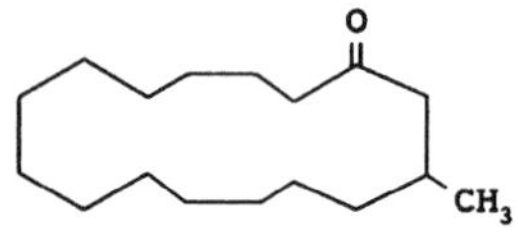

mustards: extracts of cabbage, kale, Brussels sprouts, broccoli, cauliflower, kohlrabi, mustard plants, and other members of the *Brassica* genus. They are mixtures of substances, used as flavoring agents, carminatives, counterirritants, and emetics. *See* also **nitrogen mustards** and **mustard gas**.

mustard gas: sulfur mustard; 2,2′-dichloro-diethylsulfide; a highly toxic vesicant that causes severe tissue damage, and is carcinogenic. It has been used in chemical warfare.

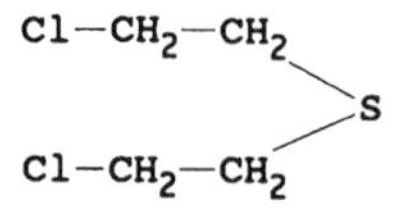

Mustela: a genus of rodents that includes ermine and mink.

mutagen: any agent that alters DNA or chromosome structure.

mutagenesis: induction of base substitutions, deletions, insertions, translocations, or other changes in DNA and chromosome structure. *See* **mutations**.

mutant: an organism with one or more genes different from the kinds present in normal ("wild-type") animals of the species. *See* **mutations**.

mutarotases: enzymes that catalyze reversible rearrangements of chemical groups around asymmetric carbon atoms, and thereby alter the optical rotation properties of solutions. One type catalyzes interconversions of β-D- and α-D-glucose. *Cf* **mutases**.

mutases: enzymes that catalyze rearrangements of chemical groups attached to some atoms of a molecule, and thereby create new kinds of molecules. *See*, for example **phosphoglucomutase**, and *cf* **mutarotases**.

mutation: a change in a genome. Mutagenic factors include X rays, ultraviolet light, chemicals, and retroviruses. Some defects arise during faulty chromosome replication, segregation and separation of chromosome segments when cells divide. The consequences depend on the kinds and locations. Limited numbers of small mutations occur spontaneously, and many of them are soon corrected by repair mechanisms. Some that do not affect viability or severely compromise cell functions are retained, and can contribute to evolutionary changes in the species. Ones that alter the kinds of proteins made affect phenotypes; and some of those cause diseases. Specific kinds of mutations are artificially imposed to study the functions of genes and their products.

mutein: a mutant protein, especially one that binds to antibodies directed against another protein made by the species.

muton: the smallest unit of DNA in which a change constitutes a mutation; one nucleotide.

mutualism: *see* **symbiosis**.

mV: millivolt; 10^{-3} volt.

μV: microvolt; 10^{-6} volt.

myasthenia: abnormal skeletal muscle weakness and/or fatigue.

myasthenia gravis: a progressive autoimmune disease in which autoantibodies directed against nicotinic type acetylcholine receptors impair neural control of skeletal muscle. The resulting weakness usually begins in the small muscles of the eyelids and the extrinsic muscles of the eyes. It later affects muscles used for speech and swallowing, and can ultimately paralyze the diaphragm. The most effective treatment is a combination of acetylcholinesterase inhibitors (which provide more neurotransmitter) and glucocorticoids (which suppress immune responses and also directly promote synthesis of new acetylcholine receptors). The condition is often associated with thymitis; and thymectomy is effective in some cases; *see* also **thymopoietin**. Many afflicted individuals additionally have other kinds of autoimmune disease.

myatonia: abnormally poor muscle tone. It can be caused by defects in muscle, or in neurotransmission mechanisms; *cf* **myotonia**.

myb: a proto-oncogene that codes for a messenger RNA which undergoes alternate splicing, and directs formation of several related 3.4-4.5K helix-turn-helix type DNA-binding nuclear transcription factors. The 3.4K form ($p75^{myb}$) predominates over the $p85^{myb}$ type, is constitutionally expressed at high levels in immature and CD^{4+} T lymphocytes, and is induced by interleukin-2. High levels are also present in liver cells, and in myelocytes. It plays essential roles in the growth and differentiation of hematopoietic cells. Overexpression has been found in colon carcinoma cells, and in individuals with some forms of leukemia. Insertion of a Moloney murine leukemia virus component leads to excessive gene activation. A mutant form (*v-myb*), made by the Abelson leukemia virus, invokes lymphosarcomas, myeloid leukemias, and plasma cell tumors in rodents. An *mbm-1* directed 34K protein inhibits the differentiation inducing effects of DMSO (dimethylsulfoxide) on Freund murine leukemia cells, whereas an *mbm-2* controlled (truncated) type, which may be a natural competitive inhibitor, enhances the differentiation. *Myb* proteins also bind to, and transactivate human immunodeficiency virus (HIV) long terminal repeats.

myc: a family of proto-oncogenes whose members regulate cell differentiation and proliferation by coding for DNA-binding nuclear proteins with leucine zipper domains that affect the transcription of many other genes. The group includes *N-myc*, which contributes to the progression of neuroendocrine and some other tumor types, and *L-myc*, initially identified in lung cancers. *V-myc* is a related oncogene made by the MC29 chicken myelomatosis virus. *C-myc* is an immediate early gene, expressed in proliferating cells and activated by numerous peptide growth factors (and by estrogen in some cell types). It is negatively controlled by its own protein product. Deregulation (which can involve gene amplification as well as overexpression) can result from insertional mutagenesis (by viruses) and chromosomal translocations that disrupt the inhibitory controls. It often invokes tumorigenesis. At least some effects are mediated via the *bcl-2* gene product. Hepatocytes, myogenic cells, and chondrocytes are among the cell types affected. Excessive amounts of c-myc protein have been found in several kinds of spontaneously developing neoplasms; and gene dysregulation is implicated in the etiology of some forms of leukemia. Burkitt's lymphoma and mouse myelomas are malignant diseases in which immature B lymphocytes undergo massive proliferation and fail to achieve terminal differentiation and the ability to synthesize LFA-1. Translocation of the *myc* coding region to a site which puts the gene under the control of an immunoglobulin promoter is a common finding. Proteins whose synthesis is directed by the gene family include plasminogen activator inhibitor-1, some cell adhesion molecules, and possibly also some heat shock types. Myc proteins also promote proliferation and acquisition of catecholamine synthesizing enzymes in neuroendocrine cells, but block their terminal differentiation. The *max* gene product forms dimers with *c-myc*. Although it has been implicated as a factor that confers specific DNA binding, max protein is also made by quiescent cells that do not express *c-myc*, and may act in them as a suppressor and/or perform other functions.

mycobacteria: tuberculosis, leprosy, and other bacteria types with cell walls that contain mycolic acids.

mycolic acids: high molecular weight, branched chain, hydroxylated fatty acid components of mycobacteria cell walls.

mycology: the study of fungi.

mydriasis: dilation of the pupils of the eyes. It occurs in response to dim light, when stress elevates norepinephrine levels (which stimulate iris radial muscle), and in response to cocaine and other sympathomimetic agents. It is opposed by acetylcholine, which stimulates the circular muscle. That neurotransmitter is released by the oculomotor nerves, and its effects usually dominate over those of norepinephrine. Deep anesthesia diminishes its influences. Homatropine and related agents are muscarinic receptor antagonists used to dilate the pupils for eye examinations.

myelin: a mostly lipid complex (with some protein), made by oligodendrocytes and Schwann cells, that forms sheaths around large nerve fibers. Its composition undergoes developmental changes, and varies with the location. In mature nervous systems, it contains cholesterol, phosphoglycerides (phosphatidylethanolamine, with smaller amounts of other phospholipids and some plasmalogens), and galactolipids (galactocerebrosides and some sulfatides) in an approximately 4:3:2 ratio. Sphingomyelins can account for 8-14% of the total lipid weight. Myelin functions as an electrical insulator, and it is essential for saltatory conduction in peripheral nerves. It inhibits neuron growth, and is destroyed in peripheral nerves undergoing regeneration.

myelin-associated glycoprotein: MAG; a nervous system cell surface glycoprotein chemically related to ICAM-1 (intercellular adhesion molecule-1) and to immunoglobulins that mediate adhesion.

myelin basic protein MBP; proteins that stabilize myelin membranes. At least 3 types made by humans are induced by epidermal growth factor (EGF). There is a critical stage of nervous system maturation during which the presence of triiodothyronine (T_3), which acts transcriptionally, and glucocorticoids (which act posttranscriptionally) are required for its production. *See* also **multiple sclerosis**. MBP is phosphorylated by mitogen activated kinases; and some enzyme assays are based on the reactions.

myelitis: inflammation of the spinal cord.

myelo-: a prefix meaning (1) bone marrow; (2) spinal cord; or (3) myelin.

myeloblasts: immature hemopoietic cells normally found only in bone marrow. They are precursors of myelocytes, and possibly also of erythrocytes. Large numbers circulate in some forms of leukemia.

myelocytes: cells that develop from myeloblasts and undergo further differentiation to granulocytic leukocytes.

myeloid: pertaining to, derived from, or resembling (1) bone marrow; (2) spinal cord.

myelomas: tumors derived from bone marrow cells. *See* also **multiple myeloma**.

myeloperoxidases: MPOs; 160K heme-containing granulocyte and macrophage lysosomal enzymes that catalyze reactions in which hydrogen peroxide oxidizes Cl^- and I^-. They are components of "metabolic burst" reactions that generate HOCl (hypochlorous acid), HOI (hypoiodous acid), and other bactericidal agents.

myf5: a gene activated specifically in muscle cells that codes for a DNA-binding nuclear protein. The product acts in conjunction with a *myf6* gene product and other factors (*see* **myoD** and **myogenin**) to promote differentiation.

Myleran: busulfan.

myo-: a prefix meaning muscle.

myoblast[s]: immature precursors of skeletal muscle fibers; *see* **myogenesis**.

myoblastin: a serine protease that contributes to myelocyte differentiation, initially identified in a human myelocytic leukemia cell line.

myocardium: the muscle layer of the **heart** (*q.v.*).

myocytes: the major components of skeletal, cardiac, and smooth muscles. Cardiac myocytes make basic fibroblast growth factor (bFGF), and are major sources of circulating atrial natriuretic hormones. *See* also ***Myo-D***.

Myo-D: a proto-oncogene that codes for a nuclear, skeletal muscle-specific helix-turn-helix type DNA binding phosphoprotein related to the *myc* gene product. It forms homodimers and heterodimers that bind to enhancer regions of genes that code for α subunits of nicotinic type acetylcholine receptors, and also to regulatory regions of creatine kinase and other muscle specific genes. It is essential for skeletal muscle development, and has been called a "molecular switch" that induces withdrawal from cell cycles as well as differentiation. High levels can also promote skeletal muscle type differentiation in dermal fibroblasts, chondroblasts, smooth muscle cells, and retinal pigmented epithelium. The effects include induction of desmin, α-actin, troponin-1, myomesin, and myosin light chain kinase. The mechanisms whereby it arrests proliferation and antagonizes the effects of mitogens in many cell types (including ones that are transformed) are independent of those that promote differentiation. High levels are present during early stages of myoblast development, but they do not inhibit proliferation, possibly because the protein is present in an inactive form. Nerve impulses inhibit its production, and transforming growth factor-β (TGFβ) opposes its influences on target cells.

myoepithelial cells: contractile cells with some smooth muscle characteristics, derived from epithelium, and present, for example in mammary glands and juxtaglomerular apparatus.

myofibrils: long, slender, threadlike components of muscle fibers composed of myofilaments arranged parallel to the long axes. *See* **muscles**.

myofilaments: fine, threadlike components of myofibrils. In skeletal muscle, the thick types contain mostly myosin, whereas thin ones contain actin, tropomyosin, and troponins. *See also* **muscles** and their components.

myogenin: one of the nuclear proteins essential for skeletal muscle differentiation. Its properties resemble those of the *MyoD* gene product.

myogenesis: formation of mature muscle fibers. The processes include differentiation of myoblasts from immature connective tissue cells, fusion of myoblasts to form myotubes, acquisition of muscle-specific proteins, organization of myofibrils, and formation of neuromuscular junctions. *See also* ***Myo-D***.

myoglobin: a component of red skeletal muscle fibers with a higher affinity for oxygen than hemoglobin. It facilitates oxygen transfer from capillary blood to muscle cells. The molecules closely resembles hemoglobin subunits. Each is composed of one globin polypeptide and one heme group.

***myo*-inositol**: the most widely distributed carbocyclic hexitol isomer in biological tissues. Usually, the term **inositol** (*q.v.*) refers to this form.

myomesin: a 165K protein of sarcomere M lines.

myometrium: the muscle layer of the **uterus** (*q.v.*).

myoid cells: contractile cells that somewhat resemble true muscle cells. They are components of ovarian follicles, seminiferous tubules, thymus glands, and other structures. Some metabolize steroids, and/or secrete hormones and enzymes.

myoneural junctions; neuromuscular junctions: functional associations between motor nerves and the muscle fibers they innervate. A junction includes the nerve terminals that store and release neurotransmitters, the membranes on the target muscle cells that hold its receptors, and the synaptic space between them. In skeletal muscle, the major messenger is acetylcholine, and the major receptors are "curariform" nicotinic types that differ from the kinds in autonomic ganglia. Responses to a single nerve impulse are brief, because acetylcholinesterase is released to the synaptic space.

myosarcomas: malignant tumors derived from muscle tissue cells.

myosin: the major skeletal muscle thick filament proteins, and components of most non-muscle contractile cells. The skeletal muscle type is an approximately 540K protein with two identical 230K heavy and four approximately 20K light polypeptide chains. Two heavy chains wind around each other to form a 1340 Å helical coiled-coiled rod ("tail"), with a 20 Å outer diameter that joins to the tail of an adjacent myosin molecule. The free end of each rod subunit terminates in a globular head region that holds the light chains, and has actin binding sites and an ATPase. Trypsin cleaves myosin into light meromyosin (LMM) fragments (two-stranded rods) and heavy meromyosin (HMM) which includes the globular heads. HMM is cleaved by papain to a rod-shaped S2 fragment plus the two S1 head regions that hold the ATPase. In nonmuscle cells, filament assembly requires phosphorylation of one of the myosin light chains; *see* **myosin light chain kinases**.

myosin light-chain kinases: MLCK; several enzymes in contractile cells (blood platelets and other nonmuscle types, as well as smooth, cardiac and skeletal muscle) that catalyze phosphorylation of myosin light chains. Nonmuscle and smooth muscle types do not use the troponin C:calcium ion interactions described for skeletal muscle fibers (*see* also **sliding filament theory**). Contraction is initiated when stimulation leads to elevation of cytosolic Ca^{2+} and calmodulin binds the ions. Ca-calmodulin then attaches to and activates the MLCK which, in turn catalyzes phosphorylation of one of the myosin light chain components. This changes the myosin configuration, permits association of myosin tails with the tails of other myosin molecules, exposes the actin binding sites, and facilitates actin activation of the myosin ATPase essential for contraction. In skeletal muscle, calmodulin is a myosin light-chain kinase subunit that, in unstimulated cells, retains the myosin ATPase in an inactivate form. When stimulation leads to elevation of cytosolic Ca^{2+}, calmodulin binds Ca^{2+}, and the Ca-calmodulin subunit activates the MLCK. At the same time, troponin C binds Ca^{2+}, and unmasks the myosin binding sites on the thin filaments. The phosphorylated light chain then facilitates actin activation of the myosin ATPase. Myosin phosphatases reverse the effects of the kinase. MLCKs are additionally regulated in various ways by kinase A. The skeletal muscle enzyme is activated when catecholamine binding to β-adrenergic receptors generates cAMP. The kinase then phosphorylates MLCK. However, in smooth muscle, kinase-A catalyzed phosphorylation mediates relaxation by weakening associations between Ca-calmodulin and the kinase.

myotendinous antigen: tenascin.

myotomes: embryonic components that give rise to somite muscle tissue.

myosis: (1) miosis; (2) formation of smooth muscle tumors (most common in the uterus).

myositis: muscle inflammation. One type is caused by Coxsackie viruses, and another by *Trichinella spiralis*.

myostatic: related to the tension of a resting muscle, or the tension generated by a myotactic reflex.

myotactic reflex: stretch reflex; contraction of a skeletal muscle in response to a tap on a tendon or muscle that stretches the **muscle spindle** (*q.v.*).

myotonia: disorders in which electrical after-discharges delay relaxation of skeletal muscles when voluntary contraction is terminated. It is attributed to muscle membrane abnormalities. One manifestation is difficulty releasing an object that has been grasped. *Cf* **myatonia**.

myotropic hormone: an uncharacterized regulator implicated as a mediator of androgen-stimulated anabolism in muscle tissue.

myotubes: the structures formed when myocytes fuse during **myogenesis** (*q.v.*).

myristic acid: *n*-tetradecanoic acid; *see* **myristoylation.**

H_3C ~~~~~~~~~ COOH

myristoylated alanine rich C kinase substrate: MARCKS; a widely distributed acidic, hydrophobic 80-87K protein, myristoylated at its *C*-terminus, that is rapidly phosphorylated by growth factor activated kinase C isozymes, and is implicated as a mediator of growth factor effects. The messenger RNA has been identified in the brain, spinal cord, spleen and lungs. Phosphorylation decreases MARCKS affinity for calmodulin.

myristoylation: covalent addition of myristic acid moieties, for example to protein amide groups. It confers lipophilic properties that mediate anchoring to membrane bilayers, and associated changes in functions. The transforming properties of pp60^{v-src} and some other oncogene products depend on plasma membrane anchoring via myristoylated terminal glycine amides. Some other proteins are myristoylated on cysteine moieties. Normal p21^{ras} is covalently linked to palmitate; and replacement with myristate confers transforming potential.

Mytilus edulis: the edible mussel, a marine bivalve mollusc with ciliated gills for filter feeding. It is used to study cilia functions.

myxedema: (1) subcutaneous accumulation of glycosaminoglycans, and of water osmotically drawn in by the molecules. The major cause is thyroid hormone deficiency effects on hyaluronic acid metabolism; (2) severe hypothyroidism in adults; *cf* **cretinism.**

N

N: (1) asparagine; (2) nitrogen; (3) norepinephrine; (4) normal, normality (of a solution); (5) the haploid number of chromosomes; (6) Newton; (7) nucleotide; G proteins were initially called N or G/N proteins because they bind guanine nucleotides.

n: nano, as in nanometer, nanogram, or nanoliter.

N.: central nervous system nucleus, as in N. ambiguous.

N-: in names of compounds, a nitrogen atom linked to another group, as in *N*-acetylglucosamine.

NA: (1) not applicable; (2) information not available.

Na: sodium.

NAAG: *N*-acetylaspartylglutamide; a dipeptide in suprachiasmatic nuclei, implicated as a mediator for synchronizing circadian rhythms with photoperiods.

Nabadial: a trade name for methandriol.

Nabolin: a trade name for methandrostenolone.

N-acetyl-: for compounds not listed under *N*-, *see N*-acetyl-.

N-acetylneuraminic acid: NANA: *see* **sialic acid**.

N-acetylserotonin: NAS; a precursor of melatonin and related regulators, made from serotonin; *see N*-acetyltransferases.

N-acetyltransferases: NATs; enzymes that catalyze reactions of the general type: R-NH$_2$ + acetyl-coenzyme A → R—NH—COCH$_3$ + CoA. In pineal glands, conversion of serotonin to *N*-acetylserotonin is rate-limiting for melatonin synthesis in many species (*see also* **hydroxyinodol-*O*-methyltransferasea**). The NAT activity is synchronized with photoperiods, and is highest during darkness in both nocturnal and diurnal animals. The pi-

neal enzyme differs from ones that act on glucoseamine and other substrates.

NAD$^+$, NADH: *see* **nicotine adenine dinucleotide**.

nadarelin: D-Nal-(2)6-GnRH; a gonadotropin releasing hormone analog that is somewhat less potent than **nafarelin** *(q.v.)*.

NAD kinase: an enzyme that catalyzes the reaction: NAD$^+$ + ATP → NADP$^+$ + ADP. The NADP$^+$ is reduced in the hexose monophosphate shunt pathway to NADPH + H$^+$, and the products are used for anabolic processess (such as fatty acid synthesis), to generate nitric oxide and some neutrophil products, and to reduce methemoglobin iron.

NADP$^+$, NADPH: *see* **nicotine adenine dinucleotide phosphate**.

NADPH diaphorases: old yellow enzyme; flavoprotein enzymes that take up electrons from substrates and can pass them to oxygen, but do not use mitochondrial electron transport chains for ATP synthesis. They stain with nitroblue tetrazolium. One function is reduction of methemoglobin iron. The nervous tissue type may be identical with neuronal nitric oxide synthase. Cells that make it are highly resistant to ischemia, and to glutamate toxicity. A similar enzyme is made in endothelium, but synthases in macrophages and in the adrenal cortex and liver are different.

NADPH oxidases: cytochrome enzymes that take up electrons from substrates, and are used by neutrophilic leukocytes to generate superoxide and other bactericidal substances. Chronic granulomatosis diseases are inherited disorders in which lesions form because X-linked or autosomal mutations severely impair resistance to pathogens by coding for ineffective enzymes.

NAF: monocyte derived neutrophil activating factor; *see* **neutrophil activating protein-1**.

nafarelin: 5-D-(2-naphthyl-alanyl)-GnRH; a long-acting gonadotropin releasing hormone agonist. The acetate is approximately 200 times as potent as GnRH, and effec-

5-oxoPro-His-Trp-Ser-Tyr——N——C——C——Leu-Arg-Pro-Gly-NH$_2$

nafarelin

tive when administered in nasal sprays. Since it desensitizes GnRH receptors, it is used to arrest precocious puberty, and to treat endometriosis, cancers of the prostate gland and breast, and other conditions in which suppression of gonadal function is beneficial.

nafoxidine: 1-[2-[4-(3,4-dihydro-6-methoxy-2-phenyl-1-naphthalenyl)phenoxy] ethyl]pyrrolidine; an agent that mimics the early effects of estrogens, and invokes one round of DNA synthesis, but then acts as anti-estrogen by interfering with estrogen receptor recycling. The hydrochloride is used to treat breast cancers.

naftopidil: 4-(2-methoxyphenyl)-α-[(1-napthalenyloxy)-methyl]-1-piperazine ethanol; an α_1 type adrenergic receptor antagonist that lowers blood pressure.

NAG: *N*-acetylglucosamine.

Naja: a genus of snakes that includes cobras. *Naja Naja* venom contains a potent acetylcholinesterase. Venoms of other species are sources of different enzymes and of lectins.

Najjar syndrome: a form of male pseudohermaphroditism with manifestations that include ambiguous genitalia, cardiomyopathy, and mental retardation.

Na$^+$/K$^+$-ATPases: sodium-potassium adenosine triphosphatases: plasma membrane enzymes that use energy released by ATP hydrolysis to drive Na$^+$ and K$^+$ exchange against concentration gradients. They are essential for maintaining resting potentials, and for repolarization. Their synthesis in various cell types is controlled by hormones, and the activities are affected by intracellular and extracellular Na$^+$ and K$^+$ levels. Renal tubule enzymes are major contributers to acid-base and water balance; *see* also **aldosterone**. In some cell types, catecholamines, triiodothyronine (T$_3$), and other hormones elevate metabolic rates by accelerating the ATP hydrolysis.

naked mole rat: *Heterocephalus glaber*; a burrowing rodent of the Batergidae family that lives underground in Kenya, Ethiopia, and some other parts of Africa. It is neither a mole, nor a rat (but in many ways closely resembles the guinea pig). Special features make it a

desirable subject for studies of behavior and thermoregulation. It is the only mammal known to depend on basking, huddling, and other activities to control its body temperature (which varies with the environment). Other than vibrissae and a few tufts around the mouth and between the toes, the body surface is almost devoid of hair or fur. It is also the only mammal known to live in social groups in which a single very large queen produces all of the progeny. Other females and nonmating males are workers, whose functions change as they mature and age. The animals subsist on underground tubers, and their digestive tracts contain microorganisms that digest cellulose. Special adaptations to the life style include small eyes, tiny ear flaps, short appendages, huge incisors, and highly developed jaw muscles.

NAL: naloxone.

Nal-: naphthyl-.

nalidixic acid: 1-ethyl-1,4-dihydro-7-methyl-4-oxo-1,8-napthyridine-3-carboxylic acid; an antibacterial agent used to treat urinary tract infections. It interferes with DNA replication and repair by attaching to DNA-binding A subunits of bacterial topoisomerase II (DNA gyrase), and causing supercoiling.

Nalline: nalorphine.

nalmefene: (5α)-17-(cyclopropylmethyl)-4,5-epoxy-6-methylenemorphinan-3,4-diol; a μ type opioid receptor antagonist, stronger than naloxone, with no partial agonist activity or known influences on other opioid receptor types. It is used to treat narcotic poisoning.

nalorphine: Nalline; allorphine; antorphine; *N*-allylnormorphine; 17-allyl-7,8-didehydro-4,5α-epoxymorphinan-3,6-α-diol; a potent μ type opioid receptor antagonist, a fairly potent partial agonist for κ receptors, and a weak partial agonist for the δ type. It is used to treat narcotic poisoning, and can invoke severe withdrawal symptoms in individuals addicted to morphine and heroine.

naloxone: Narcan; 17-allyl-4,5α-epoxy-3,14-dihydroxy-morphinan-6-one; a μ type opioid receptor antagonist with weak effects on κ and γ types. It is also a weak agonist for δ receptors, and (in high concentrations) for

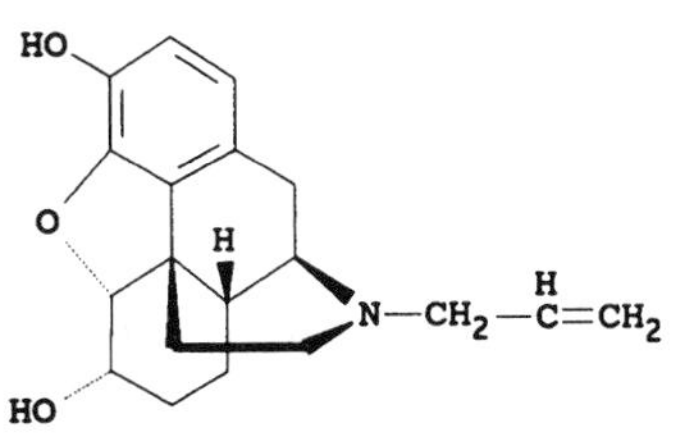

nalorphine

naltrexone

GABA types that release prolactin. Naloxone is used to counteract respiratory depression and other aspects of opioid poisoning, and is effective when substantial quantities of endogenous opioid peptides are released (for example by endotoxins, during anaphylaxis or strenuous exercise, or in response to spinal cord injury), and against the analgesic effects of placebos and acupuncture. It is incorporated into some opioid analgesic preparations administered intravenously, to antagonize the psychological effects, and thereby render them unattractive to morphine and heroine addicts, but can invoke nausea, vomiting, and cardiovascular dysfunction in susceptible individuals. Although used in laboratory studies to antagonize endorphin and enkephalin influences on the release of several hypothalamic and pituitary gland hormones, the effects vary with the species. Opioids elevate prolactin levels and suppress gonadotropin releasing hormone (GnRH) release in most mammals via mechanisms that involve dopamine inhibition, and act via cholinergic mechanisms to stimulate growth hormone release in humans and some others. Naloxone blocks all of those effects, and can also oppose the stimulatory influences of exercise and sleep on growth hormone secretion. However, it does not affect growth hormone secretion in rats, possibly because the major controls in those animals are exerted by somatostatin, and by different neurotransmitters that regulate growth hormone releasing hormone (GRH). Enkephalins inhibit the secretion of corticotropin releasing hormone (CRH) in humans, but stimulate it in rats; and high doses of naloxone inhibit both responses. Effects on thyrotropin releasing hormone (TRH) also vary with the species.

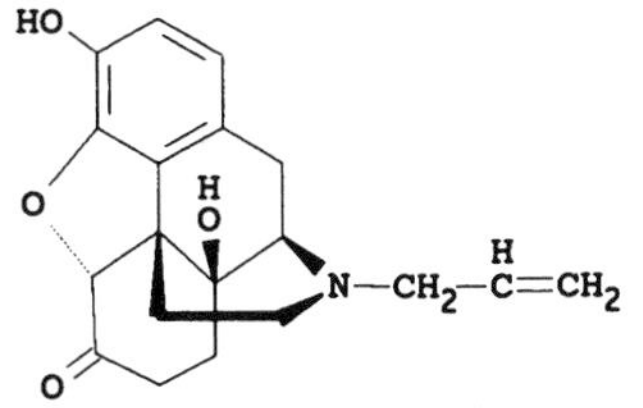

naltrexone: 17-(cyclopropyl-methyl)-4,5α-epoxy-3,14-dihydroxymorphinan-6-one; an orally effective, long-acting morphine receptor antagonist. Some properties resemble those of naloxone, but it enhances stress analgesia. It does not stimulate prolactin release, is somewhat more effective for reproductive system effects, and is not a σ agonist. Prolonged use can cause liver injury in susceptible individuals.

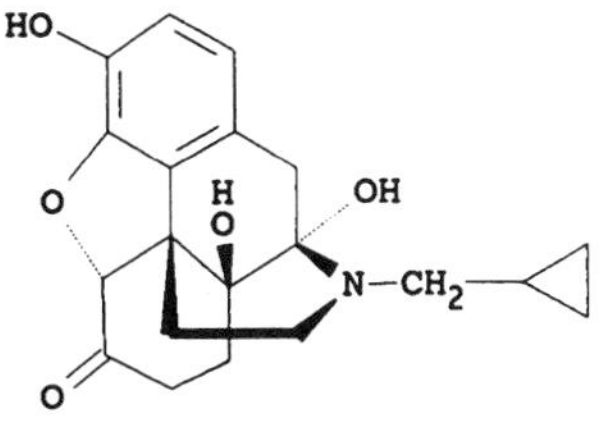

NAM: (1) *N*-acetylmuramic acid; (2) nicotinamide.

NAME: N^G-nitro-arginine methyl esters; competitive inhibitors of nitric oxide synthetase. The L isomer (L-NAME) is more potent than the D form (D-NAME).

NANA: *N*-acetylneuraminic acid; *see* **sialic acid**.

NANC: non-adrenergic, non-cholinergic; describes neurons whose functions are not affected by agents that block either adrenergic or cholinergic receptors, for example ones that release neuropeptides or other transmitters which act directly on target organs.

nandrolone: 17β-hydroxyestr-4-en-3-one; 19-nortestosterone; a testosterone analog used (often illegally by athletes) for its anabolic effects. Conjugates include the decanoate (Deca-Durabol), the *p*-hexyloxyphenylpropionate (Anador), and the phenpropionate. *See* **anabolic steroids**.

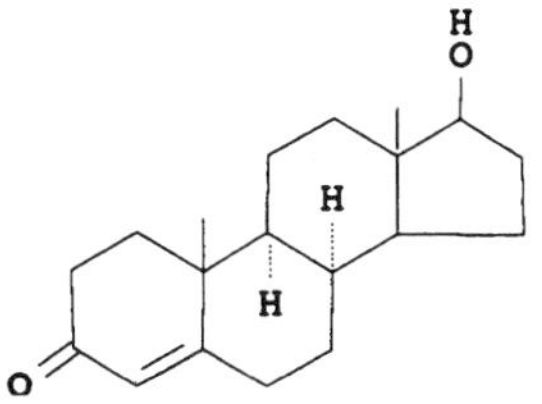

nano: 10^{-9}, as in nanogram, nanomole, and nanoliter.

NAP-1: neutrophil activating protein-1.

α-NAPAP: *N*-α-(2-naphthalenesulfonylglycyl)-4-amidino-phenylalanine piperidine; a thrombin antagonist used as an anticoagulant.

naphthalene sulfonamides: *N*-(6-aminohexyl)-chloro-naphthalene sulfonamide and *N*-(6-aminohexyl)-5-chloronaphthalene sulfonamide are potent calmodulin inhibitors. *See* **W-5** and **W-6**.

naphthoquinones: (1) members of the vitamin K family; (2) 1,4-naphthalenedione (shown below) and related plant pigments derived from naphthoquinone.

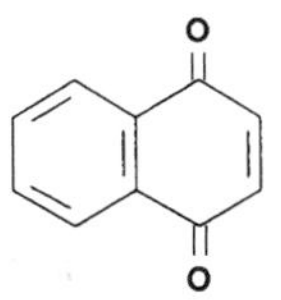

naproxen: 6-methoxy-α-methyl-2-naphthalene-acetic acid; a nonsteroidal anti-inflammatory agent that inhibits cyclooxygenase. Its antipyretic and analgesic properties are used to treat rheumatoid arthritis.

NAPS: *N*-(*p*-aminophenacetyl)-spiperidol; a selective D_2-type dopamine receptor antagonist; *see* **spiperidol**.

naproxen

narcosis: central nervous system depression associated with deep sleep or coma.

narcotics: agents that invokes narcosis, a term sometimes restricted to morphine, endogenous opioids, related compounds, and other controlled substances.

Nardil: a trade name for phenelzine sulfate.

NAS: *N*-acetylserotonin.

nasal glands: organs of some birds and reptiles that contribute to water and electrolyte balance by secreting sodium chloride. Most are regulated by aldosterone. Unlike renal excretion, the salt removal is associated with very limited water loss.

nascent: in the process of being formed, a term applied for example to a peptide attached to a ribosome that is undergoing elongation, an incompletely synthesized ribonucleic acid, or a premessenger RNA that has not yet undergone processing.

NAT: *N*-acetyltransferase.

native: usually describes (1) a species indigenous to a geographical locale (not introduced from another region); (2) a naturally occurring hormone, enzyme, or other substance (as opposed to one that has been artificially altered, or taken from another species).

natriferic: promoting sodium ion transport.

natriuresis: increased urinary excretion of sodium.

natriuretic hormones: regulators that accelerate urinary excretion of sodium (and usually also of chloride and water). The best known types are secreted by cardiac myocytes (*see* **atrial natriuretic peptides**); but others are made in the hypothalamus, adrenal medulla, and elsewhere. They contribute to control of extracellular fluid volume, acid-base balance, blood pressure, renin, aldosterone and antidiuretic hormone secretion, and calcium metabolism, and are implicated as mediators of mineralocorticoid "escape". The mechanisms include inhibition of Na^+/K^+- ATPases, augmentation of glomerular filtration rates, and the release of other hormones.

natriuretic peptides: peptides that promote urinary excretion of sodium. *See* **atrial natriuretic peptides** and **natriuretic hormones**.

natural immunity: innate immunity; natural resistance; usually, the ability to resist the effects of harmful antigens that have not previously been encountered, via mechanisms that do not involve activation of specific lymphocyte subsets. In some cases, antibodies against them are constitutionally expressed. The term *acquired immunity* refers to resistance developed after exposure to an antigen; but some authors use *natural acquired im-*

munity if the antigen is generally available (for example in foods, or as a nonpathogenic environmental component).

natural killer cells: NK cells; a heterogeneous leukocyte subset (NK1, NK2, and subgroups within them) that contributes to natural defenses against pathogens and tumorigenesis, via mechanisms that are not antigen-specific. Although secretion of tumor necrosis factor-α (TNFα) and platelet activating factor (PAF) suggest relationships to macrophages, they are not phagocytic, and several characteristis are consistent with derivation from pre-thymocytes. They express Thy-1 antigen and interleukin-2 receptors, and proliferate in response to simultaneous presentation of IL-2 and interferon-γ (IFNγ). They also express CD2, CD11b, CD56 (NKH) and other nonreceptor kinases (p60^{fyn}, and p62^{yes}), which are required for activation. Although they make CD3ζ subunit dimers that complex with CD16, they have little or no ability to transcribe CD3 α,β,δ, or γ subunits, and are mostly CD3 negative. The term *null cells* has been applied, because they lack some markers present on "typical" B and T cells. Another, *large granular lymphocytes* is not always appropriate because of marked variations in granulation. If classified as lymphocytes, they account for approximately 5% of the circulating types in human peripheral blood. Most NK cells express CD16 (FcγIII receptors), and can therefore engage in antibody-dependent cell cytotoxicity (ADCC). Some additionally bind directly to and kill virus-infected, tumor, and other cell types recognized as foreign via mechanisms independent of CD16 that involve release of perforins from their granules. Unlike killer (K) cells, they continue to function when exposed to antibodies that block CD16 effects; but NK cells that bind but cannot kill, and small numbers that cannot bind have also been described. NK cells additionally make interferon γ (and it has been suggested that high levels of IL-2 convert other lymphocytes to NK types by synergizing with the IFN). Their killer activities do not involve the kinds of antigen contact with MHC molecules that characterize those of T$_C$ cells; and they do not acquire memory. MHC proteins may, in fact, mask antigens recognized by NK cells, and thereby protect normal body components against attack. (NK cells do kill prethymocytes or other cells that cannot express the MHC molecules on their surfaces because they do not make β-microglobulin). The importance of the ability to recognize and lyse a broad spectrum of tumor and virus-infected cell types is apparent in individuals who lack them, and therefore display susceptibility for development of lymphomas and other tumors. Estrogens are reported to depress NK cell activity, at least during pregnancy; and this may be one component of mechanisms that defend embryos and fetuses. Additionally, NK or K cells may affect the production of thyroid hormones.

natural selection: changes in a population (usually associated with increased ability to survive) that result from high fecundity of individuals who possess specific allele types. Deleterious genes tend to be eliminated, and advantageous ones preserved.

nb: a gene that directs the synthesis of ankyrin.

NBD-phallicydin: a derivative of **phalloidin** (*q.v.*), used as a probe in studies of filamentous actin.

NBQX: 2,3-dihydroxy-6-nitro-7-sulfamoyl-benzo(F) quinoxaline: a selective quisqualate type glutamate receptor antagonist, more potent that DNQX and CNQX, that does not act on NMDA (*N*-methyl-D-aspartate) or glycine sites. It can protect against ischemia-invoked neural injury.

NBT: nitroblue tetrazolium.

N-CAM: neural cell adhesion molecule.

N cells: (1) gastrointestinal mucosa cells that secrete neurotensin; (2) adrenal medulla cells that secrete norepinephrine.

NCF: neutrophil chemotactic factor.

NCP: noncollagenous bone proteins.

ND: not determined (indicates that the measurements were not made).

NDGA: nordihydroguaiaretic acid.

NE: norepinephrine.

nebulin: a 600K inextensible protein attached to skeletal muscle sarcomere Z discs, and oriented in parallel with thick filaments.

NECA: 5′-*N*-ethylcarboxamido-adenosine; an A_2-type adenosine receptor agonist.

necrosin: an undefined component of exudates formed during acute inflammatory reactions that promotes necrosis.

necrosis: pathological death of cells or of parts of tissues and organs that follows infection, trauma, ischemia, exposure to toxins, or other deleterious factors, caused by release of lysosomal enzymes. The cells characteristically display pyknosis, followed by karyolysis and karyorrhexis. They can then fuse to form amorphous clumps of granular or hyaline matter. *Cf* **apoptosis**.

necrotoxins: bacterial exotoxins and other poisons that kill cells; *see* **necrosis**.

nef: a human immunodeficiency virus (HIV) gene that codes for p27 (a protein that acts in conjunction with Tat and Rev to promote formation of proviral DNA).

negative cooperativity: reduced affinity of unoccupied receptors caused by binding of small quantities of the ligands to neighboring receptors of the same kind. The mechanisms can include changes in unoccupied receptor configurations or mobilities, and can protect against sudden "bursts" of activity, for example when excessive amounts of a hormone are rapidly released (without loss of sensitivity to low levels of the regulators). *Cf* **down regulation**. Insulin, catecholamines, growth hormone (GH), and thyroid stimulating hormone (TSH) are among the ligands reported to invoke negative cooperativity.

negative feedback control: suppression of an activity or function by a product of that activity or function. For example, glucocorticoids (whose synthesis is stimulated by adrenocorticotropic hormone, ACTH) inhibit (exert negative feedback controls over) cells that make the ACTH. In a chemical reaction series of the type [A → B → C → D], B, C, or D can inhibit the enzyme that catalyzes A → B. The processes protect against overactivity. *Cf* **positive feedback controls**.

negative gene control: suppression of transcription of a gene by factors that interact (directly or indirectly) with the DNA. Repressors that bind to operons act this way.

negative staining: techniques for visualizing molecules not detected with direct staining. For electron microscopy, samples supported on thin films of carbon are sprayed with concentrated solutions of electron opaque heavy metal salts, such as sodium phosphotungstate or uranyl acetate. As the specimens dry, the salts fill crevices around the molecules, and appear as dark backgrounds that surround lighter objects.

Nelson's syndrome: conditions caused by adrenocorticotropic hormone (ACTH)-secreting tumors that develop after bilateral adrenalectomy is performed to alleviate Cushing's syndrome. Skin hyperpigmentation is a common manifestation.

NEM: *N*-ethylmaleimide.

nematodes: roundworms of the phylum *Nematoda*, which includes some parasitic organisms. *Caenorhabditis elegans* is used for studies of genetics and development, since it has a simple genome, a short life-cycle, and cells easily identified under light microscopy. Hermaphroditic adults have only 959 cells, and engage in self-fertilization. The fates of all of its embryonic cells are known.

Nembutal: a trade name for pentobarbital.

neocortex: isocortex; the most complex, and phylogenetically most recent components of the cerebral cortex.

neo-Darwinism: Charles Darwin attributed evolutionary changes to spontaneously occurring variations in phenotypic characteristics, with preferential survival of the "fittest" (who then transmit the advantages to the progeny). Neo-Darwinism links the characteristics to genes, attributes some evolutionary changes to new combinations of alleles as well as mutations, and recognizes persistence of alleles that confer no special advantage but do not seriously affect essential functions.

neoendorphins: small, biologically active opioid peptides cleaved from proenkephalin B (prodynorphin) in the brain and adrenal medulla. The first five amino acid moieties are identical with those of the leu-enkephalin. α-*neoendorphin* is Tyr-Gly-Gly-Phe-Leu-Arg-Lys-Arg-Tyr-Pro-Lys; β-*neoendorphin* is Tyr-Gly-Gly-Phe-Leu-Arg-Lys-Arg-Tyr-Pro.

neomycin: a broad-spectrum aminoglycoside antibiotic complex made by *Streptomyces fradiae*, composed of neomycins A, B (shown below), and C. Preparations are used topically for skin infections, systemically to prepare the intestines for surgery, and in the form of ear drops. The common toxic effects of systemic administration include malabsorption associated with bile salt precipitation and changes in the intestinal villi, often accompanied by lowering of blood cholesterol levels. The antibiotics can also cause renal damage, nerve deafness, and neuromuscular blockade. They are used as laboratory tools to inhibit phospholipase Cγ, and phosphatidylinositol hydrolysis.

neonatal: newborn. The term can refer to the morphological features and physiological factors characteristic of that stage of development, pathological conditions, or treatments administered soon after the time of birth.

neonatal androgenization: in rats, mice, and some other species, small quantities of androgens administered soon after birth can permanently affect development of some brain regions (*see* **organizational effects**). Neonatally androgenized females acquire male-type secretory patterns for gonadotropin releasing hormone (GnRH), growth hormone, and other regulators, and male-type hepatic and renal enzyme patterns. They do not ovulate when mature, and can display behavioral responses to gonadal steroids characteristic for the opposite sex.

neoplasia: tumor formation.

neoplasm: any benign or malignant tumor.

neostigmine: Prostigmin; (3-dimethylcarbamoxyphenyl) trimethylammonium; a potent acetylcholinesterase inhibitor. The bromide (Physostigmine) is used to treat myasthenia gravis and other conditions in which elevation of acetylcholine levels confers beneficial effects.

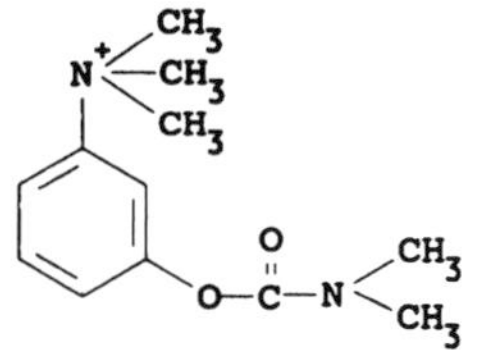

neostriatum: the part of the corpus striatum that includes the caudate nucleus and putamen; *cf* **paleostriatum**.

Neosynephrine: a trade name for phenylephrine.

neotenin: corpus allatum hormone.

neoteny: retention of larval body form in reproductively competent adults. Members of some insect and some amphibian species do not acquire the hormones patterns and/or receptors that promote metamorphosis in other animals of the same class. In mudpuppies (*Necturus*), juvenile type hormone patterns and receptors are retained, and adults are unresponsive to exogenous regulators. In contrast, the Mexican axolotlyl (*Ambystoma mexicanum*) does not undergo spontaneous changes, but does achieve metamorphosis when treated with high concentrations of thyroid hormones.

neovascularization: formation of new blood vessels; *see* **angiogenesis**.

nephrectomy: removal of the kidneys. In otherwise healthy animals, unilateral nephrectomy leads to compensatory hypertrophy of the remaining organ (which then often maintains normal functions).

nephritis: inflammation of the kidneys. It can involve glomeruli, interstitial tissue, and/or renal tubules.

nephrocalcinosis: calcium salt deposition in the kidneys, usually in the tubules. It can severely impair renal functions. The causes include hyperparathyroidism, excessive vitamin D intake, other conditions associated with high blood calcium levels, and factors that increase renal

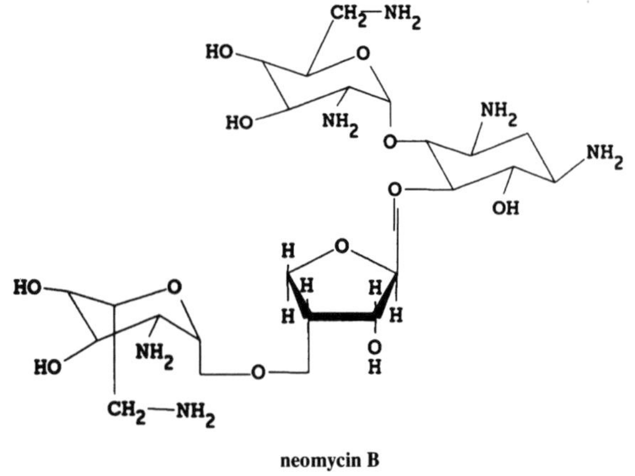

neomycin B

tubular fluid alkalinity or raise the concentrations of phosphate, oxalate, or other anions that form poorly soluble calcium salts.

nephrocystitis: inflammation of the kidneys and urinary bladder.

nephrogenesis: kidney development.

nephrogenic: originating in, or caused by factors associated with the kidney.

nephrogenic diabetes: excessive urinary loss of water caused by kidney defects such as inability to efficiently reabsorb glucose, sodium, or other substances. In *nephrogenic diabetes insipidus*, vasopressin synthesis can be adequate, but vasopressin receptors are abnormal, or are not present in sufficient numbers.

nephron: the anatomical and functional unit of the kidney. It includes a renal corpuscle, proximal convoluted tubule, Henle loop (with ascending and descending limbs), distal convoluted tubule, and (in many species) a collecting tubule. A healthy human adult kidney contains one million or more. An ultrafiltrate of blood, formed in the renal corpuscle (*see* **glomerulus**), passes through the proximal convoluted tubule (in which selective reabsorption and some secretion to tubular fluid occur), and from there through the Henle loop (a major site for regulating renal interstitial fluid osmolarity) to the distal convoluted tubule for additional processing. The nephron leads into a collecting duct, where most of the controlled water reabsorption is accomplished. The fluid (now urine) then travels to the renal pelvis, and is released to the ureters. *See* specific components and **juxtaglomerular apparatus**.

nephrosis: disorders in which degenerative changes in the kidneys impair renal function.

nereistoxin: a compound made by annelid worms that kills other worms, and also beetles and some other insects, by acting on their nervous systems; *see* **Padan**.

Nernst equation: an equation that defines the relationships between the concentration of a specific ion type and the resting membrane potential of a cell at equilibrium with an environment of constant composition, expressed as $V = RT/zF \, ln \, C_o/C_i$, where V = the equilibrium potential in volts (the internal potential minus the external potential), R = the gas constant, T = the temperature in degrees Kelvin, z = the valance of the ion, ln is the natural logarithm, C_o = its outside concentration, C_i = the inside concentration, and F is Faraday's constant.

nerve growth factor: NGF; a hormone essential for survival and maturation (but not proliferation) of newly differentiated neuroblasts that originate in the neural crests and form the major components of the sympathoadrenal system and dorsal root ganglia, and for some brain cholinergic neurons. NGF concentration gradients direct axon and dendrite growth; and the hormone induces tyrosine hydroxylase and dopamine decarboxylase (essential for catecholamine synthesis), and choline acetyltransferase (for acetylcholine synthesis in ganglion cells). Some effects of other regulators on central nervous system development require NGF. For example,

triiodothyronine (T_3) influences during critical stages include stimulation of NGF synthesis; and fibroblast growth factors induce the receptors. Deficiency early in life severely impairs development; *see* also **immunosympathectomy**. In mature nervous systems, NGF made by neuroglial and Schwann cells is taken up by axons, and undergoes retrograde transport to perikarya. It is also delivered to some organs by sympathetic nerve endings. In adrenal medulla cells (which derive from neural crests), high concentrations of glucocorticoids act on NGF-prepared cells to promote further specialization. Those cells do not have axons or dendrites, but acquire them in cultures when NGF presented. High glucocorticoid levels antagonize the effects. The hormone acts in different ways (*see* **nerve growth factor receptors**) as an essential mitogen for some cell types, including ones that form the otic vesicles and associated cochleovestibular ganglia of the developing inner ear; and excessive amounts in transfected neuroblasts invoke transformation. NGF is also synthesized in skeletal muscle, placenta, gonads, and at some other sites; and large amounts are made in the heart and spleen. In oocytes, NGF can promote germinal vesicle breakdown; and its ability to promote histamine release from mast cells in the ovary is believed to contribute to ovulation. Actions on testicular germinal cells may be needed for fertility. In the immune system, it stimulates differentiation of B lymphocytes and may perform other functions. Testosterone promotes production of large amounts in the submandibular salivary glands of male rodents. The hormone released from them during fighting is believed to mediate stress-related responses. The venom glands of moccasin snakes contain even higher concentrations. It may act there as a carrier for phospholipases, phosphodiesterases, and proteases. NGF is a member of a protein family that includes brain derived growth factor (BDGF) and neurotropic factor-3 (NF-3, NT-3). The three proteins exert some overlapping influences, compete for binding to low affinity receptors, and may interact at some sites, but have different distribution patterns in the brain. There is some homology with proinsulin and relaxin; and NGF binds to relaxin receptors. The active form is a homodimer composed of two 13.25K, 118 amino acid noncovalently associated subunits, assembled from two proNGF molecules, each of which binds a catalytic γ subunit that converts the proNGFs to NGFs. The resulting tetramer then adds two α subunits, one of which contains an esterase. The nonhormonal components are believed to protect NGF against degradation. Effects invoked in various cell types include augmented expression of *c-fos*, *c-jun*, *zif268/NGF-A1*, *nur77/NGF-B1* and other immediate early genes, increased production of ornithine decarboxylase, phosphatidylinositol-3-kinase, guanine nucleotide activating protein (GAP), guanine nucleotide exchange protein, transin, and some S-100 proteins, accelerated glucose uptake, and augmented Na^+/K^+ exchange.

nerve growth factor receptors: p^{75NGFR} is an abundant, widely distributed protein that binds NGF with low affinity. Although it may directly mediate some effects of high NGF levels, it does not possess kinase activity, is not autophosphorylated when it binds NGF, and does not exert characteristic NGF influences on terminal differentiation of neurons or on neurotransmitter synthesis. Moreover, it is made by all neurons, and by other some cell types (including some that do not respond to NGF); *see* also **neurotrophic hormones**. p140^{trk} (TRK) is a larger protein normally made in substantial amounts only by cells that cannot divide. It binds NGF with low affinity, and may directly inhibit cell proliferation. When it dimerizes with p75^{NGF}, the affinity for the hormone is approximately 100 times greater than that of either monomer; and the association is believed to confer DNA binding specificity. All cells that make both proteins respond to NGF. In its presence, the smaller component activates a tyrosine kinase in the larger one, and promotes autophosphorylation. At least some of the effects are mediated via hydrolysis of a plasma membrane glycosyl-phosphatidylinositol, and liberation of an inositol phosphoglycan that is effective when administered directly. Signal transduction involves generation of myristate-containing diacylglycerols. Targets for the ligand-activated receptor include early response genes (*see* **NGF**); and proteins subsequently phosphorylated include phospholipase Cγ, MAP-2 kinase, Raf-1, and Ras-GAP. In pheochromocytoma and some other cell types, NGF activates *nur77*, a gene that codes for a protein known as both nur77 and NGF-1B (which is also made by some cells that respond to other growth factors). NGF-B1 structurally resembles receptors of the steroid/thyroid hormone/retinoic acid family, contains response elements for estrogens and thyroid hormones, and binds DNA. It is classified as an orphan receptor (because no ligand has been identified); but it may act in special ways, since the DNA binding does not seem to involve the zinc finger component. Cells that respond to other neurotrophins (BDNF and NF-3), but not to NGF, make related proteins (TRK-B and TRK-C) that also dimerize with p75^{NGF}. All of the dimers are members of a family of transmembrane proteins that includes tumor necrosis factor receptors and B cell specific CD40.

nervonic acid: *cis*-15-tetracosanoic acid; a long-chain monounsaturated fatty acid component of several nervous system lipids, made from oleic acid.

$$H_3C-(CH_2)_7-\overset{H}{C}=\overset{H}{C}-(CH_2)_{13}-COOH$$

nesidiectomy: removal of the pancreatic islets; *cf* **pancreatectomy**.

nesidioblastomas: pancreatic islet neoplasms, believed to derive from exocrine cells.

nesidioblastosis: pancreatic islet hyperplasia.

Nessler's reagent: an aqueous solution of potassium iodide, mercuric iodide, and potassium hydroxide. It forms a product that can be measured colorimetrically when it reacts with ammonia liberated from the amino groups of proteins, and is used to determine total protein content. The procedure is conducted more rapidly than some others (such as the Kjeldahl method, in which the ammonia is steam-distilled into an excess of standard acid and titrated), but it is less precise.

N-ethylmaleimide: NEM; 1-ethyl-1*H*-pyrrole-2,5-dione; an agent that binds avidly to sulfhydryl groups and blocks the actions of many proteins, including ones that mediate translocations across plasma and internal cell membranes, and some involved in mitosis. It is used to study glucose, calcium, and phosphate transport, Golgi functions, mitosis, and protein structure. *See* also **SNAPS**.

N-ethylmaleimide sensitive proteins: NSF; cytoplasmic proteins essential for fusion of non-clathrin coated vesicles to Golgi membranes. *See* **SNAPS**.

neu: a rodent proto-oncogene that codes for p185, a transmembrane protein with a cytoplasmic tyrosine kinase domain and strong homology to the epidermal growth factor (EGF) receptor. The human counterpart is erbB2 (HER2); *see* **HER**. It does not bind EGF or transforming growth factor-α (TGFα); but it is a substrate for the EGF receptor protein kinase, and the resulting phosphorylation augments its kinase activity. The natural ligand may be a **heregulin** (*q.v.*). Some mutations code for proteins with augmented enzyme activity; and both mutated and amplified normal *neu* genes can invoke transformation. Mutated types have been identified in nitrosourea-invoked neuroblastomas and gliomas in rats; and many human mammary gland, ovarian, and other adenocarcinomas overexpress the normal human *neu* counterpart, contain abnormal related genes, or overexpress EGF.

neural cell adhesion molecules: N-CAM; immunoglobulin-like sialoglycoproteins that mediate calcium-independent homophilic and heterotypic cell-to-cell and cell-to-extracellular matrix adhesion. A single gene directs synthesis of an approximately 1000 amino acid protein that undergoes posttranslational phosphorylation, sulfation, glypiation, and/or glycosylation to yield isoforms whose expression is developmentally regulated and tissue-specific. 180K and 140K transmembrane isoforms that differ in cytoplasmic tail length, and a 120K protein that anchors to external plasma membrane surfaces via covalent linkage to a glycosyl-phosphatidylinositol component, are present in the brain. 155K and 125K nontransmembrane and 145K transmembrane proteins are made by skeletal muscle, and 150K, 140K and 130K types by cardiac muscle. Truncated forms that lack the hydrophobic groups needed for membrane attachment are secreted to cerebrospinal and other fluids. Heavily polysialated N-CAMs (PSA-N-CAM) are less adhesive than other forms, and are more prevalent during developmental stages. N-CAMs are expressed in largest amounts in embryonic brain during early stages of neural tube formation, and are essential for differentiation. Somewhat smaller ones are made later by most developing neural systems and in developing skeletal muscle, and are needed for formation of retinal structures and skeletal muscle innervation. They persist in the hypothalamus and some other brain regions, where they contribute to acquisition and regeneration of synapses, in olfactory nerves (which continue to grow into the brain), in neurohypophysis, where they play roles in morphological restructuring in response to osmotic and other factors, and in small amounts at other sites. Interactions with cytoskeleton components are believed to maintain differentiated states. In mature organisms, they are found mostly at sites engaged in restructuring.

neural crests: embryonic neuroectodermal structures that form along the peripheries of developing neural tubes. The cells migrate and give rise to dorsal root ganglia sensory components, sympathetic ganglia, Schwann, adrenomedullary, calcitonin secreting, some gastrointestinal, and some thymus gland cells, and to melanophores, melanocytes, and other APUD types. Some defects that impair migration cause immune system defects.

neural lobe: the bulbous, distal end of the neurohypophysis. It receives hypothalamo-hypophysial nerve tract terminals, and it stores and releases vasopressin, oxytocin, and their associated neurophysins to the systemic bloodstream. Other regulators identified within it include enkephalins, neuropeptide Y (NPY), cholecystokinin (CCK), thyrotropin releasing hormone (TRH), and α-amidated growth hormone releasing hormone (GRH). It has a rich capillary blood supply, and contains specialized neuroglial cells (pituicytes). *See* also **posterior pituitary gland**.

neural plate: a thick sheet of ectoderm that forms above the notochord in young vertebrate embryos (around three weeks after conception in humans). Its appearance marks the first stage of nervous system development.

neural tube: a neuroectodermal structure that forms in very young vertebrate embryos. The anterior region, which grows rapidly, gives rise to the cerebral vesicle forerunners of the brain, and the posterior part to the spinal cord. Elevated α-fetoprotein levels have been found in approximately two-thirds of pregnant women bearing fetuses with anencephaly and other neural tube defects.

neuralgia: pain in a region served by sensory nerves.

neuraminic acid: 3,5-dideoxy-5-amino-nonulsonic acid; a 9-carbon sugar aldol condensation product of pyruvic acid + mannose. Many glycoproteins and polysaccharides contain *N*-acyl- (sialic acid), and *O*-substituted derivatives. *See* also **N-acetylneuraminic acid**.

CH_2OH
$HOCH$
$HOCH$
COOH
H — O
OH
OH   H
H   H
H NH_2

neuraminidases: sialidases; enzymes that catalyze hydrolytic cleavage of glycosidic linkages between sialic acid and hexose or hexosamine moieties at nonreducing terminals of glycoprotein, glycolipid, and proteoglycan oligosaccharides. They contribute to physiological disposal of metabolites, and are used to investigate the roles of carbohydrate components of glycoprotein hormones, and of gangliosides and other glycosylated compounds. Neuraminidases on *influenza* viruses and other pathogens are antigens that invoke immune system responses.

neurexins: neuron-specific transmembrane proteins with laminin A-like extracellular domains, serine and threonine rich components similar to those of low density lipoprotein (LDL) receptors and Alzheimer precursor proteins, and epidermal growth factor (EGF)-like domains. They concentrate in synaptic regions and contribute to establishment of specific forms of neural communication by guiding axon growth and influencing cell shape and recognition events involved in synapse formation. Two sets of overlapping DNA regions direct formation of neurexins I and II. Multiple splicing events yield more than 100 different transcripts; and posttranslational processing culminates in formation of large numbers of proteins, including long (Iα and IIα) and truncated (Iβ and IIβ) types. A member of the Iα group interacts specifically with synaptotagmin (a synaptic vesicle protein), and is a receptor for α-latrotoxin.

neurilemma: neurolemma; sheath of Schwann; endoneural membrane; the flattened cells and the associated myelin-containing basement membranes that surround large peripheral nerve fibers. *Cf* **axolemma**.

neurite: (1) an axon; (2) any neuron process (axon or dendrite); (3) a process of a developing neuroblast.

neuroblasts: immature cells, capable of engaging in mitosis, that develop into neurons.

neuroblastomas: highly malignant tumors, composed mostly of undifferentiated neuroblasts.

neuroectoderm: the embryonic ectoderm that gives rise to the central nervous system, neural crests, and associated structures.

neuroendocrine: describes (1) specialized neurons that synthesize and release hormones; (2) mechanisms dependent on such cells; (3) nervous system:endocrine system interactions.

neuroendocrine cell: a neuron, or neuron-like cell that secretes one or more hormones.

neuroendocrine reflexes: processes in which stimuli perceived by neurons lead to the secretion of hormones.

neuroepithelium: epithelium specialized for reception of stimuli, present, for example in the the nasal mucosa, cochlea, and taste buds.

neurofascin: a cell surface glycoprotein that mediates physical interactions between neurons.

neurofibrillary tangles: β-amyloid containing conglomerates that accumulate in the brains of individuals with Alzheimer's disease and Down's syndrome. Smaller numbers are present in the brains of healthy infants, and in some older individuals who do not suffer abnormal memory loss.

neurofibrils: the major cytoskeletal components of neurons. They are threadlike structures composed of neurofilaments and microtubules that form cross-linked networks, course through neuron cytoplasm, and can extend along the lengths of axons or connect one dendrite with another.

neurofibromas: tumors composed of Schwann cells, fibroblasts, and neuroendocrine cells, plus collagen, and amorphous extracellular matter. Most (not all) are benign.

neurofibromatosis: disorders in which numerous fibromas develop. Von Recklinghausen's disease (neurofibromatosis type 1, NF-1), an autosomal dominant form, involves neural crest derivatives (melanocytes and Schwann cells) and other cell types. The manifestations include brown spots on the skin, cutaneous and subcutaneous tumors along nerve pathways, and nodules on the iris. Deletion of one *NF-1* gene allele (*q.v.*) and mutation of the other is a common finding. That gene is believed to confer protection against tumorigenesis by acting on cAMP-mediated suppression of Ras protein controlled cell proliferation. A different gene is implicated in the more rare neurofibromatosis II, which commonly affects the eighth cranial nerve, and sometimes also the brainstem and cervical nerve roots.

neurofilaments: fine, threadlike components of neurofibrils, composed mostly of neuroprotein "triplets" that form cross-linked helices. The amount of the protein is directly related to the axon caliber in long, myelinated peripheral nerves.

neurogenic: (1) originating in the nervous system; (2) mediated by neurotransmtters; (3) giving rise to nervous system components.

neuroglia: astrocytes, ependymal cells, oligodendrocytes, microglia, and other non-neuronal central nervous system components; *see* specific types. Schwann and satellite cells that perform related functions are sometimes called *peripheral neuroglia*.

neurohormones: hormones made by neurons. Examples include thyrotropin, growth hormone, and gonadotropin releasing hormones (TRH, GRH, and GnRH), vasopressin, and oxytocin. More hormone types are made in neurons than in endocrine glands.

neurohypophysis: the pituitary gland component that develops from neuroectoderm, and includes the neural lobe, infundibular stem, and median eminence; *cf* **posterior pituitary gland**.

neuroimmunology: interactions among the nervous and immune systems. Most also involve hormones. The thymus gland, which is innervated and controlled by humoral factors, releases regulators that affect neuron (and endocrine) functions. Lymphocytes and other immune system cells secrete mediators for both of the other systems. Dopamine controls release of prolactin (essential for some lymphocyte functions); and many other hormones and neurotransmitters contribute to the differentiation, maturation, and functions of immune and nervous system cells.

neurointermediate lobes: structures in some nonmammalian vertebrates, with components similar to those of pars intermedia and neural lobe constituents of mammalian glands.

neurokines: small, biologically active molecules released by neurons; *see* **neurokinins** and **neuromedins**.

neurokinin[s]: tachykinin type peptides released by neurons and other cell types, including substance P, neurokinins α and β (also known under different names), and amphibian peptides such as physalaemin that share a common C-terminal Phe-X-Gly-Leu-Met-NH$_2$ sequence. Very low concentrations rapidly exert influences on neurons, smooth muscle, and vascular permeability.

neurokinin α: neurokinin alpha; neurokinin A; substance K; neuromedin L: H$_2$N-His-Lys-Thr-Asp-Ser-Phe-Val-Gly-Leu-Met-CONH$_2$, a tachykinin cleaved from protachykinin B (*see* **preprotachykinins**) that acts preferentially on NK-2 type receptors, some of which couple to G proteins. It stimulates contraction of stomach, duodenal, and urinary bladder smooth muscle. It is also present in spinal cord, in thyroid glands, and at a few other sites, and is degraded by acetylcholinesterase. Neuropeptide γ and neuropeptide K are N-terminal extended isoforms in the brain that may mediate special functions.

neurokinin A: neurokinin α.

neurokinin alpha: neurokinin α.

neurokinin β: neurokinin beta; neurokinin B; neurokinin K; neuromedin K; NK; H$_2$N-Asp-Met-His-Asp-Phe-Phe-Val-Gly-Leu-Met-CONH$_2$; a tachykinin that acts predominantly on NK-3 type receptors, and promotes contraction of hepatic portal vein smooth muscle.

neurokinin B: neurokinin β.

neurokinin beta: neurokinin β.

neurokinin K: neurokinin β.

neurokinin receptors: proteins that bind neurokinins with high affinity and mediate their effects. The NK-1 type, which is widely distributed to non-neuronal as well as central nervous system cells, preferentially binds to substance P, but has some affinity for neurokinin α. NK-2 types preferentially bind neuroleukin α. The ones that predominate in duodenal and stomach smooth muscle have properties different from those of urinary bladder. NK-3 receptors preferentially bind neurokinin β, and mediate its effects on hepatic portal vein smooth muscle.

neuroleptic: (1) an agent, such as chlorpromazine, that exerts "antipsychotic" effects and/or improves faulty cognition, psychomotor activity, mood and/or behavior. Several kinds used clinically are dopamine antagonists; (2) the effects of such an agent.

neuroleukin: NL; a 56K peptide chemically similar to phosphohexoseisomerase, and to the human immunodeficiency-I virus (HIV-I) envelope glycoprotein gp[120], secreted by activated T lymphocytes, and by bone marrow, brain, kidney, salivary gland, denervated muscle, and possibly other cell types (but not by fibroblasts). It is implicated as a neurotrophic factor that promotes growth and survival of spinal cord and some sensory neurons. Although it does not directly promote cell proliferation, it enhances the mitogenic effects of other leukocyte stimulants, and also augments antibody production by B lymphocytes. Influences on monocytes, and on autocrine functions of T lymphocytes have been described.

neuromedin[s]: several peptides made by neurons that function as neuromodulators, neurotransmitters, and/or hormones. In addition to the ones cited below, the group includes peptide 7B2 (anterior pituitary peptide of the pig, APPG).

neuromedin B: Gly-Asn-Leu-Trp-Ala-Thr-Gly-His-Phe-Met-NH$_2$; a bombesin-like decapeptide chemically related to amino acids 18-27 of gastrin releasing peptide (GRP-10), made in all pituitary gland lobes, and in the hypothalamus, extra-hypothalamic brain, spinal cord, pancreas, and gastrointestinal tract. It is somewhat less potent than GRP-10, but binds to same receptors and exerts similar effects. Both peptides lower body temperature, augment secretion of gastrin, cholecystokinin, enteroglucagon, and insulin, stimulate uterine smooth muscle, and promote grooming behavior in rodents.

neuromedin C: GRP-10; *see* also **neuromedin B**.

neuromedin K: neurokinin β.

neuromedin L: neurokinin α.

neuromedin N: a peptide in gastrointestinal mucosa cleaved from the neurotensin precursor.

neuromedin U: U-8 and U-25, peptides chemically related to vasoactive intestinal peptide (VIP) and pancreatic polypeptide (PP), that stimulate uterine muscle. They are made in brain, spinal cord, thyrotrope and corticotrope cells of the pituitary gland, and intestine, and may be co-released with thyroid stimulating hormone (TSH).

neuromodulators: substances that alter neuron responses to other regulators, but do not directly affect firing rates or nerve impulse conduction. Some regulate neurotransmitter synthesis and metabolism, and/or the amounts released in response to other agents.

neuron[s]: excitable cells, specialized for rapid communication. Most are *multipolar* (have many dendrites that perceive stimuli and transmit electrical signals to the cell body (perikaryon), and an axon that extends from the other end of the perikaryon and forms one or more synapses with other neurons, or with muscle or gland cells. Some are *bipolar* (have one dendrite and one axon), and a few are *monopolar* (one process with afferent and efferent branches). Although limited numbers make electrical synapses with other neurons, most synthesize neurotransmitters, transport them in vesicles from perikarya to axons, and store the vesicles in axon terminals for release when the neuron depolarizes. *Sensory* neurons, with perikarya in dorsal root ganglia, receive stimuli from receptors (or in some cases from other neurons), and transmit information to the central nervous system. *Motor* neurons transmit from the central nervous system to effector organs. Most of their cell bodies are in the anterior horns of the spinal cord, but the ones for cranial nerves are in the brain.

neuron-glial cell adhesion factor: Ng-CAM; L1 glycoprotein; an immunoglobulin-like glycoprotein implicated (along with neural cell adhesion molecule) as a regulator of neurite development and regeneration.

neuropeptides: opioid peptides, angiotensin, cholecystokinins, neurotensin, vasoactive intestinal peptide, neuroleukins, and other regulators composed of amino acid moieties, that are released by neurons and function as hormones, neurotransmitters, and/or neuromodulators. More than fifty kinds have been identified.

neuropeptide Y: NPY: neuropeptide-tyrosine: peptides chemically related to pancreatic peptide (PP) and peptide YY (PYY), distributed throughout the central and peripheral nervous systems, with especially high concentrations in the cerebral cortex and olfactory bulbs. They are also made in megakaryocytes, peripheral blood cells, adrenal glands, heart, spleen, lungs, gonads, thymus, and pituitary gland. At various sites, they colocalize with, and can promote the release of catecholamines, function as neurotransmitters and neuromodulators, and/or act directly on some presynaptic receptors. NPYs are also potent vasoconstrictors, released by activated platelets, and are implicated as mediators of some immune system functions. Other effects include inhibition of renin, pancreatic polypeptide and insulin release, influences on the secretion of gonadotropin releasing, luteinizing, and adrenocorticotropic hormones (GnRH, LH, and ACTH), somatostatin, and glucocorticoids, and modulation of vasoactive intestinal peptide and prostaglandin E$_2$ regulation of intestinal functions. They are additionally implicated in central control of appetite. The human type is H$_2$N-Tyr-Pro-Ser-Lys-Pro-Asp-Asn-Pro-Gly-Glu-Asp-Ala-Pro-Ala-Glu-Asp-Met-Ala-Arg-Tyr-Tyr-Ser-Ala-Leu-Arg-His-Tyr-Ile-Asn-Leu-Ile-Thr-Arg-Gln-Arg-Tyr-CONH$_2$.

neurophysins: chemically similar, approximately 10K species-specific, single chain proteins cleaved from the proneurophysin precursors of several small peptide type hormones, and released with those hormones. No functions have been established, but roles in hormone storage and transport, and in lipid mobilization have been proposed. Each neurophysin type is associated with a peptide type, for example pressophysins (nicotine stimulated neurophysins) with vasopressin, estrogen stimulated neurophysins with oxytocin, and different, but closely related proteins with arginine vasotocin, mesotocin, and urohypophysial hormones.

neuropil: dense networks of neuroglia and neuron processes in the central nervous system, mostly in gray matter.

neuroproteins: intermediate filament proteins of neurofibrils, composed of three kinds of subunits that wind around each other to form helices. The largest subunits form cross-bridges. In mammals, the high molecular weight (NF-H, NF-210), intermediate molecular weight (NF-M, NF-160), and low molecular weight (NF-L, NF-68) subunits are reported to have molecular weights, respectively, of 210K, 160K, and 68K. Three different genes direct their formation. 200K, 145K, 130K, 110K, and 60K proteins have been described for other animal types.

neurosecretory cells: neuroendocrine cells; modified neurons that secrete hormones, mostly to the bloodstream.

Neurospora crassa: the common bread mold.

neurosteroids: steroids made by glial cells and neurons, including 3ß-OH—Δ^5 derivatives of cholesterol, pregnenolone, and dehydroepiandrosterone. Influences on gamma aminobutyric acid (GABA) receptors, and roles in olfaction and other functions have been suggested. Their production is not regulated by gonadal or adenohypophysial hormones.

neurotensin: NT; neuropeptides chemically related to somatostatin and substance P, believed to be mammalian homologs of avian LANT-6. They are cleaved from precursor proteins that also yield neuromedin N. The largest amounts of NT are made intestinal ileum N cells, but approximately 10% of the body content is in the hypothalamus. Lower levels occur in the stomach, duodenum, jejunum, colon, blood plasma, extrahypothalalamic brain, and pituitary gland. The distribution, circadian and meal-associated patterns for release, and the effects of administered NT are consistent with roles in digestive, circulatory, and endocrine system regulation. The peptides suppress appetite, inhibit gastric motility and emptying, and diminish the amounts of acid and pepsin released in response to lipid-rich food, but stimulate the exocrine pancreas and fatty acid transport. Their ability to invoke hyperglycemia involves both increased glucagon release and inhibition of insulin secretion. They also augment vascular permeability and lower blood pressure. Hypothalamic NT stimulates the secretion of prolactin, adrenocorticotropic hormone (ACTH) and gonadotropins, affects responses to estrogens, promotes water retention, and prolongs barbiturate sedation. Some effects have been linked with influences on acetylcholine release. The human and bovine form is *p*Glu-Leu-Tyr-Glu-Asn-Lys-Pro-Arg-Arg-Pro-Tyr-Ile-Leu-OH.

neurotoxins: agents that damage or destroy neurons or neuron components (axons or dendrites), or impair neuron functions by acting at synapses. Naturally occurring regulators that can invoke damage include high levels of glutamic and other excitatory amino acids, and nitric oxide. Some spider and snake venom components, and some synthetic agents are selective for specific neuron types, and therefore useful for studying neurotransmitter and neurohormone synthesis, metabolism, and functions. *See* **monosodium glutamate**, **capsaicin**, and 6-OH-**dopamine**.

neurotoxin NSTX-3: 2,4-dihydroxyphenylacetyl-L-asparaginyl-(L-arginyl-cadaverno-β-alanyl)-cadaverine; a toxin in the venom of the Papua New Guinea spider, *Neph-*

ilia maculata, that selectively and irreversibly blocks postsynaptic and glutamate potentials in invertebrates.

neurotransmitters: a term most often applied to regulators made by neurons that act postsynaptically on other neurons, autonomic system target cells, or skeletal muscles, and directly stimulate or inhibit. However, some act presynaptically; and a few function at other sites as hormones and/or neuromodulators. Most effects are rapidly terminated. Norepinephrine, serotonin, and some others are taken up and sequestered in the neurons that release them. Monoamine oxidases and other enzymes that degrade several kinds are present in blood, and liver, as well as in neurons and target cells.

neurotrophic: (1) supporting neuroblast survival, growth, proliferation, differentiation, and/or migration, or neuron survival and functions; (2) describes regulators that perform such functions.

neurotrophic factor-3: NF-3; NT-3; neurotrophin-4; hippocampal derived neurotrophic factor; a basic, 119 amino acid hormone identified in hind-limb motor neurons and implicated as essential for their survival. It binds with low affinity to p75^{NGF}, and with higher affinity to dimers composed of that protein plus TRK-B (a protein with tyrosine kinase activity related to p140^{NGF}); *see* **nerve growth factor** and **nerve growth factor receptors**. It is most abundant in brain, kidney, and spleen, but small amounts are expressed in most other cell types. NF-3 affects the differentiation of some neural crest derivatives that also respond to NGF, and of nodose ganglia neurons (which derive from the neural placodes). However, unlike NGF (which is present at high levels in the hippocampus), it accumulates in largest amounts in the cerebellum.

neurotrophic hormones: neurotrophic factors; (1) ciliary neurotrophic factor, neuroleukin, and other regulators that exert their most obvious effects on nervous system components, and also many hormones better known for different functions that are also neurotrophic (such as fibroblast and epidermal growth factors); (2) a specific family of regulators that includes nerve growth factor (NGF), brain derived neurotrophic factor (BDNF), neurotrophin-3, and related hormones that bind with low affinity to p75^{NGF}, and whose high affinity receptors are dimers composed of that protein plus another higher molecular weight type with a tyrosine kinase domain. They act directly on neurons that make them, and are also taken up by retrograde transport from glial cells. Although some cells respond to two or three kinds, and there are overlapping functions, the distributions differ, and some responses are restricted to certain neuron types, or to nervous system cells at specific stages of differentiation. All are additionally present in the placenta (in which they appear to be maternally-derived), and in other tissues.

neurotropic: (1) having a high affinity for neural tissue; *see* also **neurotrophic**.

neutral metalloproteinases: plasmin, collagenase, stromelysin, and other cation dependent enzymes that are active at pHs normally encountered in blood and extracellular fluids. They contribute to processes such as bone remodeling; but excessive amounts are implicated in the etiology of osteoarthritis and other degenerative diseases.

neutral mutation: a change in the DNA that does not obviously affect the phenotype.

neutral red: N^8N^8,3-trimethyl-2,8-phenazinediamine monohydrochloride; a dye taken up by Golgi components. It is used as an indicator in the pH range 6.8 (red) to 8.0 (yellow), and can exert estrogen-like effects on cultured cells.

neutropenia: inadequate numbers of neutrophilic leukocytes; *see* also **agranulocytosis**. Severe deficiencies increase the susceptibility to bacterial infections.

neutrophil[s]: cells with granules that take up both acidic and basic dyes. The term is most widely applied to neutrophilic leukocytes.

neutrophil activating protein: NAP-1; neutrophilin; monocyte-derived neutrophil chemotactic factor; MDNCF; neutrophil chemotactic factor; NCF; T cell chemotactic factor; TCf; interleukin-8; Ser-Ala-Lys-Glu-Leu-Arg-Cys-Gln-Cys-Ile-Lys-Thr-Tyr-Ser-Lys-Pro-Phe-His-Pro-Lys-Phe-Ile-Lys-Glu-Leu-Arg-Val-Ile-Glu-Ser-Gly-Pro-His-Cys-Ala-Asp-Thr-Glu-Ile-Ile-Val-Lys; an 8K heparin-binding peptide chemically related to platelet factor-4 and macrophage inflammatory proteins. It is released by macrophages and monocytes activated by *f*Met-Leu-Phe, phytohemagglutinin, tumor necrosis factor-α, skin fibroblasts stimulated by TNFα or interleukin 1α, endotoxin (lipopolysaccharide, LPS), LPS-stimulated endothelial cells, and some other hormones better known for different functions. Although named for its ability to invoke accumulation of activated neutrophilic leukocytes at sites of inflammation, it is also chemotactic for both CD4⁺ and CD8⁺ T lymphocytes, and is implicated as a mediator of cutaneous delayed hypersensitivity responses initiated by keratinocytes. Its ability to promote lymphocyte migration across high endothelial venules may be related to influences on the expression of cell surface adhesion molecules such as LFA-1. Additionally, it has serine protease activity, and can promote platelet aggregation and serotonin release. (It does not, however, affect the movements of monocytes or large granular lymphocytes, or promote lymphocyte proliferation). *See* also **interleukin-8**.

neutrophil chemotactic factor: NCF; *see* **neutrophil activating protein-1** and **interleukin-8**.

neutrophilic leukocytes: polymorphonuclear leukocytes; PMNs; leukocytes with granules that appear purple when stained with mixtures of acidic and basic dyes; *cf*

eosinophils and **basophils**. During early stages of maturation from metamyelocyte precursors, they are called band cells. They then progress to stab cells with globular nuclei. With continued maturation, the nuclei undergo segmentation; and the numbers of lobes are directly related to the cell ages. PMNs normally account for approximately 2/3 of the circulating white blood cells in humans. The total numbers (and the numbers of stab cells) rise during most acute bacterial infections. When activated, they adhere to vascular endothelium, migrate to sites of inflammation and infection, engage in phagocytosis, and undergo "respiratory bursts" that generate bactericidal agents (including hydrogen peroxide, free radicals, and proteolytic enzymes). The activators include complement component C5a, neutrophil activating protein-1, macrophage inflammatory proteins, *f*-Met-Leu-Phe, tumor necrosis factor-α, (TNFα), T lymphocyte chemotactic factor, leukotrienes, and some bacterial products.

neutrophilin: *see* **neutrophil activating protein-1** and **interleukin-8**.

neutrophil peptides: defensins such as rabbit NP-1 and human HNP-1, stored in, and released from neutrophilic leukocyte granules. In common with other defensins, they are small, cysteine-rich proteins that contribute to non-oxidative killing of bacteria, fungi, tumor cells and enveloped viruses by forming ion-permeable membrane channels that permit leakage of K⁺ and other target cell constituents.

Newton: one Newton is the force required to impart an acceleration of one meter per second per second when applied to a one kilogram mass. *See* also **joule**.

New Zealand mice: several mouse strains bred for specific kinds of investigations. New Zealand black (NZB) mice develop autoimmune hemolytic anemia and acquire low titers of anti-nuclear antibodies. New Zealand white (NZW) mice have abnormal T lymphocytes and spontaneously activated B lymphocytes. They are not overtly abnormal, but the offspring of NZB x NZW matings acquire a disease that closely resembles lupus erythematosus. New Zealand obese (NZO) mice have abnormally low pancreatic polypeptide levels, and are used for lipid metabolism studies.

nexin: (1) a protease inhibitor; *see* **protease nexins**. (2) a substance that binds, for example the 165K protein with a diameter of approximately 24 nm that links adjacent microtubule doublets in cilia and flagella.

nexus: (1) a bond; (2) a gap junction.

NF: (1) nuclear factor; (2) neurofibril protein; (3) neurofibromatosis.

NF-1: type 1 neurofibromatosis.

NF-1: a gene whose product closely resembles ras-GAP, and augments p21*ᵣᵃˢ* GTPase activity via mechanisms inhibited by arachidonic acid. It acts on neural crest derivatives (including melanocytes, and Schwann, glial, and ependymal cells), and some other cell types, and is believed to function as an anti-oncogene that suppresses tumor growth. Mutations and deletions occur in individuals with Type I neurofibromatosis.

NF-3: neurotrophic factor-3; *see* **neurotrophin-3**.

NFIII: nuclear factor III; *see* **NFA-1**.

NFA-1: nuclear factor A-1; nuclear factor III, NF-III; OTF-1: a protein product of the *oct-1* gene, made in most eukaryote cells. It binds to ATTTGCAT base sequences in promoter and enhancer regions of several genes, and accelerates transcription of small nuclear RNAs, and of messenger RNAs for histone 2B and some other proteins.

NFA-2: nuclear factor A-2; OTF-2; a product of *oct-2* genes in B lymphocytes that promotes transcription of immunoglobulin genes.

NFAT: nuclear transcription activator of T cells.

NF-H, NF-M, NF-L, NF-210, NF-160: *see* **neuroproteins**.

NFκB: p50, p55, p75, p85, a *c-rel* gene product, and related phosphoproteins that form complexes which bind to enhancer regions of many genes and viral transcription units, and accelerate transcription of kappa type immunoglobulin light chains, interleukin-2 receptor α subunits, human lymphotrophic virus I (HLTV-I) and human immunodeficiency virus-I (HIV-I) proteins, and several other inducible proteins (including some cytokines). The most potent activator appears to be a p50/p65 heterodimer or heterotetramer. In unstimulated cells, NFκB proteins reside in the cytoplasm, complexed to a 35K IκB inhibitor, and a p65 "transmodulator" that maintains the sequestration. When IκB is phosphorylated, the complexes dissociate, and the protein enters the nucleus. NFκ homodimers may also contribute to transcription regulation. Tumor necrosis factor-α (TNFα) is a potent stimulant for NFκB synthesis. Other stimuli include lipopolysaccharide (endotoxin, LPS), tumorigenic phorbol esters, and factors made by HIV-I viruses. An avian reticuloendotheliosis virus oncogene codes for p59^{v-rel}, which is believed to invoke transformation by blocking formation of p50/p65 complexes when present in either the cytoplasm or the nucleus.

NF protein: *see* **neurofibromatosis**.

Ng-CAM: neuron-glial cell adhesion factor.

NGF: nerve growth factor.

ngf-1b: *nur77*; a gene activated by nerve growth factor. Its product is currently called an "orphan receptor", since it closely resembles receptors of the steroid hormone/thyroid hormone/retinoic acid family, but no ligand has been identified.

NHPs: nonhistone proteins.

Ni: nickel.

niacin: *see* **nicotinic acid**.

niacinamide: nicotinamide.

nialamide: 4-pyridinecarboxylic acid 2-[3-oxo-3-[(phenylmethyl)amino]propyl]hydrazide; an orally effective monoamine oxidase inhibitor, used as an antidepressant.

nicardipine: 1,4-dihydro-2,6-dimethyl-4-(3-nitrophenyl)-3,5-pyridinecarboxylic acid methyl-2-[methyl-(phenylmethyl)amino]ethyl ester; a Ca^{2+} ion channel blocker used to dilate coronary blood vessels and lower blood pressure, and for studies of calcium functions. *See* **dihydropyridines**.

niche: in ecology, the place occupied by an organism in its community, its environmental requirements, and its associations with other organisms.

nick: in molecular biology, disruption of a phosphodiester bond between two adjacent nucleotides of a double-stranded DNA molecule.

nickases: enzymes that nick DNA molecules, and thereby facilitate unwinding; *see* **topoisomerases** and **endonucleases**.

nick-closing enzyme: *see* **topoisomerases**.

nickel: Ni; a metallic element (atomic number 28, atomic weight 58.69), required in trace amounts, that affects the activities of several vertebrate metalloenzymes, and a cofactor for urease. High levels of Ni^{2+} block receptor operated calcium channels (ROCC), but do not affect L type (voltage sensitive) ones.

nick translation: *in vitro* techniques for preparing radioactively labeled DNA probes. Small amounts of deoxyribonuclease I are used to nick the molecules and generate 3'-OH termini. *E. coli* DNA polymerase I then catalyzes addition of P^{32}-labeled nucleotides with bases complementary to the other strand, to the 3'-OH ends, as

nicardipine

its exonuclease activity removes nucleotides from the 5′ end.

nicotinamide: niacinamide; nicotinate; 3-pyridine carboxamide; vitamin PP; viitamin B_3 (a term also used for nicotinic acid); a component of the vitamin B complex, obtained directly from animal foods, rapidly made from plant nicotinic acid, and also synthesized from the essential amino acid, tryptophan; *see* **quinolic acid**. NAD and NADP are major coenzymes for transhydrogenation reactions; *see* **nicotinamide adenine dinucleotide** (NAD) and **nicotinamide adenine dinucleotide phosphate** (NADP). NAD also contributes to DNA repair by augmenting polyribose synthetase activity; and NADH can protect against oxidative damage invoked by streptozotocin and some other agents. **Pellagra** (*q.v.*) develops when the diet is deficient in both the vitamin and the amino acid, or when niacin deficiency is associated with impaired tryptophan transport or conditions that divert excessive amounts of the amino acid to other pathways.

nicotinamide adenine dinucleotide, NAD: a coenzyme for many transhydrogenases, formerly known as DPN, diphosphopyridine dinucleotide, and coenzyme I. The generalized reaction $[NAD^+ + RH_2 \rightarrow NADH + H^+ + R]$ describes its participation as an oxidant for substrates used for fuel and other purposes. It is essential for converting glyceraldehyde-3-phosphate to 1,3 diphosphoglycerate during glycolysis, of pyruvate to acetylcoenzyme A, for reversible interconversion of pyruvate and lactate, and for some steps in steroidogenesis, fatty acid oxidation, and the tricarboxylic acid cycle. In mitochondria, complete oxidation of each $NADH + H^+$ in the presence of molecular oxygen to $NAD^+ + H_2O$ releases enough energy to drive synthesis of 3 ATP from 3 ADP + 3 Pi. Nicotinic acid combines with 5-phosphoribosyl pyrophosphate to yield nicotinic acid mononuculeotide (NAM) + P-P. NAM (a ribonucleotide) then reacts with ATP to form desamido-NAD^+. NAD synthesis is completed by NAD synthetase, which transfers an amide group from glutamine to the nicotinate carboxyl. (The synthetase is strongly inhibited by azaserine.) The NAD kinase (NAD pyrophosphorylase) used to form the NAM also converts NAD to **nicotinamide dinucleotide phosphate** (*q.v.*).

nicotinamide adenine dinucleotide phosphate: NADP: a coenzyme for several dehydrogenases, formerly known as TPN, triphosphopyridine dinucleotide, and coenzyme II. The oxidized form is made from **nicotine adenine mononucleotide** (*q.v.*) in the reaction catalyzed by NAD-kinase: $NAD^+ + ATP \rightarrow NADP^+ + ADP$. Hexose monophosphate pathway enzymes reduce $NADP^+$ to NADPH $+ H^+$, which donates hydrogen atoms and electrons for anabolic processes such as fatty acid, cholesterol, and steroid hormone biosynthesis. NADPH also reduces glutathione, and is an essential coenzyme for some photosynthesis reactions.

nicotine amide mononucleotide: NMN: an intermediate in the pathway for biosynthesis of **nicotine adenine dinucleotide** (NAD) (*q.v.*).

nicotine: 3-(1-methyl-2-pyrrolidinyl)pyridine; an alkaloid obtained from the dried leaves of *Nicotiana tabacum*

nicotinamide adenine dinucleotide

nicotinamide adenine dinucleotide phosphate

nicotine amide mononucleotide

and *N. rustica*. It is the tobacco component that exerts the major effects on the central nervous system, and the active ingredient of chewing gums and other preparations used (in combination with other measures) to treat nicotine addiction, named for its ability to stimulate **nicotinic** type **acetylcholine receptors** (*q.v.*), and used to study them. It also affects the functions of dopaminergic neurons and of chemo-, thermo-, pain, and other receptors, and binds to brain receptors for thymopoietin. Although very high concentrations additionally act on neuromuscular junctions, the receptors at those sites are not important mediators of the sense of enhanced physical energy. Nicotine increases alertness, facilitates memory, suppresses appetite, promotes the secretion of catecholamines and other hormones, augments the activities of salivary, gastric, and bronchial, and other exocrine glands, and directly affects the medullary respiratory center, carotid bodies, and "chemotrigger" zones of the medulla oblongata. Elevation of the metabolic rate is probably secondary to catecholamine release, but the stimulatory effects on the heart and blood vessels include influences on autonomic ganglion transmission. Toxic doses can invoke nausea, vomiting, diarrhea, tremors, and convulsions. Tolerance and habituation develop in tobacco users, but prolonged exposure to very high doses depresses, and can ultimately paralyze autonomic ganglia.

nicotine

nicotine stimulated neurophysin: NSN; the neurophysin component of vasopressin precursor proteins. *See* **neurophysins**.

nicotinic acid: niacin; 3-pyridine carboxylic acid; vitamin P; P factor; pellagra prevention factor; antipellagra vitamin; antiblack tongue factor; vitamin B_3 (a term also used for nicotinamide). Niacin is a major dietary component used to make **nicotinamide** (*q.v.*). Most cells contain small amounts. Large quantities accumulate in liver, adrenal glands, milk, yeasts, and some plant tissues. Nicotinamide deficiency (usually accompanied by tryptophan deficiency or metabolic defects that affect its use) leads to the development of **pellagra** (*q.v.*). High levels of nicotinic acid decrease adenylate cyclase activity and

promote vasodilation. They lower very low, intermediate, and low density lipoprotein (VDL, IDL, and LDL) levels, but have little or no effect on the concentrations of the high density (HDL) types. This is accomplished by inhibiting lipoprotein synthesis and triacylglycerol esterification in the liver, and by augmenting plasma lipoprotein lipase activity. They also inhibit lipolysis in adipose tissue, and can lower plasma cholesterol levels, but do not directly affect cholesterol biosynthesis. Clinical use for treating some hyperlipidemias is limited by side effects that include gastrointestinal tract irritation which can lead to ulceration as well as nausea, diarrhea, and indigestion, decreased bile flow, skin reactions, glucose intolerance, eye damage, and hepatotoxicity. The vasodilation and hypolipidemic effects are not related to the vitamin functions, and are not shared by nicotinic acid amide.

nicotinic receptors: a family of acetylcholine receptors, named for the their sensitivities to nicotine, which at first stimulates, but then (especially when present in high concentrations for extended time periods) paralyzes. Various subtypes are present on postsynaptic autonomic ganglia and some brain neurons, and on adrenomedullary cells. Skeletal muscle receptors respond to only massive doses of nicotine, but are classified as nicotinic because of similar structures and postsynaptic locations. Since they are sensitive to curare and related agents, the term *curariform* is applied. The most widely studied nicotinic receptors are composed of five similar 50-65K subunits (two αs that bind the ligand, plus one β, one δ, and either one γ or one ε type). They have helical structures that span plasma membranes, form Na^+ ion channels, and regulate monovalent cation transport. Activation leads rapidly to Na^+ entry (soon followed by accelerated K^+ transport), plasma membrane depolarization, and, in most cases Ca^{2+} uptake. Genes that code for α1 and β1 subunits on skeletal muscle postsynaptic membranes, and others that code for α2, α3, α4, α7, β2, β3, and β4 types in brain have been identified; but it is not certain that all are involved in formation of functional acetylcholine receptors. α-Bungarotoxin binds tightly to muscle α subunits, and thereby blocks neuromuscular transmission. The binding is opposed by thymopoietin. Both the toxin and the hormone bind to brain α subunits, but molecules that contain the binding sites have immunological, chemical, and electrophysiological properties different from those of skeletal muscle receptors; and the toxin fails to block the brain functions. *See also* **acetylcholine**, and *cf* **muscarinic receptors**.

nictitating membrane: a third, transparent eyelid, hinged at the inner surface of the lower lid, in many vertebrates. It protects against mechanical and chemical injury and dehydration.

nidation: implantation.

nidogen: entactin.

Niemann-Pick disease: autosomal recessive disorders in which impaired production of lysosomal sphingomyelinase leads to accumulation of sphingomyelin and other lipids. The manifestations include hepatosplenomegaly, mental and physical retardation, and neurological deterioration. Afflicted infants usually die before the age of 3 years.

nifedipine: 1,4-dihydro-2.6-dimethyl-4-(2-nitrophenyl) pyridinedicarboxylic acid dimethyl ester; a Ca^{2+} channel blocker used to dilate coronary vessels and lower blood pressure, and for pharmacological studies of calcium functions; *see* **dihydropyridines**.

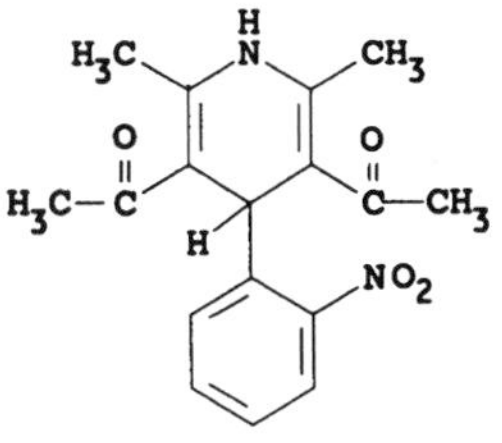

nigericin: a polyether antibiotic made by *Streptomyces hygroscopicus* that is structurally related to monensin and exerts similar effects. It is a carboxylic ionophore that promotes Na^+/H^+ and K^+/H^+ exchange, neutralizes lysosomal acidity, and affects ATPase activity.

nigrostriatal: describes bilateral nerve tracts that project on each side from the **substantia nigra** (*q.v.*) to the corpus striatum.

NIH 323 cells: easily maintained fibroblast-derived cell lines that take up and integrate foreign DNAs, and are used in gene transfer studies.

Nilevar: a trade name for norethandrolone; *see* also **anabolic steroids**.

nimodipine: 1,4-dihydro-2,6-dimethyl-4-(3-nitrophenyl)-3,5-pyridinecarboxylic acid 2-methoxyethyl-1-methylethyl ester; a dihydropyridine type voltage-sensitive (L type) calcium channel blocker. It improves cerebral blood

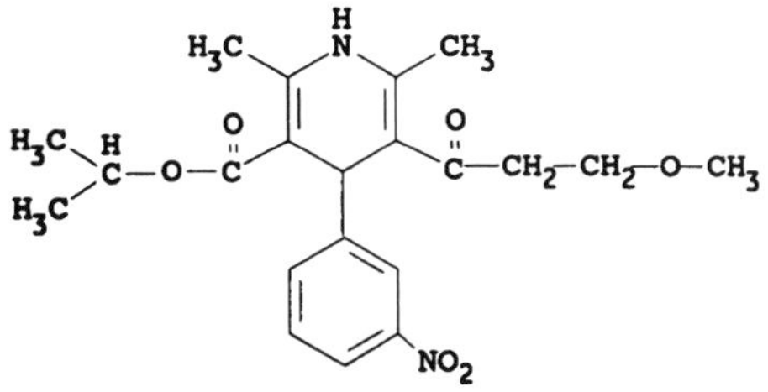

nimodipine

flow in elderly patients, and can facilitate learning in laboratory animals.

ninhydrin: 1,2,3-indatrione monohydrate; triketohydrindene hydrate; a blue dye used to locate and estimate the numbers of free amino and carboxyl groups in peptides and proteins.

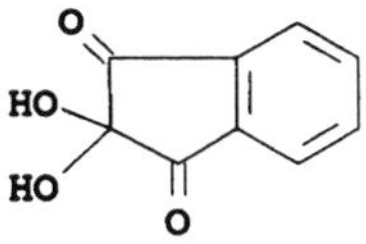

nipecotic acid: 3-piperidinecarboxylic acid; an agent that prolongs the effects of gamma aminobutyric acid (GABA) by inhibiting its uptake.

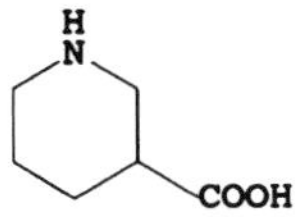

NIPS: N-(p-isothiocyanatophenethyl)spiperone: a selective, irreversible D_2 type dopamine receptor antagonist.

nisoldipine: 1,4-dihydro-2,6-dimethyl-4-(2-nitrophenyl)-3,5-pyridinedicarboxylic acid; a Ca^{2+} channel blocker used to dilate coronary vessels and lower blood pressure; *see* **dihydropyridines**.

nisoxetine: γ-(2-methoxyphenoxy)-N-methyl-benzenepropanamine; a potent, selective inhibitor of norepinephrine uptake in the brain and heart.

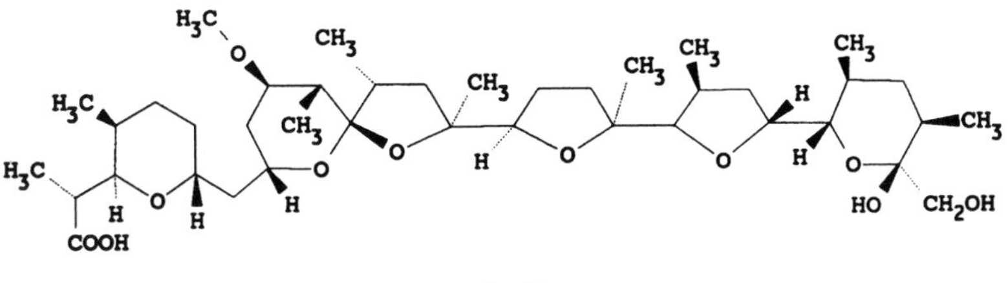

nigericin

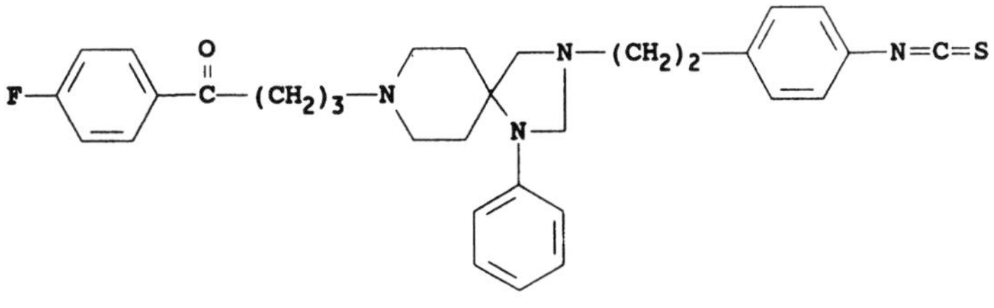

NIPS

nisoldipine

nitrendipine

nisoxetine

Nissl granules: basophilic aggregates in neuron cell bodies, composed mostly of rough endoplasmic reticulum and its associated ribosomes.

Nitella: fresh water algae of the phylum Chlorophyta, used to study cytoplasmic streaming and ion movements. They form giant, multinucleated cells.

nitrates: (1) in chemistry, compounds that contain —NO$_3$ groups. Nitrogen fixing bacteria form inorganic nitrate salts from atmospheric nitrogen. Plants and many microorganisms take it up from soil, reduce it to ammonia, and use it to make amino acids and other organic compounds. Potassium, calcium, and other nitrate salts are components of fertilizers. In animals, nitrate can be converted to nitrites and other metabolites. High concentrations inhibit iodine concentration by thyroid gland follicular cells, and are used for some thyroid hormone studies. Silver nitrate is a reagent for determination of ammonia in organic compounds, and for industrial purposes; (2) the term *organic nitrates* is applied to nitroglycerin and several other compounds used as vasodilators, mostly to treat angina pectoris. Those compounds are, in fact **nitrites** (*q.v.*).

nitrazepam: 1,3-dihydro-7-nitro-5-phenyl-2*H*-1,3-benzodiazepin-2-one: an anticonvulsant and analeptic; *see* **benzodiazepines**.

nitrendipine: 1,4-dihydro-2,6-dimethyl-4-(3-nitrophenyl)-3,5-pyridinedicarboxylic acid ethylmethyl ester; a Ca^{2+} channel blocker used to dilate coronary blood vessels and lower blood pressure; *see* **dihydropyridines**.

nitric oxide: NO; a low molecular weight gas made from arginine; see **nitric oxide synthetase**. It appears to act directly as a diffusible neurotransmitter and second messenger; but some effects may depend on conversion to longer acting nitrosamines and related compounds. Acetylcholine, bradykinin, histamine, hypoxia, and high pressure are among the stimulants for NO generation in vascular endothelial cells. NO mediates vasodilation initiated by those factors by relaxing vascular smooth muscle, and is either identical to, or the major component of endothelial cell derived relaxation factor (EDRF). Its influences are attributed to activation of soluble guanylate cyclases by binding to the enzyme heme groups. The cyclic guanosine monophosphate (cGMP) generated then hyperpolarizes and affects Ca^{2+} channels. However, not all effects are mediated in this way. At other sites, NO can affect ion channels by activating ADP-ribosyltransferase. It exerts influences on cytoskeletal proteins, activates kinase C, several proteases, and other enzymes, and induce fos, jun, and other proteins. It binds the iron of Fe-porphyrins, Fe-S containing enzymes, ferritin, and other organic molecules, can release iron from cells, forms compounds that deaminate DNA and inhibit DNA synthesis, and is a precursor of toxic ions such as peroxynitrate (OONOO$^-$), which yields hydroxyl radicals (OH•) when it decomposes. NO is a potent coronary vessel dilator, and is essential for penile erection. The probability that it contributes to generalized, tonic regulation of cardiovascular functions is consistent with observations that agents which promote its formation rapidly invoke hypotension, and synthetase inhibitors elevate systemic blood pressure. It has been suggested that dysregulation causes essential hypertension, at least in some individuals, and that overproduction contributes to cytokine mediated and septic circulatory shock. NO also acts on nonvascular smooth muscle. The large amounts in myenteric plexus neurons mediate the gastric fundus relaxation essential for accommodating food without excessive elevation of intragastric pressure; and NO released to uterine muscle may contribute to dilation associated with fetal growth. In the kidneys, it is made by mesangial cells, and may be important for macula densa mediated tuboglomerular feedback. NO delivered by bone marrow vessels directly promotes osteoclast retraction and inhibits bone resorption. In pancreatic β cells, it mediates arginine-stimulated insulin secretion. Lipopolysaccharide (LPS, endotoxin), thrombin, leukotrienes, formylated peptides, and platelet activating factor (PAF) are among the factors that promote NO formation and release by Kupffer cells, neutrophilic leukocytes, blood platelets, and mast cells. NO then kills bacteria, fungi, protozoa, helminths, and tumor cells. Some effects have been linked with inhibition of electron transport and tricarboxylic cycles. NO slows leukocyte migration, and it decreases leukocyte adhesion to postcapillary venules, and leukocyte aggregation by inhibiting the expression of some cell adhesion molecules (including lymphocyte

CD11/CD18). It also inhibits blood platelet aggregation and fibroblast mitosis (and antagonizes some effects of platelet activating factor). The effects on inflammatory and immune system responses depend on the amounts made and the microenvironments. Superoxide dismutases and catalases degrade NO, but products of the reactions can contribute to immune-complex injury. In the central nervous system, nitroxergic neurons are especially abundant in the cerebellum, and are also distributed to discrete sites of the cerebral cortex, corpus striatum, and supraoptic and paraventricular nuclei. Production there is stimulated by glutamate acting on NMDA (N-methyl-D-asparate) receptors. The gas is taken into presynaptic types via retrograde transport. There is evidence for direct involvement in synaptic plasticity, long-term synaptic depression (LTD), and other phenomena associated with learning and memory. However, some of the neurons that contribute to the processes do not make the synthetase, and in these **carbon monoxide** ($q.v.$) may be the guanylate cyclase activator that mediates the effects. Since high levels kill some neurons, NO is implicated as a major cause of the degeneration that occurs after strokes, and in Huntington's and some other nervous system diseases. Protective mechanisms that operate under normal conditions include glutamate limitation of substrate availability, via inhibition of citrulline conversion to arginine in brain tissue, and binding of NO by hemoglobin and other iron-containing compounds. Neurons that synthesize NO are resistant to its injurious effects. NO is also made in astrocytes, retinal amacrine, and adrenomedullary ganglion cells. It is believed to mediate some aspects of nervous system development, and the coupling of cerebral blood flow adjustments to neuron activity. At some sites, it co-localizes (and may be co-released) with somatostatin, neuropeptide Y, acetylcholine, and other neurotransmitters; and in a few it synergizes with prostacyclin.

nitric oxide synthases: NOS; several dioxygenases, encoded by three or more genes (at least one of which undergoes alternate splicing) that catalyze formation of nitric oxide and citrulline from arginine and oxygen, in reactions that involve reduction of 5,6,7,8-tetrahydrobiopterine (BH_4) to dihydrobiopterin (BH_2). All have binding sites for flavoproteins (FAD and FMN), as well as NADPH, and most are cytosolic. The form *constitutively* expressed in cerebellum can also function as a cytochrome P450 reductase (*see* **NADPH diaphorase**). Other constitutively expressed types with somewhat similar properties are made in astrocytes, vascular endothelium, circulating neutrophilic leukocytes, mast cells, platelets, macula densa cells, and pancreatic islet β cells. They bind, and are activated by calmodulin when Ca^{2+} levels rise. The effects of other activators vary with the cell types. Different enzymes are induced in macro-

phages, Kupffer cells, hepatocytes, mesangial cells, astrocytes, inflammatory neutrophils, articular cartilages, chondrocytes, and some cancer cells; and endothelium also contains an inducible type. The major stimulants are interferons β and γ (IFNβ and IFNγ), tumor necrosis factors α and β (TNFα and TNFβ), and interleukin-1β. Calmodulin is tightly bound to inducible types, and may be a subunit. It acts directly, and *inducible* enzymes are unaffected by changes in Ca^{2+} levels. Some anti-inflammatory influences of glucocorticoids may involve interference with the induction. Pharmacological inhibitors include N^G-methyl-L-arginine (**NMMA**) ($q.v.$), and N^G-nitro-L-arginine (shown below).

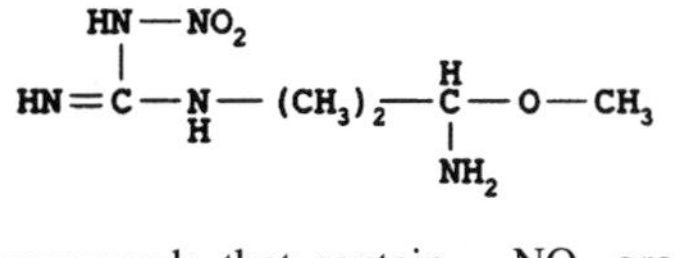

nitrites: compounds that contain —NO_2 groups. Inorganic salts are made from atmospheric nitrogen by nitrogen-fixing microorganisms; and calcium and potassium nitrates are components of fertilizers. Plants and microorganisms reduce nitrates to ammonia, which they use to make amino acids and other organic compounds. Animals can metabolize amino acids to nitric oxide and free radicals. Nitrite salts are used to cure meats, and it has been suggested that the amounts ingested with delicatessen foods can invoke mutations and/or function as procarcinogens. Nitroglycerin and some other agents used to treat angina pectoris are called "organic nitrates", but they are, in fact, nitrites. Their therapeutic effectiveness is attributed to conversion to **nitric oxide** ($q.v.$). Nitrates oxidize hemoglobin to methemoglobin. The reactions are not quantitatively important in the dosages used; and erythrocytes make a methemoglobin reductase. However, prompt administration of high concentrations of nitrite salts can combat the otherwise lethal effects of cyanide poisoning; *see* **methemoglobin**.

Nitro-BID: a trade name for nitroglycerine.

nitroblue tetrazolium chloride: nitroBT; NBT; 3,3'-(3-3'-dimethoxy4,4'-di-phenylene)-*bis*-(2-*p*-nitrophenyl)-5-(phenyl)-2*H*-tetrazolium chloride; a yellow dye used to test the respiratory burst activity of neutrophilic leukocytes, and in biological stains to detect NADPH diaphorase. It is taken up by phagocytosis and metabolized to formazan, which forms deep blue granules. NBT is also used for determinations of other dehydrogenase, threonine deaminase, and alkaline phosphatase activities, and to precipitate fibrinogen.

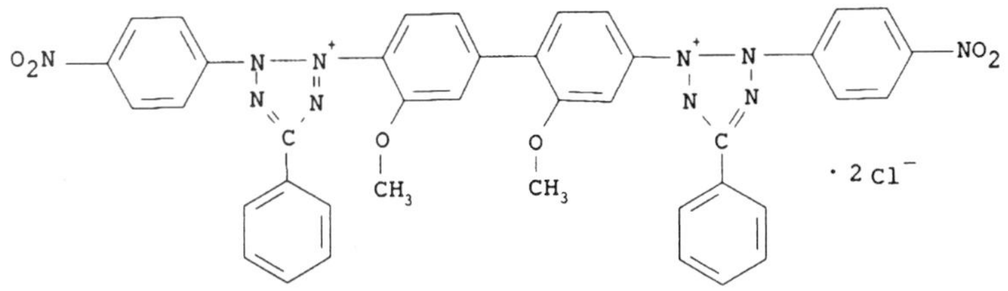

nitroblue tetrazolium chloride

nitrocellulose: an inert absorbent used to separate and concentrate macromolecules, for example as filters that retain double stranded DNA and DNA-RNA hybrids (but not single stranded molecules). Nitrocellulose paper is used in blot transfer procedures, to retain macromolecules separated by chromatography and/or electrophoresis.

nitrogen: N; an element (atomic number 7, atomic weight 14.007). At sea level (760 mm atmospheric pressure), nitrogen gas, N_2, accounts for approximately 78% of the volume of inspired air, and approximately 75% of the air in alveoli and blood plasma. Although it does not bind to hemoglobin, and is chemically inert in plants and animals (and in most *in vitro* systems), it can invoke "nitrogen narcosis" in deep sea divers when high pressure causes large amounts to dissolve in blood plasma. It is used to preserve substances that react with oxygen, and for numerous industrial purposes. Blue-green algae and some bacteria convert atmospheric nitrogen to nitrates; *see* **nitrogen fixation** and **nitrates**. The element is a component of all amines, amino acids, proteins, nucleotides, nucleic acids and many other organic molecules. Urea is the major metabolic waste product in mammals, but some creatinine and uric acid are also excreted. Uric acid is the major waste for birds and most reptiles, and ammonia for some fishes.

nitrogenase: enzyme systems that convert atmospheric nitrogen to ammonium ions (*see* **nitrogen fixation**), and can also reduce NO_2, HCN, NH_3, and some other compounds. They are 210-240K tetrameric proteins with Fe_4S_4 groups that require Mo-Fe cofactors which reduce the substrates, plus dimeric 55-50K nitrogenase reductases that also contain Fe_4S_4 and use flavoproteins and NADPH to restore the nitrogenase to its oxidized form. High levels of NH_4+ exert negative feedback control. Leghemoglobin protects both enzyme components against damage by atmospheric oxygen.

nitrogen balance: the relationship between the amount of nitrogen eaten (mostly as protein) and the amount excreted (mostly as urea). Healthy, well-nourished adult animals have equal values for the parmeters over 24-hour time periods, and are said to be in *zero* nitrogen balance. During times of food deprivation, and when glucocorticoids and other regulators accelerate protein catabolism and gluconeogenesis, excretion exceeds intake, and creates *negative* balances. *Positive* balances occur during growth, and during convalescence from debilitating diseases. Growth hormone and insulin promote nitrogen retention under many conditions.

nitrogen cycle: reactions in which atmospheric nitrogen is used to synthesize organic compounds, and is then metabolized back to free nitrogen. Nitrogen fixing microorganisms convert the gas to nitrates and ammonia, which are precursors for amino acids and other organic compounds in plants and microorganisms. Higher animals ingest many of the products (directly, or by eating other animals), use them for various biological purposes, and eventually degrade them to urea and other nitrogenous wastes. Some bacteria convert the wastes to ammonia. Soil bacteria metabolize ammonia and other nitrogenous wastes, and various nitrifying types convert them to nitrates, nitric oxide, and nitrogen. Saprophytic fungi contribute to the cycle by feeding on dead and decaying organisms and other organic matter.

nitrogen fixation: a process carried out by *Azotobacter* and some other bacteria in legume nodules, and by blue-green algae, in which energy released by ATP hydrolysis is used to convert atmospheric nitrogen to ammonium ions. **Nitrogenase** (*q.v.*) is an enzyme system that catalyzes reactions summarized as: N_2 +12 ATP + $\rightleftarrows$ electrons + 12 H_2O → 2 NH_4+ + 12 ADP + 12 Pi + $4H^+$. The product is used to make amino acids, in reactions such as α-ketoglutarate + NH_4+ + NADPH $\rightleftarrows$ glutamate + $NADP^+$ + H_2O, and pyruvate + NH_4+ → serine.

nitrogen mustard: (1) mechlorethamine; di-(2-chloroethyl)methylamine; a potent alkylating agent used to treat lymphomas and some other neoplasias, and as an immunosuppressant; (2) cyclophosphamide, melphalan, chlorambucil, and related molecules with similar properties and the general composition shown.

nitrogenous base: usually (1) a purine or pyrimidine; (2) any aromatic, nitrogen-containing compound that can accept protons.

nitroglycerine: 1,2,3-propanetriol trinitrate; a potent vasodilator, used to treat angina pectoris. Its effects are attributed to formation of **nitric oxide** (*q.v.*). Excessive amounts can invoke nausea, vomiting, headache, abdominal cramps, mental confusion, delirium, skin rashes, and methemoglobinemia, and (in extreme cases), cyanosis and death from circulatory collapse.

$$CH_2-O-NO_2$$
$$HC-O-NO_2$$
$$CH_2-O-NO_2$$

5-nitro-2-(3-phenylpropylamino)benzoic acid: NPPB; a chloride channel blocker.

nitroprusside: when administered as the sodium salt, the compound rapidly relaxes the smooth muscle of both arterioles and venules, and is sometimes used to lower

mechlorethamine

general formula

nitrogen mustard

blood pressure. It reacts with hemoglobin and with membrane bound sulfhydryl groups on proteins bound to blood vessel walls to form nitroprusside radicals that decompose to the therapeutically active derivative, **nitric oxide** (*q.v.*) plus cyanide. Usually, most of the cyanide is metabolized by rhodanase in the liver to thiocyanate (which is excreted to urine). However, infusion of large amounts of sodium nitroprusside, especially in individuals with impaired renal function, or deficient in thioglycolates (required for cyanate metabolism) can cause build-up to toxic levels. Na-nitroprusside can also accumulate when used for long time periods, and it then impairs thyroid gland function by interfering with iodide accumulation (and in very high levels, also blocks iodide organification). The properties are used for some studies of thyroid gland function.

nitrosamines: *N*-nitroso derivatives of secondary amines with the general formula shown, formed when nitrates, nitric oxide, and other nitrogenous compounds react with amines. Some decompose to mutagenic and carcinogenic alkylating agents.

5-nitroso-*N*-acetylpenicillamine: a potent vasodilator that acts by releasing nitric oxide.

S-**nitrosocysteine**: a compound formed when **nitric oxide** (*q.v.*) reacts with cysteine. It is a more potent vasodilator than, and may account for some actions attributed to NO.

nitrosoureas: compounds that contain **methylnitrosourea** moieties (*q.v.*). Most are cytotoxic. Carmustine and lomustine are among the lipophilic kinds that enter cells, and are used as antitumor agents and immunosuppressants. Streptozotocin binds tightly to pancreatic islet beta cell components, and damages the cells. It is used to induce diabetes mellitus in laboratory animals.

nitrous acid: HNO_2; a weaker acid that HNO_3 (nitric acid). It invokes mutations by deaminating cytidine and adenine bases.

nitrous oxide: N_2O; dinitrogen oxide; "laughing gas"; a colorless, nonirritating, non-explosive gas that exchanges with nitrogen, and rapidly deadens pain perception. It can invoke general anesthesia when presented alone in high concentrations, is used in this way for procedures such as tooth extraction. and in combination with other agents for general anestheisia. It is not metabolized, and does not appear to exert direct toxic effects. However, effective inhalation mixtures do not contain sufficient oxygen to sustain normal functions when used for extended time periods; and individuals who receive them often experience hallucinations and "wild" dreams.

nizatidine: Axid; *N*-[4-(6-methylamino-7-nitro-2-thio-5-axa-6-heptene-1-yl)-2-thiazolylmethyl]-*N*,*N*-dimethylamine; an H_2 type histamine receptor antagonist used to treat peptic ulcers.

NK: neurokinin K; *see* **neurokinin β**.

NK[s]: neurokinins; *see* **neurokinins**.

NK-1: (1) antigens expressed on most natural killer (NK) cells; (2) brain receptors that bind, and mediate many of the actions of substance P; *see* **neurokinin receptors**. They also interact to some extent with neurokinin α and some related tachykinins.

NK-2: antigens on some natural killer (NK) cells; (2) receptors in the stomach, duodenum, urinary bladder, and aorta that mediate the contractile effects of neurokinin β. *See* also **neurokinin receptors**.

NK-3: a receptor that mediates the contractile effects of neurokinin β on hepatic portal vein smooth muscle, and at some other sites; *see* **neurokinin receptors**.

NK$_1$, NK$_2$, NK$_3$: *see* **neurokinin receptors**.

NK cell[s]: natural killer cells.

NK cell derived inhibitory activator: NKCIA; a regulator released by natural killer cells that suppresses hemopoietic cell proliferation.

NL: neuroleukin.

N lines: regions of skeletal muscle sarcomeres that contain nebulin and other stabilizing proteins. N1 lines are in I bands, near the Z discs. N2 lines are at the ends of A bands.

***N*-linked oligosaccharides**: small glycosides covalently linked to nitrogen groups (usually of asparagine moieties) on immunoglobulins and many other glycoproteins. The functions at various sites include contributions to the conformation stability required for binding to ligands or for secretion, protection against degradation, recognition by membrane receptors that mediate intracellular transport, and slowing of metabolic clearance. Many have branched cores that contain an *N*-acetylglucosamine and three mannose moieties. High mannose types have 2-6 additional mannose groups. Complex oligosaccharides have 2-5 terminal branches composed of *N*-acetylglucosamine, galactose, and (usually) sialic acid.

NMs: neuromedins.

NMDA: *N*-methyl-D-aspartate.

NMDA receptors: excitatory amino acid receptors activated by *N*-methyl-D aspartate. They mediate glutamate and aspartate opening of Ca^{2+} ion channels, and are essential for the long term potentiation. NMR1A subunit homodimers are distributed throughout the brain. NMR1A also forms heterodimers with NMR2A, NMR2B, and NMR2C, each of which has a characteristic distribution pattern. The qualitative effects of the various dimer types are similar, but there are differences in timing (both onsets and terminations of the actions), and in susceptibilities to inhibition by Mg^{2+} ions. Excessive amounts of excitatory amino acids acting on NMDA receptors injure, and can kill some neurons (*see* **nitric oxide**); and cysteine toxicity is mediated mostly via those receptors. *Cf* **kainate** and **quisqualate receptors**.

N-methyl-D-aspartate, NMDA: an agonist that mimics the effects of excitatory amino acids on NMDA receptor subtypes, and is used to identify those receptors. High doses are excitotoxic, and can invoke a Huntington's disease-like syndrome in laboratory animals; *see* also **nitric oxide**.

NMMA: N^G-methyl arginine; an inhibitor of nitric acid synthase.

NMN: nicotinamide mononucleotide.

NMR: nuclear magnetic resonance; *see* **magnetic resonance imaging**.

NMS: *N*-methylscopolamine bromide; a muscarinic type acetylcholine receptor antagonist; *see* **scopolamine**.

NO: nitric oxide.

N₂O: nitrous oxide.

NO-711: a selective inhibitor of γ-aminobutyric acid uptake that enters the brain.

nociception: perception of pain and other unpleasant stimuli. The mediators include substance P and bradykinin.

nociceptors: receptors specialized for perception of pain and other unpleasant stimuli.

NO-711

nocodazole: 5-(2-thienylcarbonyl)-1-*H*-benzimidazole-carbamic acid methyl ester; an antibiotic used to treat some neoplasms, to study microtubule functions, and to synchronize cell division. By binding to microtubules and promoting depolymerization, it arrests mitosis in metaphase.

nocturia: excessive urine production at night, usually in quantities that interrupt sleep.

nocturnal: (1) during the night; (2) describes species that are normally most active during darkness; *cf* **diurnal**.

NOD: non-insulin dependent (type II) diabetes mellitus.

NOD mice: non-obese diabetic mice; a mutant strain whose members develop an autoimmune disease in which the pancreatic islets become infiltrated with lymphocytes that destroy the β-cells and invoke an insulin-dependent form of diabetes mellitus not associated with hyperphagia and obesity.

node: (1) a small bulge, for example one composed of a mass of tissue, as in lymph node; (2) a specialized region, as in node of Ranvier or sino-atrial node.

nodes of Ranvier: regions on large peripheral axons that are not enveloped by myelin. They have voltage-gated ion channels that mediate saltatory conduction.

nomifensine: 1,2,3,4-tetrahydro-2-methyl-4-phenyl-8-isoquninolinamine; a synthetic agent that acts indirectly as a dopamine agonist by promoting dopamine release from nerve endings and blocking its reuptake. It is no longer used an antidepressant, since it can invoke hemolytic anemia.

nonactin: monactin; 2,5,11,14,20,23,29,32-octamethyl-4,13,22,31,37,38,39,40-octaoxapen-tacyclotetracontane-3,12,21,30-tetrone; an antibiotic made by several *Strep-*

nonactin

tomyces species, used as an ionophore that selectively transports K^+ ions.

noncoding DNA: DNA that is not transcribed, for example in introns and pseudogenes. Some noncoding DNA contributes to transcription controls.

noncollagenous bone proteins: NCPs; osteocalcin, osteopontin, osteonectin, and other bone proteins that differ from collagens.

noncompetitive enzyme inhibition: usually, irreversible inhibition in which V_{max} is lowered by agents that bind to noncatalytic sites. The effects cannot be overcome by adding more substrate. *Cf* **competitive** and **uncompetitive inhibition**.

non-Darwinian evolution: formation of new species, or modification of pre-existing ones, via mechanisms other than natural selection. It can involve transmission of mutations that confer no special advantages, or of harmful ones that do not exert their effects until after reproductive competence has been attained.

nondisjunction of chromosomes: failure of homologous chromosomes or sister chromatids to separate in a normal manner during mitosis or meiosis, or failure to transmit the usual chromosome patterns to daughter cells. The progeny that survive are aneuploid. Several kinds of sex differentiation disorders are caused by nondisjunction during meiosis I or II.

nonenzymatic: describes chemical reactions that proceed spontaneously, without the assistance of enzymes, for example conversion of PGG_2 to PGH_2. *See* also **nonenzymatic glycosylation**.

nonenzymatic glycosylation: addition of carbohydrate groups to other molecules via reactions that do not require enzymes. Small amounts of glucose normally attach reversibly to amine groups of hemoglobins and other long-lived proteins and form unstable Schiff bases; and the amounts increase with advancing age. When blood glucose levels are chronically elevated, the equilibrium shifts in the direction of association, and the bases undergo Amadori rearrangements to form products that can slowly dissociate, but can also cross-link to other compounds. In time, different rearrangements lead to irreversible formation of 2-furanyl-4-(5)-2-furanyl)-1*H*-imidazole and related derivatives, collectively known as advanced glycosylation end-products (AGEs). More than 20 have been identified, most of which are yellowish to brown substances that fluoresce. Glycosylation, cross-linking, and associated changes affect the activities of enzymes and the properties of structural proteins and extracellular matrices, as well as DNA repair, transcrip-

tion, phagocytosis, and other processes, They are believed to invoke much of the pathology associated with uncontrolled diabetes mellitus, and to some of the degenerative processes associated with aging. Body components affected include collagens, crystallins, Von Willebrand factor, lipoproteins, and DNAs. Small amounts of hemoglobin A_{1c}, glycosylated on ε–lysyl moieties, are present in normal blood, and much larger ones form in individuals with recurrent or persistent hyperglycemia. The levels can be used to gauge the effectiveness of blood glucose control. (The measurements are especially useful in individuals with normal fasting glucose levels who experience bouts of hyperglycemia at irregular intervals during the day; and they provide some indication of potential damage at other sites). Although glycosylation augments hemoglobin affinity for oxygen, usually too few molecules are affected to seriously impair oxygen transport to tissue cells.

nonessential: usually describes a nutrient that can be synthesized within the organism, and is therefore not required in the diet; *cf* **essential amino** and **fatty acids**.

nonhistone proteins: NHPs; chromosomal proteins with higher molecular weights and more acidic isoelectric points than histones, including DNA polymerases and high mobility group (HMG) proteins. The latter vary in composition among species and cell types, and change during the course of development. Some are believed to mediate cell-type specific effects.

nonhomologous chromosomes: chromosomes that do not code for the same kinds of alleles, and do not pair during synapsis.

nonidentical twins: dizygotic twins; two genetically different progeny that develop during a single pregnancy. They originate from different oocytes, which are fertilized by different spermatozoa; *cf* **identical twins**.

nonionic detergents: Triton, octyl glucoside, and other detergents with uncharged heads. They are used to extract cell components, and are less likely than charged types to denature proteins, disrupt protein:protein interactions, or cause depolymerization of microtubules and microfilaments.

non-Mendelian inheritance: patterns of gene transmission that cannot be explained on the basis of segregation, independent assortment, and gene linkages. *See*, for example **cytoplasmic inheritance**, and **gene conversion**.

nonoxynols: nonoxynol is nonylphenoxypolyethoxyethanol. Related compounds with the overall formula $C_{15}H_{24}O(C_2H_4O)_n$ are named for the n values. Nonoxynol-9 is a component of several spermaticides used intravaginally for contraception. Several other derivatives are nonionic surfactants.

$$C_9H_{19} - \text{benzene ring} - (OCH_2CH_2)_n - OH$$

nootropic: enhancing cognition.

nonpolar: usually describes molecules or chemical groups that are hydrophobic and uncharged, and do not have dipole moments. They do not form hydrogen bonds, but can associate with other nonpolar substances via weak (van der Waals) forces. Phospholipids and detergents contain both polar and nonpolar groups.

nonprotein nitrogen: NPN; urea, uric acid, creatine, creatinine, amino acids, and other small nitrogen-containing compounds that circulate and are excreted to urine. Urea is the major component. *See* also **uremia**.

nonsense codons: sets of three messenger RNA bases that do not bind transfer RNA anticodons. Some provide signals for translation termination.

nonshivering thermogenesis: heat generation via processes other than skeletal muscle contraction. **Brown adipose tissue** (*q.v.*) is a major site in young and hibernating animals. The metabolic rates of many other cell types can be augmented by catecholamines, triiodothyronine, and other regulators. Food intake and exposure to cold environmental temperatures are among the factors that promote catecholamine release. Cold environments also invoke slowly developing changes in thyroid hormone functions.

nonspecific immunity: resistance to the deleterious effects of foreign substances that is not antigen-specific. *See* also **immunity** and **natural killer cells**.

nonsteroidal anti-inflammatory drugs: NSAIDs: agents other than glucocorticoids and related steroids that suppress inflammation, a term usually applied to inhibitors of eicosanoid synthesis such as aspirin, other salicylates, indomethacin, and ibuprofen. They counteract pain and fever, and can retard the destructive effects of autoimmune processes in diseases such as rheumatoid arthritis. Gastric irritation, which sometimes leads to ulcer formation, renal injury, and some other undesirable consequences of long-term use have been attributed to loss of the protective and trophic influences of prostaglandins on mucosal and other epithelial membranes. However, NSAIDs can enter cells, dissociate at normal intercellular pHs, affect plasma membrane permeabilities, and promote H^+ influx and Na^+ and K^+ efflux. They may additionally promote free radical formation by activating neutrophilic leukocytes. Buffering somewhat diminishes the gastric irritation. Prostacyclin analogs appear to protect some individuals against stomach ulceration, but to be ineffective in others. *See* also **salicylates**.

nonsteroidal estrogens: substances other than steroids that bind to estrogen receptors and mimic the effects of the hormones; *see*, for example **diethylstilbestrol**.

nonsuppressible insulin-like activity: NSILA: insulin-like activity that is not affected by antibodies directed against that hormone. Most NSILA in blood plasma is attributed to insulin-like growth factors, and especially IGF-1.

nonyl-: the chemical group shown.

$$H_3C \text{—chain—}$$

Noonan's syndrome: an autosomal dominant disease with manifestations that resemble those of females with XO Turner's syndrome (such as webbed neck, ptosis, hypogonadism, cardiac and facial defects, short stature, and mild mental retardation), attributed to defective functions of one sex chromosome in some cells. Although it can occur in 45X/46Y mosaics, and the term "male Turner's syndrome" has been applied, many afflicted males have 46 XY chromosome patterns.

nor-: a prefix that (1) indicates something is missing, as in norepinephrine (which lacks an the *N*-methyl group of epinephrine), or 19-nortestosterone (which lacks an oxygen group at position 19); (2) designates a linear structure isomeric with a branched chain type, as in norleucine.

noradrenalin: norepinephrine. The British spelling is noradrenaline.

noradrenergic: describes neurons that secrete, effects invoked by, or target cells activated by norepinephrine.

noradrenergic receptors: receptors activated by norepinephrine; *see* **adrenergic** and **norepinephrine receptors.**

norandrostenolone: nandrolone.

nordihydroguaiaretic acid: NDGA; 4,4'-(2,3-dimethyl-1,4-butanediyl)*bis*[1,2-benzenediol]; an agent that inhibits phospholipases, blocks arachidonic acid conversion to eicosanoids via cyclooxygenase, lipoxygenase, and epoxygenase pathways, and interferes with nitric oxide mediated signal transduction. It is used to inhibit thromboxane formation, and as an antioxidant.

$$HO - \text{ring} - CH_2 - \overset{CH_3}{\underset{H}{C}} - \overset{CH_3}{\underset{H}{C}} - CH_2 - \text{ring} - OH$$

norepinephrine: N; NE; 2-amino-1-(3,4-dihydroxyphenyl)ethanol; the major neurotransmitter released by postganglionic nerve terminals of the sympathetic system, a neurotransmitter for some brain neurons, and a major adrenal medulla hormone. Small amounts are also made in chromaffin tissues. It is synthesized from dopamine via a reaction catalyzed by dopamine β-hydroxylase, and stored in synaptic vesicles and secretory granules. In some cell types, phenylethanolamine-*N*-methyltransferase (PNMT) catalyzes it conversion to epinephrine (E). In common with E, it binds to β_1 type **adrenergic receptors** (*q.v.*), and invokes the same kinds of effects. Many other actions are mediated via α_1 type receptors; and it is a more potent stimulant than E at some sites. Peripherally, N augments cardiac contractile force, promotes vasoconstriction in skin, mucous membranes, and viscera, inhibits contraction of gastrointestinal smooth muscle and the secretion of digestive system hormones, decreases urine flow, accelerates lipolysis, elevates metabolic rate, promotes contraction of the spleen, invokes mydriasis and affects melatonin production. It contributes to the control of systemic blood pressure and the ability to engage in demanding skeletal muscle activity, and mediates many responses to cold environments, and to stress. Unnlike E, N does not act on β_2 receptor types which mediate vasodilation in liver and skeletal muscle. Consequently, it elevates both systolic and diastolic blood pressure, and usually thereby invokes reflex bradycardia. It exerts only limited influences on blood glucose, since it does not promote cAMP-stimulated glycogenolysis in skeletal muscle (although it can raise cytosolic Ca^{2+}; and very high concentrations can act via Ca^{2+} to augment glycogen phosphorylase activity there and in in the liver). Acetylcholine is the major stimulant for its release from both sympathetic nerve endings and adrenomedullary cells. The effects of brain norepinephrine include influences on the secretion of some hypothalamic hormones, and on food intake and other behaviors. The postsynaptic actions are short-lived, because NE is rapidly taken up by sympathetic neuron terminals, and by adrenomedullary cells. It is more slowly degraded by catecholamine-O-methyltransferase and monoamine oxidases. NE additionally acts on presynaptic α_2 receptors to exert negative feedback control over neurotransmitter release.

norepinephrine receptors: plasma membrane associated proteins that mediate norepinephrine and some epinephrine actions. See also **adrenergic receptors**. The subclasses were initially classified on the basis of location, but systems based on binding affinities for agonists and antagonists are now preferred. α_1 subtypes are located on blood vessels and other target organs, and most of the effects of ligand binding are attributed to augmented phosphatidylinositol hydrolysis, generation of inositol-1,4,5-triphosphate ($IP_{1,4,5}$, IP_3), and consequent elevation of cytosolic Ca^{2+} levels. The α_2 types are mostly presynaptic, and the inhibitory effects on norepinephrine release involve inhibition of adenylate cyclase. The β_1 types in the heart and some other structures are coupled to G_s proteins that activate adenylate cyclases.

α-methyl-**norepinephrine**: an α_1 type noradrenergic receptor agonist, used mostly for vasoconstriction. Nordefrin is the hydrochloride. Levonordefrin (the l-isomer) is more potent.

3-O-methyl-**norepinephrine**: normetanephrine.

α-methyl-norepinephrine

norethandrolone: Nilevar; 17-hydroxy-19-norpregn-4-en-3-one; a testosterone analog used for its anabolic actions; see **anabolic steroids**.

norethindrone: 19-norethisterone; Norlutin; 17-hydroxy-norpregn-4-ene-20yn-3-one; a synthetic steroid, used alone as a progestin, or as a component (with mestranol or ethinyl estradiol) of several oral contraceptive preparations.

19-**norethisterone**: norethindrone.

norethynodrel: 17-hydroxy-19-nor-17α-pregn-5(10)-en-20-yn-3-one: a synthetic progestin with some estrogen-like and androgen-like activity. It is used to treat amenorrhea, endometriosis, and some other conditions, and is a component of some oral contraceptives.

norgestimate: 17α-acetoxy-13-ethyl-17-ethynylgon-4-ene-3-one oxime; an acetate oxime of norgestrel, used as a component of oral contraceptive preparations. It appears to be more effective and less toxic than the parent compound.

norgestrel: 13β-ethyl-17-hydroxy-18,19-dinor-17α-pregn-4-3n-20-yn-3-one; a potent synthetic progestin, used alone and in combination with synthetic estrogens, in some oral contraceptive preparations.

Norlutin: a trade name for norethindrone.

normal: (1) free of defects; conforming to an established specification; (2) *see* **normality**.

normal distribution curve: a symmetrical, bell-shaped representation of the frequencies of values for a parameter in an entire population in which such measurements can theoretically be made, when all variations are random. The highest point on the Y axis represents the frequency for the mean value of X. 68.28% of the Y values fall within ± 1 standard deviation of the mean, 95.46% within ± two standard deviations, and 99.73% within ± three standard deviations. Tables constructed on the basis of such curves are used, in conjunction with statistical measurements such as Student's *t* test, or analysis of variance, to determine the probability that experimental and control groups are members of the same population. Differences between the means are said to be statistically significant if the probability falls below a specified number; *see* **statistical significance, standard deviation, standard error**, and *t* **test**.

normality: in chemistry, a measure of the numbers of gram equivalent weights of a pure solvent contained in a liter of aqueous solution. A 1N solution of any acid contains one gram equivalent weight of solute per liter, and will exactly neutralize the same volume of a 1N base. For monvalent acids, such as HCl, a 1N solution is also 1 molar. A 1 molar solution of an acid such as H_2SO_4 is 2N.

normetanephrine: 3-*O*-methyl norepinephrine; a biologically inactive norepinephrine metabolite, formed in the reaction: norepinephrine + *S*-adenosylmethionine → normetanephrine + *S*-adenosylhomocysteine, catalyzed by catecholamine-*O*-methyltransferase (COMT). It is further metabolized, mostly to vanillyl mandelic acid in peripheral tissues, and to 3-methoxy-4-hydroxy-phenylethylglycol in the central nervous system.

normo-: a prefix usually applied to values within the range for healthy individuals of the species, as in nor-moglycemia, normocalcemia, or normovolemia. It is also used in special ways; *see* **normoblast**.

normoblast: a cell type that differentiates from an erythroblast, contains some hemoglobin, and can mature to an erythrocyte. It is round, and contains a "normal" kind of nucleus (which deteriorates as the cell proceeds to the reticulocyte stage). Normoblasts do not leave the bone marrow under physiological conditions.

normocyte: an erythrocyte of normal size and shape; *cf* **normoblast**.

normorphine: desmethylmorphine; 7,8-didehydro-4,5-epoxymorphinan-3,6-diol; a narcotic analgesic, with properties similar to those of morphine.

norpseudoephedrine: *threo*-2-amino-1-hydroxy-1-phenylpropane; an amine made by the kat plant, *Catha edulis*, and by some evergreen shrubs. It appears to exert fewer undesirable central nervous system effects than amphetamines, and is used as an appetite suppressant to treat some forms of obesity.

norsynephrine: octopamine.

Northern blotting: techniques for transferring electrophoretically separated ribonucleic acids (and/or RNA fragments) from agarose gels to nitrocellulose sheets for further analysis. *Cf* **Southern blotting**.

nortriptyline: 3-(10,11-dihydro-5*H*-dibenzo[*a,d*]cyclohepten-5-ylidene)-*N*-methyl-1-propanamine; a tricyclic agent used as antidepressant, and to treat compulsive disorders. It also exerts anticholinergic effects and can alleviate some urinary system dysfunctions.

noso-: a prefix meaning disease.

nosocomial: pertaining to hospitals; it usually describes disease contracted in a hospital or other health facility.

nosology: the science of disease classification.

nosotropic: directed against disease.

notochord: an elongated, rod-shaped, dorsally located cartilaginous structure formed form mesoderm in chordate embryos that persists as a supporting structure in

novobiocin

mature members of the Cephalochordate subphylum. In vertebrate embryos, it provides temporary support, and is believed to contribute to differentiation of the axial nervous system. It then degenerates as the vertebrae form, but remnants persist as nucleus pulposus in the intervertebral disks.

novobiocin: N-[7-[[3-O-(aminocarbonyl)-6-deoxy-5-C-methyl-4-O-methyl-β-L-lyxopyranosyl]oxy]-4-hydroxy-8-methyl-2-oxo-2H-1-benzopyran-3yl]-4-hydroxy-3-(3-methyl-2-butenyl)benzamide; an antibiotic made by *Streptomyces spheroides* and *S.niveus* that blocks ATP binding to DNA gyrase, and is used on agarose columns to purify DNA-gyrase and topoisomerase II.

Novocain: a trade name for procaine hydrochloride.

N protein: (1) an obsolete term for G protein; (2) a λ bacteriophage protein essential for the early stages of infection.

NPs: neutrophilic peptides; *see* **defensins**.

NPS-: nitrophenylsulfenyl-.

NPY: neuropeptide Y.

N regions: parts of immunoglobulin and T cell receptor peptide variable regions encoded by short nucleotide segments and randomly inserted into germ line-directed polypeptides via reactions catalyzed by DNA terminal transferases. They occur 3′ or 5′ to rearranged immunoglobulin chain D segments, or at T cell receptor V-J, V-D-J, or D-D junctions.

NS: not statistically significant; a term used in conjunction with **P values**, (*q.v.*), when values for a parameter measured in one group do not differ from those measured in another to a greater extent that can theoretically be attributed to chance variations.

NSAIDs: nonsteroidal anti-inflammatory drugs.

NSFs: N-ethylmaleimide sensitive proteins; *see* **SNAPS**.

NSILA: nonsuppressible insulin-like activity.

NSP: nicotine stimulated neurophysins; the neurophysins cleaved from vasopressin precursor proteins; *see* **neurophysins**, and *cf* **estrogen stimulated neurophysin.**

NT: neurotensin.

N-**terminal**: amino terminal; the end of a peptide or protein that contains, or is closest to the region first assembled on the ribosome. It often has a free amino group, but some compounds are amidated or otherwise altered posttranslationally. *Cf* **C-terminal**.

NTF: (1) neurotrophic factor; (2) neurotropic factor.

NTPase: nuclear membrane triphosphatase.

nuclear acceptor sites: nuclear components that directly bind hormone receptors, hormone-receptor complexes, or other transcription regulators. Many are hormone response elements.

nuclear envelope: the discontinuous, concentric double membrane that encloses the nucleus of a eukaryote cell when it is not dividing. It disintegrates during the prophase of mitosis and meiosis, and new ones form in the progeny during telophase. The inner layer contains proteins that bind lamins, and is in contact with chromosomes and nuclear ribonucleoproteins. The outer one resembles, and is continuous with the endoplasmic reticulum membrane. Regulated transport of large molecules to and from the cytoplasm occurs mostly via pores in the envelope.

nuclear lamina: a fibrous protein network that lines the inner surface of the nuclear envelope. It contains lamins A, B, and C.

nuclear magnetic resonance: NMR; *see* **magnetic resonance imaging**.

nuclear matrix: nuclear scaffold; insoluble nuclear components obtained after the chromosomes, nucleoli, nuclear membranes, and nucleoplasm are extracted. They include a ribonucleoprotein network, some peripheral lamins, and some nuclear pore complexes. Certain of the proteins are similar in all nucleated cells of the organism, and consistently present. Others are cell type specific, and undergo changes during differentiation. Some associate with specific DNA base sequences and contribute to the formation of chromosomal loops, and/or bind receptors for steroid and some other hormones, and for other regulators of DNA replication and transcription. The eight proteins (matrins) that appear to be confined to the nuclear matrix include a 125K acidic matrin-3, a 105K basic matrin-4, four 60-75K proteins (matrins D-G) and matrins-12 and 13. It is believed that only actively transcribing genes attach to the matrix.

nuclear membrane triphosphatase: NTPases; nuclear enzymes that catalyzes hydrolysis of ATP and related molecules. They are required for transporting mature messenger RNAs to the cytoplasm.

nuclear scaffold: *see* **nuclear matrix**.

nucleases: enzymes that cleave nucleic acids and polynucleotides at specific sites. Cells use deoxyribonucleases (DNases) during crossing over and DNA repair, and to eliminate defective nucleotides. Ribonucleases (RNases) are essential for processing primary gene transcripts to mature messenger RNAs, and for destroying the mRNAs that are no longer needed. *See* also **restriction endonucleases**, **endonucleases**, and **exonucleases**.

nuclease sensitive sites: DNA regions easily cleaved by nucleases. They are the major (possibly the only) sites engaged in transcription.

nucleation: initiation of processes, such as microtubule polymerization, fiber organization, or mineral deposition, that lead to subsequent events which involve addition of more components. It is usually the slowest and most energy-consuming step of the assembly.

nucleic acids: large nucleotide polymers; *see* **ribonucleic acids** and **deoxyribonucleic acids**.

nucleocapsid: a virus coat and the genome it encloses.

nucleolar organizers: DNA loops with several genes that code for ribosomal RNAs.

nucleolin: a 713 amino acid, 92K eukaryote nucleolar protein, formerly called C23, that regulates chromatin structure. Each molecule binds to a nucleosome and (when not phosphorylated) inhibits transcription. After kinase A-mediated phosphorylation and cleavage by a proteolytic enzyme, it promotes nucleosome decondensation (in part by releasing histone H1), affects DNA: protein interactions, confers RNA polymerase specificity, and may control RNA polymerase I activity. It also binds to primary (preribosomal) RNA transcripts, and regulates RNA maturation.

nucleolus [nucleoli]: one or more dark-staining spherical structures within a cell nucleus, in which RNA polymerase I catalyzes assembly of preribosomal RNAs, and other enzymes process the molecules to mature rRNAs.

nucleon: an atomic nucleus particle.

nucleoplasm: karyoplasm; the gel-like component of cell nuclei.

nucleoplasmin: an acidic 105-110K pentameric nuclear protein with 29K subunits essential for nucleosome assembly. It binds histones H2A and H2B and translocates them to the DNA. Although it functions as a nuclear chaperone, it does not attach directly to either DNA or nucleosome core particles.

nucleosides: molecules composed of sugars (usually ribose or deoxyribose) covalently linked to purine or pyrimidine bases. Examples include cytosine and deoxyadenosine. The corresponding phosphorylated derivatives (nucleotides) are, respectively, cytidylate (cytidylic acid) and deoxyadenylate.

nucleosin: *see* **thymopoietin**.

nucleosome: a bead-like component of a eukaryote chromosome, approximately 10 nm in diameter, composed of a DNA segment (usually with 140 base pairs) wrapped around a disk-like core. It is connected to adjacent nucleosomes by a linear (linker) DNA segment that binds histone H1. The core is an octomer composed of two molecules each of histones H2A, H2B, H3, and H4. Groups of adjacent nucleosomes and their linkers form spiral solenoids.

nucleotidases: enzymes that catalyze cleavage of nucleotides to nucleosides and inorganic phosphate. Since 5′-nucleotidases, which act on RNAs, occur only in plasma membranes, they are used as markers in cell fractionation studies.

nucleotides: molecules composed of purine or pyrimidine bases covalently linked to sugars (usually ribose or deoxyribose) which are, in turn, covalently linked to one or more phosphate groups; *cf* **nucleosides**. Examples include adenosine-triphosphate, guanosine-diphosphate, and inosine-monophosphate (ATP, GDP, and IMP). RNAs and DNAs are nucleotide polymers.

nucleus [nuclei]: (1) a cell nucleus. In a typical eukaryotic cell that is not dividing, it is the largest organelle. It contains chromosomes, one or more nucleoli, nucleoplasm and nuclear matrix, and is separated from the cytoplasm by a double nuclear envelope with pores. Mature erythrocytes do not contain nuclei (and therefore cannot replicate or make new RNAs). Macrophages and osteoclasts among the types that contain two or more. Skeletal muscle fibers are elongated, multinucleate syncytia. Prokaryote cells do not have circumscribed nuclei. In most types, the cytoplasm contains a single, circular chromosome; (2) a cluster of structurally similar, functionally related neuron cell bodies within the central nervous system; *see*, for example **paraventricular nuclei**; (3) the part of an atom that contains the protons and neutrons; (4) an organizing center.

nucleus accumbens: N. accumbens; nucleus accumbens septi; a neuron cell body cluster in the floor of the anterior horn of the brain lateral ventricle, implicated in mediation of some dopamine functions. It is an extension of the corpus striatum, and is associated with the septum and olfactory tubercle.

nucleus ambiguous: N. ambiguous; a neuron cell body cluster in the ventrolateral region of the medulla oblongata, between the inferior olivary complex and the spinal nucleus of the trigeminal nerve. It receives afferent fibers from the mucosa and muscles of the pharynx and larynx (via the vagus, trigeminal, and glossopharyngeal nerves), and extends efferent fibers to glossopharyngeal, vagus and spinal accessory nerves.

nucleus:cytoplasmic ratio: the relative volumes of the nucleus and cytoplasm within a cell. High values are associated with high nucleic acid synthesis rates.

nucleus tractus solitarius: NST; a collection of nerve fibers in the dorsomedial part of the medulla oblongata. The axons originate in heterogenous perikarya, in which thirty or more neurotransmitters and neurohormones have been identified. The neurons engage in two-way communication with most parts of the central nervous system, including the limbic system, the paraventricular and arcuate nuclei, and the spinal cord; but no efferent nerves extend to the periphery. The NST is a major integration site for autonomic nervous system functions, contains synapses for baroreceptor reflexes, and is involved in control of blood pressure, chemoreception, gustation, gastrointestinal activity, and other functions.

nude mice: a mutant strain that carries an autosomal recessive *nu* gene. Homozygotes are almost devoid of body hair. They are used to study immunological functions, and as recipients for tumors and other tissues that do not grow in normal counterparts, because their thymus glands do not mature. The mice lack most of the T lymphocyte populations present in normal mice that are essential for cell-mediated immunity, are unable to make antibodies directed against most pathogens, and do not reject allografts or xenografts. They do, however, have natural killer (NK) cells and B lymphocytes.

null allele: an allele that does not direct formation of a functional product.

null cells: circulating lymphocytes that do not express the surface markers characteristic for either T or B types. They mature into large granular lymphocytes, some of which may be natural killer (NK) or killer (K) cells.

null hypothesis: a working hypothesis which states that the differences for a parameter measured in two groups are no greater than random variations within a single population. Statistical methods (which involve considerations of sample size as well as test values) are used to evaluate the differences. If the differences are statistically significant (*see* **P values**), the hypothesis is disproved.

Nuprin: a trade name for ibuprofen.

nuptial: associated with mating. The term can refer to secondary sex characteristics that affect partner choice, behavioral patterns, or chemical sex attractants.

nur/NGF-B: a gene activated by, and believed to mediate some of the effects of nerve growth factor (NGF).

nurse cells: cells that support the survival, differentiation, and/or functions of other cells; *see*, for example **Sertoli cells**.

nyctalopia: night blindness; faulty vision in dim light. The most common cause is vitamin A deficiency.

nycto-: a prefix meaning night, as in nyctohemeral or nyctalopia.

nyctohemeral: describes processes or phenomena that occur during the night (or during the dark phases of photoperiods).

nymph: the wingless, sexually immature stage of some insects.

nystagmus: spontaneous rapid eye movements of the kinds that characteristize REM sleep. *Optokinetic* nystagmus occurs in normal individuals when they follow moving objects, or watch stationary ones while they are moving. Vestibular dysfunctions, some gastrointestinal diseases, and some kinds of visual impairment are among the pathological conditions that cause nystagmus at other times.

nystatin: a mixture of three polyene type antifungal agents made by *Streptomyces aureus* and *S. noursei*, with actions similar to those of amphotericin B. It is used topically, but the toxicity precludes systemic administration. The structure of Nystatin A_1 is shown.

NZB: New Zealand black mice.

NZO: New Zealand obese mice.

NZW: New Zealand white mice.

Nystatin A_1

O

o: (1) ovine when used in acronyms, as in oPRL; (2) outside the cell, when used as a subscript, as in Ca_o^{2+} for extracellular Ca^{2+}.

O: oxygen.

o-: ortho-.

OA: okadaic acid.

OAF: osteoclast activating factor.

OB: osteoblast.

ob/ob **mice**: homozygotes of a mutant mouse strain that become hyperphagic and develop a form of obesity associated with supersensitivity of the paraventricular nuclei to norepinephrine, exaggerated responses to glucocorticoids, impaired thermogenesis, and other defects.

obesity: conditions in which excessive amounts of adipose tissue accumulate. It is usually (but not necessarily) associated with hyperphagia and higher than normal body weight. Some forms can be invoked in strains of laboratory animals that are otherwise lean by force-feeding, providing unlimited quantities of "cafeteria" type or high-fat diets, injecting appetite stimulants, or creating hormone imbalances. In most previously healthy types, body weights decline (although not always to normal levels) when the stimuli are removed. (There is some evidence for long-term persistence of new adipocytes formed while the obesity was developing.) Gonadectomized adult animals usually become moderately obese because they are less active than their intact counterparts, and tend to be somewhat hyperphagic. Several kinds of stress invoke hyperphagia by elevating glucocorticoid levels and/or affecting brain regions that contribute to the control of food intake. Animals with mild forms of thyroid hormone deficiency can gain weight because of low metabolic rates and generalized sluggishness; but severe hypothyroidism usually depresses the appetite. Insulin stimulates lipogenesis, and inhibits lipolysis. Some "**hypothalamic obesity**" (*q.v.*) is caused in part by hyperinsulinism. The appetite-stimulating effects have been linked with influences on blood glucose levels. In contrast, high insulin levels in the brain inhibit by acting on specialized neurons, if euglycemia is maintained. Catecholamines elevate metabolic rates; and failure to release sufficient amounts in response to food intake accounts for some forms of obesity. Cholecystokinin (CCK) is one of several identified physiological appetite suppressants. Other regulators of food intake, metabolic processes, gastrointestinal functions, and/or lipogenesis include corticotropin releasing hormone (CRH), opioid peptides, growth hormone (GH), prolactin, oxytocin, and neuropeptide Y. Obesity develops spontaneously in several

animal strains with mutations that affect Na^+/K^+-ATPase activity, glycerol kinase, mitochondrial functions, or other processes; *see*, for example *ob/ob* mice and *fa/fa* rats. In some, food restriction lowers body protein, but not fat content.

O blood type: the blood type in which erythrocytes do not express either A or B type antigens, but the plasma contains antibodies directed against both of them. Heterozygotes with A + O, or B + O alleles have A and B blood types, respectively.

OC: (1) osteoclast; (2) osteocalcin; (3) oral contraceptives.

Occam's razor: the concept that the simplest plausible hypothesis is preferred, even when other (more complex) explanations seem reasonable. It is seldom applicable to mechanisms of hormone action.

ocellus: (1) an eyespot, for example of a microorganism; (2) a simple eye located near the compound eye of an insect.

occludens junction: zonular occludens; *see* **tight junctions**.

oct: a set of genes that codes for family of transcription regulators with common 75-amino acid segments. The gene products are homeodomain proteins that bind ATTTGCAT (octamer) sequences of DNA molecules, and function as promoters or enhancers. *Oct-1* is expressed in all eukaryote cell types, and is a component of many genes. *Oct-2* directs production of nuclear factor NFA-2 by B lymphocytes. One function is control of immunoglobulin synthesis. The *oct-3* gene is expressed at highest levels in totipotent and pluripotent stem, germ, and embryonal cancer cells. It is essential for vertebrate development, including progression from the one-cell zygote stage. Unlike most other members of the group, its activity declines as cells undergo spontaneous or retinoic acid-mediated differentiation. *Oct-4* is an alternate term for *oct-3*. The *oct-6* products (SCIP, Tst-1) are made by proliferating (but not mature) Schwann cells, and in the testes. *See* also **POU domains**.

octapressin: felypressin; a lysine vasopressin analog used for its vasoconstrictor properties. The cysteine moieties in the sequence shown are joined: Cys-Phe-Phe-Gln-Asn-Cys-Pro-Lys-Gly-NH₂. *See* also **vasopressins**.

Octatensine: a trade name for guanethidine.

octopamine: norsynephrine; *p*-hydroxyphenylethanolamine; a biogenic amine formed by β-hydroxylation of tyramine. It is synthesized in octopus salivary glands, and is a major neurotransmitter for some invertebrates. In vertebrates, the small amounts made under normal conditions in pineal glands and at some other sites may perform special functions; but larger quantities formed when monoamine oxidase inhibitors and other factors that alter catecholamine metabolism are administered are **false transmitters** (*q.v.*).

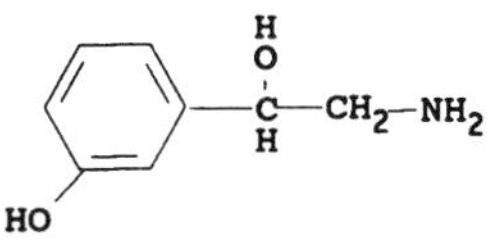

octopine: N^2-(1-carboxyethyl)-L-arginine; a metabolite made by some invertebrates from arginine and pyruvate; *see* **opines**.

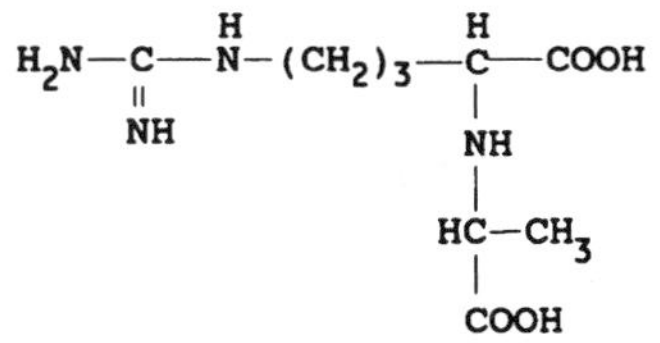

octoxynol: Triton X; polyethyleneglycol *p*-isooctylphenyl ether; a nonioninc detergent, used as an emulsifier, dispersing agent, and spermaticide.

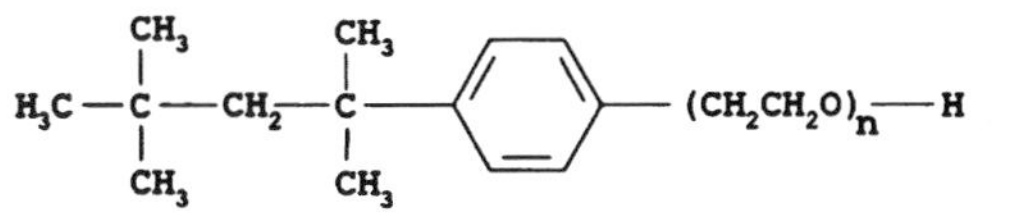

octreotide: Sandostatin; SMS 201,995; a long-acting somatostatin analog that inhibits the secretion of hydrochloric acid, growth hormone, and several gastrointestinal tract and pancreatic hormones. It is used to treat peptic ulcers, and to depress the secretory activities of pancreatic tumor cells and vipomas. It also constricts splanchnic blood vessels, and can alleviate orthostatic and postprandial hypotension. Doses effective for other purposes exert only minimal influences on insulin secretion.

octyl-β-glucopyranoside: octyl-β-glucoside; OG; a nonionic detergent used to reconstitute biological membranes, and to prepare lipid vesicles.

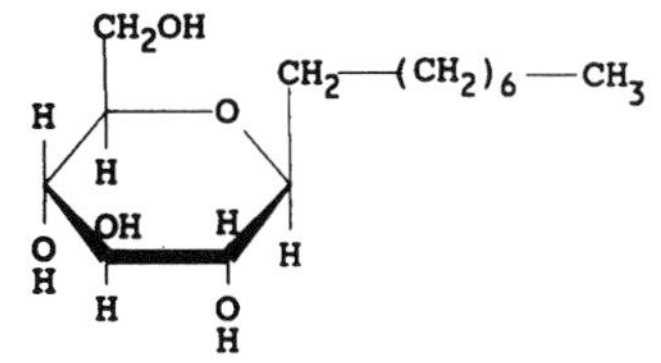

O.D.: optical density.

ODC: ornithine decarboxylase.

odontoblasts: cells that make and deposit dentin.

oe-: the British equivalent for many chemical terms that begin with e-, as in oestrogen.

OFAG: orthogonal field agar gel electrophoresis.

OG: octyl-β-glycopyranoside.

OGF: ovarian growth factor.

OIF: osteoinductive factor.

okadaic acid: a toxic polyether fatty acid initially isolated from the marine sponge *Halochondria okadaii*, but also made by *Prorocentrum lima* and some other marine dinoflagellates. Related dinoflagellate toxins include dinophysistoxin-1 (which has an additional methyl group), and acanthifolicin (an episulfide derivative). The toxins are the major causes of sea-food poisoning associated with diarrhea. OA invokes gastroenteritis, and causes prolonged contraction of vascular smooth muscle by augmenting Ca^{2+} currents and sustaining myosin phosphorylation (but it can relax as well as stimulate the aorta). The effects on muscle are not antagonized by inhibitors of acetylcholine, serotonin, histamine, or epinephrine receptors. Okadaic acid also blocks protein synthesis by indirectly augmenting elongation factor EF-2 phosphorylation. Although it indirectly enhances MPF activity and promotes the growth of some tumors, it can reverse the transformation caused by *raf* and some other

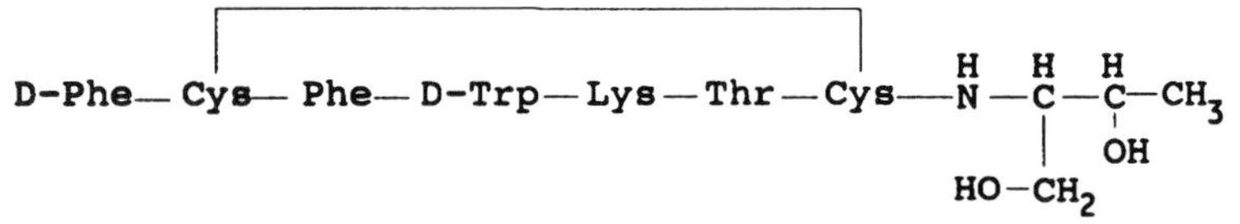

octreotide

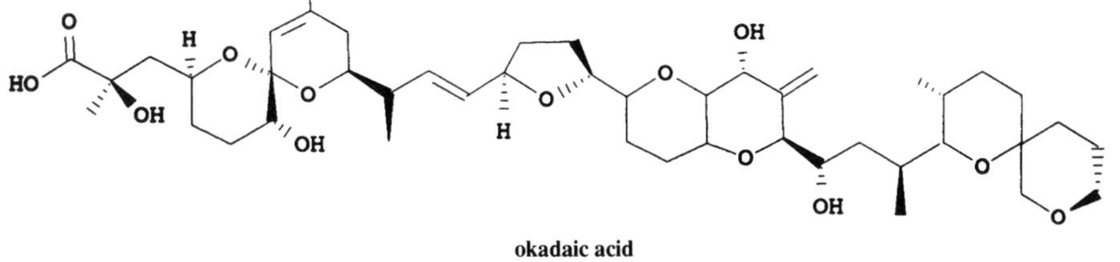

okadaic acid

509

oncogenes. Other effects include stimulation of glucose transport. It is a laboratory tool for specifically inhibiting serine-threonine type protein phosphatases 1 and 2A (PP1 and PP2A). In the concentrations employed, it does not affect the activities of tyrosine specific protein phosphatases such as calmodulin dependent PP2B, Mg^{2+}-dependent PP2C, or CD45, and exerts no discernible influences on several protein kinases, or on enzymes that dephosphorylate pyruvate dehydrogenase, inositol triphosphatase, or acid and alkaline phosphatases.

OK antibodies: monoclonal antibodies that recognize specific glycoproteins on human cells involved in immune system functions, and on their murine counterparts. The molecular species bound by some types are shown in brackets.

OKM1: [CD11b (Mac-1)]

OKM5: [CD36]

OKM9 and OKM10: [CD 11 components]

OKT1: [CD5 (lyt1, leu1), T1$_A$]

OKT3: [CD3 δ subunits of human T lymphocyte receptors (leu4, T3$_A$)]

OKT4: [CD4 (leu3a, leu3b, T4$_A$)]

OKT5: [CD8 (leu2)]

OKT6: [CD1 (leu6)]

OKT8: [CD8 (leu2a, leu2b)]

OKT9: [CD9 (transferrin receptor)]

OKT11: [CD2 (leu5, leu9.6, T11]

Okazaki fragments: 1000-2000 base polynucleotides segments, formed during discontinuous replication of DNA lagging strands, and then joined by DNA ligase catalyzed reactions. *See* **DNA replication**.

OKC: an opossum kidney cell line with proximal tubule characteristics, including ability to perform Na^+-coupled hexose sugar transport. They have receptors for parathyroid hormone (PTH), but not for calcitonin or vasopressin.

OKY-046: ozagrel.

-ol: indicates the presence of an alcoholic (—OH) group, as in ethanol, estradiol, or cholesterol.

olefins: hydrocarbons with double bonds joining carbon atoms (—C=C— groups).

oleic acid: *cis*-9-octanoic acid; a nonessential, monounsaturated fatty acid component of olive oil and other foods, used as a biological fuel, and for the biosynthesis of fats, phospholipids and other compounds. The *trans* isomer is elaidic acid.

olfaction: sense of smell, usually conscious perception via the main olfactory bulbs; *cf* **accessory olfactory bulbs** and **vomeronasal organs**. Some receptors in olfactory epithelium are coupled to a special kind of G protein (G$_{olf}$) that augments adenylate cyclase activity. Signal transduction by some others involves generation of cyclic guanosine monophosphate (GMP); *see* also **carbon monoxide**. Neurosteroids and carnosine are implicated as regulators. Some genes identical to the kinds active in olfactory epithelium have been identified in testes.

olfactory system: structures that mediate perception of and responses to odors, including not only nasal olfactory epithelium and primary pathways to the cerebral cortex involved in conscious perception of highly volatile molecules, but also vomeronasal organs that sense less volatile agents (such as pheromones) that are sniffed or ingested and send messages to the limbic system and pineal gland. Both pathways communicate with other brain regions, and they affect body rhythms, emotions, some forms of behavior, reproduction, and other functions.

oligo-: a prefix meaning (1) a few, as in oligosaccharide; (2) an insufficient number or amount, as in oligocythemia.

oligodendrocytes: oligodendrogliocytes; non-neural central nervous system cells derived from neuroectoderm. They are smaller than astrocytes, and extend fewer cytoplasmic processes. Most wrap around axons, and synthesize myelin.

oligolecithal: describes egg cells with very little yolk substance; *cf* **macrolecithal**.

oligomenorrhea: subnormal menstruation frequency and/or volume.

oligomers: tetramers, pentamers, and other molecules with small numbers of subunits.

oligomycin: several macrolide antibiotics made by *Streptomyces* strains, used mostly as fungicides. The structure of oligomycin A is shown. Oligomycin B, 28-oxooligomycin, is a laboratory tool that uncouples oxidative phosphorylation by binding to an ATP synthetase component.

oligonucleotides: polymers composed of small numbers of nucleotides.

oligosaccharides: trisaccharides, tetrasaccharides, and other compounds composed of several sugar units held together by glycoside bonds.

oligosaccharins: plant cell wall fragments that exert hormone-like effects.

oleic acid

elaidic acid

oligomycin A

oligospermia: production of inadequate numbers of spermatozoa.

*O***-linked oligosaccharides**: sugars and sugar derivatives held together by glycosidic bonds, that are linked to oxygen atoms on amino acid moieties of glycopeptides or glycoproteins; *cf* **N-linked oligosaccharides**. Most commonly, *N*-acetylgalactosamine binds to an asparagine, serine, or threonine residue; but some oligosaccharides bind to hydroxylysine. Many *O*-linked types also contain sialic acid moieties.

omeprazole: Prilosec; 5-methoxy-2[[(4-methoxy-3,5-dimethyl-2-pyridinyl)methyl]sulfinyl]-1*H*-benzimidazole; an H^+/K^+-ATPase inhibitor that decreases gastric hydrochloric acid production. It is used to treat Zollinger-Ellison syndrome and peptic ulcers. The original trade name, Losec was discarded to avoid confusion with Lasix (furosemide).

OMF: oocyte maturation factor.

OMI: oocyte maturation inhibitor.

oncofetal antigens: molecules expressed on the surfaces of normal fetal, and on some tumor cells; *see* for example α**-fetoprotein** and **carcinoembryonic antigen**.

oncogenes: tumor promoting genes; genes that code for products capable of invoking uncontrolled cell proliferation, transformation, and tumorigenesis. The types designated by *v-* are components of retroviral genomes derived from normal eukaryote proto-oncogenes (for which the prefix *c-* is used). Many can insert into host DNAs and undergo replication. Various types initiate tumor growth or stimulate progression by affecting processes such as signal transduction, enzyme activation (or inhibition),

transcription, translation, and RNA and protein stability. Some alter cytoskeletal structure, the expression of cell surface molecules (including adhesion factors and hormone receptors), growth factor synthesis and release, and/or the production and degradation of extracellular matrix components. The protein products include truncated forms of hormone receptors that act like host counterparts but do not require ligand binding to function, constitutively active enzymes, and mutated forms of growth or transcription factors. DNA segments transcribed from viral RNAs can also alter host genome structure in ways that lead to amplification of normal genes, or impair the usual constraints over excessive expression (or expression at inappropriate times). In some cases, one oncogene cooperates with others to achieve the effects. Related events can be initiated in uninfected eukaryote cells by exposing them to X-rays, ultraviolet rays, and chemicals that damage DNA and/or interfere with DNA repair. More than 50 kinds of oncogenes have been identified in malignant tumors. *See* individual types under alphabetical listings that follow *c-* or *v-*.

oncogenic: causing uncontrolled cell proliferation, transformation, and/or tumor growth.

oncology: the study of tumors.

oncolytic: capable of destroying cancer cells.

oncorna viruses: oncoviruses; tumor causing viruses of the Retroviridae family, including types that invoke leukemias, sarcomas, and other malignancies; *see* also **retroviruses**.

oncostatin M: a 28K glycoprotein cytokine made by activated monocytes and T lymphocytes that inhibits the growth of melanomas and some other solid tumors, and promotes differentiation of myeloid leukemia cells to macrophages, but does not affect normal fibroblasts. It is structurally similar to, and shares some amino acid sequences with granulocyte colony stimulating factor (G-CSF), and with **leukemia inhibitory factor** (*q.v.*). A 150-160K receptor with properties that suggest roles in hematopoiesis has been identified.

oncotic pressure: the effective osmotic pressure of the blood. It is directly related to the concentrations of large molecules (especially albumin) that do not diffuse across endothelial cell plasma membranes.

ondansetron: 1,2,3,9-tetrahydro-9-methyl-3-[(2-methyl-1*H*-imidazol-1-yl)methyl]-4*H*-carba-zol-4-one; a 5HT$_3$ type serotonin receptor antagonist, used to control vomiting in patients receiving chemotherapy.

one cell/one hormone hypothesis: the concept that a single cell makes and secretes just one kind of hormone. It has been discarded, since two, three, or more are made by many cell types. They can be products of the same gene, or synthesized from unrelated messenger RNAs. In some cases, chemically unrelated types are sequestered in common secretory granules, and are co-secreted.

ontogeny: development of an individual from conception to maturity.

oocyesis: ovarian pregnancy.

oocytes: ovocytes; female germ cells that differentiate from oogonia; *see* **primary** and **secondary oocytes** and **ovum**.

oocyte maturation factor: OMF; one or more undefined factors made in the ovaries that stimulate resumption of meiosis in primary oocytes. Progesterone is effective (at least *in vitro*) for amphibian types. It has been proposed that maturation is accomplished in mammals by antagonizing the effects of **oocyte maturation inhibitor** (*q.v.*).

oocyte maturation inhibitor: OMI; oocyte meiosis inhibitor: one or more uncharacterized small peptides believed to be secreted by granulosa cells that arrest oocyte meiosis during the follicular phases of the ovarians cycle. The presence of OMI, and a decline in its production during the late follicular phase, are suggested by observations that immature oocytes resume meiosis if removed from the follicles, that arrest is maintained if the entire follicle is explanted, and that follicular fluid extracts obtained from sows and some other mammals can arrest meiosis *in vitro*. Müllerian duct inhibitor (MDI) and gonadocrinin are proposed candidates. Follicle stimulating hormone (FSH) and the cAMP it generates may induce or activate OMI. Oocytes destined to advance to preovulatory stages acquire large numbers of luteinizing hormone (LH) receptors; and LH may antagonize the effects of the peptides. The potential use of OMIs to achieve contraception without invoking the hormone imbalances imposed by estrogen-progestin preparations has been suggested. *See* also **cytostatin** and **MPF**.

oogenesis: processes involved in formation of secondary oocytes from germinal cell precursors (including vitellogenesis in some species).

oogonium [oogonia]: a diploid cell type formed from a gonocyte precursor in embryonic and fetal ovaries. It can divide by mitosis to yield more cells of the same kind, or mature to a primary oocyte. In most mammals (including humans), all oogonia either mature or are lost via degeneration or extrusion across ovarian surfaces before birth. In a few species (such as domestic cats), limited numbers persist in juveniles.

oolemma: the oocyte plasma membrane.

ootid: a mature ovum. (Since meiosis is not completed before fertilization in most vertebrates, the ootid contains the male pronucleus.)

oophorectomy: ovariectomy.

OP: osmotic pressure.

opal codon: UGA; the triplet (three-base messenger RNA sequence) that codes for "stop" (termination of peptide chain elongation). In some mutant bacterial strains, the synthesis of certain proteins is prematurely terminated if a UGA sequence replaces a triplet that binds to a transfer RNA-amino acid complex. Opal suppressors are aminoacyl-tRNA molecules that support chain elongation in bacteria by facilitating insertion of amino acids at UAG sites.

OPC-21268: 1-{1-[4-(3-acetylaminopropoxy)benzoyl]-4-piperidyl}-3,4-dihydro-2(1*H*)-quinoline; a potent and specific, orally effective V_1 type vasopressin receptor antagonist.

open reading frame: ORF; usually, (1) a DNA segment that can be transcribed; (2) an RNA segment that directs translation.

operator: in molecular biology, a DNA base sequence, downstream from a gene coding sequence, that overlaps with or immediately follows an RNA polymerase binding site, and controls the expression of adjacent genes by interacting with repressors and/or activators.

operculum: a covering membrane or lid, such as a trophoblast component that closes over an implantation site, or a flap that covers the gills of a bony fish.

operon: A bacterial DNA unit composed of two or more coordinately regulated, tandemly arranged genes that directs formation of a single messenger RNA species, plus elements that control transcription by binding to activators and/or repressors.

ophio-: ophi-; a prefix meaning snake or snake-like.

ophthalmic: pertaining to the eye.

opiates: (1) substances derived from opium poppies; (2) compounds with similar properties that invoke narcosis; (3) substances used to induce sleep; (4) opioid peptides.

opines: octopine (*q.v.*), synthesized from arginine, alanopine from alanine, and other imino acids made by many invertebrates via anaerobic pathways of the general type: pyruvate + amino acid + NADH + H$^+$ → opine + NAD$^+$ + H$_2$O.

opioid[s]: compounds that resembles opium in chemical structure and/or biological properties; *see* also **opioid peptides**.

opioid peptides: endorphins, dynorphins, enkephalins, and related peptides whose actions are mediated via one or more kinds of **opioid receptors** (*q.v.*). Animals make

EOPs (endogenous opioid peptides). Various types affect pain perception, mood and mental functions, smooth muscle contraction, and the secretion of hypothalamic, adenohypophysial, gonadal, and other hormones. Some central responses involve interactions with receptors for dopamine and other neurotransmitters, whereas many peripheral ones contribute to fine controls of processes regulated by other hormones, by acting via paracrine and/or autocrine mechanisms. For example, by inhibiting the secretion of gonadotropin releasing hormone (GnRH) in the hypothalamus, EOPs lower luteinizing hormone (LH) and testosterone levels. Ones made in testicular Leydig cells directly affect Sertoli cell functions and indirectly inhibit steroidogenesis. LH and follicle stimulating hormone (FSH) promote EOP release, testosterone antagonizes their actions, and both corticotropin releasing hormone (CRH) and glucocorticoids modulate their effects. Inhibitory influences on tumor growth have also been described.

opioid receptors: proteins that mediate the biological actions of morphine, opioid peptides, and related agents. Major subtypes that differ from each other in affinities for agonists and antagonists, and involvements in various functions have been identified, but both the ligands and the receptors display overlapping properties and species differences in distributions. Attempts to classify the receptors with pharmacological agents are further complicated by the presence of enzymes that cleave them to smaller molecules with different properties. *Mu* (μ) types bind β-endorphin, morphine and metorphamide with high affinity, and also interact with metenkephalin, metenkephalin-Arg-Phe, peptide E, and dynorphin 1-8. They are widely distributed throughout the brain and spinal cord, and occur in high concentrations in guinea pig ileum. DAGO (an enkephalin analog) and dermorphins are selective agonists. Mu receptors mediate analgesia, respiratory depression, addictive responses, and smooth muscle contraction. They may also contribute to euphoria, and are implicated as tonic inhibitors of corticotropin releasing, gonadotropin releasing, corticotropic and thyroid stimulating hormone (CRH, GnRH, ACTH, and TSH) secretion. The mechanisms involve influences on K^+ channels, and inhibition of adenylate cyclases. "Addicted" cells compensate by making more adenylate cyclase, and transiently generate excessive amounts of cAMP. Subtypes, such as μ_1 for analgesia, and μ_2 for respiratory depression, have been proposed. *Delta* (δ) types are named for the high levels in mouse vas deferens, and their abilities to promote contraction of reproductive tract smooth muscle. However, they are also abundant in hindbrain; and the ones in the limbic system may affect emotions. In common with μ types, they alter K^+ channel activity, and can contribute to analgesia. In brain neurons, they display the highest affinity for leu-enkephalin, but also bind metenkephalin, metenkephalin-Arg-Phe, metenkephalin-Arg-Gly-Leu, several dynorphin peptides, β-neoendorphin and β-endorphin. DPDPE is the most selective agonist. DADLE [(D-Ala^{2}D-Leu)]-enkephalin is more potent, but also displays considerable affinity for μ receptors. Nalorphine and pentazocine are partial agonists. Antagonists include naltrexone, naloxone, and ICI 174,864. *Epsilon* (ϵ) types are abundant in the rat vas deferens. They bind β-endorphin with high affinity, and also peptides E and F, and mediate contraction of some kinds of smooth muscle. *Kappa* (k) types are named for their binding to ketocyclazocine and related agonists (such as ethylketocyclazocine and bromazocin). The natural ligands appear to be dynorphins, neoendorphins, and peptide E. U50,488 is a highly selective agonist, and pentazocine is a partial agonist. Nalorphine is also an agonist, whereas high concentrations of naloxone and naltrexone antagonize. Kappa receptors mediate morphine induced hallucinations, dysphoria, sedation, miosis, anorexia, and possibly also respiratory depression, and are implicated in inhibition of corticotropin releasing and corticotropic hormone (CRH and ACTH) secretion. Receptors in the neural lobe may exert negative feedback controls over vasopressin release. Many of the effects are exerted on Ca^{2+} channels. Some classification systems include a *sigma* (σ) type, proposed to mediate certain morphine effects on the autonomic nervous system, and to invoke dysphoria and hallucinations. However, the sigma types bind haloperidol and PCP (phencyclidine). Most investigators do not regard them as true opioid receptors.

opium: the dried exudate of unripe capsules of *Papaver somniferum* and related poppy species. It is the major source of morphine, and also contains codeine, papaverine, thebaine, and some other alkaloids.

opportunist infections: infections that flourish mostly when normal resistance is impaired, for example in individuals with defective immune systems, or in ones using antibiotics that kill off protective microorganisms.

opsins: 20-40K transmembrane proteins that combine with vitamin A derivatives to form light-sensitive molecules, including the scotopsins of vertebrate retinal rods (*see* **rhodopsin**), photopsins of vertebrate cone cells, bacteriopsins used for photosynthesis, invertebrate visual pigments, and related compounds made by some microorganisms that serve as photosensors and affect movements toward or away from light sources.

opsonins: substances that facilitate phagocytosis by binding particulate antigens on the surfaces of bacteria and other cell types. Some also coat viruses. Most mammalian types are immunoglobulins or complement fragments; but some are lysozymes or other enzymes. The binding of IgG1, IgG3, and IgM Fab fragments exposes Fc regions that are recognized by phagocytic cell receptors. Neutrophilic leukocytes respond to antigen-antibody complexes that contain fragment C3b (released during complement activation); and macrophages are affected by complexes that contain C3d.

opsonization: changes on the surfaces of bacteria and other cells invoked by opsonin binding.

optic chiasma: the part of the brain where the optic nerves cross.

optic nerves: bilateral nerve tracts composed of retina ganglion cell axons that connect the retinas with the optic tracts. The central fibers cross to the opposite side in the optic chiasma, whereas the peripheral fibers do not.

optic tracts: axon bundles that connect the optic nerves to specific brain regions. The *primary* optic tracts, which terminate in the lateral geniculate nuclei of the thalamus, are essential for visual perception. *Accessory* optic tracts travel to the midbrain and carry messages for pupillary and accommodation reflexes, and for eyeball movements. Fine *retinohypothalamic* tracts relay information essential for synchronizing body rhythms with photoperiods to the hypothalamus and pineal gland, but do not contribute to conscious perception; *see also* **suprachiasmatic nuclei**.

optical activity: ability to rotate the plane of polarized light. It is related to molecular asymmetry, and can be used to measure the concentrations of some pure solutes. *See* also **optical isomers**.

optical density: OD; absorbance. The relationship between the amount of light absorbed by a pure solute in a specified solvent under controlled conditions, and its concentration is defined by the Beer-Lambert law equation: $E = \log_{10} I_o/I = kcb$, in which E = the optical density, I_o = the intensity of the incident monochromatic light, I = the intensity of the transmitted light, k is a constant determined by the temperature, the light wavelength, and the solvent properties, c = the concentration of the solute, and b = the length of the path through the solution.

optical isomers: pairs of molecules that are mirror images with identical numbers of each atom type. The dextrorotary (*d*) form rotates polarized light to the right, and the *l* (levorotary) form to the left. *Cf* L and D configurations.

oral: by or of the mouth.

oral contraceptives: orally effective agents used to control fertility. Most contain a synthetic estrogen such as ethinyl estradiol or mestranol, and a progestin, both of which resist degradation by hepatic enzymes. Norethindrone, norethynodrel, or norgestrel were the progestins used for many years, but newer "third generation" agents such as desogestrel, gestodene, and norgestimate appear to be more effective and less toxic. The major mechanism is interference with the mounting of LH (luteinizing hormone) surges that are required for ovulation; but they also affect ovarian follicle growth, endometrium preparation for implantation, cervical mucus production, and oviduct motility. Several preparations that differ from each other in dosage levels as well as steroid types are taken for 21 consecutive days, during which the superficial layers of the endometrium grow, specialize, and undergo vascularization. No pill (or a placebo) is taken for the next 7 days, during which menstruation occurs. The steroid combinations are almost 100% effective in individuals who rigidly adhere to the schedules. Methods that employ varying levels of progestins (for example 0.5 mg of norethindrone for the first seven days, 0.75 or 1.0 for the next nine, and 0.5 mg for the following five), in combination with an unchanging, relatively low dose of ethinyl estradiol, were introduced in attempts to more closely mimic physiological

conditions. However, not all observers agree that they provide any special advantage, and some report greater toxicity. All combination preparations can invoke unpleasant "side-effects" such as nausea, body weight gain, and mood changes. The incidence of toxicity is low, but serious effects that include cerebrovascular accidents and liver dysfunction occur in susceptible individuals; and the risks are apparently greater in women who are older and in those who smoke. "Minipills", which contain only progestins, were advocated when it was believed that the major toxicities are caused by estrogens. However, they also invoke side effects that most commonly include psychic depression, excessive menstrual bleeding, and some intermediate metabolism defects. The progestins exert most of their inhibitory influences on cervical mucus production, implantation and gamete transport. Since ovulation can occur, the "failure" rates are higher. They have been recommended for nursing mothers (to avoid estrogen transfer to milk). Synergism with the antifertility effects of prolactin and other factors related to lactation has been suggested.

oral hypoglycemic agents: orally effective agents that lower blood glucose levels and exert other actions useful for treating some forms of diabetes mellitus. Sulfonylurea types stimulate insulin secretion, and are effective only in individuals with functioning pancreatic β cells. The mechanisms involve inhibition of ATP-regulated K^+ channels, β cell depolarization, and elevation of cytosolic Ca^{2+} levels. Biguanide types mimic some insulin actions, but are generally more toxic. Indications of higher death rates from cardiovascular and other causes in recipients, as compared with patients receiving insulin, have led to a decline in oral hypoglycemic agent use. However, recently developed agents are safer than the ones initially introduced; and the pills are especially advantageous when blindness or other physical problems impair the ability to inject hormone preparations. *See* also **phenformin**, **glibenclamide**, and other specific types.

orange II: 4-(2-hydroxy-1-naphthylazo)benzenesulfonic acid sodium salt; a biological stain used alone for keratins, and in combination with other dyes (such as fast green, safranine, and crystal violet) for other cell and/or matrix components. It changes from yellow to red over the pH range 11.0-13.0, and can be used as an indicator.

orange G: 7-hydroxy-8-(phenylazo)1,3-napthalenedisulfonic acid sodium salt; a dye used alone to stain connective tissue fibers, and to identify some cell types (*see*, for example **orangeophils**). It is also a component of Mallory's triple, Papanicolaou, and some quadruple stains.

orangeophils: aurantophils; acidophilic adenohypophysial cells with granules that take up orange-G dye and appear orange-colored or golden. Pre-staining and stain-

orange G

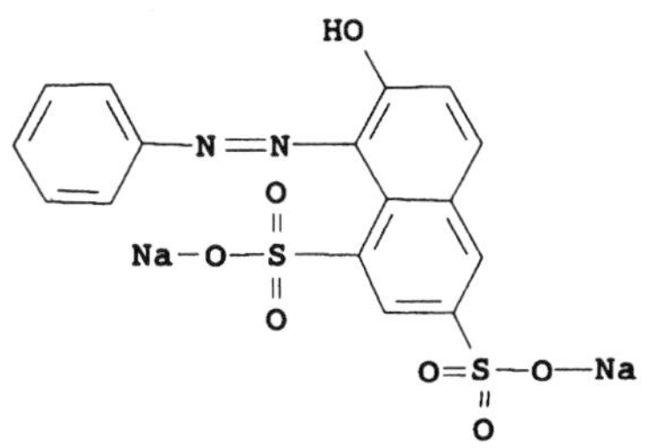

ing techniques can be varied to identify either somatotropes or lactotropes (but *see* also **mammosomatotropes**).

orcein: a brown dye initially obtained from lichens, that contains α-aminoorcein (shown below) and several related compounds. It is used to stain elastic fibers.

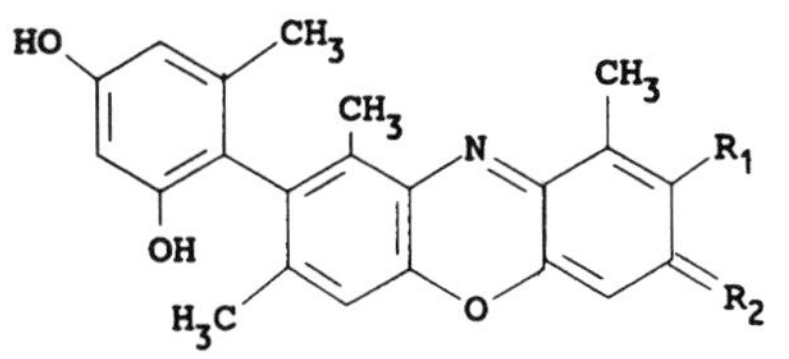

orchiectomy: orchidectomy: surgical removal of the testes.

orcinol: orcin: 5-methyl-1,3-benzenediol; a light-sensitive reagent used for determinations of arabinose, pentoses, and some other sugars.

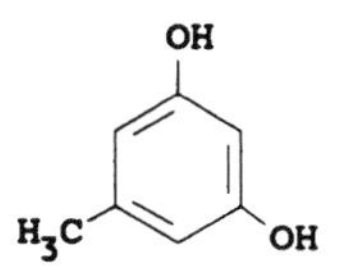

orectic: (1) having an appetite; (2) an agent that enhances the appetite; *cf* **anorectic**.

Oreton: a trade name for testosterone propionate.

orexia: appetite.

ORF: open reading frame.

organ: organum; an organized structure composed of two or more tissue types that cooperate to perform a special function, for example a heart, kidney, liver, or ovary.

organelle: a membrane-enclosed structure within a cell, such as a nucleus, mitochondrion, or lysosome. *Cf* **cell inclusion**.

organic: describes (1) chemical compounds that contain carbon and hydrogen. The simplest one is methane (CH_4). Most organic compounds additionally contain nitrogen, oxygen and/or other kinds of atoms. Although made by living organisms, carbon dioxide and carbon monoxide are generally regarded as inorganic; (2) living entities or their dead counterparts; (3) substances made by living or dead organisms.

organism: an entire living individual. It can be a single-celled entity, or a complex animal or or plant.

organizational actions of hormones: effects exerted early in life that affect development, and then influence behavior, responses to regulators, or other functions when maturity is attained. They are usually irreversible and associated with structural changes. Examples include influences of embryonic or fetal regulators on neuron survival, establishment of specific kinds of synapses, and acquisition of receptors for hormones and neurotransmitters. *Cf* **activational actions**.

organizer: (1) a part of an embryo that directs the development of other parts; (2) an entity that directs assembly of a complex structure, for example a microtubule organizing center.

organogenesis: organ development.

organotherapy: insertion of organs or administration of organ extracts for therapeutic purposes.

organum vasculosum of the lamina terminalis: OVLT; a circumventricular organ associated with the third ventricle of the brain that contributes to the control of thirst, vasopressin release, and some reproductive system processes. It contains cells that make gonadotropin releasing hormone (GnRH), somatostatin, and other regulators, and receptors for angiotensin II and other ligands.

ornithine: α,δ-diaminovaleric acid; an amino acid that is not incorporated into proteins, but is needed for growth, and for the metabolism of other amino acids. It can be converted to glutamate (*see* **ornithine aminotransferase**), and is a precursor of polyamines (*see* **ornithine decarboxylase**). The cholesterol lowering effects of high concentrations are attributed to formation of polyamines that accelerate lipolysis. In mammals, ornithine is classified as non-essential, because it can be made in the first step of the urea cycle via a reaction catalyzed by arginase: arginine + H_2O → ornithine + urea. In the second step of the cycle, ornithine transcarbamoylase catalyzes: ornithine + carbamoyl phosphate → citrulline + Pi. Citrulline metabolism yields fumarate for the tricarboxylic acid cycle and arginine (which is incorporated into proteins or used for nitric acid synthesis and other functions). Excessive ornithine is converted to ornithuric acid and excreted. In birds, nicotinic and other aromatic amino acids are excreted as diacyl-ornithines. Some bacteria synthesize ornithine from glutamate and convert it to proline.

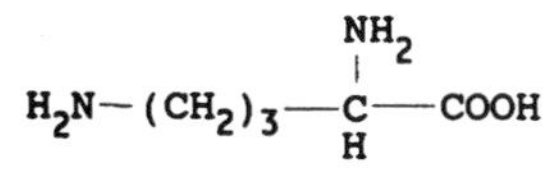

ornithine aminotransferase: a mitochondrial enzyme that catalyzes the reaction: ornithine + α-ketoglutarate → glutamate 5-semialdehyde + glutamate. Its activity is augmented by epidermal growth factor (EGF). Some forms of retinal atrophy are attributed to genetic defects that impair synthesis of the enzyme, and consequent accumulation of toxic amounts of ornithine.

ornithine decarboxylase: ODC; an enzyme that catalyzes conversion of ornithine to putrescine, and of arginine to spermine and spermidine. The polyamines contribute to cell growth and proliferation. ODC deficiencies impair growth, and can cause protein intolerance and ammonia accumulation. The enzyme levels are highest in rapidly dividing cells, for example in embryos, regenerating liver, cardiac muscle undergoing hypertrophy, intestinal mucosa (which requires continuous cell renewal), injured tissue undergoing repair, and some tumors. The activity rises before RNA and DNA synthesis accelerate in response to stimulants. Although the polyamines associate with nucleic acids, the mechanisms whereby they promote growth are not known. X chromosomes direct formation of a precursor protein that is processed in, and used by mitochondria. Prolactin, growth hormone, insulin, insulin-like growth factors (IGFs), triiodothyronine (T_3), thyroid stimulating, luteinizing, and parathyroid hormones (TSH, LH, and PTH), glucagon, cAMP, testosterone, high protein diets, and tumorigenic phorbol esters augment ODC synthesis in various cell types.

ornithine transcarbamoylase: OTC; an enzyme of the urea cycle that catalyzes the reaction: ornithine + carbamoyl phosphate → citrulline. Its production is directed by a gene on the X chromosome. Inherited defects lead to accumulation of NH_3, which invokes neurological damage and can cause death during infancy.

ornithuric acid: $N^{2,N5}$-dibenzoylornithine; a metabolic waste product formed when ornithine condenses with benzoic and phenylacetic acids.

oro-: a prefix meaning mouth, as in oropharynx.

orosomucoid: α_1-acidic glycoprotein.

orotate phosphoribosyltransferase: an enzyme that catalyzes the reaction: orotate + PRPP → orotidylate + Pi; *see* **orotic acid**.

orotic acid {orotate}: animal galactose factor; vitamin B_{13}; uracil-6-carboxylic acid; a pyrimidine intermediate of pathways for the biosynthesis of uridine triphosphate (UTP) and cytidine triphosphate (CTP). Aspartate transcarbamoylase catalyzes the reaction: carbamoyl phosphate + aspartate → N-carbamoyl aspartate. The product is dehydrated to form dihydroorotate via a reaction catalyzed by dihydroorotase. Dihydroorotate dehydrogenase then catalyzes: dihydroorotate + NAD^+ →NADH + orotate. The latter combines with 5-phosphoribosylpyrophosphate (PRPP) in a reaction catalyzed by orotate phosphoribosyltransferase to form Pi + orotidylate. Finally, decarboxylation and phosphorylation yield UTP, which is used directly, or after reacting with glutamine to make CTP. Orotate salts are used to accelerate uric acid excretion in individuals with gout. Tritium-labeled orotate is a tool for monitoring RNA synthesis.

orotidine: 6-carboxyuridine; an intermediate in the pathway for biosynthesis of UTP and CTP; *see* **orotic acid**.

orphan drugs: agents used to treat disorders that affect only small numbers of individuals, so named because pharmaceutical companies hesitate to invest in their development.

orphan receptors: cell components that closely resemble receptors for hormones and other regulators, whose ligands have not been identified. Ligands for a few types were discovered after the receptors were categorized as orphan. However, some of the "receptors" appear to function in different ways, for example by directly interacting with specific kinds of DNA segments.

ortho-: a prefix that can mean (1) normal or correct, as in orthochromic; (2) upright, as in orthostatic; (3) straight, as in orthodactylous (having straight fingers or toes). In chemistry, it can refer to the oxide hydration, and specify the most common form of a compound, as in orthophosphoric acid (H_3PO_4), or describe the sites of substitutions on cyclic compounds, for example ones at positions 1 and 2 of benzene rings (as in *ortho* dichlorobenzene [1,2-dichlorobenzene]). The prefixes *m*- (meta), and *p*- (*para*) are used for corresponding compounds with different amounts of hydration, as in metaphosphoric acid (HPO_3), or for substitutions at other positions.

orthochromatic: having a single color, a term that usually refers to biological stains, or to the appearance of specimens treated with them; *cf* **metachromatic**.

orthogonal: at right angles. Confluent fibroblasts in culture, and collagen fibrils are among the entities that tend to form orthogonal arrays.

orthograde: in the correct or usual direction; used, for example to describe transport from a neuron cell body outward along an axon; *cf* **retrograde**.

Ortho-Novum: a trade name for several oral contraceptive preparations that contain norethindrone plus either mestranol or ethinyl estradiol. The numbers refer to the dosages. For example, each Ortho-Novum 1/50 pill contains 1 mg of norethindrone and 50 µg of mestranol, and each Ortho-Novum 1/35 pill 1 mg of norethindrone plus 35 µg of ethinyl estradiol.

orthophosphoric acid: H_3PO_4. It is more stable than metaphosphoric acid (HPO_3), which tends to form $(HPO_2)_n$ polymers.

orthostatic: pertaining to or caused by assumption of upright posture.

orthostatic hypotension: postural hypotension; a fall in blood pressure to levels that comprise blood flow to the cerebral cortex and can cause fainting, in susceptible individuals when rapidly assuming upright posture or standing. Predisposing factors include diabetes mellitus associated with neuropathy (which impairs baroreceptor reflexes), anemia, and chronically subnormal diastolic blood pressure. It can also occur in healthy individuals who stand motionless for prolonged time periods, especially when environmental temperatures are high, and under special conditions (such as suddenly arising to answer a telephone when not fully awake).

orthotopic: describes placement of an organ or tissue at a site it normally occupies; *cf* **ectopic**.

orthovanadate: *see* **vanadium**.

os [**ossa**]: (1) a bone; (2) an opening, usually at the proximal end of a tubular structure.

Os: osmium.

oschea: scrotum.

oscilloscopes: instruments that record cathode ray deflections on fluorescent screens. When used to follow action potentials, the screens are often marked off in vertically arranged units that correspond to millivolts, and horizontal ones for time periods.

osculum: a small opening.

-ose: a suffix for naming sugar types (as in glucose or mannose), and for indicating the numbers of carbon atoms (as in hexose or pentose), the kinds of reducing groups (as in aldose and ketose), or the ring structures (as in pyranose and furanose).

-osmia: a suffix that refers to the sense of smell, as in anosmia.

osmiophilic: describes substances that bind osmium tetroxide, reduce it to a lower oxide, and appear black in electron micrographs.

osmium: Os; an element (atomic number 76, atomic weight 190.2). The tetroxide is used to fix specimens for electron microscopy. The name derives from the pungent odor emitted by the oxide.

osmo-: a prefix that (1) refers to osmotic pressure; (2) means smell, as in osmoreceptor.

osmol: *see* **osmole**.

osmolality: osmoles of solute per kilogram of solvent.

osmolarity: osmoles of solute per liter of solution.

osmole: osmol; a measure of the numbers of osmotically active solute particles per liter of aqueous solution at a pressure of 1 atmosphere. For compounds such as glucose (which do not dissociate) 1 gram molecular weight of solute per liter equals 1 osmole. For NaCl (which yields two osmotically active ions per molecule, 1 GMW = 2 osmoles. At pH levels that cause H_3PO_4 to dissociate to three H^+ and one PO_4^{3-}, 1GMW = 4 osmoles. In biological studies, a more convenient unit is milliosmole. *See also* **osmotic pressure**.

osmophores: molecular components that invoke perception of specific kinds of odors. The effects are directly related to the spatial arrangements of the atomic groups.

osmoreceptors: neurons, or other cell types specialized for sensing extracellular solute concentrations. They rapidly gain or lose water when the concentrations change.

osmosis: diffusion of water across a semipermeable membrane that blocks solute passage. It is a major determinant of water movements into and out of cells and blood capillaries. *See also* **hypertonic**, **hypotonic**, and **osmotic pressure**.

osmotaxis: cell movement directed by environmental solute concentration gradients.

osmotic pressure: OP; the pressure required to oppose the diffusion of water across a semipermeable membrane. Its value is directly related to the concentration of solute particles that cannot cross the membrane. A 1 molar (1M) solution of a compound such as sucrose that does not ionize exerts one osmole of pressure at a pressure of 1 atmosphere; *see* also **osmole**. Since some solutes (such as urea) cross plasma membranes and draw water into cells, a solution hyperosmotic with respect to cytoplasm (tested with a membrane that does not permit its diffusion) can be hypotonic for cells.

osmotic shock: procedures in which hypoosmotic solutions are used to lyse cells or organelles (by promoting swelling and membrane rupture).

osmotherapy: use of hypertonic solutions to reduce edema and dehydrate tissues.

osseo-: osteo-.

osseomucin: the homogeneous "ground substance" of bone matrix.

osseous: composed of, or resembling bone.

ossicle: a very small bone, for example one of the middle ear.

ossification: bone formation. The term describes normal processes (*see* **endochondral** and **intramembranous ossification**), as well as heterotopic or metaplastic kinds (in which bone deposits at sites where it does not normally occur).

osteitis: bone inflammation.

osteitis deformans: Paget's disease; a bone disease in which overactive osteoclasts promote excessively rapid bone resorption, and indirectly stimulate excessive osteoblast-mediated bone formation. It may be initiated by a slow virus. The manifestations can include pain, weakness, and deformities. Calcitonin and etidronate are among the agents used to treat it.

osteitis fibrosa cystica: von Recklinghausen's disease of bone; osteitis and fibrous degeneration of bone, with cyst and nodule formation, usually caused by hyperparathyroidism.

osteo-: osseo-; a prefix meaning bone.

osteoarthritis: chronic, progressive, degenerative joint diseases in which degradation of articular cartilage exposes bone ends and leads to deposition of new bone in the form of spurs that reduce the sizes of join cavities. Some osteoarthritis occurs in all elderly humans. Injury is a major cause in younger ones. *Cf* **rheumatoid** and **gouty arthritis**.

osteoblasts: bone-forming cells. They differentiate from osteoprogenitor cells, synthesize $\alpha 1(I)$ collagen, osteocalcin, matrix Gla protein, osteonectin, osteopontin, sialoproteins, and other matrix components, and large amounts of alkaline phosphatase (an enzyme required for bone formation and repair that is used as a marker for the cell type). They actively promote mineralization, communicate with each other via gap junctions, and modulate to osteocytes when surrounded by calcified matirx. The cells have receptors for parathyroid hormone (PTH), 1,25-dihydroxyvitamin D, insulin-like growth factor-I (IGF-I), epidermal growth factor (EGF), androgens, estrogens, progesterone, glucocorticoids, growth hormone, prostaglandin E_2, interleukin 1β, retinoic acid, estrogens, and other regulators. They make numerous paracrine and autocrine growth factors (including IGF-I) that affect their growth and functions, and release interleukins 1 and 6, tumor necrosis factors α and β (TNFα and TNFβ), and other regulators that act on osteoclasts and couple new bone formation with old bone resorption. Continuous remodeling is essential for growth of bones with normal contours and marrow cavities, and also for repair, adjustments to changing needs, and calcium homeostasis. The bone-forming activities are enhanced by mechanical pressure, which is believed to affect stretch-sensitive ion channels. Some humoral regulators apparently also affect those channels. By taking up calcium from surrounding fluids, osteoblasts protect against hypercalcemia and store mineral reserves. This activity declines when plasma calcium concentrations fall to suboptimal levels. Protection against hypocalcemia is, however, mediated mostly by osteocytes and osteoclasts.

osteocalcin: OC; bone Gla protein; BGP; species-specific, 56-65K (36-50 amino acid), vitamin K-dependent, acidic, calcium binding extracellular matrix proteins made by osteoblasts and odontoblasts. The human type, with 49 amino acids, is the most abundant noncollagenous bone protein (NCP). It normally accounts for 1-2% of the total protein content. Fragments, including BGP 37-49, with the sequence NH_2-Gly-Phe-Gln-Glu-Ala-Tyr-Arg-Arg-Phe-Tyr-Gly-Pro-Val-OH, and BGP 7-18, with the sequence H-Gly-Ala-Pro-Val-Pro-Tyr-Pro-Asp-Pro-Leu-Glu-Pro-Arg-OH, are used to study its location and functions. OC binds to hydroxyapatite, is chemotactic for mononuclear phagocytic cells, and is implicated in controls for bone formation and resorption. Small amounts are secreted; and blood levels vary directly with the rates of new bone formation and remodeling. 1,25-dihydroxyvitamin D accelerates osteocalcin synthesis, and its effects are augmented by insulin and insulin-like growth factor-I (IGF-I). Other hormones that regulate include epidermal growth factor (EGF) and calcitonin. OC is also made at ectopic calcification sites, and may be involved in the metastatic migration of cancer cells to bone. Parathyroid hormone inhibits OC secretion in normal tissue, but promotes formation of the messenger RNA in some osteosarcoma cells. Different gla proteins are made by cartilage, kidney, liver, and placental cells.

osteoclast[s]: OCs; phagocytic bone-resorbing cells that differentiate from a subpopulation of bone marrow cells similar to, but not identical with macrophage precursors (although macrophage colony stimulating factor acts on both types). They are distinguished histochemically by their tartrate resistant acid phosphatase (TRAP) content, and by their ability to rapidly take up acridine orange (a fluorescent dye). Parathyroid hormone stimulates their migration and fusion to multinucleate "giant" cells, and it, along with 1,25-dihydroxyvitamin D_3, paracrine regulators released from osteoblasts, and other local factors increase their activities. Some effects are indirect, and a few are mediated by prostaglandin E_2 (PGE$_2$). When activated, osteoclasts form "ruffled borders" by extending microvilli, carve resorption pits (Howship's lacunae) that become highly acidic, and secrete several proteolytic enzymes and other factors. The clear cell regions adjacent to the borders mediate attachments to bone, and seal off resorption sites. They contain vinculin and talin, and have vitronectin receptors. The resorption contributes to long-range maintenance of extracellular fluid calcium and phosphate levels (but *see* **osteocytes** and **osteoblasts**). In mammals (but not in birds), calcitonin promotes rapid withdrawal of microvilli and exerts other inhibitory effects. The coupling of bone resorption to new bone formation is attributed to exchange of messengers between osteoclasts and osteoblasts.

osteoclast activating factor: OAF; a term applied to factors released by immune system cells during chronic inflammation that stimulate osteoclasts and thereby promote bone resorption and invoke hypercalcemia. Substances with such activity are made by activated T lymphocytes, are present in spleen extracts of animals treated with concanavalin A and some other stimulants, and are released by some antigen-stimulated peripheral blood leukocytes, and by some kinds of tumor cells. Factors known to exert the effects *in vivo* include interleukin 1β (IL-Iβ) tumor necrosis factor-α (TNFα), tumor growth factors (TGFs), and prostaglandin E_2 (PGE$_2$). A different, uncharacterized agent that acts directly on cultured cells, and is antagonized by calcitonin, PGE$_2$ and interferon γ (IFNγ) has been described.

osteocytes: the most numerous bone cells. They modulate from osteoblasts, and are enclosed in lacunae surrounded by mineralized matrix, but communicate with each other via cytoplasmic processes that pass through canaliculi. The cells have receptors similar to the kinds described for osteoblasts, and at least some engage in limited osteogenesis when plasma calcium levels are adequate. A subpopulation with large numbers of parathyroid hormone (PTH) receptors has been described, and is believed to rapidly release small amounts of calcium (and some phosphate) when the levels fall. (By promoting bone resorption, osteoclasts exert sustained influences of greater magnitude, but there is a much longer latent period.)

osteodystrophy: several diseases in which defective bone formation is associated with other abnormalities. The manifestations appear during childhood, and can include mental retardation, obesity and impaired growth, as well as combinations of the kinds of defects described for osteomalacia, osteoporosis, osteitis fibrosa cystica, and in some cases osteopetrosis. The term *Albright's hereditary osteodystrophy* is usually restricted to conditions in which pseudohypoparathyroidism is caused by impaired ability to make normal parathyroid hormone or functional PTH receptors. In some other forms, the major problem is pseudohypoparathyroidism in which PTH binding to its receptors does not effectively couple with G protein transducers that augment adenylate cyclase activity. In *renal osteodystrophy*, chronic loss of phosphate to the urine lowers blood Ca^{2+} levels, invokes secondary hyperparathyroidism, and in some cases also causes problems related to 1,25-dihydroxyvitamin D formation and actions.

osteogenesis: bone formation.

osteogenesis imperfecta: several inherited bone disorders attributed to synthesis of defective type $\alpha 1(I)$ collagen. The manifestations include osteoporosis and bone fractures.

osteogenic: (1) bone forming; (2) derived from bone, or initiated by bone factors.

osteogenin: approximately 50K, microheterogeneous heparin-binding proteins in extracellular matrices of bone, cartilage, and fibroblasts that closely resemble bone morphogenetic protein. They stimulate fibroblast proliferation, and they induce sulfated proteoglycans in chondroblasts and chondrocytes, and alkaline phosphatase, collagen, and noncollagenous proteins in bone. They also augment parathyroid hormone-stimulated cAMP generation, and are implicated as inducers of bone cell differentiation.

osteoid: unmineralized bone matrix.

osteoinductive factor: OIF; a heavily glycosylated 22-28K glycoprotein present in low concentrations in bone tissue, but released during bone resorption and believed to be a major physiological regulator of balances between bone formation and resorption. Minute amounts synergize with transforming growth factor-β (TGFβ) to inhibit osteoclast formation and functions, promote osteoblast precursor cell proliferation, augment alkaline phosphate production, and also ectopic bone formation. High levels can directly exert similar actions. Since OIF does not augment the effects of high calcitonin levels, it may share common mechanisms.

osteomas: tumors that contain bone tissue.

osteomalacia: disorders in which bone pain and skeletal muscle weakness are associated with softening of the bones. They are attributed to impaired mineralization and/or overproduction of osteoid. Since they usually develop after bone growth is completed, they do not cause the kinds of deformities that characterize rickets. The major causes are vitamin D-deficient diets and 1,25-dihydroxyvitamin D receptor defects. Others include intestinal conditions that impair vitamin D absorption, hepatic dysfunctions that decrease vitamin D conversion to its 25-hydroxylated derivative or decrease production of the bile salts essential for vitamin D absorption, and renal disorders that slow conversion of 25-hydroxyvitamin D to 1,25-dihydroxyvitamin D, affect calcium and phosphate conservation, invoke uremia, and/or lead to metabolic acidosis (which affects bone directly and also accelerates calcium loss to the urine). When caused by barbiturates, phenytoins, or other anti-convulsants, the problems can be overcome with vitamin D supplements. High aluminum levels do not cause osteomalacia, but the amounts of the mineral that deposit in bones of patients on renal dialysis can block healing that would otherwise be accomplished by administering phosphates. Some cancers produce factors that inhibit the renal 1α-hydroxylase. (Many others invoke different problems by making a parathyroid hormone-like protein.)

osteomyelitis: inflammation of bone and bone marrow, initiated by infections.

osteon: Haversian system; the basic structural unit of mature, compact bone, composed of concentric rings of osteocytes (lamellae) that surround a central canal through which blood vessels enter.

osteonectin: a 287-amino acid, 32K, phosphorylated acidic glycoprotein of bone and dental tissue extracellular matrices that is also made in the central nervous system, and by blood platelets, fibroblasts, endothelium, and some cancer cells. It is very similar to or identical with SPARC (sialyated acidic protein of mouse endoderm) and it shares amino acid sequences with ovomucoid. Osteonectin is constitutively made by bone cells, in which it binds fibronectin with high affinity. Its presence in newly formed osteoid, high affinity for hydroxyapatite, and ability to bind calcium and collagen suggest roles in matrix assembly and mineral nucleation.

osteopenia: diminished bone mass, a term sometimes restricted to disorders in which the existing bone is normal in appearance. The causes include factors that impair bone matrix production or promote more rapid degradation than synthesis. Diabetes mellitus, hyperthyroidism, hyperparathyroidism, severe malnutrition, and hematological disorders associated with bone marrow hypertrophy are among the conditions in which it occurs.

osteopetrosis: marble bone disease; disorders in which bone is excessively dense. Some are inherited. The causes of acquired types include heavy metal or fluoride poisoning, metastatic cancer, and Paget's disease. A related condition has been invoked by viral infection in birds, and there is evidence for viral involvement in some human cases. Bone growth that narrows nerve channels can cause hearing and visual impairment and other neurological problems; and bone impingement on marrow cavities can interfere with hematopoiesis.

osteopontin: a bone matrix sialoglycoprotein synthesized in and secreted by osteoblasts, and also made in kidney and placenta. It contains an RGD (Arg-Gly-Asp) sequence, and binds collagen and hydroxyapatite. Regulators affecting its synthesis include parathyroid hormone, 1,25-dihydroxyvitamin D_3, and transforming growth factor-β (TGFβ).

osteoporosis: decreased bone mass associated with increased fragility, caused by more rapid resorption than new bone formation. Some reduction in bone mass accompanies normal aging; and the processes accelerate when gonadal steroid levels fall (under natural conditions or following gonadectomy). The terms *senile* and *postmenopausal* are applied, respectively, when excessive loss occurs in elderly perons, or following cessation of ovarian cycles. One predisposing condition is inadequate bone formation during childhood, adolescence, and/or early adulthood. Although bone mass is controlled to a considerable extent by genetic factors, poor nutrition (for example inadequate calcium, vitamin, and/or protein intake), very strenuous exercise, renal disorders that invoke metabolic acidosis and some other imbalances, and excessive amounts of some hormones exert negative influences. High levels of glucocorticoids (secreted by individuals with Cushing's syndrome, or taken in pharmacological doses for conditions such as rheumatoid arthritis) accelerate bone resorption. Other endocrine imbalances that reduce bone mass include hyperthyroidism, hyperparathyroidism, diabetes mellitus, and gonadal steroid deficiencies. Estrogen treatment instituted around the time of menopause can slow bone loss; but the processes accelerate when the treatment discontinued. Estrogen is also reported to augment bone mass when used in combination with other forms of therapy. Beneficial influences on lipid metabolism that reduce the risk for heart attacks have also been described; but the steroid can invoke nausea and water retention, cause anemia in some recipients by depressing hematopoiesis and re-instituting menstrual bleeding, and increase the risks for thrombosis and endometrial cancer. Progesterone has been given in combination with estrogens to reduce the cancer risk; and it may additionally directly stimulate bone formation. However, it does not appear to protect against (and may even exacerbate) the danger of developing breast cancers in susceptible individuals; and it can increase menstrual blood volume and negate the effects on the cardiovascular system. Calcitonin transiently slows bone resorption, but responsivity soon diminishes.

It also secondarily slows new bone formation. Calcium and vitamin D supplements are useful when they correct deficiencies; but excessive amounts lower the levels of parathyroid hormone (essential for osteoprogenitor cell proliferation) and slow conversion of vitamin D to its 1,25-dihydroxy derivative. Very high calciferol levels can also accelerate bone resorption, and cause hypercalcemia and metastatic calcification. Fluorides augment bone mass, but the new bone displays low resistance to fracture. Some other forms of therapy, such as intermittent administration of etidronates, and the use of estrogens or other agents during intervals when it is not given, are reported to confer benefits.

osteoprogenitor cells: periosteal cells that differentiate from fibroblasts and mature to osteoblasts. They divide by mitosis and are essential for maintaining bone cell populations. Parathyroid hormone is a major stimulant.

osteosarcoma: highly malignant cancers composed mostly of bone forming cells. Truncated forms of *met* genes, and loss of normal *Rb* gene function have been demonstrated for some. Some cell lines derived from the tumors are used to study osteoblast functions.

osteosarcoma derived growth factor: *see* **platelet derived growth factor**.

ostium [ostia]: a small aperture or pore.

OT: oxytocin.

OTC: ornithine transcarbamylase.

oto-: a prefix meaning ear, as in otoscope, ototoxicity, otosclerosis, or otolith.

OTF1, OTF2: *oct* gene transcription factors 1 and 2; *see* nuclear factors **NFA-1** and **NFA-2**.

ouabain: G-strophanthin; 3-[(6-deoxy-α-L-mannopyranosyl)oxy]-1,5,11α,14,19-pentahy-droxycard-20(22)-enolide; an alkaloid derived from the seeds of *Strophanthus gratus*, initially used as an arrow poison. It inhibits plasma membrane Na^+/K^+-ATPases, thereby elevates intracellular Na^+ levels, and is used to study the functions of those enzymes. It acts more rapidly than digitalis, and can alleviate acute congestive heart failure and some forms of tachycardia.

Ouchterlony technique: double immunodiffusion procedures for identifying and estimating the concentrations of specific antibodies in test sera, in which both antigens and antibodies diffuse through gels and form precipitation lines at sites of antigen-antibody complex formation. The widths of the lines vary with the antibody concentrations. In the first example shown, solutions containing equal quantities of purified antigen A are introduced into two wells on an agar plate, and serum that contains anti-A antibody (Xa) is in the other well positioned mid-point between the first two. Since the antibody combines equally with the antigens in both wells, an *identity* pattern of precipitating lines is formed. The convergence indicates the presence of an antibody that specifically binds to a single kind of epitope in both antigen wells. (No precipitin line would form if the serum did not contain anti-A; and a different pattern would be obtained if the two A wells were not identical). In the second example, one well contains antigen A, the second holds an unrelated antigen B, and the serum contains both anti-A and anti-B (Xb). The crossed lines *(nonidentity pattern)* indicate no cross-reactivity (anti-A binds only A, and anti-B binds only B). In the third example, an antigen with two epitopes, C and D (CD) is placed in one well, an antigen with just the C epitope in the second. The serum contains both anti-D (Xd) and an antibody directed against both C and D epitopes (Xcd). The *partial identity* precipitin pattern indicates the presence of two antibodies, only one of which binds to both epitopes.

Oudin technique: a method for separating antigens, in which an aqueous antigen mixture is layered over a gel column that contains the antibodies. After diffusing through the gel, each antigen forms its own precipitation line with the corresponding antibody.

outbreeding: mating of individuals who (1) are genetically less closely related than the usual mating pairs in that population; (2) share few genetic loci.

ova: plural of ovum.

ovalbumin: a 45K glycoprotein that accounts for approximately 75% of the white of a bird's egg. Estradiol stimulates differentiation of oviduct cells that synthesize the protein as well as ovalbumin synthesis, and also induces progesterone receptors. Progesterone augments the synthesis in estrogen-primed cells.

ovolarviparous: describes females of some parasitic species who retain and nurture hatched larvae in their uteri before delivering them to the hosts.

ovarian: pertaining to, or derived from the ovaries.

ovarian cycles: regularly recurring changes in the ovaries of reproductively competent females that are essential for production of gametes. All cycles in mammals include a *follicular* phase, during which follicle stimulating hormone (FSH) promotes growth and maturation of granulosa cells, partial maturation of oocytes, synthesis of some specific proteins, and estrogen secretion. This is followed by an *ovulatory* phase, during which one or more secondary oocytes and the surrounding cells are discharged. The *luteal* phase, in which progesterone is secreted, begins soon afterward. There are marked species variations in the durations of the phases, the numbers of oocytes prepared for ovulation, the hormone levels and their behavioral effects, and the control mechanisms. *See* **LH surge, estrus cycles, spontaneous ovulators** and **reflex ovulators**.

ovarian dysgenesis: faulty or incomplete ovarian development. *See* **Turner's syndrome**.

ovarian follicle: a structure composed of an oocyte and surrounding granulosa cells. *See* **primordial, primary, secondary, vesicular,** and **preovulatory follicles**.

ovarian growth factor: OGF; an uncharacterized peptide (different from adenohypophysial gonadotropins) that promotes growth and survival of ovarian follicles. Autocrine and paracrine regulators made in the ovaries known to contribute to growth include basic fibroblast growth factors (bFGF), insulin-like growth factor-I (IGF-I), and transforming growth factors.

ovarian stroma: ovarian tissue peripheral to the follicles. Some of the cells are precursors for the theca layers. Others that are not incorporated into follicles synthesize and metabolize steroid hormones, and are sources of androgens in postmenopausal women.

ovariectomy: oophorectomy; surgical removal of ovaries. Bilateral ovariectomy is performed when the organs are diseased or have the potential to become cancerous, to eliminate the sources of gonadal hormones in women bearing tumors whose cells are stimulated by those hormones, and in laboratory studies of reproductive system functions and feedback mechanisms. Unilateral excision is performed when one ovary is diseased, and to study compensatory hypertrophy or the effects of altered gonadal hormone levels on processes such as gonadotropin secretion.

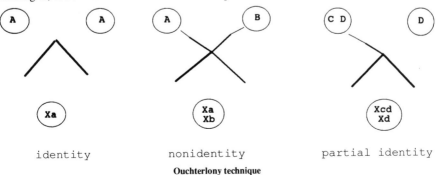

identity   nonidentity   partial identity

Ouchterlony technique

ovaries: female gonads; the sites for oocyte development. Normal mammalian ovaries secrete estrogens, progesterone and related steroids, inhibin, relaxin, oxytocin, some growth factors, and small amounts of androgens. *See* also **ovarian follicles**, **ovarian stroma**, and **corpora lutea**.

oviducts: fine, bilateral tubular structures attached at their lower ends to the uterus (usually called Fallopian tubes in mammals). The walls contain longitudinal and circular smooth muscle whose contraction is regulated by catecholamines. The lumens are lined by mucous membranes with ciliated and secretory cells, regulated mostly by ovarian steroids. Fimbria (mobile, finger-like projections) at the upper ends lie close to the ovaries around the time of ovulation and direct oocytes and their surrounding cells to the ostia. Cilia, secreted fluids, and muscle contractions promote downward transport of oocytes to the fertilization site (just above the ampullary-isthmic junction in most species). The tubes also contribute to upward transport of spermatozoa. Estrogen stimulates secretion of fluids that provide an environment conducive to sperm suvival and capacitation around the time of ovulation. Later, progesterone directs production of fluids that support development of zygotes to the blastocyst stage. Smooth muscle contractions then assist delivery of conceptuses to the uterine lumen. In birds, oviduct components include shell glands.

ovine: derived from or characteristic of sheep and related animals.

oviparous: describes females that lay eggs with protective coatings, in which embryos use stored nutrients and develop to free-living stages; *cf* **viviparous** and **ovoviparous**. The reproductive pattern, which predominates in vertebrate species that produce very large numbers of progeny, averts problems related to the increases in maternal size and weight associated with intrauterine development, such as reduced mobility and a prolonged time period during which there is continuous need for large quantities of water and nutrients (both of which increase the vulnerability to predators). Although various mechanisms are employed to protect the eggs and larvae, considerable numbers of most species die from exposure to enivronmental factors or are eaten by other animals. Most birds maintain body temperatures too high to support intrauterine development of the embryos.

oviposition: egg-laying.

OVLT: organum vasculosum of the lamina terminalis.

ovogenesis: oogenesis.

ovocyte: oocyte.

ovomucoid: (1) an approximately 28K glycoprotein in egg white that inhibits several serine proteases, including kallikreins. Its synthesis is stimulated by estrogens and progesterone; (2) a term applied to other glycoproteins with similar physical properties.

ovotestis: a gonad that contains both male and female type germinal cells. *See* also **hermaphroditism**.

ovotransferrin: conalbumin.

ovoviparous: describes females that retain eggs with protective coatings in their uteri for extended time periods after fertilization, and support development of embryos to the hatching stage, but do not form true placentas. Most of the nutrients are provided by the yolks. Some reptiles, fishes, and insects are ovoviparous. *Cf* **oviparous** and **viviparous**.

OVT: $[d(CH_2)_5Tyr(OMe)^2,Orn^8]$-vasotocin: an ornithine-substituted vasotocin analog, used as an oxytocin receptor antagonist.

ovulation: release of a mature secondary oocyte and its surrounding cells from a mature ovarian follicle (or release of two or more from separate follicles). In mammals and some other species, ovulation requires, and is preceded by an LH surge. *See* also **spontaneous** and **induced ovulators**.

ovum [ova]: an egg cell. The term is commonly applied to mature secondary oocytes. Since meiosis II is completed *after* fertilization in most species, a true ovum (with maternally derived haploid chromosomes) contains a male pronucleus.

oxalic acid {oxalate}: ethaneioic acid; a component of some plant foods that avidly binds Ca^{2+} and some other metallic ions. High concentrations impair the intestinal absorption of minerals. Calcium oxalate can also precipitate in ureters and kidney tubules. Sodium oxalate added to blood drawn for some chemical analyses blocks coagulation by binding the Ca^{2+}. (However, it interferes with some chemical reactions. Heparin is preferred for some procedures; and citrate salts are used for blood that will be transfused.)

$$CH_2-COOH$$
$$|$$
$$CH_2-COOH$$

oxaloacetic acid {oxaloacetate}: an intermediate in several biochemical pathways. In the tricarboxylic acid cycle, it is formed via the reaction catalyzed by malate dehydrogenase: malate + $NAD^+ \rightarrow$ oxaloacetate + NADH + H^+. During gluconeogenesis, it is synthesized in the reaction catalyzed by pyruvate carboxylase: pyruvate + CO_2 + ATP $\rightarrow$ oxaloacetate + ADP + Pi + $2H^+$, and the product is converted to phosphoenol pyruvate. Citrate synthase catalyzes: oxaloacetate + acetyl-CoA $\rightarrow$ citrate + acetyl CoA-SH + H^+. Oxaloacetate also participates in transamination reactions, in which it accepts NH_2 groups from amino acids and is converted to aspartate.

$$O=C——COOH$$
$$|$$
$$CH_2-COOH$$

oxalosuccinic acid {oxalosuccinate}: an unstable intermediate of the tricarboxylic acid cycle, formed in the reaction: isocitrate + $NAD^+ \rightarrow$ oxalosuccinate $\rightarrow$NADH + H^+. It is not released, since the isocitric dehydrogenase enzyme complex immediately drives the next reaction: oxalosuccinate + $H^+ \rightarrow$ α-ketoglutarate + CO_2.

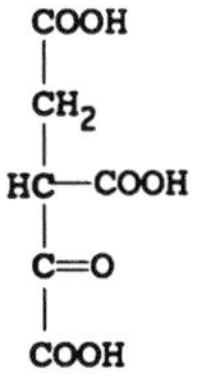

oxalosuccinic acid

oxandrolone: Anavar; 17β-hydroxy-17-methyl-2-oxa-5α-androstan-3-one; an androgen analog used for it anabolic effects; *see* **anabolic steroids.**

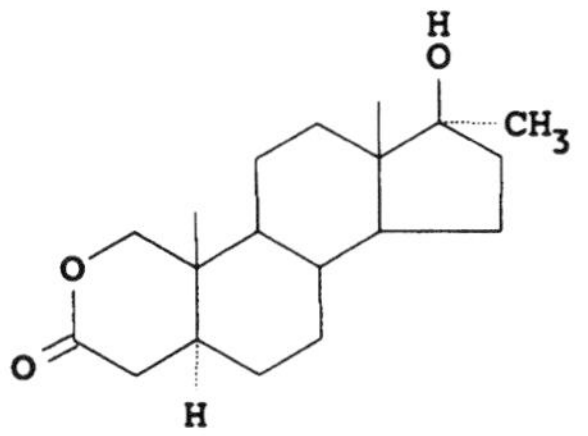

oxazepam: 7-chloro-1,3-dihydro-3-hydroxy-5-phenyl-2H-1,4-benzodiazepin-2-one; a benzodiazepine type anxiolytic agent.

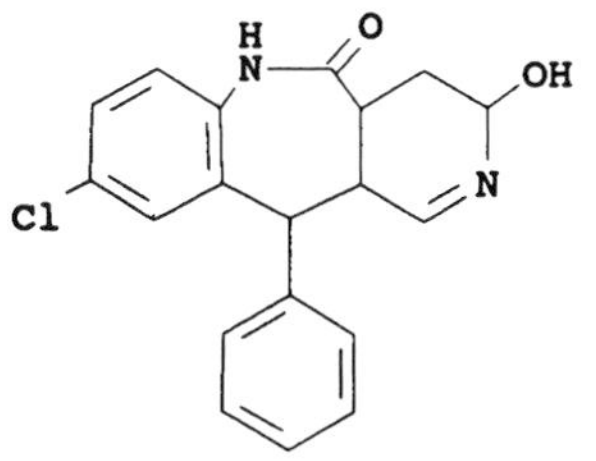

oxidases: flavoproteins and some other oxo-reductases that catalyze reactions in which hydrogen atoms and electrons are passed to molecular oxygen, and hydrogen peroxide is formed. Examples include amino acid, glucose, xanthine, and ascorbic acid oxidases. *Cf* **dehydrogenases** and **peroxidases.**

oxidation: loss of electrons; *see* **oxidation-reduction reactions.**

β-oxidation: the major pathway for degrading long-chain fatty acids to shorter ones. It proceeds in cycles, in which the carbon atom in the β position is oxidized, the product reacts with coenzyme A, and the fatty acid is cleaved to one with two fewer carbons, plus a molecule of acetyl-coenzyme A. *See* **fatty acid oxidation.**

oxidation-reduction reactions: oxido-reduction; reactions in which electrons donated by one substrate are accepted by another. Many require coenzymes that simultaneously transfer hydrogen atoms, as in $XH + NAD^+ \rightarrow X + NADH + H^+$ (in which X is oxidized and NAD^+ is reduced), or $NADH + H^+ + FAD \rightarrow NAD^+ + FADH_2$. In electron transport chains, cytochrome iron atoms undergo reversible oxidation-reduction: Fe^{3+} + electron $\rightleftarrows Fe^{2+}$. Molecular oxygen is the final electron acceptor: $O + 2$ electrons $\rightarrow O^{2-}$.

oxidative phosphorylation: reactions in mitochondria, in which hydrogen atoms and electrons donated by coenzymes are transferred through a series of intermediate steps to molecular oxygen, and much of the energy released is trapped to drive synthesis of ATP from ADP + Pi. (Some energy is lost as heat.) *See* **electron transport chains.** When the initial donor is NADH+H$^+$, coupling of electron transport to phosphorylation can yield 3 ATP for each molecule of coenzyme that passes its hydrogen and electrons to oxygen. Oxidation of a flavoprotein coenzyme molecule can yield 2 ATP. *Cf* **substrate-linked phosphorylation.**

oxido-reductases: peroxidases, dehydrogenases, and oxidases that catalyze transfers of electrons from one substrate to another.

oxonium: H_3O^+; a highly reactive ion formed in some oxidative reactions. It can kill microorganisms, and damage body cells.

oxotremorine: 1-[4-(1-pyrrolinidyl)-2-butynyl]-2-pyrrolidinone; an M_1-type muscarinic receptor agonist that stimulates cyclic guanosine monophosphate (cGMP) formation, inhibits adenylate cyclases, and can accelerate phosphatidylinositol hydrolysis. Large doses act on basal ganglia, invoke a Parkinson's-like syndrome, and are used to study the disease. Oxotremorine also acts on receptors in the hippocampus and some other brain regions.

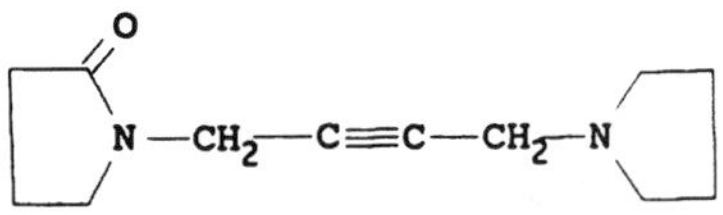

oxprenolol: 1-(isopropylamino)-2-hydroxy-3-[o-(allyloxy)phenoxy]propane; a β$_1$-type adrenergic receptor antagonist, used to lower blood pressure and to treat angina pectoris and cardiac dysrhythmias.

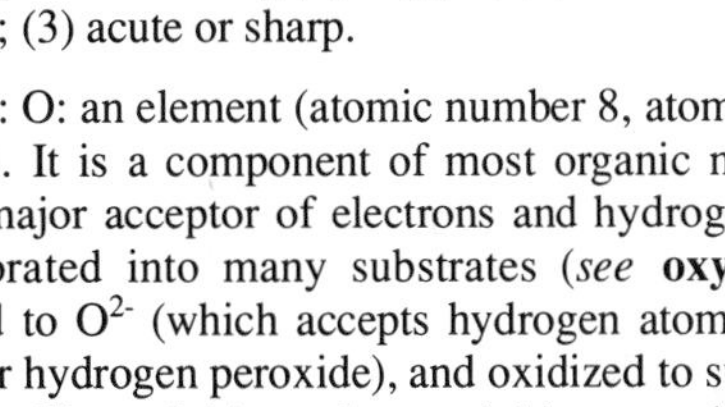

oxy-: a prefix meaning (1) oxygen; (2) acid or sour, as in oxyntic; (3) acute or sharp.

oxygen: O: an element (atomic number 8, atomic weight 16.000). It is a component of most organic molecules, and a major acceptor of electrons and hydrogen atoms, incorporated into many substrates (*see* **oxygenases**), reduced to O^{2-} (which accepts hydrogen atoms to form water or hydrogen peroxide), and oxidized to superoxide radicals. Hemoglobin and myoglobin carry it with no oxidation or reduction. Oxygen is administered to individuals with pulmonary diseases that impede respiratory gas diffusion, to patients who have recently suffered heart attacks (to decrease the muscular work involved in breathing), and to treat carbon monoxide poisoning. Excessive amounts slow the movements of tracheal mucus, constrict pulmonary arterioles, increase alveolar permeability, and invoke inflammation. Prolonged administration can damage the lungs, and cause death from pulmonary edema. In premature infants, excessively high levels cause retrolental fibroplasia. [18]O is a stable isotope used in metabolic studies.

oxygenases: enzymes that catalyze insertion of oxygen atoms into organic molecules. *Monooxygenases* (also called hydroxylases and mixed function oxidases) donate one atom to each molecule of substrate. The second usually accepts hydrogen atoms and electrons from a coenzyme and ends up in a water molecule, but is in some cases transferred to another substrate. *Dioxygenases* insert both atoms of O_2 into the substrate.

oxygenation: reversible, noncovalent addition of oxygen molecules, for example to hemoglobin or myoglobin; *cf* **oxidation**.

oxymetholone: Anapolon; Anadrol; 17-hydroxy-2-(hydroxymethylene)-17-methylandrostan-3-one; a synthetic steroid used for its anabolic effects; *see* **anabolic steroids**.

oxymorphone: 14-hydroxydihydromorphinone; a semisynthetic morphine analog administered rectally for its analgesic actions. In common with morphine, it is an addictive narcotic.

oxytetracycline: hydroxytetracyclin; a broad spectrum antibiotic made by *Streptomyces rimosus*. In common with other tetracyclins, it inhibits protein synthesis by binding to bacterial ribosome 30S subunits and blocking aminoacyl-tRNA attachment. Very high concentrations also affect eukaryotic ribosomes. The side-effects are similar to those of tetracycline.

oxythiamine: 3-[(1,4-dihydro-2-methyl-4-oxo-5-pyrimidinyl)methyl]-5-(2-hydroxyethyl)-4-methylthiazolium chloride; a thiamine analog that antagonizes the actions of the vitamin. It is used in metabolic studies.

oxyntic cells: stomach gland parietal cells that secrete **hydrochloric acid** (*q.v.*). They have acetylcholine, gastrin and H_2 type histamine receptors.

oxyntomodulin: glucagon-37; H_2N-His-Ser-Gln-Gly-Thr-Phe-Thr-Ser-Asp-Tyr-Ser-Lys-Tyr-Leu-Asp-Ser-Arg-Arg-Ala-Gln-Asp-Phe-Val-Gln-Trp-Leu-Met-Asn-Thr-Lys-Arg-Asn-Lys-Asn-Asn-Ile-Ala-OH; a peptide identical to amino acids 33-69 of glicentin, made by intestinal L cells. It reacts with anti-glucagon antibodies, and glucagon can be cleaved from it. However, it is a weak agonist for most of the receptors. Its primary targets may be the oxyntic cells of the stomach, in which it stimulates cAMP production and inhibits pentagastrin-stimulated acid secretion.

oxyphil cells: acidophils; cells with granules that stain with acid dyes, for example adenohypophysial cells that make growth hormone and prolactin, and some parathyroid gland cells whose functions have not been determined.

oxytocin, OT: a mammalian nonapeptide structurally similar to **vasopressin** (*q.v.*), but with the amino acid sequence: Cys-Tyr-Ile-Gln-Asn-Cys-Pro-Leu-Gly-NH_2. It is cleaved from a precursor protein that also yields estrogen-stimulated neurophysin. OT is best known as a hormone that is synthesized in hypothalamic magnocellular nuclei, stored in the neural lobe, and released to the bloodstream during parturition and for some time afterward. It contributes to delivery of the newborns by acting on hormone-prepared uterine smooth muscle, and then protects against excessive blood loss by stimulating contractions of uterine muscle that compress the blood vessels. Later, it promotes physiological involution of the uterus. Since laboratory animals with hypothalamic lesions that block oxytocin delivery to the bloodstream can deliver young, it has been suggested that OT is not absolutely required for parturition. However, other findings are inconsistent with the concept. OT levels rise slowly throughout the gestation period, and they increase rapidly in response to reflexes initiated by uterine cervix stretch receptors; and gonadal hormones released during pregnancy accelerate the formation of oxytocin receptors. Moreover, OT is made in endometrial epithelial cells, and the levels can rise 150-fold just prior to parturition onset in laboratory animals. The numbers of OT receptors also rise sharply before marked changes in blood levels can be detected. Uterine OT may therefore contribute in major ways to initiation of labor. The circulating hormone appears to be more important for later stages, and for delivery of the placenta. In animals that cannot secrete it, parturition is prolonged, and often associated with excessive bleeding, retention of placentas, and death of some of the young. In women, exogenous OT can hasten labor that is progressing too slowly. OT has also been called "milk let-down factor". It is released in response to suckling stimuli, and then promotes contraction of the mammary gland myoepithelial cells required to discharge preformed milk. OT additionally promotes the release of prolactin (a hormone required for milk synthesis), and prolactin, in turn, appears to facilitate OT release. Ergonovine (which mimics OT actions on the uterus) is given to women who do not nurse their infants, to control post-partum bleeding, and to promote shrinking of the uterus to a size appropriate for the non-pregnant state. Oxytocin additionally performs other functions. It is synthesized in the reproductive tracts of both males and females, in corpora lutea, and at other sites where it appears to function as a paracrine and/or autocrine regulator. The known effects include stimulation of gamete transport and penile erection. High concentrations promote lipolysis, inhibit gonadotropin stimulation of steroidogenesis in the gonads, augment prostaglandin release, and invoke corpus luteum regression. Its release from the hypothalamus is coordinated with that of vasopressin in response to osmotic and cardiovascular stimuli, nociception, and several forms of stress, and it is believed to contribute to stress responses. Factors that invoke nausea, abdominal distention, or satiety promote OT release with no simultaneous effect on vasopressin, and cholecystokinin (CCK) is also an effective stimulant. OT can lower blood pressure, accelerate sodium excretion to the urine, and augment glucagon release. In the extrahypothalamic brain, OT functions as a neurotransmitter that invokes maternal, mating, and grooming behavior, and yawning in laboratory animals, and is proposed to favorably affect interpersonal relationships in humans. Factors that promote oxytocin secretion include estrogens, corticotropin releasing hormone (CRH), and the neurotransmitters norepinephrine, dopamine, serotonin, and acetylcholine acting, respectively on α_1-type adrenergic, D_1, $5HT_2$, nicotinic and muscarinic receptor types. Additional stimulants include excitatory amino acids (evidently via both NMDA and non-NMDA mechanisms), and angiotensin II. The inhibitors include catecholamines acting on β_2 type receptors, gamma aminobutyric acid (GABA), and endogenous opioid peptides.

8-deamino-oxytocin: a synthetic oxytocin analog that acts like the hormone but is more potent.

[Ile^8]-**oxytocin**: mesotocin.

[Ser^8,Ile^8]-**oxytocin**: isotocin.

oxytocin neurophysin: estrogen stimulated neurophysin; a peptide cleaved from the precursor protein that yields oxytocin. It may contribute to hormone packaging and protection against degradation. Although co-secreted, it is not essential for oxytocin actions. *See* also **neurophysins**.

oxytocinases: nonspecific aminopeptidases in uterine and placental tissues that degrade oxytocin and vasopressin by cleaving peptide tyrosyl-cysteinyl bonds.

ozagrel: OKY-46; 3-[4-(1*H*-imidazol-1-yl-methyl)phenyl-2-propenoic acid; an inhibitor of thromboxane and leukotriene synthesis, used to block cerebral and pulmonary blood vessel spasms, and to protect against intravascular blood coagulation.

P

P: (1) phosphorus; (2) proline; (3) substance P; (4) progesterone; (5) properdin; (6) probability; *see* **statistical significance**.

p-: (1) porcine, as in pLH; (2) the short arm of a chromosome; it can be preceded by the chromosome number and followed by the locus, as in 7p12; (3) pico; 10^{-12}, as in pM (picomolar) or pL (picoliter); (5) protein, when used with the molecular weights or other indicators, as in p36. (6) partial pressure, as in pCO_2. *See* also **pp**.

p-: (1) *para*, as in *p*-aminobenzoic acid; (2) pyro-, as in *p*Glu (pyroglutamic acid).

P1: perforin.

P$_1$: in genetics, the parents of an F_1 generation. P_2 and P_3 are used, respectively for the grandparents and great grandparents.

P$_4$: progesterone.

p11: an S-100 protein that binds to and inhibits phosphorylation of calpactin protein p36.

p21^{ras}: *see ras*.

p34^{cdc}: *see* **MPF**.

p35, p36: *see* **calpactins**.

p53: the product of the mammalian tumor suppressor genes most frequently mutated or deleted in colorectal and several other kinds of cancers; *see* **Li-Fraumeni syndrome**. It is a predominantly nuclear protein that binds CAAT binding proteins, blocks DNA synthesis, suppresses transcription of *c-fos*, *c-myc* and other genes that contribute to replication, and of some viral transforming types, and arrests division in G1 phases of cell cycles. It also increases production of heat shock protein 70s, induces differentiation in B lymphocytes and certain other cell types, and can initiate apoptosis in a few. The levels are generally low under normal conditions; and a p95 protein, interleukin-6, some other growth factors, and some viral gene products are among the factors that bind to it and block its effects. The levels rise in cells with damaged DNA; and one function may be to arrest division until the DNA is repaired. Another may be mediation of the effects of cytokines that promote differentiation and suppress proliferation, or slowing of abnormal processes in cells that have escaped the usual inhibitory controls. Point mutations that alter protein configurations may be more effective than gene deletions for permitting uncontrolled growth. Animals that lack the gene can develop normally, but tend to form numerous tumors at early ages.

p55, p70: the α and β subunits, respectively, of interleukin-2 receptors.

p56^{lck}: *see* **lck**.

p59^{fyn}: a tyrosine kinase associated with antigen receptors (CD3s) of T lymphocytes that make α and β type polypeptide chains.

p60^{src}: *see src*.

p81: a protein identified in intestinal cell brush border villi.

P-170: *see* **P glycoprotein**.

p185: insulin receptor substrate-1.

p185^{neu}: *see* **erbB**.

p210: *see* **Philadelphia chromosome**.

P-450: *see* **cytochrome-P450**.

P680, P700: the forms of chlorophyll with light absorption maxima at wavelengths of 680nm and 700 nm, respectively.

p150,95: Leu M5; a dimeric cell adhesion protein of the LFA-1 (lymphocyte function antigen-1) family, with a 150K α subunit identical to CD11c and a 95K β subunit identical to CD18. It is expressed on macrophages, monocytes, granulocytes and some T_C and T_H lymphocytes, and stored in granulocyte granules. It contributes to defenses against microorganisms by binding complement fragment C3bi. Tumor necrosis factor-α (TNFα) and some other mediators of inflammation accelerate its synthesis.

PA: (1) plasminogen activator; (2) phosphatidic acid; (3) pernicious anemia.

PABA: para-aminobenzoic acid.

PACAP: pituitary adenylate cyclase activating peptide.

pacemaker: a rate-regulating component of a system, for example the sino-atrial node of the heart, or the suprachiasmatic nuclei of the hypothalamus.

pachy-: a prefix meaning thick.

pachynema: pachytene.

pachytene: the stage of meiosis that follows zygotene and precedes diplotene, during which chromosomes shorten, thicken, and separate into tetrad sister chromatids, and crossing over occurs.

packing ratio: the ratio of the length of a DNA molecule to the length of the fiber in which it is contained.

pactamycin: 2-hydroxy-6-methylbenzoic acid[5-[(3-acetylphenyl)amino]4-amino-3-[[(dimethylamino)-carbonyl]amino]-1,2-dihydroxy-3-(1-hydroxyethyl)-2-methycyclopentyl]-methyl ester; an antibiotic and antineoplastic agent made by *Streptomyces pactum* that inhibits transcription initiation and promotes release of RNAs from polysomes.

Padan: cartap; carbamothioc acid; an agent derived from a defense protein made by the marine annelid, *Lumbrineris heteropoda* that kills other worms. It is a potent insecticide that affects neuromuscular transmission.

PADGEM: *see* **CD62** and **selectins**.

paedo-: the British spelling for pedo-.

PAF: PAF-acetether: *see* **platelet activating factor**.

PAF-1: peroxisome assembly factor-1; a 35K integral protein of peroxisome membranes essential for assembly of the organelles; *see* also **Zollweger syndrome**.

PAG: pineal antigonadotropin.

PAGE: polyacrylamide gel electrophoresis.

Paget's disease: (1) osteitis deformans; (2) Paget's disease of the skin, a condition characterized by formation of carcinomas with mucus-secreting cells. Mammary gland nipples are the most common sites, but some tumors form in anogenital and other regions.

PAH: para-aminohippuric acid.

PAI: plasminogen activator inhibitors.

pair feeding: procedures in which the food presented to control animals is limited to the amounts voluntarily ingested by experimental groups. It is used to avoid artifacts related to malnutrition in the experimental group, but can impose stress on the controls.

pairing: synapsis.

paleo-: a prefix meaning old.

Paleocene: the geological epoch that extended from 63 to 58 million years ago, during which primitive mammals (insectivores and now extinct species related to modern carnivores and ungulates) evolved. It is part of the Cenozoic era, which also includes the Eocene, Oligocene, Miocene, and Pliocene epochs.

Paleolithic: the era from 500,00 to 10,000 years ago, during which humans obtained food by hunting, fishing, and gathering, named for the first use of unpolished stones. It was followed by the Neolithic period, during which food was cultivated, and stones were made into tools.

paleontology: the study of extinct forms of life. It is used to obtain information on ancestors of modern forms, and on interrelationships between organisms and their environments.

paleostriatum: globus pallidus, the phylogenetically older component of the corpus striatum; *cf* **neostriatum**.

Paleozoic: a geological era that extended from 600 to 225 million years ago. Some organisms that evolved during each of the six periods are cited in brackets: Cambrian [marine algae, trilobites, sponges, jellyfish, brachiopods]; Ordovician [fish-like vertebrates, bivalve and coiled mollusks, corals]; Silurian [marine arachnids, wingless insects, lungfishes, cephalopods, primitive land plants]; Devonian [amphibians, armored fishes, mosses, giant ferns]; Carboniferous [first reptiles, new insects, horseshoe crabs]; and Permian [new reptiles, modern insect types, conifers].

palindromes: base sequences on complementary strands of double stranded DNAs that are identical (or nearly so) when one is read in the $5' \rightarrow 3'$ direction, and the other $3' \rightarrow 5'$. They are recognition sites for restriction enzymes, RNA polymerases, and many proteins that regulate gene expression.

paling: blanching of amphibian larvae (young tadpoles) that occurs in response to dark environments, attributed to melatonin release and consequent consperion of melanosomes. Frogs and most other older amphibians in dark environments release α-melanocyte stimulating hormone (α-MSH, which promotes melanosome *dispersion*.

palisade zone of the median eminence: the external layer or the median eminence. The hypothalamo-hypophysial portal vessels pass through this region.

palmitic acid: hexadecanoic acid; cetylic acid; a long-chain saturated fatty acid component of triacylglycerols, phospholipids, cholesterol esters, and other lipids. Pancreatic enzymes catalyze its release from food lipids, and bile salts assist its uptake by intestinal cells that incorporate it into chylomicron lipids. When liberated by lipoprotein lipases, it can be used directly as a fuel (*see* **fatty acid oxidation**). Insulin accelerates its release from the chylomicrons, and its incorporation into triacylglycerides for storage in adipose tissue; but limited amounts circulate, mostly in loose association with albumins. Norepinephrine and some other hormones liberate it within cells by activating lipolytic enzymes. Some palmitic acid is synthesized in the liver from acetyl-coenzyme A and shorter fatty acids. Hepatocytes incorporate it into low density lipoprotein (LDL) lipids, and use it to make other fatty acids (including monounsaturated, but not polyunsaturated types). They also oxidize substantial amounts, and use some to synthesize other lipids. By binding covalently, palmitic acid anchors some proteins to phospholipid bilayers in a manner that affects the functions.

palmitic acid

palmitoleic acid: *cis*-9-hexadecenoic acid; a monounsaturated fatty acid with properties and uses similar to those described for, and convertible to **palmitic acid** (*q.v.*), but somewhat more reactive (and not used directly as a protein anchor).

palpebra: eyelid.

PAM: (1) peptidyl-glycine α-amidating monooxygenase; (2) pulmonary alveolar macrophage.

L-**PAM**: 4-[bis(2-chlorethyl)amino]-L-phenylalanine; a nitrogen mustard type antineoplastic agent that is toxic to bone marrow. The D-L mixture is also known as **melphalan** (*q.v.*) and sarcolysine, and the D form as medphalan and D-sarcolysine.

2-**PAM chloride**: praloxidime chloride; 1-methyl-2-formylpyridinium chloride; an agent that reverses the effects of acetylcholinesterase inhibitors. The iodide analog has similar properties.

pampiniform: resembling vine shoots and tendrils.

pampiniform plexus: a tendril-like arrangement of blood vessels. The ovarian plexus lies within the broad ligament, and facilitates arterio-venous countercurrent exchange of steroid hormones. The spermatic cord plexus provides a nonpulsatile arterial blood supply to the testis and epididymis. It is cooled as it travels towards the scrotum, and warmed as it returns to the abdomen.

pan-: a prefix meaning all, whole, or complete, as in pancytopenia.

Pan: a genus of anthropoid apes that includes chimpanzees and gorillas.

pancreas: a gland associated with the digestive system, composed mostly of acinar cell groups that secrete pancreatic juice. Although some exocrine cells secrete pancreatic polypeptide, somatostatin, and other regulators (*see* **exocrine pancreas**), the major endocrine functions are performed by the **pancreatic islets** (*q.v.*) scattered within the acinar tissue. The two components

share common blood vessels, and they interact in several ways. Neurotransmitters that regulate the functions include acetylcholine, norepinephrine, vasoactive intestinal peptide (VIP), and neurotensin.

pancreastatin: PST; peptides of the secretin family, cleaved from chromogranin A in pancreatic islet β and δ cells, that inhibit glucose-stimulated insulin secretion. Peptides composed of amino acid moieties 240-288, and 243-294, 250-301, and others with overlapping segments have been reported to exert the activity. A human pancreastatin has the sequence: H-Gly-Glu-Ser-Arg-Ser-Glu-Ala-Leu-Ala-Val-Asp-Gly-Ala-Gly-Ala-Gly-Lys-Pro-Gly-Ala-Glu-Glu-Ala-Gln-Asp-Pro-Glu-Gly-Lys-Gly-Glu-Gln-Glu-His-Ser-Gln-Gln-Lys-Glu-Glu-Glu-Glu-Glu-Met-Ala-Val-Val-Pro-Gln-Gly-Leu-Phe-Arg-Gly-NH$_2$. A porcine type is H$_2$N-Gly-Trp-Pro-Gln-Ala-Pro-Ala-Met-Asp-Gly-Ala-Gly-Lys-Thr-Gly-Ala-Glu-Glu-Ala-Gln-Pro-Pro-Glu-Gly-Lys-Gly-Ala-Arg-Glu-His-Ser-Arg-Gln-Glu-Glu-Glu-Glu-Glu-Thr-Ala-Gly-Ala-Pro-Gln-Gly-Leu-Phe-Arg-Gly-NH$_2$. Related peptides are made in the adrenal medulla (*see* **chromostatin**), in parathyroid glands (*see* **parastatin**), in pituitary and thymus glands, in exocrine pancreas, duodenum, stomach, and elsewhere in the body, and by some tumor cells. Some inhibit insulin and somatostatin responses to moderate rises in glucose concentrations; but very high sugar levels reverse the effects. PSTs also inhibit DNA synthesis and cell proliferation, possibly by lowering polyamine levels. Their release is augmented by cAMP and high cytosolic Ca^{2+} (which synergize), and by protein kinase C isozymes.

pancreatectomy: surgical removal of the pancreas. Since the consequences include loss of essential digestive system enzymes and islet cell hormones, attempts are made to conserve as much normal tissue as possible when tumors are excised. Total pancreactectomy cannot be accomplished in many species without serious damage to blood vessels and other structures, because the tissue is diffuse and adherent; *see* **alloxan** and **streptozotocin**.

pancreatic islets; islets of Langerhans; small, organized, innervated endocrine glands within the exocrine parts of the pancreas. All contain α cells that secrete glucagon, β cells that secrete insulin, and either somatostatin secreting δ (D$_1$), or pancreatic polypeptide secreting F (D$_2$) cells. At least some islets have additional endocrine components. Gastrin has been identified in fetal glands and in islet cell tumors. The parasympathetic innervation exerts mostly stimulatory influences, whereas sympathetic nerves mediate mostly inhibition. The cells also respond to other neurotransmitters, and to changing levels of glucose, certain amino acids, and some small lipid compounds. *See* also **insulin**, **glucagon**, **somatostatin**, and **pancreatic polypeptide**.

pancreatic juice: the aqueous fluid made by exocrine pancreas cells. It contains enzymes essential for digestion of all major dietary macromolecules, including amylase, lipases, and phospholipases, and also sodium bicarbonate (which neutralizes acid chyme and provides the a pH suitable for the enzyme action) and substantial amounts of calcium. The cells also secrete trypsinogen and chymotrypsinogen (converted in the intestine to trypsin and chymotrypsin, respectively), DNases, RNases, and elastase.

pancreatic polypeptide: PP; species specific peptides made by pancreatic islet F cells, some gastrointestinal tract cells, and possibly other cell types. Human PP has the amino acid sequence: Ala-Pro-Leu-Glu-Pro-Val-Tyr-Pro-Gly-Asp-Asn-Ala-Thr-Pro-Glu-Gln-Met-Ala-Gln-Tyr-Ala-Ala-Asp-Leu-Arg-Arg-Tyr-Ile-Asn-Met-Leu-Thr-Arg-Pro-Arg-Tyr-NH$_2$. Very similar peptides are made by other mammals. PPs are chemically related to neuropeptide Y (NPY) and peptide YY (PYY), but do not act on receptors for those regulators. They are secreted in response to food ingestion (but not intravenous administration of nutrients). The blood levels also rise during exercise, after prolonged fasting, during acute hypoglycemia, and following administration of acetylcholine, secretin, cholecystokinin, and bombesin or gastrin releasing peptide. Hyperglycemia, somatostatin, and high levels of free fatty acids inhibit. Since exogenous PP decreases exocrine pancreas secretion and bile release, and indirectly stimulates intestinal motility (via effects exerted on enterocytes), roles in conservation of digestive system secretions have been suggested. PP also depresses appetite. The secretory responses to meals are diminished in some forms of obesity; and New Zealand obese mice (which are hyperphagic) have very few F cells. PP has also been identified in the adenohypophysis, in which high levels inhibit gonadotropin release, and it (or a closely related substance) is present in mammalian suprachiasmatic nuclei. Additional targets may include brain, liver, spleen, and bone marrow. Different peptides are cleaved from the same precursor protein, but it has not been determined that are hormones. Avian PP differs both chemically and biologically from the mammalian types. It can accelerate hepatic gluconeogenesis and inhibit lipolysis.

pancreatic trypsin inhibitor: a 6K protein that binds tightly to, and inhibits trypsin.

pancreatin: an enzyme mixture extracted from the pancreas (*see* **pancreatic** juice), used to prepare amino acid hydrolysates, and to aid digestion in individuals with impaired exocrine pancreas function.

pancreozymin: PZ; *see* **cholecystokinin-pancreozymin**.

pancytopenia: aplastic anemia; Fanconi syndrome; deficiency of all blood cell types. The causes include autoimmune processes and some pharmacological agents.

pandemic: describes diseases that occur simultaneously in many geographical locales and spread rapidly.

Paneth cells: intestinal epithelial cells within crypts of Lieberkühn that make peptidases and store them in secretory granules.

pangamic acid: "vitamin B$_{15}$"; an uncharacterized mixture obtained from the seeds of apricots and other plants, purported to exert beneficial effects.

pangenesis: the outmoded concept that small hereditary particles (pangenes) made in various body parts replicate,

travel via the bloodstream, diffuse into gametes, and provide "seeds" for development and mechanisms for transmitting acquired characteristics.

panhypopituitarism: deficiency of all adenohypophysial, or of all pituitary gland hormones, usually caused by genetic defects or by initiated by injury.

pannus: (1) vascularized granulation tissue that contains fibroblasts, lymphocytes, and macrophages, formed from degenerating synovial membranes in individuals with rheumatoid arthritis; (2) granulation tissue in inflamed corneas.

pantetheine: 2,4-dihydroxy-*N*-[3-[2-mercaptoethyl) amino]-3-oxopropyl]-3,3-dimethylbutanamide; a component of coenzyme A. *See* **pantothenic acid**.

$$\text{HO—CH}_2\text{—}\underset{\underset{\text{CH}_3}{|}}{\overset{\overset{\text{CH}_3}{|}}{\text{C}}}\text{—}\underset{\text{OH}}{\overset{\text{H}}{\text{C}}}\text{—}\underset{\text{O}}{\overset{\text{O}}{\text{C}}}\text{—}\overset{\text{H}}{\text{N}}\text{—CH}_2\text{—CH}_2\text{—}\underset{\text{O}}{\overset{\text{O}}{\text{C}}}\text{—}\overset{\text{H}}{\text{N}}\text{—CH}_2\text{—CH}_2\text{—SH}$$

pantothenic acid {**pantothenate**}: D(+)-*N*-(2,4-dihydroxy-3,3-dimethylbutyryl)-β-alanine; a component of the vitamin B complex, variously known as vitamin B$_3$ (a term more commonly applied to nicotinamide), vitamin B$_5$, vitamin B$_x$, Factor II, anti-gray hair factor, chick anti-dermatitis factor, chick anti-pellagra factor, and anti-chromotrichia factor, synthesized by plants and microorganisms. Reactions that require four ATP and a cysteine yield, successively, 4′-phosphopantethenate, 4′-phosphopantothenyl-cysteine, 4′-phosphopantetheine, dephospho-coenzyme A, and finally coenzyme A (with release of 1 ADP and 1 P-P). Since most foods contain the vitamin, isolated deficiencies have not been observed. 3-Methylpantothenic acid blocks its actions and invokes fatigue, headaches, sleep disturbances and gastrointestinal symptoms in humans, and neuromuscular degeneration along with adrenocortical hormone deficiency in laboratory animals.

$$\text{HO—CH}_2\text{—}\underset{\underset{\text{CH}_3}{|}}{\overset{\overset{\text{CH}_3}{|}}{\text{C}}}\text{—}\underset{\text{OH}}{\overset{\text{H}}{\text{C}}}\text{—}\underset{\text{O}}{\overset{\text{O}}{\text{C}}}\text{—}\overset{\text{H}}{\text{N}}\text{—CH}_2\text{—CH}_2\text{—COOH}$$

PAP: (1) peroxidase-antiperoxidase; (2) platelet activating proteins.

PAP-I: PAP-I, PAP-II, PAP-III, and PAP-14 are identical, respectively, to annexins V, IV, III, and II.

papain: a 23.4K pepsin-like protease extracted from the green fruit and leaves of *Carica* papaya that acts preferentially on peptide bonds formed by lysine, arginine, and glycine moieties. It is used topically to promote wound healing and prevent adhesion formation, to kill some helminths, and as a meat tenderizer.

Papanicolaou stain: a hematoxylin, Orange G, phosphotungstic acid, light green, Bismarck brown, and eosin Y mixture used to determine differentiation stages and detect malignant and premalignant cells in vaginal, cervical, and endometrial tissue.

papaverine: 6,7-dimethoxy-1-veratrylisoquinoline; an opium alkaloid that does not act centrally, but is a mild analgesic. It inhibits catechol-*O*-methyltransferase (COMT), cyclic nucleotide phosphodiesterases in many cell types, and renin release. It also directly slows conduction in the heart, prolongs refractory periods, and relaxes arterial smooth muscle in the coronary, cerebral, and pulmonary circuits. The hydrochloride and sulfate are used to alleviate some cardiac dysrhythmias.

paper factor: a substance in paper towels that exerts juvenile hormone-like effects on insects.

Papez circuit: a neuron pathway of the limbic system that connects the cingulate gyrus, hippocampus, and mammillary region of the hypothalamus, and is implicated in mediation of emotional experience and expression.

papilla: a small, finger-like projection, such as a taste bud, or a projection of dermis into epidermis.

papillomas: benign skin or mucus membrane neoplasms derived from epithelium. Skin warts are the most common types. The tumors can also form in the urinary bladder, nasal cavity, breast, reproductive organs, and elsewhere. Many extend finger-like projections into surrounding tissues.

papillomavirus: papovaviruses that cause warts and other papillomas.

papovaviruses: papilloma, polyoma, vacuolating (SV40), and other small DNA viruses.

PAPP: *p*-aminophenylethyl-*m*-trifluoromethylphenyl piperazine; a selective 5-HT$_{1A}$ type serotonin receptor agonist.

PAPP-A: pregnancy associated plasma protein A.

Pappenheim stain: a mixture of methyl green and pyronin that stains DNA blue-green, and RNA red.

PAPS: 3′-phosphoadenosine-5′-phosphosulfate; a compound made from ATP + SO$_4^{2-}$ that donates sulfate in sulfokinase catalyzed reactions.

PAPS

PAP test: use of **Papanicolaou stain** (*q.v.*) to search for malignant and premalignant cell types, usually in vaginal smears.

para-: a prefix meaning (1) beside or bordering, as in parafollicular; (2) beyond, or apart from, as in paracentesis; (3) resembling, but not identical to, as in paracholera; (4) disordered, or diseased, as in paracusis.

-para: a suffix that refers to birth, as in primipara. (It can be used with Roman numerals that indicate the numbers of births, as in para II.)

para-: *p*-; (1) describes substitutions at the 1 and 4 positions of benzene rings, as in *para*-chlorophenylalanine; *cf* ***ortho-*** and ***meta-***.

para-aminobenzoic acid: PABA; vitamin B$_x$; bacterial vitamin H[1]; chromotrichia factor; anti-chromotrichia factor; rat anti-gray hair factor; a nutrient in vitamin B complexes, required by some microorganisms, but not by most mammals. Sulfonamide type antibiotics inhibit bacterial enzymes that catalyze its use for folic acid synthesis. It absorbs ultraviolet radiation and is used in sunscreen lotions.

para-aminohippuric acid: PAH; a metabolically stable compound, filtered by glomeruli and secreted by renal tubules. It is used to assess renal blood plasma flow and nephron tubule functions.

para-aminosalicylic acid: PAS; 4-amino-2-hydroxybenzoic acid; an antimetabolite used to treat tuberculosis infections. Its mechanism of action is similar to that of para-aminobenzoic acid, but it is also effective against organisms that tolerate PABA.

parabiosis: surgical joining of two animals. Since the pairs establish interconnecting blood vessels, they are used to investigate effects of substances secreted by one member on the other. The procedure is usually employed when there are indications that a circulating factor mediates a specific response, but its chemical nature and/or source are unknown.

paracentesis: insertion of a fine, hollow needle into the abdominal cavity to draw fluid for diagnosis, or to remove excess fluid.

paracentric inversion: inversion of a DNA segment that is outside the centromere region.

parachloromercuriphenyl sulfonic acid: PCMBS; an agent that inhibits cysteine proteases.

parachlorophenylalanine: PCPA: an agent that inhibits tyrosine and tryptophan hydroxlases, used a laboratory tool used to block serotonin synthesis.

paracholera: a disease that resembles cholera but is caused by a microorganism other than *Vibrio cholerae*.

parachordal: situated along the notochord.

paracortex: usually, the mid-cortical region of a lymph node (between the subcapsular cortex and the medullary cords) in which T lymphocytes accumulate.

paracrine: describes control mechanisms in which hormones or other regulators act on neighboring cells different from the kinds that secrete them (with no transport through the bloodstream); *cf* **autocrine, endocrine,** and **intracrine.**

paracusis: (1) hearing impairment; (2) an unusual auditory phenomenon, such as a hallucination; (3) the apparent ability of some partially deaf persons to hear speech better in noisy surroundings, attributed to the tendency for speakers to raise their voices.

paracyclic ovulation: oocyte release at an unusual time of an ovarian cycle. It can be invoked by psychological factors, some pharmacological agents, and large doses of some hormones, and may account for the high pregnancy rate following rape, and for some of the failures of "rhythm" method contraception.

paradidymis: a small collection of convoluted tubules, with ciliated, columnar epithelium, situated above the epididymis, and often attached to the spermatic cord. It is a vestigial structure, formed in male embryos from mesonephric caudal tubules.

paradigm: a pattern, example, or model.

paradipsia: ingestion of fluids in quantities unrelated to body water requirements.

paraendocrine: describes hormone formation by body components not traditionally included in the endocrine system. The term can refer to ectopic production, or to processes such as angiotensin I conversion to angiotensin II in the lungs.

paraffin: mixtures of solid hydrocarbons with the general formula C_xH_{2X+2}. Specimens to be viewed under light microscopy are commonly embedded in paraffin for sectioning and staining.

parafollicular cells: cells external to follicles, such as calcitonin types in mammalian thyroid glands.

paraganglia: usually, (1) clusters of chromaffin cells outside the adrenal medulla, most of which secrete norepinephrine and/or epinephrine. Some are located along the aorta and its major branches. Others are associated with sympathetic system neurons in retroperitoneal regions, or in the kidney, liver, heart, gonads, and other internal organs; (2) structures derived from embryonic neural crests, composed of cells that synthesize neurotransmitters.

paragenesis: (1) artificial modification of embryonic development; (2) production of hybrids.

paragenetic: describes changes in gene expression caused by conditions that do not directly alter the DNA allele composition.

parageusia: disordered taste perception.

parahormone: usually, (1) a regulator such as carbon dioxide that exerts some hormone-like effects but is produced by many cell types. Some authors include prostaglandins, histamine, and other widely distributed substances; (2) a hormone or hormone-like substance that acts via paracrine or autocrine mechanisms.

paralactins: prolactin-like hormones made by fishes.

parallel evolution: acquisition of similar traits, or occurrence of similar changes in two or more unrelated populations.

paramesonephric ducts: Müllerian ducts.

paramesonephros: an embryonic structure that forms near the mesonephros and gives rise to the Müllerian duct on that side.

paramethasone: 6α-fluoro-11β,17,21-trihydroxy-16α-methylpregna-1,4-diene-3,20-dione. The acetate is an orally effective synthetic glucocorticoid.

Paramecium: a genus of small, cigar-shaped, ciliated protozoa. The organisms inhabit stagnant freshwater ponds, feed on bacteria, and reproduce by binary fission. Various strains are used to study morphogenesis, host-predator relationships, feeding mechanisms, taxis, genetics, ecology, and other biological phenomena.

parameter: a population characteristic that can be measured, such as height, weight or glucose concentra-

paramethasone

tion, or one that can be calculated (for example a mean or standard deviation). In statistics, parametric methods are used for data that conform with normal, binomial, Poisson or other defined probability distributions.

paramutation: (1) the effects of one (paramutagenic) allele on the expression of another (paramutable) allele, manifested when both are present in a heterozygote; (2) a heritable mutation that can undergo reversible inactivation.

paramylon: a storage polysaccharide made by *Euglena* and some other microorganisms.

paramyosin: tropomyosin-A; 200-220K proteins in the thick filaments of mollusc and annelid muscle fibers.

paraneuron: a cell with some neuron-like characteristics (such as ability to make and release neurotransmitters), but different morphological and other properties. The term is applied to some pineal gland cells.

parapatric: describes populations that occupy adjacent, overlapping geographical locales, within which hybridization often occurs.

parapedesis: secretion or excretion through an abnormal channel; *cf* **diapedesis**.

paraphilias: psychosexual disorders in which unusual conditions are required to achieve arousal or gratification, for example fetishism, exhibitionism, or pedophilia.

paraphysis: an evagination of the diencephalon roof anterior to the pineal gland that forms during embryonic development, and persists as a permanent structure in some nonmammalian vertebrates. It usually disappears during fetal life in humans.

parapineal: frontal organ; Stirnorgan; a pineal complex component in some submammalian vertebrates. Most parapineals contain photoreceptors that sense changes in environmental light, but are not involved in vision.

paraplegia: spastic or flaccid paralysis of both lower limbs; *cf* **hemiplegia** and **quadriplegia**.

parapraxia: defective performance of purposeful movements.

parapsychology: study of relationships between individuals and their environments that do not involve known natural laws or principles, such as telepathy or clairvoyance.

parapsychosis: a transitory psychotic episode.

parasitism: a form of **symbiosis** *(q.v.)*, in which an individual (or a population) lives intracellularly or extracellularly at the expense of its host.

parastatin: a peptide cleaved from chromogranin A (CGA) in parathyroid glands that inhibits parathyroid hormone secretion, and may function as an autocrine or paracrine regulator. Its amino acid sequence (identical to CGA 251-294), is: Glu-Ser-Arg-Ser-Glu-Ala-Leu-Ala-Val-Asp-Gly-Ala-Gly-Lys-Pro-Glu-Ala-Glu-Glu-Ala-Gln-Asp-Pro-Glu-Gly-Lys-Gly-Glu-Gln-Glu-His-Ser-Gln-Gln-Glu-Lys-Glu-Glu-Glu-Glu-Met-Ala-Val.

parasympathetic system: the division of the autonomic nervous system most active during nutrient digestion and rest. Most preganglionic neuron cell bodies originate in the brain and sacral spinal cord, extend long axons, and synapse with postganglionic neurons in or near the target organs. Acetylcholine, which acts on muscarinic type receptors, is the major neurotransmitter released by postganglionic axons. The targets include the heart, gut, lungs, kidneys, urinary bladder, genitalia, and several endocrine and exocrine glands. *Cf* **sympathetic system**.

parathion: diethyl-*p*-nitrophenyl monothiophosphate, DNTP; a potent acetylcholinesterase inhibitor, used as an insecticide and ascaricide.

parathormone: parathyroid hormone.

parathyrin: parathyroid hormone.

parathyroid glands: small endocrine glands in mammals, birds, reptiles, and amphibians (but not fishes) that contain chief cells which secrete parathyroid hormone and parathyroid secretory protein (PSP, chromogranin A); *see* also **parastatin**. Some additionally have oxyphil cells of unknown function. The secretory cells originate in the neural crests. In humans and some other mammals, most migrate to, and are incorporated within the thyroid gland capsules; but a few sometimes colonize the thymus gland, esophagus, and/or trachea. In some other species, the glands regularly reside in the thymus, or along the sides of the aorta. Humans, rats, and many others usually have two well-defined glands. Guinea pigs and ruminants and are among the species that typically have four.

parathyroid hormone: PTH; parathormone; parathyrin; species-specific 84-amino acid hormones that regulate calcium and phosphorus metabolism. The parathyroid glands are the major (and possibly sole) sources of circulating PTH, but a related regulator is made in the skin and brain; *see* **parathyroid-like polypeptide**. The human type has the amino acid sequence: Ser-Val-Ser-Glu-Ile-Gln-Leu-Met-His-Asn-Leu-Gly-Lys-His-Leu-Asn-Ser-Met-Glu-Arg-Val-Glu-Trp-Leu-Arg-Lys-Lys-Leu-Gln-Asp-Val-His-Asn-Phe-Val-Ala-Leu-Gly-Ala-Pro-Leu-Ala-Pro-Arg-Asp-Ala-Gly-Ser-Gln-Arg-Pro-Arg-Lys-Lys-Glu-Asp-Asn-Val-Leu-Val-Glu-Ser-His-Glu-Lys-Ser-Leu-Gly-Glu-Ala-Asp-Lys-Ala-Asp-Val-Leu-Thr-Lys-Ala-Lys-Ser-Gln. The first 34 amino acids bind to the receptor and exert the known actions. In bone, PTH stimulates osteoprogenitor cell proliferation, inhibits osteoblast synthesis of collagen, alkaline phosphatase, and other proteins, and promotes generation and/or release of messengers that act on osteoclasts. It can rapidly augment the osteolytic activities of osteocytes, in part by accelerating glycolysis and inhibiting isocitric dehydrogenase; and it accelerates osteoclast precursor cell migration and fusion. Although physiological amounts are required to maintain bone cell renewal, high levels support bone resorption; and excessive amounts can cause metastatic calcification. In the kidneys, it induces cholecalciferol-1α-hydroxylase (an enzyme required for formation of 1,25-dihydroxyvitamin D), promotes phosphate and bicarbonate excretion, facilitates calcium reabsorption, and stimulates gluconeogenesis. The net effects on blood plasma include elevation of both Ca^{2+} levels and Ca:P ratios, and lowering of inorganic phosphate levels. PTH also affects magnesium levels; and high concentrations can invoke metabolic acidosis. Additionally, it regulates milk calcium content, dilates visceral blood vessels, promotes lipolysis, and stimulates mitosis in lymphocytes. The mechanisms involve increased cell Ca^{2+} uptake, cAMP generation, and phosphatidylinositol hydrolysis. High circulating Ca^{2+} inhibits PTH release and accelerates hormone destruction in parathyroid glands. Parastatin and calciferol hormones also inhibit the secretion, whereas calcitonin stimulates.

parathyroid hormone-like polypeptide: PTH-LP; parathyroid hormone related protein, PTHrP; humoral hypercalcemic factor of malignancy, HHM; large peptides, initially identified as secretory products of squamous cell carcinomas that invoke hypercalcemia and hypophosphatemia. At least three forms (with 139, 141, and 173 amino acid moieties) have been identified in human blood. The two longer ones contain all of the 139 residues of the shortest type, and are believed to be derived via differential splicing of a single premessenger RNA. The first 13 *N*-terminal moieties are similar to those of PTH; and the peptides activate parathyroid hormone receptors. However, although equipotent with PTH for bone, they are less effective in kidney assay systems, and it has been suggested that they act physiologically on different receptors. Small amounts of PTH-LP circulate in healthy humans; and renal disease leads to accumulation of *C*-terminal fragments. Substantial amounts are made by epidermal stratum spinosum keratinocytes, in which PTH-LP appears to be an autocrine stimulant of growth and differentiation. It is also made by parathyroid and adrenal glands, and in the central nervous system, and is present in bone and gastrointestinal epithelium. Lactation induces the peptide in mammary glands, with milk concentrations 1000-10,000 times those of blood. PTH-LP stimulates mammary gland growth, accelerates calcium absorption in nursing infants, and may regulate other aspects of calcium metabolism. In the placenta, PTH-LP promotes calcium transfer from maternal to fetal blood, and is present in developing fetal gastrointestinal

tract, liver, kidney, smooth and striated muscle, thyroid and parathyroid glands, and bone cells (both osteoblasts and osteocytes). High concentrations can transform cells.

parathyroid secretory protein: PSP; a 70K acidic glycoprotein similar to or identical with chromogranin A, made in parathyroid glands. It is the precursor of **parastatin** (*q.v.*). Although stored in secretory granules that contain PTH, its release does not parallel that of parathyroid hormone. It may directly regulate intracellular transport of pro-parathyroid hormone, and inhibit PTH secretion.

paratope: the component of an immunoglobulin to which an antigen epitope binds.

paraventricular nuclei: PVN; usually, (1) bilateral neuron cell body clusters in hypothalamic regions that border the third ventricle of the brain. They contain magnocellular neurons that secrete vasopressin, oxytocin, and the related neurophysins, and parvicellular types that secrete thyrotropin releasing hormone (TRH) and other regulators, and contribute to the regulation of food intake, autonomic nervous system activities, gonadotropin secretion, growth hormone secretion (via somatostatin), and other functions; (2) neuron clusters in the dorsomedial ventricular wall of the thalamus.

paraxanthine: 1,7-dimethyl xanthine; a ligand for adenosine receptors that also binds to D_1 dopamine types.

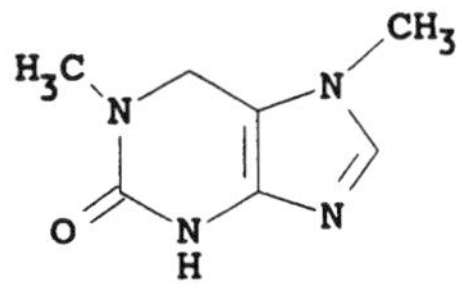

parenchyma: the components of an organ that perform its major functions, for example the hepatocytes of the liver, or the secretory (as opposed to the duct wall or blood vessel components) of a gland; *cf* **stroma**. Typically, the cells are thin-walled, with abundant cytoplasm, and are supported by vascularized connective tissue.

parenteral: by some route other than the mouth; describes, for example intravenous, intraspinal, subcutaneous, or intramuscular administration.

paresis: weakness; partial paralysis.

paresthesias: sensations unrelated to external stimuli, for example "pins and needles".

pargyline: *N*-methyl-*N*-2-propynylbenzenemethanamine; an inhibitor of both A and B type monoamine oxidases that crosses the blood-brain barrier. Its ability to lower blood pressure is attributed to influences on $α_2$-type noradrenergic receptors. By disrupting catecholamine metabolism, it augments prolactin production. When injected into neonatal rodents, it facilitates androgenization and advances puberty in females, and impairs organizational effects of androgens on mating behavior in males.

parietal lobes: bilateral lobes of the cerebrum, located posterior to the frontal, anterior to the occipital, and supe-

pargyline

rior to the temporal lobes. The parietal cortex contains the somesthetic areas.

parietal cells: usually (1) the oxyntic, hydrochloric acid producing cells of the stomach; (2) peripherally located cells, for example in the walls of an organ.

parietal eyes: "third eyes" of lizards and some other nonmammalian vertebrates. They are pineal complex components with photoreceptors that mediate effects of environmental light on thermoregulation and other functions, but are not involved in visual perception.

parity: refers to the numbers of successful pregnancies. A women of parity 0 has borne no live infants (but may have been pregnant). Parity 1 indicates that a single successful pregnancy has led to the birth of one or more live infants.

Parkinsonism: symptoms resembling those of Parkinson's disease that are invoked by prolonged use of "antipsychotic" agents that block dopamine receptors, or by other chemicals; *see* **MPTP**. In some cases, they abate when the medication is discontinued.

Parkinson's disease: a progressive neurological disease attributed in part to degeneration of dopaminergic neurons within the substantia nigra. The symptoms include muscle rigidity, excessive salivation, tremors, and involuntary movements. *See* also **dihydroxyphenylalanine**, and **selegiline**.

Parlodel: bromocriptine mesylate; *see* **bromocriptine**.

parotid glands: large salivary glands, located below the ears, that produce mostly watery secretions (with little or no mucus). They receive postganglionic fibers from the parasympathetic otic, and sympathetic superior cervical ganglia.

parotid hormone: a parotid gland product proposed to retard tooth decay, and to be regulated by a hypothalamic parotid hormone release factor. It may be related to, or the same as parotin.

parotin: an acidic globulin made by parotid glands that stimulates growth of mesenchyme-derived tissues and tooth calcification, promotes leukocytosis, and invokes hypocalcemia.

paroxysmal nocturnal hemoglobinuria: a form of hemolytic anemia, in which red blood cells are fragile, and hemoglobin intermittently enters the urine at night. It can be caused by deficiency of decay accelerating factor (an inhibitor of the complement activation pathway), LFA-3 (lymphocyte function associated antigen-3), FcγRIII (the complement receptor on several cell types), or other glycophospholipid anchored proteins.

pars: a division or part.

pars distalis: the largest component of the adenohypophysis, located farthest from the brain. It derives mostly from Rathke's pouch, but contains neuroendocrine cells that migrate in from neural tissue. Morphological features, staining properties, and binding to antibodies directed against specific hormones are used to distinguish somatotropes, corticotropes (corticolipotropes), thyrotropes, gonadotropes, and lactotropes. However, some cell types do not contain visible secretory granules, some secrete more than one kind of hormone (*see* **somatomammotropes**), a few bind three or more kinds of antibodies, and specialized gonadotropes that secrete just one of the gonadotropins have been described (*see* **folliculotropes** and **interstitiotropes**). It has been proposed that mature types develop from stem cells capable of differentiation along two or more pathways, and that microenvironments affect the processes. In many species, a distinct **pars intermedia** (*q.v.*) develops. It is mostly under neural control. Hormones made in the hypothalamus and delivered via hypothalamo-hypophysial portal blood vessels regulate the morphology and secretory functions. Most stimulate (*see* table, and **hypothalamic releasing hormones**); but a few (marked by asterisks) inhibit. Adenohypophysial hormones travel via the bloodstream to target glands. Hormones made by them exert mostly inhibitory influences on the adenohypophysis, and some additionally act on the hypothalamus (which is also controlled by numerous neurotransmitters). Adenohypophysial cells also make paracrine regulators that act on neighboring types; and there are many interactions with the immune system. *See* also **anterior pituitary** and **folliculo-stellate cells**.

pars intermedia: a component of the adenohypophysis that develops from the part of Rathke's pouch that contacts developing hypothalamic neurons, and contains cells that synthesize and secrete α-MSH, β-endorphin, and other regulators; *see* also **corticotropin like intermediate peptide**. It has a limited blood supply and is regulated mostly by dopamine and other neurotransmitters that inhibit MSH release; *see* also **melanocyte inhibiting** and **melanocyte stimulating hormones**. The pars intermedia is large in camels, llamas, and other mammals that are highly resistant to water deprivation. It never forms in birds and some other vertebrates in which no brain contact is made during development. In humans, it is believed to function during fetal life, but it deteriorates as the gland matures, and is represented by cells scattered within other parts of the hypophysis. *See* also **neurointermediate lobe**.

pars nervosa: usually (1) the neural lobe of the pituitary gland; (2) the neurohypophysis.

pars recta: a straight part, such as the nonconvoluted portion of a nephron tubule.

pars tuberalis: a component of the adenohypophysis that forms a collar around the infundibulum. The hypothalamo-hypophysial blood vessels pass through it and provide functional connections with the hypothalamus. It contains cells that secrete gonadotropins and other hormones, and have melatonin receptors.

Cell Type	Major Hormones	Major Hypothalamic Regulators	Target Hormones
Thyrotrope	TSH	TRH	T_3
Corticotrope	ACTH β-endorphin	CRH	Glucocorticoids
Somatotrope	GH	GRH, Somatostatin*	IGF-I
Gonadotrope	FSH, LH	GnRH	Androgens Estrogens Inhibins (Activins stimulate)
Lactotrope	PRL	PIF* GAP* VIP	
Folliculo- Stellate	bFGF, Interleukins		
Melanotropes	α-MSH	neurotransmitters	

parthenogenesis: parthogenesis; development of an individual from an unfertilized ovum. This form of reproduction is used by some reptiles and many insect species; and it occurs spontaneously (to a limited extent) in turkeys and other birds. It can be accomplished in amphibians by subjecting oocytes to nonspecific stimuli such as pin pricks. (Mammalian oocytes similarly stimulated go through several cleavage stages, but the embryos die because placenta formation requires sperm DNA.) When only a secondary oocyte is involved, all alleles are identical with ones of the parent cell, but the individual can be diploid if the chromosomes replicate prior to cleavage. (Some lizards are triploid.) Nondisjunction can lead to mosaicism, and incorporation of a polar body to chimerism. In amphibians with XX/XY chromosome patterns, only an X is derived from the oocyte, and all progeny are female. In birds, a Z chromosome is essential for survival, and all progeny are male (since they can develop only from oocytes with Z chromosomes). In insect species in which sex determination depends on the relative numbers of autosomes as compared with sex chromosomes, the parthenogenetic progeny are male. *See* also **gynogenesis**.

partial pressure: the contribution of one component to the total pressure exerted by a gas mixture. For example, if air at atmospheric pressure is 20.7% oxygen, the partial pressure of oxygen (pO_2) is 157.3mm (20.7% of 760mm). Partial pressures are useful for estimating diffusion rates of individual gas types in mixtures. Oxygen is expected to undergo net diffusion from outside air to lung alveoli, because the pO_2 of atmospheric air (157.3 mm in the example cited) is much higher than the pO_2 in lungs (approximately 100mm). Carbon dioxide is expected to diffuse outward more rapidly, since the pCO_2 of alveolar air is around 40 mm, whereas that of atmospheric is around 0.3 mm.

partial thromboplastin time: PTT; a sensitive test for the ability of blood to coagulate. The sample is treated with citrate (which prevents clotting by binding Ca^{2+}), and is then mixed with phospholipids. The time required to form clots after calcium salts are added is measured.

particulate: containing discrete particles, a term applied to enzymes and other compounds in cell homogenates that are bound to plasma, endoplasmic reticulum, or other membranes.

partition coefficient: the ratio, after equilibrium is attained, of the concentration of a solute in one solvent to its concentration in another. Differences in solubility are used to separate molecules (*see* **chromatography**). When one solvent is hydrophobic and the other hydrophilic, the ratio provides a measure of the ease of penetration through membrane lipid bilayers.

partricin: a heptaene macrolide antibiotic complex made by *Streptomyces aureofaciens* that disrupts membrane transport, and is used to treat benign prostatic hypertrophy. In the structure shown, R = CH_3 for partricin A, and H for partricin B.

parturition: the process of giving birth; labor and the associated uterine contractions, delivery of the fetus, and expulsion of the placenta.

parvalbumin: a 12K calcium-binding protein in fish muscle related to calmodulins.

parvicellular: parvocellular; having small cells; *cf* **magnocellular**. The term describes clusters of small neuron cell bodies in the brain. Some in hypothalamic parvicellular nuclei synthesize and release thyrotropin, gonadotropin, corticotropin, and growth hormone releasing hormones (TRH, LRH, CRH, and GRH), and other regulators.

Parvoviridae: a class of pathogenic DNA viruses. Some have single-stranded genomes and require helper viruses to replicate.

PAS: (1) periodic acid-Schiff; (2) para-aminosalicylic acid.

passenger: in molecular biology, a DNA segment that is spliced and inserted into a vehicle for cloning.

passenger cells: B lymphocytes, monocytes, macrophages, and Langerhans cells that express class II histocompatibility antigens and contribute to graft rejection. Some migrate from the graft to lymph nodes, where they release molecules that invoke immune system reactions.

passive: describes processes such as diffusion that do not require energy input (*cf* **active transport**). *See* also **passive immunity**.

passive cutaneous anaphylaxis: PCA; localized responses induced when intradermal injections of sera from sensitized animals with antibodies that bind to mast cell IgE receptors are followed after some time by intravenous injections of the associated antigens. Antigen-antibody complexes that form at the skin sites cause release of histamine, which augments blood vessel permeability. A dye such as Evans blue administered along with the antigens leaks from the vessels.

passive hemolysis: complement-mediated destruction of antibody-coated erythrocytes.

passive immunity: ability to mount immune system attacks against microorganisms and toxins, via mechanisms available before the antigen is encountered; *cf* **active immunity**. The mediators can be constitutively produced antibodies or other substances that initiate responses, or ones acquired by ingestion or injection.

passive transfer: initiation of an immune response (or part of one) by administration of substances from another individual of the same species. *Adoptive* transfer, mediated by lymphocytes from sensitized donors, can invoke delayed hypersensitivity in recipients injected with the same antigen. *Humoral* transfer is accomplished with donor antibodies.

passive transport: diffusion of molecules or ions down concentration gradients. It can be mediated by carriers, but does not require outside energy sources. *Cf* **active transport**.

Pasteur effect: the slowing of glycolysis that occurs in the presence of oxygen, attributed to ATP and citrate inhibition of the associated enzymes.

patch clamping: several techniques for studying electrical activities of cells that involve formation of seals with high electrical resistance between micropipettes and small portions of plasma membranes. If the cytoplasmic face of a seal is totally surrounded by membrane, current that enters the pipette via ion channels within the region can be recorded. Changes in the whole cell are observed if the seal is ruptured by suction to establish continuity between the cell interior and the pipette fluid. If the pipette is then pulled away from the cell, membrane fragments organize around the pipette tip to form an "outside-in" patch whose properties can be studied in solutions of various ion concentrations. An "inside-out" patch forms if the pipette is withdrawn without suction, since a segment of the membrane then folds over the pipette. *See* also **voltage clamping**.

patching: passive, ligand-mediated redistribution of membrane proteins that leads to formation of large clusters of molecules capable of establishing cross-links. Many ligands promote receptor patching that contributes to (or is essential for) the actions. In some cases, lectins and divalent antibodies mimic the effects of the ligands. *See* also **capping**.

patch tests: procedures for identifying agents that invoke allergic contact dermatitis. Substances suspected of causing the reactions are applied to the skin (on supports, such as cotton or filter paper). After 24-48 hours, the sites are examined for erythema, vesiculation, and edema.

pathogen[s]: disease-producing microorganisms.

pathogenic: describes conditions or agents that cause disease.

pathogen related proteins: PR; proteins that contribute to plant defenses against microorganisms and feeders. *See* **hypersensitive responses**, **phytoalexins**, **jasmomic acid**, and **systemin**.

pavementing: leukocyte adherence to inflamed blood vessel epithelia.

Pb: lead.

PBI: protein bound iodine.

PBL: peripheral blood lymphocytes.

PBN: phenyl *N-tert*-butylnitrone; *N-tert*-butyl-α-phenyl-nitrone; a spin trapping agent that protects against oxidative damage by combing with free radicals and by

partricin

increasing the activities of neutral proteases that destroy oxidized proteins.

PBN

PBZ: tripelennamine.

PC: phosphatidylcholine.

PC1, PC2, PC3: enzymes that cleave prohormones at specific sites to yield the active products; *see* **prohormone convertases**.

PC12: a rat cell line derived from a pheochromocytoma, used to study catecholamine and nerve growth factor functions, hormone receptors, and stimulus-secretion coupling.

PCA: passive cutaneous anaphylaxis.

P-cadherin: *see* P-**cadherin**.

PCB: polychlorinated biphenyls.

P cells: (1) Paneth cells; (2) cells that secrete substance P; (3) persisting cells; (4) "principal cells" of renal collecting duct epithelium.

PCGF: P cell growth factor; persistent cell stimulating factor; *see* **interleukin-3**.

P cell growth factor: PCGF; *see* **interleukin-3**.

pCi: picocurie.

PCMBS: parachloromercuriphenyl sulfonic acid.

PCNA: proliferating cell nuclear antigen.

PCOD: polycystic ovary disease.

PCP: phencyclidine.

PCPA: parachlorophenylalanine.

PCR: polymerase chain reaction.

PCSF: persistent cell stimulating factor; *see* **interleukin-3**.

PDA: (-)*cis*-2,3-piperidine dicarboxylic acid; a broad-spectrum excitatory amino acid receptor antagonist. The *trans* form is an agonist.

PDE: phosphodiesterases.

PD-ECGF: platelet-derived endothelial cell growth factor.

PDGF: platelet-derived growth factor.

PDI: peptidyl-disulfide isomerases; enzymes that catalyze formation of disulfide bonds.

PE: (1) phenylethylamine; (2) persistent estrus; (3) potential energy.

peanut agglutinin: PNA: a lectin obtained from peanuts that binds terminal *N*-acetylgalactosyl moieties. It is used to identify PN^+ immature thymocytes of the thymus gland cortex, and to isolate lymph node germinal cells. PN^- cells of the thymus medulla are Thy-1^+, glucocorticoid-resistant, rich in 20α-steroid dehydrogenase, and insensitive to interleukin-3.

PECAM: *see* **CD31**.

pectinate; pectiniform: having tooth-like projections.

pectins: (20-400K) plant cell wall polysaccharides. Most are heteropolymers composed of rhamnose, galactose, arabinose, fucose, and other sugar moieties, as well as sugar acids (some of which are methylated) and other sugar derivatives. Specific terms that identify the major components include galactans, arabinans, and galacturonans.

pectoral: pertaining to the chest.

ped-: pedi-; pedo-; prefixes meaning (1) foot or foot-like; (2) child, as in pediatrics.

pederasty: anal intercourse with a boy as the receptive partner.

pedicel: podocyte; foot plate; foot process; a cytoplasmic extension expanded at the site of contact with a basement membrane. *See* also **Bowman's capsule**.

pedigree: a diagramatic representation of the inheritance of a family trait or phenotype. Horizontal lines connect symbols for the parents (circle for female and square for male), and vertical lines projecting downward from their centers display the progeny (with diamonds if the sex is not known). A fully shaded symbol indicates homozygosity for, or expression of the trait. One-half is shaded for a heterozygote, and a dark circle within a clear symbol shows a carrier. When the inheritance of an individual is not known because of early death, a cross within a symbol is used.

pedo-: ped-.

pedogenesis: paedogenesis; sexual maturation of the larval form of a species that is capable of undergoing metamorphosis. It occurs in axolotls and some insects. *Cf* **neoteny**.

pedomorphosis: acquisition by adult members of a population of characteristics that resemble those of ancestral juveniles.

pedophilia: paraphilia, in which a prepubertal child is essential for sexual gratification.

PEG: polyethylene glycol.

α₁-**PEG**: *see* **plasma protein 14**.

pelage: the hair or fur that covers an animal.

P elements: transposable elements of *Drosophila melanogaster* that mediate a form of hybrid dysgenesis. Some are incorporated into germ line chromosomes.

pellagra: black tongue; a disease commonly attributed to nicotinamide deficiency that is probably caused by combined vitamin and tryptophan deficiency. (Diets inadequate for one are usually poor in the other.) The manifestations include skin rashes, swelling of the tongue and changes in its surface, diarrhea, polyneuropathy, irritability, and, in severe cases, delirium and psychotic symptoms.

pellicle: (1) the outer coating of a protozoan; (2) a skin or thin membrane; (3) a film of coagulated matter on the surface of a liquid.

pemphigus: several autoimmune diseases in which blisters form within the epidermis and/or mucous membranes.

penetrance: in genetics, the proportion of individuals of a genotype that, under specified conditions, acquires an expected phenotype.

D-**penicillamine**: 3-mercapto-D-valine; β,β-dimethylcysteine; an agent obtained by hydrolytic degradation of penicillin that chelates copper, zinc, mercury, and lead. It is used to treat heavy metal poisoning and liver disorders associated with metal accumulation. It also complexes with and promotes cystine excretion, and exerts some inhibitory influences on immune system cells. The L isomer also chelates, but is not used clinically because it inhibits enzymes that use pyridoxal cofactors.

L-**penicillamine**: *see* D-**penicillamine**.

penicillic acid: 3-methoxy-5-methyl-4-oxo-2,5-hexadienoic acid; an antibiotic made by some *Penicillium* and *Aspergillus* strains. It undergoes reversible cyclization, and is carcinogenic.

penicillin[s]: antibiotics made by several *Penicillium* strains, and semi-synthetic derivatives. All contain fused thiazolidine and beta-lactam rings. The various types differ in the kinds of side-chains peptide bonded to the beta-lactam groups. Penicillin G potassium (shown) is [2S-(2α,5α,6β)]-3,3-dimethyl-7-oxo-6-[(phenylacetyl)-amino-4-thia-1-azabicyclo[3.2.O]heptane-2-carboxylic acid monopotassium salt. Penicillins rupture bacterial cell membranes by activating autolysins. They also acetylate, and thereby irreversibly inhibit a glycopeptide transpeptidase required to cross-link peptidoglycan strands during a final stage in cell wall synthesis. Although effective against many gram positive organisms, some spirochetes and fungi, the kinds initially used do not penetrate the capsules and lipopolysaccharide layers that surround gram negative types. Many bacteria make penicillinases; and some strains acquire resistance to the autolysis activation. Broad spectrum, hydrophilic antibiotics, such as ampicillin, do penetrate membranes; and some semi-synthetic derivatives resist degradation. Types easily degraded are used to harvest resistant mutants from mixed cultures.

penicillinases: β-lactamases; 50K enzymes with varying specificities that catalyze hydrolysis of β-lactam bonds. They are made by *Staphylococci* and many other bacteria, and account for much of the resistance to penicillins and cephalosporins. Some types are membrane-bound; others are released from the cells.

penile: pertaining to, or affecting the penis.

penillic acids: 2,3,7,7a-tetrahydro-2,2-dimethylimidazol[5,1-*b*]thiazole-3,7-dicarboxylic acid derivatives that differ in the R side-chain shown. They are degradation products formed during acid hydrolysis of penicillins.

penis: phallus; the male copulatory organ, comprising in mammals a root attached to the pubic arch, a body (corpus) covered by skin, and a broader, tactile-sensitive glans at the distal end. The body contains two corpora cavernosa and a corpus spongiosum, which become engorged with blood during erection. The blood vessels are controlled by autonomic system neurotransmitters; and nitric oxide (or a closely related derivative) is the major vasodilator. The penile urethra passes through the spongiosa and terminates in a pore in the glans. The organ differentiates from the embryonic genital tubercle and part of urogenital sinus. Both its development and reproductive functions require dihydrotestosterone.

pennate: penniform; feather-like; a term applied to some skeletal muscles.

penta-: a prefix meaning five.

pentagastrin: Boc-β-Ala-Tyr-Met-Asp-Phe-NH$_2$; a synthetic gastrin receptor agonist with the four terminal amino acids of the hormone. It is used to assess stomach gland functions.

penicillic acid

pentamidine isethionate

pentamidine isethionate: an NMDA receptor antagonist that protects against excitatory amino acid toxicity. It also displays antimicrobial activity, and is used to treat acquired autoimmune deficiency syndrome (AIDS)-associated *Pneumocystis carinii* pneumonia.

pentazocine: 1,2,3,4,5,6-hexahydro-6,11-dimethyl-3-(3-methyl-2-butenyl)-2.6-methano-3-benzazocin-8-ol; a benzomorphan derivative used as an analgesic. It is a partial agonist for δ and κ type opioid receptors that affects the functions of K$^+$ channels. In common with morphine, it promotes sedation, affects gastrointestinal tract and reproductive system functions, and can invoke respiratory depression; but it tends to accelerate cardiac rate and elevate blood pressure, and is less addictive.

pentobarbital sodium : Nembutal; 5-ethyl-5-(1-methyl-butyl)-2,4,6(1*H,3H,5H*)-pyrimidinetrione monosodium salt; a moderately long-acting central nervous system depressant (*see* also **barbiturates**). Low doses promote sedation, and higher ones invoke sleep. Nembutal is used as a general anesthetic for laboratory animals, and in large doses for euthanasia. Closely matched individuals display considerable variation in responses to a specific dosage, even when adjustments are made for body weight and other factors.

pentolinium tartrate: 1,1′-pentamethylene-*bis*(1-methyl-pyrrolidinium) hydrogen tartrate; a ganglionic blocking agent used to treat hypertension.

pentosans: polysaccharides in which the major repeating units are 5-carbon sugars.

pentoses: 5-carbon sugars, such as ribose, deoxyribose, xylose, and arabinose.

pentose pathway: *see* **hexose monophosphate shunt**.

pentosuria: a benign, autosomal recessive disease, in which impaired production of NADP-xylitol dehydrogenase causes loss of large amounts of L-xylulose to the urine.

penultimate: next to the last.

PEP: (1) phosphoenol pyruvate; (2) progesterone-associated endometrial protein.

PEP-19: a developmentally regulated calcium-binding cerebellar protein.

Pepcid: a trade name for famotidine.

PEPCK: phosphoenol pyruvate carboxykinase.

pepsins: 34.5K proteolytic enzymes formed in gastric juice from pepsinogen. They initiate digestion of food proteins by converting them to proteoses and peptones, and are most effective for catalyzing hydrolysis of peptide bonds in which the —C=O donor is phenylalanine, tryptophan, or tyrosine (but also act on bonds with leucine moieties). The optimum pH range is 1.5-2.0. Purified preparations are used to improve digestion in individuals who do not make sufficient enzyme.

pepsinogen: 40K proenzymes secreted by stomach chief cells. Cleavage to pepsins is initiated by hydrochloric acid, but then becomes autocatalytic (is catalyzed by pepsin).

pepstatins: pentapedites made by some *Streptomycin* strains that inhibit pepsin, renin, cathepsin D, and other acid proteases. Pepstatin A is *N*-[(3-methyl-1-oxobutyl)-L-valyl-L-valyl-4-amino-3-hydroxy-6-methylheptanoyl-L-alanyl]-4-amino-3-hydroxy-6-methylheptanoic acid. Pepstatins B and C are, respectively, *N*-n-caproyl, and *N*-iso-caproyl derivatives. The enzymes are used to treat peptic ulcers, and to block peptide degradation by endogenous enzymes in biological tissues and fluids.

peptic: pertaining to pepsin, gastric juice, or the stomach.

peptidases: enzymes that cleave CO—NH bonds; *see* **endopeptidases, exopeptidases, proteinases**, and specific types.

peptide[s]: molecules composed of relatively small numbers of amino acids joined by peptide bonds. Qualifying prefixes that refer to the sizes include di-, tri-, penta-, oligo-, and poly-. Compounds with 100 or more moieties are usually called proteins.

peptide A: H$_2$N-Val-Ala-Pro-Ser-Asp-Ser-Ile-Gln-Ala-Glu-Glu-Trp-Tyr-Phe-Gly-Lys-Ile-Thr-Arg-Arg-Glu-OH; a synthetic peptide used to inhibit tyrosine kinases.

peptide B: an opioid peptide cleaved from proenkephalin A in adrenal glands. The bovine type has the sequence: H₂N-Phe-Ala-Glu-Pro-Leu-Pro-Ser-glu-Glu-Glu-Gly-Glu-Ser-Tyr-Ser-Lys-Glu-Val-Pro-Glu-Met-Glu-Lys-Arg-Tyr-Gly-Gly-Phe-Met-Arg-Phe-OH.

peptide 7B2: APPG; anterior pituitary peptide of the pig; a 180K peptide homologous to secretin, duck proinsulin, and Rous sarcoma virus transforming protein, initially identified in the hypothalamus and in all pituitary gland lobes of swine. It is co-released with luteinizing hormone (LH), and is implicated as a regulator of gonadotropin secretion. Since it is also present in spinal cord, pancreas, thyroid and adrenal glands, and in gastrointestinal and urinary tract cells, it probably performs other functions.

peptide bond: CO—NH; the covalent bond that links amino acid moieties of peptides and proteins, formed mostly during translation via dehydration synthesis, in which the amino group of one moiety joins the carboxyl group of another, and water is released (*see* **peptidyl transferases**). Some proteases act on many substrates; others preferentially cleave bonds formed by specific kinds of amino acids.

peptide E: adrenal peptide E; Tyr-Gly-Gly-Phe-Met-Arg-Arg-Val-Gly-Arg-Pro-Glu-Trp-Trp-Met-Asp-Tyr-Gly-Gly-Phe-Leu; a peptide cleaved from proenkephalin A in the adrenal medulla. It exerts metenkephalin like actions, but is more potent.

peptide F: an opioid peptide cleaved from proenkephalin A in the adrenal medulla that contains two metenkephalin components, one at each end. Its analgesic properties are similar to those of peptide E.

peptide histidine-isoleucine: peptide histidine isoleucinamide; PHI-27; a porcine peptide with properties similar to those of human **peptide histidine-methionine** *(q.v.)*. It contains lysyl and isoleucinyl moieties at positions 12 and 27, respectively.

peptide histidine-methionine: PHM-27; PHM; His-Ala-Asp-Gly-Val-Phe-Thr-Ser-Asp-Phe-Ser-Lys-Leu-Leu-Gly-Gln-Leu-Ser-Ala-Lys-Lys-Tyr-Leu-Glu-Ser-Leu-Met-NH₂; the human fuctional equivalent of porcine peptide histidine-isoleucine (PHI-27), cleaved from a protein precursor which also yields vasoactive intestinal peptide (VIP). It is co-secreted by some cells, interacts with some VIP receptors, and competes with VIP for binding. PHM is also chemically related to gonadotropin releasing hormone (GRH). It is made in neurons that release corticotropin releasing hormone (CRH) and/or enkephalin, and in other parts of the central nervous system, in the gastrointestinal and urogenital tracts, and in thyroid glands, ovaries, and some tumor cells. It potentiates CRH stimulation of adrenocorticotropic hormone (ACTH) secretion and suckling-associated prolactin secretion. It also accelerates amylase, glucagon, and insulin release, augments steroidogenesis, and relaxes tracheal and gall bladder smooth muscle. It additionally stimulates cAMP generation and water transport in the small intestine (but the watery diarrhea caused by VIPomas is attributed to co-release of VIP).

peptide I: an opioid peptide cleaved from proenkephalin A in adrenal glands. It contains one internally located metenkephalin sequence, and one *C*-terminal leu-enkephalin moiety.

peptide T: Ala-Ser-Thr-Thr-Thr-Asn-Tyr-Thr; an amino acid sequence contained in human immunodeficiency virus (HIV) envelope protein gp120, named for its high threonine content. It is chemically related to thymosin α_1, and to vasoactive intestinal peptide (VIP), exerts some VIP-like effects, and is chemotactic. Since it blocks *in vitro* binding of gp120 to the CD4 receptor on T lymphocytes, it is under investigation for treatment of acquired immunodeficiency syndrome (AIDS).

peptide YY: PYY; Tyr-Pro-Ala-Lys-Pro-Glu-Ala-Pro-Gly-Glu-Asn-Ala-Ser-Pro-Glu-Glu-Leu-Ser-Arg-Tyr-Tyr-Ala-Ser-Leu-Arg-His-Tyr-Leu-Asn-Leu-Val-Thr-Arg-Gln-Arg-Tyr-NH₂; a peptide chemically related to avian type pancreatic polypeptide and to neuropeptide Y, named for the tyrosyl (Y) moieties at both ends. It is made in neurons and in intestinal mucosa, and is released to the gastrointestinal tract following meal ingestion. PYY inhibits secretin and cholecystokinin (CCK)-stimulated pancreatic juice production, depresses jejunum and colon motility, constricts intestinal blood vessels, and raises systemic blood pressure. Opioid peptides inhibit its release.

peptidoglycans: chemically related cross-linked macromolecules of Gram negative bacterial inner cell walls, composed of *N*-acetylglucosamine-*N*-acetylneuraminic acid polymers and peptide chains with 4-10 amino acid moieties. They confer mechanical support and protect against cell rupture. *See* also **penicillins**.

peptidyl-glycine α-amidating monooxygenase: PAM; a copper and ascorbic acid dependent enzyme that catalyzes reactions in which molecular oxygen is used to amidate terminal glycyl moieties of peptides. It contributes to posttranslational processing of several prehormones, and acts on some finished products. Hormones that exist in amidated forms include POMC derivatives (such as α-melanocyte stimulating hormone, α-MSH), proenkephalin A cleavage products, vasoactive intestinal peptide (VIP), galanin, substance P, gastrin and pancreastatin. PAM isozymes are generated via differential splicing of the pre-messenger RNA; and enzyme production is developmentally and tissue-specifically regulated by glucocorticoids, triiodothyronine (T₃), and other hormones. High levels are made in pituitary glands (especially intermediate and neural lobes), and lower ones in heart, frog skin, and elsewhere.

peptidyl lysine hydroxylase: an enzyme that catalyzes hydroxylation of lysyl moieties during collagen synthesis; *see* **lysyl hydroxylase**.

peptidyl-proline *cis-trans* isomerase: PPI; cyclophilin; an enzyme that catalyzes the rate-limiting step required for the folding of some proteins; *see* **rotamase**.

peptidyl site: P site; a component of ribosome small subunits essential for beginning translation, and for peptide chain elongation. It forms an **initiation complex**

(*q.v.*) with factor eIF, GTP and Met-tRNA in eukaryotes (and with *f*-Met-tRNA and related factors in prokaryotes). When the met-tRNA anti-codon attaches to the start codon of the messenger RNA, the small ribosome subunit links to a large one, and the next amino-acyl-tRNA binds to the A site. The methionine t-RNA is released, methionine is transferred to the A site, and a peptide bond is formed with the second amino acid (*see* also **peptidyltransferase**). The second t-RNA is then released, the dipeptide is translocated to the P site, and the vacated A site is free to accept the third amino-acyl-tRNA.

peptidyltransferases: enzyme components of large ribosomal subunits essential for peptide chain elongation during translation. When the first amino acid attaches to the **P site** (*q.v.*), and the second to the A site, the enzyme catalyzes transfer of the first to the A site, formation of a peptide bond, and translocation of the dipeptide to the P site. The third amino acid then attaches to the A site, and the enzyme promotes transfer of the dipeptide to the A site for formation of the second peptide bond. The process is repeated until the stop codon is reached.

peptones: fragments formed during partial digestion of proteins by gastric juice pepsin and hydrochloric acid. They are further degraded by pancreatic juice proteases.

per-: a prefix used for molecules that contain more than the usual amount of oxygen (or of some other component), as in peroxide and permanganate.

percentile: the rank in a system in which variables are divided into 99 groups of ascending (or descending) magnitude. If a value in a distribution falls within the thirtieth percentile, there are 29 lower, and 70 higher ranks.

perchlorate: ClO_4^-; an anion that competes with iodide for active transport across thyroid gland follicular cell membranes. When administered after a dose of radioactive iodine, it promotes release of iodine that has not been incorporated into thyroglobulin, and is used to study some thyroid gland functions. It also inhibits thyroid hormone synthesis, but is not used to treat hyperthyroidism (since it can cause fatal aplastic anemia).

Percoll: a trade name for a colloidal suspension of silica, used in density gradient centrifugation.

percutaneous: through the skin.

perforins: P1; pore forming proteins; cytolysins; 70-75K proteins induced by interleukin-2, and stored in the granules of cytotoxic T lymphocytes and natural killer (NK) cells. The human type has 534 amino acid moieties. When activated cells attach to their targets, they release the granules, and the proteins undergo Ca^{2+}-dependent binding to target cell plasma membrane components. They then polymerize to form plasma membrane channels (approximately 10 nm in diameter), and this leads to target cell lysis. Perforins display homologies to C9 and other complement attack complex proteins. The functions of domains similar to the kinds in epidermal growth factor (EGF), thrombospondin, and low density lipoprotein (LDL) receptors are not known. Physiological inhibitors of the cytolytic effects have been identified.

performic acid: peroxyformic acid; an agent used to oxidize the sulfhydryl groups of cysteine, methionine, and other organic molecules.

$$H-\overset{\overset{\text{O}}{\|}}{C}-O-OH$$

perfusion: sending fluids through organs or tissues (via blood vessels, or in other ways *in vitro*); *cf* **perifusion**. The fluids used for various purposes can contain hormones, ions, substrates, dyes, or fixatives.

pergolide: 8-[(methylthio)methyl]-6-propylergoline; a highly potent dopamine receptor agonist, more effective on D_2 than on D_1 types. It is used to inhibit excessive growth hormone and prolactin secretion. Although it can invoke nausea and orthostatic hypotension, it is used to treat Parkinson's disease resistant to other forms of medication.

Pergonal: a trade name for a preparation from the urine of postmenopausal women. It has high follicle stimulating hormone (FSH) activity, and is used to promote maturation of multiple secondary oocytes for *in vitro* fertilization. It can also improve fertility in men unable to produce adequate numbers of spermatozoa because of FSH deficiency. Pergonal was formerly used to increase the probability of conception in women with low fertility, but it is difficult to determine the optimum dosage, and it tends to promote formation of more conceptuses than can be accommodated in the uterus and brought to term; *cf* **clomiphene**.

peri-: a prefix meaning around, about, or near.

periarteritis nodosa: polyarteritis nodosa; a disease in which neutrophils infiltrate into and initiate necrotic destruction of blood vessels. It is attributed to formation of abnormal immune complexes, and is often associated with Hepatitis B infections or rheumatoid arthritis.

pericardium: a fibromembranous sac composed of parietal and visceral layers, that surrounds the heart and the roots of the pulmonary trunk and aorta. A small quantity of serous pericardial fluid normally present between the layers functions as a lubricant.

pericentric inversion: a chromosomal rearrangement in which the inverted segment includes centromere components.

pericentriolar region: the amorphous region that surrounds the centriole of an animal cell. It contains the major microtubule organizing center.

perichondrium: the membrane that surrounds cartilage. It contains blood vessels, nerve endings, and cells that give rise to chondroblasts.

pericytes: pericapillary cells; Rouget cells; precapillary sphincter cells; adventitial cells; small, contractile cells in the connective tissue that surround and form sphincters for some blood capillaries and metarterioles.

perifusion: bathing cells or tissues with continuously renewed fluids.

perikaryon: usually (1) the cell body of a neuron; (2) the region that surrounds a cell nucleus.

perilipin: an adipocyte phosphoprotein rapidly converted from a 62K to more heavily phosphorylated 65-67K forms by isoproterenol and other kinase A activators. It is used to assess kinase A activity in those cells.

perilymph: the fluid that separates the bony labyrinth of the internal ear from the membranous labyrinth (which contains endolymph).

perinatal: around the time of birth, a term that can refer to the time periods shortly preceding and soon following birth, to events that occur then, or to treatments administered at such times.

perineum: the area between the thighs and below the pelvic diaphragm that extends from the coccyx to the pubis. It includes the scrotum in males, and the vulva in females.

periodic acid-Schiff: PAS; a procedure for staining carbohydrates and identifying glycogen, neutral glycosaminoglycans, glycoproteins, and cells (such as thyrotropes and gonadotropes) that make substantial quantities of such compounds. The specimens are treated with periodic acid (HIO_4), which oxidizes alcoholic groups to aldehydes. The aldehydes then react with nitrogen groups of the Schiff reagent (basic fuchsin decolorized by sulfurous acid) to form magenta-colored products. *See* also **Schiff base**.

periodicity: (1) recurrence at regular intervals, a term often modified by others (such as diurnal or lunar) that relate to the time period for one cycle; (2) the time interval between between a specific phase of one cycle and the corresponding phase of the next one; (3) in molecular biology, the numbers of base pairs per turn of a DNA helix; (4) the distance between repeating units of a complex molecule.

periosteum: connective tissue membranes that cover bone surfaces. They contain blood vessels, nerves, and osteoprogenitor cells; *cf* **endosteum**.

peripheral lymphoid tissue: lymphoid system components other than bone marrow or thymus gland, for example lymph nodes, tonsils, spleen, appendix, and Peyer's patches.

peripheral membrane proteins: proteins that are not totally integrated within phospholipid bilayers. They can be bound to integral membrane proteins, or be anchored to bilayers by fatty acid and other hydrophobic moieties, and can project to either the cytoplasm or the external environment.

peripheral nervous system: PNS; all nervous system components outside the brain and spinal cord; *cf* **central nervous system**.

peripheral neuritis: inflammation of tissue that surrounds peripheral nervous system cells.

peristalsis: successive waves of contraction and relaxation along tubular muscular organs, such as the intestine or ureters. Relaxation of circular, and contraction of longitudinal smooth muscle, which dilates segments and facilitates filling, alternates with contraction of circular, and relaxation of longitudinal muscle, which then propels luminal components towards the ends of the tubes.

peritoneum: a double serous membrane composed of a parietal layer that lines the walls of the abdominal and pelvic cavities, and a visceral layer that covers and adheres to the internal organs. Peritoneal fluid between them provides moisture and mechanical protection, and reduces friction during movements. Non-irritating aqueous substances injected intraperitoneally are rapidly absorbed into blood vessels. Irritants and other agents are used to invoke special responses, such as recruitment of leukocytes that can be aspirated with peritoneal fluid.

peritubular cells of the testis: cells that lie outside the seminiferous tubules. Myoid types contribute to hormone controls and sperm release.

permeability: the extent to which a membrane permits the passage of specific kinds of molecules or ions.

permeability coefficient: the rate at which a substance diffuses across a membrane under specified conditions, expressed, for example in millimeters per second. The values vary with the sizes, lipid solubilities, and electrical charges of the penetrating substances, the membrane characteristics, and the temperature.

permeases: agents that accelerate diffusion across (but do not damage) membranes (for example some aldosterone-induced proteins). Bacteria use several types to take up specific kinds of nutrients.

permissive action: a change brought about by a regulator that does not directly invoke a response, but supports the actions of another agent. For example, glucocorticoids exert only minor direct effects on vascular smooth muscle contraction, but their presence is essential for sizeable, rapid responses to norepinephrine. Some "permissive hormones" induce (or covalently modify) enzymes or receptors activated by other regulators, slow second messenger degradation, or promote formation of messenger RNAs that are stabilized by other regulators.

permissive conditions: environmental temperatures and other conditions that support survival and/or responses.

permissive hosts: organisms in which viruses can complete lytic cycles.

pernicious: having a severe, progressive course that can lead to a fatal outcome.

pernicious anemia: very severe forms of anemia, usually associated with other defects. The term is often applied to the kind caused by vitamin B_{12} deficiency (which affects the nervous system). In most cases, the vitamin is available, but is not absorbed from the gastrointestinal tract because little or no **intrinsic factor** (*q.v.*) is made. The condition can be alleviated by parenteral administration of the vitamin.

Peromyscus: a genus that includes deer mice (*P. maniculatus*) and at least 40 related species.

per os: by mouth.

perosis: a bone disease in chickens, attributed to deficiencies of trace elements, vitamins, or other essential nutrients.

peroxidases: heme-containing enzymes that catalyze reactions of the general type: $H_2O_2 + XH_2 \rightarrow X + 2H_2O$, in which hydrogen peroxide is reduced to water and a substrate is oxidized. Specific kinds are essential for the synthesis of some regulators (such as iodinated thyroid hormones and eicosanoids), for oocyte cortical reactions, and for the operation of glyoxylate cycles and other processes; and H_2O_2 is one of the bactericidal agents released by activated neutrophilic leukocytes. Small amounts of hydrogen peroxide are also generated in reactions that involve transfers of hydrogen atoms and electrons from flavoproteins to molecular oxygen, catalyzed by different kinds of enzymes. Although it can directly damage cells by oxidizing fatty acids and other compounds, H_2O_2 is less toxic than superoxide anions ($O_2^- \bullet$), which are also made by neutrophils during inflammatory reactions, and to some extent in electron transport chains. Superoxide dismutase degrades it to the less toxic product via: $O_2^- \bullet + 2H^+ \rightarrow H_2O_2$. *See* also **horse radish peroxidase**, **lactoperoxidase**, **thyroperoxidase**, and **peroxidase-antiperoxidase method**.

peroxidase-antiperoxidase method: PAP; a technique for detecting antigens in tissue sections. After incubation with a specific rabbit antibody, an excess of rabbit IgG immunoglobulin is added. The section is then treated with a horseradish peroxidase-rabbit antiperoxidase complex (which binds via IgG to antibody-bound antigen). The resulting PAP complex is then stained with a chromogen.

peroxide: (1) any compound with the general formula X-O-O-Y (in which X and Y can be identical); (2) hydrogen peroxide.

peroxisomes: organelles morphologically similar to lysosomes (bounded by single membranes), in most eukaryotic cells and especially abundant in the livers and kidneys of higher animals. They are also called microbodies (a term additionally applied to glyoxisomes and related plant cell organelles). Their enzymes use molecular oxygen to remove hydrogen atoms from substrates, and are required for oxidation of very long chain fatty acids, and for conversion of cholesterol to bile acids. Very long chain fatty acid synthetase (VLCFA-Co A synthetase) initiates β-oxidation of hexacosanoate (C26:0), docosanoate (C22:0), erucic acid (C22:1) and related long-chain saturated and monounsaturated acids. Other enzymes include acyl-CoA oxidases, flavin linked oxidases that generate hydrogen peroxide, catalases that

degrade H_2O_2, amino acid and urate oxidases, and others for plasmalogen synthesis. The organelles are self-replicating, but do not contain DNA or ribosomes. Inability to synthesize peroxisome assembly factor-1 impairs development, and leads to plasmalogen deficiency and accumulation of very long chain fatty acids. Individuals with Zellweger syndrome have dysmorphic features, neurological abnormalities, hepatomegaly, and renal cysts. *See* also **peroxisome proliferators** and **peroxisome proliferator activated receptors**.

peroxisome proliferator[s]: diverse chemicals (including some agents used to lower blood lipid levels) that increase the numbers of hepatic peroxisomes by acting on peroxisome proliferator activated receptors (PPARs). The consequences include accelerated transcription of genes for β-oxidation of very long-chain fatty acids, and of others that code for members of the cytochrome P_{450} IV family. The enzymes lower circulating lipid levels and catalyze formation of large quantities of hydrogen peroxide. They degrade some toxins, but initiate the growth of hepatic tumors by causing oxidative stress that damages DNA.

peroxisome proliferator activated receptors: PPARs; cell components that closely resemble receptors for steroid hormones, calciferols, retinoids, and thyroid hormones. When activated by peroxisome proliferators, they function as transcription factors that stimulate formation of large numbers of peroxisomes.

perphenazine: PZC; 4-[3-(2-chlorophenothiazin-10-yl)-propyl]-1-piperazine ethanol; a dopamine receptor antagonist, used as a tranquilizer, "antipsychotic" agent, and anti-emetic, and as a component of some pre-anesthetic preparations. In common with other **phenothiazines** (*q.v.*), it can invoke undesirable pyramidal and autonomic nervous system effects. Its ability to promote marked, sustained hyperprolactinemia in rodents is used to study hormone-dependent mammary gland tumors.

persistent estrus: PE; constant estrus; conditions in which follicles mature and secrete large quantities of estrogen, but ovarian cycles are arrested at the estrus stage. The term can apply to **induced ovulators** (*q.v.*), in which LH (luteinizing hormone) surges and ovulation require vulval stimulation, and to spontaneous ovulators subjected to procedures which interrupt normal mechanisms for LH release. PE can be invoked in rats and some other rodents by neonatal androgenization, exposure to continuous bright light, or injection of pharmacological agents that block gonadotropin releasing hormone (GnRH) release; and it can be terminated by mating or artificial stimulation. *See* also **paracyclic ovulation**.

persistent Müllerian duct syndrome: retention, usually with some development, of embryonic Müllerian ducts in a genotypic and otherwise phenotypic male, attributed to failure to produce adequate amounts of Müllerian duct inhibitor at a critical stage of fetal development, or (more rarely) inability to respond to that hormone.

persisting cells: P cells; cells that survive in bone marrow cultures maintained on conditioned media that contain interleukin-like factors, but lack growth factors essential for supporting the survival, proliferation, and differentiation of other cell types. Most are pluripotential stem cells.

persisting cell stimulating growth factor: P cell stimulating factor; PCSF; P cell growth factor; PCGF; a regulator made by T lymphocytes that promotes P cell proliferation and induces Thy-1 antigen. It appears to be identical with interleukin-3.

pertechnetate: $^{99}\text{TcO}_4^-$: a radioactive ion taken up and concentrated by thyroid gland follicular cells, but not incorporated into thyroglobulins. It is used to assess iodide transport rates, and to visualize hormone-producing thyroid tumors. The atomic weight of stable **technetium** (Tc, *q.v.*) is 98.

pertussis toxin: PTTX; PTX; islet activating protein; IAP; a 117K hexameric protein made by *Bordetella pertussis*, the organism that causes whooping cough. The B pentamer (composed of 23K, 22K, 11.7K and 9.3K peptide chains) binds to cell membranes and facilitates insertion of the 28K A subunit, a single polypeptide chain. The A subunit catalyzes ADP-ribosylation of several kinds of G protein α subunits, including $G_{\alpha o}$, $G\alpha_{\alpha i1}$, $G_{\alpha i2}$, and $G_{\alpha i3)}$, all of which covalently link to plasma membranes via myristate and serve as transducers for hormones and neurotransmitters. Some mediate inhibitory influences on adenylate cyclases; others affect phospholipases, and /or ion channels. ADP-ribosylation impairs their functions by lowering α subunit affinity for GTP. Since it does not affect $G_{\alpha s}$ subunits (*cf* **cholera toxin**) and some other types, it is used to ascertain the kinds of G proteins involved in specific hormone actions. PTX promotes persistent insulin secretion by pancreatic β cells; but very high insulin levels block PTX-catalyzed ADP-ribosylation of $G_{\alpha i}$. Other effects include down-regulation of α_2 adrenergic, cholinergic, and some other receptor types, interference with adenosine inhibition of glutamate release, and with neutrophil activation, and influences on several immune system functions.

PEST: Pro-Glu-Ser-Thr; an amino acid sequence common to many calmodulin binding proteins that affects susceptibility to calpain-mediated degradation.

petite mutants: dwarf yeast colonies with mutations that arise spontaneously or can be induced by ethidium bromide, studied most intensively in *S. cerevisiae*. Since some organisms lack mitochondrial DNA, and others have insufficient or altered forms, growth retardation is attributed to dependence on anaerobic respiration.

Petromyzon: the lamprey eel, a jawless, parasitic, aquatic vertebrate of the class Agnatha. It is in many ways more primitive than most other members of the vertebrate subphylum, but more advanced than the **hagfish** (*q.v.*).

Peyer's patches: clumps of lymphatic tissue in the submucosal layer of the intestine that contribute to gut-associated immunity and perform functions in mammals comparable to those of the bursa of Fabricius in birds. They contain antigen presenting M cells (Peyer's patch type), T lymphocytes (with mostly δγ type receptor subunits), and large numbers of B lymphocytes that produce IgA class antibodies. Their high endothelium venules express cell adhesion molecules that bind B cell homing receptors.

P face: the cytoplasmic half of a plasma membrane lipid bilayer; *see* **freeze fracture**.

PFGE: pulsed field gel electrophoresis.

PFK: phosphofructokinase.

PG: prostaglandin.

3-**PG**: 3-phosphoglycerate.

PGA, PGB, PGC, PGD, PGE: *see* **prostaglandins** A, B, C, D, and E.

PGF: plerocercoid growth factor.

PGF$_{1\alpha}$, PGF$_{2\alpha}$: *see* **prostaglandins**.

2,3-dinor-6-keto-**PGF$_{1\alpha}$**: a prostacyclin degradation product. The amounts made are more dependable indicators of prostacyclin synthesis rates than 6-keto-PGF$_{1\alpha}$ levels.

6-keto-**PGF$_{1\alpha}$**: a biologically inactive prostacyclin degradation product. The amounts made reflect the amounts of prostacyclin synthesized; but *see* 2,3-dinor-6-keto-**PGF$_{1\alpha}$**.

PGG2: prostaglandin G_2; an endoperoxide intermediate in the pathway for biosynthesis of prostaglandins and thromboxanes. It very rapidly and spontaneously converts to PGH2.

PGH2: a hydroxyendoperoxide intermediate in the pathway for biosynthesis of prostaglandins and thromboxanes. The immediate precursor is PGG$_2$. Although short-lived, it acts on thromboxane receptors and

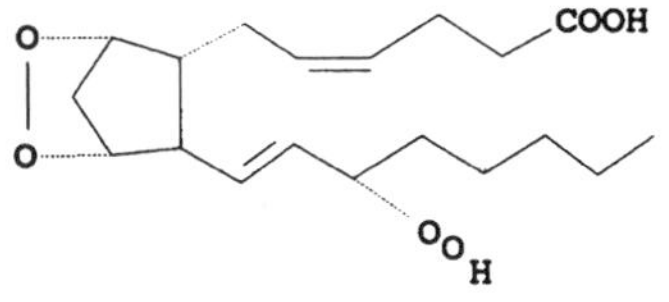

PGG2

mediates platelet aggregation and contraction of vascular smooth muscle.

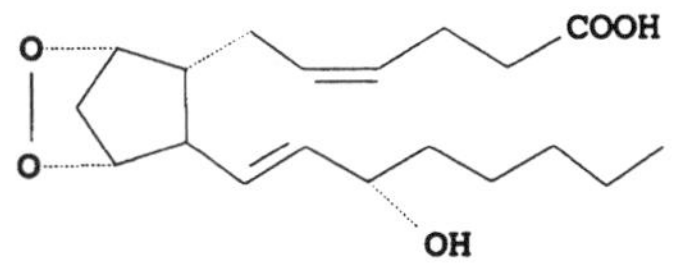

PGH2

PGI$_2$: prostacyclin.

PGJ: *see* **prostaglandin J**.

P Glycoprotein: P-170: 130-200K phosphorylated glycoproteins that mediate multidrug resistance by inserting into membranes, binding ATP, and using energy liberated by ATP hydrolysis to drive extrusion of several kinds of chemicals. Changes in fluidity and other membrane properties have also been observed. Some cell types respond to antineoplastic agents or to factors that augment kinase C activity by amplifying and/or activating their *mdr* genes. There are at least three types. Under more normal conditions, P-170s are believed to function as physiological regulators of endogenous peptide and protein export. The proteins, composed of two homologous halves, both of which bind the ATP, are members of a superfamily that includes cystic fibrosis transmembrane conductance regulator (CTFR), the product of the *S. cerevisiae* gene that mediates α-factor pheromone effects, and a product of the *Plasmodium falciparum* gene that confers resistance to chloroquine.

Pgp-1: phagocyte protein 1; *see* **CD44**.

PGX: an obsolete term for **prostacyclin**.

pH: the negative logarithm to the base 10 of the hydrogen ion concentration in moles per liter. Under standard conditions, the product of the hydrogen and hydroxyl ion concentrations in water is 10^{-14} M. Since water and neutral aqueous solutions have equal numbers of H$^+$ and OH$^-$ ions, the pHs = 7. Acidic solutions have more H$^+$ than OH$^-$, and therefore lower pH values. The stronger the acid, the lower the pH (and the greater the alkalinity, the higher the pH). The pH of 10^{-3} HCl is 3. Since the [H$^+$] of 10^{-3} M NaOH = $(10^{-14} - 10^{-3})$, its pH =11. Normal blood is in the 7.35–7.45 range, and most body fluids and cell cytoplasms maintain slightly alkaline levels. In contrast, the interiors of lysosomes are acidic; and values for gastric juice can be 1 or less. Since the activities of some enzymes are more markedly affected by small changes than others, deviations from normal ranges change balances. Many growth factors elevate the levels by activating Na$^+$/H$^+$ exchanges. Acidity more effectively activates catabolic than anabolic enzymes; and hypoxia mediates destruction in part by lowering cytoplasmic pH. *See* also **buffers, acidosis**, and **alkalosis**.

PHA: (1) posterior hypothalamic area; (2) phytohemagglutinin.

phaclofen: 3-amino-2-(4-chlorophenyl)propylphosphonic acid; a GABA$_B$ type gamma aminobutyric acid receptor antagonist.

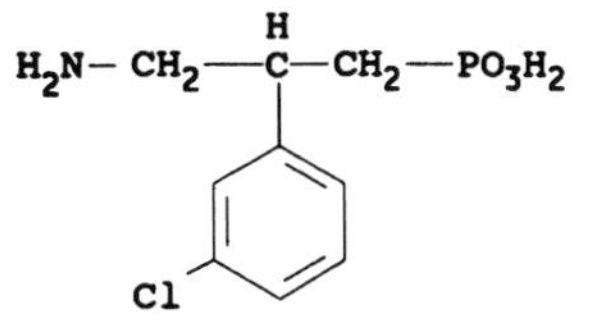

phaeo-: pheo-: a prefix meaning brown or dark.

phaeochromocytoma: pheochromocytoma.

phaeomelanins: pheomelanins; red, yellow, and light-brown pigments in skin and skin derivatives such as hair, fur, and feathers. They are chemically related to **eumelanins** (*q.v.*), but contain sulfur. Phenylalanine-3.4-quinone (dopaquinone), derived from tyrosine, condenses with cysteine to yield the major component of the phaeomelanin polymer, cysteinyl-DOPA.

phage: *see* **bacteriophage**.

phagocytes: neutrophilic leukocytes, macrophages, osteoclasts, and other cells that engulf particulate matter (such as microorganisms, other cells, macromolecular nutrients, or debris).

phagocytosis: cell ingestion of particulate matter. It begins with extension of pseudopods toward, and then around the particles. The pseudopod ends soon join to

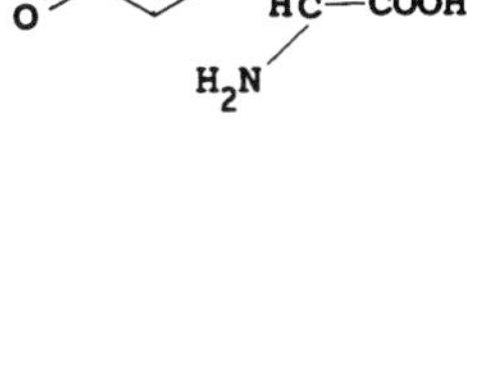

phenylalanine-3,4-quinone

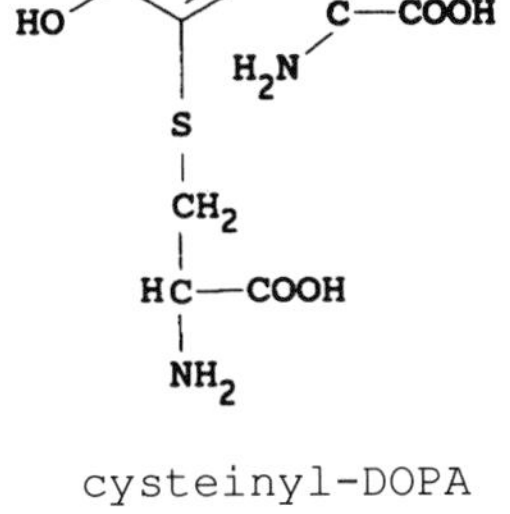

cysteinyl-DOPA

form a phagosome, which is internalized when the pseudopod membranes fuse with the plasma membrane from which they formed. In most cases, the phagosome fuses with a lysosome, in which digestion occurs. The processes are used to dispose of microorganisms and other cells foreign to the body, dead cells and their fragments, and other debris, and for functions such as bone resorption and thyroid hormone synthesis.

phagolysosomes: organelles formed when phagosomes fuse with lysosomes. Lysosomal enzymes degrade substances taken up by phagocytosis.

phagosomes: membrane-enclosed vesicles that surround matter taken up by phagocytosis.

phakomatosis: phacomatosis; hereditary disorders in which eye, skin, and/or glial cells proliferate excessively and form tumors that are not malignant but can cause damage. Examples include neurofibromatosis, tuberous sclerosis, and ataxia-telangiectasia.

phalloidin: phalloidine: a heat-stable 789K cyclic peptide obtained made by *Amanita phalloides* mushrooms that binds to and stabilizes F actin. Accidental ingestion causes vomiting, diarrhea, and convulsions. Although chemically related to α-amanitin made by the same fungi, and potentially lethal, phalloidin acts more rapidly, via different mechanisms, and is somewhat less toxic.

phallus: an externally protruding, tactile-sensitive reproductive system organ. The term usually refers to a penis or closely related male structure that delivers sperm, but can designate a clitoris or genital tubercle.

pharmacodynamics: the study of the mechanisms of drug action on living organisms.

pharmacogenetics: the study of genetically controlled factors that affect responses to exogenous agents.

pharmacokinetics: the study of drug absorption, distribution, metabolism, and excretion.

pharmacological dose: a quantity of a naturally occurring or closely related agent that raises cell, tissue or body fluid concentrations to levels higher than those encountered under physiological conditions. Large doses of hormones and other regulators are administered when

barriers limit absorption, when the agents are rapidly degraded, sequestered, and/or excreted, to exaggerate responses in laboratory animals, and for certain therapeutic purposes. Supraphysiological amounts can act on targets not affected by their endogenous counterparts.

pharyngeal hypophysis: pituitary tissue that has migrated to the pharynx. It can maintain connections to the adenohypophysis and contain cells that secrete growth hormone and/or prolactin.

pharyngeal pouches: soft structures that evaginate along the lateral pharyngeal walls of chordate embryos. They develop clefts, and mesoderm organizes around them to form pharyngeal arches. In fishes and some lower chordates, the clefts open and become gill slits. In humans and some other mammals, the most anterior (mandibular) pouch on each side gives rise to the incus and malleus bones of the inner ear, part of the mandible, and some associated muscles. The second pair forms the stapes and parts of the temporal and hyoid bones. The third and fourth contain the origins of the carotid bodies and most of the laryngeal cartilages. The fates of the other structures vary with the animal types and species. In most mammals and birds, thymus gland tissue originates in the fourth pouches (although some may come from the third), but thymus precursors are more widely distributed in lower vertebrates. The fourth and fifth pouches are the major sources of parathyroid precursor cells in amphibians, birds and mammals, and the sixth provide the aortic bodies. The most posterior pouch is the source of calcitonin-secreting cells, which are incorporated into ultimobranchial bodies of most vertebrates, and into thyroid glands of mammals.

phase: (1) a specific component of a phenomenon that changes with time, for example a proliferative, growth, or recovery phase. The term can refer to morphological, biochemical, or functional features, as in prophase and interphase, or to components of regularly recurring cycles, as in dark or light phase; (2) a physically distinct component of a mixture, as in liquid or solid phase.

phase-contrast microscopy: a form of interference microscopy in which differences in the lengths of light paths through the various components of the specimen are visualized as differences in light intensities. The path lengths are affected by refractive indices as well as by object thicknesses.

phalloidin

phaseolin: 6bR-cis-6b,12b-dihydro-3,3-dimethyl-3H, 7H-furol[3,2-c:5,4f']bis[1]benzopyran-10-ol; an antifungal phytoalexin made by the *Phaseolus vulgaris* bean in response to attack by fungi and some other forms of stress.

phe: F; *see* **phenylalanine**.

Phe-Met-Arg-Phe-amide: FMRF amide; a neuropeptide made by some invertebrates that inhibits acetylcholine release from presynaptic nerve endings by impeding Ca^{2+} uptake and decreasing responsivity to Ca^{2+}.

phenacetin: acetophenetidin; *p*-ethoxyacetanilide; an agent used for its analgesic and antipyretic effects. It lacks the anti-inflammatory properties of aspirin and other salicylates, and is less likely to irritate the gastric mucosa. Although well tolerated by most humans, it is more toxic than acetaminophen. Small amounts cause skin rashes in susceptible individuals; and habitual ingestion of large doses can damage the liver and kidneys, and cause methemoglobinemia. Toxic concentrations are carcinogenic, and can cause cardiac arrest.

phenalzine: phenelzine.

phenanthrene: a coal tar hydrocarbon; *see also* **cyclopentanoperhydrophenanthrene**.

1,10-phenanthroline: a metal chelator that binds iron, and is used to inhibit formation of free radicals.

phenazocine: 1,2,3,4,5,6-hexahydro-6,11-dimethyl-3-(2-phenethyl)-2,5-benzazocin-8-ol; a synthetic, benzomorphan type opioid narcotic and analgesic (available in the United Kingdom but not in the United States). It is less potent than morphine, but has a more favorable analgesic:side effect ratio, and a lesser tendency to cause addiction.

phenazone: antipyrine; 1,2-dihydro-1,5-dimethyl-2-phenyl-3H-pyrazol-3-one; an analgesic and antipyretic agent, no longer used clinically because of its toxicity.

phencyclidine: PCP; 1-(1-phenylcyclohexyl)piperidine. The hydrochloride is a potent analgesic and anesthetic, but is no longer used for those purposes because it alters sensory perception and can invoke hallucinations and long-lasting psychological disturbances. A street preparation ("angel dust") is used to elevate mood. PCP acts on σ type receptors that bind haloperidol and were once believed to be opioid subtypes. The major effect on the central nervous system may be blockage of glutamate-activated Ca^{2+} channels via interactions with NMDA (*N*-methyl-D-aspartate) receptors.

phendimetrazine: 3,4-dimethyl-2-phenylmorpholine; an agent with properties similar to those of phenmetrazine.

phene: a genetically determined characteristic.

phenelzine; phenalzine: Nardil; β-phenylethylhydrazine; an inhibitor of B type **monoamine oxidases** (*q.v.*), used as an antidepressant.

Phenergan: a trade name for promethazine.

phenformin: 1-phenylethylbiguanide; one of the first biguanide type oral hypoglycemic agents used to treat type II diabetes mellitus. It can cause lactacidosis, and has been replaced by less toxic preparations.

phenindione: Hedulin; 2-phenyl-1,3-indandione; a vitamin K antagonist, used clinically as an anticoagulant.

pheniprazine: Catron; 1-phenyl-2-hydrazinopropane; an inhibitor of type B monoamine oxidases. It is used to treat hypertension, and for studies of catecholamine functions.

pheniramine: 3-phenyl-3-(2-pyridyl)-3-*N,N*-dimethylpropylamine; an H_1 type histamine receptor antagonist.

phenmetrazine: Preludin; 3-methyl-2-phenylmorpholine; a sympathomimetic agent that stimulates the central nervous system. It has been used as an appetite suppressant, but can cause habituation, sleep disturbances, hypertension, and psychological dysfunction.

phenobarbital: Luminol; 5-ethyl-5-phenylbarbituric acid; a long-acting central nervous system depressant. Low dosages invoke sedation. Chronic use to combat insomnia leads to habituation and disruption of normal sleep patterns, with decreases in REM (rapid eye movement) phases. High doses exert phenytoin-like effects. They are hypnotic and anticonvulsant, and can lower thyroid hormone levels. In laboratory animals, they suppress gonadotropin releasing hormone (GnRH) release.

phenocopy: (1) isophan; a phenotype that resembles a genetically determined form, but is induced by environmental factors (2) an individual that displays the phenotype.

phenobarbital

phenol: carbolic acid; an agent that coagulates tissue proteins, and is used mostly to sterilize equipment, and for industrial purposes, but to a limited extent as a topical antiseptic and antipruritic agent, and to destroy warts. Ingestion of even minute amounts can invoke nausea, vomiting, necrosis, circulatory collapse, convulsions, and coma.

phenolphthalein: 3,3-*bis*-4-hydroxyphenyl)-1-(3*H*)-isobenzofuranone; an indicator that changes from colorless at pH 8.5 to pink at pH 9, and to deep red in very alkaline solutions. It stimulates intestinal muscle, and is a component of some laxatives.

phenolphthalin: decolorized phenolphthalein; phthalin; 4',4″-dihydroxytriphenylmethane; a reagent used to assay oxidases, peroxidases, oxidases, copper, and cyanide.

phenol red: phenolsulfonphthalein.

phenolsulfonphthalein: PSP; P.S.P.; phenol red; 4,4'-(3*H*-2,1-benzoxathiol-3-ylidine)-*bis*-phenol *S,S*-dioxide; an agent transported across nephron tubules that imparts a bright red color to urine, and is used to assess renal tubular function. It is also an indicator for monitoring acidity in cell and tissue studies, but exerts estrogen-like effects.

phenothiazines: (1) a class of tricyclic tranquilizer and "antipsychotic" agents that includes chlorpromazine, trifluoperazine, and perphenazine and other dopamine

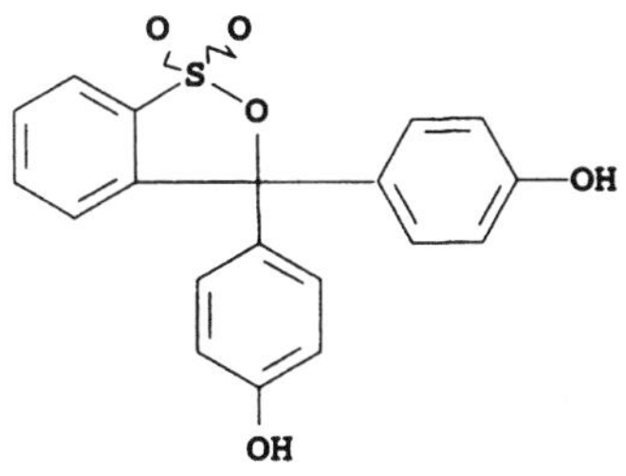

phenolsulfonphthalein

receptor antagonists; (2) when used in the singular, dibenzothiazine (*see* structure), an agent used to kill helminths, as an insecticide, and as laboratory tool that antagonizes calmodulin-regulated processes (*see* also **calmidazolium**). Antiverm and Helmetina are trade names.

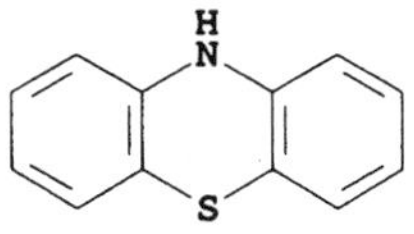

phenothiazine

phenotype: the physical, biochemical, and/or physiological attributes manifested by an individual (including genetically determined factors that can be modified by nutrition, environmental conditions, and life-style); *cf* **genotype**.

phenoxybenzamine: *N*-phenoxyisopropyl-*N*-benzyl-β-chloroethylamine; a haloalkylamine type irreversible α_1 adrenergic receptor antagonist, used to treat pheochromocytoma and some forms of hypertension not caused by tumors. Since it inhibits catecholamine uptake by synaptic vesicles, some transient agonist-like effects can precede the beneficial ones. Phenoxybenzamine also decreases the hyperreflexia that follows spinal cord transection. High concentrations block responses to serotonin, histamine, and acetylcholine. Toxic doses are carcinogenic. The effects on receptors in the urinary bladder and prostate gland can alleviate problems caused by obstruction in individuals with benign prostatic hypertrophy; but the drug also inhibits ejaculation; and long-term use leads to aspermia.

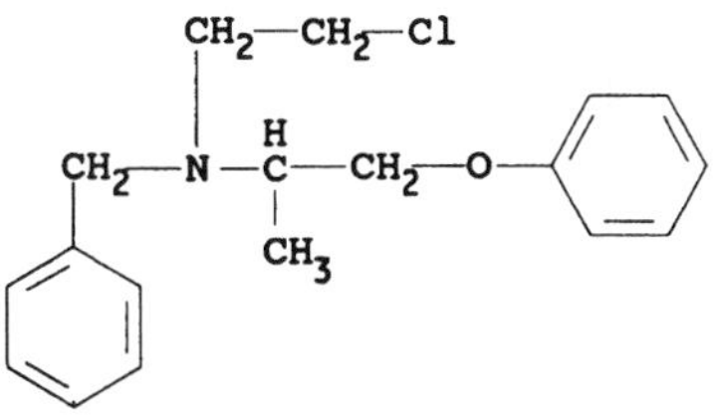

phenoxypropazine: (1-methyl-2-phenoxyethyl)hydrazine; an agent formerly used as a monoamine oxidase inhibitor.

phentolamine: 2-(*N*-*p*-tolyl-*N*′-*m*-hydoxyphenylaminomethyl)-2-imidazoline: an imidazoline type, nonspecific competitive α_1 and α_2 adrenergic receptor antagonist that lowers blood pressure. It also exerts some histamine-like effects, some cholinergic ones (for example on gastric

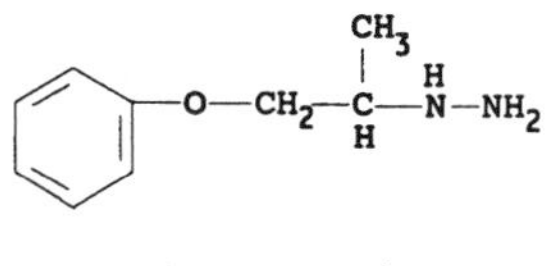

phenoxypropazine

acid secretion and gut motility) that can be blocked with atropine, and some influences on serotonin receptors, but is not effective against certain neurotransmitter invoked responses that are blocked by phenoxybenzamine. It is used to alleviate excessive vasoconstriction, and as a pharmacological tool.

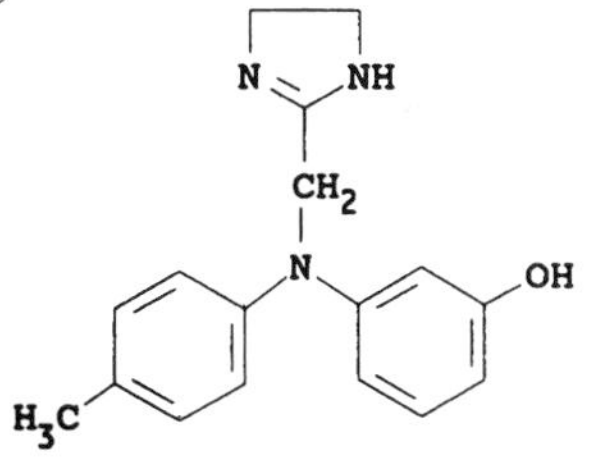

phenylalanine: Phe; F; an essential amino acid, incorporated directly, or after conversion to tyrosine, into many peptides and proteins. It is a precursor of catecholamines and related amines; but very high levels compete with tyrosine for plasma membrane transport systems, and can inhibit tyrosine hydroxylase. The degradation products include fumarate and acetoacetate. *See* also **homogentisate** and **phenylketonuria**.

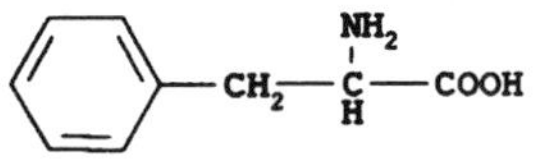

phenylalanine hydroxylase: phenylalanine 4-monooxygenase; an enzyme that catalyzes the reaction: phenylalanine + O_2 + tetrahydrobiopterin $\rightarrow$ tyrosine + H_2O. (Tetrahydrobiopterin is formed from dihydrobiopterin via a reaction in which NADPH + H^+ supply the hydrogen atoms and electrons; and it is subsequently reduced to the quinoid derivative by donating electrons and H^+ to NADH). Since most diets contain more phenylalanine than tyrosine, enzyme defects lead to accumulation of phenylalanine and several of its metabolites (*see* **phenylketonuria**), and to tryptophan deficiency.

phenylalkyloxirane carboxylic acid: POCA; an agent used to inhibit carnityltransferase.

3-**phenylamino**-L-alanine: a contaminant of L-tryptophan preparations that are made by microorganisms and used as nutritional supplements (or to treat insomnia). It is implicated as a cause of eosinophilia myalgia syndrome; *see* also **tryptophan**.

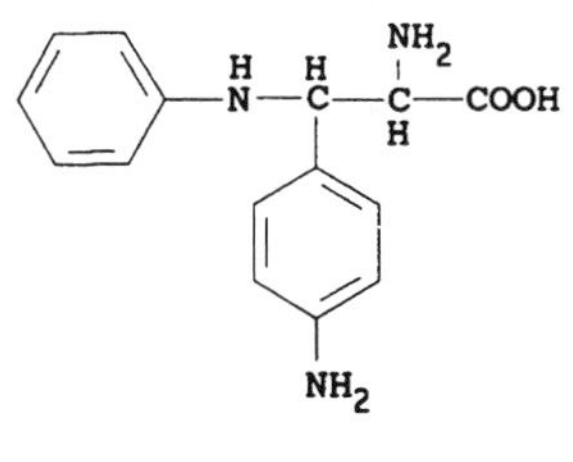

N-phenylanthranilic acid: diphenylamine-2-carboxylic acid; a chloride channel blocking agent.

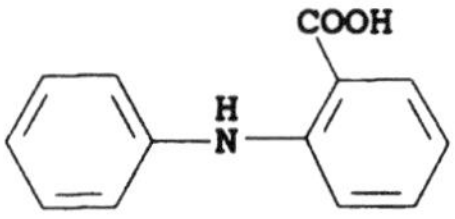

COOH

H
N

phenylbiguanidine: *N*-phenyl-imidocarbonimidic diamide; a 5HT$_3$-type serotonin receptor agonist.

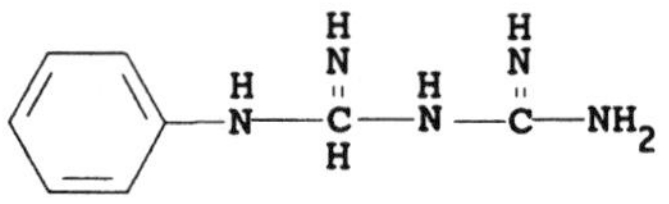

H   H
N   N
H   ‖   H   ‖
N——C——N——C——NH$_2$
H

phenylbutazone: 4-butyl-1,2,diphenyl-3,5,pyrazolidine-dione: a cyclooxygenase inhibitor used for its analgesic, anti-inflammatory, antipyretic, and uricosuric effects. Since it can damage the bone marrow, liver, and kidneys, and impair thyroid hormone synthesis, it is usually used only for short-term treatment of conditions such gout and rheumatoid arthritis that responds poory to salicylates.

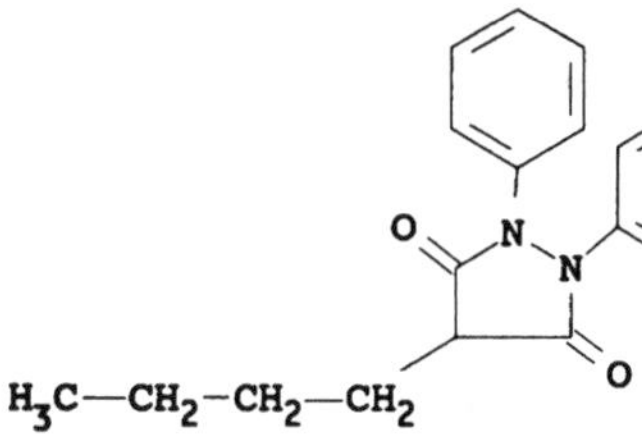

O   N
N
H$_3$C——CH$_2$—CH$_2$—CH$_2$
O

phenylephrine: *m*-methylaminoethanol; an α$_1$ type adrenergic receptor agonist. It is a potent vasoconstrictor that can elevate blood pressure. The *l*-isomer hydrochloride (Neo-synephrine) is a component of ophthalmic and nasal preparations used to reduce congestion. High concentrations also activate β$_1$ receptors.

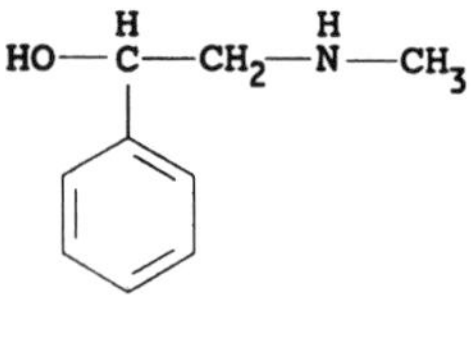

H   H
HO——C——CH$_2$——N——CH$_3$

phenylethanolamine: an agent chemically related to catecholamines that acts on α$_1$ receptors. The sulfate is used as a topical vasoconstrictor.

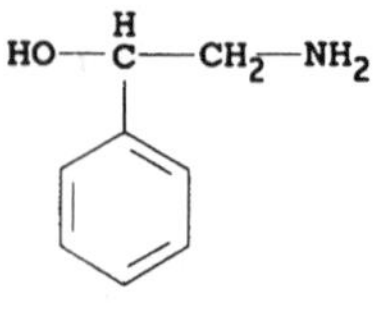

H
HO——C——CH$_2$——NH$_2$

phenylethanolamine-*N*-methyltransferase: PNMT: an enzyme that catalyzes conversion of norepinephrine to epinephrine, and some other reactions of the general type: *S*-adenosylmethionine + X → *S*-adenosylhomocysteine + X-CH$_3$. Blood vessels that drain the adrenal cortex supply the high glucocorticoid concentrations required to induce the enzyme in the adrenal medulla.

phenylethylamine, PE: an amine normally synthesized in small amounts from phenylalanine in catecholamine secreting cells, and implicated as a factor that elevates mood when released in larger amounts during physical exercise. Monoamine oxidase inhibitors, and other factors that alter catecholamine metabolism can cause accumulation of excessive quantities. When administered systemically, high doses act as false transmitters that affect behavior in laboratory animals. It has been suggested that PE accumulation invokes psychological dysfunction in humans, and that it contributes to the manifestations of schizophrenia in some individuals. It is is used topically as a vasoconstrictor.

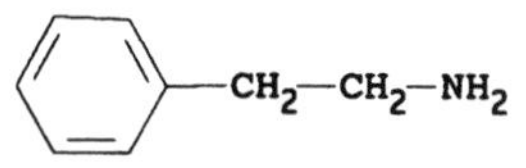

CH$_2$—CH$_2$—NH$_2$

phenylhydrazine: a hemolytic agent, used to invoke anemia in experimental animals for studies of erythropoietin synthesis and functions, and other hematological processes.

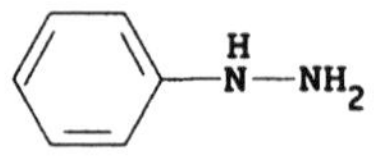

H
N——NH$_2$

N^6-phenylisopropyladenosine: an agent used to inhibit adenylate cyclases.

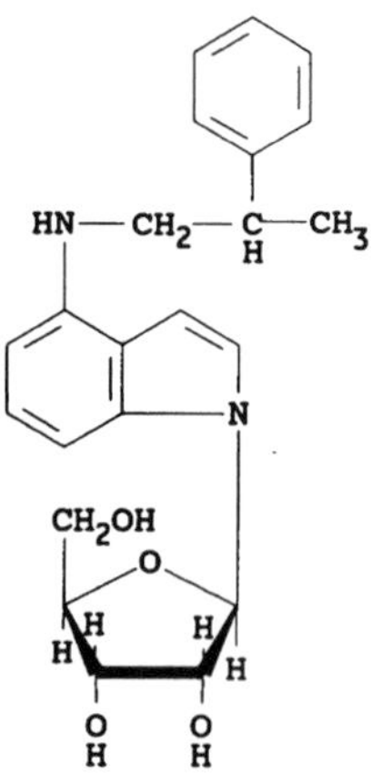

HN——CH$_2$——C——CH$_3$
H

N

CH$_2$OH
O
H   H
H   H
O   O
H   H

phenylisothiocyanate: a reagent used in the Edman degradation method for determining amino acid sequences. The *N*-terminal moiety of the peptide or protein reacts with the reagent, and is released as a phenyl-thiohydantoin (PTH) derivative.

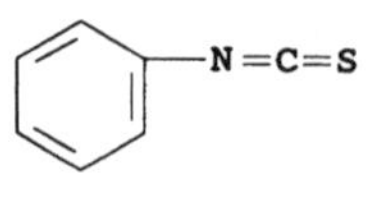

N=C=S

S
N——C
NH
O——C
H   CH$_3$

phenylisothio-
cyanate

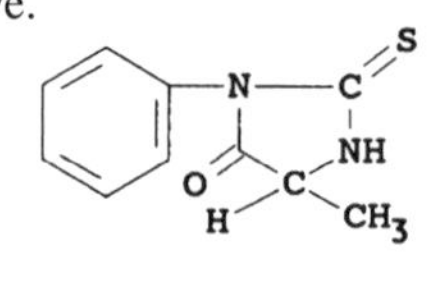

PTH-alanine

phenylketonuria: PKU; an autosomal recessive disorder in which brain development and functions are impaired by phenylalanine hydroxylase deficiency and consequent accumulation of large quantities of phenylalanine and phenylpyruvic acid. The symptoms can be averted with phenylalanine deficient diets.

phenylmethylsulfonyl chloride: tosyl chloride; this agent, and phenylmethyl sulfonyl fluoride (PMSF), are used to inhibit serine proteases.

$$CH_2-\overset{\overset{O}{\|}}{\underset{\underset{O}{\|}}{S}}-Cl$$

phenylpropanolamine: α-hydroxy-β-aminopropylbenzene; an α_1 type adrenergic receptor agonist The hydrochloride is used as a nasal decongestant, and as a component of some "diet pills" used to suppress appetite.

$$HO-\overset{\overset{}{\underset{H}{C}}}{}-\overset{\overset{NH_2}{\underset{H}{C}}}{}-CH_3$$

3-phenylpropylargylamine hydrochloride: a potent dopamine β-hydroxylase inhibitor.

$$C\equiv C-CH_2-NH_2 \cdot HCl$$

8-phenyltheophylline: 1,3-dimethyl-8-phenylxanthine; a selective A_1 type adenosine receptor antagonist.

phenylthiocarbamide: PTC; *see* **phenylthiourea**.

phenylthiohydantoin: PTH; *see* **phenylisothiocyanate**.

phenylthiourea: phenylthiocarbamide; PTC; an agent sensed as bitter by most humans, but tasteless by those homozygous for a recessive gene that affects taste perception. It is used for genetics studies.

$$\overset{}{\underset{}{N}}-\overset{\overset{}{}}{\underset{\underset{NH_2}{|}}{C}}=S$$

phenytoin: Dilantin; 5,5-diphenyl-2,4-imidazolidinedione; an anticonvulsant used to treat epilepsy and to control some cardiac arrhythmias. It affects ion transport (and especially Na^+ uptake), but does not invoke generalized central nervous system depression. Although it accelerates glucose oxidation in many cell types, it can invoke hyperglycemia and alleviate hyperinsulinemia by decreasing pancreatic β cell sensitivity to glucose. It lowers T_4 affinity for thyronine binding protein (TBG), and can invoke hypothryoidism by accelerating hepatic uptake and degradation of the hormone and antagonizing some of its actions.

pheo-: phaeo-; a prefix meaning brown or yellowish-brown, as in pheochromocytes.

phenytoin

pheochromoblasts: immature cells that develop into pheochromocytes.

pheochromocytes: chromaffin cells of the adrenal medulla, sympathetic paraganglia, and pheochromocytomas.

pheochromocytomas: encapsulated chromaffin cell tumors, usually in the adrenal medulla or associated with sympathetic system ganglia. Most are benign, but secrete quantities of norepinephrine (and in some cases also epinephrine) that invoke paroxysmal hypertension, sweating, pallor or flushing, vomiting, pain, headaches, and anxiety.

pheresis: procedures in which blood is withdrawn, and one or more components are subsequently returned to the body. In *plasmapheresis*, the formed elements are returned, to avert anemia and leukopenia in the donors. It is used to obtain certain components from healthy individuals, such as clotting factors for hemophiliacs, and also to remove undesirable substances in individuals with severe kidney diseases.

pheromones: regulators released externally that act on other members of the species. Some are made by microorganisms; *see* **mating types**. The term *releaser* describes alarm pheromones, sex attractants, and other volatile chemicals made by insects and some other invertebrates that act rapidly on the nervous systems of recipients and invoke stereotyped behavior. *Primer* is used for honeybee queen substance and related kinds, sensed by olfactory receptors, that act over long time periods on endocrine systems to influence reproduction. Some are ingested by the recipients. Vertebrates make some perceived as odors, but most types are sensed by vomeronasal organs. A few act rapidly on nervous systems, but (since the responses are more complex, less reproducible than insect types, and affected by the context in which they are received) the term *activational* is preferred to releaser. Examples include ones that arouse interest in members of the opposite sex, the kinds used to mark territories, and some that attract suckling infants to their mothers. Primer types can initiate complex responses; *see*, for example **Bruce**, **Vandenberg**, and **Whitten effects**, and **copulin**. Hormones regulate the biosynthesis, and some of the products are chemically related to gonadal steroids, A few are identical to hormones that also act internally. Others are are simpler alcohols, aldehydes, acetates, or mixtures of several related substances. *Cf* **allomones**, **kairomones**, and **synonomes**.

PHI: PHI-27; *see* **peptide histidine-isoleucine**.

-**phil**: -phile; *see* -**philia**.

Philadelphia chromosome: an abnormal chromosome in bone marrow cells of humans with chronic myelogenous leukemia, formed by a reciprocal translocation, (t9:22) (q34:q11), in which the *abl* oncogene of the short arm of chromosome 9 fuses head to tail with the end of a broken chromosome 22 long arm. In some cases, chromosome 22 splits at its major break cluster region (*bcr*); in others the break is at the first intron. Fused *bcr-abl* genes code for abnormal, heavily phosphorylated proteins (p190 and p210) with persistent tyrosine kinase activity that resemble the p160$^{gag-v-abl}$ viral protein whose synthesis is directed by the *v-abl* oncogene. In some humans with chronic myelogenous leukemia, more complex translocations that involve chromosome 17 have been described; and different rearrangements have been linked with erythroid leukemias.

philanthotoxin: *S-N*-[3-[[4-[(3-aminopropyl)amino]butyl]amino]propyl]-4-hydroxy-α-[(1-oxobutyl)amino]-benzenepropanamide; a synthetic analog of a wasp venom toxin that blocks NMDA-gated ion channels.

-**phile**: a suffix used for individuals to whom the suffix -philia applies.

-**philia**: -phile: a suffix meaning (1) excessive fondness for, or attraction to, as in paedophilia, or (2) excessive numbers or amounts, as in neutrophilia.

philo-: a prefix meaning love of, or craving for, as in philogyny (love of females).

phimosis: constriction or narrowing of an opening, for example of the vaginal orifice or prepuce. It can be caused by genetic defects, inflammation, or injury followed by scar formation.

phleb-: a prefix meaning vein, as in phlebotomy or phlebitis (inflammation of a vein).

phloretin: 3-(4-hydroxyphenyl)-1-(2,4,6-trihydroxy-phenyl)-1-propane; the aglucone of **phloridzin** *(q.v.)*.

phloridzin: phlorizin; phloretin glucoside: 1-[2-(β-D-glucopyranosyloxy)-4,6,-dihydroxy-phenyl]-3-(4-hydroxyphenyl)-1-propane; a glycoside in apple tree bark used for metabolism studies. It inhibits active glucose transport across renal, intestinal cell, and erythrocyte plasma membranes by binding to the carriers. The effects on proximal convoluted tubules lead to glycosuria.

PHM: peptide histidine-methionine.

phocomelia: developmental disorders in which the proximal portions of one or more limbs fail to develop (so that hands or feet are attached to the trunk by a single

phloridzin

bone). They can be caused by autosomal recessive gene defects, or are induced during fetal life by adverse conditions and pharmacological agents such as thalidomide.

phon-, **phono-**: a prefix meaning (1) sound, as in phonocardiograph; or (2) voice, as in phonation.

phorbol: 1,1a,1b,4,4a,7a,7b,8,9,9a-decahydro-4a,7b,9,9a-tetrahydroxy-3-(hydroxymethyl)-1,1,6,8-tetramethyl-5*H*-cyclopropa[3,4]benz[1,2-e]azulen-5-one; a complex polycyclic alcohol component of croton oil, expressed from the seeds of *Croton tiglium*. Although not effective in this form, diester derivatives such as PMA and TMA are highly potent inflammatory agents and co-carcinogens. They are diacylglycerol analogs that promote tumor formation by intercalating into plasma membranes and activating protein kinase C isozymes. The effects persist for long time periods, because the compounds are not rapidly degraded; and they invoke long-range secondary effects that include induction of transcription factors, interactions with MAP-1 (mitogen activated kinase-1), and changes in cell morphology. The consequences vary with the cell types. The esters can inhibit the binding of epidermal growth factor (EGF), somatostatin, thyrotropin releasing hormone (TRH), and other regulators to their receptors, activate some tyrosine kinases, and promote phosphorylations of receptors for EGF, insulin, insulin-like growth factors (IGFs) and other hormones, and of cytoskeletal components such as vinculin. They affect gap junctions, promote cytosol alkalinization by activating H$^+$/Na$^+$ exchange, accelerate internalization of receptors for EGF, somatostatin, and transferrin, promote the synthesis and turnover of phospholipids, prostaglandins, polyamines, proteins, and RNAs, and can induce cell differentiation and/or proliferation. By promoting phosphorylation of CD2, CD3, and other transmembrane proteins, they facilitate expression of interleukin-2 receptors, and can also stimulate degranulation of neutrophils, mast cells, and blood platelets. However, when continuously present for extended time periods, a major delayed effect is "down-regulation" of kinase C isozymes. Different phorbol esters that do not exert the

philanthotoxin

552

described actions (such as 4-α-phorbol-12,13-dideca-noate) are used as controls, but are potentially carcinogenic when presented for long time periods.

phorbol

phorbol 12-myristate-13-acetate: PMA; a highly potent co-carcinogen that activates kinase C isozymes; *see* **phorbols**.

phosgene: carbonyl chloride; a highly toxic gas generated in some industrial processes that can severely damage lung tissue, and has been used in chemical warfare.

phosphamidon: 2-chloro-2-diethylcarbamoyl-1-methyl-vinyl dimethyl phosphate; an insecticide that inhibits cholinesterases.

phosphagens: compounds with one or more high energy phosphate bonds that can be transferred to ADP and related molecules. Examples include creatine phosphate in vertebrate, and phosphoarginine in invertebrate muscle, both of which contain phosphoguanido groups.

phosphatases: enzymes that catalyze hydrolytic cleavage of phosphate ester bonds and release inorganic phosphate or pyrophosphate; *cf* **phosphodiesterases**. Some act on just one, or a limited number of related substrates, whereas others have broad specificities. The kinds that participate in intermediary metabolism are usually named for their substrates, as in glucose-6- and fructose-6-phosphatase. A few, such as *tartrate resistant acid phosphatase* are distinguished by special properties; *see* also **acid** and **alkaline phosphatases**. The substrates for phosphoprotein phosphatases (*see* **protein phosphatases**) include other enzymes, such as glycogen synthase (which is activated by loss of phosphate groups), glycogen phosphorylase (which is inactivated), as well as regulatory proteins that mediate signal transduction or are involved in protein synthesis, cell cycle control, and other major functions. For some types, the effects of dephosphorylation at one molecular locus are very different from those at another. Many molecules dephosphorylated by the enzymes are substrates for tyrosine and or/serine-threonine kinases.

phosphate: (1) inorganic phosphate, represented in equations as P or Pi; (2) ions such as orthophosphate (PO_4^{3-}) and metaphosphate (HPO_3^{2-}), and compounds formed from them, including inorganic salts such as Na_3PO_4 and or Na_2HPO_4, and organic compounds of the general type $X-OPO_3H_2$. (Compounds with two covalently linked phosphate groups are pyrophosphates.) The most common inorganic ion in biological fluids is HPO_4^{2-}. *See* also **phosphorus**, **phosphatases**, and **phosphorylases**.

phosphate bond energy: chemical energy stored in a phosphate ester bond that can be released by hydrolysis, for example the energy stored in the two terminal phosphate bonds of adenosine and guanosine triphosphates (ATP and GTP), and related nucleotides, and in compounds such as creatine-phosphate and phosphoenol-pyruvate (PEP). The high energy content is related to electrostatic repulsions caused by the presence of four negative charges, and to bond resonance. The amount of free energy released by hydrolysis varies with the chemical nature. Approximate values in Cal/mole are 14.8, 7.3, and 3.3, respectively for PEP, the γ bond of ATP, and glucose-6-phosphate.

phosphatidal cholines: plasmalogens in cardiac and nervous tissue, and also present in small amounts in circulating blood. Each molecule contains an α,β-unsaturated fatty acid linked to carbon 1 of glycerol by an ether bond, a second fatty acid linked to carbon 2 by an acyl bond, and phosphorylcholine attached to carbon 3. *Cf* **phosphatidylcholines**.

phosphatidic acids {**phosphatidates**}: PA; diacyl-glycerol-3-phosphates; compounds composed of two long-chain fatty acids linked by ester bonds to carbons 1

phorbol 12-myristate-13-acetate

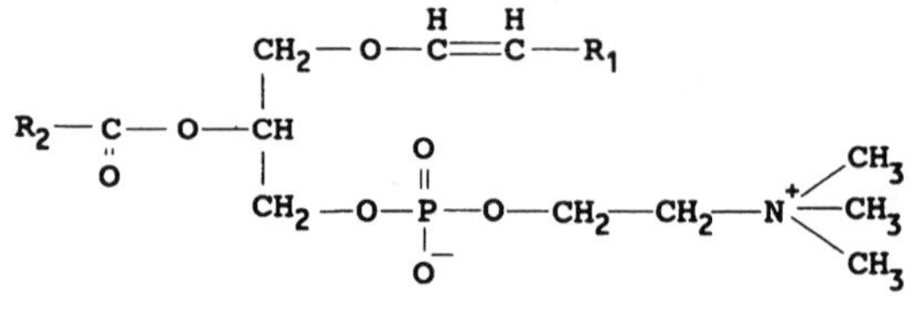

phosphatidal cholines

and 2 of glycerol, and a phosphate group linked to carbon 3. They are intermediates in pathways for biosynthesis of triacylglycerols, most phospholipids, and some other lipids. Their formation is accomplished in two steps: glycerol-3-phosphate + fatty-acyl-CoA → lysophosphatide + CoA, followed by lysophosphatide + fatty-acyl-CoA → PA + CoA. PAs are liberated from membrane phospholipids by phospholipase D-catalyzed reactions, and are metabolized to yield free fatty acids (including eicosanoid precursors). Although most effects are mediated by the products, PAs directly activate kinase C isozymes; and at least two PA-dependent kinases (one of which is Ca^{2+}-independent) induce c-myc and c-fos proteins, platelet derived growth factor (PDGF), and other proliferation stimulants, and promote blood platelet aggregation, superoxide generation by neutrophilic leukocytes, steroid hormone synthesis, and release of aldosterone, insulin, and parathyroid hormone.

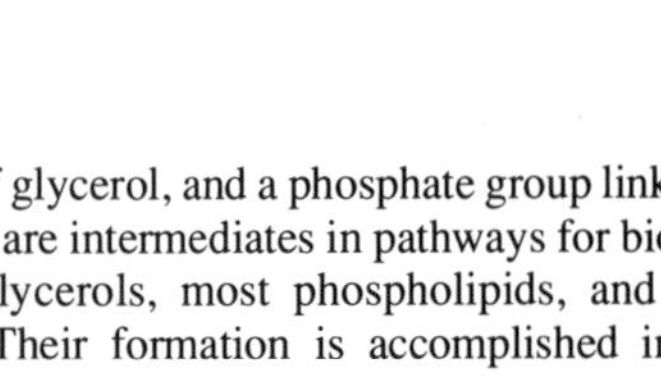

phosphatidic acids

phosphatidylcholines: PC; lecithins; vitellin; the most abundant phospholipid types in eukaryote cell plasma membranes. In most kinds, the fatty acid attached to the first carbon of the glycerol component is stearic, palmitic, or oleic. PCs are also components of bile, and of egg yolk and other foods. Since they are amphipathic, their surfactant properties are used in food preparation and other processes. The biosynthesis is accomplished via: phosphorylcholine + CTP (cytidine triphosphate) → CDP-choline + P-P, followed by CDP-choline + diacylglycerol → PC + CMP. Cells also make PCs from other membrane phospholipids, for example in reactions in which phosphatidyl ethanolamine accepts three methyl groups from *S*-adenosyl-methionine (and 3 *S*-adenosylhomocysteines are liberated). *See* also **phospholipases**.

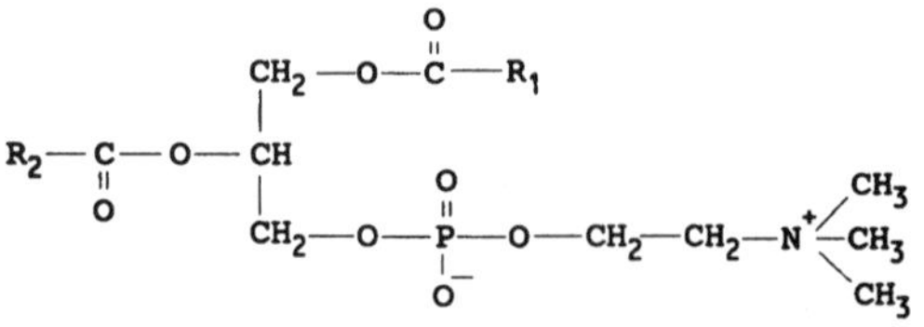

phosphatidylethanolamines: PE; phospholipids in which the alcoholic group is ethanolamine, synthesized via pathways similar to those for phosphatidylcholines, and also derived from those molecules via demethylation, or from phosphatidylserines via decarboxylation of the amino acid moieties. PEs are more abundant than phosphatidylcholines in prokaryotic plasma membranes and internal membranes of eukaryotic cells, and are the major myelin phospholipids.

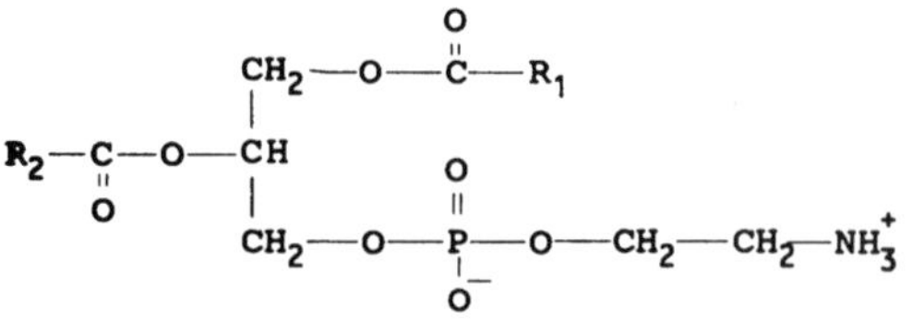

phosphatidylinositols: PtdIns; PIs; phospholipids (*q.v.*) in which *myo*-inositol is the alcoholic moiety. The fatty acid attached to carbon 2 of glycerol is usually unsaturated. PIs are present in much smaller amounts than other plasma membrane phospholipids, and function primarily in signal transduction and cell cycle control after conversion to **phosphatidylinositol phosphates** (*q.v.*). *See* also **phosphoinositidase** C and **phosphatidylinositol glycans**.

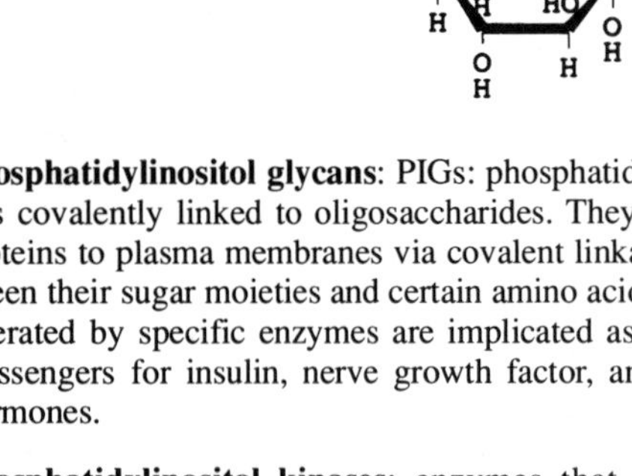

phosphatidylinositol glycans: PIGs: phosphatidylinositols covalently linked to oligosaccharides. They anchor proteins to plasma membranes via covalent linkages between their sugar moieties and certain amino acids. PIGs liberated by specific enzymes are implicated as second messengers for insulin, nerve growth factor, and other hormones.

phosphatidylinositol kinases: enzymes that convert phosphatidylinositol to **phosphatidylinositol phosphates** (*q.v.*). *See* also **phosphoinositidase** C and **inositol phosphates**.

phosphatidylinositol phosphates: PtdInsPs; PIPs; phosphorylated, inositol-containing membrane phospholipids derived from phosphatidylinositols via reactions catalyzed by phosphatidylinositol kinases. Ptdlns (1,4) biphosphate is cleaved to **inositol(1,4,5) triphosphate** ($IP_{1,4,5}$, *q.v.*) and **diacylglycerols** (*q.v.*). $IP_{1,4,5}$ is a major second messenger that recruits intracellular Ca^{2+} from non-mitochondrial sequestration sites, and a substrate for kinases that convert it to $Ins(1,3,4,5)P_4$ and other derivatives. The diacylglycerols activate kinase C isozymes, and are substrates for lipases that release arachidonate. An inositol lipid 3-kinase converts $PtdIns(4,5)P_2$ to $PtdIns(3,4,5)P_3$. The product is not cleaved by phosphoinositidase C, but is acted on by phosphatases to yield $PtdIns(3,4)P_2$ and $PtdIns(3)P$. The products of those reactions are believed to function as receptors on the inner faces of plasma membranes that bind as yet unidentified ligands and contribute to cell cycle controls. Many hormone-receptor complexes that couple to G proteins activate phosphoinositidase C isozymes. The enzymes are also activated by ligands for epidermal growth factor (EGF), platelet derived growth factor (PDGF), and other receptor types that possess intrinsic tyrosine kinase components, and by src-related tyrosine kinases (including T lymphocyte $\alpha\beta$-CD3-p59^{fyn} antigen receptors).

phosphatidylserines: PS; negatively charged membrane **phospholipids** (*q.v.*) in which serine is the alcoholic group, synthesized from CDP-diacylglycerols in reactions of the kinds shown for phosphatidylcholines. They can be methylated to phosphatidylcholines. PSs bind Ca^{2+} and other divalent ions, and contribute to activation of some protein kinase C isozymes and to the control of some adenylate cyclases and other enzymes.

phosphoarginine: an invertebrate muscle phosphagen with functions analogous to those of creatine phosphate in vertebrate muscle.

phosphocreatine: creatine phosphate.

phosphodiester[s]: compounds in which two oxygen atoms of a phosphate group form covalent bonds. Examples include cyclic adenosine and guanosine monophosphates (cAMP and cGMP), and nucleic acids. In the diagram, B = a nitrogens base, and S a sugar.

phosphodiesterases: PDEs: cyclic nucleotide phosphodiesterases, endonucleases, and other enzymes that cleave single covalent phosphate bonds of phosphodiesters. Unlike phosphatases, they do not liberate Pi.

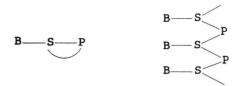

phosphodiesters

Some act on numerous substrate types, whereas others have more restricted specificities.

phosphoenolpyruvic acid {**phosphoenolpyruvate**}: PEP; an intermediate of several biochemical pathways. It is made from 2-phosphoglycerate, and its irreversible conversion to pyruvate is an energy-yielding step that "pulls" glycolysis to completion. During gluconeogenesis, it is made from oxaloacetate (*see* **phosphoenolpyruvate carboxykinase**). In some plants, it is generated via: pyruvate + ATP + P → PEP + AMP + P-P + H$^+$. In bacteria, it contributes to glucose transport by donating its phosphate group to glucose.

phosphoenolpyruvate carboxykinase: PEP carboxykinase: PEPCK; an enzyme that catalyzes the reaction of the gluconeogenesis pathway: oxaloacetate + GTP → phosphoenolpyruvate + GDP + CO_2. It is induced by glucocorticoids and triiodothyronine (T_3), and its activity in liver is augmented by glucagon.

phosphofructokinases: PFK; isozymes that catalyze: fructose-6-phosphate + ATP → fructose-1-6-biphosphate + ADP. The reaction is irreversible under physiological conditions, and it "pushes" the substrate into the glycolysis pathway. ATP is a negative allosteric regulator whose effects are reversed by AMP. Other negative regulators include high H^+ and citrate levels. The liver isozyme is a 340K tetramer strongly affected by fructose-2-6-biphosphate (which increases affinity for the substrate and diminishes the effects of ATP). Insulin activates the enzyme via dephosphorylation; glucagon (which promotes phosphorylation) inhibits.

phosphoglucomutase: an enzyme that catalyzes reversible interconversion of glucose-1-and glucose-6-phosphate. The direction is controlled mostly by substrate concentrations. An intermediate, glucose-1,6-biphosphate, is formed but not released from the enzyme. Glucose is converted directly to Glu-6-P, the metabolite that enters the glycolysis and hexose monophosphate pathways. Glu-1-P is the form needed for glycogen synthesis (*see* **glycogen synthetase**). It is also the product of glycogen phosphorylase reactions, and of ones in which galactose-P epimerizes to glucose phosphate.

6-**phosphogluconate**: a metabolite of the hexose monophosphate pathway. Glucose-6-phosphate dehydrogenase catalyzes: glucose-6-phosphate + NADP$^+$ → 6-phosphoglucono-δ-lactone, and the product is then hydrolyzed to 6-phosphogluconate. The next step, catalyzed by 6-phosphogluconate dehydrogenase, is 6-phosphogluconate +

$NADP^+ \rightarrow$ ribulose-5-phosphate. $NADPH + H^+$ is made in both reactions.

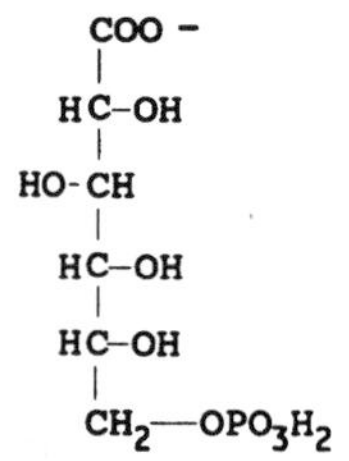

$$
\begin{array}{c}
COO^- \\
|\\
HC{-}OH \\
|\\
HO{-}CH \\
|\\
HC{-}OH \\
|\\
HC{-}OH \\
|\\
CH_2{-}OPO_3H_2
\end{array}
$$

6-phosphogluconate

3-**phosphoglyceraldehyde**: glyceraldehyde-3-phosphate: an intermediate in the glycolysis pathway, formed (along with dihydroxyacetone-phosphate) from fructose-1,6-biphosphate in a reaction catalyzed by aldolase. Glyceraldehyde-3-phosphate dehydrogenase then catalyzes its oxidation to 1,3-bisphosphoglycerate. It can also be made from, and converted to dihydroxyacetone phosphate, the direct precursor of the glycerol-3-phosphate used for triacylglycerol synthesis.

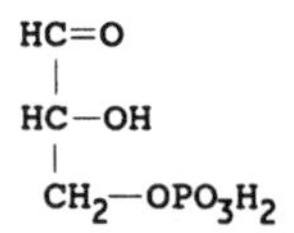

$$
\begin{array}{c}
HC{=}O \\
|\\
HC{-}OH \\
|\\
CH_2{-}OPO_3H_2
\end{array}
$$

3-**phosphoglyceraldehyde dehydrogenase**: *see* **glyceraldehyde-3-phosphate dehydrogenase**.

phosphoglycerate dehydrogenase: an enzyme that catalyzes: 3-phosphoglycerate $+ NAD^+ \rightarrow$ phosphohydroxypyruvate $+ NADH + H^+$. Phosphohydroxypyruvate reacts with glutamate to yield 3-phosphoserine $+$ α-ketoglutarate; and phosphoserine phosphatase releases serine $+$ Pi.

phosphoglycerate kinase: an enzyme that catalyzes the reversible reaction: 3-phosphoglycerate $+$ Pi $\rightarrow$ 1,3-diphosphoglycerate. The reaction proceeds to the right in the glycolysis pathway, and to the left in gluconeogenesis.

3-**phosphoglyceric acid** {3-**phosphoglycerate ion**}: 3-PG; one of the two intermediates of the glycolysis pathway formed in substrate linked phosphorylation reaction: 1,3-bisphosphoglycerate $+$ ADP $\rightarrow$ 3-PG $+$ ATP. In the next step, 3-PG is converted to 2-phosphoglycerate (the precursor of phosphoenolpyruvate). In gluconeogenesis, 3-PG is phosphorylated to 1,3-biphosphoglycerate. 3-PG is also made (via enediol and hydroperoxide intermediates) from ribulose-5-phosphate. Phosphoglycerate dehydrogenase catalyzes: 3-PG $+ NAD^+ \rightarrow NADH + H^+$ $+$ phosphohydroxypyruvate (an intermediate in pathways for biosynthesis of serine and glycine).

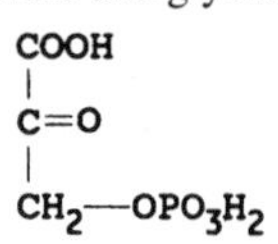

$$
\begin{array}{c}
COOH \\
|\\
C{=}O \\
|\\
CH_2{-}OPO_3H_2
\end{array}
$$

phosphoglycerides: phosphatidic acid, phospholipids, and other compounds with glycerol moieties covalently linked to phosphate groups. Most have fatty acids linked via ester bonds to carbons 1 and 2 of the glycerol.

phosphoglyceromutase: an enzyme that catalyzes the reversible reaction of glycolysis and gluconeogenesis pathways: 3-phosphoglycerate $\rightleftarrows$ 2 phosphoglycerate, via a 2,3-diphosphoglycerate intermediate that is not released.

phosphohexoseisomerase: an enzyme that catalyzes the reversible reaction used in both glycolysis and gluconeogenesis: glucose-6-phosphate $\rightleftarrows$ fructose-6-phosphate.

phosphohydroxypyruvate: an intermediate in the pathway for biosynthesis of serine from 3-**phosphoglycerate** (*q.v.*).

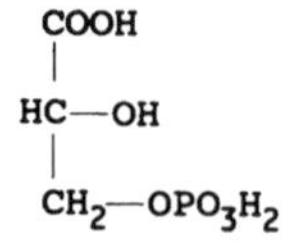

$$
\begin{array}{c}
COOH \\
|\\
HC{-}OH \\
|\\
CH_2{-}OPO_3H_2
\end{array}
$$

phosphoinositidases: phospholipase C isozymes specific for phosphatidylinositol substrates. Their activities are regulated by several hormones. The products are diacylglycerols and inositol-phosphates. *See* also **phosphatidylinositol phosphates**.

phospholamban: PLN; an integral sarcoplasmic reticulum protein of cardiac, smooth, and slow-twitch skeletal muscles (but not fast-twitch muscles or of plasma membranes), composed of five identical, 6.1K peptides that can assume several configurations. Each of the peptide chains contains sequences for selective kinase A and calmodulin kinase mediated phosphorylations. The unphosphorylated form binds to calcium-free Ca^{2+}-ATPase in the endoplasmic reticulum, inhibits the enzyme, and mediates muscle relaxation. High Ca^{2+} and phosphorylation relieve the inhibition. Phospholamban is formed when adrenergic agents acting on β_1 type receptors generate cAMP.

phospholipases: enzymes that catalyze hydrolytic degradation of phospholipids; *see* **phospholipases A$_1$, A$_2$, C,** and **D, phosphoinositidases**, and **phospholipids**. The diagram shows the cleavage sites for the various types. Isozymes within each class differ from each other in chemical make-up, distribution, and sensitivities to regulators. The activities are modified by hormones with receptors that are coupled to G proteins or contain tyrosine kinase components. The reaction products include several second messengers and messenger precursors.

phospholipase A$_1$: enzymes that catalyze Ca^{2+}-dependent cleavage of phospholipid acyl bonds at carbon 1 positions of glycerol moieties. Each molecule yields a biologically active lysophosphatidic acid and a free fatty acid, both of which affect membrane properties. Most of the liberated fatty acids are long-chain saturated types.

phospholipase A$_2$: enzymes that catalyze Ca^{2+}-dependent cleavage of phospholipid acyl bonds at carbon 2 positions of glycerol moieties. Each phospholipid mole-

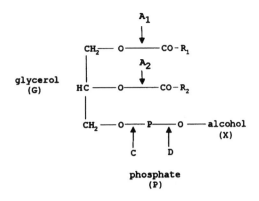

glycerol
(G)

$$CH_2 - O \xrightarrow{A_1} CO-R_1$$
$$HC - O \xrightarrow{A_2} CO-R_2$$
$$CH_2 - O \xleftarrow[C]{} P \xleftarrow[D]{} O - \text{alcohol (X)}$$

phosphate
(P)

$PLA_1 \rightarrow$ R_1—COOH + lysophosphatidic acid *

$PLA_2 \rightarrow$ R_2—COOH + lysophosphatidic acid **

PLC $\rightarrow$ diacylglycerol *** + alcohol phosphate ****

PLD $\rightarrow$ phosphatidic acid ***** + alcohol

phospholipases

cule yields a lysophosphatidic acid and a free fatty acid. Arachidonic is the major type, but some phospholipids release homogammalinoleic or other fatty acids. Class I types act mostly on molecules associated with membranes or micelles, and are activated by hormones and other regulators. The Formosan cobra (*Naja naja atra*) and some related species make enzymes similar to the 14K type in pancreatic acinar cells. Mammals usually make only minute amounts of secretory (class II) enzymes; but mediators of inflammatory reactions promote their accumulation in exudates, and the ones in synovial fluids of individuals with rheumatoid arthritis are believed to initiate pathological changes. The venom of the diamond back rattlesnake, *Crotalus atrax* contains a similar enzyme. Chemically different, incompletely characterized forms are present in blood platelets and in bee venoms. Glucocorticoids stimulate the synthesis of lipocortins, which indirectly inhibit by binding the substrates; and they also inhibit enzymes that promote conversion of arachidonic and other polyunsaturated fatty acids to eicosanoids.

phospholipase B: a term formerly applied to enzymes believed to possess both phospholipase A_1 and phospholipase A_2 activities, and to ones that cleave lysophosphatidic acids to phosphatidic acids + free fatty acids. More specific terms, such as lysolecithinase, are now used.

phospholipase C: enzymes that cleave phospholipid acyl bonds at the carbon 3 position. Both products (diacylglycerols and phosphorylated alcohols) are biologically active. At least five different genes code for immunologically distinct types with only limited amino acid sequence homologies. They differ in distributions and properties such as calcium dependence. Three are specific for phosphatidylinositols and their phosphorylated derivatives; *see* also **phosphatidylinositol phosphates**. 65K and 68K proteins of this group, isolated from sheep seminal vesicles and rat liver, respectively, were initially called type I are but are now known as type α. They resemble a 62K protein from guinea pig uterus that was initially called type II. The terms β_1, β_2, and β_3 have been proposed for 150-154K, 130K, and 100K isozymes identified in bovine brain, and γ for a 145K isozyme in brain and elsewhere. The platelet isozyme appears to differ from the others. Phospholipase $C_{\beta1}$ is activated when acetylcholine binds to M1 type muscarinic receptors which couple to G proteins, and the enzyme, in turn, augments the GTPase activity of the G protein α subunit. Phospholipase Cγ isozymes are the major types activated by hormones that promote generation of **inositol phosphates** (*q.v.*).

phospholipase D: enzymes that cleave phospholipid phosphate-alcohol bonds. The products are phosphatidic acids and free alcohols (mostly choline, serine, and ethanolamine).

phospholipids: amphipathic compounds composed of fatty acid, alcoholic, and phosphate moieties. Phosphatidylcholines, phosphatidylserines, phosphatidylethanolamines (named for their alcoholic groups) are essential components of all cell membrane bilayers, and precursors of biologically active derivatives. They affect properties such as fluidity and the activities of many enzymes. Some are sources of second messengers and other cell regulators. Phosphatidylinositols, which are present in smaller amounts, serve primarily as sources of second messengers, and possibly also as receptor precursors. All of the preceding have two fatty acid moieties linked to carbons 1 and 2 of glycerol, a phosphate linked to the third carbon, and an alcohol linked to the phosphate. Sphingomyelins, which predominate in nervous tissues, contain sphingosine bonded to a single fatty acid, plus a phosphorylcholine moiety. *See* also **plasmalogens** and **platelet activating factor**.

phospholipid bilayer: the major component of biological membranes, composed of two layers of phospholipid molecules oriented as shown in the diagram, with hydrophobic tails (fatty acid chains represented by wavy lines) directed inward towards each other. The hydrophilic heads (charged regions represented by circles) of one layer face the cytoplasm, and those of the other contact the external environment. Integral membrane proteins and cholesterol reside within the bilayer. Some peripheral proteins have covalently linked hydrophobic groups that insert into it; others are anchored at one end via bonds to integral proteins.

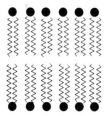

phosphomycin: phosphonomycin.

phosphonates: nonhydrolyzable compounds that contain R—C—P— or P—C—P— bonds. They bind calcium, and can affect bone mineralization; *see*, for example **etidronate**.

phosphonoacetic acid: an agent that inhibits the DNA-dependent DNA polymerases (and thereby DNA replication) of *Herpes* viruses and cytomegalovirus.

phosphonoacetic acid

phosphonomycin: phosphomycin; fosfomycin; (2-*R-cis*)-(3-methyloxiranyl)-phosphonic acid; an antibiotic made by some *Streptomyces* strains. It is a phosphoenolpyruvate analog that blocks incorporation of lactyl groups into muramic acids.

phosphoproteins: pp; proteins with one or more amino acid moieties covalently linked to phosphate groups, a term also applied to types that can undergo reversible dephosphorylations catalyzed by phosphatases. The most common phosphorylation sites are serine, threonine, and tyrosine moieties.

phosphoprotein phosphatases: *see* **protein phosphatases**.

phosphoramidon: *N*-[α-rhamnopyranosyloxyhydroxyphosphinyl]-Leu-Trp; an antibiotic obtained from bacteria that inhibits thermolysin, collagenases, and enkephalinases.

5-phosphoribosyl-1-pyrophosphate: PRPP; the ribose-phosphate donor for nucleotide biosynthesis, and an essential intermediate for bacterial synthesis of tryptophan and histidine, made in the reaction: ribose-5-phosphate + ATP → PRPP + AMP. It reacts with orotate to yield orotidylate + P-P. In other reactions that liberate P-P, it combines with glutamine to yield 5-phosphorylribosyl-1-amine + glutamate, with anthraniliate to form a tryptophan precursor, and with ATP to form a histidine precursor.

PRPP

orotodylate

phosphoribosyl transferases: enzymes that catalyze reactions of the general type: X + 5-phosphoribosyl pyrophosphate (PRPP) $\rightarrow$ X-P + P-P, where X is a nucleotide precursor. Mammalian types include adenine and hypoxanthine-guanine transferases, and an orotidate type that additionally displays orotidine decarboxylase activity. Bacteria make some kinds not present in higher animals, for example one specific for uracil.

phosphorolysis: reactions of the general type: X—O—Y + $H\text{-}OPO_3H_2$ $\rightarrow$ X—OH + $Y\text{—}OPO_3H_2$, in which X is organic; *cf* **hydrolysis**. One example is $glycogen_{n\ glucose}$ + Pi $\rightarrow$ $glycogen_{(n\text{-}1)\ glucose}$ + glucose-1-phosphate.

phosphorus: P; an element (atomic number 15, atomic weight 30.794). It is an essential component of hydroxyapatite, nucleic acids, ATP, cAMP, cGMP, phospholipids, phosphoproteins, metabolic intermediates such as glucose-phosphates, some oligosaccharides, and other biologically important compounds; and it affects most physiological functions either directly or via interactions with calcium. Many enzymes are activated by phosphorylation at specific sites, and others are inactivated in that way. Since it forms poorly ionized calcium salts, inorganic phosphate is a major determinant of the amount of calcium present as free Ca^{2+} ion. It is sequestered in mitochondria as amorphous, inactive $Ca_3(PO_4)_2$. Since the precipitate is made in the reaction: 2 Ca^{2+} + 2 HPO_4^{2-} $\rightarrow$ $Ca_3(PO_4)_2$ + 2 H^+, it lowers cytoplasmic phosphate, and also cytoplasmic pH (since the H^+ is released). (The reverse changes occur when the calcium phosphate is recruited). $[^{32}]P$, a radioactive isotope with a half-life of 14.3 days, is widely used in metabolic studies, and to label nucleic acids and other compounds.

phosphorylases: enzymes that catalyze reactions of the general type XY + $H\text{-}OPO_3H_2$ $\rightleftarrows$ XH + $Y\text{-}OPO_3H_2$. Although theoretically reversible, most proceed in just one direction in cells. For example, glycogen phosphorylase converts a glycogen molecule branch with *n* sugar moieties to one with *n−1* moieties, and liberates a glucose phosphate. (Glycogen chain elongation is accomplished via a different pathway, in which a uridyl transferase catalyzes formation of uridine-diphosphate glucose [UDPG], and glycogen synthetase promotes transfer of the glucose component of that molecule to the end of a glycogen chain.) Unlike **kinases** (*q.v.*), phosphorylases do not use ATP or related energy donors; and unlike phosphatases, they do not use water. However, the term *phosphorylation* can apply to any reaction in which phosphate is added to a substrate, and *dephosphorylation* to any in which phosphate is removed (*see* also **phosphotransferases**, and **oxidative** and **substrate-linked phosphorylations**).

phosphorylase kinases: enzymes that catalyze transfers of phosphate groups from ATP or related high energy phosphate donors to phosphorylase enzymes; *see*, for example **glycogen phosphorylase *b* kinase**, and *cf* **phosphorylases**.

phosphorylase phosphatases: enzymes that cleave phosphate groups from phosphorylases and release inorganic phosphate.

phosphorylation: any reaction that involves covalent addition of phosphate groups to other molecules, including ones catalyzed by phosphorylases, phosphotransferases, and kinases. The reactions can affect surface charges, affinities for cations, nucleic acids, and other substances, molecular configurations, and enzyme activities. *See* also **oxidative phosphorylation** and **substrate-linked phosphorylation**.

phosphorylcholine: an intermediate in the pathway for biosynthesis of phospholipids and related molecules, and a product formed when phospholipase C type enzymes degrade phosphatidylcholine.

phosphotransferases: enzymes that transfer phosphate groups from one organic molecule to another, or from one position to another within the same molecule.

phosvitin: phosphovitellin; a 40K egg yolk protein cleaved from vitellogenin; *see* **lipovitellin**. It is used as an anticoagulant.

photoactivation: changing the properties of molecules by exposing them to light (usually in the ultraviolet range). Compounds that enter cells and undergo such activation are used as markers to study the functions of cations and other cell components. *See* also **photoaffinity labeling**.

photoaffinity labeling: techniques for identifying molecules with marker compounds which, when activated by light (usually in the ultraviolet range) covalently link to the substances investigated. Most markers are radioactive or fluorescent. Since they can promote tight bonding of molecules that otherwise form loose physical associations, the markers are also used to identify the points of contact.

photallergens: substances that invoke allergic reactions when sensitized individuals are exposed to light.

photoauxotrophs: organisms that use light energy to convert inorganic molecules to metabolic fuels and cell components, and therefore do not require organic nutrients made by other organisms.

photobleaching: light-induced loss of the ability to absorb light of specific wavelengths.

photochromogenic: describes substances that form colored derivatives when exposed to light.

photodensitometry: quantitative measurements (usually with photoelectric cells) of the darkening of processed photographic or X-ray films, by determining the amounts of light transmitted through various regions.

photodermatitis: allergic skin reactions invoked by photoallergens.

photodisintegration: atomic emission of neutrons or charged particles induced by high-energy radiation.

photoelectric effect: acquisition of kinetic energy by molecules subjected to photons that promote ejection of electrons.

photoelectron: an electron ejected from its orbit by collision with a photon.

photogenesis: light production, for example by bioluminescent organisms.

photogenic: in science, (1) produced by light; (2) producing or emitting light.

photohaptens: substances produced when compounds altered by exposure to light (usually in the ultraviolet range) combine with skin proteins to form photoallergens.

photoluminescence: fluorescence or other light emission induced by exposure to light rays.

photolysis: light-induced cleavage of chemical bonds. Reactions of this type are used in photosynthesis.

photon: an uncharged quantum of electromagnetic radiation that travels at the speed of light.

photoperiod: the duration of the light phase of a light-dark cycle.

photoperiodism: regularly recurring responses of living organisms to cyclical changes in the wavelengths, intensities, and/or durations of environmental light. The activities of several "biological clocks" are synchronized by photoperiods; *see*, for example **suprachiasmatic nuclei**. Examples of animal responses include diurnal rhythms for body temperatures, locomotor activity, renal excretion of ions, and the release of gonadotropins, growth hormone, glucocorticoids, and other humoral regulators, as well as seasonal rhythms that, in some species, markedly affect reproductive system functions and fur color. Enzymes affected include ones involved in melatonin synthesis, and the kinds that determine whether plants are "long day" (flower when the hours of daylight increase during spring and summer) or "short day" types.

photophosphorylation: usually, reactions in chloroplasts in which light provides the energy for ATP synthesis. In *non-cyclic* photophosphorylation, electrons released by photolysis of water generate proton gradients, and $NADP^+$ is converted to $NADPH + H^+$. In *cyclic* photophosphorylation, proton gradients are generated, but the electrons are recycled and $NADP^+$ is not reduced.

photopic vision: light perception and associated sequelae, mediated by retinal cones. It requires bright light, and is used to visualize colors and fine detail; *cf* **scotopic vision**.

photopsins: visual pigments of retinal cones; *cf* **scotopsins**. *See* also **transducins**.

photoreactivation: reversal, by light in the visible range, of injury caused by ultraviolet radiation.

photoreceptors: cells specialized for perceiving light and transmitting signals to other cell types (usually neurons). Examples include the light-sensitive components of vertebrate retinal rods, cones, and pineal glands, the ommatidia of invertebrates, and the eye-spots of some microorganisms. Some signals in animals lead to conscious visual perception. Others affect processes such as contraction of iris muscles, hormone production rates, and synchronization of body rhythms with photoperiods. *See* also **primary**, **accessory**, and **retinohypothalamic tracts**.

photosynthesis: processes by which green plants, algae, and some bacteria absorb radiant energy from the sun and use it to synthesize organic compounds. It begins with light absorption by carotenoids and chlorophyll in chloroplast thylakoid membranes (or by chlorophyll related and accessory substances in microorganisms). When light energy activates, hydrogen and electrons are transferred from donor to acceptor molecules. In plants, the donor is water, and molecular oxygen is released. In sulfur bacteria, the donor is hydrogen sulfide (H_2S), and sulfur is released. (The *Hill reaction*, in which isolated illuminated chloroplasts cleave water, release oxygen, and pass electrons to ferricyanide, has provided insights into the processes.) The *light phase* in plants employs two pathways. *Photosystem I* has P_{700}, which absorbs wave lengths of up to 700 nm, and passes electrons along a ferredoxin-containing chain, which (with water) promotes reduction of $NADP^+$, and also sends electron along chains similar to those of mitochondria which generate ATP from ADP + Pi. *Photosystem II* contains P_{680}, which passes electrons along pathways that reactivate P_{700}, and others that lead to ATP synthesis. Light reactions provide the energy for the *dark phase* of plant photosynthesis (*Calvin cycle*), in which ribulose-1,5-biphosphate molecules incorporate CO_2 to form intermediates, each of which yields two molecules of 3-phosphoglycerate. The 3-phosphoglycerate is then converted to glucose in several reactions that require ATP and NADPH. Regeneration of ribulose 1,5-biphosphate also requires ATP energy. The overall pathway for the dark reaction can be summarized as: $6\ CO_2 + 18\ ATP + 12\ NADPH + 12\ H_2O \rightarrow C_6H_{12}O_6 + 18\ ADP + 18\ Pi + 12NADP^+ + 6\ H^+$.

photosystems I and **II**: *see* **photosynthesis**.

phototaxis: light-directed movement (*positive* if toward, and *negative* if away from the light source), The term can refer to the activities of motile whole organisms, or to cells within an organism whose movements affect growth patterns; *see* also **phototropism**.

phototropes: organisms that depend on light energy to synthesize fuels and body constituents.

phototropism: usually, *positive phototropism*, in which the parts of a stationary organism grow towards a light source. For example, the cells of plant shoots most shaded from sunlight elongate more rapidly than those exposed to the light source, and the structure as a whole bends toward the light. The uneven growth is attributed to higher auxin levels on the shaded side. In *negative phototropism*, the parts of an organism exposed to the most light grow more rapidly, and the structure bends away from the light source.

phreno-: a prefix meaning (1) mind or brain; (2) diaphragm or phrenic nerve.

phrenosins: membrane galactocerebrosides, composed of *N*-[1-[β-D-galactopyranosyloxy)-methyl]-2-hydroxy-3-heptadecenyl]-2-hydroxytetracosanamide covalently linked (at the position indicated by R) to a long-chain fatty acid (2-hydroxystearic, cerebronic or lignoceric). They are most abundant in the central nervous system, and especially in myelin sheaths; but minute amounts are present in liver and other organs.

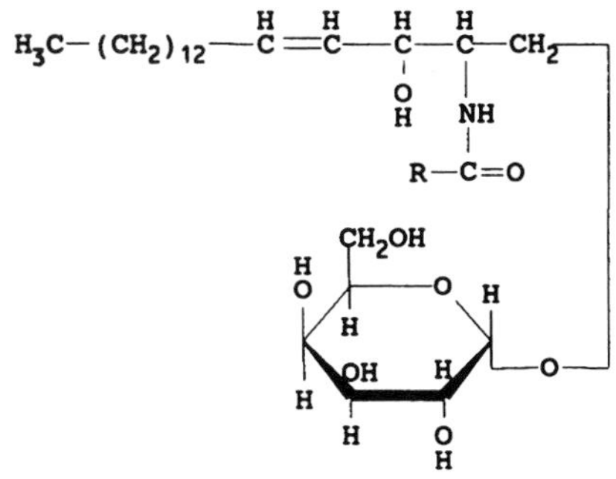

phthalic acid: 1,2-benzenedicarboxylic acid; a compound used in industry. High concentrations of the salts can invoke narcosis.

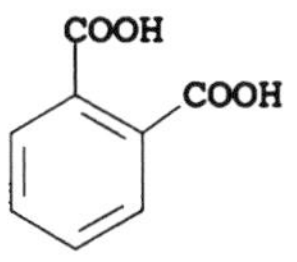

phycobilins: phycocyanobilin, phycoerythrobilin, and related porphyrin pigments made by algae that contribute to photosynthesis. They absorb light and attach to proteins; *see* **phycobiliproteins**.

phycobiliproteins: phycobilins linked to proteins. They assemble into phycobilosomes, absorb light, and transfer it to chlorophylls. Two examples of pigments linked to cysteine moieties are shown. Since the proteins fluoresce and attach to nucleic acids, enzymes, vitamins, and other biological molecules, they are used to label DNA probes, in fluorescence immunoassays of enzymes and other proteins, in microscopy, and to count T and B lymphocytes.

phycocyanins: several chemically related plant porphyrins; *see* **phycobilins** and **phycobiliproteins**.

phycoerythrins: several chemically related plant porphyrins; *see* **phycobilins** and **phycobiliproteins**.

phycomycetes: fungi that form nonseptate hyphae.

phyla: plural of **phylum** (*q.v.*).

phylaxis: defense against infection.

-phylaxis: a suffix for terms that describe reactions to exogenous substances, as in tachyphylaxis, anaphylaxis, and prophylaxis.

phyllo-: a prefix meaning leaf.

phyllomedusin: *p*Glu-Asn-Pro-Asn-Arg-Phe-Ile-Gly-Leu-Met-NH$_2$; a tachykinin chemically and biologically related to substance P and physalaemin, isolated from the skins of the Amazonian frog *Phyllomedusa bicolor* and related species.

phylloquinone: vitamin K.

Leu[8]-**phyllotorin**: *p*Glu-Leu-Trp-Ala-Val-Gly-Ser-Leu-Met-NH$_2$; a tachykinin chemically and biologically related to ranatensins and neuromedin B, isolated from the skin of the frog *Phyllomedusa sauvagei*.

Phe[8]-**phyllotorin**: *p*Glu-Leu-Trp-Ala-Val-Gly-Ser-Phe-Met-NH$_2$; a tachykinin biologically related to ranatensins and neuromedin B, isolated from the skin of the frog *Phyllomedusa sauvagei*.

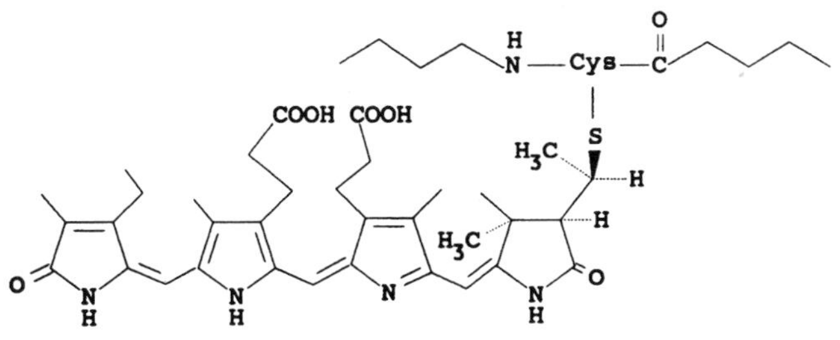

phycocyanobilin-peptide

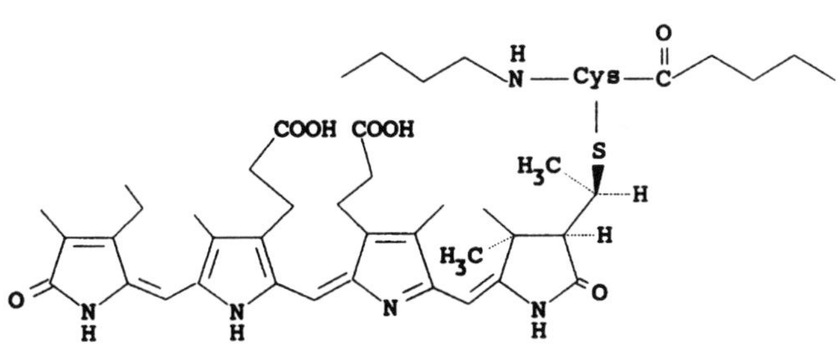

phycoerythrobilin peptide

phylogeny: the evolutionary history of a group of organisms, and the associated relationships to other organisms.

phylum [phyla]: a major subdivision of systems for classifying organisms. The Phylum Chordata is included in the subkingdom Metazoa, of the kingdom Animalia and the superkingdom Eukaryotes. It includes the Sub-phylum Vertebrata (or Craniata) which can be divided into classes Mammalia, Aves (birds), Reptilia, Amphibia, Osteichthyes (bony fishes), Chondrichthyes (cartilaginous fishes), and Cyclostomata (jawless vertebrates); but some systems classify fishes and other aquatic vertebrates in different ways. The class Mammalia includes Prototheria (egg laying mammals), Metatheria (Marsupials) and Eutheria (placental mammals). The subclasses are further divided into orders, and the orders into families. For example, humans, apes, monkeys, and related animals are members of the order Primates; rats, guinea pigs and others of the order Rodentia; and rabbits of the order Lagomorpha. *See* also **genus** and **species**.

physalaemin: physalamin; pGlu-Ala-Asp-Pro-Asn-Lys-Phe-Tyr-Gly-Leu-Met-NH$_2$; a tachykinin chemically and biologically related to substance P, isolated from the skin of some frogs (including *Physalaemus bigilonigerus* and *Physalaemus fuscumaculatus*).

physiological: occurring under natural conditions in healthy organisms; *cf* **pharmacological** and **pathological**.

physiological color changes: rapid changes in coloration mediated by chromatophore granule dispersion or conspersion, and by processes that affect the positions of reflecting components. Hormones effecting such changes in various species include α-melanocyte stimulating hormone (α-MSH), melatonin, and catecholamines. *Cf* **morphological color changes**.

physiological conditions: environmental or organismic states associated with normal function. The term is usually not applied when organisms are exposed to the kinds of stress that can be encountered under natural conditions.

physiological dose: a quantity of substance that, when administered, provides concentrations in biological systems comparable to ones that occur under normal conditions. A physiological dose of an agent can be used to replace a component that the organisms lacks or possesses in insufficient amounts. *Cf* **pharmacological dose**.

physiological saline: isotonic salt solutions used to maintain normal cell hydration. Sodium chloride is usually the major solute; but some solutions also contain glucose or other nutrients, buffers, and/or small quantities of K$^+$, Ca^{2+}, Mg^{2+}, HPO$_4^{2-}$ and other ions. When present alone, 0.85% NaCl is isotonic for mammalian and some other cells, and 0.7% for the cells of many amphibians. *See* also **Ringer's solution**.

physostigmine: eserine; 1,2,3,3a,8,8a-hexahydro-1,3a,8-trimethylpyrrolol[2,3-*b*]indol-5-ol-methylcarbamate; an alkaloid extracted from calabar beans (*Physostigma venenosum*). It is a potent acetylcholinesterase inhibitor, used as such, and in the form of sulfate and salicylate esters, to combat the effects of anticholinesterase drug overdosage, to treat myasthenia gravis, and (since it promotes miosis), to treat glaucoma.

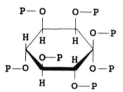

phytagglutinins: phytoagglutinins; plant lectins that promote cell agglutination. *See* also **phythemagglutinin**.

phythemagglutinin: (1) any plant lectin that promotes erythrocyte clumping; (2) phytohemagglutinin.

phytic acid {phytate}: inositol hexaphosphate; a compound made by plant cells that accumulates in seeds, in which it serves as a storage vehicle for phosphate groups. It binds minerals, and is used in humans to remove heavy metals and lower calcium levels. Large quantities in foods impair intestinal absorption of calcium. In the structure shown, P = PO$_3$H$_2$.

phytoalexins: phaseolin, pisatin, and other substances made by plants in response to attacks by pathogens, and to other forms of stress. They are toxic to bacteria and fungi.

phytohemagglutinin: PHA; a lectin obtained from red kidney beans (*Phaseolus vulgaris*) that binds to oligosaccharide pentamers composed of galactose, *N*-acetylgalactosamine, and mannose (Gal-Gal*N*Ac-Man-Gal*N*Ac-Gal) moieties on erythrocytes of all human and several other blood types, and to T lymphocytes. It agglutinates red blood cells, and stimulates T cell mitosis.

phytohormones: auxins, gibberellins, cytokinins and other hormones made by plant cells. The term is not usually applied to different kinds of regulators made by plants that are chemically and/or biologically related to animal hormones. *See* also **hypersensitive responses**.

phytol: 3,7,11,15-tetramethyl-2-hexadecen-1-ol; an alcohol chemically related to carotene and xanthophyll that binds covalently to chlorophyll and is used for the synthesis of vitamins A and E.

phytosterols: sitosterol, stigmasterol, campesterol, and other sterols made by higher plants. Many are similar to, but not identical with animal sterols.

phytotoxic: toxic to plants.

phytotoxin: a general term for substances made by plants that exert toxic effects on animals. Examples include ricin and abrin. *See* also **hypersensitive responses**.

pI: isoelectric point; the pH at which a substance does not move in an electrical field because its net surface charge = 0.

PI: (1) phosphatidylinositol; (2) protamine insulin.

Pi: inorganic phosphate.

pia: soft, as in pia mater.

PIA: phenylisopropyl-adenosine isomers are used to identify adenosine receptor types. *R*-PIA binds with high affinity to A_1 types, and *S*-PIA to A_2 forms.

pico-: a prefix meaning (1) very small; (2) 10^{-12} (one trillionth), as in picogram or picomolar.

picolinic acid: a thiamine isomer formed during tryptophan catabolism.

picocurie: a unit of radioactivity equivalent to 3.7×10^{-12} becquerel.

picornaviruses: polio-, entero-, rhino-, Coxsackie, and other very small, single-stranded RNA viruses with ether-resistant icosahedral capsules.

picogram: pg; one trillionth of a gram; 10^{-12} gram.

picramic acid: 2-amino-4,6-dinitrophenol; an industrial agent that is rapidly absorbed through intact skin and respiratory epithelium, and exerts effects similar to those described for dinitrophenol. It can cause dermatitis, cataracts, granulocytopenia, hypermetabolism, and circulatory collapse.

picric acid: 2,4,6-trinitrophenol; a toxic, explosive agent used in industry, to preserve tissues for histological studies, and topically to treat burns and some skin infections. It stains the skin and can invoke skin eruptions. The systemic effects can include vomiting, diarrhea, convulsions, and stupor.

picrotin: [1*aR*-[1*α*,2*a*β,3β,698,6αβ,8*aS*,8*b*β,9*S*)]-hexahydro-2*a*-hydroxy-9-(1-hydroxy-1-methylethyl)-8*b*-methyl-3,6-methano-8-*H*-1,5,7-trioxacyclopenta[*i,j*]-cyclaprop[*a*]azulene-4,8(3*H*)-dione. *See* **picrotoxin**.

picrotoxin: a complex in the seeds of *Anamirta cocculus*, composed of one molecule of picrotoxinin and one of picrotin. It stimulates the central nervous system by blocking presynaptic inhibition, and has been used to treat poisoning by barbiturates and some other drugs. Since it is toxic, and can invoke convulsions, it is now employed mostly as an investigative tool.

picrotoxinin: picrotoxin alkaloid; [1*aR*-[1*α*,2*a*β,3β, 698.8*aS*,8*b*β,9*R*)]-hexahydro-2*a*-hydroxy-8*b*-methyl-9-(1-methylethenyl)-3,6-methano-8-*H*-1,5,7-trioxacyclopenta[*i,j*]-cyclaprop[*a*]azulene-4,8(3*H*)-dione. The major biologically active component in the seeds of *Anamirta cocculus*; *see* **picrotoxin**. It is a potent receptor antagonist that blocks $GABA_A$ gated chloride channels.

piebald: describes (1) skin or fur with colored patches, or an animal with such fur. The condition is inherited, and is normal for some animal strains. In others, it is caused by mutations, and is a marker for different kinds of mutations; (2) in humans, piebaldism (partial albinism) is a rare hereditary condition in which patches of skin lack pigment.

piezoelectricity: electricity generated by mechanical pressure. Naturally occurring and artificially induced piezoelectric currents stimulate bone growth.

PIF: prolactin inhibitory factor.

pig: swine; members of the genus *Sus*. Without qualifying terms (such as wild) the term usually applies to domesticated species. Minipigs are small animals bred for laboratory use that are easier to handle, and cheaper to maintain. Because of resemblances to humans, pigs are used to study circulatory systems functions, and also to investigate ovarian functions, pregnancy, pheromone production, and other processes.

PIGs: phosphatidylinositolglycans.

pigment cells: chromatophores; cells that produce colored substances; *see*, for example **melanosomes**, **melanophores**, and **erythrophores**.

pili: plural of pilus.

piliform: hair-like.

pilin: the protein that aggregates to form the major component of bacterial pili; *see* **pilus**.

"pill": *see* **oral contraceptives**.

pilocarpine: 3-ethyldihydro-4-[(1-methyl-1*H*-imidazol-5-yl)methyl]-2-(3*H*)-furanone; an alkaloid from *Pilocarpus jaborandi*. It is a muscarinic type acetylcholine receptor agonist, used directly and in the form of hydrochloride and nitrate derivatives as an investigative tool, and clinically to treat glaucoma, stimulate gastrointestinal tract muscles, or invoke sweating for diagnostic purposes.

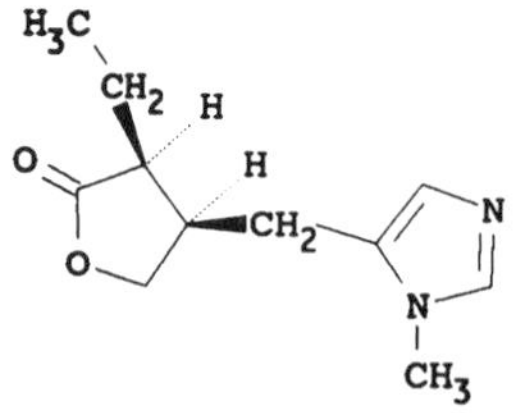

piloerection: elevation of hair or fur by contraction of skin arrectores pilorum muscles. It is invoked by norepinephrine, and occurs in response to cold exposure and some other forms of stress, and when strong emotions are experienced. In heavily furred animals, it decreases heat loss from body surfaces, and can contribute to defenses against predators by making animals appear larger.

pilomotor: producing or relating to movement of hair; *see* also **piloerection**.

pilus [**pili**]: (1) a hair; (2) a hair-like process; (3) a filamentous hollow appendage (conjugation tube) that extends from the surface of a bacterial cell.

pimelic acid: heptane dioic acid; a bacterial metabolite used to cross link cell wall peptides.

$$HOOC-(CH_2)_5-COOH$$

pim-1: pim1; a small protein related to mammalian **RCC1** (*q.v.*) that interacts with the *ran* proto-oncogene product (a small ras-related guanine nucleotide binding protein), and contributes to cell cycle control. Mutants undergo premature chromatin condensation (before replication is completed).

pimelo-: a prefix meaning fat or fatty.

pimozide: 1-[1-[4,4-bis(4-fluorophenyl)butyl]-4-piperidinyl]-1,3-dihydro-2*H*-benzimidazole-2-one; a D$_2$ type dopamine receptor antagonist, used a tranquilizer and "antipsychotic" agent, and to inhibit calmodulins.

pinacidil: *N*-cyano-*N'*-pyridinal-*N''*-(1,2,2-trimethylpropyl)-guanidine; a potassium channel activator that lowers blood pressure.

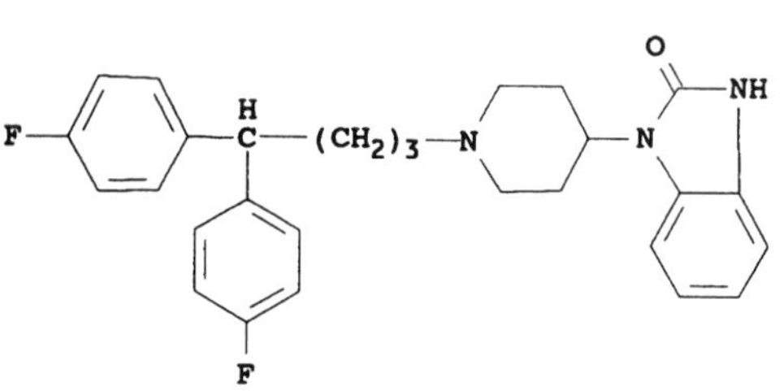

pimozide

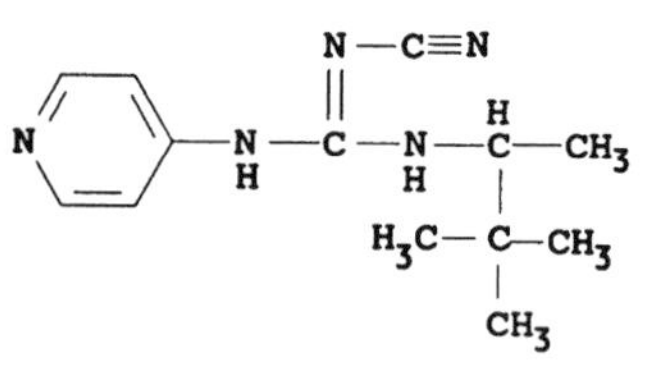

pinacidil

pinazepam: 7-chloro-1,3-dihydro-5-phenyl-1-(2-propynyl)-2*H*-1,4-benzodiazepin-2-one; a benzodiazepine type central nervous system depressant, used as an anxiolytic.

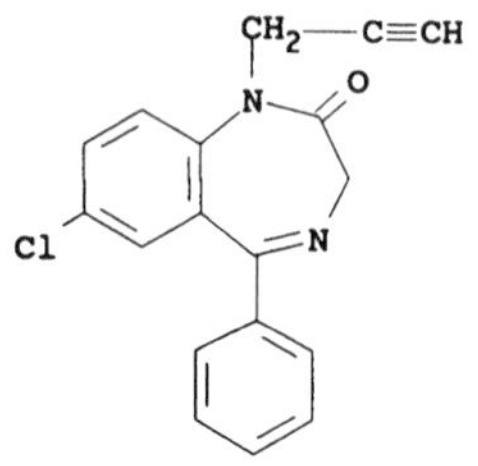

pindolol: 1-I1*H*-indol-4-yloxy)-3-[(1-methylethyl) amino]-2-propanol; an orally effective adrenergic antagonist that acts on both β$_1$ and β2 receptor subtypes, but is a weak, partial agonist in the heart, and directly dilates blood vessels. It is used to block excessive increases in cardiac output invoked by muscular activity. Derivatives labeled with radioactive iodine are used to identify and isolate the receptors.

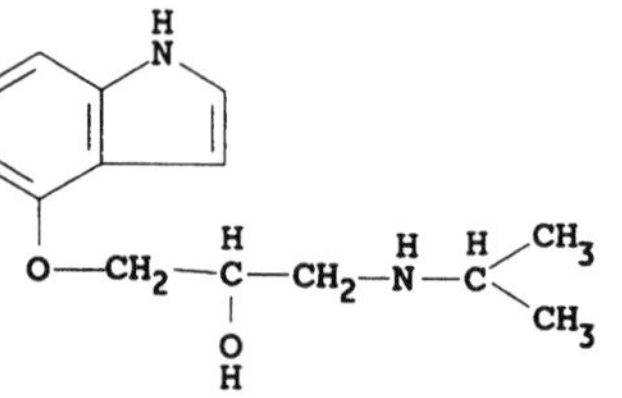

pineal antigonadotropin: PAG; an uncharacterized peptide in pineal gland extracts that inhibits gonadotropin secretion. It differs from some other, chemically defined peptides with similar actions, but may be identical to gonadotropin inhibitory substance (GIS).

pineal complex: the pineal gland, and structures associated with it in some nonmammalian vertebrates, such as fish parapineal glands, amphibian frontal organs, and lizard parietal eyes.

pineal gland: epiphysis cerebri; corpus pineale; a small gland within the brain that undergoes cyclical changes in hormone production, and is a major regulator of several circadian and annual rhythms. In mammals, it differentiates from an evagination of the diencephalon roof and later occupies a groove between the right and left superior colliculi of the midbrain. Although it remains attached to the epithalamus via a short stalk, it receives its major innervation from postganglionic fibers of the superior cervical ganglia (SCG). Messages from the suprachiasmatic nuclei affect norepinephrine release, and thereby melatonin (MLT) synthesis. The SCG also receive inputs from olfactory system and other brain components. A less important cholinergic innervation is present in at least some species; and other neurotransmitters and/or modulators identified include serotonin, vasoactive intestinal peptide (VIP), vasotocin, oxytocin, somatostatin, and taurine. The responses to regulators are affected by cyclical changes in pineal gland receptor numbers. In some other vertebrates, the gland is associated with additional structures (*see* **pineal complex**), and can contain photoreceptors. Environmental light inhibits MLT synthesis in both nocturnal and diurnal species. More is made at night than during the day, and (in locales distant from the equator), more in winter than in summer. The hormone enters cerebrospinal fluid as well as circulating blood, and affects reproductive system functions, as well as cyclical changes in body temperature, sleep, locomotor activity, mood, and skin and fur pigmentation. 5-Methoxytryptophol, other melatonin metabolites, threonyl-serine-lysine (TSL), and some uncharacterized peptides, such as pinealin and pineal antigonadotropin are also made in the glands, and are implicated as humoral regulators.

pinealocytes: the major nonneural cells in pineal glands. There are marked morphological and functional variations across species; and a single gland can have two or more kinds. Most (but not all) are believed to secrete hormones. Some respond directly to light.

pinealin: an uncharacterized protein made in pineal glands and implicated as a regulator of pineal gland functions.

ping pong reaction: a double-displacement reaction of the general type A + B ⇄ C + D, catalyzed by a single enzyme complex, in which the first substrate (A) initially binds alone to the enzyme (E). AE then transforms to an intermediate complex (EFC) that releases C. The remaining component of the intermediate complex (F) then binds to the second substrate (B), and EFB transforms to a different intermediate (EFD) that releases D and restores the enzyme to E (the condition in which it can bind more A). Transamination catalyzed by glutamic-aspartic transaminase, and acetyl-CoA carboxylase catalyzed conversion of acetyl-coenzyme A to malonyl coenzyme A are examples.

pinocytosis: "cell drinking"; uptake of liquids and small, dissolved solutes via endocytosis. The processes are similar to those described for phagocytosis.

pinosomes: fluid-filled vesicles formed during pinocytosis.

pinpoint depolarizations: minute changes in neuron membrane electrical properties that augment responses to

stimulants, but do not directly invoke neurotransmitter release.

PIP[s]: PtdInsPs; *see* **phosphatidylinositol phosphates**. Cells make at least half of the possible 63 isomeric linear types, along with some cyclic molecules.

L-**pipecolic acid**: S(-)piperidine-2-carboxylic acid; a lysine metabolite. Large amounts may invoke neurological dysfunctions.

piperidine-4-sulfonic acid: a gamma aminobutyric acid agonist, specific for postsynaptic receptor types.

piperonal: heliotropin; 3,4-(methylenedioxy)benzaldehyde; a light-sensitive, aromatic agent used in the perfume industry, and as a pediculicide.

piperoxan: 2-piperidinomethyl-1,4-benzodioxan; an adrenergic blocking agent with properties similar to those of phentolamine, formerly used to diagnose pheochromocytomas and to block the associated hypertensive episodes.

PIPES: 1,4-piperazine-*bis*(ethanesulfonic acid); a zwitterion buffer for the pH range 6.1-7.5.

pipsyl chloride: *p*-iodobenzenesulfonyl chloride; a reagent that binds to sulfhydryl groups and is used in protein analysis.

pirenpirone: 3-[2-[4-(4-fluorobenzoyl)-1-piperidinyl] ethyl-2-methyl-4*H*-pyrido-[1,2-a]pyrimidin-4-one; a selective M₁ type muscarinic receptor antagonist.

pirenzepine: 5,11-dihydro-11-[(4-methyl-1-piperazinyl) acetyl]-6*H*-pyridol-[2,3-*b*][1,4]benzo-diazepin-6-one; an M₁-type muscarinic type acetylcholine receptor antagonist that inhibits gastric acid secretion, and is used to treat peptic ulcers. It invokes dry mouth and blurred vision in some individuals, but does not enter the brain.

piriform: pear-shaped.

piroxicam: Feldene; 4-hydroxy-2-methyl-*N*-2-pyridinyl-2*H*-1,2-benzothiazine-3-carboxamide1,1-dioxide; an orally effective agent that blocks eicosanoid production, and acts via different pathways to inhibit neutrophil activation. Its anti-inflammatory, antipyretic, and analgesic effects are used to treat severe forms of rheumatoid arthritis, osteoarthritis, postoperative pain, gout, dysmenorrhea, ankylosing spondylitis, and some acute musculoskeletal disorders. In common with most other nonsteroidal anti-inflammatory agents (NSAIDs), it can irritate gastrointestinal mucosa, alter platelet function, and cause bronchoconstriction in sensitive individuals.

pisatin: a phytoallexin made by the garden pea, *Pisum sativum* (*q.v.*).

Pisum sativum: the garden pea, a subject of Gregor Mendel's genetics studies, now used to investigate photosynthesis and phytoalexin production, and as the source of a lectin that binds to terminal α-D-mannose and α-D-glucose moieties.

Pit-1: pituitary factor-1; GHF-1 (growth hormone factor-1) or that protein plus other very closely related ones, made in pituitary glands are essential for differentiation of specific cell types and the synthesis of their hormones. In common with Oct-1, Oct-2, and Unc-86, the compo-nents are approximately 33K *trans*-activating transcription factors with homeobox and POU domains. GHF-1 transcripts can be detected soon after Rathke's pouch forms; and the protein product appears in developing somatotropes and somatolactotropes (mammosomatotropes) around the time when growth hormone (GH) is made. It binds to two sites on GH promoters, and induces GH in those cells (and in other cell types following transfection). Pit-I is both induced and autoregulated by cAMP, which is generated by growth hormone releasing hormone (GRH) and acts via CREB (cyclic AMP regulated DNA binding protein). Although initially reported to be made in lactotropes that do not secrete GH, there is evidence for control of lactotrope differentiation and functions by a different protein with very similar properties and an identical 19K subunit, variously called LSF-1 (lactotroph stimulating factor-1) and Puf-1 (prolactin upstream factor-1). It is expressed by lactotropes of dwarf mice that have few or no somatotropes, and little or no GH-1 or GH. (GH-1 can, however, bind to and activate prolactin promoters when present in very high concentrations.) There are controversies concerning whether GH-1 or a third closely related factor is essential for acquisition of the ability to synthesize thyroid stimulating hormone (TSH) in response to thyrotropin releasing hormone (TRH). Pars distalis and pars intermedia cells that secrete proopiomelanocortin (POMC)-derived regulators do not appear to make the factors.

pithing: destruction of the spinal cord and brain by inserting a blunt probe through the central canal and cranium. It abolishes pain perception and spinal reflexes. For some kinds of studies (for example of spinal reflexes), only the brain is destroyed.

Pitocin: an oxytocin preparation extracted from pituitary glands.

Pitressin: a vasopressin preparation extracted from pituitary glands.

pituicytes: neuroglia type cells in neural lobes, implicated as contributors to the nourishment and support of the nerve terminals that store and release vasopressin and oxytocin, to their repair, and to the control of hormone release.

pituitary adenylate cyclase-activating factor: PACAP; several closely related peptides in the cerebral cortex, cerebellum, basal ganglia, hypothalamus, brainstem, pituitary gland, and some peripheral tissues. The most active form has 38 amino acid moieties, but similar effects are invoked by 28 amino acid and 27 amino acid amide types. All display homologies with vasoactive intestinal peptide (VIP), but are more potent stimulants of cAMP generation. They augment prolactin secretion *in vivo*. In superfused rat pituitary glands, high levels additionally promote growth hormone (GH), adrenocorticotropic hormone (ACTH), and luteinizing hormone (LH) release. Astrocytes, pancreatic acinar cells, and lymphocytes are among the targets that contain receptors.

pituitary gland: hypophysis; *see* **adenohypophysis, neurohypophysis, anterior pituitary**, and **posterior pituitary**.

Pituitrin: a pituitary gland extract that contains both vasopressin and oxytocin.

pizotifen: a sulfated cyproheptadine analog that stimulates appetite by acting on serotonin receptors.

pK: the negative logarithm to the base 10 of the ionization constant of an acid. Its relationship to pH is defined by the **Henderson-Hasselbalch equation** (*q.v.*).

PK: protein kinases.

pKa protein: a protein identified in rats that stimulates mammary gland differentiation. It may be the rat counterpart of a protein 18A2 described for other species.

PKA: protein kinase A.

PKC: protein kinase C.

PKG: protein kinase G.

PKU: phenylketonuria.

PLs: placental lactogens.

PL017: N-MePhe^3-D-Pro^6-casomorphin: a μ-type opioid receptor agonist.

placebo: a pharmacologically inert agent used for its psychological effects. In studies of drug actions, toxicities, and potential therapeutic benefits in humans, subjects assigned to control groups are given placebos, and neither they nor the ones receiving the active compounds are informed of the nature of the agents administered. In double-blind procedures, the individuals who directly study the effects are also not told which subjects received the active agent. Placebos are sometimes given to patients for potential benefits associated with knowledge that they are receiving treatment.

placenta [placentae, placentas]: complex, vascularized structures that develop during pregnancy from endometrial and trophoblast components in eutherian and some metatherian mammals. They synthesize and metabolize hormones, transport nutrients, oxygen, and regulators from the mother to the fetus(es), deliver wastes and hormones to the maternal blood, and contribute to protection against immunological rejection of the conceptuses. The types vary with the species, and range from *epitheliochorial* (which involves little disruption of the maternal endometrium) through *syndesmochorial*, to *hemochorial* (in which there is extensive invasion and blood vessel destruction). The hormones synthesized can include chorionic gonadotropins, placental lactogens, gonadal steroids, several kinds of growth factors, and also peptides similar to or identical with ones made in the

hypothalamus and hypophysis. *See* also **cytotrophoblast**, **syncytiotrophoblast**, and **feto-placental unit**.

placental anticoagulant protein: a 33K annexin made in placentas. It is identical to lipocortin 5, endonexin II, and chromobindin 5 or 7.

placental lactogens: somatomammotropins: hormones chemically and biologically related to prolactin and growth hormone, synthesized by syncytiotrophoblastic cells of chorionic villi, and delivered to maternal blood. They are made in largest amounts by primates (and are also secreted by some tumor cells). Human placental lactogen (hPL) is a 21.8K, 191 amino acid protein that can be detected in the syncytiotrophoblast 5-10 days postconception (12-17 days after implantation), and in maternal blood two weeks later. Carbohydrate-free forms predominate, but glycosylated molecules are also made. The levels rise during midpregnancy in parallel with the numbers of cells that produce them, remain elevated until term, and are positively correlated with fetal weight. The human type acts on growth hormone receptors, but its potency is only 1% that of pituitary GH activity in mature individuals. In contrast, it stimulates amino acid uptake, DNA synthesis, mitogenesis, and IGF-I synthesis in fetal tissues unresponsive to GH. It is a weak prolactin agonist that promotes mammary gland maturation and protein synthesis, but does not stimulate milk production. Since it competes with prolactin for PRL receptors, one function may be antagonism of prolactin stimulation. Maternal levels rise during times of fasting, and it then accelerates lipolysis and inhibits glucose oxidation. It may therefore be important for maintaining glucose (and possibly amino acid and mineral) delivery to conceptuses, especially when maternal food intake is suboptimal. Gestational diabetes mellitus is a usually transient condition that may be caused by high levels. hPL also stimulates lipogenesis following food intake, and is proposed to promote accumulation of triacylglycerol reserves (to provide energy for subsequent lactation). According to some observers, it is not an important regulator in well-nourished women, since women with genetic defects that block its synthesis have delivered healthy infants. The hormones of some other species are more like prolactins; and some are luteotropic.

placental lactogen-1, placental lactogen-2: two prolactin-like hormones identified in placentas of several non-primate vertebrate species, named for their order of appearance in mice.

placental protein 12: PP12: a 34K protein secreted by endometrium and present in amniotic fluid. It binds insulin-like growth factors, but not insulin.

placental protein 14: pregnancy associated endometrial $α_2$-globulin; $α_1$PEG; a progesterone-regulated protein chemically related to β-lactoglobulins, made by uterine (but not placental) cells of pregnant women, and present in amniotic fluid. Since it is also the major protein secreted by endometrium during luteal phases of ovarian cycles, and the largest amounts are made during the first trimester of pregnancy, roles in decidualization have been proposed. Assays are used as indices of the condition of the endometrium.

placenta previa: conditions in which implantation occurs too close to the cervical os, and the placenta covers or impinges on the os. It causes bleeding during late pregnancy and/or excessive bleeding during parturition.

placentation: placenta formation.

placentomas: neoplasms that develop from placental tissue retained after spontaneous or induced abortions.

placode: a broad, flat object or plate, for example the neuroectodermal structures in embryos that give rise to eye and ear components.

plakalbumins: fragments cleaved from ovalbumin via reactions catalyzed by subtilisin.

plakoglobins: 83K polypeptide components of desmosomes, and chemically related smaller cytoplasmic peptides.

planaria: a phylum of flatworms. Some species are used to study tissue and organ regeneration, and effects of electrical fields and other environmental factors on development.

Plantae: a phylum that includes all multicellular eukaryotes that use energy derived from sunlight to synthesize organic nutrients. Most members are anchored to soil or other substrata, but have moveable parts. Some produce motile male gametes.

plant growth regulators: phytohormones and other factors that regulate plant growth and differentiation; *see* **auxins, cytokinins, gibberellins**, and **ethylene**.

plant lectins: carbohydrate-binding proteins derived from plants. *See* **lectins** and specific types, such as peanut agglutinin, pokeweed mitogen, and soy bean lectins.

plaque: (1) a patch or flat area; (2) a lesion that takes this form, for example an atheromatous blood vessel type; (3) an opaque conglomerate surrounded by a clear area, such as a collection of bacteria surrounded by a region in which the organisms have been killed by a virus, a cluster of erythrocytes surrounded by a region in which hemolysis has occurred, or a group of cultured cells surrounded by a region in which lysis has been invoked by activated complement or other factors; (4) a dental plaque. *See* also **adhesion plaque** and **hemolytic plaque assays**.

plaque forming assays: *see* **hemolytic plaque assays**.

plaque forming cells: (1) antibody-secreting cells that act with complement components to lyse erythrocytes and other cell types; (2) components of the immune system that promote plaque formation by directly attacking target cells.

-plasia: a suffix meaning molding or forming, and in hyperplasia.

plasm: the genetic substance of germ cells.

-plasm: (1) a suffix used for fluid or semi-fluid substances, as in cytoplasm or nucleoplasm.

plasma: (1) blood plasma; the clear fluid obtained when the formed elements are removed from uncoagulated blood; *cf* **serum**; (2) the fluid component of lymph; (3) a fluid or semi-fluid substance.

plasmablast: a cell type formed when an activated B lymphocyte is in the process of modulating to a plasma cell.

plasma cells: plasmacytes; cells formed when B lymphocytes undergo terminal differentiation in response to antigen stimulation. They accumulate in the spleen and lymph nodes, secrete large quantities of antibodies specific for the antigens, and lose surface receptors for complement.

plasmacrit: the volume of blood plasma relative to the volume of formed elements, usually expressed as a percentage (calculated by taking the total volume in the tube as 100%, and subtracting from it the per cent of the volume occupied by the formed elements.)

plasmacytes: plasma cells.

plasmacytomas: usually (1) malignant tumors derived from plasma cells that can develop into myelomas. They can be induced in rodents with Freund's complete adjuvant; *see* also **hybridomas**. (2) plasma cell aggregations.

plasmacytoma growth factor: PGF; hybridoma-plasmacytoma growth factor; *see* **interleukin-6**.

plasmacytosis: (1) the presence of plasma cells in circulating blood; (2) unusually large numbers of plasma cells in bone marrow or at other sites.

plasmalemma: plasma membrane.

plasmalogens: phospholipids synthesized from dihydroxyacetone phosphate, fatty acyl coenzyme As, and phosphorylated alcohols that differ from the more common types in that an an *ether* bond links the fatty acid to

plasmalogens

the first carbon of the glycerol moiety. An NAD$^+$ dependent desaturase catalyzes formation of the ether bond. The structure shown is a choline plasmalogen. The highest concentrations are in myelin sheaths. Blood platelets and muscle cell membranes contain small amounts.

plasma membrane: the living, semi-permeable membrane that defines the outer limits of a cell, composed of a phospholipid bilayer into which proteins (and usually also cholesterol) are inserted. Although water, oxygen, carbon dioxide, and other gases diffuse across it in both directions, the typical membrane has carriers for passive uptake of glucose and some other small nutrients, different kinds for amino acids, regulated channels for several kinds of ions, and ATPases that supply energy for active transport. Some take up and release larger molecules via endocytosis and exocytosis, respectively. Many have externally directed receptors, and filaments that transmit the effects of surface changes to cytoskeletal components. Specializations at various sites include microvilli, gap junctions, desmosomes, and tight junctions.

plasmapheresis: removal of blood, followed by return of the formed elements to the body, performed for diagnostic purposes, or to obtain specific blood plasma components such as antibodies and coagulation factors.

plasma proteins: albumins, globulins, coagulation factors, and other proteins in blood plasma. Most (including hormone carriers) are made in the liver. *See* specific types.

plasma renin activity: PRA; nanograms of angiotensin I generated per hour when 1 ml of blood plasma is incubated with a renin substrate under standardized conditions. It is used as an indicator of *in vivo* renin activity; but incubation is usually performed at pHs of 5.5-5.7, and artificial substrates are commonly used.

plasmids: genetic elements in some bacteria that replicate independently of the chromosome, and can be transferred to other cells via conjugation or transduction. Most contain cyclic, double-stranded DNA that codes for factors advantageous to the organisms but not essential for survival under ordinary conditions. (Some products degrade toxins). Restriction endonucleases open the DNA at specific sites and form complementary, single stranded molecules with cohesive ends. DNA ligases then catalyze DNA chain bonding. Vertebrate DNA fragments obtained with the same kinds of enzymes, and annealed to the ends of the single strands, are taken up by bacteria. They are used to direct the synthesis of mammalian messenger RNAs and proteins, such as human type growth hormone, insulins, interferons, and other substances not easily obtained from vertebrate tissues, or to study the roles of specific gene types. Host cells that contain the vertebrate DNA can be identified if other genes are linked to the ones for the desired proteins. For example, if the linked genes confer resistance to tetracycline, only cells that contain the artificially constructed plasmids survive when the antibiotic is added to the culture system. Tumor-inducing (Ti) plasmids are injected into plant cells to study gene functions, improve crop yields, change the colors of flowers or the qualities of fruits and vegetables, or confer resistance to fungi, bacteria, insects, or other feeders.

plasmin: fibrinolysin; broad-spectrum serine proteases that degrade fibrin, fibrinogen, blood coagulation factors V and VII, kininogens, and several other proteins. Plasminogen activators cleave them from proenzymes (plasminogens). Plasmins affect several platelet functions, dissolve blood clots, and contribute to complement activation. They also function in ovulation, implantation, spermiation, bone formation and resorption, cartilage formation and destruction, removal of cells no longer needed (for example in mammary glands when lactation is terminated), the activities of basement membranes and extracellular matrices, and other processes. Additionally, they affect cell migration during development, and are implicated as facilitators of metastasis. Some effects are attributed to activation of collagenases. *See also* **seminal plasmin**.

plasminogens: single chain polypeptide proenzymes cleaved at Arg-Lys or S-S sites to yield plasmins, via reactions catalyzed by plasminogen activators, thrombin, and kallikreins. They are made by several cell types; but most circulating proenzyme originates in the liver.

plasminogen activators: PAs; serine proteases that convert plasminogens to plasmins, and act on several other proteins. Secreted types are present in most biological fluids (including blood plasma, milk, saliva, tears, and seminal fluid). Endothelial cells that are damaged or actively engaged in angiogenesis, cells transformed by Simian sarcoma and some other viruses, and activated monocytes can release large amounts. Production at most sites is regulated by hormones. The broad range of molecular weights results from fragmentation of large precursors. Urokinase is a PA made in the kidney, released to the blood, and excreted to the urine. Some *tissue* type plasminogen activators (tPAs) resemble urokinase, whereas others differ in amino acid make-up, and bind more avidly to fibrin than fibrinogen. Streptokinase and some other bacterial enzymes resemble the second type, and are used to prevent coronary thrombosis.

plasminogen activator inhibitors: PAIs; enzymes that block the actions of plasminogen activators. Type I (PAI-1) binds to blood platelets.

Plasmodium: a genus of sporozoan parasites that includes *P. malariae* and *P. falciparum*, both of which infect erythrocytes.

plasticity: usually, the ability to undergo prolonged (often adaptive) functional modifications. Neuron plasticity, which is needed for long-term memory, involves changes in membrane properties, synaptic connections, and neurotransmitter release. In embryos, plasticity affects neuron survival and contributes to nervous system development.

platelets: blood platelets; thrombocytes; disc-like bodies 2-4 nanometers in diameter, formed by fragmentation of megakaryocytes. Most circulate, but substantial numbers accumulate in the spleen. Interleukin-3 is the major stimulant for megakaryocyte maturation, but thrombopoietin may control the rate of fragment release to the bloodstream. Platelets lack nuclei, but have mitochondria, lysosomes, *dense granules* that contain adenine nucleotides, serotonin, catecholamines, calcium ions, and pyrophosphate, and α *granules* that contain platelet-derived growth factor (PDGF), transforming growth factor β (TGFβ), a hepatocyte growth factor, connective tissue activating peptide III, platelet factor 4, β-thromboglobulin, thrombospondin, fibronectin, albumin, platelet fibrinogen, coagulation factor V, von Willebrand factor (vWf), plasminogen, $α_2$-plasmin inhibitor, C-1 esterase inhibitor, and other biologically active molecules. They also contain several low molecular weight GTP-binding proteins; and the membranes hold receptors for adenosine diphosphate (ADP), catecholamines, serotonin, antigen-antibody complexes, collagen, thrombin, fibrinogen, laminin, fibronectin, thrombospondin, vWf, and other molecules. The membranes additionally contain platelet factor 3 and other coagulation factors, and several enzymes (including adenylate cyclase and phospholipases). Glycoprotein-rich glycocalyces that surround the surfaces attract fibrinogen, coagulation factors V and VIII, and other blood proteins. Small blood vessels are frequently injured under normal conditions, and this exposes collagen and other proteins otherwise covered by endothelium. Endothelial cells are then stimulated to release regulators that include vWf; and small amounts of plasma prothrombin are converted to thrombin. Hemostasis begins with contraction of the vessels walls, and vWf mediated platelet adhesion to the inner surfaces. The platelet plugs that form are often sufficient for arresting bleeding when the injuries are small; but platelet activation is required for larger breaks. It is a complex process mediated by many factors from blood vessel cells and circulating plasma, as well as the platelets themselves, and it involves G proteins, messengers generated by activation of phospholipase C and A isozymes, elevation of cytosol Ca^{2+}, synergisms, cascades and positive feedback mechanisms, and translocation of platelet receptors from interiors to surfaces. The early, reversible phases are initiated by platelet membrane glycoprotein Ia binding to collagen and glycoprotein Ib binding to thrombin. Fibrinogen is essential for adherence, and binding to fibronectin facilitates the process. Some GPIIb/IIIA then appears at platelet surfaces, and mediates additional effects essential for platelet aggregation. Changes in the cytoskeleton lead to rounding of the disks, and extension of pseudopods. If the stimuli persist, ADP and other substances released, and circulating thrombin, epinephrine, platelet activating factor, vWf, vasopressin, neutrophilin,

and thromboxane A_2 (TXA_2) and other eicosanoids (generated by Ca^{2+}-mediated enzyme activation) modify the cell surface properties. Ca^{2+}-mediated stimulation of the platelet actin-myosin system leads to irreversible changes in morphology, and granule discharge. Release of thromboplastin initiates coagulation cascades. Later, platelets promote syneresis, and also dissolution of blood clots that are no longer needed. Physiological inhibitors include prostacyclin (PGI_2), cAMP, and prostaglandin E_2 (PGE_2), made by platelets, and also nitric oxide (NO), and heparin. Thrombocytopenia is invariably associated with internal bleeding; but excessive numbers of platelets and inadequately controlled activity can cause intravascular clotting and tissue damage. Platelets also contribute to wound healing by releasing growth factors, and to inflammation by generating and releasing several other mediators.

platelet activating factor: PAF; PAF-acetether; AGEPC; acetyl-glyceryletherphosphorylcholine; 1-*O*-alkyl-2,3-acetyl-glycerol-3-phosphorylcholine; an ether phospholipid released by activated macrophages, neutrophils, monocytes, basophils, mast cells, and endothelial cells. It is also present in kidneys, lungs, liver, reproductive system organs, retinas, nervous tissue, and amniotic fluid. PAF facilitates hemostasis by promoting platelet adhesion to blood vessel walls, aggregation, serotonin release, and leukotriene synthesis. It also plays roles in inflammation which contribute to body defenses; but high levels can invoke allergies, anaphylaxis, and several kinds of tissue damage. It is a chemoattractant for eosinophils, and it promotes eosinophil adhesion to vascular epithelium, with release of eosinophilic basic proteins. Additionally, it directly promotes vasodilation, augments vascular permeability, and can thereby invoke hemoconcentration and hypotension, reduce cardiac output, and cause circulatory collapse. In the kidneys, it slows renal blood flow, contracts mesangial cells, and invokes proteinuria. Toxic amounts cause necrotizing lesions of the intestine, and gastric ulcers, and invoke respiratory distress by promoting bronchoconstriction and pulmonary edema. In the liver, PAF accelerates glycogenolysis and glucose release. Under physiological conditions, PAF is involved in implantation, parturition, and neural function control. The receptors interact with pertussis toxin sensitive G protein $α_i$ subunits. Some effects have been linked with activation of phospholipase A_2 and consequent generation of eicosanoids, and with release of histamine and other mediators (although prostaglandins antagonize some of its influences). Others are attributed to activation of phospholipase C isozymes, phosphatidylinositol hydrolysis, and generation of diacylglycerol and inositol phosphates.

platelet activating factor

platelet adhesion receptor glycoprotein: glycoprotein IIb/IIIa; GPIIb/IIIA: a complex composed of two glycoproteins made by **blood platelets** (*q.v.*) and exposed on their surfaces following activation. It is similar to or identical with VLA-2 (very late antigen-2) and shares amino acid sequences with the β-subunit of LFA-1 (lymphocyte function associated antigen-1). GPIIb/IIIa functions as a receptor that facilitates platelet adhesion and aggregation by mediating binding to fibrinogen, fibronectin, von Willebrand factor, and possibly also thrombospondin; and it promotes adhesion to vitronectin.

platelet basic protein: a GRO-related protein made by blood platelets that interacts with β-thromboglobulin and connective tissue activating factor, and contributes to hemostasis.

platelet-derived endothelial cell growth factor: PD-ECGF; 45-49K proteins made by blood platelets and placental cells that stimulate endothelium growth and proliferation, and are chemotactic for some cell types (but do not affect smooth muscle). They contribute to embryogenesis, wound healing, and cell regeneration. Excessive amounts cause formation of pathological lesions. *Cf* **platelet-derived growth factor**.

platelet-derived growth factor: PDGF; approximately 32K proteins composed of two disulfide linked subunits, made by platelets, fibroblasts, macrophages, endothelial cells, smooth muscle, and cytotrophoblast, initially identified as the major mitogens of whole blood plasma (but not serum) that support the proliferation of several kinds of cultured cells, and especially ones of mesodermal origin. A and B subunits, 40% homologous, derive from different, separately regulated genes, and assemble into AA, AB, and BB dimers. Variations in subtype composition have been described. Some cells make more than one kind; and species differences within analogous cell types are known. For example, human platelets make mostly AB, whereas BB predominates in porcine types. The peptides promote angiogenesis and wound healing. They are competence factors that stimulate cell cycle advance from G_1 to S, and block return to G_0. They activate *c-myc*, *c-fos* and other genes, promote growth of fibroblast, smooth muscle, and glial cells, facilitate cell migration, and invoke vasoconstriction. They also activate plasma membrane Na^+/H^+ pumps, promote amino acid uptake, accelerate synthesis of cholesterol, prostacyclins, and several proteins, and exert influences on receptors for low density lipoproteins (LDLs), epidermal growth factor (EGF), serotonin, and luteinizing hormone (LH). There are controversies concerning whether the major responses are linked to activation of phospholipases, protein kinase C, or phosphatidylinositol hydrolysis. PDGF dysfunction is implicated in the etiology of atherosclerosis, arthritis, scleroderma, and bone marrow fibrosis. PDGFs and closely related peptides are made by several kinds of tumor cells. The *sis* proto-oncogene that directs B subunit synthesis closely resembles the *v-sis* oncogene product; and B subunits tightly associated with membranes invoke transformation when they and their receptors are present in excessive amounts. (Some AA dimers are secreted, but AA types predominate in osteosarcomas). Other names

include osteosarcoma-derived growth factor, glioma-derived growth factor, transforming protein of Simian sarcoma virus, and fibroblast-derived growth factor (different from fibroblast growth factors). *See* also **platelet derived growth factor receptors**.

platelet derived growth factor receptors: PDGF receptors; 180-190K, immunoglobulin-like glycoproteins on fibroblasts, smooth and skeletal muscle cells, glial and mesangial cells, and in cytotrophoblast and fetal brain. The α type binds both A and B type subunits, whereas the β binds only B. An α linked to AA can associate covalently with another α-AA; and both α-ABs and α-BBs can form α-β as well as α-α complexes. Some cell types make PDGF A subunits but β receptors. Presumably, this protects them against undesirable paracrine or intracrine stimulation when they synthesize and release the peptides. Ligand binding activates receptor tyrosine kinase activity and promotes autophosphorylation. There is also some evidence for direct activation of PDGF receptors by mitogen-associated protein kinases in the absence of the ligand.

platelet factor 3: a platelet plasma membrane associated glycoprotein that interacts with other factors to form thromboplastin.

platelet factor 4: a small protein secreted by platelets, chemically related to macrophage inflammatory protein-2 and β-thromboglobulin, that is chemotactic for leukocytes and is implicated as a mediator of inflammation. It can accelerate blood coagulation by binding to and inactivating heparin.

platelet glycoprotein Ia/IIa: *see* blood **platelets** and **very late antigens**.

platelet glycoprotein IIb/IIIa: *see* **platelets** and **platelet adhesion receptor**.

platinum: Pt; a metallic element (atomic number 78, atomic weight 195.08) It does not react with most chemicals, but platinum salt dusts irritate the respiratory tract and can cause dermatitis. Pt is a component of cisplatin and some other agents used to treat neoplasms.

platy-: a suffix meaning flat or broad.

Platyhelminthes: a phylum of flatworms that includes **planarians** (*q.v.*), tapeworms, and flukes.

"pleasure centers": brain regions purported to mediate pleasure sensations and promote reward seeking behavior. The concept that such phenomena can be linked to restricted neuron clusters and pathways is not widely accepted. If electrodes are implanted into specific sites within the limbic systems of rats, and switches to activate them are provided, the animals display extremely strong motivation for self-stimulation, even when this involves considerable muscular effort and/or interferes with food ingestion, sleep, and other processes.

pleiotropic: capable of eliciting several different kinds of responses. The term can refer to genes that direct production of several seemingly unrelated proteins, to hormones and other regulators that exert diverse influences, or to cells that can modulate to various functional forms. *See also* **pluripotent**.

pleomorphism: capable of existing in more than one form. The term is applied to whole organisms and cells, and also to molecular species that display microheterogeneities.

plerocercoid: the second or final larval stage of development of some tapeworms.

plerocercoid growth factor: PGF; a substance derived from tapeworm larvae that does not bind to growth hormone receptors, but invokes effects similar to those of insulin-like growth factor I (IGF-I). It is used in laboratory animals to distinguish direct actions of GH on target cells from ones that involve production of secondary mediators.

plethysmographs: instruments that measure changes in the blood supply and volumes of body parts.

pleura: a double serous membrane composed of a visceral layer that adheres to the lungs, and a parietal layer that lines the thoracic cavity. A small quantity of pleural fluid between the layers reduces friction during breathing.

plexus: network, a term that usually refers to arrangements of veins, lymphatic vessels, or nerve fibers.

PLF: proliferin.

plica: a fold.

plicamycin: mithramycin.

PLN: phospholamban.

ploidy-: a suffix used with terms that relate to the chromosome numbers, as in aneuploidy, euploidy, and polyploidy. *See also* **diploid** and **haploid**.

PLP: pyridoxal-5-phosphate.

plumbism: lead poisoning.

Plummer's disease: hyperthyroidism associated with toxic nodular goiter.

pluriglandular endocrine deficiency; polyglandular endocrine deficiency: autoimmune diseases that destroy or impair the functions of more than one kind of endocrine gland. The adrenal and thyroid glands are the ones most commonly affected; but some syndromes involve parathyroid, gonadal, and/or pituitary cells. The conditions can be associated with other autoimmune disorders such as pernicious anemia or myasthenia gravis. *Cf* **multiple endocrine neoplasia**.

pluripotent: having many capabilities, a term that usually refers to undifferentiated or incompletely differentiated cell types, for example the kinds in bone marrow that can give rise to several kinds of progeny. *See also* **pleiotropic**.

PMA: plasminogen activator.

PMN: *see* **polymorphonuclear leukocytes**.

P-ModS: 56K P-ModS(A), and 59K P-ModS(B), made by peritubular myoid cells of the testis. They stimulate Sertoli cell production of androgen binding protein, transferrin, and inhibin, and are believed to play major roles in both differentiation and maintenance of the morphology and functions. They augment cGMP production and amplify the effects of androgens. Their production is stimulated by androgens released from the interstitial cells.

PMP: pyridoxamine phosphate; *see* **pyridoxal phosphate**.

PMS: premenstrual syndrome.

PMSF: phenylmethyl sulfonyl fluoride; *see* **phenylmethyl sulfonyl chloride**.

PMSG: pregnant mare's serum gonadotropin.

PN: protease nexin.

PN-II: protein nexin II; *see* **amyloid precursor protein**.

PNA: peanut agglutinin.

pneumocytes: alveolar cells; pulmonary epithelial cells; flat, *type I* (membranous) cells that cover alveolar surfaces, and rounder, granular, *type II* cells that synthesize surfactant.

pneumothorax: air in the pleural cavity, caused by entry through a chest lesion, or induced by injection to collapse and immobilize a lung segment and thereby facilitate healing of a tuberculosis infected region.

PNMT: phenylethanolamine-*N*-methyltransferase.

PNP: purine nucleoside phosphorylase.

POA: preoptic area.

POCA: phenylalkyloxirane carboxylic acid.

podocytes: specialized Bowman's capsule cells that extend cytoplasmic processes (foot processes, pedicels) which closely appose glomerular capillary basement membranes and interdigitate with processes of adjacent podocytes to form filtration slits.

podophyllotoxin: 5,8,8*a*,9-tetrahydro-9-hydroxy-5-(3,4,5,-trimethoxyphenyl)furo[3′4′):6,7]naphthol[2,3-d]1,3-dioxol-6-(5*aH*)-one; a toxic glucoside from *Podophyllum peltatum* rhizomes, and a component of **podophyllum resins** (*q.v.*), used as a laboratory tool that binds to tubulin, blocks its polymerization, and arrests cells at metaphase. It causes catharsis and neuropathy if ingested, and skin ulceration if applied topically.

podophyllum: India May apple root; mandrake root; a mixture of toxins from the rhizomes and roots of *Podophyllum peltatum* that includes podophyllotoxin and related glycosides, quercetin, lignols, and flavonols. It is used in veterinary medicine as a purgative.

podophyllum resin: podophyllin; an alcoholic extract of *Podophyllum peltatum* roots that contains podophyllotoxin and other substances, used topically (alone, and in combination with cantharidin and salicylic acid) to remove warts, and to treat keratoses and some other skin

podophyllotoxin

conditions. It is a strong irritant that can cause skin ulceration and damage mucous membranes. If ingested, it is a potent cathartic, and can invoke neuropathy.

Poecilia: a genus of minnows used for genetics and endocrine system studies.

-poiesis: a suffix meaning formation, as in erythropoiesis and leukopoiesis.

-poietin: a suffix for regulators that promote proliferation and/or differentiation of specific cell types, as in erythropoietin and thymopoietin.

poikilo-: a prefix that designates irregular or unusual, as in poikilocyte, or refers to processes in other animal types that differ from those of humans and other mammals, as in poikilothermy.

poikilocytes: cells with unusual shape, a term usually applied to misshapen erythrocytes in the blood of individuals with pernicious and some other forms of anemia.

poikilotherms: exotherms; heterotherms; animals whose body temperatures vary in parallel with environmental factors such as air or water temperature, and/or ultraviolet radiation. They are said to be "cold blooded" because their body temperatures are usually lower than those of mammals and birds. The term *ectotherm* is now preferred. *Cf* **endotherm** and **homeotherm**.

poikilothermy: (1) body temperature regulation in heterotherms; (2) deviations of 2°C or more from normal body temperature levels in homeotherms. Injury to or dysfunction of the posterior hypothalamic and/or pre-optic brain regions can disrupt normal responses to environmental temperature changes.

point mutations: mutations in which a single nucleotide base is replaced by another. Some occur under natural conditions. The effects vary with the locations and kinds of substitutions. Artificially induced types that invoke physiologically significant changes in protein synthesis are used to identify gene, RNA, or protein regions essential for specific functions.

Poiseuille's law: the principle that the flow rate of a liquid through a tube varies directly with the pressure decline along the tube and the fourth power of the radius, and is inversely proportional to the viscosity of the fluid and the length of the tube.

poison glands: structures that produce and release substances toxic to other organisms. Some amphibian skin poison glands also make thyrotropin releasing hormone (TRH) and other peptides similar to or identical with kinds synthesized in mammalian nervous systems and gastrointestinal tracts.

Poisson distribution: a statistical function that defines the probability an event will occur in a finite set of independent trials, in which the chances of occurrence do not vary from trial to trial.

pokeweed mitogen: PWM; a lectin extracted from the pokeweed, *Phytolocca americana*, that binds to oligosaccharide β-*N*-acetylglucosamine moieties. It stimulates B lymphocyte proliferation and differentiation.

pol: polymerase; *see* **DNA** and **RNA polymerases**. Numbers that follow pol, as in pol I and pol II, refer to specific enzyme types.

pol: a gene made by viruses that directs synthesis of a reverse transcriptase. The *gag-pol* gene can direct formation of either a gag protein (which is cleaved to four core types), or a gag-pol protein from which the transcriptase is derived.

polar bodies: When a primary oocyte completes meiosis I, the products are a secondary oocyte (which receives most of the cytoplasm) and a *first polar body*, which contains two copies of a haploid set of chromosomes, and degenerates or soon afterward (directly or after giving rise to *third* and *fourth* polar bodies). Meiosis II yields a large ovum and a *second polar body*, both of which are haploid. Under abnormal conditions, a polar body survives and adheres to a secondary oocyte, and is sometimes fertilized; *see* **sex differentiation disorders**.

polar compounds: molecules with unevenly distributed electrical charges. Water dipole moments promote hydrogen bond formation. The negative OH ends of sugar molecules account for their water solubility.

polarization: (1) establishment of potential differences across membranes. A typical "resting" cell plasma membrane is highly permeable to K^+ ions but sharply limits Na^+ entry from extracellular fluids and contains an Na^+/K^+-ATPase that extrudes Na^+ in exchange for K^+. Negatively charged proteins and other large molecules that cannot leave attract K^+; but the concentration gradient (high K^+ inside and low outside) causes outward diffusion of those ions. Since extracellular fluids have a high Na^+ content, Na^+ ions accumulate along the outer surface of the membrane. Consequently, the inside of the membrane becomes electronegative with respect to the outside. Most stimuli invoke *depolarization* by opening Na^+ channels. Afterward, cells undergo *repolarization* by closing the Na^+ channels and actively extruding the Na^+. *See* also **action potentials** and **hyperpolarization**; (2) *see* **polarized cell**; (3) *see* **animal** and **vegetal poles**.

polarized cell: a cell (1) that has undergone electrical **polarization**, *see* definition 1; (2) with directionally oriented components, for example a membrane highly permeable to one or more ions on one side, and ATPases that fuel extrusion pumps at the other.

polidexide

polidexide: DEAE Sephadex; poly [2-(diethylamino)-ethyl] polyglycerylene dextran hydrochloride; an anion exchange resin that binds to bile acids, and is used to lower blood cholesterol levels by impeding lipid absorption in the small intestine.

polioencephalitis: inflammation of brain gray matter.

poliomyelitis: inflammation of the gray matter of the spinal cord.

poliomyelitis virus: poliovirus; (1) a virus of the *Enterovirus* genus of the Picornaviridae family; (2) any virus that causes poliomyelitis.

poly-: a prefix meaning many, as in polypeptide.

poly-A: *see* **polyadenylate**.

polyacrylamide gel electrophoresis: PAGE; *see* **electrophoresis**.

polyadenylate: poly-A; a chain of up to 250 adenine nucleotides, synthesized in reactions catalyzed by polyadenylate polymerases, and added as a "tail" to the 3′ end of a pre-messenger RNA. The tails are believed to contribute to RNA stabilization, and to more efficient transcript processing, transport to the cytoplasm, and translation. However, although most transcripts have them, ones for histones and a few other proteins do not; and some protein synthesis does proceed when agents such as cordycepin block their addition.

polyadenylate polymerase: *see* **polyadenylate**.

polyamine[s]: ornithine, putrescine, spermine, spermidine, and other small linear molecules with two or more —NH$_2$ groups. The positive charges at physiological pHs promote associations with negatively charged regulatory molecules that mediate many of their actions; *see* also **polyamine dependent kinase**. Polyamines affect DNA, RNA and protein synthesis, and the activities of inositol phosphate kinases, protein kinase C isozymes, nuclear kinases, acetyltransferases, deacetylases, poly (ADP) ribosyl synthetase, demethylases, and other enzymes. They are essential for optimum growth and proliferation of normal cells, and for organ regeneration following injury. They also function as autocrine stimulants for some kinds of tumors and as second messengers for the anabolic actions of insulin, prolactin, gonadotropins, estrogens, and some other hormones. The levels rise shortly before cells enter rapid phases of growth and proliferation. In some cell types, two or more hormones cooperate to accomplish the synthesis of special kinds. Prolactin accelerates ornithine synthesis by activating arginase and ornithine decarboxylase; and it regulates polyamine transport. Cortisol promotes ornithine conversion to spermidine. Some effects of that hormone are attributed to formation of hypusine, which is derived from spermidine.

polyamine dependent kinase: protein kinase NII; casein kinase G; a protein with two 38K α and two 27K β subunits that accelerates transcription and translation by phosphorylating RNA polymerases, a high mobility group protein, and eIF-2. Spermidine activates it directly, and also binds to and inactivates a proteoglycan inhibitor. Insulin and some other hormones activate the enzyme indirectly.

polyandry: usually (1) reproductive strategies in which females mate with more than one male; *cf* **polygyny**; (2) polyspermy.

polyanions: nucleic acids, other macromolecules, and some resins that carry many negative surface charges.

polyarteritis: vasculitis, an autoimmune disease in which small and medium-sized arteries are infiltrated with neutrophils, and eventually become necrotic. It is often associated with rheumatoid arthritis, rheumatic disease, lupus erythematosus, or other connective tissue disorders. *See* also **polyarteritis nodosa**.

polyarteritis nodosa: Kussmaul's disease; a form of **polyarteritis** *(q.v.)* that can affect the heart, gastrointestinal tract, muscles, kidneys, and other organs, but is not associated with rheumatic disease. It may be initiated by viral infections.

polyarthritis: inflammation of many joints. Benign forms persist for short time periods and heal without residual damage. Chronic ones lead to permanent degenerative changes.

polycations: polylysine, other macromolecules, and some resins that carry many positive charges.

polycentric: having two or more centers, a term applied to some chromosomes.

polychlorinated biphenyls: PCBs; mixtures of organic compounds with the general structure shown, in which X can be either H or Cl. They can cause gastrointestinal tract, skin, mouth, and eye damage, liver hypertrophy, and hepatocellular carcinoma, and are classified as environmental pollutants.

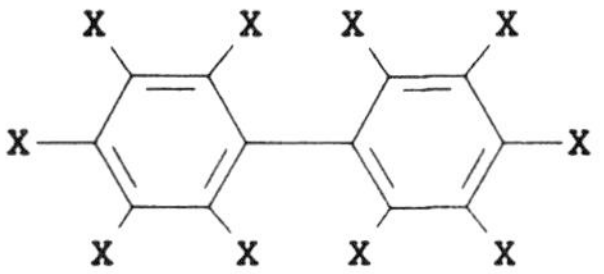

polychromasia: excessive numbers of circulating immature erythrocytes with high RNA content that avidly bind Romanowsky stains and form blue products.

polychromatic: having many colors.

polycistronic mRNAs: messenger RNAs transcribed from two or more linked, tandemly arranged genes.

polyclonal: describes colonies that derive from more than one cell type, or molecular species obtained from more than one source. *See* also **polyclonal antibodies**.

polyclonal antibodies: immunoglobulin preparations obtained from more than one B lymphocyte subset (or other source), with affinities for two or more antigens; *cf* **monoclonal antibodies**.

polycystic ovary: PCO: *see* **polycystic ovary disease**.

polycystic ovary disease: PCOD; polycystic ovary syndrome: several disorders in which the ovarian stroma hypertrophies and produces excessive amounts of androgens, cysts form, and large numbers of atretic follicles accumulate. The term *Stein-Levinthal syndrome* is used as a synonym by some authors, and to designate one form of the disease by others. In some cases, ovarian follicle maturation is incomplete; in others, follicles mature, but ovulation does not follow. Menstrual cycles are initiated, but are usually irregular; and oligomenorrhea or amenorrhea (or more rarely menorrhagia and dysmenorrhea) commonly develop afterward. Abnormal gonadotropin releasing hormone (GnRH) and luteinizing hormone (LH) rhythms, high LH:FSH ratios, and hyperprolactinemia are common findings. The causes include hypothalamic defects that impair adenohypophysial functions. In some cases, neuron defects appear to alter negative feedback by gonadal steroids; in others, neurotransmitter control over those neurons may be deranged. Different kinds of defects more directly invoke hyperandrogenism by affecting ovarian and/or adrenocortical steroidogenesis, impairing androgen metabolism, decreasing production of sex hormone binding globulins, or causing formation of abnormal androgen receptors. Androgen-secreting ovarian and adrenocortical tumors are rare, but it has been suggested that some arise in response to endocrine imbalances at the time of adrenarche. High LH levels can stimulate production of sufficient androgen (mostly androstenedione, but also testosterone and dehydroepiandrosterone) by stromal and thecal cells to invoke hirsutism and other signs of virilization, hyperinsulinism, insulin resistance, and obesity. High intraovarian androgen causes follicle atresia and relative increases in stromal mass. Granulosa cell depletion limits intraovarian estrogen synthesis. Some androgen is converted peripherally to estrone, which augments gonadotropin sensitivity to GnRH, and can thereby further augment LH secretion. Estrogen-progesterone type contraceptives, medroxyprogesterone, GnRH analogs that desensitize gonadotropes, and antiandrogens can alleviate the symptoms; and RU-486 is reported to exert beneficial effects. Ovulation can often be induced with clomiphene; and it has been known to be stimulated by sexual intercourse; *see* **induced ovulation**.

polycythemia: excessive numbers of circulating blood cells (usually *polycythemia vera*, in which the cells are erythrocytes). The resulting increase in viscosity impairs blood flow through small vessels. Severe dehydration elevates red blood cell counts, but true polycythemia in humans is usually caused by tumors that release hematopoietic growth factors, or by hypoxia. It can be invoked in laboratory animals by exposure to high altitudes, oxygen deprivation, or erythropoietin injections.

polydeoxyribonucleotide synthases: DNA ligases; enzymes that catalyze formation of phosphodiester bonds between 5′-phosphoryl and 3′-hydroxy ends of DNA molecules. Some require ATP as a cofactor, and others NAD^+. They are used for DNA replication, recombination, and repair.

polydipsia: excessive drinking, usually associated with polyuria. The major cause is vasopressin deficiency (*see* **diabetes insipidus**). Others include diabetes mellitus, renal defects, and psychological disorders.

polyendocrinoma: *see* **multiple endocrine neoplasia**.

polyenes: compounds with many conjugated double bonds.

polyene antibiotics: amphotericin, nystatin, and some other polyene antibiotics derived from *Streptomyces* species that damage and kill fungi by binding to sterols and altering transport and other cell membrane functions. Most do not affect bacteria. Some kinds are used to study hormone influences on ion transport.

polyergic: capable of acting in several different ways.

polyergin: the Simian form of transforming growth factor β_2.

polyestrous: having more than one estrous cycle per season.

polyethylene glycol: PEG; mixtures of ethylene oxide/water polymers with the general composition: α-hydro-w-poly(oxy-1,2-ethanediyl). They are used as stationary phases for gas-liquid chromatography, as lubricants, and to promote fusion of cultured cells (to achieve transfection or produce hybridomas). Numbers after the names refer to approximate weights. Polyethylene glycol 200 (carbowax) has a molecular weight of 190-210, with an average value of 4 for n, whereas values for PEG 6000 are, respectively 7000-9000 and 158-204.

polyethylene p-octyl phenol: a Triton X type detergent.

polygamy: polyandry or polygyny; mating with more than one partner; *cf* **monogamy**.

polyglandular endocrine deficiency: *see* **pluriglandular endocrine deficiency**.

polygalactia: excessive milk production.

polygenic: describes traits controlled by the combined effects of two or more genes.

polygyny: (1) reproductive strategies in which one male mates with more than one female; *cf* **polyandry**; (2) union of two or more female pronuclei with one male pronucleus.

polykaryocyte: a giant cell with several nuclei, such as a megakaryocyte, macrophage, or skeletal muscle fiber.

polylysines: large peptides composed of lysine moieties, synthesized *in vitro*. When applied to glass or plastic substrates, they facilitate anchoring and growth of cultured cells. They interact with G proteins (especially $G_{\alpha s}$ types), and with clathrin associated protein 2. Low levels increase, and higher ones inhibit adenylate cyclase activity. Other effects on some cell types include stimulation of phosphatidylinositol hydrolysis, and activation of some protein kinases.

polymastia: the presence of more than the usual number of mammary glands.

polymenorrhea: too frequent menstrual cycles; *cf* **metrorrhagia**.

polymers: polysaccharides, nucleic acids, and other compounds composed of large numbers of covalently linked monomers. *Homopolymers* such as glycogen contain a single kind of repeating unit, whereas *heteropolymers* such as glycosaminoglycans, can contain two or more types.

polymerases: enzymes that catalyzes assembly of monomers into polymers; *see*, for example **DNA** and **RNA polymerases**, **polyadenylate**, and **polymerase chain reaction**.

polymerase chain reaction: PCR; powerful *in vitro* techniques for deriving large quantities of specific DNA sequences from minute amounts of starting materials. The DNA strands are separated by warming, and then used (in systems that contain primers, nucleotides and a bacterial DNA polymerase) to synthesize complementary DNA segments. The process is repeated many times with initial plus newly synthesized DNA segments. 200,000 fold amplification can be achieved within hours. *Taq* polymerase, from *Thermus aquaticus* was used initially, but *Pfu* (from *Pyrococcus furiosus*) and Vent (from *Thermococcus litoralis*) are reported to have superior properties.

polymorphic: occurring in more than one form. The term can refer to variants of a molecular species (for example of histocompatibility antigens), structures that change during development or in response to environmental factors, or phenotypes within a population.

polymorphonuclear leukocytes: PMNs; usually (1) the most numerous kinds of circulating white blood cells in most species, named for their nuclear forms. When released to the bloodstream, they have U-shaped nuclei and are called stab cells. As the curves straighten, they become *band cells*. With advancing age, constrictions lead to the formation of lobes connected by short chromatin strands. The oldest cells can have as many as seven. PMNs are also called *neutrophils*, because their granules bind both acidic and basic dyes. Large numbers enter the blood during most bacterial infections. They express cell adhesion molecules on their surfaces, and receptors for chemotaxins and other regulators. When activated, they migrate across blood vessels via diapedesis, accumulate at sites of infection and inflammation, phagocytose small microorganisms, and release numerous enzymes, superoxide radicals, and other bactericidal agents. Excessive amounts, and/or inadequate controls by enzyme inactivators and other regulators can damage normal body cells. PMNs also bind to fibrin and contribute to blood clot dissolution; (2) any leukocyte of myelocyte lineage with a lobed nucleus, such as a basophil or eosinophil.

polymyxin: an antibiotic complex (which includes polymyxins A, B_1, B_2, C, D, E, F, K, M, P, S, and T), made by some aerobic spore-forming soil bacteria, and

polyethylene p-octyl phenol

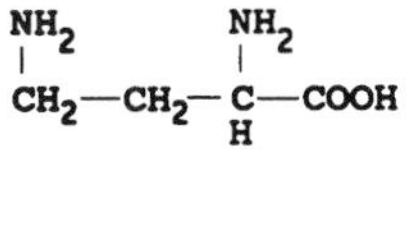

$$NH_2 \quad NH_2$$
$$CH_2-CH_2-\underset{\underset{H}{|}}{C}-COOH$$

α-γ-GAM

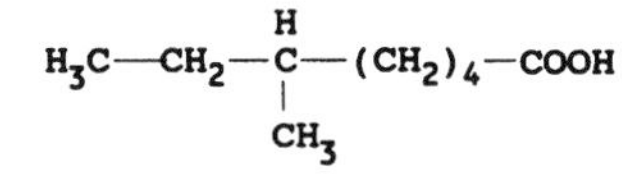

$$H_3C-CH_2-\underset{\underset{CH_3}{|}}{\overset{\overset{H}{|}}{C}}-(CH_2)_4-COOH$$

6-methyl-octanoyl

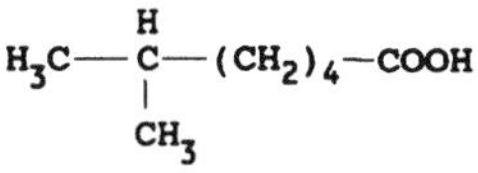

$$H_3C-\underset{\underset{CH_3}{|}}{\overset{\overset{H}{|}}{C}}-(CH_2)_4-COOH$$

6-methyl-heptanoyl

$$R-L\text{-}DAB-X-L\text{-}DAB\Big\langle{\begin{array}{l}L\text{-}DAB-Y-Z\\ \\ X-L\text{-}DAB-L\text{-}DAB\end{array}}$$

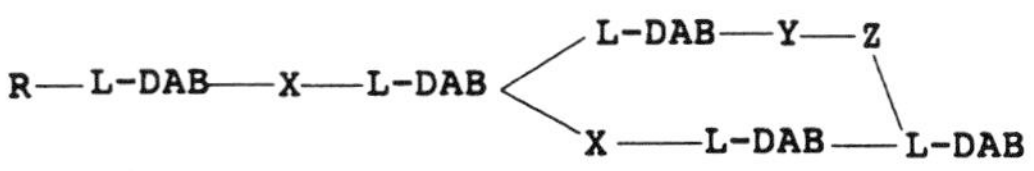

polymyxins

especially by various *Bacillus polymyxa* strains. Polymixin E (Colistin) is usually obtained from *Aerobacillus colistinus*. The components share the common structure shown, in which DAB = α,γ-diaminobutyric acid, R is a 6-methyloctanoyl, 6-methylheptanoyl, or a related fatty acid moiety, and X, Y, and Z are amino acids. All polymyxins have both hydrophilic and hydrophobic groups that interact with phospholipids, and disrupt membrane structure. They are applied topically to treat skin, eye, and ear infections. B types, in which X, Y, and Z are, respectively, L-threonine, D-phenylalanine, and L-leucine, bind and inactivate endotoxin (lipopolysaccharide, LPS) by attaching to the lipid A component, and are used to counteract endotoxin effects and remove LPS from some *in vitro* systems. They also inhibit protein kinase C isozymes, and promote catecholamine release. Although effective against many kinds of gram-negative bacteria, potential kidney damage and other serious toxic effects preclude systemic use, except under special conditions.

polyneuritis: inflammation of many peripheral nerves.

polynucleotides: linear sequences of covalently linked nucleotides.

polynucleotide kinase: T₄PNK; an enzyme from T-4 phage infected *E. coli* bacteria that catalyzes transfers of γ phosphate groups from ATP to the 5′-hydroxy termini of DNAs and RNAs (and also has 3′-phosphatase activity). It is used to end-label nucleic acids with ^{32}P, and to phosphorylate synthetic linkers and nucleic acid fragments prior to ligation.

polynucleotide phosphorylase: an enzyme that covalently links ribonucleotides. It is used for RNA synthesis, and to produce artificial mRNA molecules.

polyol pathway: the biochemical pathway in which **aldose reductase** (*q.v.*) converts glucose to sorbitol (a sugar alcohol that does not rapidly diffuse out of cells and can therefore osmotically draw water into them). Cataracts, neuropathy and some other devastating effects of chronic hyperglycemia are attributed, in part to sorbitol accumulation in eye lenses, Schwann cells, neurons, and elsewhere. *Myo*-inositol can attenuate, and even partially reverse the effects, possibly by competing with glucose for transport systems, or by correcting a *myo*-inositol deficiency caused by the subnormal Na⁺/K⁺-ATPase activity commonly associated with diabetes mellitus. Inositol also contributes to plasma membrane

structure, lowers the activities of some kinase C isozymes augmented by glucose, is lipolytic, and is an essential growth factor for at least some species.

polyomavirus: a genus of small DNA tumor viruses of the *Papaoviridae* family whose members induce several kinds of neoplasias when injected into infant mice and some other infant rodents, but do not cause obvious disease during spontaneous infections in adults of the same strains. The virus replicates in and kills mouse cells infected *in vitro*. In contrast, the cells of hamsters and some other animal types undergo abortive infections, with only small numbers transformed.

polyovular: describes species in which two or more oocytes are regularly prepared for fertilization during a single ovarian cycle.

polyps: mostly benign growths that project from mucous membranes or other surfaces.

polypeptides: moderate sized compounds composed of amino acids moieties linked by peptide bonds. Molecules with more than 100 amino acid groups are usually called proteins. Those with fewer are called oligopeptides, or named for the numbers, as in decapeptide or pentapeptide.

polyphenism: the presence of several phenotypes in a population that do not derive from genetic differences.

polyphosphatidylinositidases: *see* **phosphatidylinositidases**.

polyploidy: the presence of three or more copies of each chromosome type. The numbers of copies are usually indicated, as in triploidy or tetraploidy. *Cf* **euploidy**.

polyprotein: a protein that can be cleaved to several products; *see*, for example **proopiomelanocortin** (POMC).

polyribosomes: polysomes.

polysaccharides: starches, glycogens, cellulose, inulin, and other homopolymers composed of repeating units of a single sugar type, pectins and other sugar heteropolymers, and some large molecules that contain uronic acids and other sugar derivatives, some of which are *N*-acetylated and/or sulfated. The complex cell wall polysaccharides of most bacteria are antigenic in higher animals.

polysome: polyribosome; a structural unit composed of multiple ribosomes that can move along a common messenger RNA, and rapidly direct formation of large numbers of identical protein molecules. Globins and some other abundant proteins are constitutively translated in this way. Insulin, triiodothyronine (T_3), and many other hormones promote monosome assembly into polysomes.

polysomy: the presence of more than two chromosomes of one kind in a diploid organism. The numbers and locations are usually indicated, as in trisomy 21. The extra chromosomes often exert deleterious influences.

polysorbates: polymers of ethylene oxide moieties linked to sorbitol and sorbitol esters. Polysorbate 80 and some others are used as surfactants.

polysorbate 80: Tween 80; derivatives of sorbitan mono-9-octodecanoate-poly(oxo-1,2-ethanediyl). They are surfactants, used as emulsifying and anti-foaming agents. In the structure shown, $R = C_{17}H_{33}COOH$, and the sum of w, x, y, and z = 20.

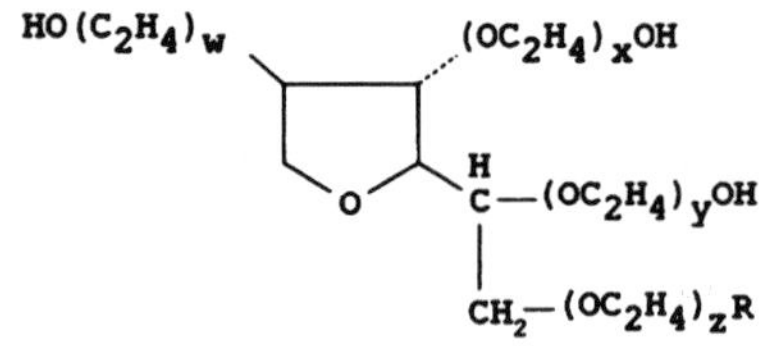

$$HO(C_2H_4)_w \quad (OC_2H_4)_x OH$$
$$\underset{O}{\overset{H}{C}}-(OC_2H_4)_y OH$$
$$CH_2-(OC_2H_4)_z R$$

polyspermy: usually (1) fertilization of an oocyte by more than one spermatozoan; (2) release of more than the usual numbers of spermatozoa.

polysynaptic: multisynaptic; involving functional interactions between three or more neurons (or between at least two and a neuromuscular junction or other structure across which transmitters are sent).

polytene chromosomes: giant chromosomes of some insect and plant cells, composed of up to 1000 identical chromatids aligned in parallel. They are formed by successive replications of homologous chromosomes pairs that do not separate. When stained, the aligned genes show up as vertical bands. Ecdysone and other factors that direct embryogenesis and maturation regulate the formation of puffs (expanded regions at transcription sites essential, but not sufficient for gene activation) during various stages of development. The puffs can also be induced by heat shock, and by exogenous ecdy-sone. *Drosophila* salivary gland giant chromosomes are the most widely studied kinds.

polythelic: having more than the usual number of breast nipples.

polytocous: giving birth to multiple young following a single pregnancy.

poly U: polyuridine.

polyunsaturated fatty acids: linoleic, linolenic, arachidonic, and other fatty acids with two or more double bonds separated by methylene groups. They are classified as essential because most animals cannot synthesize them. (Animals can, however, shorten and lengthen chains, and in other ways convert some types to others.)

In the structure shown, R_1 and R_2 are carbon chains that can contain additional unsaturated bonds.

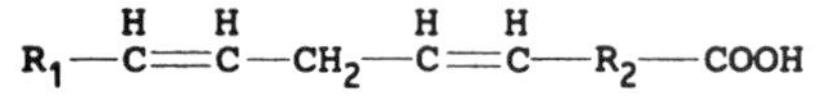

$$R_1-\overset{H}{\underset{}{C}}=\overset{H}{\underset{}{C}}-CH_2-\overset{H}{\underset{}{C}}=\overset{H}{\underset{}{C}}-R_2-COOH$$

polyuria: formation of excessive amounts of urine. Usually, the water loss leads to thirst and polydipsia. A major cause is vasopressin deficiency. Others include formation of abnormal vasopressin receptors, and conditions such as diabetes mellitus in which osmotically active molecules in renal tubular fluids draw water to the urine.

polyuridylic acid: poly U; an artificial polynucleotide in which all the nitrogenous bases are uracil. In cell-free translation systems, it directs formation of peptides composed exclusively of phenylalanine moieties.

POMC: proopiomelanocortin.

POMP: prednisone, oncovin (vincristine), methotrexate, and 6-mercaptopurine, a drug combination used to treat some neoplastic diseases.

Pompe disease: glycogen storage disease II, a severe, autosomal recessive disorder in which synthesis of α1 → 4-glycosidase (an enzyme that acts on branched carbohydrate chains and is required for efficient glycogen catabolism) is impaired. Glycogen accumulation in the nervous system, heart, and other sites causes mental and motor retardation during infancy, and usually, early death from heart failure.

ponderal: pertaining to body weight.

ponderal index: height in centimeters divided by body weight in kilograms.

Pongidae: the primate family that includes all anthropoid apes.

pons: usually (1) the part of the brainstem anterior to the cerebellum (with which it communicates via the middle cerebellar peduncles), and superior to the medulla oblongata. It contains the pneumotaxic and apneustic areas, and nuclei for the trigeminal, abducens, facial, and vestibulocochlear cranial nerves; (2) a bridge.

P:O ratio: the number of ATP molecules that can theoretically be synthesized from ADP + Pi for each oxygen atom that accepts two hydrogen atoms and two electrons in a mitochondrial electron transport chain. The value is 3 when the hydrogen and electron donor is NADH + H^+, and 2 when it is $FADH_2$.

porcine: characteristic of, or derived from domestic pigs (*Sus scrofa*) and related species, represented by *p* in acronyms, as in *p*ACTH (porcine adrenocorticotropic hormone).

porins: 37K proteins that traverse the outer membranes of eukaryote mitochondria and the outer cell membranes of bacteria, so named because the molecules have pores that function as channels for the passage of ions and small (<10K), hydrophilic molecules. *Cf* **perforins**.

porosis: cavity formation. The term can refer to a disease of chickens caused by a vitamin deficiency, or used as a suffix, as in osteoporosis.

porphins: cyclic compounds with four pyrrole rings linked by methine bridges; 21*H*,23*H*-porphine is shown. *See* also **porphyrins**.

porphobilins: several porphin-related pigments, including some hemoglobin degradation products. Minute amounts are excreted to the urine under normal conditions, and larger ones by individuals with porphyria.

porphobilinogen: 2-aminomethylpyrrol-3-acetic acid 5-propionic acid; an intermediate in the pathway for porphyrin biosynthesis, made in the reaction: 2 δ-aminolevulate → porphobilinogen + 2 H_2O. Four porphobilinogen molecules polymerize to yield polypyrryl methane, a linear tetrapyrrole.

porphobilinogen deaminase: an enzyme used for hemoglobin biosynthesis that converts porphobilinogen (a linear tetrapyrrole) to cyclic uroporphyrinogen III, with release of NH_3.

porphyria: several disorders in which large quantities of porphyrin compounds are excreted to the urine. When unqualified, the term usually refers to *acute intermittent porphyria*, an autosomal dominant inherited disease attributed to porphobilinogen deaminase deficiency. The manifestations include recurrent abdominal pain, tachycardia, postural hypotension, urinary retention, sweating, vomiting, constipation, and severe neurological dysfunction. *Congenital erythropoietic porphyria* is a rare autosomal recessive disorder characterized by hemolytic anemia, cutaneous photosensitivity with blistering, keratosis and scarring of the skin, and conjunctivitis. Other porphyrias are caused by some hepatic and hemolytic diseases.

porphyrins: porphin compounds in which some hydrogen atoms are replaced by methyl, vinyl, propionyl, or other small chemical groups. δ-aminolevulinate synthetase is the major enzyme required for the biosynthesis. The nitrogen atoms chelate Fe in **heme** (*q.v.*) and Mg in chlorophylls. Zn and other metals attach to different, biologically active porphin derivatives. *See* also **porphobilinogen**.

porphyrinogens: hexahydroporphyrins, such as uroporphyrinogen, an intermediate in the pathway for biosynthesis of hemoglobin and related compounds.

porphyropsin: 11-*cis*-dehydroretinal (vitamin A_2) bound to scotopsin, the retinal photoreceptor pigment of lampreys, fresh water fishes, and some amphibians.

portal system: an anatomical arrangement in which venules collect blood from one set of capillaries and deliver it to a second set; *see*, for example **hypothalamo-hypophysial** and **hepatic portal systems**. Similar arrangements occur in kidneys (in which blood from efferent arterioles enters peritubular capillaries), and in adrenal glands (where blood leaving the cortex enters capillaries of the medulla).

positive control: (1) describes systems in which transcription is initiated by the binding of a regulatory protein to an operator; (2) *see* **positive feedback controls**.

positive cooperativity: usually, increased affinity of unoccupied receptors for their ligands, initiated by binding of the same kind of ligand to adjacent receptors.

positive feedback controls: regulatory mechanisms in which something created by a system enhances the activity of the system, for example ones in which an intermediate or product of a biochemical pathway increases the activity of a rate-limiting enzyme of the same pathway, or in which secretion of a tropic hormone is stimulated by a different hormone released from its target cells. The term is also applied when a hormone induces its own receptors. Positive feedback is used to accomplish processes such as ovulation and parturition, in which very high hormone levels are needed for finite time periods, or when something must be rapidly made. *Cf* **negative feedback controls**.

positive interference: the tendency for a chromosome crossover event to suppress occurrence of a second crossover by the same chromosomes.

positron: a positively charged atomic particle with a mass equivalent to that of an electron.

postabsorptive state: in adequately nourished individuals, the metabolic condition during times of fasting (when dietary nutrients are not absorbed, and all fuels and metabolic building blocks are drawn from stored reserves). Lipolysis, fatty acid oxidation, glycogenolysis, and gluconeogenesis proceed at high rates, driven in part by glucagon and glucocorticoids; but the metabolic rate declines. Insulin levels are low, lipogenesis and glycogenesis proceed slowly, and only minimal amounts of glucose are taken up by skeletal muscle and other cell types with insulin-regulated transport systems. Although growth hormone concentrations are usually high, very little insulin-like growth factor I (IGF-I) is made; and inhibitors diminish its effectiveness. Since the fuel mixture oxidized by healthy humans is known, oxygen consumption equivalents can be calculated for measurements of **basal metabolic rate** (*q.v.*). The tests are usually performed in the morning, 12 or more hours after the last meal.

postcoital contraceptives: interceptives; agents that promote extrusion of newly formed conceptuses and/or block implantation. Very large doses of estrogens stimulate contraction of uterine and oviduct smooth muscle, but often invoke nausea, cramping, and other unwanted effects; and there is some evidence that repeated use can damage hypothalamic mechanisms for controlling gonadotropin releasing hormone (GnRH) secretion patterns. Prostaglandin $F_2\alpha$ is also a good stimulant, but it must be infused (because it is rapidly degraded). Longer-lasting analogs, some of which are effective orally exert similar actions, but they (and $PGF_{2\alpha}$) cause abdominal pain, diarrhea, nausea, and other undesirable effects. *See* also **mifepristone**.

post coitum: after mating.

posterior: toward the back, a term roughly equivalent to dorsal in humans and other upright animals, and caudal in tetrapods. *Cf* **anterior** and **ventral**.

posterior hypothalamic area: PHA; a brain region that contains neurons involved in thermoregulation and control of other sympathetic system functions.

posterior pituitary: posterior pituitary gland; the hypophysial component left behind in an experimental animal when the more easily removed anterior components are excised. It usually includes the pars intermedia (if one is present), and some of the pars tuberalis, as well as the entire neural lobe. The term is used synonymously with neural lobe by some authors. *See* also **neurohypophysis**.

postganglionic: describes (1) neurons that originate in autonomic nervous system ganglia and extend axons towards target organs, or (2) events that follow stimulation of such neurons. *Cf* **preganglionic**.

postmitotic: describes (1) cells that have undergone terminal differentiation and have lost the ability to divide; (2) events that occur immediately following mitosis or soon thereafter.

postpartum: following parturition.

postpartum hemorrhage: excessive bleeding following parturition. Oxytocin released during and soon after parturition, and during lactation, stimulates the contraction of uterine muscle, and protects by compressing blood vessels. Ergonovine is routinely administered to mimic the effects in women who do not nurse their infants.

postreceptor defects: dysfunctions caused by inability to respond in the usual ways to the ligand-receptor complexes, even when both components are normal in structure and present in adequate amounts. It can be caused by defective transduction mechanisms, inability to make the enzymes and/or other cell components involved in the responses, or severe nutritional deficiencies.

postsynaptic: describes (1) a neuron that synapses with and is activated (or inhibited) by another neuron, or a target cell (such as a muscle fiber) activated by a neurotransmitter; (2) an event initiated by release of a neurotransmitter at a synapse.

postsynaptic potentials: the electrochemical properties of the membranes of postsynaptic neurons that are not generating nerve impulses. When presynaptic neurons release subthreshold amounts of stimulatory neuro-

transmitters, they invoke excitatory presynaptic potentials (EPSPs) by promoting partial depolarizations, and they thereby augment the sensitivities of the targets to stimulants. Inhibitory neurotransmitters invoke post synaptic inhibitory potentials (IPSPs) by promoting hyperpolarizations that decrease the sensitivities.

postthymic cells: T lymphocytes that have completed maturation in, and have left the thymus gland.

posttranscriptional: occurring after formation of a primary RNA transcript. The term can refer to RNA processing (such as capping, intron excision, and polyadenylation), RNA stabilization or degradation, or RNA transport. (It is not usually applied to translation or posttranslational events).

posttranslational: occurring after protein synthesis on ribosomes has been completed. The term can refer to processes such as selective peptide bond cleavage, changes in the composition of oligosaccharides added after translation, or covalent modifications such as phosphorylation, amidation, acetylation, sulfation, or oxidation.

potassium: K; a metallic element (atomic number 19, atomic weight 39.102). K^+ is the major intracellular cation. It is attracted into cells by negatively charged cytoplasmic proteins, enters via diffusion and/or potassium channels, and is taken up when Na^+/K^+-ATPases exchange it for Na^+. The movements are opposed by high intracellular:extracellular concentration gradients; *see* also **polarization** and **Nernst equation**. Intracellular K^+ contributes to the regulation of cell pH and water balance, affects the activities of several enzymes, and is an essential cofactor for pyruvate kinase and some others. Extracellular K^+ is a physiological vasodilator and myocardial depressant. Excessively high concentrations can invoke hypotension and diastolic arrest. Supraphysiological levels can depolarize cells and promote the release of many hormones and neurotransmitters. K^+ levels at both sites also affect the activities of plasma membrane Na^+/K^+-ATPases. Aldosterone accelerates renal excretion of the ions and facilitates K^+ extrusion by muscle fibers and other cell types. Epinephrine and some other regulators promote cell upake. [42]K is a radioactive isotope with a half-life of 12.4 hours used for transport studies.

potassium channels: plasma membrane complexes with pores for exchange of K^+ ions between cells and their microenvironments. Constitutively active "leak channels" that permit entry and exit of K^+, but not of Ca^{2+} or Na^+, contribute to polarization and some aspects of depolarization and repolarization. *Voltage gated* types open in response to cell depolarization. In some neurons, rapid transmission of impulses is accomplished via A-type ("early") K^+ channels that open almost immediately following Na^+ entry. Delayed kinds open a short time later, and contribute to both repolarization and long-range processes such as memory. In some cells, elevation of cytoplasmic Ca^{2+} is required for delayed types. *Receptor operated* (ligand gated) kinds respond to hormones and other regulators. A single kind of neurotransmitter can exert diverse effects. For example, when acetylcholine acts on nicotinic type receptors in skeletal muscle and some other cells, and promotes depolarization, voltage gated channels respond. In cardiac muscle, it acts via inhibitory G proteins to open ligand gated K^+ types that are insensitive to membrane voltage changes. *See* also **tetraethylammonium**.

potassium iodide: KI; a component of **Lugol's solution** (*q.v.*), used to treat some thyroid gland dysfunctions. KI also augments sensitivities to some fungicides. Large amounts can invoke lacrimation, nausea, vomiting, acne, and skin lesions; and long-term use facilitates goiter growth; *see* **Wolff-Chaikoff effect**.

potato lectin: a lectin extracted from the potato, *Solanum tuberosum*, that binds to *N*-acetylglucosamine moieties of oligosaccharides.

potentiation: (1) describes interactions between two agents that, when presented in combination, elicit greater effects than the sum of the responses to either presented alone; *cf* **additive effects**. Usually, this indicates that the agents act via different mechanisms; i.e. the actions of one facilitate those of the other on a common end point. Potentiation can be achieved, for example if one agent is a ligand for plasma membrane receptors and the other promotes receptor translocation to the membrane, or if one promotes synthesis of a messenger RNA, and the other inhibits degradation of the RNA or activates its translation product; (2) a term sometimes used synonymously with synergism.

potentiometers: instruments with devices for controlling electrical resistance, used to measure small voltage differences at two points, or to maintain constant voltages.

potomania: dipsomania; ingestion of excessive quantities of fluid. The term can describe the behavior of individuals with psychological disorders or brain lesions that affect the drive to ingest water or other fluids, but has also been applied to ones who ingest very large quantities of beer.

POU domain genes: *Pit-1*, *Oct*, *Unc-8*, and other homeotic genes that direct synthesis of proteins with POU domains. The products are 76-78 amino acid transcription factors that function as "molecular switches" for control of differentiation and of some activities of mature cells by binding to similar octamer DNA segments of promoters and enhancers, and selectively activating other genes. Some POU genes are ubiquitously expressed; others function in just a few cell types.

POU-I: a POU domain gene required for pituitary gland development. It codes for Pit-1, a protein in somatotropes and somatomammotropes that directs differentiation of those cells, and may also promote precursor cell proliferation. It binds to growth hormone gene promoters and stimulates growth hormone synthesis. It, or a closely related Prl-1 binds to prolactin promoters and stimulates prolactin synthesis. A third subtype that augments thyroid stimulating hormone (TSH) synthesis by affecting thyrotrope sensitivity to thyrotropin releasing hormone (TRH), and a fourth transiently expressed in developing neural tubes have been described.

POU-II: a POU domain gene that directs the synthesis of Oct-1 and related proteins. *Oct-1* is expressed in many cell types, including some thalamic and cerebellar neurons. The protein product is identical to nuclear factor-1 (NF-1), which regulates the expression of many genes (including ones that code for histone 2B). Oct-2 protein is abundant in developing nervous systems, in which it plays essential roles in neurogenesis. In mature animals, high levels are restricted to B lymphocytes, where they regulate immunoglobulin synthesis. Oct-3 protein (also known as Oct-4 protein and nuclear factor A3) in one-cell zygotes is essential for progression to the two-cell stage. It is later expressed at highest levels in totipotent and pluripotent hematopoietic stem and germ cells; and large amounts are made by embryonal cancers.

POU-III: a set of closely related POU domain genes that direct the synthesis of Brn-1, Brn-2, Tst-1, and SCIP proteins, all of which contribute to nervous system development. Brn-1 and Brn-2 are expressed in many brain regions, whereas Tst-1 is restricted to a few sites, and is also made in testes. Tst-1 appears to be a fragment of SCIP (suppressed cAMP-induced POU), a protein made by immature, proliferating Schwann cells and by Schwann cells of mature organisms that proliferate in response to peripheral nerve injury. Unlike other POU proteins, it is a transcription repressor that promotes dedifferentiation.

POU-IV: a POU domain gene that directs the synthesis of Brn-3 protein in rat brain, and unc-86 protein in *Caenorhabditis elegans*. Br-3 is required for nervous system development, but its expression is limited to a few sites in the brain.

povidone: polyvinylpyrrolidone; polymers of 1-ethinyl-2-pyrrolidinone with the repeating unit shown, used as dispersing and suspending agents. Iodine complexed with povidone is a topical anesthetic that slowly releases iodine.

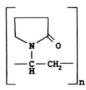

Poxviridae: a class of large, complex DNA viruses that includes *vaccinia*, *variola*, and *myxoma* types. They establish nucleus-like structures in host cytoplasm, and use them for proliferation.

P-P: pyrophosphate.

PP: pancreatic polypeptide.

PP-1, PP-2A, PP-2B PP-2C: *see* **protein phosphatases**.

PP-12: placental protein-12.

PP-14: placental protein-14.

pp: phosphoprotein; numbers that follow usually indicate known, estimated, or approximate molecular weights; superscripts can refer to the source, as in pp60^{src}.

p.p.: postpartum.

pp30$^{c\text{-mos}}$: *see* **cytostatic factor**.

pp60^{src}: *see* **Rous sarcoma virus**.

pp80: an 87K phosphoprotein substrate for protein kinase C.

PPACK: D-Phe-L-Pro-L-Arg-CH$_2$Cl; D-phenylalanyl-L-prolyl-L-arginine chloromethylketone: a reversible inhibitor of thrombin, used to measure plasma thrombin levels, to study blood clotting, and as an anticoagulant.

PPCA: proserum prothrombin conversion accelerator; blood coagulation factor VII; *see* **coagulation**.

PP cells: D cells; cells that secrete pancreatic polypeptide.

PPI: peptidyl-protein *cis-trans* isomerase; *see* **rotamase**.

ppm: parts per million.

PPP: platelet poor plasma.

3-PPP: preclamol; 3-(3-hydroxyphenyl)-*N*-(1-propyl) piperidine; a dopamine autoreceptor agonist and post-receptor antagonist, and a partial agonist for α_1 and α_2 adrenergic receptors, that also binds with high affinity to σ types.

PPT: preprotachykinins.

PRA: plasma renin activity.

practolol: 1-(4-acetamidophenoxy)-3-isopropylamino-2-propanol; a β_1 type adrenergic receptor antagonist used to treat cardiac dysrhythmias.

PRAD-1: a proto-oncogene amplifed in some breast, squamous cell, and parathyroid gland adenomas. Its product is cyclin D1.

Prader-Labhart-Willi Syndrome: *see* Prader-Willi syndrome.

Prader-Willi Syndrome: inherited disorders, most common in the progeny of aging mothers, in which hypogonadism is associated with short stature, obesity, mental retardation, impaired responses to growth hormone and insulin, and failure to display normal hormone rhythms. Gonadotropin secretion is deficient in many, but not all cases. Most afflicted individuals have cytogenetically visible deletions of paternally derived chromosome #15, or lack the entire chromosome. Some have two maternally derived copies.

pralidoxime: 2-[(hydroxyimino)methyl]-1-methylpyridinium; pyridine-2-aldoxime methyl chloride; *see* 2-**PAM**.

prandial: pertaining to meals. The term is also used as a suffix, as in postprandial.

pravastatin: 3β-hydroxycompactin; a 3-hydroxy-3-methyl-glutaryl-coenzyme A (HMG-CoA) reductase inhibitor with chemical and biological properties similar to those described for **mevastatin** (*q.v.*) and lovastatin.

praxis: ability to perform skilled movements.

prazepam: 7-chloro-1-(cyclopropylmethyl)-1,3-dihydro-5-phenyl-2*H*-1,4-benzodiazepin-2-one; an orally effective diazepam type sedative and tranquilizer.

prazosin: 1-(4-amino-6,7-dimethoxy-2-quinazolinyl)-4-(2-furanylcarbonyl)piperazine; a potent α_1-type adrenergic receptor antagonist used to treat some forms of hypertension.

practolol

prazosin

PRC: plasma renin concentration.

PRE: progesterone response element; *see* **progesterone receptors**.

preadaptation: mutations that effect changes which are not immediately apparent, but prove useful to later generations exposed to different environmental factors.

preadipocytes: cells that have begun, but have not completed differentiation to adipocytes.

prealbumin: a plasma protein fraction that migrates more rapidly than albumin in electrophoresis fields. It contains thyroxine binding prealbumin.

preantral follicles: vesicular ovarian follicles that have undergone partial maturation (including vesicle formation), but have not yet acquired antra.

precipitins: antigens that promote aggregation and formation of visible precipitates when they bind to specific antibodies.

precocial: describes animals sufficiently mature at birth or hatching to move about independently, survive with minimal maternal care, and perform other functions developed postnatally by other animals of the same class.

precocious: maturing at an earlier age than is characteristic of the species.

precocious puberty: sexual maturation at an earlier age than is characteristic for the species, in which the hypothalamus acquires adult type gonadotropin releasing hormone (GnRH) and gonadotropin release patterns. The causes include hormone-secreting tumors and head injuries. *Cf* **pseudoprecocious puberty**.

precocious pseudopuberty: *see* **pseudoprecocious puberty**.

prediabetes: a condition in which no overt symptoms of diabetes mellitus are manifested, but glucose tolerance and other laboratory tests reveal carbohydrate metabolism abnormalities, some of which may be associated with high blood insulin levels. It occurs most commonly in close relatives of individuals with diabetes mellitus, and can be followed by development of the overt symptoms.

prednisolone: 11,17,21-trihydroxypregnan-1,4-diene-3-one; Δ^1-hydrocortisone; a synthetic glucocorticoid with greater anti-inflammatory, and lower mineralocorticoid potency than hydrocortisone. It, and several esters (such as the acetate, phosphate, succinate, and tebutate) are used to treat rheumatoid arthritis, allergies, bursitis, some neoplastic diseases, some blood dyscrasias, and

other disorders. Excessive amounts invoke Cushing's syndrome.

prednisone: 17,21-dihydroxypregna-1,4-diene-3,11,20-trione; an orally effective synthetic steroid that does not directly bind to glucocorticoid receptors but is rapidly converted to prednisolone.

preeclampsia: disorders that develop during pregnancy and subside after parturition, in which hypertension, proteinuria, and usually also edema are associated with swollen renal glomerular epithelial and capillary cells, diminished renal blood flow, and impaired glomerular filtration rate. They usually begin during the second trimester of a first pregnancy, when an immature uterine vasculature causes uteroplacental ischemia, but can develop earlier, or in later pregnancies. Trophoblastic disease, preexisting hypertension, blood vessel damage related to diabetes mellitus, or large placental masses associated with two or more fetuses are implicated in some cases. The symptoms have been attributed to exaggerated responses to high maternal estrogen levels, impaired negative feedback controls over renin substrate, angiotensin II, aldosterone, and/or prostaglandin production, and prostacyclin deficiency.

preformation: an outmoded idea that ova and zygotes contain preformed, miniature versions of adult structures which serve as precursors for the mature ones. *Cf* **epigenesis**.

preganglionic: describes (1) autonomic system neurons with cell bodies in the brain or spinal cord, and axons that terminate in ganglia; (2) processes mediated by such neurons, or events attributed to their activities. *Cf* **postganglionic**.

pregnancy: the condition of a mother from the time of conception (or implantation) to parturition. The duration varies with the species, and is related to nervous system complexity, neonate size and maturity, and the numbers of conceptuses simultaneously nurtured. When counted from conception, it ranges from 16 days in hamsters and some marsupials to more than 600 in elephants, and averages 266 days in women.

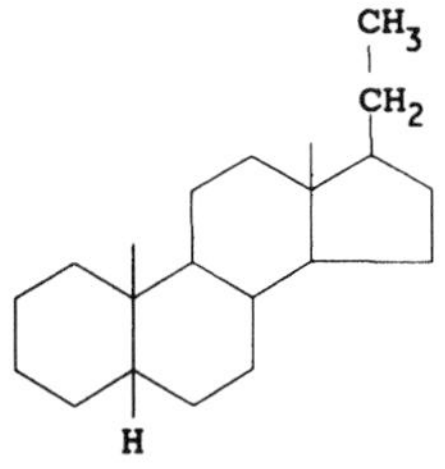

pregnane

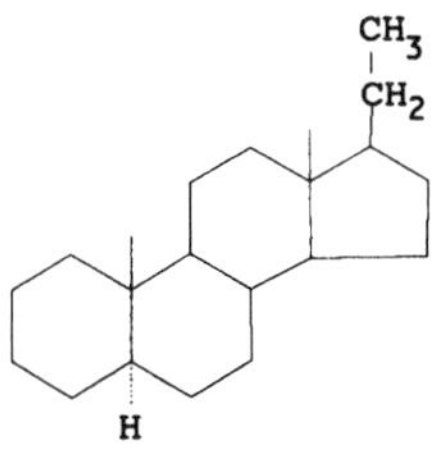

allopregnane

pregnancy associated endometrial α₂-globulin: α_2-PEG; a 56K monomeric, microheterogeneic glycoprotein closely related to β-lactoglobulin, that may be identical with placental protein-14. It is induced by progesterone, appears in uterine and amniotic fluids during early pregnancy, and is implicated as a mediator of implantation and the events that follow soon afterward. Since it is the most abundant endometrial secretory protein at that time, and small amounts enter the maternal bloodstream, it is used to assess endometrial functions.

pregnancy associated plasma protein A: PAPP-A; one of several proteins made by decidual and trophoblastic cells and released to maternal blood. It is also made in some mammary gland carcinomas.

pregnancy specific β₁-glycoprotein: SP_1: the major placental glycoproteins of humans and some other primates, synthesized by syncytiotrophoblast, amniotic epithelium, and placental cells. At least 12 closely related types, all members of the immunoglobulin superfamily, are encoded by multiple genes. Small amounts are made by fibroblasts, and low levels are present in the blood and cerebrospinal fluid of men and nonpregnant women. Progesterone induced decidual fibroblast differentiation may account in part for the increases during pregnancy. One suggested function is immunosuppression that protects against maternal rejection of conceptuses. Since they are easily detected soon after conception, and the levels rise afterward, SP_1s are used as a markers for pregnancy, and to monitor fetal growth. In laboratory animals, antibodies directed against them terminate pregnancies. SP_1 is also made by hydatidiform moles and choriocarcinoma cells; and changing levels can indicate the success of treatment regimes.

pregnancy tests: most tests in women depend on detection of hCG (human chorionic gonadotropin) in maternal urine. Older procedures, based on the luteinizing hor-

mone (LH)-like or LH plus follicle stimulating hormone (FSH)-like properties include the Aschheim-Zondek, Friedman, and Galli-Mainini types. Immunological methods are more reliable, less time-consuming, and less expensive; and they do not require the use of laboratory animals. Most are based on the ability of free hCG in the specimen to displace labeled hCG from a complex with anti-hCG. A radioreceptor assay for hCG can be performed at an earlier time on blood, but it demands special equipment and expertise. Cross-reactivity with LH is a problem, but antibodies can be raised against the hCG component not present in the pituitary hormone.

pregnane: 5β-pregnane; 17β-ethyletiocholane; a saturated, 21-carbon compound used for steroid hormone nomenclature. Small amounts of the 5α isomer (allopregnane) are made and excreted to urine.

pregnanediols: 5β-pregnan-3α,20α-diol is the major progesterone degradation product excreted to urine in women and some other mammals during luteal phases of ovarian cycles, and during pregnancy. No biological activity is known. 5α-pregnan-3α,20α-diol (allopregnanediol) is an isomer in the urine of pregnant women.

3,20-**pregnanedione**: a progesterone degradation product excreted to the urine by several mammalian species.

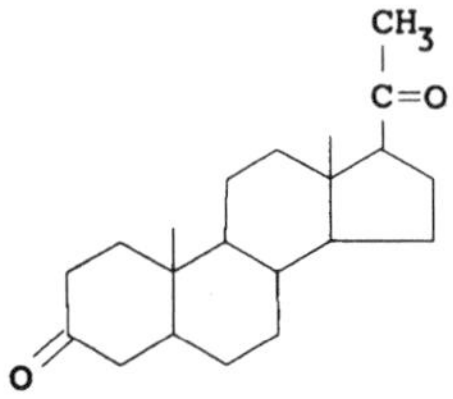

pregnanetriols: several trihydroxylated steroid hormone degradation products in blood and urine. 5β-pregnane-3α,17α,20α-triol, the major type derived from pro-

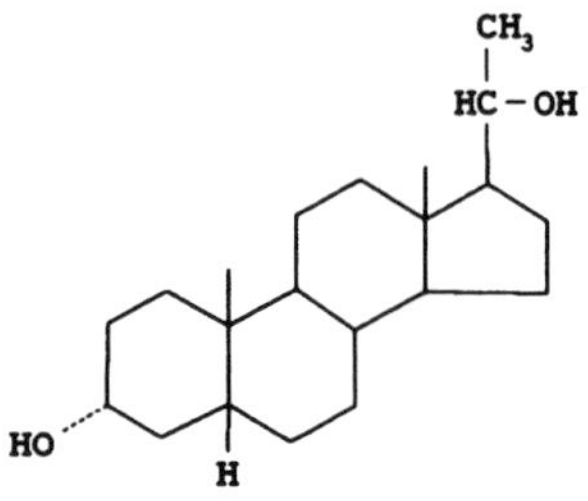

5β–pregnane–3α,20α–diol

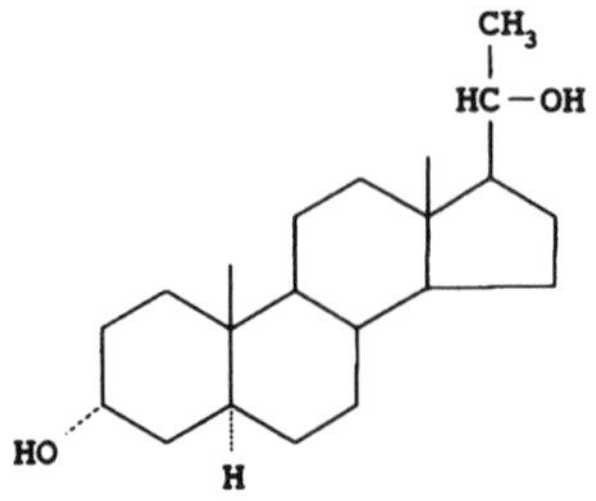

5α–pregnane–3α,20α–diol

584

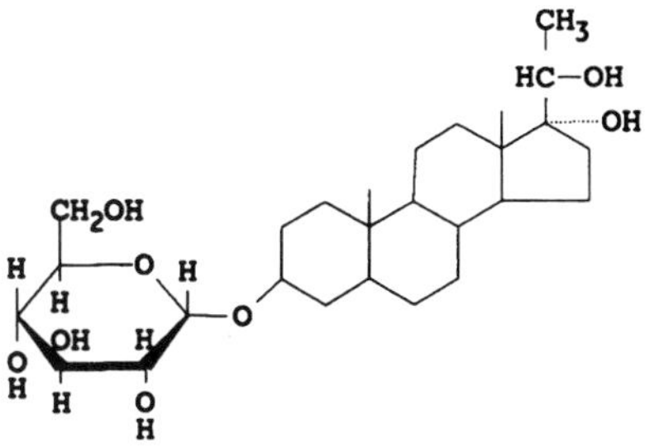

5β-pregna-3α,17α,20α-triol
glucuronide

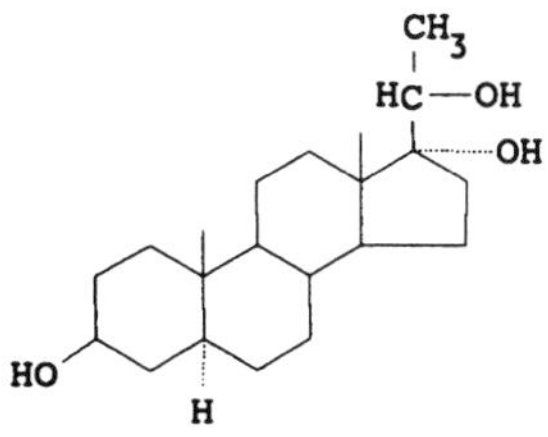

5α-pregna-3α,17α,20α-triol

pregnanetriols

gesterone, is excreted mostly as a glucuronide conjugate. Large amounts of 5α-pregnan-3α,17α,20α-triol, formed mostly from adrenocortical steroids, accumulate in individuals with 21-hydroxylase deficiency.

pregnant mares' serum gonadotropin: PMSG; a glycoprotein with FSH-like and LH-like properties obtained from the blood of pregnant mares. Its long half-life is attributed to its high carbohydrate content (40% by weight).

pregnenes: Δ^4 and Δ^5 unsaturated steroid structures used for steroid hormone nomenclature.

pregnenolone: 3β-hydroxypregn-5-ene-20-one; an intermediate in the pathway for biosynthesis of progesterone and related steroids from cholesterol; *see* **pregnenolone synthase**.

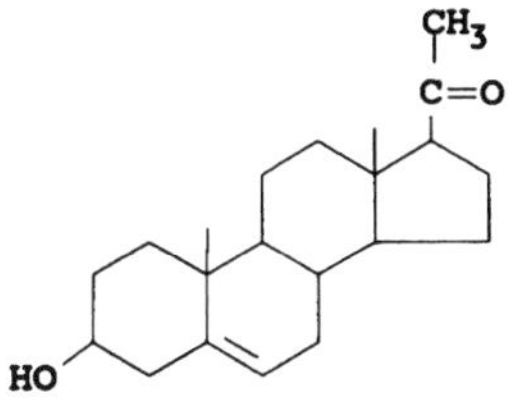

pregnenolone-sulfate: a steroid synthesized mostly from pregnenolone; but some derives from cholesterol-sulfate. It can be converted to pregnenolone, or serve as a precursor of sulfated steroid hormones. Small amounts are excreted to the urine.

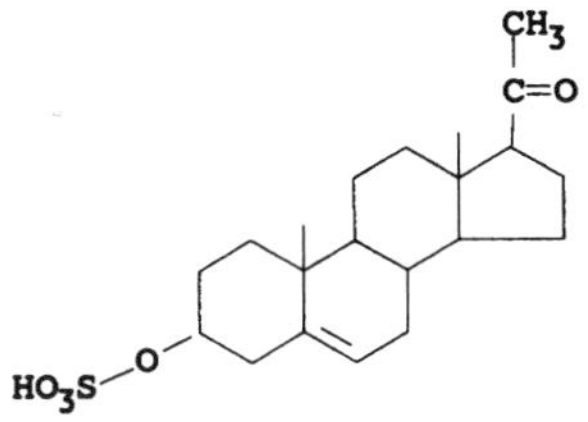

pregnenolone synthase: pregnenolone synthetase: desmolase; an enzyme system on inner mitochondrial membranes surfaces essential for the biosynthesis of glucocorticoids, mineralocorticoids, androgens, and estrogens. Its activity is augmented by luteinizing hormone (LH) in the gonads, hCG (human chorionic gonadotropin) in the placenta, and adrenocorticotropic hormone (ACTH) in the adrenal cortex. It is a mixed function oxidase that comprises a non-heme iron-sulfur protein (adrenodoxin in the adrenal cortex), an NADPH-dependent flavoprotein (adrenodoxin reductase in the adrenal cortex), and a substrate-specific heme protein (cytochrome P-450$_{scc}$). Cholesterol is oxidized at positions 20 and 22, and the product is cleaved to pregnenolone + isocaproylaldehyde (which is rapidly oxidized to isocaproic acid).

17α-hydroxy-**pregnenolone**: an intermediate in the pathway for biosynthesis of cortisol, progestins, androgens, and estrogens, and the direct precursor of 17α-hydroxy-progesterone and dehydroepiandrosterone (DHEA). It is made mostly from pregnenolone, but can also be formed from 17-α-hydroxycholesterol.

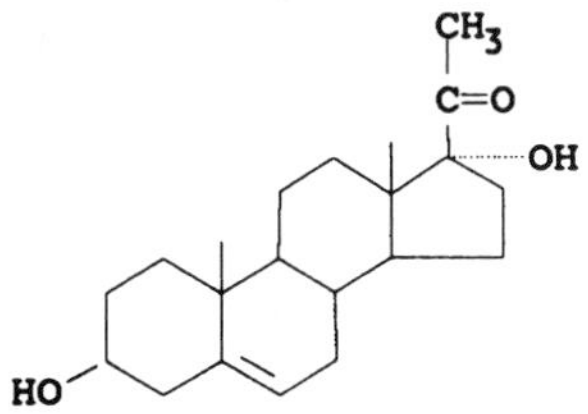

20α-hydroxy-**pregnenolone**: a minor pregnenolone metabolite.

Pregnyl: a commercial preparation of gonadotropins from the urine of pregnant women.

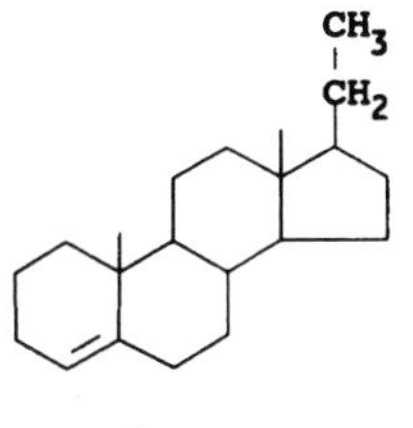

Δ^4-pregnene

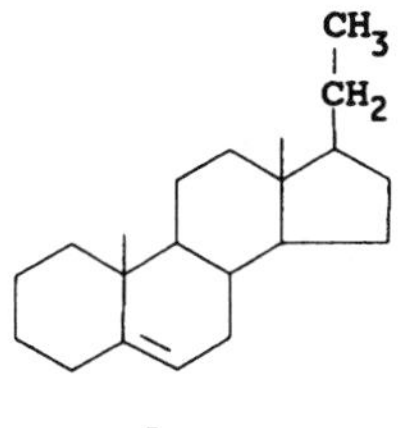

Δ^5-pregnene

585

20α-hydroxy-pregnenolone

pregranulosa cells: small, flattened epithelial cells that surround the oocytes of primordial follicles, and can maturate to granulosa cells.

prehormones: hormone precursor proteins with signal sequences. They cannnot be recovered directly from eukaryote cells, because the signal sequences are cleaved before translation is completed. However, they can be made in cell free systems that contain the messenger RNA and other essential factors, but lack the enzymes for cleaving the signal sequence. *Cf* **preprohormones** and **prohormones**.

prehypertensin: an obsolete term for renin substrate.

prekallikreins: proenzymes that are cleaved to yield kallikreins.

Premarin: a trade name for preparations derived from the urine of pregnant mares, composed of estrone sulfate (50-65%), sodium equilin sulfate (20-35%), and small amounts of equilenin sodium salts, 17α-estrone and 17-dihyroequilenin. Orally effective, injectable, and vaginal cream types are used to treat estrogen deficiency states and other conditions (such as postmenopausal osteoporosis) in which elevation of estrogen levels is deemed beneficial.

premenstrual syndrome: PMS: severe distress that recurs regularly in some women during the late luteal phases of their menstrual cycles. The symptoms, which vary from one individual to another, and within the same individual at different times, can include psychic depression, irritability, short attention span, water retention, edema, abdominal bloating, nausea, headache, and carbohydrate craving. The suggested causes include several forms of hormone imbalance (such as exaggerated declines in ovarian steroid output immediately preceding the onset). High progesterone levels have not been consistently demonstrated, but some women given progesterone after menopause have experienced the symptoms; and progesterone is known to be capable of invoking water retention and psychic depression. Salt restriction, exercise, vitamin supplements, gonadal steroids, gonadotropin releasing hormone (GnRH) analogs, cyclooxygenase inhibitors, and tranquilizers are among the treatments purported to afford relief. Although estrogen-progestin type contraceptives and some others appear to alleviate the symptoms in selected cases, they are no more effective than placebos in others.

premessenger RNAs: primary transcripts that undergo processing to yield mature mRNAs.

premonocyte: promonocyte.

premorbid: occurring before the onset of pathological signs or symptoms.

premyeloblast: promyeloblast.

premyelocyte: promyelocyte.

prenalterol: (-)(*S*)-1-(*p*-hydroxyphenoxy)-3-(isopropylamino-2-propanol; a β₁ type adrenergic receptor agonist used as a cardiac stimulant.

preneoplastic: usually describes cells or tissues with abnormal properties, and the potential for developing into neoplasms.

pre-Sertoli cells: embryronic gonad cells that respond to testis determining factor, differentiate to types that surround prespermatogonia, align to form spermatic cords, and inhibit progression of prespermatogonia to spermatogonia. After puberty onset, they mature to **Sertoli cells** (*q.v.*). Postpubertal types are initially highly responsive to the growth promoting effects of follicle stimulating hormone (FSH), but sensitivity soon declines.

prespermatogonia: germinal cells of the immature testis whose progression to spermatogonia is inhibited by pre-Sertoli cells. They resume maturation after puberty.

prenylamine: *N*-(1-methyl-2-phenylethyl)-γ-phenylbenzenepropanamine; a diphenylalkamine type Ca²⁺ ion channel blocker used to dilate coronary blood vessels. High doses also block Na⁺ ion channels.

preoptic area: POA; a region anterior or superior to the optic chiasma, anatomically part of the forebrain, but physiologically related to the hypothalamus. In laboratory mammals, it contains receptors for gonadal, adrenocortical, and other hormones, and contributes to the control of estrous cycles, reproductive behavior, sleep-wake cycles, and body temperature. Sexual dimorphism is invoked by gonadal steroids during critical stages of development. Fish preoptic nuclei synthesize neurohypophysial hormones.

preosteoblast: (1) an osteoprogenitor cell; (2) an incompletely differentiated osteoblast.

preovulatory follicles: Graafian follicles; mature ovarian follicles fully prepared for ovulation. They have large, fluid-filled antra, and their granulosa cells have luteinizing hormone (LH) receptors. The secondary oocyte is arrested in meiotic metaphase II, and is surrounded by a closely apposed cumulus oophorus.

prepriming: the first stages of DNA replication, during which a helicase unwinds the DNA at a replication fork, and proteins bind to the separated strands. An RNA primer then attaches, and the complex (*primosome*) initiates DNA synthesis at the 3′ end of the primer. The proteins then released travel along unwound DNA and facilitate initiation at other sites. The primer is later excised.

preproenkephalins: *see* **proenkephalin A**, **proenkephalin B**, and **preprohormones**.

preprohormones: hormone precursors with signal sequences. They cannot be recovered from eukaryote cells, because the signal sequences are cleaved before translation is completed (and only prohormones are released from the ribosomes). They can be made in cell free systems with the messenger RNAs and other essential factors, but no enzymes for signal sequence cleavage. Some prohormones have limited biological activities. An additional cleavage is required to yield the "true" hormones. Most protein and peptide hormones are made form precursors with pro- sequences; but a few are not (*see* **prehormones**).

preprotachykinin gene: a DNA sequence that directs formation of both protachykinin A and protachykinin B. Preprotachykinin A (A-PPT, α-PPT) predominates in the nervous system. Preprotachykinin B (B-PPT, beta-PPT) is made in thyroid glands and other peripheral organs.

prepuce: usually (1) the foreskin fold that covers the glans penis; (2) an analogous structure that surrounds the clitoris.

preputial glands: modified sebaceous glands that flank the penis (and also the clitoris in many species). In at least some mammals, they secrete pheromones. Androgens stimulate their growth, maturation, and secretory functions.

preribosmal RNAs: primary transcripts that are processed to yield mature rRNAs.

presby-: a prefix that relates to old age, as in presbyopia.

presbycusis: gradual diminution of hearing acuity, associated with aging and attributed to sensory cell degeneration.

presbyopia: gradual, age-associated loss of the ability to accommodate for close vision that involves weakening of the ciliary muscles, and changes in lens structure that impair ability to assume a spherical form.

pressophysins: neurophysins cleaved from the prohormones that yield vasopressins.

pressor: tending to elevate blood pressure, usually by contracting arteriolar smooth muscle.

pressoreceptors: baroreceptors; cells specialized to respond to changes in pressure. Most are in blood vessels, but others are present in the lungs and elsewhere. Some

transmit message components of neuronal reflexes. Others directly promote release of norepinephrine, vasopressin, renin, and other factors that contribute to blood pressure control.

presumptive: describes an embryonic structure expected to develop along a specific pathway.

presynaptic: describes (1) neurons with axons that release neurotransmitters to synapses in brain, spinal cord, autonomic ganglia or neuromuscular junctions; (2) events initated by those neurons.

presynaptic receptors: receptors on presynaptic neuron dendrites or perikarya. Some respond to the regulators released by their terminals. For example, when norepinephrine is released in large amounts from sympathetic neurons, and when levels of circulating catecholamines are high, activation of α$_2$-type presynaptic adrenergic receptors inhibits the release of additional neurotransmitter. This protects against overstimulation.

prethymocytes: prethymic cells: subsets of immature lymphocytes released from bone marrow that migrate to thymus glands. Some develop into T lymphocytes; but large numbers die within the gland.

previtamin: a vitamin precursor, such as carotene or provitamin D.

previtamin D$_3$: a secosteroid formed when ultraviolet light acts on provitamin D$_3$. It spontaneously transforms to vitamin D$_3$ (*see* **cholecalciferol**). *Cf* **provitamin D**.

PRF: prolactin releasing factor; a term that describes the biological activity in hypothalamic extracts that accounts for increased secretion of prolactin, for example during lactation. Vasoactive intestinal peptide (VIP) and some other hypothalamic factors possesses such activity. Thyrotropin releasing hormone can also promote PRL release, but this effect may not be physiologically important.

priapism: persistent, often painful, erection, unrelated to sexual stimulation, and usually caused by venospasm.

Pribnow box: a noncoding promoter component of a prokaryote gene, located approximately 10 base-pairs upstream from the RNA synthesis initiation site. It binds RNA polymerase and is essential for transcription initiation. The most common base sequence is TATAAT (*cf* **TATA box**).

prickle cells: large, flattened keratinocytes of the epidermis stratum spinosum that project fine spines when treated with fixatives (which act on the desmosomes). They are the major sources of parathyroid hormone-like polypeptide.

primaquine: N^4-(6-methoxy-8-quinolinyl)-1,4,-pentadiene; an agent that kills malaria parasites, at least in part by acting on mitochondria. It invokes methemoglobinemia and hemolysis in individuals with glucose-6-phosphate dehydrogenase deficient erythrocytes.

primary cultures: cultures started with cells, tissues or organs taken directly from animals or plants. Most con-

pre-vitamin D₃   vitamin D₃

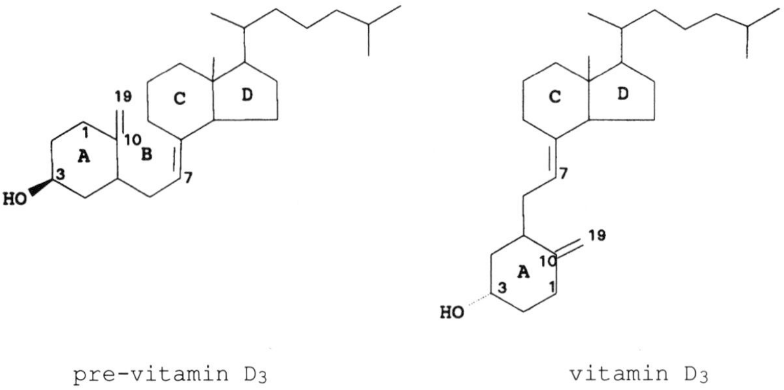

previtamin D₃

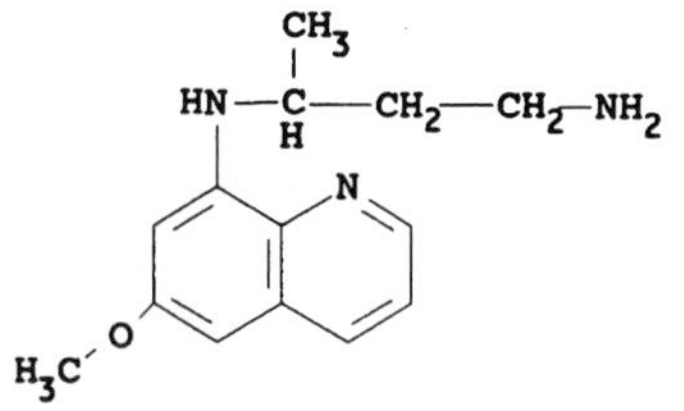

primaquine

tain more than one kind of cell. In some cases, specific types are selected for secondary cultures.

primary follicle: a primary oocyte surrounded by one or more concentric layers of granulosa cells, with receptors for follicle stimulating hormone (FSH) and estrogen. In humans, some develop from primordial follicles during the third trimester of fetal life, whereas others can do so as late as the fourth, fifth, or even sixth decade after birth. Large numbers of primary follicles undergo atresia; but some advance to secondary and tertiary stages, and serve as estrogen-secreting cohorts. A few complete maturation to to the preovulatory stage. The major events are similar in other mammals, but the timing varies widely with the species.

primary germ layers: three sets of cells formed in young embryos that give rise to fetal and more mature structures. *See* **ectoderm**, **mesoderm**, and **endoderm**.

primary immune responses: transient immune system reactions that follow the first exposures to foreign antigens. Lymphocyte subsets with receptors for those antigens are activated, and memory cells form. *See* also **cellular** and **humoral immunity**, and *cf* **secondary immune responses**.

primary oocytes: diploid cells that differentiate from oogonia during fetal life in most species. Some are extruded from ovarian surfaces soon after formation. Others enter the prophase of meiosis I and are incorporated into primordial follicles. A few grow and and complete meiosis I in more advanced follicles. Each then yields one secondary oocyte and one first polar body.

primary protein structure: *see* **proteins**.

primary reproductive organs: structures that produce gametes. In animals, testes and ovaries; *cf* **accessory reproductive organs** and **secondary sex characteristics**.

primary sex ratio: the ratio of males to females at the time of conception. In most species, including humans, more males than females are conceived, but more male than female embryos and fetuses die.

primary spermatocytes: diploid cells that differentiate from spermatogonia. They undergo several maturational stages before entering meiosis and giving rise to secondary spermatocytes.

primary transcripts: premessenger, preribosomal, and other RNA molecules formed during transcription. Most are processed to yield mature, functional messenger, ribosomal, or transfer RNAs. Many premessenger types contain two or more exons, and some undergo cell type specific splicing to yield two or more products, each of which directs formation of its own kinds of proteins.

primases: RNA polymerases that catalyze formation of short RNAs complementary to DNA segments; *see* **prepriming** and **primers**.

primates: members of the order Primates, which includes humans as well as monkeys, apes, lemurs, marmosets, and related animal types. Features that characterize subgroups include cerebral cortex development, limb structure, digital mobility, stereoscopic vision, and dentition.

primers: entities that must be present to accomplish macromolecule biosynthesis or other complex processes, such as glycogenin for glycogen synthesis and primososomes for DNA synthesis.

primer pheromones: *see* **pheromones**.

primidone: 2-dexoyphenobarbital; an agent metabolically converted to phenobarbital. It is used to treat some forms of epilepsy.

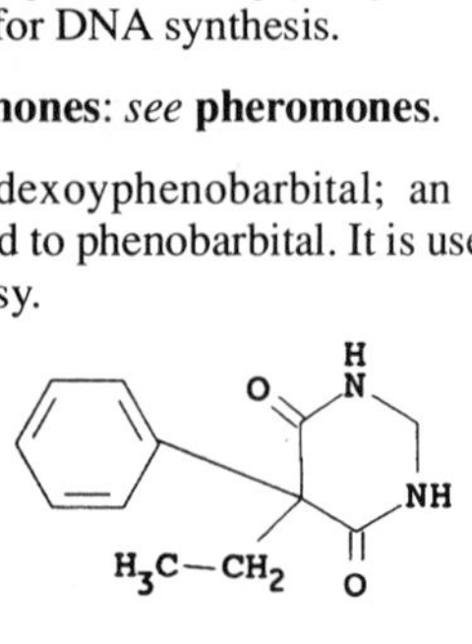

primigravid: describes a woman undergoing a first pregnancy.

priming: establishing conditions that facilitate or are essential for achieving other processes. Estrogens "prime" some cells for subsequent responses to estrogens and/or progesterone, in part by inducing new hormone receptors. Exposure to specific antigens primes immune systems for more rapid and more vigorous responses if the same antigens are presented at a later time. *See* also **primer**, and **pheromones**.

primipara: a women who has completed one pregnancy, during which one or more fetuses matured to a state consistent with survival outside the uterus.

primitive: describes (1) an early stage in the evolutionary history of a class of organisms; (2) an early stage in the development of a structure that undergoes further maturation; (3) a simple structure functionally related to a more complex one in other species.

Primobolan: a trade name for methenolone.

primordial follicle: a single layer of flat pregranulosa cells that surrounds an immature primary oocyte. Primordial follicles begin to form during the third trimester of fetal life in humans. Many degenerate, but substantial numbers mature to primary follicles.

primordium: a cluster of progenitor cells, usually in an embryo, that can give rise to a specific kind of mature structure.

primosomes: *see* **prepriming**.

primulin: direct yellow 59; a dye neurons take up via retrograde transport. It is used to study axon branching.

prions: infectious proteins that can be transmitted to other individuals (including types that cause scrapie and Creutzfeldt-Jakob disease). They do not contain DNA or RNA, but can invoke changes in host cell proteins that affect nucleic acid synthesis.

pristane: 2,6,10,14-tetramethylpentadecane; an agent used to stimulate hybridoma growth, and as a biological marker.

privileged site: a region such as the anterior chamber of the eye in which allografts are protected against immune rejection. Some have poor lymphatic drainage, which limits antigen release.

pro-: a prefix meaning precursor, as in prohormone or proparathyroid hormone.

Pro: P; *see* **proline**.

proaccelerin: accelerator globulin; blood coagulation factor V; a cofactor for prothrombin conversion to thrombin.

proacrosin: a proenzyme in the head region of a spermatozoan. It is converted to acrosin during the acrosome reaction that precedes fertilization.

probability: *see* **P value**.

proband: propositus; the first family member known to display a specific inherited trait. Information on inheritance patterns for specific diseases can be obtained by constructing genetic trees that show the incidences of the traits in parents, grandparents, siblings, and other family members of afflicted individuals.

probes: agents that bind tightly to, and can therefore be used to identify or isolate genes, proteins, or other specific kinds of molecules. They are usually labeled with radioactive isotopes, fluorescent substances, or other markers.

probenecid: Benemid; *p*-(dipropylsufamyl)benzoic acid; an agent that accelerates uric acid excretion by inhibiting the carrier-mediated organic acid transport system in renal tubules, used to treat gout. By inhibiting tubular secretion, it slows loss of penicillins and some other therapeutic agents to the urine, and can serve as an adjunct for maintaining high blood levels. It also slows the transport of serotonin sulfates and some other acidic molecules in nervous tissue.

Probolin: a trade name for methandriol dipropionate.

probucol: Lorelco; 4,4'-(isopropylidenedithio)-*bis*[2,6-di-*tert*-butylphenol]; an agent used for its anti-atherogenic effects, and to reduce xanthomas in individuals with severe hypercholesterolemia. It somewhat lowers low density lipoprotein (LDL) and total cholesterol levels, but also reduces the numbers of high density lipoproteins (HDLs). The beneficial effects are attributed to mostly to decreased formation of toxic LDL oxidation products. Undesirable ones can include nausea, abdominal pain, and diarrhea. In monkeys fed high fat, high cholesterol diets, it invokes cardiac dysrhythmias.

procainamide hydrochloride: Pronestyl hydrochloride; 4-amino-*N*-[2-(diethylamino)ethyl]-benzamide hydrochloride; an orally effective cardiac depressant that slows Na$^+$ uptake and conduction through Purkinje fibers, exerts weak effects on autonomic ganglia, blocks transmission of impulses along sensory nerves, and is degraded

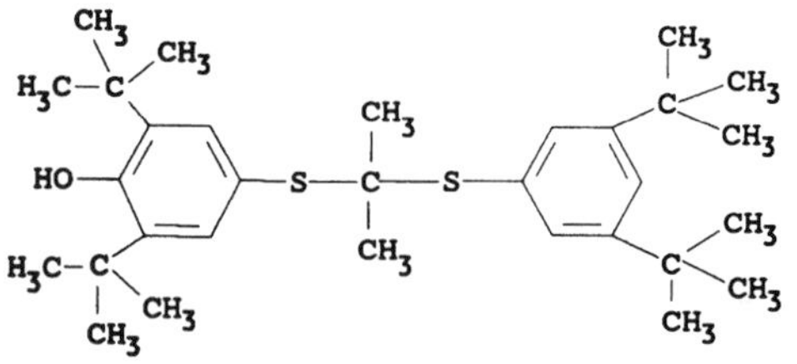

probucol

by acetylcholinesterases. It is used to treat some cardiac dysrhythmias, and for subarachnoid anesthesia.

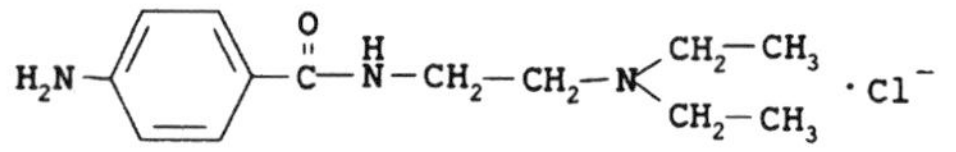

procaine: 4-aminobenzoic acid 2(diethylamino)ethyl ester: an agent that blocks nerve conduction, mostly be decreasing Na^+ uptake. Novocaine (procaine hydrochloride), and some other salts are used as local anesthetics.

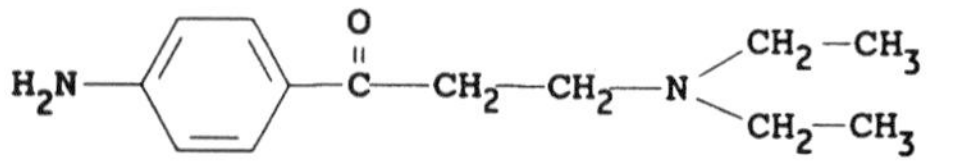

procalcitonin: *see* **calcitonin genes**.

procallus: granulation tissue that develops in the region of a healing bone fracture, and is soon replaced by a true callus.

procarcinogens: agents that become carcinogenic after metabolic conversion to active products.

Procardia: a trade name for nifedipine.

procaryote: prokaryote.

proceptivity: estrogen-dependent behavior manifested towards the end of the proestrus phase of an ovarian cycle by a nonprimate female mammal. In addition to displays of interest in, and extension of sexual invitations to males, it can include increased motor activity, ear-wiggling, and other forms of behavior characteristic of the species. *Cf* **receptivity**.

prochirality: describes molecules with asymmetries recognized by enzymes, but with structures that appear symmetric when represented on paper. Examples include citric acid and NADH; *see* also **stereoisomerism**.

prochlorperazine: Compazine; 2-chloro-10-[3-(-1-methyl-4-piperazinyl)propyl]phenothiazine; a phenothiazine type "antipsychotic" agent, used to control vomiting in paitents receiving radiation or chemotherapy.

procoagulant: (1) a blood coagulation factor precursor; (2) a substance that promotes coagulation. Prothrombin fits both definitions.

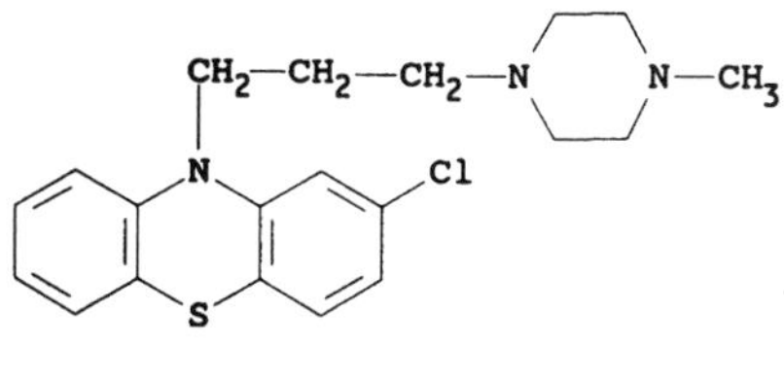

prochlorperazine

procodazole: 1*H*-benzimidazole-2-propanoic acid; a nonspecific immune system stimulant used to augment resistance to bacterial and viral infections.

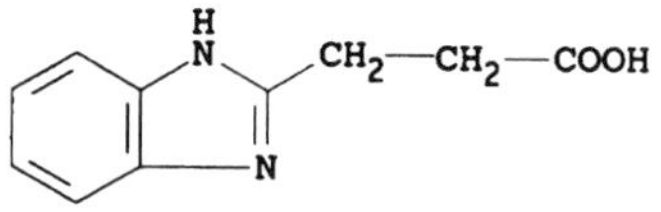

procollagens: collagen precursors made and secreted by osteoblasts, chondroblasts, fibroblasts, and some other cell types. Conversion to collagens involves selective proteolytic cleavage and removal of some covalently linked moieties that protect against intracellular polymerization.

proconvertases: proteases that cleave precursor proteins to more mature types; *see* also **prohormone converting enzymes**.

proconvertin: blood coagulation factor V; *see* **coagulation**.

proconceptives: agents or processes that facilitate, or increase the probability of conception.

proctodone: a hormone secreted by anterior intestinal cells of some insects that terminates diapause.

proctolin: Arg-tyr-Leu-Pro-Thr: a neurotransmitter made by some insects. It is used as a substrate for measuring vitamin K dependent carboxylase activity.

prodrome: an early symptom that precedes the onset of a disorder, or suggests that one is likely to follow.

prodynorphin: proenkephalin B; a widely distributed precursor of leu-enkephalin, dynorphin A, dynorphin B (rimorphin, prodynorphin 228-240, dynorphin 1-13), dynorphin 1-8, peptide E, α-neoendorphin, β-neoendorphin, and some other opioid peptides that is not biologically active prior to cell type specific processing (which involves cleavages at various sites catalyzed by enkephalin converting enzymes). Its synthesis is directed by a single gene.

proecdysis: the stage of an arthropod molting cycle during which minerals and organic substances are resorbed from the exoskeleton which will be shed, and deposited into the newly forming shell.

proelastins: linear proteins that undergo cross-linkage reactions to yield elastins.

proenkephalin: a term used for both proenkephalin A proenkephalin B.

proenkephalin A: a widely distributed opioid peptide precursor encoded by a gene different from the one that directs prodynorphin synthesis. It undergoes cell type specific processing to yield metenkephalin, leu-enkephalin, peptide F, and peptide I, and some other opioid peptides.

proenkephalin B: prodynorphin.

proenzymes: zymogens; peptides or proteins that undergo selective proteolytic cleavage to yield active enzymes. Since they possess little or no activity, they do not digest the cells that make them. Examples include pepsinogen, trypsinogen, and prekallikreins.

proestrus: the phase of the estrous cycle that precedes estrus, during which estrogen levels rise, and proceptivity can be manifested. It is followed by estrus.

profilactin: a profilin-actin complex that interacts with inositol phosphates; *see* **profilin**.

profilagrin: a protein made by keratinocytes, stored in keratohyaline granules, and converted to profilin.

profilins: 12-15K microfilament proteins of nonmuscle cells, including at least two subtypes (profilins I and II) with somewhat different properties. They are believed to play major roles in signal transduction, and in the coupling of surface receptor activation to changes in the cytoskeleton. In unstimulated cells, profilin II binds membrane-bound clusters of phosphatidylinositol-phosphate (PIP$_2$) molecules, and in this way blocks their hydrolysis by unphosphorylated phospholipase Cγ1. When receptors for epidermal and platelet derived growth factors (EGF and PDGF), and some other growth promoting hormones dimerize and undergo autophosphorylation, they attach to and catalyze phosphorylation of the phospholipase. The phosphorylated enzyme then promotes dissociation of profilin-PIP$_2$ complexes, catalyzes PIP$_2$ hydrolysis, and releases profilin for interaction with actin. EGF, PDGF and some other growth promoting hormones also activate Na$^+$/H$^+$ exchange mechanisms, and the resulting cytoplasmic alkalinization further facilitates profilin-PIP$_2$ dissociation. Prolfilins bind actin monomers directly in 1:1 ratios. It was initially believed they block monomer polymerization; but the amounts present are small compared with those of actins; also, the binding affinity is low, and neither Ca^{2+} nor phosphorylation dependent. Moreover, since profilins bind to the ends of rapidly elongating filaments and promote exchange of monomer-bound ADP for ATP, and since ATP-actins polymerize faster and form stiffer filaments, profilins may, in fact accelerate filament elongation. In yeast cells, the *N*-terminal of an adenylate cyclase associated protein (CAP) is required for normal responsiveness to activated RAS protein, and the *C*-terminal contributes to the control of cell morphology. It can bind both profilins and actins; and exogenous profilins normalize functions of mutants that are CAP-deficient. Profilins are also made by many other organisms, including plants; and roles in plant fertilization have been proposed. Some plant types invoke allergic reactions in susceptible individuals who make IgE type antibodies directed against them.

proflavine: 3,6-diaminoacridine; an acridine dye used as a topical anesthetic. It attaches to DNAs, and is a laboratory tool for invoking frame-shift mutagenesis.

progabide: 4[[(4-chlorophenyl)(5-fluoro-2-hydroxyphenyl)methylene]amino]butanamide; a gamma aminobutyric acid (GABA) receptor antagonist, used to alleviate spasticity, and under investigation for the treatment of forms of epilepsy resistant to more commonly used agents.

progenitor: a parent or ancestor of an individual, gene, molecular species, organelle, or other entity that has undergone evolutionary changes.

progeny: (1) offspring; descendants of a mating pair, or daughter cells formed when a parent cell divides.

progeria: premature aging.

progestagen: progestogen; progestin; a compound (usually a steroid) that exerts progesterone-like actions. Since progesterone and other naturally occurring types are rapidly degraded by hepatic enzymes, analogs that resist degradation and are orally effective are used to treat deficiency conditions, and as components of contraceptive preparations.

progestational: prepared for implantation; describes the condition of the luteal phase endometrium that has been conditioned by estrogens and progesterone.

progesterone: P$_4$; pregn-4-ene-3,20-dione; a steroid hormone made from pregnenolone via a reaction catalyzed by 3β-hydroxysteroid dehydrogenase/4,5-isomerase. Small amounts discharged from preovulatory ovarian follicles facilitate the rapid, massive release of luteinizing hormone (LH surge) required for ovulation. Much larger ones are secreted by corpora lutea and placentas. P$_4$ contributes to endometrial preparation for implantation by promoting specialization of estrogen-primed cells, and is essential for maintaining pregnancy. In rabbits, sheep, and some other mammals, it depresses myometrial muscle excitability, blocks the mounting of organized contractions, and protects against premature parturition. (In many other species, relaxin is more important; but progesterone exerts some indirect effects by inhibiting the synthesis of prostaglandin PGF$_{2\alpha}$). P$_4$ also contributes to the maturation of mammary gland alveoli; but high levels inhibit lactose synthesis during pregnancy. Other targets include vaginal and Fallopian tube cells, and neurons involved in reproductive, maternal, locomotor and feeding behaviors, and body temperature. In humans, P_4 affects mood; and very high levels are central nervous system depressants. P_4 additionally affects carbohydrate and lipid metabolism, contributes to the control of receptor numbers for some steroid hormones, and exerts some anabolic influences on bone. Although most effects are initiated by interactions with intracellular progesterone receptors (many of which are induced by estrogen), some (for example on amphibian oocyte maturation) involve different mechanisms. In birds, P_4 contributes to oviduct maturation and functions, production of ovalbumin, and hepatic synthesis of vitellogenin. Progesterone is converted to deoxycorticosterone and other steroids in the adrenal cortex, to androgens in the gonads (see Δ^4 **pathway**), and to some other steroids in feto-placental units. It is a weak agonist for mineralocorticoid receptors that can, in high concentrations, compete with aldosterone for receptor binding.

5α-dihydro-progesterone: a progesterone metabolite formed in several target cells via a reaction catalyzed by 5α-reductase. Some progesterone effects are attributed to competition with androgens for the same enzyme; but the product can also augment the reductase activity. A role in decreasing vascular smooth muscle sensitivity to angiotensin II during pregnancy has been suggested.

3α-hydroxy-progesterone: a progesterone metabolite made in Sertoli cells that inhibits both basal and gonadotropin releasing hormone (GnRH)-stimulated secretion of follicle stimulating hormone (FSH), and may play roles in the timing of puberty onset.

16α-hydroxy-progesterone: a steroid hormone made in substantial amounts by fetuses, and in small ones by Sertoli cells. No special functions are known.

17α-hydroxy-progesterone: a steroid hormone made from 17α-hydroxy-pregnenolone and progesterone that exerts several progesterone-like actions. It is secreted in limited amounts by steroidogenic tissues, and is a major precursor of cortisol, dehydroepiandrosterone, testosterone, estradiol and other steroids in many species.

progesterone-associated endometrial protein: PEP; one of several proteins secreted by the endometrium during pregnancy (when maternal progesterone levels are high). The amounts formed have been used an indicators of endometrial function.

progesterone receptors: some progesterone effects (for example the ones on amphibian oocytes, and others on neurons) are mediated via as yet uncharacterized plasma membrane receptors. However, most are initiated by high-affinity binding to intracellular phosphoproteins that closely resemble the receptors for other steroid hormones (and for secosteroids, retinoids, and triiodothyronine, T_3). Ligand binding promotes release of hsp90 and other proteins, and invokes changes that facilitate hormone-receptor complex attachment to progesterone response element components of specific genes; see also **steroid hormone receptors** and **mifepristone**. In endometrium, vagina, mammary gland, and some other target tissues, estrogens induce progesterone receptors.

progestins: progestogens; see **progestagens**.

proglucagon: the prohormone for **glucagon** (q.v.) and some related peptides; see also **glicentin**.

proglumide: 4-(benzoylamino)-5-(dipropylamino)-5-oxopentanoic acid; a gastrin and cholecystokinin (CCK) receptor antagonist used to treat peptic ulcers.

progoitrin: a component of cabbage, kale, and some other vegetables that is converted *in vivo* to **goitrin** (*q.v.*).

programmed cell death: *see* **apoptosis**.

progression factors: regulators that promote completion of mitosis or meiosis after cells have entered the S phases of their cycles. Insulin and epidermal growth factor (EGF) are examples for some cell types. *See* also **MPF**; and *cf* **competence factors**.

Progynon: a trade name for some estradiol preparations. Progynon-B is estradiol benzoate.

prohormone[s]: compounds that can be metabolically processed to one or more hormones. The term is most commonly applied to proteins and polypeptides, such as proparathyroid (pro-PTH) and proinsulins, from which amino acids sequences must be cleaved to yield the products. Since cells lack mechanisms for direct cytoplasmic synthesis of small proteins and polypeptides, and there are minimum sizes for proteins made on ribosomes, synthesis in this way appears to be essential. However, prohormones serve other purposes. Some undergo cell-type specific processing to liberate two or more active products (*see*, for example **proopiomelanocortin**). Prohormones are usually resistant to rapid intracellular degradation, in part because their extra amino acid groups mask enzyme combining sites. Some have hydrophobic surfaces that facilitate transport. Many have little or no intrinsic activity, and therefore do not act on the cells that make them. For some, the pro sequences are needed to maintain three-dimensional conformations essential for correct positioning of internal S-S and other covalent bonds. Additionally, since protein synthesis takes time, but prohormone cleavage is rapidly accomplished, they can serve as readily recruitable storage forms for the active regulators. The term can also be used for compounds such as pregnenolone and 25-hydroxy-cholecalciferol (precursors of steroid hormones and 1,25 dihydroxycholecalciferol), testosterone (convertible to estrogens and 5α-dihydrotestosterone), and dopamine (convertible to norepinephrine and epinephrine).

prohormone convertases: PCs; enzymes that cleave protein and peptide prohormones at specific sites to yield active hormones. At least some are closely related to yeast kex-2 proteins and bacterial subtilisins. **Furins** (*q.v.*) are Golgi components of most cell types that contribute to the processing many kinds of proteins, including receptors for insulin, and nerve growth factor and some prohormones. They act mostly on Lys/Arg bonds of Arg-X-(Lys/Arg)-Arg sequences. More specific enzymes expressed only in neural and endocrine cells act mostly on Arg-Arg, Arg-Lys or Lys-Lys bonds. The group includes PC1 (also called PC3), and PC2. However, they additionally perform other functions, for example during embryonic development. A closely related PC4 enzyme, expressed only in spermatocytes and spermatids, is believed to play roles in gamete maturation.

proinsulins: approximately 9K species-specific single chain peptides with three S-S bonds that serve as precursors (prohormones) for insulins. They display very weak insulin-like activity, are stored in secretory granules, and can be released by exocytosis. Each molecule also yields a C peptide, and two dipeptides. *See* **insulin** for structure. The striped and clear circles represent, respectively, the amino acid moieties of insulin A and B chains, and the black ones the moieties of the C peptide.

prokaryotes: procaryotes; bacteria and other organisms that lack nuclear membranes and some other organelles characteristic of eukaryotes. The DNA is contained within a single chromosome. The ribosomes resemble the kinds in eukaryote mitochondria.

prolactin: PRL; lactogenic hormone; mammotropin; species-specific, multifunctional hormones, best known for their ability to stimulate mammary gland growth and maturation, and the synthesis of casein, lactalbumin, lactose, fatty acids, and other milk components. The major type in mammals is a 23K protein secreted by lactotropes and mammosomatotropes that tends to form dimers and oligomers. Variants include a 25K glycosylated form, and biologically active 16K and 18K cleavage products. A specific transcription factor that promotes PRL synthesis has been identified in the glands (*see* also **Pit-1**). Estrogens are major stimulants for lactotrope proliferation and PRL synthesis. Adenohypophysial secretion occurs in two phases. The first converts PRL from a storage to a releasable form, and the second accomplishes extrusion from the cells. *See* also **prolactin inhibitory factors**, **prolactin releasing factors**, **suckling reflex**, and **hyperprolactinemia**. Within the gland, PRLs exert paracrine inhibition of gonadotropin release. PRLs are also present in ovaries, seminal fluid, and amniotic fluid; and related proteins are made in placentas, the central nervous system, and at some other sites. They are members of a superfamily that includes growth hormones and placental lactogens. In some species, they interact with growth hormone receptors and exert GH-like effects; but in humans the potency is very low. In a few they can oppose certain GH actions. The functions, which vary with the species, include regulation of receptor numbers for many hormones, influences on steroid hormone synthesis and metabolism in the adrenal glands and gonads, modulation of carbohydrate and lipid metabolism, corpora lutea maintenance, roles in maternal and reproductive behavior, stimulation of fetal growth, and direct influences on the proliferation and functions of some immune system cells. (PRL is present in T lymphocyte nuclei, and appears to be essential for the effects of interleukin-1.) In birds, PRL stimulates crop sac growth, maturation and secretory activity. In mature amphibians, it acts on the skin to invoke water drive; and in larval forms it counteracts the metamorphosis-promoting effects of thyroid hormones. In euryhaline fish, PRL-like regulators contribute to adaptations for fresh water by inhibiting Na^+/K^+-ATPases (thereby accelerating uptake of both Na^+ and Ca^{2+}), and via influences on mucus production and Cl^- excretion. Related effects are exerted on water transport across the placentas of mammalian fetuses; and roles in electrolyte and water metabolism of mature mammals have been described. Only some of the mechanisms are known. In at least some cell types, phospholipase C isozymes are activated; but the receptors do not display tyrosine kinase activity. Fetal growth is partially mediated via induction of insulin-like growth factors, *c-fos* and *c-mos* gene products, and of ornithine decarboxylase and other enzymes.

prolactin inhibitory factor: PIF; a term initially applied to an uncharacterized component of hypothalamic extracts that inhibits prolactin (PRL) secretion. Unlike other adenohypophysial cell types, which depend on stimulatory hypothalamic regulators, PRL is tonically inhibited under most physiological conditions. Several observations led to the concept that dopamine is *the* PIF. The amine made in tuberoinfundibular neurons enters hypothalamohypophysial portal blood vessels, and is present in the extracts. Moreover, D_2 type receptors are abundant on lactotropes, DA antagonists increase PRL secretion, DA agonists inhibit, and the effects of some stimulatory hormones (*see* **prolactin release factors**) involve dissociation of DA from its receptors. Some DA actions are mediated via G proteins that inhibit adenylate cyclases, whereas others have been linked with inhibitory influences on phosphatidylinositol hydrolysis and Ca^{2+} channels. However, DA affects just one of the secretory phases (*see* **prolactin**), and vasoactive intestinal peptide (VIP) can stimulate in its presence. One inhibitory component of dopamine-free hypothalamic extracts appears to be gonadotropin releasing hormone associated peptide (GAP), which is cleaved from a precursor that yields LH. Gamma aminobutyric acid (GABA) can also inhibit.

prolactin releasing factors: PRF; regulators that promote prolactin (PRL) secretion. Although PRL release is tonically inhibited under most physiological conditions (*see* **prolactin inhibitory factor**), it is rapidly discharged in response to suckling and some other stimuli, including some forms of stress. Vasoactive intestinal peptide (VIP), which acts via a G protein to augment adenylate cyclase activity, appears to be a major PRF associated with lactation. The effects take some time to develop, and can occur in the presence of dopamine. Thyrotropin releasing hormone (TRH) is a potent stimulant that acts rapidly. Its effects are attributed mostly to influences on dopamine dissociation from its receptors. Although additive with VIP, it is probably not a major contributor to suckling induced PRL release. Thyroid stimulating hormone (TSH) levels do not rise in parallel with PRL at such times, and TRH antisera do not block the effects of VIP. Other PRL secretion stimulants include oxytocin, angiotensin II, and bombesin-like peptides. Estrogens can lower dopamine levels and accelerate PRL release. They also increase the numbers of PRL-secreting lactotropes.

proliferating cell nuclear antigen: PCNA; a cofactor for DNA polymerase III (DNA polymerase δ) that acts in part by down-regulating p53. It associates with cyclins D1, D2, and D3 during G1 phases of cell cycles.

proliferin: PLF; an approximately 24K glycoprotein that shares amino acid sequences with the prohormone for prolactin, initially identified in mouse placenta and called mitogen-related protein. It is secreted by trophoblast cells, present in amniotic fluid and maternal blood, and implicated as a growth factor for maternal and/or fetal tissues. PLF is also made by stimulated fibroblast cells in culture. Basic fibroblast and platelet derived growth factors (FGF and PDGF) promote its synthesis. Transforming growth factor-β (TGF-β) antagonizes its actions.

proliferin related protein: a secreted placental hormone that shares amino acid sequences with proliferin.

proline: Pro; P; 2-pyrrolidinecarboxylic acid; an imino acid, often referred to as an amino acid. It is classified as nonessential, since animals synthesize it. Glutamate reacts with ATP + NADPH to form glutamic-γ-semialdehyde, which is dehydrated to Δ'-pyrroline-5-carboxylate. NADPH mediated reduction then yields proline. A reverse pathway converts proline to α-ketoglutarate, which enters the Krebs cycle or provides oxaloacetate for gluconeogenesis. Proline is a major constituent of collagens (*see* also **hydroxyproline**), and a component of protamines and some other proteins, in which it is an important determinant of the three-dimensional configuration.

Proluton: a trade name for some progestins, including the 17α-hydroxyprogesterone caproate incorporated into long-acting depot preparations. Proluton C is ethisterone.

prolyl hydroxylase: a dioxygenase that converts collagen prolyl moieties to 3- and 4-hydroxyprolyls, and is essential for the biosynthesis of normal collagens. It requires ascorbic acid as a co-factor. Many of manifestations of of scurvy are caused by impaired function of the enzyme.

promazine: *N-N*-dimethyl-10*H*-phenothiazine-10-propanamine; a tricyclic antidepressant, used as a tranquilizer and "antipsychotic" agent.

glutamate-γ-semialdehyde   Δ'-pyrroline-5-carboxylate   proline

promazine

promecarb: 3-methyl-5-(1-methylethyl)phenol methylcarbamic acid; a cholinesterase inhibitor used as an insecticide.

promegestone: RU 5020; 17α-methyl-17-propionylestra-4,9-dien-3-one; a potent progestagen devoid of androgenic potency.

promethazine: *N,N,*α-trimethyl-10*H*-phenothiazine-10-ethananamine; a potent H₁ type histamine receptor antagonist and central nervous system depressant, used as an antiemetic.

promoter: usually (1) a gene segment that includes a TATA or Pribnow box plus a second conserved base sequence approximately 35 base pairs upstream from the start site, both of which contribute to transcription initiation by binding RNA polymerase and transcription factors; (2) an agent that augments responses to carcinogens; (3) a catalyst or inducer.

promyelocytes: premyelocytes; partially committed, immature bone marrow cells that can differentiate to granulocytic leukocytes.

pronase: a mixture of trypsin-like and chymotrypsin-like proteases derived from *Streptomyces griseus* that digests most proteins to amino acids over a broad pH range, but does not act on glutamate:glutamate or glutarate:aspartate bonds, and does not disrupt the structures of amino acids and other small molecules. It is used to remove proteins from double stranded DNAs, liquefy mucins, isolate living chondrocytes, and improve the staining properties of starches.

pronephron: one of the functional units of a pronephros.

pronephros: the first kidney-like organ made by vertebrate embryos. It functions in fishes, but is rudimentary and soon replaced by a mesonephros in higher vertebrates. In birds and mammals, the mesonephros is replaced by a metanephros.

Pronestyl: a trade name for procainamide hydrochloride.

pronethalol: 2-isopropylamino-(1-(2-naphthyl)ethanol; a β-type adrenergic receptor antagonist, used to treat angina, cardiac dysrhythmias, and hypertension.

pronucleus: a haploid nucleus formed when meiosis II is completed.

proofreading: in molecular biology, mechanisms used to recognize and repair nucleic acid defects.

proopiomelanocortin: POMC; a prohormone most abundant in the adenohypophysis, but also synthesized in the hypothalamus, reproductive tract, placenta, male and female gonads, and elsewhere. The major cleavage products in corticolipotropes are adrenocorticotropic hormone (ACTH), β-lipotropin and d β-endorphin; but some γ-MSH may also be released. Pars intermedia cells cleave most of the ACTH component to corticotropin-like intermediate peptide (CLIP) and α-melanocyte stimulating hormone (α-MSH), and much of the latter is amidated. They also make β-endorphin. In other cell types, the β-endorphin component is processed to smaller peptides. POMC contains the amino acid sequences for met-enkephalin, but that peptide is derived *in vivo* from proenkephalin A. The most important regulators of POMC gene expression in the pars distalis are corticotropin releasing hormone (CRH, which stimulates), and glucocorticoids (which inhibit). Gonadotropins appear to be primary regulators in the gonads.

propantheline bromide: β-diisopropylaminoethyl 9-xanthenecarboxylate methobromide; a muscarinic type acetylcholine receptor antagonist that diminishes gastric hyperacidity and hypermotility, and is used to treat gastric ulcers.

properdin: factor P; a circulating 441 amino acid, 223K glycoprotein that contributes to nonspecific defenses against infection, in part by activating complement systems. It complexes with C3b, and stabilizes the C3 convertase of the alternate pathway. The term *properdin pathway* refers to non-antigenic mechanisms for complement activation (for example ones initiated by endotoxin).

properidine: 1-methyl-4-phenyl-4-piperidinecarboxylic acid 1-methylethyl ester; a narcotic analgesic and antispasmodic agent.

prophage: a lysogenic phage genome that integrates into bacterial DNA and replicates with the host genome.

prophase: the stage of cell division preceded by interphase and followed by metaphase, in which chromosomes condense, the nuclear membrane disintegrates, and the centrioles begin migration to opposite poles. *See* also **mitosis** and **meiosis**. Meiosis I prophase is divided into leptotene, zygotene, pachytene, diplotene, and diakinesis. Meiosis II prophase is similar in many respects to mitosis prophase, but it very rapidly follows completion of meiosis I, and involves haploid chromosomes.

propionic acid: propanoic acid; a glucogenic fatty acid made by bacteria, and absorbed and metabolized by ruminants. It is a component of cheeses and some other foods. *See* also **propionyl-coenzyme A**.

$$CH_3 - CH_2 - COOH$$

propionyl-coenzyme A: a compound made from ingested propionic acid and coenzyme A, a degradation product of methionine and isoleucine, and an intermediate formed during β-oxidation of odd chain fatty acids. Propionyl CoA carboxylase is a biotin dependent enzyme that catalyzes its reaction with ATP to yield malonyl-CoA + AMP + P-P. Methylmalonyl-CoA mutase, which uses a vitamin B_{12} derived cofactor, then promotes formation of succinyl-CoA.

propiophenone: 1-phenyl-1-propanone; a catechol-*O*-methyltransferase (COMT) inhibitor, used as a precursor for industrial synthesis of ephedrine, and in the manufacture of perfumes.

propositus: *see* **proband**.

propranolol: 1-(isopropylamino)-3-(1-naphthyloxy)-2-propanol; a nonspecific β_1 and β_2-type adrenergic receptor antagonist used to treat some cardiac dysrhythmias, and as a laboratory tool. Its ability to alleviate some forms of hypertension is attributed in part to inhibition of norepinephrine release. High concentrations are weak local anesthetics.

propressophysin: a prohormone cleaved to yield vasopressin and its associated neurophysin.

proprioception: awareness of body position, movement, or balance.

propylthiouracil: 6-*n*-propylthiouracil; PTU; 2-thio-4-oxo-6-propyl-1,3-pyrimidine; an inhibitor of thyroid peroxidase (an enzyme that catalyzes iodide oxidation, iodine incorporation into thyroglobulins, and the coupling reaction required for iodothyronine formation). It also inhibits a deiodinase in many cell types that converts thyroxine (T_4) to triiodothyronine (T_3); *cf* **methimazole**. PTU is used to treat Graves' disease, in which it lowers T_4 and T_3 levels, and can decrease production of immunoglobulins that stimulate the thyroid gland. The immunosuppresssion may be secondary to the influences on thyroid hormone synthesis. It is sometimes used alone to control the symptoms; but maximal effects are not achieved until preformed iodinated thyroglobulin stores are depleted. In others cases, the primary therapeutic objective is attenuation of hyperthyroidism to a level compatible with ability to withstand the stress of thyroid gland surgery, or preparation of the patient for administration of radioactive iodine (which destroys thyroid tissue). The side-effects can include allergic reactions and bone marrow damage. Under normal conditions, thyroid stimulating hormone (TSH) made by thyrotropes is the major stimulant for thyroid gland growth and secretory functions. Thyrotropes cells take up circulating T_4 and convert it to T_3, the major intracellular inibitor of TSH synthesis and secretion. PTU impairs the negative feedback control, and is used to promote goiter formation in laboratory animals. However, since it does not inhibit the *thyrotrope* deiodinase, thyroidectomized animals receiving it but maintained on very low T_4 dosages can have low circulating T_3 levels (and hypothyroidism) without developing goiters. The antithyroid effects on metabolic rate have been used to promote fattening of farm animals.

propylure: 10-propyl-5,9-tridecadien-1-ol acetate; an insect sex-attractant pheromone.

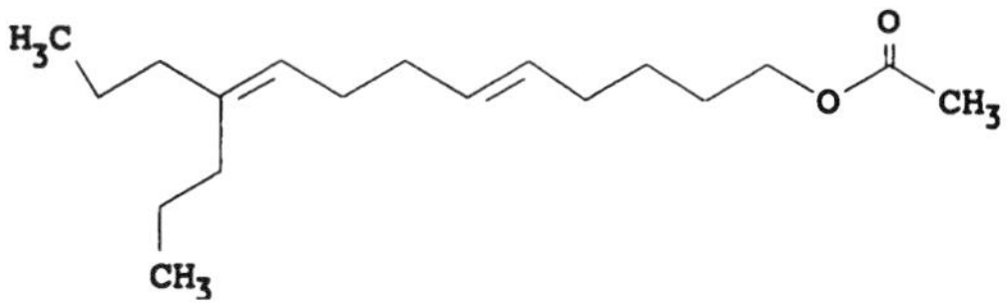

prorenins: glycoproteins in blood plasma, kidney, and elsewhere that can be activated (by freezing and thawing, acids, kallikreins, or other means) to display renin-like activity. The major form, with 383 amino acid moieties, originates in the kidneys.

prosimians: members of a primate suborder that includes lemurs, tree shrews and tarsiers.

PROST: pronuclear ovum stage transfer; an *in vitro* fertilization procedure.

prostacyclin: PGI$_2$; (5Z, 9α,11α,13E,15(S)6,9-epoxy-11,15-dihydroxyprosta-5,13-dien-1-oic acid; an eicosanoid made by endothelial, renal, immune system, and many other cell types that relaxes the smooth muscle of blood vessels, bronchioles, and myometrium. It protects against thromboxane toxicity by inhibiting platelet aggregation and thrombus formation, and against angiotensin excess by inhibiting renin release. It also stabilizes lysosomal membranes, decreases immune system reactivity, reduces gastric acidity, and augments renal blood flow. In fetuses, it appears to be essential for maintaining the patency of the ductus arteriosus. The major stimuli for its production include interleukin-1 and platelet derived growth factor (PDGF). In common with other eicosanoids, the rate-limiting reaction is release of free arachidonic acid (mostly from phospholipids). A cyclooxygenase catalyzed reaction forms prostaglandin H$_2$ (PGH$_2$); *see* prostaglandins. Prostacyclin synthetase then converts the product to PGI$_2$. Since it is rapidly degraded to 6α-keto-PGI$_2$, the effects are transient if synthesis does not continue. Many have been linked with activation of adenylate cyclases.

prostaglandins: PGs; several eicosanoids made from essential fatty acids. Except for prostacyclin (included by some authors), all have similar chemical structures whose

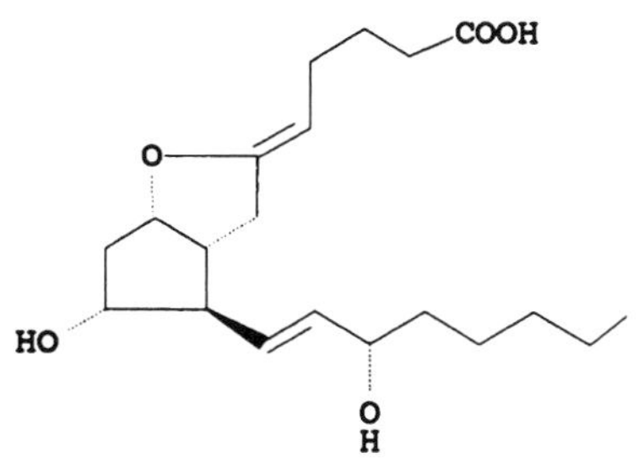

prostacyclin

trivial names are based on **prostanoic acid** (*q.v.*). They are distinguished from each other by Roman capital letters that define the ring structures (*see* below), subscript numbers which indicate the numbers of side-chain double bonds, and Greek letters that designate the stereoisomeric forms. The rate-limiting factor for biosynthesis is the availability of free substrate. Many regulators provide it by activating phospholipases; but some act on lipases or cholesterol esterases. Low density lipoproteins (LDLs) are good sources; and arachidonic acid (AA, the major substrate) acts in conjunction with LDL receptors to exert negative feedback controls over PG synthesis. Nonspecific stimuli that liberate fatty acids from plama membranes include hypoxia, excess pressure, and trauma. Arachidonic acid products (PG$_2$s) have two side-chain double bonds. PGs with one and three double bonds are derived mostly from dihomo-γ-linoleic, and eicosapentaenoic acid, respectively. All are metabolized along similar pathways. A consistently available cyclooxygenase system catalyzes the initial step, in which AA is converted to the endoperoxide, prostaglandin G$_2$ (PGG$_2$), a short-lived intermediate that transforms spontaneously to the hydroendoperoxide, PGH$_2$. Prostacyclin synthetase, endoperoxide E-isomerase, and endoperoxide D-isomerase in various cell types then catalzye formation of PGI, PGE$_2$, and PGD$_2$, respectively. Some products can be converted to others. The fatty acid precursors can also be oxidized without enzymes when activated macrophages and other cell types that generate free oxygen radicals. The kinds and amounts formed vary with the cell types. Although rapidly degraded, PGs exert profound influences on almost all known physiological functions, by acting directly, promoting the release of other

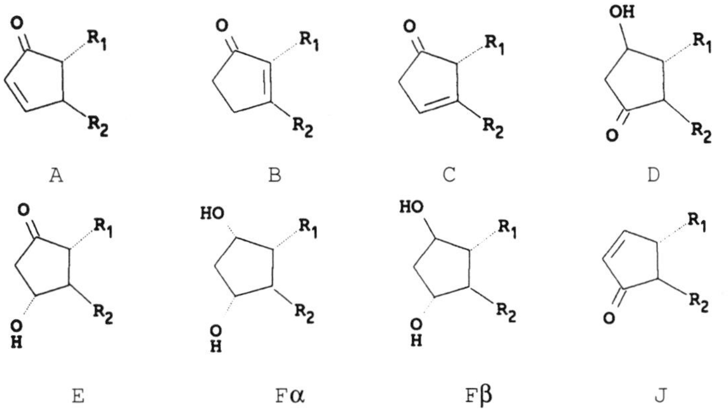

prostaglandin ring structures

PGA₁ ... PGA₂

regulators, or affecting blood flow; *see* specific types, and especially PGEs. Several nonsteroidal anti-inflammatory agents reversibly inactivate the cyclooxygenase system; and aspirin acts irreversibly by acetylating the enzyme. However, one consequence of actions confined to this system is increased production of leukotrienes, lipoxins, and other unsaturated fatty acid products made in pathways catalyzed by lipoxygenases and related enzymes. In contrast, inhibitors of phospholipases and other substrate liberators affect the synthesis of all eicosanoids. The anti-inflammatory effects of glucocorticoids are mediated in part via **lipocortins** (*q.v.*). The gastrointestinal irritation (and in some cases ulceration) caused by prolonged use of most anti-inflammatory agents has been attributed to prostaglandin deficiency; but *see* **misoprostol** and **salicylates**.

prostaglandin A: PGA₁ (13E, 15S)-15-hydroxy-9-oxaprosta-10-13-dien-1-oic acid), and PGA₂ ((5Z, 13 E)-15-hydroxy-9-oxoprosta-5,10,13-trien-1-oic acid) enter cell nuclei, suppress *c-myc* expression, liberate heat shock protein hsp70, arrest cell proliferation, and promote differentiation of some kinds of leukemia cells. They are inactivated by conjugation to cysteine and glutathione. Although PGA₂ can lower blood pressure, and was once believed to be a major renal medulluary hormone that regulates this function, it is now known that the large amounts in some kidney extracts derive from artifactual, nonenzymatic conversion of PGE₂ to PGA₂.

prostaglandin B₂: PGB₂; (15Z,9α,13E,15S)9,15-dihydroxy-11-oxoprosta-5,13-dien-1-oic acid; a prostaglandin made mostly in the nervous system, reported to exert influences on behavior. Its formation from PGE₂ can proceed without enzymes, in the pathway: PGE₂ → PGA₂ → PGC₂ → PGB₂. Prostaglandin B₁, (13E,15S)-15-hydroxy-9-oxoprosta-8[2],13-dien-1-oic acid, made in minute amounts, has similar properties.

prostaglandin D₂: PGD₂; (15Z,9α,13E, 15S)9,15-dihydroxy-11-oxoprosta-5,13-dien-1-oic acid; a prostaglandin synthesized from PGH₂ via a reaction catalyzed by endoperoxidase D-isomerase that regulates bone and immune system functions, and is implicated as a major physiological mediator of sleep. When released from activated mast cells, it promotes contraction of bronchial muscle and constriction of lung blood vessels, and contributes to the development of asthma. Although it diminishes blood flow to the kidneys, it relaxes small blood vessels in some other areas. PGD₂ also stimulates gastrointestinal muscle and promotes blood platelet aggregation.

prostaglandin E₁: PGE₁; (11α,13E,15S)11,15-dihydroxy-9-oxoprost-13-en-1-oic acid; a prostaglandin made in small amounts that relaxes vascular and respiratory system smooth muscle, and inhibits gastric acid production and blood platelet aggregation. It augments adenylate cyclase activity in certain cell types, but inhibits the adipocyte enzyme and antagonizes the lipolytic effects of epinephrine and some other hormones. It is also one of the factors that promotes neuroblast differentiation.

prostaglandin E₂: PGE₂; (15Z,11α,13E,15S)11,15-dihydroxy-9-oxoprosta-5,13-dien-1-oic acid; the most abundant of the prostaglandins. Its effects vary with the target cell types, and in some cases with the concentrations. Some are mediated via adenylate cyclase activation; but many are secondary to influences on blood flow and the release of other regulators. It is also converted by 9-ketoreductase to PGF₂α, and nonenzymatically to prostaglandins A₂, C₂, and B₂. PGE₂ directly promotes vasodilation at many sites, and can thereby lower systemic blood pressure; but it augments renin release and exerts variable influences on sympathetic neurons. When released from activated monocytic phagocytes, it contributes to inflammatory reactions by increasing the permeabilities of small blood vessels, elevating body temperature (via both lipolysis and direct effects on neurons), and mediating perception of pain and other nociceptive stimuli; but it inhibits T lymphocyte growth and the expression of class II histocompatibility antigens on macrophage and T lymphocyte cell surfaces, antagonizes the platelet-aggregating effects of thromboxane A₂, and counteracts the somnogenic effects of PGD₂. Depending on prevailing conditions and concentrations, it can either stimulate or relax uterine smooth muscle (*cf*

prostaglandin E₁

prostaglandin $F_{2\alpha}$). It stimulates in the respiratory tract. In the gastrointestinal tract, it stimulates longitudinal, but relaxes circular muscle. PGE_2 also decreases HCl production in the stomach, and exerts protective and trophic effects on gastric mucosa. In the endocrine system, it antagonizes vasopressin mediated water conservation, inhibits glucose stimulated insulin release, promotes glucagon secretion, facilitates the release of adrenocorticotropic, luteinizing and thyroid stimulating hormones (ACTH, LH, and TSH), and mediates some effects of those hormones on their target glands. Additionally, it potentiates the effects of some factors that promote bone resorption, and is implicated as a major contributor to joint damage associated with rheumatoid arthritis.

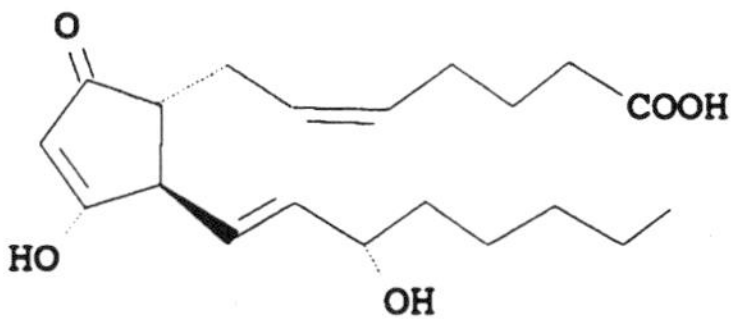

prostaglandin E_3: PGE_3; a prostaglandin with properties similar to those described for prostaglandin E_2.

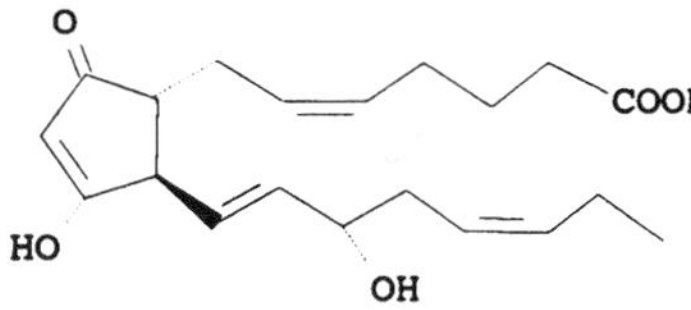

prostaglandin endoperoxide[s]: short-lived eicosanoids made from essential fatty acids. The major types are PGG_2 and PGH_2. PGG_2 is almost immediately converted to PGH_2. The latter is also short-lived, and rapidly converted to different prostaglandins, thromboxanes, and other eicosanoids; but it directly stimulates smooth muscle and accelerates blood platelet aggregation.

prostaglandin endoperoxide synthetase: prostaglandin endoperoxide synthase; *see* **cyclooxygenase**.

prostaglandin $F_{1\alpha}$: $PGF_{1\alpha}$; $(9\alpha,11\alpha,13E,15S)9,11,15$-trihydroxy-prost-13-en-1-oic acid; a prostaglandin made from dihomo-γ-linolenic acid that exerts effects similar to those described for prostaglandin $F_{2\alpha}$.

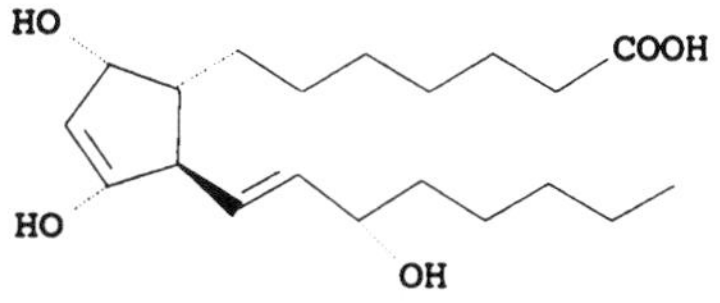

prostaglandin $F_{2\alpha}$: $PGF_{2\alpha}$; a major prostaglandin, made from PGE_2, and also directly from PGH_2. It is a potent stimulant for most smooth muscle, and thereby raises systemic blood pressure. It can invoke bronchoconstriction, uterine cramps, and gastrointestinal tract distress, and is implicated as a primary cause of dysmenorrhea. It plays essential roles in parturition, ovulation, and luteolysis, and is used in some cases to induce abortion, or to accelerate parturition. Many of its actions have been linked with adenylate cyclase inhibition. It also facilitates the release of adrenocorticotropic hormone (ACTH), prolactin, and gonadotropins.

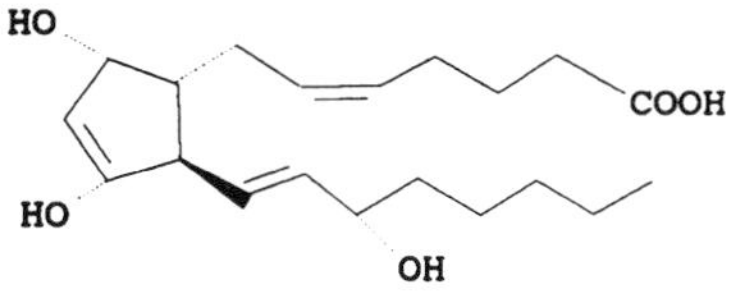

prostaglandin G_2 (PGG_2) and prostaglandin H_2 (PGH_2): *see* **prostaglandin endoperoxides**.

9,11-epoxymethano-prostaglandin H_2: a prostaglandin H_2 analog that resists degradation, and is used to study prostaglandin H_2 effects.

Δ^{12}-prostaglandin J_2: a prostaglandin concentrated in cell nuclei that induces heat shock protein hsp68 and can arrest the growth of some murine leukemia cells.

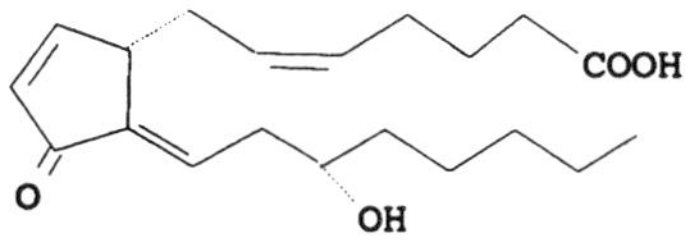

6-keto-prostaglandin 1α: *see* **6-keto-PGF1α**.

prostanoic acid: a compound used for prostaglandin nomenclature.

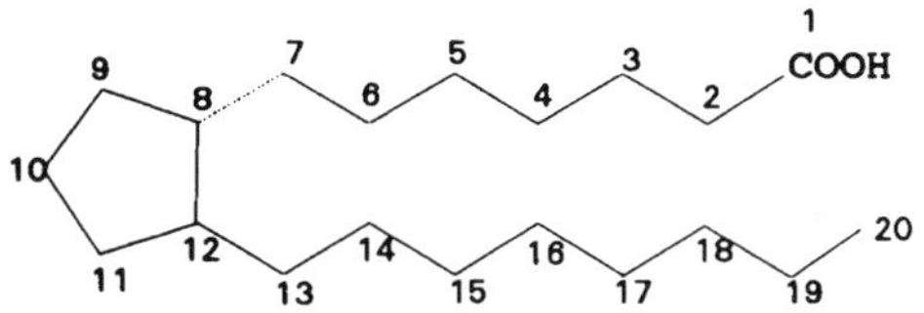

prostate glands: accessory reproductive organs in most male mammals that differentiate from urogenital sinuses, and surround the urethras. They provide several seminal fluid components, including water, buffers, nutrients, and coagulation enzymes. The development, maturation, and secretory functions are androgen-dependent, and require testosterone conversion to 5α-dihydrotestosterone. In castrated laboratory animals, prostate gland growth can

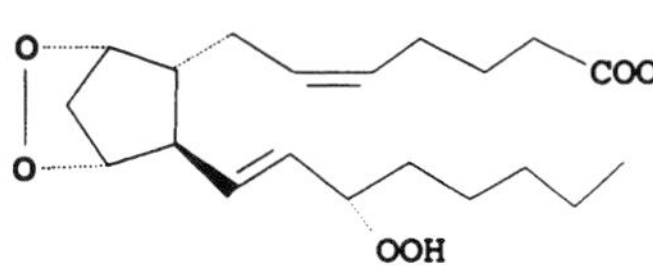

PGG$_2$

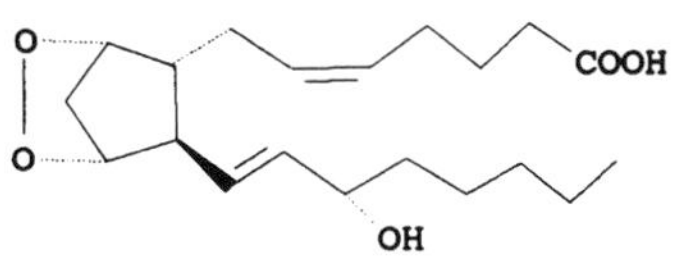

PGH$_2$

be reversibly stimulated in a dose-related manner by injecting androgens; and regression follows hormone withdrawal. In humans, dogs, lions, and some other species, the gland enlarges late in life. The incidence of benign prostatic hypertrophy has been estimated at 50% for men at age 50, and at close to 100% at age 80. Some glands undergo neoplastic changes that do not invoke symptoms. Androgens have been implicated in the etiology of prostatic cancer, and in some cases surgical or chemical castration, and/or administration of 5α-reductase inhibitors can exert beneficial effects. However, age-related changes occur at a time when testicular production of the hormone declines. (Blood levels do not fall as much, because the clearance rate slows.) Factors proposed to accelerate prostatic growth in older individuals include augmented production of, or responses to autocrine stimulants such as epidermal growth factor (EGF) whose receptors are induced by androgens, diminished production and/or effectiveness of inhibitors, and changes in testosterone metabolism (including more rapid conversion to estrogens, which induce DHT receptors). Increased prolactin production may contribute to the stimulation. *See* also **prostatic growth factor** and **prostatotropin**.

prostatein: a steroid-binding prostate gland protein. Androgens augment its synthesis and release.

prostate specific antigen: PSA; a protein made in prostate glands and released to the bloodstream in amounts related to the gland size. Since serum levels are high in individuals with prostatic carcinoma, it has been proposed that measurements can be used as indicators of the presence of cancer cells. However, the concentrations are also high in those with benign prostatic hypertrophy. The determinations are more useful for following the effectiveness of prostatectomy and other therapies than for initial diagnosis.

prostatic growth factor: PGF; a mitogen related to or identical with a basic fibroblast growth factor, implicated as a stimulant for prostate gland cells.

prostatotropin: a heparin-binding mitogen related to or identical with an acidic fibroblast growth factor. It promotes prostate gland growth, and is also made in neural tissues.

prosthetic group: a non-protein component that associates with an enzyme or other protein and is essential for its functions, for example a coenzyme or a heme group.

Prostigmin: a trade name for neostigmine.

protachykinins: prohormones cleaved to several neuropeptides that share the *C*-terminal amino acid sequence Phe-X-Gly-Leu-Met-NH$_2$, in which X can be Phe-, Val-, Ile-, or Tyr-; *see* **protachykinin A**, **protachykinin B**, and **preprotachykinin**.

protachykinin A: α-protachykinin; a prohormone for substance P.

protachykinin B: a prohormone for substance P and neurokinin A (substance K).

protamines: 4-5K basic proteins, high in arginine content, that also contain alanine and serine, but no tyrosine or tryptophan. They are most abundant in sperm, in which they replace the histones of most other cell types. The ones in fish spermatozoa include salmine, clupein, and iridine. Protamines bind nucleic acids, neutralize the acidity conferred by phosphate groups, facilitate DNA compaction, and inhibit protease nexins, and also lipoprotein lipases, plasminogen activators, and some other enzymes. They suppress angiogenesis, and can act alone as anticoagulants, but complex with and antagonize heparin effects on clot formation. Although used to precipitate some other proteins, they are incorporated into insulin preparations to prevent aggregation of the hormone molecules.

protandry: a form of sequential hermaphroditism, in which male type gonads differentiate first (and the individual acquires a male phenotype), after which female structures and the associated characteristics emerge. Oysters sea-slugs, some fish and some frog species follow this pattern; *cf* **protogyny**.

protease[s]: enzymes that degrade proteins and large peptides to smaller molecules by catalyzing hydrolytic cleavage of peptide bonds. Digestive system enzymes break down dietary proteins, lysosomal and others destroy proteins that are damaged (*see* also **ubiquitins**), no longer needed, or metabolized for fuel and other purposes in nutrient deprived cells, and specialized types act at specific sites to convert proenzymes to enzymes, prohormones to hormones, and cell-bound molecules to secreted forms. Collagenases and elastases are among the kinds named for their substrates. Others names such as pepsin describe functions. *Endopeptidases* attack internal bonds, whereas *exopeptidases* (carboxypeptidases and aminopeptidases) act at the termini. A different nomenclature (which includes terms such as serine proteinases and cysteine proteases) is based on the amino acid types contained within the active sites. Metalloproteases require inorganic cation cofactors.

protease nexins: PNs; peptides secreted by fibroblasts, muscle, epithelial, and central nervous system cells that bind covalently to and inhibit thrombin, trypsin, plasmins, and other proteases. They act at cell surfaces, protect the integrity of extracellular matrices, and block metastasis of some tumor cells. PN-I (protein nexin-I), also known as glia-derived neurite promoting factor and glia derived protease inhibitor, is developmentally regulated. It antagonizes thrombin inhibition of astrocyte and astrocyte precursor cell proliferation, stimulates neurite growth, and affects embryonic neuronal cell migration. Protease nexin-II (P-II) made by fibroblasts, inhibits chymotrypsin-like enzymes. It binds the γ-subunit of nerve growth factor (NGF), and forms complexes with a pro-EGF processing serine esterase. Amyloid precursor proteins APP770 and AP751 contain a protease nexin II sequence; and the secreted form of APP in Alzheimer disease plaques is identical with that nexin. (Extremely low levels of PN-I have been found at autopsy in the brains of individuals with Alzheimer's disease.) The protein complexes are internalized and degraded by the cells. Protamines and some tumor cell products antagonize their effects. *Cf* **nexins**.

protein[s]: molecules composed of large numbers of amino acid moieties joined by peptide bonds. (Compounds with fewer than 100 amino acids are usually called peptides or polypeptides.) When the molecular weight is known, a protein can be represented by p followed by a number, as in p26. The properties are related to *primary structures* (numbers and kinds of amino acid moieties and orders in which they are arranged), *secondary structures* (coiling, bending, and/or other configuration assumed in surrounding media, mostly because of hydrogen bonds), *tertiary structures* (folding or other three-dimensional arrangements stabilized by covalent bonds, for example between sulfur atoms), and, for some, also *quaternary structures* (stable interactions between two or more peptide chains). Proteins are major factors that account for species differences and distinguish one cell type within an organism from another. They are also components of extracellular matrices. Most enzymes and many hormones and prohormones are proteins.

protein II: *see* **calpactins**.

protein 4.1: an erythrocyte protein composed of two almost identical subunits that links spectrin filaments to plasma membranes, and spectrin-actin complexes to glycophorin.

protein 7B2: APPG; a 180K protein chemically related to duck proinsulin, secretin, and the transforming protein of Rous sarcoma virus, identified in pituitary glands, hypothalamus, extra-hypothalamic brain, spinal cord, ileum, colon, pancreas, urogenital tracts, thyroid glands, and adrenal glands. It colocalizes with gonadotropins, and its secretion is stimulated by gonadotropin releasing hormone.

protein A: a constituent of *Staphylococcus aureus* cell walls, linked to peptidoglycans, that binds Fc regions of all IgG type immunoglobulins except IgG3, and Fab regions of some IgM and IgA classes. It may contribute to the ability of the organisms to evade immune attacks by covering antigenic determinants (but is a potent mitogen for B lymphocytes). The Cowan strain type is used to identify and isolate immunoglobulins and antigen-antibody complexes, and to remove them from serum. *Cf* **protein G**.

proteinases: usually, endopeptidase type proteases.

protein bound iodine: PBI; iodine in serum protein and plasma protein fractions. Since much of it is thyroxine associated with the plasma proteins, PBI measurements have been used to estimate circulating T_4 levels, and as indices of thyroid gland secretory functions. However, the fractions also contain biologically inactive iodothyronines. Butanol extracted iodine (BEI) contains fewer inactive molecules. Both methods have been largely replaced by direct assays for thyroxine and triiodothyronine (T_3), and by other procedures for assessing cell activities.

protein C: a 62K circulating proenzyme, also known as blood coagulation factor XIV, that contains a γ-carboxyglutamate (gla) moiety. When converted to its active form, it catalyzes proteolytic degradation of coagulation factors V and VII, and may contribute to protection against intravascular clotting.

protein G: a constituent of the cell walls of some *Streptococci* that binds Fc regions of most IgG molecules, but does not bind to IgA or IgM type immunoglobulins; *cf* **protein C**. Protein G sepharose is used to separate immunoglobulin subclasses.

protein glycation: non-enzymatic binding of sugars to proteins; *see* **nonenzymatic glycosylation**. It accelerates when glucose levels are elevated, and is believed to cause some of the pathology associated with diabetes mellitus. The amounts of hemoglobin A converted to the A_{1c} are used as indicators for bouts of hyperglycemia not detected in standard measurements of blood glucose levels. *Cf* **protein glycosylation**.

protein glycosylation: usually, enzyme-catalyzed covalent addition of sugars to proteins. Some groups bind during translation, but most additions and modifications are accomplished in the Golgi apparatus. Carbohydrate moieties affect protein configurations, surface charges, binding properties, and metabolic clearance rates. Some are essential for the functions of the affected molecules; *see*, for example **gonadotropins** and **thyroid stimulating hormone**.

protein K: protein kinase NII; *see* **polyamine dependent kinase**.

protein kinases: PKs; numerous enzymes that catalyze transfers of terminal phosphate groups from ATP (and to a lesser extent from GTP and other nucleotides) to mostly serine, threonine, or tyrosine moieties of proteins. (*Kinase* is a broader term that also applies to enzymes which transfer the phosphate groups to small molecules such as glucose.) Most PK substrates are enzymes, enzyme inhibitors, cytoskeletal components, plasma membrane molecules, or other regulatory compounds whose functions are changed by additions at specific positions. Some are components of cascades, in which activation of one enzyme leads successively to activation of several others. Kinases A and G, calcium-calmodulin dependent (Ca-CaM) kinases, and RNA-dependent kinases are among the types named for their activators. Numbers have been assigned to a few. For example, kinase 2a is a specific type activated by double stranded RNAs. (It is induced by interferons α and β, and it then augments production of the IFNβ messenger RNA). Glycogen phosphorylase kinase, myosin light-chain kinases, and histone kinases and others are named for their substrates. Many kinases are activated by high Ca^{2+}; and phosphorylation can augment Ca^{2+} sensitivity to the point where ordinary cytoplasmic levels become effective. The receptors for insulin, insulin like growth factor-I (IGF-I), platelet derived growth factor (PDGF), and other growth stimulants contain tyrosine kinase components that are activated by ligand binding. Activators for other types include diacylglycerols and arachidonic acid. *See* also **SH2 domains**. Ones with broad specificities include Ca^{2+}/CaM kinase II (kinase II), which acts on synapsin I, tryptophan hydroxylase, skeletal muscle glycogen phosphorylase, and some microtubule-associated proteins; and EF-2 kinase may be a calcium-calmodulin isozyme. Casein kinases (PKI, PKII, PKIII) are identified by their abilities to promote phosphorylations of certain acidic proteins. Several protein kinases have overlapping substrate specificities, and in some cases one enzyme acts at a specific position within a substrate, and another phosphorylates at a different site. In certain cell types, one hormone receptor activates a protein kinase, and a different receptor for the same hormone affects another kinase. Dual function kinases require phosphorylations on both serine-threonine and tyrosine moieties to achieve full activity. Kinase mediated phosphorylation affects intermediate metabolism, cell cycle initiation and progression, DNA, RNA, and protein synthesis, signal transduction, vision, olfaction, cell morphology, embryonic development, and other functions. Protein kinase activities are closely regulated under physiological conditions; and their effects are antagonized by protein phosphatases. Defective controls over some lead to transformation (and the effects of some oncogenes are directly linked with persistent activation). *See* also **mitogen activated kinases**, **MPF**, **cyclins**, and **tyrosine kinases**.

protein kinase A: cAMP-activated protein kinase; *see* **kinase A**.

protein kinase C: *see* **kinase C**.

protein kinase G: cGMP dependent protein kinase; *see* **kinase G**.

protein kinase inhibitors: several peptides made by cells that interact with, and decrease the activities of protein kinases. Some are regulated by protein kinases or protein phosphatases. A peptide isolated from rabbit tissues that acts mostly on kinase A has the amino acid sequence: Thr-Thr-Tyr-Ala-ASp-Phe-Ile-Ala-Ser-Gly-Arg-Thr-Gly-Arg-Arg-Asn-Ala-Ile-His-Asp-. **H-7, H-8, H-9** (*q.v.*) are examples of types synthesized for laboratory use. Different kinds are present in some venoms, some of which preferentially act on kinase C enzymes. Some structures are shown below.

protein kinase N: *see* **kinase N**.

protein kinase NII: protein K; *see* **polyamine dependent kinase**.

protein kinase P: polypeptide dependent protein kinase; *see* **kinase P**.

protein phosphatases: phosphoprotein phosphatases; enzymes made by all nucleated cells that catalyze hydrolytic cleavage of covalent bonds between amino acid moieties of proteins and phosphate groups. The substrates include other enzymes (some of which are protein kinases), enzyme inhibitors, ribosomal proteins, transcription factors, hormone receptors, ion channel components, and other regulatory molecules. Dephosphorylations affect surface charges and configurations. The consequences include activation of some intermediary metabolism enzymes (such as glycogen synthase), inhibition of others (for example triacylglycerol lipases and glycogen phosphorylase), and influences on signal transduction, neurotransmitter release, skeletal, smooth and cardiac muscle contraction, sperm motility,

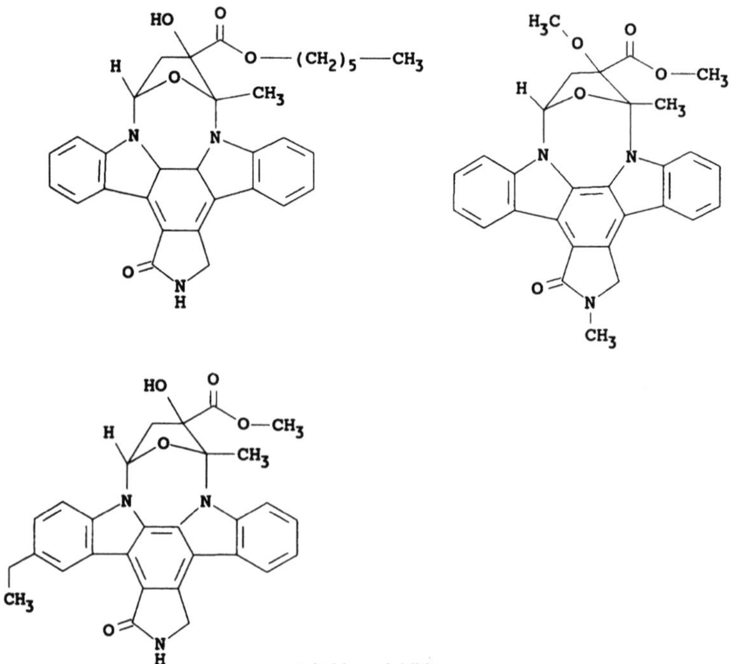

protein kinase inhibitors

mitochondrial functions, DNA replication, cell cycle progression, RNA and protein synthesis, fertilization, oocyte maturation, embryonic development, water and ion transport across renal tubules, inflammation, cell morphology, adhesion to extracellular matrices and motility, immune system responses, and melanocyte movements. In some cases, dephosphorylation of an amino acid moiety at one locus within a protein has end effects opposite in direction to those caused by dephosphorylation of the same molecule at other sites. The large numbers of protein phosphatases, the overlapping substrate specificities, and complex interactions make classification difficult. One scheme divides them into nuclear, mitochondrial, transmembrane, cytoskeleton-associated, and "cytoplasmic" types (most of which associate with intracellular membranes). Some are constitutionally active, and are believed to continuously protect cells against hyperphosphorylation by **protein kinases** (*q.v.*). A different classification is based on factors such as substrate specificities and responses to regulators. Numbers and letters have been assigned to four major groups that act preferentially on non-mitochondrial proteins. *Type 1A (PP-1A)* enzymes catalyze serine and/or threonine dephosphorylation of phosphorylase kinase β-subunits, and of glycogen synthetase, and are inhibited by phosphatase inhibitors 1 and 2. The activities of those inhibitors are also affected by phosphorylation-dephosphorylation reactions; *see* also **dopamine and cAMP regulated phosphoprotein**. They are not dependent on divalent cations for activation, and are not activated by calmodulins. Most are associated with membranes and inhibited by heparin. Another set, *type 1B (PP 1-B)* differs from the others in that it dephosphorylates tyrosyl moieties (*see* also **tyrosine phosphatases**). Those enzymes are major antagonists for insulin, insulin-like growth factors, epidermal growth factor, and other growth stimulants; and complex systems for protection against tumor formation and growth invoked by protein kinases have been described. *Type 2* enzymes dephosphorylate the α-subunits of phosphorylase kinase, and are not affected by inhibitors 1 and 2. The subgroups include *2A (PP-2A)*, whose members are neither cation-dependent nor affected by calmodulins, *2B (PP-2B)*, which require Ca^{2+} and are activated by calmodulins and include calcineurins, and *2C (PP-2C)*, which are Mg^{2+}-dependent and not activated by calmodulins. CD45 (common leukocyte antigen) is a hematopoietic system phosphatase essential for T lymphocyte activation and interleukin-2 production. It activates kinase p56^{lck} by dephosphorylating a regulatory subunit.

protein S: a 69K, vitamin-K dependent monomeric protein cofactor for protein C of the blood coagulation system.

proteinuria: excessive amounts of proteins in urine. Albumin leakage from glomeruli occurs transiently during demanding exercise, fevers, and some other forms of stress. Glomerular damage is a major cause of persistent albuminuria. Other causes include renal tubular and urinary tract infections. *See* also **Bence-Jones protein**.

proteoglycans: glycosaminoglycans covalently linked to protein cores. They form viscous solutions that coat the surfaces of most cell types, and accumulate in substantial amounts in connective tissue matrices, mucus, synovial fluid, and vitreous humor. Most of the molecules have sulfate or other acidic groups that attract water. Some contain linker protein components that stabilize large complexes.

proteoliasin: a 230K monomeric acidic protein that, in the presence of Ca^{2+}, binds to oocyte vitelline layers and promotes translocation of ovoperoxidase from intracellular sites to extracellular matrices.

proteolysis: protein degradation by any means (including cleavage by strong acids, bases, and other chemicals, as well as by enzymes).

proteoses: large peptides formed during partial digestion of proteins. Pepsin promotes their formation in the stomach lumen, and further degrades them to peptones and polypeptides that are subsequently acted on by pancreatic juice enzymes.

prothionine sulfoximine: an agent used to inhibit glutathione synthesis.

prothoracic glands: insect glands derived from ectodermal epithelium that migrate to the thoracic region and secrete ecdysones. They are ring gland components in some species.

prothoracicotropic hormones: PTTH; peptide hormones secreted by insect brain neurosecretory cells that act on prothoracic glands and stimulate ecdysone secretion.

prothrombin: procoagulation factor II; 69-74K vitamin K-dependent plasma proteins with carboxyglutamate (gla) and sugar moieties, secreted by the liver. They are proenzymes made from prothrombinogens and converted in the presence of Ca^{2+} to thrombins by phospholipids, factor X_a and factor V.

prothrombinase: thrombokinin; coagulation factor X_a.

prothrombinogens: coagulation factor VII; proteins made in the liver and converted in the presence of vitamin K to prothrombins.

prothrombin time: the time required for coagulation to occur after Ca^{2+} is added to a mixture of citrated blood plasma and tissue thromboplastin. It is prolonged if extrinsic pathway coagulation factors are deficient or defective, or if excessive amounts of inhibitors are present. *See* also **partial thromboplastin time**.

prothymocytes: immature cells that begin differentiation in bone marrow, and then migrate to the thymus gland. Some complete maturation to T lymphocytes, but many die within the gland.

prothymosin α: *see* **thymosins**.

Protista: a term used to classify organisms. In one system, it is a kingdom that comprises all simple animal-like and plant-like eukaryotes. In another, it is a phylum that includes just protozoa.

protocollagens: molecules formed from tropocollagens when hydroxylation defects impair conversion to procollagens.

protogyny: a form of sequential hermaphroditism, in which female type gonads (and phenotypes) develop, and are later replaced by male type structures; *cf* **protandry**. The pattern occurs regularly in a few fish species. In some Coral fishes, animals that would otherwise go through life as females retain the potential for conversion to males. When all males are removed from a population, one female realizes that potential.

protomer: a single polypeptide chain (subunit) of a multimeric protein, or a single microtubule precursor.

proton: a positively charged particle of an atomic nucleus with a mass 1836 times that of an electron. The atomic number of an element is determined by the numbers of protons (and the atomic weight by the sum of the weights of the protons and neutrons). Hydrogen ions are protons.

proton pumps: enzyme systems that use energy to transport hydrogen ions across membranes. The electrochemical gradients created can drive active transport of molecules and other ions. In mitochondria, H^+ transport from the matrix to the intermembrane space is driven by energy released when electrons travel down transport chains. The gradients facilitate phosphate uptake and ATP synthesis from ADP + Pi. Plasma membranes of aerobic bacteria contain comparable elements. Chloroplasts have photic pumps, in which light is used to energize electrons. Different proton pumps that derive energy from ATP hydrolysis are used to acidify lysosomes and other organelles, produce hydrochloric acid in the stomach, and support nutrient uptake under anaerobic conditions in bacteria.

protonophores: agents that facilitate passive proton transport across membranes. They can dissipate the effects of proton pumps, and thereby uncouple oxidative phosphorylation in mitochondria, or interfere with organelle acidification.

proto-oncogenes: cellular genes that play major roles in growth, differentiation, and other functions, but have the potential for invoking transformation and tumor growth stimulation if overexpressed or expressed at inappropriate times. Their activities in normal cells are tightly regulated, by inhibitors or the availability of transcription stimulants. The protective mechanisms can be disrupted by proto-oncogene amplification, translocations that shift controls over coding regions to constitutionally active promoters, or mutations to forms that function independently of stimulants or are unaffected by the inhibitors. Oncogenes are mutated or misplaced forms that are constitutionally active or unresponsive to the protective mechanisms. Some arise spontaneously. Others are introduced by retroviral nucleic acids (initially obtained from eukaryote cells) that integrate into host DNA.

protoplasm: the living substance of a cell, including both cytoplasmic and nuclear components.

protoplast: usually (1) a bacterial cell deprived of its cell wall, for example one grown in a medium that contains antibiotics which block peptidoglycan synthesis; (2) a plant cell deprived of its cell wall, usually by exposure to enzymes that degrade wall components.

protoporphyria: conditions in which excessive amounts of protoporphyrins accumulate. The most common form is an autosomal dominant defect that impairs the final step in heme biosynthesis. The manifestations include cutaneous photosensitivity, and progressive hepatic disease.

protoporphyrins: porphins with methyl, vinyl, carboxyethyl, and other substitutions for porphyrin hydrogen atoms. Protoporphyrin IX, 3,7,12,17-tetramethyl-8,13-divinyl, 2,18-porphinedipropionic acid (shown below) is the precursor of hemoglobin and of some plant pigments.

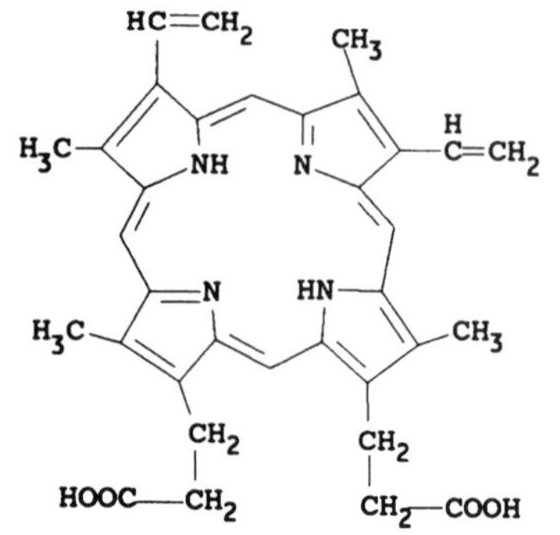

Prototheria: a suborder of mammals that contains the most primitive species; *see* **monotremes**.

prototrophs: (1) microorganisms that can survive and grow on defined media. They can be harvested from mixed cultures, since bacterial strains unable to synthesize one or more essential enzymes die; (2) organisms that can subsist on inorganic compounds and a carbon source. (Most bacteria require glucose, whereas plants require CO_2). *Cf* **autotroph**.

Protozoa: a subkingdom that comprises all single-celled animals (including some colonial types).

provirus: a virus that integrates into a host genome and can be transmitted to the cell progeny when the host cell replicates, but does not cause cell lysis.

provitamin: a substance that can be converted to a vitamin. Examples include some carotenes (which are also called previtamins) and provitamin D.

provitamin D_3: 7-dehydro-cholesterol. It is made in the liver and small intestine, and accumulates in skin. Ultraviolet radiation converts it to previtamin D_3, which spontaneously transforms to vitamin D_3.

proximal: nearer to the body center, or closer to the site of attachment. For example, the elbow is proximal to the wrist. *Cf* **distal**.

proximal convoluted tubules: nephron components that receive glomerular filtrates from Bowman's capsules, process them, and send the products to descending Henle

provitamin D₃

previtamin D₃

loop limbs. The walls are composed of a single layers of interdigitating "brush border" cells, with numerous villi that face the lumens, and tight junctions at their luminal borders. They actively reabsorb glucose, amino acids, ketones, some salts, some vitamins, and other filtrate constituents. Under normal conditions, a large fraction of the filtered Na^+ is returned to the blood, and passive reabsorption of 60-70% of the filtered water results in delivery of a reduced volume of isotonic fluid to the Henle loops. Proximal tubules also contribute to urine acidification by secreting H^+ and reabsorbing bicarbonate ions.

Prozac: a trade name for fluoxetine.

PRPP: 5-phosphoribosyl-1-pyrophosphate.

PS: phosphatidylserine.

PS2 protein: an estrogen-induced 84 amino acid poly-peptide identified in mouse mammary gland tumors and implicated in tumorigenesis. An identical or closely related peptide that does not respond to estrogens is made in gastric mucosa; *see* also **trefoil proteins**.

psammoma bodies: calcareous concretions (acervuli) that accumulate with advancing age in pineal glands.

pseudo-: a prefix meaning false, as in pseudopregnancy.

pseudoalleles: functionally related, closely associated genes that behave like, but are not true alleles. They can be separated during crossing over.

pseudoautosomal: describes components of sex chromosomes, identical in males and females, that behave like autosomes.

pseudocholinesterases: enzymes that, unlike "true" acetylcholinesterases, catalyze hydrolysis of succinylcholine and some other substrates in addition to acetylcholine. Some are present in blood plasma.

pseudocyesis: false pregnancy; manifestation of pregnancy-associated symptoms, such as weight gain, mammary gland changes, and "morning sickness" in women who are not carrying conceptuses. The causes can include excessive secretion of prolactin and/or gonadal hormones, or other hormone imbalances. Psychological factors (such as strong, unfulfilled desire for pregnancy) can affect hypothalamic control of pituitary gland functions. *Cf* **pseudopregnancy**.

pseudodominance: phenotypic expression of a recessive allele that occurs when the associated dominant allele on the homologous chromosome is deleted or does not function.

pseudoendocrinopathies: endocrine system disorders in which normal amounts of the associated hormone are secreted; see, for example **pseudohypoparathyroidism**. The causes include abnormal or inappropriate numbers of hormone receptors, signal transduction defects, deficiencies of enzymes or other cellular factors required for the responses to the signals, hepatic, or renal disorders that alter hormone metabolism, and production of substances that exert antagonistic actions, compete for hormone receptors, or impair hormone-receptor binding to acceptor molecules.

pseudogamy: parthenogenetic development that follows stimulation of an oocyte by a male gamete which does not penetrate and donate DNA.

pseudogene: a DNA region with base sequences similar to those of a functioning gene that is not transcribed, or directs formation of a primary transcript that is not processed to a messenger RNA. Pseudogenes in normal cells that lack promoters include members of the growth hormone gene superfamily, some clusters similar to the ones that direct β-globulin synthesis, and DNA segments with sequences that code for steroid 21-hydroxylase. Some are believed to have arisen during the course of evolution via inaccurate gene duplication, reverse transcription, or incorporation of viral genomes into host DNA. Additions, deletions, and translocations of DNA fragments are among the factors can block transcription.

pseudoglobulins: globulins sparingly soluble in water. (Euglobulins are insoluble.)

pseudohermaphrodite: an individual with some male and some female type reproductive system organs, but just one kind of gonad; *cf* **hermaphrodite**. Classification into male and female types is usually based on sex chromosome patterns or gonad types. The conditions can occur in XY individuals with defects that impair Müllerian duct regression or normal development of male structures, and in XX individuals exposed prenatally to excessive androgen levels. *See*, for example **feminizing testis** and **adrenogenital syndrome**.

pseudohypoaldosteronism: a condition in which aldosterone is secreted, but defective receptors impair responses to the hormone. Affected individuals lose excessive amounts of sodium to the urine and display other signs of aldosterone deficiency.

pseudohypoparathyroidism: conditions in which parathyroid hormone is secreted, but affected individuals develop PTH deficiency symptoms. In some types, the hormone binds to its receptors, but G protein defects block signal transduction. Other causes include abnormal PTH receptors, and renal defects that impair responses.

Pseudomonas: a genus of motile, rod shaped Gram negative bacteria, present in soil and water. Some strains cause plant diseases. *P. aeruginosa* (a soil type) is pathogenic in immunodeficient humans. It can also infect wounds and burned areas, and cause formation of blue pus in otherwise healthy individuals.

pseudoprecocious puberty: premature sexual maturation caused by production of excessive quantities of gonadal and/or adrenocortical steroids, with no elevation of gonadotropin or gonadotropin releasing hormone levels; *cf* **precocious puberty**. The causes include adrenocortical or gonadal tumors and/or enzyme defects that affect hormone biosynthesis.

pseudopregnancy: conditions in which symptoms associated with pregnancy (such as abdominal swelling, mammary gland growth, and altered behavior patterns) occur in females that are not carrying conceptuses. Progesterone and prolactin levels are often elevated. The term *pseudocyesis* is usually not applied when the initiating factors are hormonal. In many species with estrous cycles, pseudopregnancy can be induced by mating with a sterile male, or by mechanically stimulating the uterine cervix and vulval region.

pseudopod: pseudopodium; a temporary cytoplasmic extension, used for locomotion by some leukocytes, and by amebae and other single-celled organisms. Somewhat similar structures are formed during phagocytosis.

pseudorenins: proteins that cleave renin substrates and release angiotensin peptides, but differ chemically from true renins. Most have lower pH optima.

pseudostratified: describes epithelia in which the cells appear to exist in layers, but are actually single layers of various sizes, all of which rest on basement membranes.

pseudouridine: 5-ribosyluracil; Ψ; a pyrimidine ribonucleoside, in which the sugar is attached via a C—C bond to the nitrogenous base. It is formed by post-transcriptional modification of uridine, and is a component of transfer RNAs.

pseudovirions: synthetic viruses, each composed of a protein coat from one virus and a nucleic acid from another. They are used in transduction studies.

psilocin: 4-hydroxy-*N*,*N*-dimethyltryptamine: a lysergic acid diethylamide (LSD)-like hallucinogen made in small amounts by the *Psilocybe mexicana* mushroom, and derived metabolically from psilocybin (which is present in greater amounts). It has been suggested that some human psychological disorders are caused by impaired tryptophan and serotonin metabolism that leads to formation of such amines.

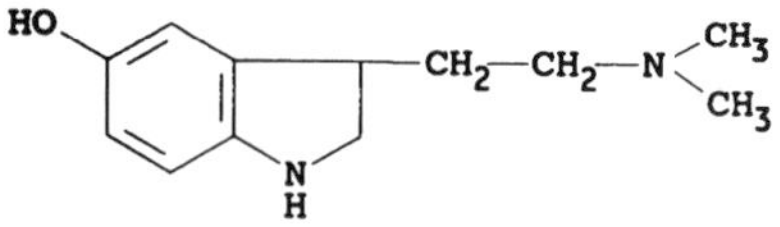

psilocybin: *O*-phosphoryl-4-hydroxy-*N*-*N*-dimethyltryptamine; *see* **psilocin**.

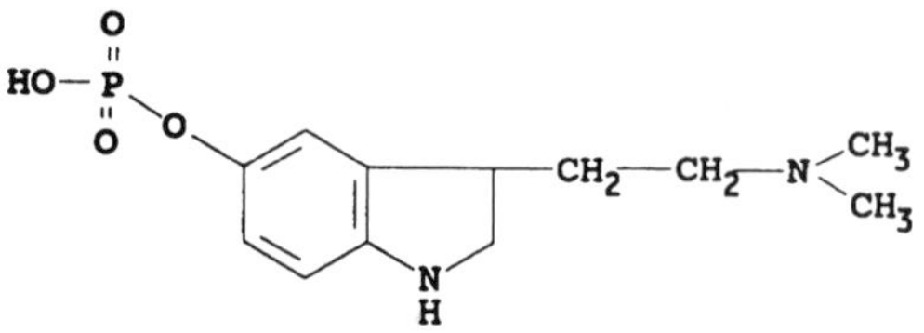

P site: peptidyl-tRNA binding site. When translation begins on a ribosome, the P site binds the initiating aminoacyl-tRNA complex (met-tRNA in eukaryotes and *f*-met-tRNA in prokaryotes). A second aminoacyl-tRNA then binds to the A site, and the amino acid moiety on the P site is transferred to the *N*-terminal of the second amino-acyl-tRNA; and the first tRNA is released. After the first peptide bond is formed, the dipeptidyl-tRNA is transferred to the P site for the next round of elongation.

psoralens: 6-hydroxy-5-benzofuranacrylic acid δ-lactone, chemically related phytoalexins made by *Psoralen coryfolia* and several other plants (including limes, cloves, celery, parsnips. parsley, and figs), and synthetic derivatives such as methoxsalen (Oxsoralen), 8-methoxypsoralen, and Trioxsalen (trimethyoxypsoralen). In the dark, they intercalate into DNA but do not form covalent bonds. After exposure to ultraviolet light, they form adducts with pyrimidine bases on one or both

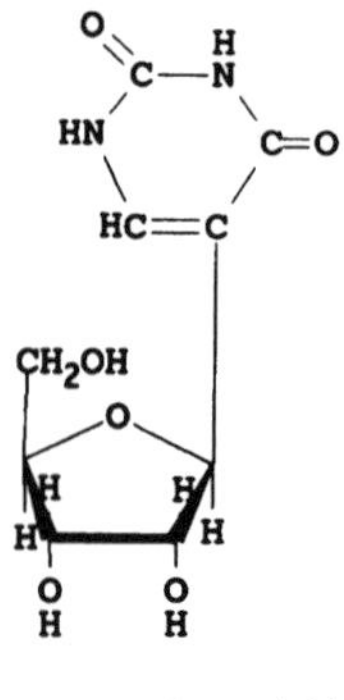

pseudouridine

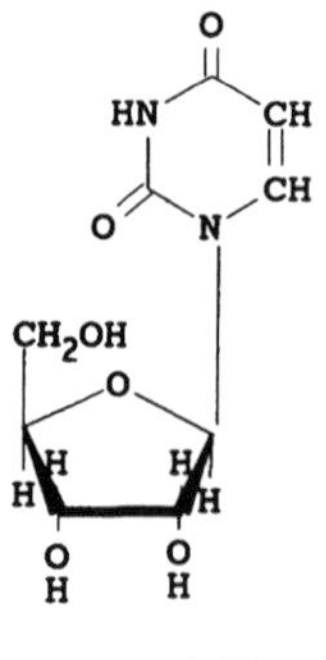

uridine

psoralen   8-methoxypsoralen   Trioxalen

strands, and inhibit DNA replication, after which they react with oxygen to form free radicals (oxygen singlets and superoxide ions). Small amounts are incorporated into "suntan lotions", to enhance ultraviolet light-stimulated melanin production and the transfer of the pigments from hair follicles to epidermal layers. Larger amounts are used both topically and systemically to treat vitiligo and other skin disorders; *see* also **PUVA**. They additionally alter lymphocyte distribution, augment the activities of suppressor types, and damage some others. These effects probably account for their ability to attenuate contact hypersensitivity. However, they can cause phototoxic dermatitis with blistering; and long-term use increases the risk for developing skin cancers. Moreover, they are absorbed into the bloodstream, can cause cataracts, and are metabolized to hepatotoxic derivatives.

psoriasis: a cutaneous disease in which cells proliferate excessively, keratinocytes become hyperactive, dull red or salmon-pink plaques covered with silvery scales form, and incompletely matured cells are shed from the epidermis. There is evidence for autoimmune involvement and genetic predisposition. Vitamin A derivatives and psoralens are used to treat the condition; *see* also **PUFA**.

PSP: (1) parathyroid secretory protein; (2) phenolsulfonphthalein; (3) porcine spasmolytic protein; *see* **trefoil proteins**.

P.S.P.: phenolsulfonphthalein.

PST: pancreastatin.

psychopathy: any mental disorder.

psychosis: any severe mental disorder in which comprehension of reality is distorted. The manifestations can include incoherent thinking, delusions, hallucinations, bizarre behavior, and catatonia. Several types (including paranoia and manic-depressive illness) have been described. Some are known to be caused by organic factors, and it is suspected that others are caused by defects that affect the kinds and amounts of neurotransmitters produced, neurotransmitter metabolism, and/or the distributions of neurotransmitter receptors.

Pt: platinum.

PTA: plasma thromboplastin antecedent; blood coagulation factor XII; *see* **coagulation**.

PTC: (1) phenylthiocarbamide, phenylthiourea; (2) plasma thromboplastin component.

pteridine: pyrimidine-4′,5′:2,3-pyrazine; a lipid-soluble component of plant pteridophores, butterfly wings, bird feathers, and some other pigmented structures. Pteridine obtained from foods is used to synthesize bihydro-

pteridine cofactors for tyrosine hydroxylase, tryptophan hydroxylase, and some other enzymes. *See* also **pteroic acid**.

pteridophores: xanthophores, erythrophores, and other chromatophores that contain pteridines and/or carotenes, and impart yellowish or reddish colorations.

pteroic acid: *p*-[(2-amino-4-hydroxy-6-pteridylmethyl)-amino]-benzoic acid; a food component used for folic acid synthesis.

pteroylglutamic acid: folic acid.

PTH: (1) parathyroid hormone; (2) phenylisothiohydantoin.

PTH peptides: *see* **phenylisothiocyanate**.

PTH-LP: PTH-rP: parathyroid hormone-like peptide: *see* **parathyroid hormone-like peptide**.

ptomaines: cadaverine, muscarine, neurine, putrescine, and related amino acid decarboxylation products made by bacteria, that cause some forms of food poisoning.

PTTH: prothoracicotropic hormone.

PTTX: PTX; *see* **pertussis toxin**.

PTU: propylthiouracil.

PTX: parathyroidectomy.

ptyalin: an obsolete term for salivary amylase.

Pu: purine.

pubarche: the first manifestations of sexual maturation, especially the first appearance of pubic hair.

puberty: (1) attainment of the ability to produce mature gametes; (2) the time period during which reproductive organs and secondary sex characteristics mature to adult forms; (3) the body changes associated with sexual maturation.

pudendum [**pudenda**]: the external genitalia, a term usually applied to female structures.

PUF-1: *see* **Pit-1**.

PUFA: psoralen-ultraviolet-vitamin A regime; a topical treatment for psoriasis. The vitamin promotes cell differentiation and inhibits proliferation. Psoralens exposed to ultraviolet light inhibit DNA synthesis and suppress some immune system responses.

puff: *see* **chromosomal puff**.

puffer fish: fugu fish; a fish eaten in Japan that must be carefully prepared because some of its organs contain tetrodotoxin.

pulmonary: pertaining to the lungs.

pulmonary emphysema: a disease in which dilation of pulmonary alveoli and destruction of some alveolar walls diminishes the surface area for respiratory gas exchange, and thereby impairs oxygen delivery and carbon dioxide removal.

pulse chase: techniques used to determine the times required for synthesizing specific substances, and for following metabolic pathways, in which amino acids, thymidine, or other precursors labeled with radioactive isotopes are presented for brief time periods, then removed and replaced by non-labeled compounds of the same kind, or with ones labeled with different isotopes.

pulsed field gel electrophoresis: PFGE; *see* **electrophoresis**.

punctate: having the appearance of points or dots, a term applied, for example to some skin eruptions. *See* also **melanophore index**.

punctuated equilibrium: the concept that large, functionally important genetic changes (macromutations) that can involve regulatory elements occur rapidly in geographically restricted locales, and that populations of individuals with genes that confer advantages expand and replace the native species of surrounding regions. *Cf* **gradualism**.

Punnett squares: diagrams used to predict and illustrate the genotypes of progeny when very large numbers of individuals of a species with known allele types are mated, no mutations or crossing overs occur, and inheritance follows patterns for random assortment. The female allele types are displayed horizontally above the square, and the male types vertically to the left. When both parents are homozygous, inheritance is fully predictable (since only one kind of allele is transmitted by each). When one or both are heterozygous, the diagrams represent the relative numbers of each kind of offspring predicted for a very large population (but not for any one mating, since it is not known which allele is carried by a given gamete). In the example shown, A and *a* represent dominant and recessive alleles, respectively for a single trait. The female is heterozygous (Aa), whereas the male is homozygous dominant (AA). *See* also **crossing over** and **genetic linkge**.

♂ ♀ →	A	a
A	AA	Aa
A	AA	Aa

pupa: a holometabolous insect in the developmental stage between the final larval instar and the imago (adult).

purines: Pu; 7*H*-imidazo[4,5-*d*]pyrimidine (shown below), and related substances; *see*, for example **adenine**, **guanine**, **xanthine**, **hypoxanthine**, **uric acid**, and methyl substituted compounds such as **caffeine**, **theophylline** and **theobromine**.

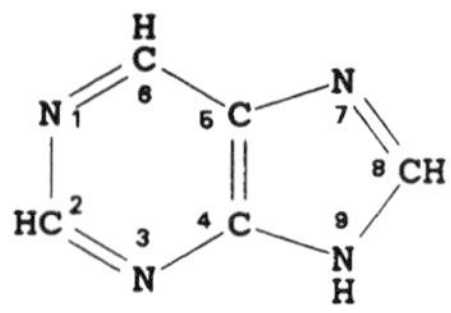

purine nucleosidases: enzymes that catalyze hydrolysis of *N*-ribosylpurines to free purines + ribose.

purine nucleoside phosphorylase: PNP; a trimeric enzyme in all nucleated cells composed of 32K subunits that acts on guanosine, deoxyguanosine, and inosine, and catalyzes reactions of the general type: purine nucleoside + Pi → purine + ribose-1-phosphate. Severe combined immunodeficiency is an autosomal recessive disorder in which mutant forms of the enzyme lead to accumulation of guanosine, deoxyguanosine, GTP, and deoxy-GTP. High levels of dGTP impair T lymphocyte functions by inhibiting ribonucleoside diphosphate reductase (an enzyme required for DNA synthesis).

purinergic: describes (1) neurons that synthesize and release adenine and other purines or purine derivative neurotransmitters; (2) effects mediated by those regulators.

Purkinje cells: a single row of very large neurons that forms the middle (Purkinje) layer of the cerebellar cortex. The dendrites and somas receive excitatory inputs from both climbing fibers (axons that originate in the contralateral inferior olive) and parallel fibers (granule cell axons), and also inhibitory ones from basket and stellate neurons. They convey inhibitory signals to deep cerebellar and lateral vestibular nuclei. *Cf* **Purkinje fibers**.

Purkinje effect: Purkinje shift; Purkinje phenomenon; increased sensitivity to short wave-lengths that occurs during scotopic vision and accounts for the brighter appearance of blue light under those conditions.

Purkinje fibers: specialized fibers within the heart that convey signals from the atrioventricular (A-V) node to ventricular muscle.

Purkinje shift: Purkinje effect.

puromycin: 3-(α-amino-*p*-methoxyhydrocinnamamido)-3-deoxy-*N*,*N*-dimethyladenosine; an antibiotic made by *Streptomyces alboniger*. It is an aminoacyl-tRNA analog that binds to ribosome A sites, forms peptide linkages with peptide chains, prematurely terminates translation, and promotes the release of nascent (uncompleted) peptide chains. It is used to arrest the growth of some neoplasms and as a laboratory tool for determining which cell responses require the synthesis of new proteins. *Cf* **cycloheximide**.

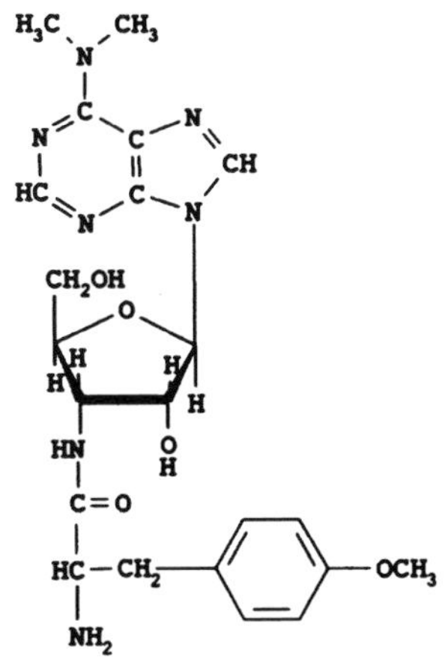

puromycin

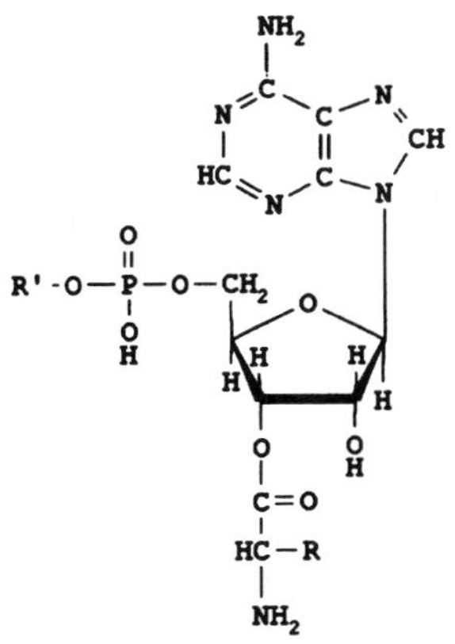

aminoacyl-tRNA

purple membrane protein: bacteriorhodopsin; a 26K retinal-containing protein that functions as a light-driven proton pump for oxidative phosphorylation in halobacteia.

purple phosphatase: the tartrate-resistant acid phosphatase (TRAP) made by, and used as a marker for osteoclasts.

purple protein: an iron-transporting protein secreted by the uterus of the pregnant sow.

purpura: the purple appearance of skin caused by small hemorrhages from dermal blood vessels. The condition occurs in individuals with allergic reactions, autoimmune diseases, or thrombocytopenia.

purpurin: (1) a 20K heparin binding protein released by cultured chick neural retinal cells; (2) neutral red; natural red; 1,2,4-trihydroxyanthroquinone; a dye used to stain nuclei, and to detect insoluble calcium salts within cells.

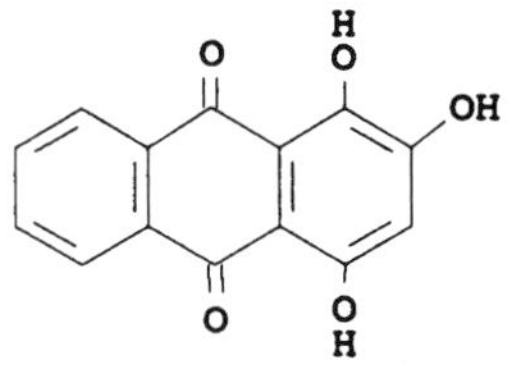

purulent: consisting of, containing, or contributing to the production of pus.

pus: an exudate formed during inflammatory reactions composed of living and dead leukocytes, cell debris, and protein-rich fluid.

putamen: a basal ganglia component that forms the external shell of the lenticular nucleus.

putrescine: 1,4-butanediamine; a DNA-binding metabolite formed in vertebrates and microorganisms via a reaction catalyzed by ornithine decarboxylase. It is a growth factor for some cell types in culture. An aminopropyl transferase catalyzes a reaction in which it combines with

S-(5-adenosyl)-3-methylmercaptopropylamine to yield spermidine. *See also* **polyamines** and **ptomaines**.

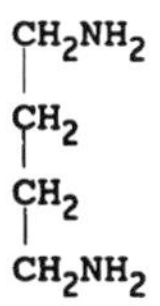

P value: a measure of the probability that the differences between the means for measured parameters do not exceed differences that could arise from random sampling of a common population. In some kinds of studies, a P value of $<.05$ is accepted as an indication that the difference could not occur by chance, and is therefore said to be statistically significant. For other studies, in which values of $<.01$ or $<.001$ are more appropriate, $<.05$ can be regarded as "probably significant".

PVN: paraventricular nucleus.

PWM: pokeweed mitogen.

Py: pyrimidine.

pycnosis: pyknosis; a form of cell degeneration that begins with nuclear condensation, and proceeds to nuclear destruction; *cf* **apoptosis**.

Pyd: pyridinoline: *see* **hydroxylsine**.

pyel-: pyelo-; a prefix that refers to the renal pelvis.

pyemia: septicemia; invasion of the bloodstream by microorganisms.

pyknosis: pycnosis.

pyle-: a prefix that refers to the hepatic portal vein; *cf* **pyel-**.

pylorus: the terminal region of the stomach that includes the smooth muscle of the pyloric sphincter, and the pyloric orifice that leads to the duodenum.

pyocyanine: 1-hydroxy-5-methylphenazinium hydroxide inner salt; a blue-green pigment made by *Pseudomonas aeruginosa* that is toxic to some microorganisms.

pyocin: bacteriocins made by *Pseudomonas aeruginosa*.

pyogenic: pus forming.

pyramid: (1) any pyramid-shaped anatomical structure; (2) specific components with this appearance in the medulla oblongata or kidney; *see* also **pyramidal cells**.

pyramidal cells: large, conical or pyramid-shaped neurons with small dendrites and large axons. They are the most prominent types in the cerebral cortex. Similar ones occur in the hippocampus.

pyramidal tracts: cerebrospinal tracts; nerve tracts that originate in cerebral cortex primary motor area pyramidal cells, descend to motor neurons, and mediate voluntary movements. Most cross in the pyramids of the medulla oblongata.

pyranose: a ring structure composed of one oxygen and six carbon atoms, assumed by glucose, galactose, and other aldohexose sugars in aqueous solutions. α-D-glucopyranose is shown. *Cf* **furanose**.

pyrazinamide: a synthetic nicotinamide analog that blocks the actions of NAD-dependent enzymes. It is used to treat tuberculosis, but the toxic effects can include liver damage, fever, gastrointestinal disturbances, and arthralgias. It can also precipitate acute attacks of gout by inhibiting uric acid excretion.

pyrazine: 1,4-diazine; a heterocyclic ring structure component of flavins, pteridines, and some other biologically important compounds.

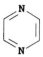

pyrenoids: small, starch forming bodies in some chloroplasts.

pyrethrins: jasmolins; insecticides obtained from pyrethrum flowers that exert DDT-like effects on neuron membranes and commonly invoke allergic reactions in humans. Pyrethrin-1 is 2,2-dimethyl-3-(2-methyl-1-propenyl)cyclopropanecarboxylic acid 2-methyl-4-oxo-3-(2,4-pentadienyl)-2-cyclopenten-1-yl ester.

pyrethrum flowers: preparations of *Pyrethrum cineraiefolium* and *P. coccineum* chrysanthemum flowers, used as insecticides, to treat scabies infections, and (in veterinary medicine) to kill ectoparasites. *See* also **pyrethrins**.

pyrexia: fever; heat stroke.

pyribenzamine: PBZ; *see* **tripelennamine**.

pyridine: a component of tobacco and some foods. It is used as a solvent for electrophoresis, in chromatography, and in industrial processes. Toxic amounts can invoke gastrointestinal disorders, and also liver and kidney damage. Pyridine components of NAD^+ and $NADH^+$ coenzymes are hydrogen and electron acceptors and donors.

pyridine nucleotides: *see* **NAD+** and **NADH**.

pyridinoline: *see* **hydroxylysine**.

pyridostigmine bromide: 3-(dimethylcarbamyloxy)-1-methylpyridinium bromide; an acetylcholinesterase inhibitor used to treat myasthenia gravis, and to reverse the effects of curare-like muscle relaxants.

pyrethrin-1

pyridoxal: a form of vitamin B_6; *see* **pyridoxal phosphate** and **pyridoxine**.

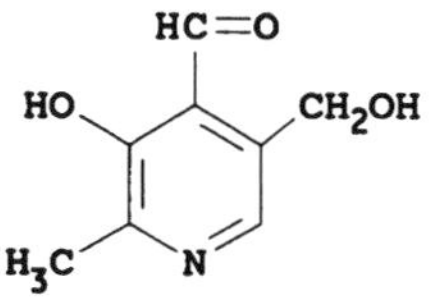

pyridoxal kinase: an enzyme that catalyzes formation of pyridoxal-5-phosphate from pyridoxal + ATP.

pyridoxal-5-phosphate: PLP: 3-hydroxy-5-(hydroxymethyl)-2-methylisonicotinaldehyde; a coenzyme synthesized from pyridoxal via a reaction catalyzed by pyridoxal kinase. PLP participates in glycogenolysis by binding to glycogen phosphorylase and donating protons to inorganic $H_2PO_4{}^{2-}$. The protonated inorganic phosphates then attach to sugar moieties at the ends of glycogen chains. When glucose-1-phosphates are released, the glycogen chains are shortened by one sugar moiety, and the coenzyme molecules regain their protons. PLP aldehyde groups activate some enzymes by forming Schiff bases with their lysine amino groups at specific loci. When linked to deaminases, PLP converts to pyridoxamine by accepting amino groups: α-amino acid + PLP → α-keto-acid + pyridoxamine phosphate. The aminated enzymes can then donate amino groups to other α-keto acids. PLP is also a coenzyme for tryptophan metabolism, in which it attaches to kynureninase (which catalyzes cleavage of kynurenine to anthranilic acid, and 3-hydroxykynurenine to 3-hydroxyanthranilic acid). It is additionally required for the functions of tryptophan, tyrosine, glutamate, and other decarboxylases (and therefore for neurotransmitter biosynthesis), and for conversion of methionine to cysteine. It contributes to some racemization reactions, and it modulates the actions of steroid hormones by interacting with steroid-receptor complexes.

pyridoxamine: one form of vitamin B_6; the others are pyridoxal and pyridoxine (pyridoxol). *See* also **pyridoxal phosphate**.

pyridoxamine-5-monophosphate: PMP; the amide formed when pyridoxal-5-phosphate accepts an amino group in amino acid transferase reactions.

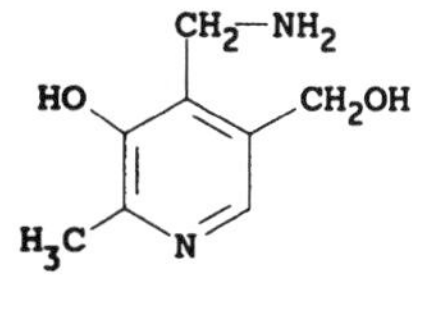

pyridoxamine

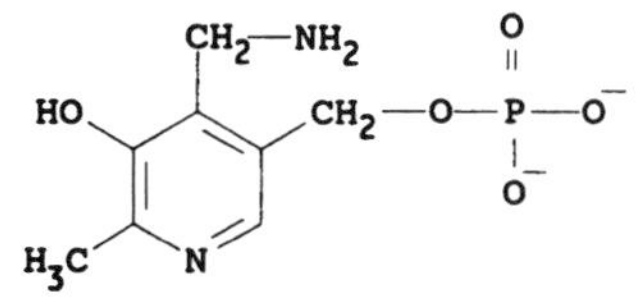

pyridoxamine-5-monophosphate

pyridoxine: pyridoxol; 5-hydroxy-6-methyl-3,4-pyridinemethanol; one form of vitamin B_6. (The others are pyridoxal and pyridoxamine.) The hydrochloride is used in vitamin pills, and is present in cereals, liver, and other foods. *See* also **pyridoxal phosphate**. The effects of vitamin B_6 deficiency include seborrhea-like skin lesions, glossitis, stomatitis, and peripheral neuritis. Convulsions that develop in severe cases are attributed to subnormal gamma aminobutyric acid (GABA) levels. Excessive amounts can invoke neuritis. They also decrease the effectiveness of L-DOPA treatment for Parkinson's disease by accelerating its peripheral conversion to dopamine.

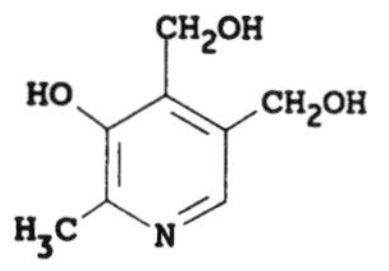

4-deoxy-pyridoxine: a competitive inhibitor of pyridoxine-dependent reactions, used to invoke vitamin B_6 deficiency in laboratory animals.

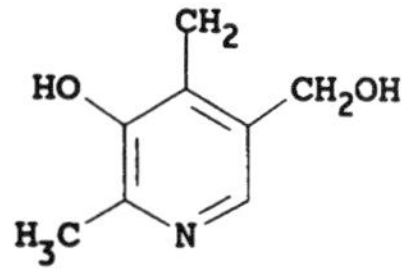

pyridoxol: pyridoxine; *see* also **pyridoxal phosphate**.

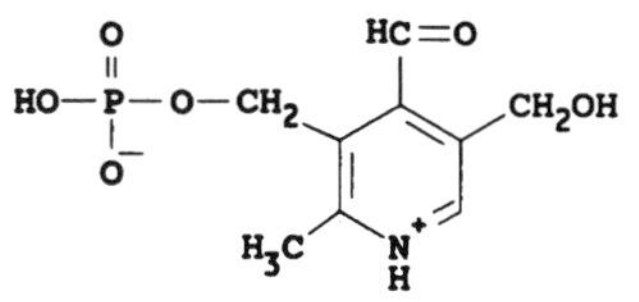

PLP 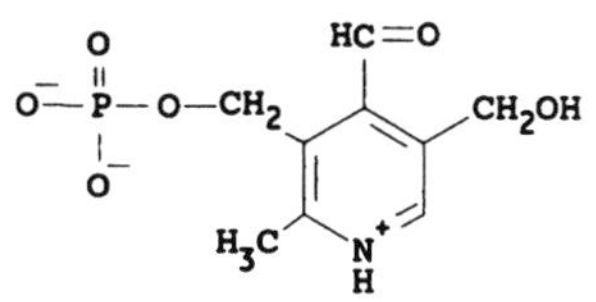   deprotonated PLP 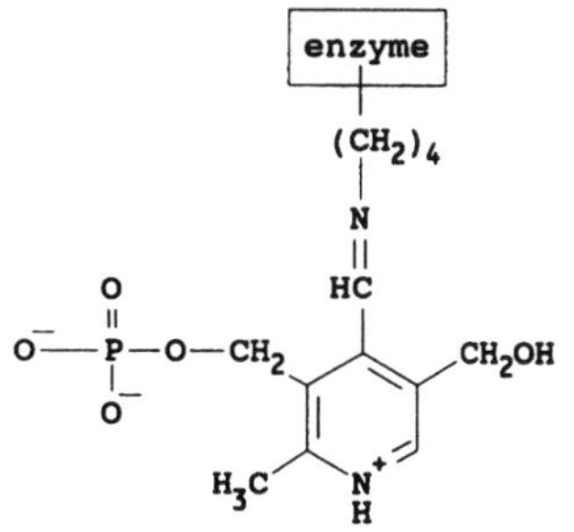   PLP-enzyme Schiff base

pyrilamine: mepyramine; *N*-[(4-methoxyphenyl)methyl]-*N'*,*N'*-dimethyl-*N*-2-pyridinyl-1,2-ethanediamine; an H$_1$-type histamine receptor antagonist used to treat allergies.

pyrimethamine: Chloridin; Daraprim; 2,4-diamino-5-(*p*-chlorophenyl)-6-ethylpyrimidine; an antibiotic that synergizes with sulfonamides and is effective against malaria parasites.

pyrimidines: Py; 1,3-diazine (shown) and its derivatives; *see also* **guanine**, **thymine**, and **uracil**. Pyrimidine biosynthesis in mammals requires **CAD** (a multifunctional enzyme complex, *q.v.*). Aspartate transcarbamoylase catalyzes: carbamoyl phosphate + aspartate → *N*-carbamoylaspartate. Dihydroorotase hydrolyzes the product to dihydroorotate, which is then oxidized by NAD$^+$-dependent dihydroorotate dehydrogenase to orotate, the precursor of orotidylate and other nucleotides.

pyro-: a prefix (1) meaning heat. *p*- is used for amino acids with internal bonds formed by dehydration reactions, as in *p*-Glu (pyroglutamic acid).

pyrogallol: 1,2,3-benzenetriol; a catecholamine-*O*-methyltransferase (COMT) inhibitor that is also used to remove oxygen from air. It is absorbed by skin; and large amounts can invoke renal and hepatic damage, hemo-

lysis, methemoglobinemia, circulatory collapse, and convulsions.

pyrogens: fever-causing agents; *see* for example **interleukin-1** and **prostaglandin E$_2$**.

L-pyroglutamic acid: *p*-Glu; 5-oxo-L-proline; a component of thyrotropin releasing hormone (TRH) and some other biologically active peptides. It is used *in vitro* to resolve racemic mixtures of amines.

L-*trans*-pyrollidine-2,4-dicarboxylic acid: a selective inhibitor of glutamate uptake.

pyrolysis: heat-mediated degradation.

pyronine B: 3,6-*bis*(diethylamino)xanthylium chloride; a biological stain for bacteria, molds, and ribonucleic acids.

pyronine Y: 3,6-*bis*-(dimethylamino)xanthylium chloride; a dye used in alkaline solutions to stain bacteria. In 2M MgCl$_2$ at pH 5.7, it is specific for undegraded RNA.

pyronine B

pyrophosphate: P-P; a byproduct of reactions such as ATP → cAMP + P-P, and UTP + glucose → UDPG + P-P, and an inhibitor of bone mineralization. It is used as a buffer in some systems.

pyrophosphatases: enzymes that rapidly hydrolyze pyrophosphate to orthophosphate.

pyrophosphorolysis: reactions of the general type $R_1—O—R_2 + P—P → R_1OH + P—O—R_2$.

pyrophosphorylases: enzymes that catalyze reversible reactions of the kind shown for pyrophosphorolysis, for example glucose-1-phosphate uridyltransferase, which catalyzes the reaction: UDPG + P-P $\rightleftharpoons$ UTP + glucose-1-phosphate.

pyrrole: a heterocyclic ring component of heme, chlorophyll, many pigments, and some other compounds.

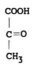

pyruvic acid {pyruvate}: 2-oxanopropionic acid (2-oxanopropionate): the end-product of glycolysis. It can be converted to lactate (for example in contracting skeletal muscle), to acetyl coenzyme A (in mitochondria), to glucose (in the liver), to alanine (in transaminase reactions), and to ethanol by some microorganisms.

$$\begin{array}{c} COOH \\ | \\ C=O \\ | \\ CH_3 \end{array}$$

pyruvate carboxylase: an enzyme that catalyzes: pyruvate + CO_2 + GTP → oxaloacetate + GDP + Pi, the first step in the gluconeogenesis pathway that converts pyruvate to glucose. Glucagon is the major stimulatory regulator.

pyruvate dehydrogenase: an enzyme complex that catalyzes the overall pathway: pyruvate + NAD^+ + coenzyme A → acetyl coenzyme A + NADH + H^+ + CO_2. The cofactors include thiamine pyrophosphate (for oxidative decarboxylation of pyruvate), lipoamide (for transfer of the derived acetyl groups to coenzyme A), and FAD (to regenerate the oxidized form of lipoic acid). Insulin activates pyruvate dehydrogenase by promoting its dephosphorylation, and AMP is another activator. Glucagon inhibits by activating a protein kinase. The products exert negative feedback controls.

PYY: peptide YY.

PZ: pancreozymin; *see* **cholecystokinin**.

PZC: perphenazine.

PZI: protamine zinc insulin.

Q

Q: (1) glutamine; (2) ubiquinone.

q: the long arm of a chromosome; *cf* **p**. A number after the q (as in q21) indicates the position of a gene on the long arm.

Q_{10}: a temperature coefficient for determining how much the rate of a process increases under standard conditions for each $10°C$ rise in temperature, expressed as a multiple of the initial rate. For example, if $Q_{10} = 2$, the rate doubles for a $10°$ rise.

QA: quisqualic acid.

Qa antigens: class 1-like mouse proteins on the surfaces of some T lymphocytes, small numbers of B lymphocytes, and liver cells, encoded by genes located close to the major histocompatibility complex (H-2). They may be recognized by natural killer cells. The types are identified by numbers (Q-1 through Q-10).

Qa genes: mouse genes adjacent to the histocompatibility complex that code for Qa antigens.

Qβ: a bacteriophage with a single + (plus) strand circular RNA genome that infects *E.coli* and is used to produce large quantities of messenger RNAs. It directs synthesis of viral proteins, and can serve as a template for the synthesis of - strands to form double-stranded RNAs. A replicase then promotes synthesis of new + strands.

Q bands: stripes observed when chromosomes are stained with fluorochrome dyes such as quinacrine dihydrochloride and viewed under ultraviolet light. The bright ones correspond roughly to dark G bands, but are useful for studying Y chromosomes and detecting polymorphisms not easily observed with G banding procedures.

Q_{CO_2}: the rate of carbon dioxide production per unit time under standard conditions, usually expressed as microliters per milligram dry tissue per hour.

Q coenzyme: coenzyme Q: *see* **ubiquinones**.

Q enzyme: enzyme Q; α-glucan branching glycosyltransferase; an enzyme used in glycogen biosynthesis (and obtained commercially from potatoes) that promotes branching by catalyzing transfers of parts of 1,4-glycosan chains from 4 to 6 positions.

QH_2-cytochrome c reductase: an enzyme complex on inner mitochondrial membranes that contains cytochromes b and c_1, and iron-sulfur proteins. It catalyzes transfers of electrons from reduced coenzyme Q to cytochrome c.

QNB[^{3}H]: tritium-labeled quinuclidinyl benzoate; a ligand used to identify muscarinic type acetylcholine receptors; *see* **quninuclidine**.

q.n.s.: quantity not sufficient.

Q_{O_2}: the rate of oxygen use under standard conditions, usually expressed as microliters per milligram dry tissue per hour.

Q protein: a lambda phage protein essential for phage gene expression.

QRS: the component of an electrocardiograph associated with ventricle depolarization.

quadrigeminal: in four parts. The corpora quadrigemina of the midbrain is composed of right and left superior, and right and left inferior colliculi.

quadriplegia: paralysis and loss of sensations in all four limbs; *cf* **paraplegia**.

quadrivalent: describes (1) associations of four homologous chromatids; *see* **meiosis**; (2) cations with four positive charges or anions with four negative ones.

quail: a small galliform bird used for studies of embryonic development and immune system functions. The cells are easily distinguished from chicken types when grafted to chicken embryos. *Coturnix coturnix japonica* is the species most commonly used.

quaking locus: a segment of mouse chromosome #17 that codes for factors required for survival of male embryos, and for regulation of myelination and spermiogenesis. Several kinds of mutations (spontaneous, or induced by radiation or with ethyl nitrosourea) are used for genetics studies, since the manifestations are easily recognized. Non-lethal types can cause sterility, and/or large tremors and other severe neuromuscular disorders.

quantal response: an all-or-none reaction that either does or does not occur. A stimulus stronger than an effective one invokes no greater response.

quantasomes: photosynthetically active particles of chloroplast grana.

quantum yield: the numbers of photons required for photosynthetic production of one oxygen molecule.

quasidiploid: having two sets of chromosomes, but an abnormal distribution; for example when one chromosome of a homologous pair is replaced by a different type that has undergone duplication.

quasidominant: pseudodominant; describes recessive traits that appear to be inherited as dominant types. They are expressed in homozygous recessives, when dominant alleles have been deleted, and in some progeny of those with deletions mated with heterozygotes.

quaternary structure: *see* **proteins**.

quazepam: 7-chloro-5-(2-flurophenyl)-1,3-dihydro-1-(2,2,2-trifluoroethyl)-2*H*-1,4-benzo-diazepine-2-thione; a diazepam type hypnotic and sedative.

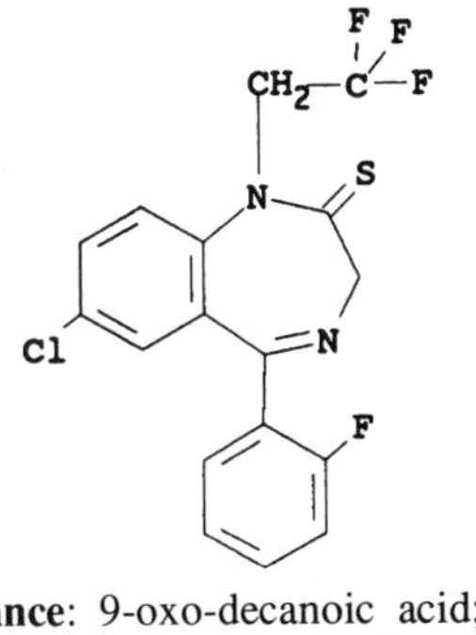

queen substance: 9-oxo-decanoic acid; a pheromone secreted by the mandibular glands of queen honey bees of *Apis mellifera* and related species that inhibits development of worker bee ovaries, attracts males to the queen, and inhibits queen cell formation. Purported beneficial effects of "royal jelly" which contains it, have not been substantiated.

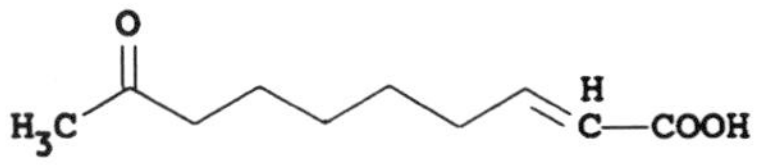

quenching: decrease in intensity, or loss of a property, a term that usually refers to changes in fluorescence.

quercetin: meletin; sophoretin; 2-(3,4-dihydroxyphenyl)-3,5,7-trihydroxy-4*H*-1-benzopyran-4-one; a yellow bioflavinol plant pigment, usually present as a glycoside such as quercitrin or rutin. It inhibits histamine release, and is used to decrease blood capillary fragility; but high concentrations are mutagenic. It additionally inhibits tyrosine kinases and phosphodiesterases, and also lactate transport and glycolysis in Ehrlich tumor cells.

quercitrin: quercitroside; quercetin-3-L-rhamnose; a glycoside of **quercetin** (*q.v.*).

Questran: a trade name for cholestyramine.

quiescent: not active; describes cells in the G_o phases of their cycles.

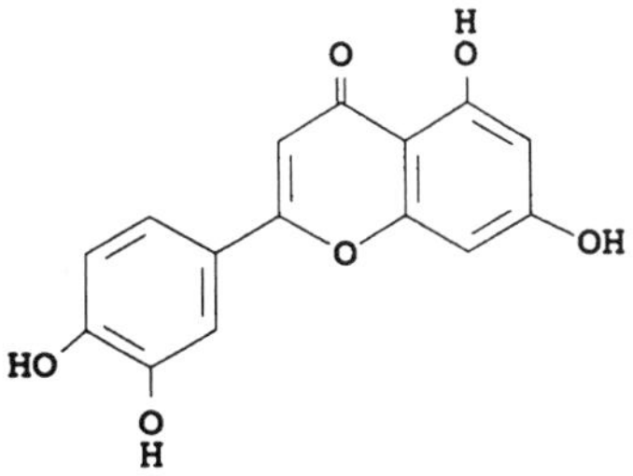

quercitin

Quin 2: 2-[(2-amino-5-methylphenoxy)methyl]-6-methoxy-8-aminoquinolone-N,N,N′,N′-tetraacetic acid. The tetrapotassium salt is an indicator highly specific for Ca^{2+} that undergoes a shift in its ultra-violet spectrum and fluoresces when it binds Ca^{2+}; *see* also **Quin 2-AM**.

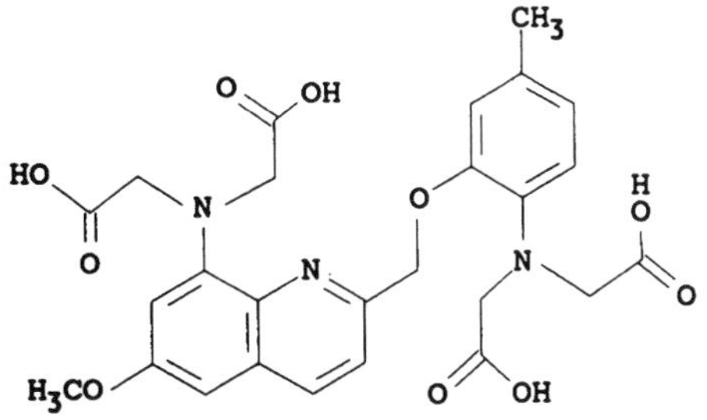

Quin 2-AM: tetrakis(acetoxymethyl)-8-amino-2-[(2-amino-5-methylphenoxy)methyl]-6-methoxyquinoline-N,N,N′,N′-tetraacetate; a lipophilic ester of **Quin-2** (*q.v.*) that crosses plasma membranes and is rapidly hydrolyzed to the free, active form. It is used to monitor intracellular Ca^{2+} concentration changes.

quinacrine: mepacrine; N^4-(6-chloro-2-methoxy-9-acridinyl)-N^1,N^1-diethyl-4-pentanediamine; an agent that inhibits D-amino acid oxidases by competing for FAD, and also inhibits phospholipase A_2s. The hydrochloride (Atabrin) arrests the growth of some neoplasms. Although it kills some parasites, it is no longer used to control malaria because it is toxic, and is ineffective against some forms of the disease. When injected into the uterus, it promotes sclerotic occlusion of Fallopian tubes, and has been used to achieve sterilization. Since it fluoresces under ultraviolet light, the hydrochloride is employed as a probe for acetylcholine-activated synaptic membranes. *See* also **Q-bands**.

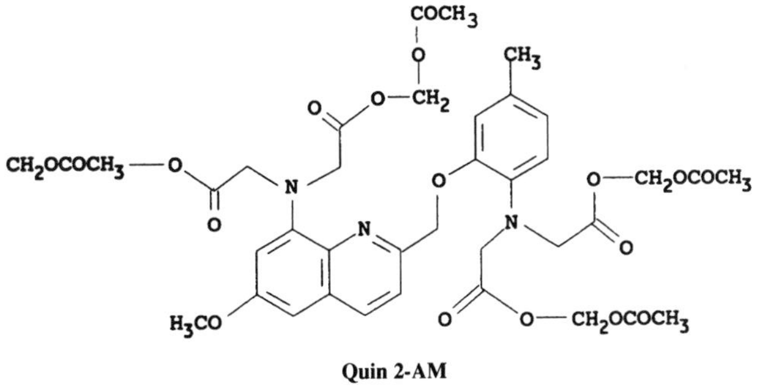

Quin 2-AM

615

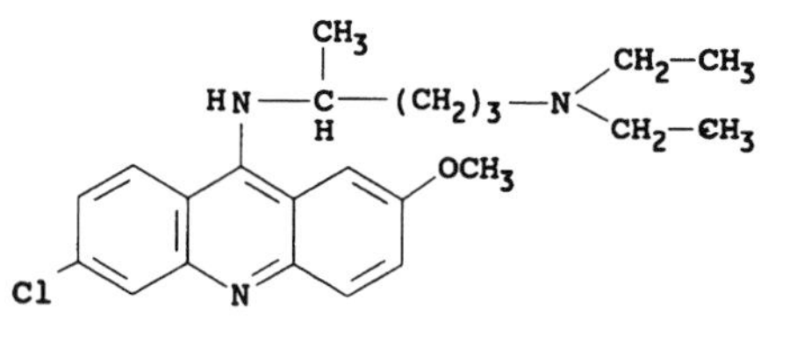

quinacrine

quinaldic acid: quinaldinic acid; xanthenic acid; quino-line-2-carboxylic acid; a tryptophan degradation product, made by oxidation of kynurenic acid, and excreted to urine. It is used as a reagent for determinations of copper, zinc, and uranium.

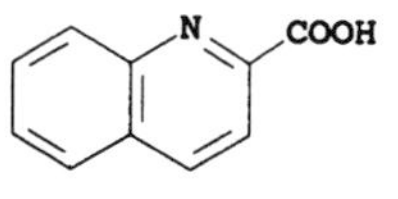

quinaldine blue: pinacyanol chloride; 1,1'-diethyl-2,2'-trimethinequinocyanine chloride; a biological stain for chromosomes.

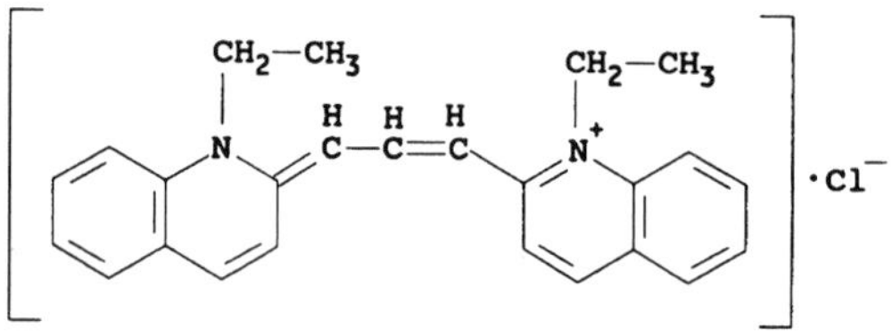

quinaldine red: 2-(p-dimethylaminostyryl)quinoline ethiodide: an indicator, colorless at pH 1.4 and red at pH 3.0.

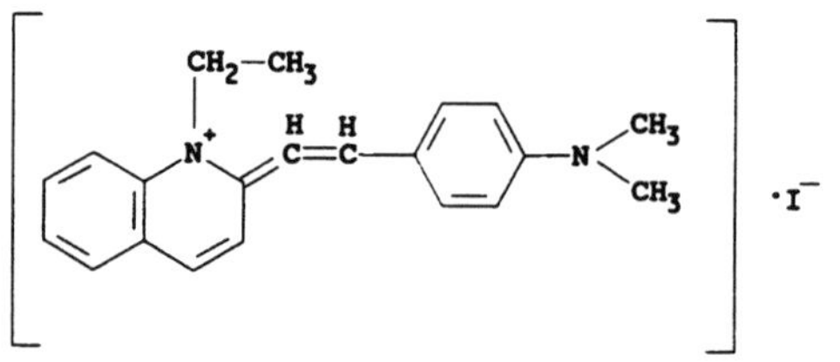

quinbolone: 1-dehydrotestosterone 17-cyclopent-1'-enyl ether; a long-acting anabolic steroid stored in, and slowly released from adipose tissue.

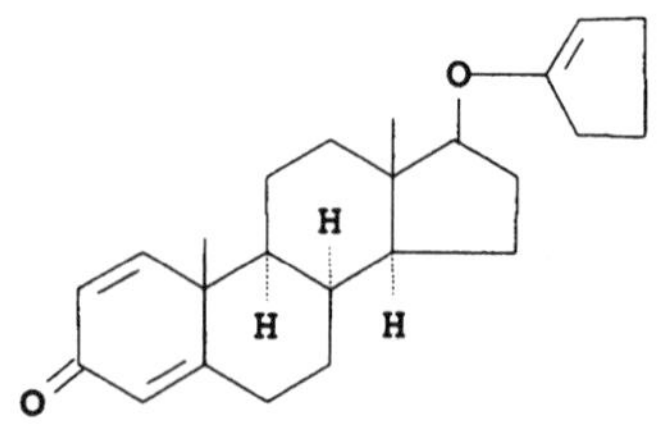

quinestrol: 3-(cyclopentyloxy)-19-nor-17α-pregna-1,3, 5(10)-trien-20-yn-17-ol; a long-acting synthetic estrogen stored in, and slowly released from adipose tissue.

quinethazone: Hydromox; Aquamox; 7-chloro-2-ethyl-1,2,3,4-tetrahydro-4-oxo-6-quin-azolinesulfonamide; an orally effective, long-acting loop diuretic that promotes Na$^+$ excretion, but does not inhibit carbonic anhydrases and has little effect on chloride excretion. It is used to

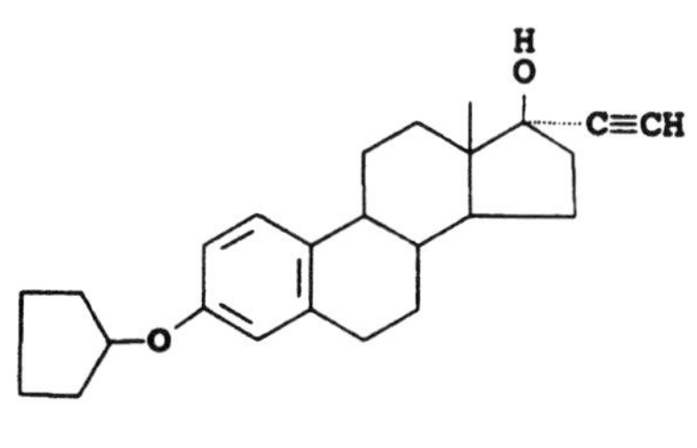

treat some forms of hypertension, and also edema caused by cardiac, renal, or hepatic dysfunction.

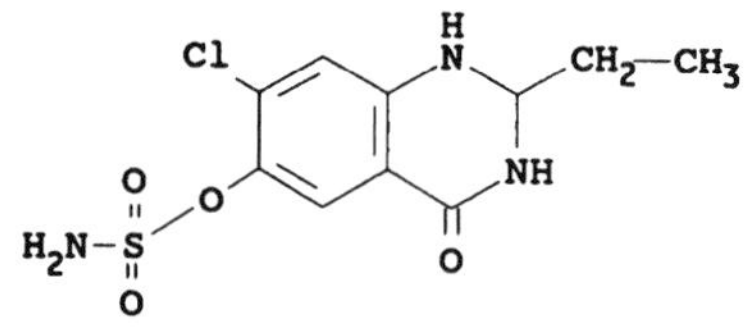

quinestrol

quinethazone

quingestrone: 3-(cyclopentoxy)pregna-3-5-diene-20-one; an orally effective, long-acting synthetic progestin.

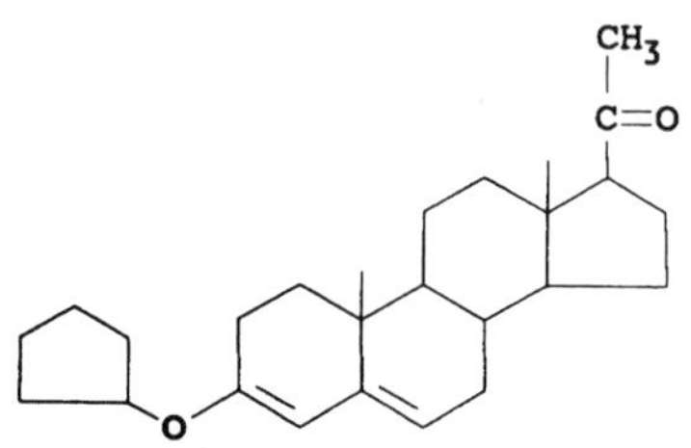

quinic acid: kinic acid; 1,3,4,5-tetrahydroxycyclohexane carboxylic acid; an alkaloid in *Cinchona* bark, tobacco and carrot leaves, apples, pears, plums, peaches, and other plant components that is reversibly oxidized to quinone.

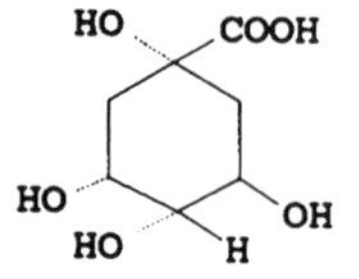

quinidine: 6-methoxycinchonan-9-ol; quinine dextro-isomer; an alkaloid made by several *Cinchona* species. It is a myocardial depressant that slows conduction along Purkinje fibers, It is used to treat some cardiac dysrhyth-mias, but can cause thrombocytopenia. It also has anal-gesic, anti-malarial, antipyretic, and oxytocin-like properties.

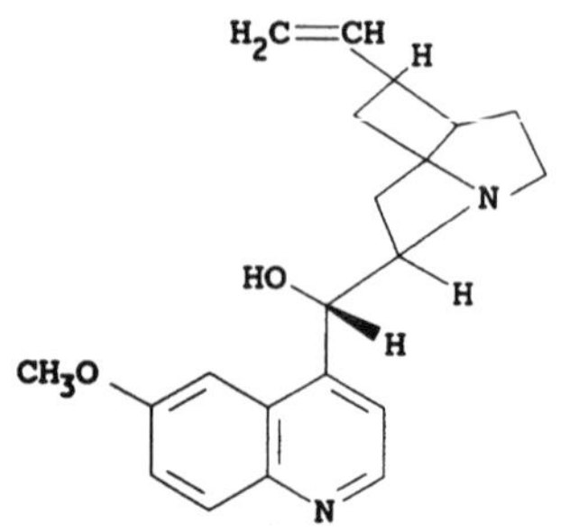

quinine: 6′methoxycinchonan-9-ol; an alkaloid chemically and biologically related to quinidine, made by several *Cinchona* species, and used to treat malaria. It also stimulates insulin secretion and can invoke hypoglycemia.

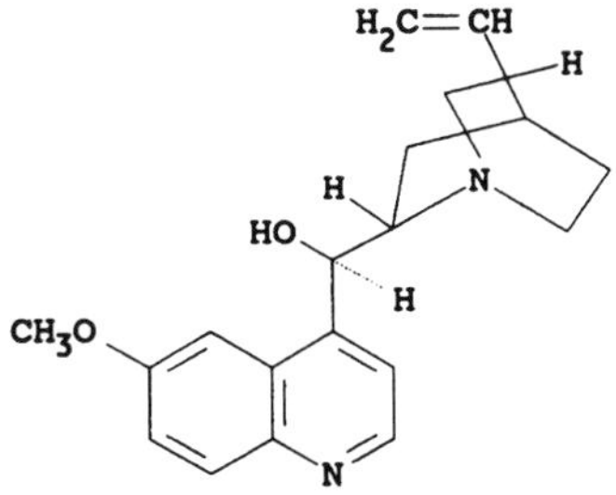

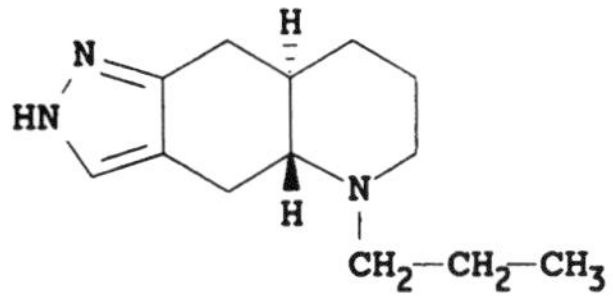

quinpirole

quinuclidine

quinolinic acid: 2-3-pyridine dicarboxylate; an endogenous neurotoxin derived from tryptophan that selectively kills gamma aminobutyric acid (GABA)-secreting neurons in some brain regions, and is a weak agonist for NMDA (*N*-methyl-D-aspartate) type excitatory amino acid receptors. It is implicated in the etiology of Huntington's disease.

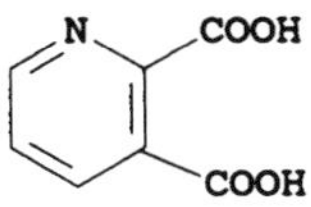

quinupramine: 10,11-dihydro-5-(3-quinuclidinyl)-5*H*-dibenz[*b*,*f*]azepine; an analog of **imipramine** (*q.v.*), with similar biological properties.

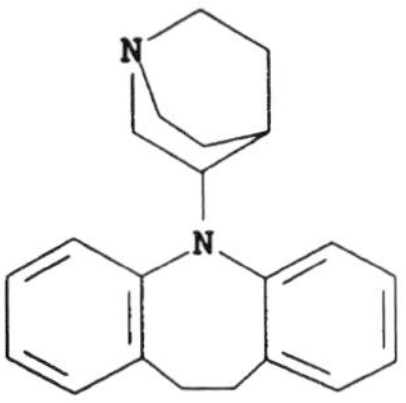

quinolones: **nalidixic acid** (*q.v.*), and several related synthetic antibiotics that block DNA synthesis and transcription by binding to DNA gyrase.

quinone: 2,5-cyclohexadiene-1,4-dione; a compound that undergoes reversible oxidation-reduction. It converts hemoglobin to methemoglobin and acts on other Fe^{2+}-containing substrates. Ubiquinone is a dimethoxy-carbonyl derivative in electron transport chains.

quinoxalinediones: CNQX (6-cyano-7-nitroquinoxaline-2,3-dione), DNQX (6,7-dinitroquinoxaline-2,3-dione), and related excitatory amino acid antagonists that act preferentially on quisqualate receptor subtypes, and can protect against excitatory amino acid toxicity in the brain (but do not affect glycine binding sites). NBQX (2,3-dihydroxy-6-nitro-7-sulfamoyl-benzo(F)quinoxaline), is more potent than the others.

quinpirole: LY17155; *trans*(-)4a*R*-4,4a,5,6,7,8,8a9-octahydro-5-propyl-1*H*-pyrazole-[3,4-*g*]-quinoline; a selective D_2-type dopamine receptor agonist.

quinuclidine: 1,4-ethylenepiperidine; the benzilate ester is used as a muscarinic type acetylcholine receptor antagonist, and (when labeled with tritium) a ligand for identifying and isolating those receptors.

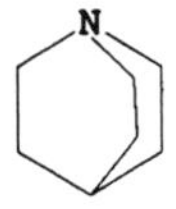

quipazine: a serotonin receptor antagonist most effective for $5HT_3$ types, that also binds $5-HT_{1B}$ and $5-H_2$ forms. It can elevate serotonin levels by acting presynaptically to augment its release, and by inhibiting postsynaptic uptake into nerve terminals. Some effects are attributed to $GABA_B$ type aminobutyric acid and muscarinic receptor antagonism, and to release of substance P and somatostatin. Others have been linked with histamine receptor stimulation, where it is more potent for H_2 than H_1 subtypes. Its appetite suppressing effects may be secondary to ones on mood.

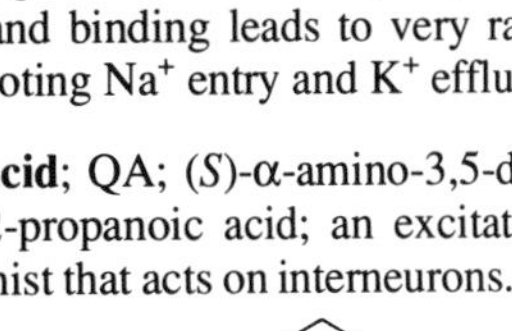

quisqualate receptors: excitatory amino acid receptors with much higher affinities for quisqualic acid than for kainate. Ligand binding leads to very rapid depolarization by promoting Na^+ entry and K^+ efflux.

quisqualic acid: QA; (*S*)-α-amino-3,5-dioxo-1,2,4-oxadiazolidine-2-propanoic acid; an excitatory amino acid receptor agonist that acts on interneurons. Very low levels

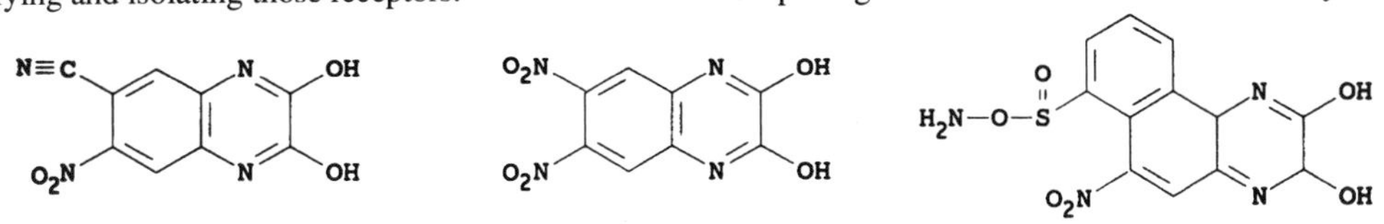

CNQX

DNQX

NBQX

quinoxalinediones

hyperpolarize neurons stimulated by glutamic and aspartic acids, moderate ones depolarize, and toxic concentrations destroy the cells. QA also blocks cysteine transport.

quisqualic acid

quotidian: recurring on a daily basis.

q.v.: *quo vide*; which see.

R

R: (1) arginine; (2) a member of a group of closely related chemical structures; for example, R in R-COOH can be any fatty acid moiety; (3) a regulatory subunit of an enzyme; (4) Roentgen; (5) the gas constant (1.987 calories per mole, 8.4144 joules per mole, or 0.82 liter atmospheres per degree per mole); (6) a plasmid that confers bacterial resistance to one or more antibiotics.

R: defines a three-dimensional configuration; *see* **stereoisomerism**.

r: (1) correlation coefficient; (2) a ring chromosome, used after a number or type as in Xra; (3) reproductive potential.

ρ: the Greek letter rho, used for (1) correlation coefficient; (2) electrical charge density; (3) mass density.

R 5020: RU 5020; *see* **promegestone**,

RA: retinoic acid.

Ra: radium.

rab: *ras*-related mammalian proto-oncogenes that code for at least 19 small (p21), prenylated guanine nucleotide binding proteins which function in endocytosis, exocytosis, and intracellular trafficking of molecules. They bind with lower affinities to inner faces of plasma membranes than most other members of the superfamily, and are not known to invoke transformation. Rab4p attaches to early endosomes, is regulated in part via p34^{cdc2} catalyzed phosphorylations, and is believed to account for the endocytosis arrest associated with cell division. Rab7p binds to late endosomes, and rab5p localizes to luminal fluid phases.

rabbits: several species of small, long-eared, furry animals, distinguished from rodents by their dentition. They deliver relatively mature young after long gestation periods. *Oryctolagus cuniculus* is the species most widely used in laboratory studies.

rabbit test: *see* **Friedman test** for pregnancy.

rac: genes that code for 58K protein kinases related to kinases A and C. They are amplified in some tumor types.

race: a phenotypically and/or geographically distinct subspecies or division of a subspecies. It can be defined by biochemical or immunological properties that do not affect the external appearance.

racemases: enzymes that promote formation of racemic mixtures by catalyzing enantiomer interconversions.

racemic mixture: a solution that contains both D and L enantiomorphs of an organic compound. If the isomers are present in equal amounts, the solution is optically inactive (even if each member is active when present alone).

racemose: possessing several dilated parts; resembling a bunch of grapes.

rachitic: affected with, caused by, or related to rickets.

RACKS: 30-33K receptor activated proteins that translocate kinase C isozymes to plasma membranes.

rad: radiation absorbed dose; a unit of ionizing radiation equivalent to 100 ergs per gram or 0.1 joules per kg.

radiation: divergence from a center. The term can describe a morphological characteristic, or refer to light, heat, ionizing radiation, or sound.

radiation chimera: an experimental animal in which a cell, tissue, organ or other component is destroyed by ionizing radiation and replaced by a corresponding one from another animal. Donor hemopoietic stem and some other cell types proliferate in radiated hosts.

radiation sickness: syndromes caused by exposure to high dosages of radiant energy. Early manifestations include nausea, vomiting, and diarrhea. Hair loss, blood cell depletion, high susceptibility to infections, and sterility soon follow. Rapidly proliferating cells (for example in bone marrow, gastrointestinal mucosa, gonads, thymus, and skin) are highly vulnerable to injury and account for most of the effects. Since many kinds of cancer cells are killed, whereas normal types can be restored after the treatments are completed, damaging but sublethal doses are administered to patients with neoplastic cells that cannot be surgically removed.

radical: an ion group, such as PO_4^{-3}, HCO_3^-, or SO_4^{2-} that functions as a unit in chemical reactions. *See also* **free radical**.

radical scavengers: substances that bind free radicals with high affinity, and can thereby protect against oxidative damage.

radioactive atoms: atoms that spontaneously disintegrate to stable types with different numbers of protons, and give off radiant energy (alpha particles, beta particles, positrons, and/or gamma rays). They are used to label molecules for metabolic studies and analytical procedures, and to destroy cells for therapeutic or experimental purposes. High concentrations are mutagenic.

radioactive decay: disintegration of unstable atom nuclei, accompanied by emission of energy (*see* **radioactive atoms**). The half-life (t/2) is the time period during which one-half of the unstable atoms are expected to disintegrate. It varies with the atom type, and can range from a fraction of a second to thousands of years.

radioactive iodine: [125]I or ^{131}I; *see* **iodine**.

radioautography: *see* **autoradiography**:

radioimmunoassays: RIAs: procedures for measuring substances present in low concentrations. The component of the test material, which serves as an antigen, is incubated under standardized conditions with a complex that contains the same antigen, labeled with a radioactive marker such as ^{125}I linked to its specific antibody. Since the labeled antigen dissociates from its complex, it can be displaced by the unlabeled component of the specimen. Then, either the amount of labeled antigen displaced, or the amount still linked to the complex is measured, and the quantity of test substance is determined from curves constructed with a series of predetermined antigen concentrations. In some cases, an enzyme such as horseradish peroxidase is used to visualize the molecules; *see* **ELISA**. The methods can be applied to steroids, cyclic nucleotides, and other compounds that do not directly bind antibodies, but attach to specific kinds of proteins. The values obtained with radioimmunoassays do not necessarily match those from bioassays, since different parts of the test substance molecules are involved.

radioimmunodiffusion: highly sensitive techniques for identifying antigens or antibodies in which one of the components is labeled with radioactive atoms; *see* **immunodiffusion**.

radioimmunoelectrophoresis: *see* **electrophoresis**.

radioisotopes: unstable atoms with the same numbers of protons and electrons as their stable counterparts, but different numbers of neutrons; *see* **radioactive decay**. The conventional representation is a superscript with the atomic weight enclosed in a bracket, followed by the symbol for the element, as in ^{131}I, but symbols followed by superscripts (as in I[131]) are also used. Generally, the chemical and most physical properties are almost identical to those of stable types. However, because of marked differences in mass, tritium (^{3}H) behaves differently from the common form of hydrogen in biological systems.

radiomimemtic chemicals: compounds such as nitrogen mustards that invoke mutations and other damage comparable to the kinds caused by ionizing radiation.

radionuclide: the nucleus of a radioactive atom.

radioreceptor assays: immunological methods similar to radioimmunoassays, but based on displacement of hormones from hormone-receptor complexes by components of the specimens. The major advantage is high sensitivity, but the procedures are expensive, time-consuming, and difficult to perform; and cross-reactivity can be a problem. One application is determination of circulating hCG (human chorionic gonadotropin) levels within days after possible conception in women whose health can be severely threatened by pregnancy, or when the presence of a trophoblastic tumor is suspected. In some procedures, luteinizing hormone (LH) binds to the same receptors.

radioresistance: low vulnerability to the damaging effects of radiation, a term applied to bacteria that can excise and replace ultraviolet light-induced thymine dimers.

radium; Ra; a radioactive element (atomic number 88, atomic weight 226.05) with a half-life of 1622 years. It emits alpha particles and disintegrates to radon. Inhalation, ingestion, or body surface exposure can invoke lung cancer, osteogenic sarcomas, skin lesions, and blood dyscrasias. Radium salts are applied to restricted sites to destroy some kinds of neoplastic cells.

radon: Rn; a gaseous radioactive element (atomic number 86, atomic weight 222) with a half-life of 3.83 days), formed when radium undergoes radioactive decay. It emits alpha particles, gamma rays, and products that also emit beta particles. Radon can accumulate in poorly ventilated buildings.

raf: proto-oncogenes that code for 72-74K proteins, including Raf-1, a cytoplasmic serine-threonine protein kinase induced by GM-CSF (granulocyte-macrophage colony stimulating factor), interleukins 2 and 3 (but not 4), and some other mitogens. It is overexpressed in some kinds of tumor cells. In unstimulated normal types, an *N*-terminal region maintains Raf-1 in an inactive form until phosphorylated by Ras-GTP, kinase C isozymes, or tyrosine kinases. The proteins cooperate with *ras* products to promote cell proliferation. *V*-Raf is a related oncogene product that is truncated and constitutively active. A related oncogene in mice infected with 3611 murine sarcoma virus codes for a p75$^{gag\text{-}raf}$ protein, and one in chickens infected with avian carcinoma virus MH2 codes for p100$^{gag\text{-}raf}$. The viral forms can invoke transformation even when *ras* functions are blocked. *See* also **Sos**.

raffinose: melitose; melitriose; β-D-fructofuranosyl-*O*-α-D-galactopyranosyl-(1→6)-α-D-glucopyranoside; an edible non-reducing trisaccharide in sugar beets, cottonseeds, and some other plant foods.

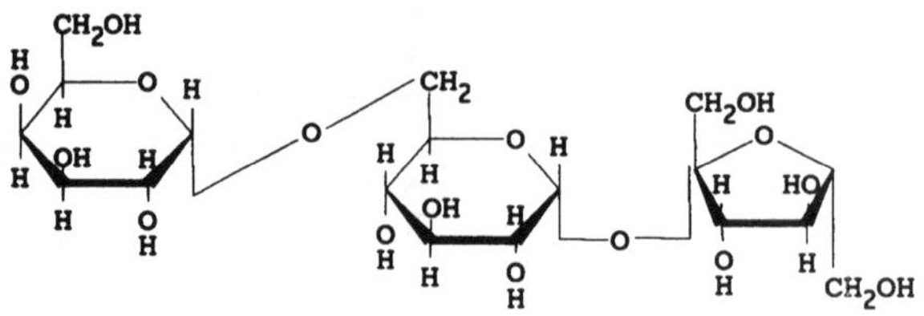

raffinose

Raji cells: lymphoblastoid cells derived from a patient with Burkitt's lymphoma with defects that affect β2-microglobulin synthesis. They lack surface immunoglobulins, but have Fcγ, complement 1, complement 2, and C1q receptors. Their ability to displace ligands from radiolabeled aggregated IgG type immunoglobulin binding sites is used to detect immune complexes.

ral: a *ras*-related mammalian proto-oncogene that codes for a guanine nucleotide binding p21 protein which attaches to the inner faces of plasma membranes, but does not invoke transformation.

ramus: a branch, for example of a blood vessel, lymphatic vessel, neuron, or nerve tract.

ran: proto-oncogenes that code for ras-related 25K guanine nucleotide binding proteins that function as negative regulators of cell division by binding p34^{cdc2} and other proteins (including some mammalian types as well as Pim-1 made by *S. pombe*).

Rana: a genus of frogs that includes *Rana pipiens* (the common leopard frog) and *Rana catesbiana* (the bullfrog), as well as species used for special characteristics (such as *Rana temporaria* and *Rana esculenta*).

ranatensins: several species specific tachykinins isolated from frog skin with the common *N*-terminal sequence -Gly-His-Phe-Met-NH$_2$. When used without qualification, the term usually refers to the type made by *Rana pipiens*, in which the tetrapeptide amide sequence is preceded by *p*Glu-Val-Pro-Gln-Trp-Ala-Val-. In ranatensin C from *Rana catesbiana*, the tetrapeptide is preceded by *p*Glu-Thr-Pro-Trp-Ala-Thr-.

random coils: configurations assumed by most polypeptide chains in aqueous solutions after treatment with 8M urea, 6M guanidine, or other agents that disrupt covalent bonds.

random mating: systems in which gametes with all chromosome combinations normal for the species have equal opportunities to engage in fertilization. Genetic diversity is thereby maintained in large populations.

random walk: the path followed by a cell or particle when there are no impediments to its movements.

random X inactivation: *see* **Lyon hypothesis**.

ranitidine: Zantac; *N*-[2-[[[-5-[(dimethylamino)methyl]-2-furanyl]methyl]thio]ethyl]-*N*′-methyl-2-nitro-1,1-ethenediamine; an H$_2$-type histamine receptor antagonist used to decrease gastric HCl production and thereby promote healing of peptic ulcers.

rap: *ras*-related mammalian proto-oncogenes. The 88K Rap-1 product binds to upstream regulatory components of many genes. It functions in some cases as an activator, and in others as a silencer of transcription. The genes affected include some that code for glycolytic pathway enzymes and others needed to make ribosomal proteins. In neutrophilic leukocytes, it associates with cytochrome *b* and accelerates superoxide ion generation. It also shortens chromosome telomeres, possibly by affecting conformations and augmenting susceptibilities to attacks by teleomerases. It is phosphorylated by kinase A. Its ability to suppress *ras*-invoked transformation and promote reversion to normal phenotypes is attributed to its GAP (GTPase) activity, and possibly also to competition for some ras binding sites. However, when overexpressed in *S. cerevisiae*, it accelerates meiotic recombination and promotes gene conversions.

rapamycin: an immunosuppressant under investigation for treating autoimmune diseases and preventing organ transplant rejection. Although chemically unrelated to **FK 506** (*q.v.*), it complexes with some FK 506 binding proteins (*see* **FKBPs** and **immunophilins**), and inhibits

rapamycin

rotamases different from the enzymes affected by cyclosporin A. Its ability to block IgE immunoglobulin-mediated exocytosis in mast cells may be related to influences on a common signal transduction pathway. However, unlike FK 506 (which acts early in cell cycles and inhibits calcineurins involved in T lymphocyte activation), it inhibits the proliferation of hematopoietic cells mediated by interleukins 2, 3, and 4, erythropoietin, granulocyte-macrophage stimulating factor (GM-CSF) and some other cytokines, and also blocks insulin-stimulated p70 S6 (but not p185) kinase activity and some other growth factor effects associated with phosphorylations.

raphe: a seam; usually a visible site where bilateral structures have joined.

raphe of brainstem: a region in the pons that contains high levels of serotonin, and substantial amounts of histamine and other regulators. The neurons communicate with other brain regions, including some that control hypothalamic releasing hormone secretion.

rapid eye movements: REM; rapid, involuntary movements of the eyeballs that occur normally during REM sleep, deep anesthesia, when observing moving objects, and when moving subjects fix on stationary objects. *See* also **nystagmus**.

RARs: a set **retinoic acid receptors** (*q.v.*).

rare bases: ribothymidine, 5,6-dihydrouridine, 5-ribosyluridine (pseudouridine), inosine, 1-methylinosine, 1-methylguanosine, dimethylguanosine, and other purine and pyrimidine nucleoside phosphates in transfer and some ribosomal (but not messenger) RNAs. They are formed posttranscriptionally from the more common nitrogenous bases.

RAS: (1) renin-angiotensin system; (2) reticular activating system.

ras: proto-oncogenes that code for p21, prenylated guanine nucleotide binding proteins with GTPase activity that insert into inner faces of plasma membranes, and contribute to signal transduction. *H-ras*, *K-ras*, and *N-ras* are related oncogenes of Harvey rat sarcoma, Kirsten murine sarcoma, and neuroblastoma viruses. Normal *ras* genes play essential roles in the proliferation of hematopoietic and some other normal cell types, in spermatogenesis, and probably also in oocyte maturation, neuronal differentiation, and the functions of post-mitotic neurons. At least some effects involve phospholipid turnover, diacylglycerol generation, and the activities of inositol-phosphate 3-kinase and kinase C isozymes. The genes can be direct targets for chemical carcinogens; and some forms with point mutations interact with other genes to invoke transformation. Altered H-ras proteins have been identified in benign skin papillomas, and in malignant carcinomas of the skin, mammary glands, and liver. Mutant K-ras proteins occur in many pancreatic, colon, and lung cancers, and mutant N-ras types in neuroblastomas and breast cancers, and the bone marrows of individuals with acute myeloid and lymphatic leukemias. The transforming potential has been linked with persistent activation unaffected by normal regulatory processes, because of loss of the GTPase activity or accelerated GTP exchange for GDP. Gene amplification without mutation has been demonstrated for H-ras in some human urinary bladder cancers, and for K-ras in some human lung, bladder and ovarian cancers, and in some mouse lung cancers. Cooperation with genes that code for platelet derived and epidermal growth factors (PDGF and EGF), and/or other mitotic stimulants, appears to mediate malignancy in some cases, whereas tumor suppressor gene deletions are evidently important in others. RAS1 and RAS2 are related, somewhat larger (40K) proteins that activate adenylate cyclase in *S. cerevisiae* (but not in mammals), at least one of which must be present to accomplish cell division. *Ras* related genes include *rab*, *ral*, *rho*, and also *rap-1*, which suppresses *ras*-induced transformation.

rat: when used alone, any of several small rodents of the genus *Rattus* (*q.v.*). The "**naked mole rat**" (*Heterocephalus glaber*) (*q.v.*) is an ectothermic mammal with no body fur or sweat glands and very little subcutaneous fat, that lives in colonies in which behavior patterns have been likened to those of insects. The kangaroo rat is a small marsupial.

rate-limiting enzymes: major determinants of the reaction rates of metabolic pathways over wide substrate concentration ranges. They are usually present in limited amounts, and commonly provide the sites for hormonal control. Regulators can affect transcription of the associated genes, messenger RNA stability, translation rates, protein degradation, intracellular translocations, posttranslational modifications that alter the activities, and/or the synthesis and activation of inhibitors. *See* also **rate-limiting reactions**.

rate-limiting reactions: steps in biochemical pathways that determine the rates for end-product production. The amounts of **rate-limiting enzymes** (*q.v.*) in active forms are major control factors; but some reactions are regulated by substrate availability or product removal.

Rathke's pouch: an evagination of the ectoderm of the roof of the mouth of a vertebrate embryo. Further growth of the ectoderm leads to formation of a vesicle that separates from the mouth and gives rise to major components of the adenohypophysis. In most vertebrates (but not in birds or in whales and a few other mammals), the pouch contacts the floor of the third ventricle of the developing embryonic brain, an association essential for formation of a pars intermedia.

rat kangaroo: *Potorous tridactylis*; a small marsupial used for genetics studies. It has a small number of easily distinguishable chromosomes.

Rattus: a genus of rodents that includes black (*R. rattus*), and Norway (*R. norvegicus*) rats. Most laboratory strains (for example Wistar, Fischer, and Sprague-Dawley albino, and Long-Evans hooded) are *R. norvegicus* descendants.

Raudixin: the powdered whole root of *Rauwolfia*; *see* **reserpine**.

Rauwolfia serpentina: a small tropical shrub used for medicinal purposes; *see* **reserpine** and α-**yohimbine**.

Rb: rubidium.

R bands: chromosome regions that stain with dyes after heat treatment in phosphate buffers. R banding is used to identify gene loci.

RBC: red blood cells; *see* **erythrocytes**.

Rb **gene**: *see* **retinoblastoma** and **osteosarcoma**.

RBPs: retinol binding proteins.

RCC1: regulator of chromatin condensation; a protein that binds DNA, interacts with *ran* proto-oncogene products, recognizes incompletely replicated DNA, and prevents cell cycle progression from S to mitosis if replication is not completed. The human type has 421 amino acids. Very similar proteins are made by other vertebrates. Related types include pim-1 and PRP20, made, respectively by *S. pombe*, *S. cerevisiae*, and BJ1 made by *Drosophila*. Although abundant in dividing cells, RCC1 levels do not vary directly with the cell cycles. The proteins may additionally contribute to formation of nuclei after chormosome separation, initiation and termination of transcription, pre-messenger RNA splicing, and mRNA export to the cytoplasm.

RCE: retinoblastoma control elements.

rDNA: (1) recombinant DNA. When inserted into plasmids, it can undergo massive amplification in the oocytes of amphibians, some insects, and some other animal types; (2) ribosomal DNA, the DNA that directs synthesis of rRNA.

reabsorption: usually, transport of substances derived from the blood back to the bloodstream, for example return of renal tubular fluid components to peritubular capillaries, or of bile components to hepatic portal vessels. *Cf* resorption.

reactive blue 2: 1-amino-4-[[4-[[4-chloro-6-[[3(or4)-sulfophenyl]amino]-1,3,5-triazin-2-yl]amino]-3-sulfophenyl]amino]-9,10-dihydro-9,10-dioxo-2-anthracenesulfonic acid; an antagonist for ATP ativated ion channels.

reading frame: sets of nucleotide triplets that direct insertion of specific amino acid types into nascent peptide chains during translation; *see* also **open reading frame**.

reading frame shift: a change in the positions of some messenger RNA nucleotide bases, caused by deletion or insertion of one or two nucleotides. If translation can proceed through and beyond the shift site, abnormal proteins may be synthesized. For example, the sequence ..AUA-GGA-CAG-UUA... codes for ...-Ile-Glu-Gln-Leu... Loss of the first G shifts the triplets to ..AUA-GAC-AGU-AA.., which codes for ..Ile-Asp-Ser-... Loss of the first A causes use of UAG, the "stop" codon that terminates translation. Since the genetic code is degenerate, some frame shifts have lesser effects.

reading error: insertion of a wrong amino acid during translation.

readthrough: (1) transcription that continues beyond the usual termination signal, caused, for example by failure of the RNA polymerase to recognize the termination signal; (2) translation that continues beyond the usual termination point.

reagin: an IgE type immunoglobulin that mediates immediate hypersensitivity reactions.

recapitulation theory: the concept that embryonic development in higher animals passes through short, sequential phases during which structures resembling those of evolutionary precursors appear, and are replaced by ones resembling those of more modern ancestors. Although some embryonic structures roughly conform, the "ontogeny recapitulates phylogeny" concept is no longer accepted in its original form.

receptivity: in females with estrous cycles, acceptance of the sexual advances of a male. The behavior is estrogen-dependent, and is manifested during periovulatory phases of the cycles. *Cf* **proceptivity**.

receptor: a cell component that binds a hormone or other regulator with high affinity and specificity, and thereby contributes to initiation of responses.

receptor-gated ion channels: receptor operated ion channels; ROC; plasma membrane channels whose opening (and/or closing) is regulated by hormones, neurotransmitters, or other ligands. *Cf* **voltage-gated ion channels**.

receptor-mediated endocytosis: endocytosis *(q.v.)* initiated by the binding of a specific ligand (such as ferritin, an LDL, or a hormone) to its receptor on a cell surface. The ligand-receptor complex is incorporated into a vesicle and internalized, after which its components usually dissociate. Some receptors are recycled to the

reactive blue 2

membranes; others are degraded; *see* also **down regulation**.

receptor operated ion channel: ROC: *see* **receptor gated ion channel**. The acronym ROCC refers to receptor operated calcium ion channels.

receptor potential: (1) the electrical properties of a target cell plasma membrane; (2) changes in that potential invoked by effective stimuli.

receptosomes: endosomes; intracellular transport vesicles formed during receptor-mediated endocytosis. The internal pH (usually around 4.5-5.0), facilitates dissociation of the ligands from their receptors. The vesicles then translocate to the Golgi, after which some endosomes transfer both components to lysosomes for degradation (*see* also **down regulation**). Other endosomes send only ligands to lysosomes, whereas receptors are recycled to plasma membranes. A third type sends both ligands and receptors to exocytotic vesicles for recycling.

recess: a small hollow or space.

recessive genes: genes whose phenotypic expression is realized only in homozygotes; *cf* **dominant genes**.

recidivation: recurrence, for example of a diseased state, or of addictive or other abnormal behavior patterns.

Recklinghausen's disease: neurofibromatosis.

Recklinghausen's disease of bone: osteitis fibrosa cystica.

recombinant DNAs: rDNAs; synthetic deoxyribonucleotide polymers composed of DNA segments from two different sources, made by cleaving DNA molecules at specific sites with restriction endonucleases, and joining the derived segments with ligases. rDNAS with easily controlled promoters are incorporated into plasmids and used to direct the synthesis of large quantities of associated messenger RNAs and their protein products.

recombinant inbred strain: an animal strain obtained by mating members of two different inbred strains.

recombination: (1) crossing over; exchange of DNA segments by adjacent chromosomes during meiosis; (2) any change in chromosome makeup that results from exchange of segments from one DNA for those of another.

recon: the smallest DNA unit capable of recombination.

recoverin: a 23K protein, present in rod and cone photoreceptors in amounts 1/250 those of rhodopsin and related pigments, and also in pineal glands. It functions in photoreception and receptor stabilization. During darkness, cyclic guanosine monophosphate (cGMP) maintains Na^+ ion channels in partially open states (*see* also **transducins**). Calcium ions then enter via Ca^{2+} channels (and are extruded more slowly via Na^+/Ca^{2+} exchange). When the cytoplasmic Ca^{2+} levels rise sufficiently, recoverin binds Ca^{2+} and is inactivated. Light indirectly accelerates cGMP hydrolysis and closes the channels. When Ca^{2+} levels fall sufficiently (because entry, but not efflux, is blocked), recoverin dissociates from Ca^{2+}, and

then promotes "recovery" of the dark current by activating the guanylate cyclase. It is again inactivated when the Ca^{2+} concentrations return to the steady state darkness levels.

recrudescence: reawakening, resurgence; reappearance; (1) restoration of reproductive capability and the associated body changes in seasonal breeders whose organs undergo atrophy during quiescent periods; (2) reappearance of a diseased state after a remission.

recruitment: enlisting of several similar entities to accomplish a response, for example spatial summation in the nervous system, or formation of sufficient numbers of cohort follicles to achieve adequate estrogen levels during ovarian cycles; *cf* **selection**.

rectal glands: organs located at the posterior ends of the gastrointestinal tracts of some species that contribute to water and electrolyte balance.

rectus: straight.

red muscle: skeletal muscle that appears red because it has a good blood supply and is rich in myoglobin. It contracts more slowly than white muscle, and is more resistant to fatigue.

red nuclei: bilateral ovoid neuron clusters in the midbrain that contribute to extrapyramidal system functions.

redox potential: oxidation-reduction potential; reduction potential; the electromotive force (EMF) generated when a solution that initially contains 1M concentrations of both oxidized and reduced forms of a compound is connected via an agar bridge to another that contains 1M H^+ in equilibrium with hydrogen gas at 1 atmosphere. The potential is negative for strong reductants such as NADH (with lower affinities for electrons than H_2), and positive for strong oxidants.

5α-reductases: enzymes that reduce steroids to their 5α derivatives by transferring hydrogens and electrons from NADPH + H^+. The reactions are irreversible under cell conditions. 5α-dihydrotestosterone (DHT) binds more effectively than testosterone to most androgen receptors. Its formation is essential for development of the external genitalia in male mammalian embryos, and for many other androgen actions. Testosterone is a major inducer of the enzymes (which also act on progesterone and other substrates). *Cf* 5β-**reductases**.

5β-reductases: enzymes that reduce steroids to their 5β derivatives by transferring hydrogen atoms and electrons from NADPH + H^+. The reactions inactivate some hormones; but *see* 5β-**dihydrotestosterone**.

20α-reductases: enzymes that reduce progesterone and other steroids to their 20α derivatives, and thereby contribute to hormone inactivation.

reduction: gain of electrons; *see* **oxidation-reduction reactions**.

reduction division: cell division in which diploid parent cells give rise to haploid progeny; *see* **meiosis**.

Reed Sternberg cells: Sternberg Reed Cells; Hodgkin cells; giant CD30$^+$ cells with multilobed or multiple nuclei and large nucleoli, in individuals with Hodgkin's disease.

reflectosomes: chromatophores in the skin of some fishes and other poikilothermic vertebrates that contain purine pigment plates. When exposed to light in the visible spectrum, they impart a white or iridescent appearance. Melanocyte stimulating hormones are major regulators of their functions in some species.

reflex: an unlearned, stereotyped response to a stimulus.

reflex ovulator: induced ovulator; a female in which ovarian follicle maturation is accomplished by endogenous mechanisms, but ovulation requires mating-associated stimuli. Rabbits, cats, and ferrets are among the animal types that normally display this form of control. *Cf* **spontaneous ovulators**.

refraction: bending, for example of light rays passing through a medium.

refractive index: the ratio of light velocity in a vacuum to its velocity in a specified medium.

refractory period: the *absolute* refractory period is the time period during which a neuron or other excitable cell that has been stimulated cell cannot respond to another stimulus (usually because it is depolarized). Repolarization then begins, and sensitivity is gradually recovered during the *relative* refractory period. Before it is completed, the cell responds to stimuli of greater intensity than are required in the "resting" state.

regeneration: restoration of an organ or organ part that has been lost. Examples include re-establishment of normal cell numbers in the liver after hepatic injury in mammals, and replacement of severed limbs in some amphibians.

Regitine: a trade name for phentolamine.

regression: (1) return to an earlier (usually less mature) state; (2) the tendency to re-establish parameter values to levels formerly most prevalent in a population; or the tendency for progeny to acquire characteristics closer to the population average than to those of parents with very high or very low values; (3) the statistical relationship between a dependent variable (Y, something that is measured, such as height) and a selected independent variable (X, for example age). **Linear regression** is a procedure for deriving the most appropriate straight line for the slope of a graph when Y is plotted against X.

regression coefficient (ρ): a statistical measure of the relationship between two variables (*see* **regression**, definition 3). A consistent increment in one directly proportional to an increment in the other yields a coefficient of +1 (perfect positive correlation); and a consistent decrement in the first as the second rises yields a coefficient of −1 (perfect negative correlation). Neither positive nor negative values provide information on causes and effects. A coefficient of 0 indicates no consistent association between the values of the two parameters.

regulator gene: a gene that controls the expression of other genes, for example by directing formation of a repressor or activator; *cf* **structural gene**.

regulatory enzymes: enzymes whose activities determine the rates of biochemical pathways. Some directly catalyze rate-limiting reactions; others control the activities of other enzymes.

regulatory sequences: DNA segments that control the expression of one or more structural genes. *See* also **operators, promoters**, and **enhancers**.

regulatory subunit: a component of a dimeric or multimeric enzyme that controls the activity. For example, the R subunit of kinase A inhibits the catalytic subunit.

regulon: a set of noncontiguous genes controlled by a common regulator gene.

Reifenstein's Syndrome: several X-linked sex differentiation disorders in human males with 46XY chromosome patterns. The manifestations can include hypospadias, incompletely fused scrotums, cryptorchism, undeveloped Wolffian duct-derived accessory reproductive organs, and gynecomastia. Typically, androgen production is subnormal, but gonadotropin levels are high. Some individuals make adequate amounts of androgens, but have too few or defective androgen receptors.

reiterated genes: multiple copies of genes clustered in tandem on a chromosome, for example genes that direct the formation of ribosomal RNAs, transfer RNAs, and histones.

rejection: *see* **immunological rejection**.

rel: c-rel proto-oncogenes universally expressed in oocytes, embryos, and some mature cell types that code for cell-type specific transcription activators, and for some morphogens, and are essential for embryonic development. Phosphorylation affects the activities of the proteins, and their translocations to nuclei. One mammalian type is the 65K subunit of NF-Kb; and a rel-associated 40K protein is functionally related to IkB (an NF-Kb inhibitor). V-rel oncogene products are mostly truncated mutant forms with weaker transcription activation properties that invoke transformation, in part by blocking c-rel functions. One type, made by a turkey reticuloendotheliosis virus (strain T) rapidly invokes fatal leukemia in birds.

relaxed form of hemoglobin: R hemoglobin; it avidly binds oxygen. Reversible shifts in peptide chain positions yield T (tense) hemoglobin, which delivers O_2 to tissue cells.

relaxin: RLX; hormones with disulfide linked A and B chains that are chemically related to proinsulin and insulin like growth factor I (IGF-1), and more distantly to epidermal growth factor (EGF). They are best known for relaxing the myometrium during pregnancy, and facilitating parturition by softening and dilating the uterine cervix and loosening symphysis pubis ligaments. Most species have a single RLX gene. Humans have nonallelic H1 and H2 types; but only the second is known to be expressed. There are substantial species differences in amino acid makeup, sites of synthesis, blood concentrations, and control mechanisms. The diagram (with one letter representations of the amino acids) shows the posi-

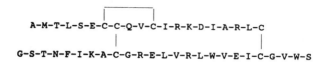

A–M–T–L–S–E–C–C–Q–V–C–I–R–K–D–I–A–R–L–C

G–S–T–N–F–I–K–A–C–G–R–E–L–V–R–L–W–V–E–I–C–G–V–W–S

relaxin

tion of the A chain S-S bond, and the cysteine moieties that link it to the B chain in the porcine type. The A chain is: Arg-Met-Thr-Leu-Ser-Glu-Lys-Cys-Cys-Glu-Val-Cys-Ile-Arg-Lys-Asp-Ile-Ala-Arg-Leu-Cys, and the B chain: Glu-Ser-Thr-Asn-Asp-Phe-Ile-Lys-Ala-Cys-Gly-Arg-Leu-Val-Arg-Leu-Trp-Val-Glu-Ile-Cys-Gly-Val-Trp-Ser. Human relaxins have similar three-dimenstional configurations. One human A chain is: *p*glu-Leu-Tyr-Ser-Ala-Leu-Ala-Asn-Lys-Cys-Cys-His-Val-Gly-Cys-Thr-Ser-Lys-Arg-Ser-Leu-Ala-Arg-Phe-Cys-. B chains with 20-27 amino acids have been described. One is H_2N-Asp-Ser-Trp-Met-Glu-Glu-Val-Ile-Lys-Leu-Cys-Gly-Arg-Glu-Leu-Val-Arg-Ala-Gln-Ile-Ala-Ile-Cys-Gly-Met-Ser-Thr-Trp-Ser. Maternal blood levels rise soon after conception in most mammals, and roles in implantation have been suggested. In some, there is a much greater rise several days before parturition, followed by an abrupt fall shortly before the onset of labor that is believed to facilitate myometrium contraction. In others, high levels persist to the time of birth, and in these RLX may contribute to fetal membrane rupture. The corpora lutea of pregnancy are major sources, but RLX is also made by cytotrophoblast and endometrium. It is implicated as a stimulant of uterine and vaginal growth, uterine vascularization, and also of mammary gland growth and maturation. Insulin-like actions have additionally been described. The stimuli for RLX synthesis include hCG (human chorionic gonadotropin), estrogens, and prostaglandin $PGF_{2\alpha}$. In nonpregnant females, small amounts made by ovarian follicle theca cells are believed to contribute to ovulation by enhancing the activities of collagenase and plasminogen activator. Luteinizing hormone (LH) may be the primary stimulant. Although not known to circulate in males, small amounts are made in prostate glands and released to seminal fluid. They may contribute to sperm motility and fertilization. High affinity binding sites have been identified in many brain regions (including the olfactory system, neocortex, hypothalamus, and medulla oblongata); and the hormone may gain access to neurons via circumventricular organs. It inhibits oxytocin and vasopressin release, and appears to interact with brain angiotensin II to regulate blood pressure and volume. RLX is used to treat dysmenorrhea and, in some cases to arrest premature labor.

release factors: usually, hypothalamic extract components that affect the secretion of adenohypophysial hormones. Terms such as corticotropin release factor (CRF), and thyrotropin release factor (TRF) were introduced when the chemical structures were unknown. Most (but not all) authors now prefer corticotropin releasing hormone (CRH), thyrotropin releasing hormone (TRH), and related terms.

releaser pheromones: signalling pheromones; regulators released externally that act rapidly on the nervous systems of other individuals and affect their behavior; *see* **pheromones**.

releasing hormones: *see* **release factors** and **pheromones**.

rem: roentgen equivalent in man; the dose of ionizing radiation that invokes the biological effects of one X-ray rad.

REM sleep: rapid eye movement sleep (*q.v.*); paradoxical sleep; the stage of sleep during which rapid eye movements and dreams occur, and skeletal muscle relaxes. Although causes and effects have not been established, growth hormone secretion declines during REM sleep, and increases during **slow wave sleep** (*q.v.*).

renal: pertaining to the kidney.

renal corpuscle: the nephron component that includes Bowman's capsule and the glomerular capillary tuft. Glomerular filtrate derived from the capillary blood enters Bowman's capsule, from which it is transported to the proximal convoluted tubule.

renal diabetes: excessive urine volume caused by renal factors such as damaged or inadequate numbers of nephrons, or inability to respond to vasopressin and some other regulators. *Cf* **diabetes mellitus** and **diabetes insipidus**.

renal hypertension: high blood pressure secondary to kidney dysfunction. The major causes are narrowing of renal arteries or other factors that lower the blood pressure in afferent arterioles that supply the glomeruli, and consequent release of excessive quantities of renin (*see* **renin-angiotensin system**). Less common ones include inadequate production of kallidin or other vasodilators.

renal osteodystrophy: renal rickets; pseudorickets; bone disorders initiated by renal dysfunction and consequent phosphate retention. The major symptoms are bone pain and skeletal muscle weakness (and growth failure in children). Since phosphate forms poorly ionized calcium salts, hyperphosphatemia decreases the amount of calcium available as free ion. This leads secondarily to excessive secretion of parathyroid hormone (PTH). The hormone imbalance accounts for some of the early effects on bone, and for metastatic calcification in some individuals. Later, inhibition of renal 1α-hydroxylase activity in the kidney by high phosphate concentrations assumes greater importance. The consequences can include osteitis fibrosa cystica, osteopenia, osteoporosis, osteopetrosis, osteomalacia, and rickets.

renaturation: return of a denatured protein or nucleic acid to its native three-dimensional configuration.

renins: species specific 42K glycoproteins with aspartyl proteinase activity that liberate angiotensin I (A-I) from renin substrates by cleaving leucine-leucine bonds near the *N*-terminals. A-I is rapidly converted to angiotensin II, and most effects of renin release are mediated by that peptide. The major human form of renin has 347 amino acid moieties. Most circulating enzyme originates in renal juxtaglomerular cells; and the amounts released to the bloodstream are major determinants of plasma angiotensin levels. Low pressure in the glomerular afferent arterioles, and catecholamines acting on β-type adrenergic receptors, directly accelerate renin release. Low blood volume usually decreases the pressure, and low blood Na^+ levels act indirectly (*see* **macula densa**). Although parathyroid hormone stimulates renin release, high intracellular Ca^{2+} has been reported to inhibit. Small amounts of renin are also synthesized in blood vessels, brain, adrenal cortex, gonads, reproductive tract organs, and elsewhere, and used locally; and some tumor cells secrete the enzymes. In rodents, *ren-1*, expressed in kidneys, and a non-allelic *ren-2* gene that is more widely distributed have been identified; and those animals make substantial amounts of the enzyme in their salivary glands. An abnormal type in a strain of Dahl rats is implicated as a factor in the hypertension that develops when the animals are fed high-salt diets. Isorenins made outside the kidney catalyze similar reactions, but differ somewhat in chemical makeup and pH optima. *See* also **plasma renin activity**, **prorenin**, and **pseudorenin**.

renin-angiotensin systems: RAS; body components that generate angiotensins and control their levels. **Angiotensin II**, an octatpeptide (*q.v.*) is the major active component. Renin released to the bloodstream by juxtaglomerular cells cleaves a circulating substrate that yields angiotensin I (a decapeptide). During a single passage through the lungs, A-I is converted to A-II. RAS systems that produce small amounts of A-II for local use are widely distributed. *See* also **juxtaglomerular apparatus**, **renins**, **renin substrates**, **angiotensin converting enzymes**, and **kallidins**.

renin substrates: angiotensinogens; 57K α_2-globulins cleaved by renins to yield angiotensin I. The major human type, which is made in the liver and secreted to the bloodstream, contains 453 amino acid moieties. Carbohydrate accounts for 13% of the molecular weight. Its production is increased by estrogens and some other hormones. Smaller amounts are made at several other sites in which **renins** (*q.v.*) are produced.

rennin: chymosin; an enzyme made in the stomachs of bovine calves that coagulates milk proteins; *cf* **renins**. (Commercial preparations are used to make puddings.)

reno-: a prefix that refers to the kidneys.

renocortin: one of the terms used for the **lipocortins** (*q.v.*) made in the kidneys.

renotropic: traveling towards, or stimulating the growth and/or functions of the kidneys.

renotropin: an uncharacterized factor that promotes kidney regeneration after injury or removal of a portion, and compensatory hypertrophy of the remaining organ after unilateral nephrectomy. Fibroblast growth factors (which affect many cell types) are renotropic. Exogenous AMP and ADP can also promote renal growth.

reoviruses: several double-stranded RNA viruses that reside in respiratory and gastrointestinal tracts, but are not known to directly cause disease.

repair nucleases: endonucleases and exonucleases that excise defective DNA segments and replace them with normal ones.

repetitive DNA: large numbers of identical DNA sequences within a genome. In mammals, hundreds of tandemly arranged identical genes code for histones and some other proteins. Millions of copies of others, concentrated in centromeric regions, contribute to chromosome alignment during mitosis and meiosis.

replacement therapy: administration of naturally occurring hormones (or other substances with similar actions) in amounts that correct deficiencies. Many forms of therapy employ **pharmacological doses** (*q.v.*). For example, the quantities of glucocorticoids used to treat severe forms of rheumatoid arthritis and some leukemias can invoke Cushing's disease symptoms.

replacement vector: a phage cloning vector in which a foreign DNA segment is substituted for a part of the genome. The vectors are used to obtain many copies of the foreign DNA.

replicases: DNA polymerases, RNA polymerases, or other enzymes that catalyze formation of molecules identical to ones initially present.

replication: formation of a new substance identical in composition to one initially present. The term usually refers to the DNA synthesis that precedes cell division.

replication fork: a structure formed when the strands of DNA segments separate in preparation for replication. The leading strand then serves directly as a template for 3′ to 5′ replication, whereas Okazaki fragments build up on the lagging strand.

replicon: an autonomously functioning genetic unit that can replicate independently. It contains a DNA initiation sequence (which binds RNA polymerase), a termination sequence, and a DNA polymerase; but it requires an RNA polymerase to direct formation of an RNA primer. The single chromosome in a bacterium is a replicon. Eukaryote chromosomes contain hundreds of replicons arranged in series.

replisome: a bacterial structure that assembles at a replication fork and initiates DNA synthesis. It contains a DNA polymerase and other enzymes.

replitase: a large multienzyme complex used for DNA synthesis that includes a DNA polymerase and a ribonucleotide reductase.

repolarization: re-establishment of a resting membrane potential following depolarization.

reporter genes: DNA segments that direct formation of cell components which confer easily recognizable characteristics, such as resistance to specific kinds of antibiotics. They are attached to other DNA segments that direct the synthesis of different kinds of messenger RNAs. The effects of the reporter genes are used to identify the cells of a mixed population that contain the other DNA segments.

repression: inhibition; the term can refer to the effects of a repressor, or of a biochemical pathway component that exerts negative feedback control over the rate-limiting step.

repressors: cell components that arrest gene transcription by interacting (directly or indirectly) with specific DNA segments. Most are proteins whose synthesis is directed by regulator genes. Their abilities to bind to operators (located upstream from initiation sites) and to thereby block initiation of messenger RNA synthesis by RNA polymerases, can be enhanced by corepressors and diminished by inducers.

reproduction: formation of new cells or individuals with genetic elements that derive from parent cells. In mitosis, the major form of *asexual* reproduction, a single cell replicates its DNA and transmits identical copies to each of two daughter cells. Higher animals use the process for growth, hematopoiesis, formation of gamete precursors, and to replace cells of the skin, liver, gastrointestinal tract, and other organs. Budding and fission are alternate forms of asexual reproduction in small organisms. *Sexual* reproduction, which is used to form new individuals, requires genetic components from two different parent cells. In most species, it involves production of haploid gametes (each of which contains just half the DNA of the parent cell), and the joining of gametes from two individuals to form zygotes that differ genetically from both of the parents. In some unicellular organisms and some plants, genetic elements are exchanged during conjugation.

reproductive success: the numbers of offspring produced by an individual that survive to an age when they are capable of reproduction.

RER: rough endoplasmic reticulum.

RES: reticuloendothelial system.

resact: Cys-Val-Thr-Gly-Ala-Pro-Gly-Cys-Val-Gly-Gly-Gly-Arg-Leu-NH_2; a species-specific peptide released by *Arabacia punctulata* sea urchin oocytes that attracts sperm, stimulates sperm motility, initiates acrosome reactions, and may contribute to fertilization. It binds to a 160K receptor on the sperm plasma membrane surface, and activates a guanylate cyclase. This is rapidly followed by H^+ efflux. Closely related peptides include speract (made by other sea urchins), and sand dollar mosact.

reserpine: 11,17β-dimethoxy-18β-[(3,4,5-trimethoxy-benzoyl)oxy]-3β-α-yohimban-16β-carboxylic acid methyl ester; an alkaloid from the roots of *Rauwolfia serpentina* that inhibits catecholamine and serotonin uptake by nerve terminals and secretory granules, and thereby transiently prolongs the effectiveness of those amines. Since amines that are not taken up are rapidly degraded, prolonged administration depletes the stores. The delayed effects are used to achieve tranquilization and to lower blood pressure.

residual bodies: usually (1) minute particles of sperm cytoplasm retained by Sertoli cells during spermiation, implicated as negative regulators of spermatogenesis; (2) secondary lysosomes; (3) particulate matter left over after a process is completed.

residual lumen: hypophysial cleft; the remnant of the lumen of Rathke's pouch that persists in a mature adenohypophysis. *See* also **anterior pituitary**.

resinferatoxin: 6,7,-deepoxy-6,7-didehydro-5-deoxy-21-dephenyl-21(phenylmethyldaphnetoxin,20-4-(4-hydroxy-3-methoxybenzene acetate); an extremely potent neurotoxin that destroys capsaicin-sensitive cells.

resins: mixtures of carboxylic acids and terpenes obtained from plant exudates or made synthetically. Many bind specific substances with high affinity and are used to remove them from other materials. *See* **cholestyramine** and **ion exchange resins**.

resistance vessels: blood vessels (mostly arterioles and small arteries) that contribute to the control of systemic blood pressure and blood flow by undergoing constriction and dilation; *cf* **capacitance vessels**.

resorcinol: 1,3-benzenediol; a topical antipruritic and antiseptic. When absorbed, it interferes with the synthesis of iodinated thyroid hormones.

resorption: removal of an entity previously formed or secreted. The term is applied to the actions of osteoclasts on bone, the disposal of debris by phagocytic cells, and the processes by which degenerating embryos and fetuses

reserpine

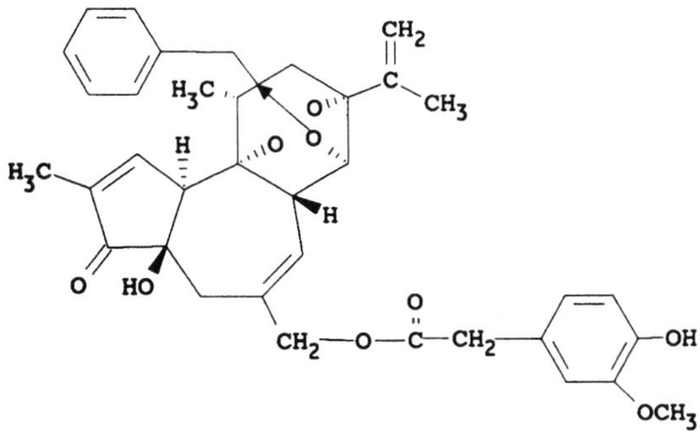

resinferatoxin

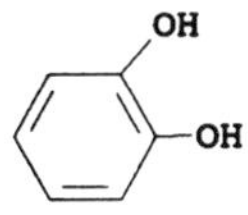

resorcinol

are degraded and the products are absorbed by maternal blood vessels.

respiration: the terms *external* and *internal* respiration refer to CO_2 and O_2 exchange between alveolar air and pulmonary capillaries, and between systemic capillaries and tissue cells, respectively; *cf* **ventilation**. *Cellular* respiration (oxidation of fuels) includes glycolysis and other anaerobic processes, as well as biochemical pathways in which oxygen serves as the electron acceptor.

respiratory acidosis: subnormal blood pH associated with a low $NaHCO_3$:$HHCO_3$ ratio, usually caused by impaired ventilation that leads to carbon dioxide retention; *cf* **metabolic acidosis**. In *compensated* respiratory acidosis, Na^+ retention leads to $NaHCO_3$ accumulation and pushes the ratio closer to normal values.

respiratory alkalosis: excessively high blood pH associated with elevation of the $NaHCO_3$: $HHCO_3$ ratio. It

is usually caused by hyperventilation and consequent CO_2 depletion; *cf* **metabolic alkalosis**. In *compensated* respiratory alkalosis, accelerated $NaHCO_3$ excretion lowers the ratio.

respiratory burst: metabolic burst; rapid release of oxidizing agents by activated neutrophilic leukocytes.

respiratory quotient: R.Q.; the ratio of the volume of CO_2 produced to the volume of O_2 consumed. It varies with the kind of fuel used, and is 1.0 for carbohydrates, 0.7 for fats, 0.8 for most proteins, and approximately 0.87 for the metabolic mixture used by humans in the postabsorptive state. The metabolic rate (in Calories) can be calculated from oxygen consumption measurements if the R.Q is known.

restriction endonucleases: enzymes that recognize specific 4-8 base pair palindromic sequences on double stranded DNA molecules, and cleave phosphodiesterase bonds. Microorganisms use the enzymes to destroy defective or foreign (phage) DNA. Their own DNA is protected by methylation at those sites. Approximately 100 bacterial types have been characterized and given names with three letters for the organisms in which they originate, and Roman numbers which indicate the order in which they were discovered. Some are shown below,

Endonuclease	Origin	Cleavage site
EcoRI	*Escherichia coli*	↓ 5'... G—A*—A—T—T—C... 3' 3'... C—T—T—A—A—G... 5' ↑
BamHI	*Bacillus amyloliquefaciens H*	↓ 5'...G—G—A—T—C—C...3' 3'...C—C—T—A—G—G...5' ↑
HpaI	*Hemophilus parainfluenzae*	↓ 5'...G—T—T—A—C—C...3' 3'...C—C—A—T—T—G—..5' ↑

restriction endonucleases

and others are listed under their names. The A* in the first example is methyl-adenine. Type I enzymes bind to the recognition sites, but make random cuts. Type II enzymes cut within the recognition sites on both strands. They generate sticky ends, and are used to analyze chromosome structures (see **finger-printing**), determine base sequences of long DNAs, and isolate genes. Since any fragment produced by the action of a specific endonuclease can be annealed to any other fragment obtained in the same way, artificial DNAs can be constructed and inserted into plasmids for cloning.

restriction fragment: a DNA fragment obtained by endonuclease digestion.

restriction fragment length polymorphisms: RFLPs: variations in the lengths of restriction fragments obtained when DNAs of a species are cleaved by specific restriction endonucleases. Since the DNA of each individual generates a characteristic pattern, RFLPs can provide information on the identity of individuals from whom the DNA was derived (*see* **footprinting**). Certain patterns also indicate the presence mutations.

restriction map: a linear array of DNA segments obtained by restriction endonuclease cleavage.

restriction point: the stage of the G_1 phase of the cell cycle in which all protein components critical for progression to S have been synthesized, and essential amino acids are no longer required for advancement to the next phase.

ret: a proto-oncogene that codes for a protein of the cadherin family with tyrosine kinase activity, believed to function in signal transduction.

reticular activating system: RAS; the central nervous system component essential for arousal, and for maintaining alertness; *see* **reticular formation**.

reticular formation: a diffuse neural network in the gray matter of the thalamus, hypothalamus, midbrain, pons, medulla oblongata, and spinal cord that receives inputs from several kinds of receptors. It functions as the reticular activating system, and contributes to cerebellar functions and controls over the release of some hormones.

reticulin: (1) a scleroprotein with an amino acid composition similar to that of type III collagen. Carbohydrate accounts for approximately 4% of the weight, and lipid (mostly myristate) for 11%. It occurs mostly in fine connective tissue, and is especially abundant in renal glomeruli and tubules, and in the lungs; (2) hydroxystreptomycin, an antibiotic made by *Streptomyces reticuli* with properties similar to those of streptomycin. In the structure shown, R = —HC—N—.

reticulocytes: cells that differentiate from bone marrow erythroblasts and develop into mature erythrocytes, named for the network-like appearance of fragmented nuclei. Small numbers circulate under normal conditions. Although they contain less hemoglobin than mature red cells, their oxygen carrying capacity assumes physiological importance under conditions in which **reticulocytosis** (*q.v.*) occurs.

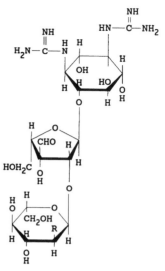

reticulin

reticulocytosis: increased numbers of reticulocytes in circulating blood. It occurs in response to hypoxia, for example in some forms of anemia, following hemorrhage, or soon after ascent to high altitudes.

reticuloendothelial system: RES; a network of phagocytic cells that includes microglia, Kupffer cells, and macrophages of the spleen, lungs, bone marrow, and connective tissues. It removes degenerating cells and their products (including hemoglobin), debris, bacteria, and some chemicals.

reticuloendotheliosis: several reticuloendothelium system disorders, including a rare form of leukemia in which the spleen enlarges, and "hairy" cells accumulate in the bone marrow, lymph nodes and spleen.

reticulosis: any benign or malignant proliferative disorder of the reticuloendothelial system.

reticulum [reticula]: a network.

retina: the innermost tunic of the eyeball. It contains a pigment layer, photoreceptors (rods and cones in humans and many other species), blood vessels, and several kinds of neurons (bipolar, amacrine, horizontal, and ganglion). Retinal pigment cells mediate transport of water, ions, nutrients, and macromolecules between the photoreceptors and the blood vessels of the choroid plexus. They store retinyl esters, convert all *trans*-retinol to all 9-*cis*-retinal, regenerate visual pigments, phagocytose shed photoreceptor outer segment tips, and have both muscarinic and β-adrenergic receptors. ON type bipolar neurons are depolarized by light (and are hyperpolarized in the dark), whereas OFF bipolar neurons are hyperpolarized by light. Both these and amacrine cells are interneurons that communicate with photoreceptors and ganglion cells. The optic nerves convey messages from the retinas to the primary and accessory optic tracts (essential for vision and reflexes, respectively) and to the retinohypothalamic tracts (which mediate synchronization of body rhythms with photoperiods). Neurotransmit-

11-*cis*-retinal

all-*trans*-retinal

ters that regulate the functions, including gamma aminobutyric acid (GABA), substance P and melatonin, use at least seven different G protein transducers. *See* also **transducin**.

retin-A: tretinoin; *see* **retinoic acid**.

retinal: (1) pertaining to the retina; (2) retinaldehyde; retinene; vitamin A aldehyde; 3,7-dimethyl-9-(2,6,6-trimethyl-1-cyclohexen-1-yl)-2,4,6,8-nonatetraen-1-al; any of 16 carotenoid isomers related to vitamin A (vitamin A_1 in mammals). In mammalian photoreceptors, the Δ^{11}-*cis*-retinal isomer combines with scotopsin to form **rhodopsin** *(q.v.)*, and with photopsins for cone visual pigments. It is converted to all-*trans*-retinal when light decomposes rhodopsin. The *trans* form released from the protein is then reduced to retinol. A reversible reaction catalyzed by an isomerase restores the *cis* form. Retinal is also irreversibly oxidized to retinoic acid, and is a precursor of 3,4-didehydroretinoic acid, several retinyl esters, and other biologically important compounds.

retinal binding protein: CRALBP: cellular retinal binding protein; a 36K intracellular protein that binds retinal with high affinity and is believed to function in visual cycles (*see* also **retinal**). It differs from a 140K intercellular retinol binding protein (IRBP), which also binds retinol, and appears to function primarily as an intracellular retinol transporter. *Cf* **retinoic acid binding proteins**.

retinaldehyde: *see* **retinal**, definition 2.

retinal isomerase: a retinal enzyme that catalyzes conversion of all-*trans*-retinal aldehyde to 11-*cis*-retinal, which then combines with opsins. *See* also **retinol dehydrogenase**.

retinene: *see* **retinal**, definition 2.

retinitis: inflammation of the retina.

retinitis pigmentosa: a progressive autosomal recessive disease in which melanin granules released from degenerating epithelial cells of the pigment layer migrate through the retina, deposit on blood vessel walls, and eventually cause blindness.

retinoblastoma[s]: malignant tumors derived from immature retinal cells (retinoblasts). Childhood types, usually manifested before the age of 4 years, are attributed to inherited defects in which one *Rb* allele is deleted or defective, and the second subsequently undergoes mutation.

retinoblastoma gene: *Rb*: autosomal genes that exert negative control over cell cycles and protect against tumorigenesis and transformation. Retinoblastomas, testicular tumors, and some osteosarcomas, small cell lung, urinary bladder, endometrial, prostate gland, and breast carcinomas develop in individuals who lack a functioning Rb gene (because both alleles are mutated, or one is mutated and the other deleted). Transfection of a normal gene can reverse the effects in some cultured cell types. Impaired transcription of apparently healthy genes has also been described. *Rb* directs formation of p105, a nuclear protein that is continuously made, but is normally hypophosphorylated in G_o and G_1 phases of cell cycles and phosphorylated as cells pass through the G_1/S boundary. The hypophosphorylated form interacts with an Rb control element (RCE) in promoter regions of *c-fos* and several other genes that contribute to the control of cell proliferation and differentiation, and it suppresses AP-1 activity. Some tumor promoters (including an SV40 component) bind to and inactivate the hypophosphorylated form. Since transforming growth factor-β1 (TGFβ1) blocks the phosphorylation, and *Rb* up-regulates TGFβ1 in a few cell types, some effects on differentiation are attributed to interactions with that regulator. Others have been linked with *Rb* inhibition of interleukin-6 production.

retinohypothalamic tracts: fine bilateral nerve tracts that originate in optic nerves, travel directly to the hypothalamus, innervate the suprachiasmatic nuclei, and make functional connections with the pineal gland. They mediate synchronization of body rhythms with photoperiods, but are not involved in visual perception.

retinoic acids: RAs; retin-A and tretinoin are all-*trans* 3,7-dimethyl-9-(2,6,6-trimethyl-1-cyclohexen-1-yl)-2,4,6,8-nonatetraenoic acid, a hormone made from vitamin A via both irreversible oxidation of retinol and in pathways in which the alcohol is not formed. By acting directly, and after conversion to other isomers, RAs play essential roles in development of the heart, vascular system, limb buds, and epithelial structures. They also maintain the differentiated states of both moist type mucociliary epithelium (in the trachea and other structures), and dry type squamous epithelium (in skin), and are believed to protect against tumorigenesis in respiratory, buccal, stomach, mammary gland and skin tissue. Additionally, they contribute to controls over hematopoietic cell proliferation and differentiation; and high concentrations are effective for treating promyelocytic leukemias. It has been stated that RAs cannot replace retinol for support of gametogenesis, but some observed differences in responses relate to poorer RA penetration across cell membranes. Although the effects are concentration dependent (and both deficiencies and excessive can cause malformations), the hypothesis that they act directly in a gradient-dependent manner as morphogens (embryonic

all-*trans*-retinoic acid

9-*cis*-retinoic acid

13-*cis*-retinoic acid

inducers) has been replaced by more complicated concepts that involve binding to several receptor isoforms whose numbers are developmentally regulated, and to at least two kinds of nonreceptor retinoic acid binding proteins that are induced by RAs, as well as interactions with transforming growth factors β1 and β2 (TGFβ1 and TGFβ2), bone morphogenetic protein-2 (BMP-2), and other growth regulating hormones. The receptors can directly attach to c-fos and c-jum proteins; and receptor binding to retinoic acid response elements is modified by the receptors for glucocorticoids, 1,25-dihydroxyvitamin D_3, triiodothyronine, and other factors. Various target cell types selectively degrade RA or convert it to other biologically active compounds, including 3,4-didehydroretinoic acid (which can also derive directly from vitamin A), and 9-*cis*-retinoic acid (retinoid X). RAs regulate genes that code for growth hormone, laminin B1, complement factor H, osteocalcin, $β_2$-macroglobulin, type IV collagen, alcohol dehydrogenase, phosphoenolpyruvate carboxykinase and other compounds, and they exert posttranscriptional influences on some homeobox types.

retinoic acid binding proteins: several cytoplasmic proteins similar to, but distinguishable from cell retinol binding proteins that bind retinoic acid with high affinities, but differ from retinoic acid receptors. 15-16K types (CRABP-I and CRABP-II) regulate cell retinoic acid concentrations, and can deliver RA to nuclear receptors. A more important function may be limitation of the concentrations of free RA available for transfer. Since they are selectively induced by RAs, they may be components of negative feedback loops that protect cells against excessive amounts. (The 9-*cis* form is specific for CRABP-II.) However, some cell types that do not make the proteins respond to RA. Two 20K epididymal fluid proteins related to CRABPS may have different functions.

retinoic acid receptors: RARs; proteins of the steroid and thyroid hormone receptor superfamily that bind retinoic acid with high affinity and mediate its effects by interacting with nuclear retinoic acid response elements (RAREs). RARα, RARβ, and RARγ classes are encoded by separate genes. Two major α, three major β, and two major γ subtypes are generated by alternate mRNA splicings; and selective activation of multiple promotors as well as posttranslational processing give rise to at least seven isoforms for each subtype. All RARα, RARβ, and

RARγ proteins are structurally similar, with identical DNA binding sites; but they have different *N*-terminal amino acid sequences that affect binding affinities for RAs. RARα types have the highest affinity for all-*trans*-retinoic acid, and the β classes the lowest. The α types also bind 9-*cis*-retinoic acid. An aberrant form in human promyelocytic leukemia cells may function only in the presence of supraphysiological RA concentrations, since administered tretinoin can promote differentiation and suppresses proliferation. Most cell types constitutively make RARαs. RARβs have been identified in tracheobronchial, intestinal, and genital tract epithelium, and in fetal and adult brains. RARγs appears to be confined to embryos, and to differentiated skin and lung cells. The kinds made vary with the states of maturation; and both RARα and RARβ types are induced by RA at various sites. In addition to forming homodimers that bind directly to RAREs of many genes, RA-RAR complexes dimerize with other receptor proteins of the superfamily; and their transactivating activities vary with the dimer types. Different effects may involve direct protein:protein interactions with transcription regulators that affect the abilities of those proteins to act on DNA. For example, RARαs are believed to block AP-1 stimulation by directly binding to c-fos proteins. The effects of RA-RAR complexes are modified by receptors for several other hormones. Thyroid hormone receptors directly activate RAREs on growth hormone genes in some cell types, and block RAR access to RAREs in some others. Glucocorticoids bound to their own receptors antagonize some effects, but augment others. The primary ligand for RXRα (which does not bind all-*trans*-RA with high affinity) appears to be 9-*cis*-RA, made from the *trans* isomer in the liver, kidney, and some other cell types.

retinoic acid response elements: RAREs; nucleic acid sequences that bind retinoic acid-RAR complexes and mediate many of the effects of retinoids by serving as enhancers for several genes. Some also bind receptors for thyroid hormone and calciferols. *See* **retinoic acid receptors**.

retinoid: (1) resembling the retina; (2) a general term applied to vitamin A-related compounds, including retinal, retinol, retinoic acids, and 3,4-didehydro-retinoic acid.

retinoid X: 9-*cis*-retinoic acid; *see* **retinoic acids** and **retinoic acid receptors**.

retinol: vitamin A$_1$; vitamin A alcohol (*see* also **vitamin A** and **vitamin A$_2$**); 3,7-dimethyl-9-(2,6,6-trimethyl-1-cyclohexen-1-yl)-2,4,6,8-nonatetraen-1-ol; a regulator obtained from β-carotene in vegetables and retinyl esters in animal foods, absorbed by enterocytes, esterified (mostly with saturated, long-chain fatty acids), and incorporated into chylomicrons that enter the lymph. Hepatocytes take up the chylomicrons and transfer much of the retinol to perisinusoidal stellate cells for storage, and for subsequent release (in association with retinol binding proteins) to the bloodstream. Small amounts of retinol are also liberated from chylomicrons by lipoprotein lipases; and some retinol esters are taken up by lipoprotein receptors. Most cell types irreversibly oxidize retinol to retinoic acid (RA); and many effects depend on that conversion. (Retinol cannot substitute for retinoic acid in systems that lack the oxidating enzymes.) RA can prevent necrotic death of activated immune system cells, but retinol cannot. Retinol is also the precursor of retinal (required for photoreception, but not obtained from RA), and of 14-HRR (14-hydroxy-4,14 *retro*-retinol), a growth-promoting metabolite formed in a different metabolic pathway. Although reported to exert some effects in vitamin-A deprived animals (for example on spermatogenesis, pregnancy maintenance, and hatching) that are not achieved with RA administration, its ability to more rapidly traverse plasma membranes may explain some of observations. Toxic levels impair some membrane functions.

retinol binding proteins: RBPs; the major type is a 21K polypeptide that resembles β-lactoglobin and binds most of the circulating retinol. It facilitates retinol transport, and is believed to protect cells against excessive levels of the free alcohol (which can disrupt cell membrane structures and functions). 21K RBP associates with circulating transthyretin (prealbumin) and protects it against loss to glomerular filtrates. Four additional 22K proteins made by uterine cells in pigs (and probably other species) facilitate retinol transport to fetuses. *Cellular* retinol binding proteins (CRBPs I and II) are 15-16K cytoplasmic compounds derived from the gene that directs synthesis of the 21K type. They contribute to the control of intracellular retinol transport and esterification. By concentrating intracellular retinol, they provide the major sources of retinoic acid and other metabolites. CRBP II also binds retinal, but not retinoic acid.

retinol dehydrogenase: an NADP$^+$-dependent enzyme that oxidizes all-*trans*-retinol to its corresponding aldehyde. The product is a substrate for retinal isomerase, which is needed to make 11-*cis*-retinal.

retinopathy: noninflammatory retinal disease. Microaneurysms, minute hemorrhages, and blood vessel proliferation occur in many individuals with diabetes mellitus.

retinylphosphate-mannose: a retinoic acid metabolite believed to regulate sugar transport.

retrochiasmatic area: a region of the anterior hypothalamus that contributes to control of gonadotropin secretion. Melatonin implants inhibit hormone release.

retrocytosis: unidirectional transport of hormones and other substances from intracellular sites to cell surfaces or extracellular spaces.

retrograde transport: transport in a direction opposite the one usually expected, for example from axon endings to neuron cell bodies. Nerve growth factor and some other regulators are taken up in this way.

retroposons: *see* **retrotransposons**.

retrotransposons: retroposons; repetitive DNA sequences whose synthesis is directed by reverse transcriptases. They lack introns, but have 3′ polyadenosine tails and transcribable segments that code for new reverse transcriptases. Retroviral types can integrate into and replicate with host chromosomes, and are believed to contribute to evolution by affecting controls over pre-existing genes, deleting stop codons, invoking insertional mutagenesis, and forming pseudogenes. *See* also **retroviruses** and **transposons**.

retroviral oncogenes: genes introduced into host cells that invoke transformation. *See* **retroviruses**.

retroviruses: RNA viruses that use reverse transcriptases to generate DNA molecules which integrate into host chromosomes and replicate when the host cells prepare for division. They can take up proto-oncogenes from host eukaryotic cells and convert them to transforming oncogenes.

rev: genes that regulate virion protein expression and promote accumulation of *gag-pol* and *env* viral messenger RNAs.

reverse hemolytic plaque assays: techniques for identifying cells that hold specific kinds of proteins on their surfaces, or secrete them, including single cells surrounded by different types. Erythrocytes are coated with antigens that bind the proteins. Complement factors are then added to generate zones of hemolysis at the binding sites.

reverse mutation: a change in a mutant gene that restores normal function.

reverse T$_3$: rT$_3$; 3,3′5′-triiodothyronine; a thyroxine metabolite with little or no physiological activity. Starvation, carbohydrate deprivation, febrile illnesses, and other conditions that slow T$_3$ synthesis elevate rT$_3$: T$_3$ ratios. By decreasing availability of the active hormone, diversion of T$_4$ to the rT$_3$ pathway can reduce fuel wastage when the supply is short, and protect against excessive body temperature elevation. *See* also **deiodinases** and **triiodothyronine**.

reverse transcriptases: RNA-dependent DNA polymerases made by retroviruses. They direct synthesis of complementary DNA sequences in host cells.

reverse triiodothyronine: *see* **reverse T$_3$**.

reward areas: brain regions said to confer sensations of pleasure when stimulated, and to affect motivation and contain receptors for addictive drugs. The concept derives in part from the behavior of laboratory animals provided with switches they can operate to activate electrodes inserted into the median forebrain bundle, nucleus accumbens, ventral tegmentum, and some other brain loci; *see* **"pleasure centers"**.

R_f: in paper chromatography, the ratio of the distance traveled by the solute to the distance traveled by the solvent. It varies with the physical properties of both solute and solvent.

RF: (1) releasing factor (as in CRF); (2) rheumatoid factor; (3) recombination frequency.

ρ **factor**: rho factor.

RFLP: restriction fragment length polymorphism.

RGD: *see* **Arg-Gly-Asp**.

Rh: rhodium.

rhabdo-: a prefix meaning rod-shaped.

rhabdomyoblasts: immature skeletal muscle cell precursors.

rhabdomyomas: benign, striated (cardiac or skeletal) muscle cell tumors.

rhabdomyosarcomas: malignant rhabdomyoblast tumors.

Rhabdoviridae: rabies, vesicular stomatitis, and other viruses whose genomes contain single negative-stranded RNA associated with virus-specific RNA polymerases.

rhamnose: 6-deoxy-L-mannose; a hexose component of poison sumac and some other plant glycosides, and of some gram-negative bacteria cell walls. Rhamnogalacturons bind pectins in plants, and are minor components of some animal oligosaccharides.

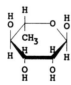

rheo-: a prefix meaning flow or current.

rheotaxis: movement of a cell component or organism towards or against the direction of the flow of its surrounding liquid.

Rhesus blood groups: C, D, and E antigens on the surfaces of most human erythrocytes. D types are the strongest antigens. *See* **Rh factor**.

Rhesus monkey: *Macaca Rhesus*; a small, short-tailed monkey used to study behavior, reproduction, immune system responses, and other biological functions.

rheumatic fever: autoimmune diseases that causes joint inflammation and irreversible heart valve damage, in which antibodies made against streptococcal antigens act on host cells. The autoimmune reactions are usually self-limiting, but the damage persists. *Cf* **rheumatism** and **rheumatoid arthritis**.

rheumatism: an imprecise term applied to tendinitis, bursitis, some forms of arthritis, and other undefined

conditions that affect ligaments or bone, or cause muscle or joint pains.

rheumatoid arthritis: chronic, progressive, systemic diseases attributed to autoimmune processes, in which synovial membranes are inflamed, macrophages, neutrophilic leukocytes, lymphocytes and plasma cells accumulate in numerous joints, and granulation tissue forms (*see* **pannus**). The processes may be initiated by an antigen modified by macrophages that invokes proliferation of cytotoxic lymphocyte subsets, release of interleukin-1, and secondary release of other cytokines and prostaglandins. In severe cases, there is extensive destruction of joint cartilage, and joints become immobilized by fusion of the exposed ends. The systemic manifestations include low-grade fevers and malaise. Nonsteroidal anti-inflammatory agents (NSAIDs) suppress the inflammation and pain, mostly by inhibiting prostaglandin synthesis, and can control the symptoms in mild cases. Glucocorticoids, which additionally inhibit neutrophil activities and the release of other cytokines, are more effective; but long-term use invokes Cushing's syndrome toxicity. *See* also **rheumatoid factor**.

rheumatoid factor: autoantibodies to IgG and/or IgA type immunoglobulins, in approximately 70% of individuals with rheumatoid arthritis, and in some with other autoimmune diseases. Sera containing them agglutinate IgG or IgA coated latex particles.

Rh factor: Rhesus factor; D type Rhesus blood group antigens on the surfaces of most human erythrocytes, initially identified in Rhesus monkeys. Individuals who express them (and their blood) are said to be Rh⁺. Those with Rh⁻ blood make IgG type anti-Rh antibodies when exposed to the antigen. Problems arise when an Rh⁻ mother carries an Rh⁺ fetus, since both the antigens and antibodies can cross the placenta. Usually, the low antibody titers formed during a first pregnancy do little damage; but large amounts of antigen released during parturition are strong stimulants that can affect subsequent pregnancies. High antibody levels destroy the erythrocytes of Rh⁺ fetuses, and invoke erythroblastosis fetalis. *See* also **Rh₀(D) immunoglobulin**.

rhin-: rhino-: a prefix meaning nose.

rhinencephalon: the anterior region of the brain that includes olfactory nerves, bulbs and tracts, and parts of the limbic system. It mediates conscious olfactory perception and pheromone effects, and is involved in the control of emotions, behavior, some aspects of learning, and the secretion of gonadotropin releasing hormone (GnRH).

rhinoviruses: at least 100 single-stranded viruses of the *Rhinovirus* genus (Picornaviridae family), including agents that cause common colds.

rhizopod: an ameba of the superclass Rhizopoda.

rhizotomy: division of a spinal nerve root.

rhod-: rhodo-: a prefix meaning red.

rhodamines: several triphenylmethane-derived dyes that bind to proteins and emit red to orange fluorescence

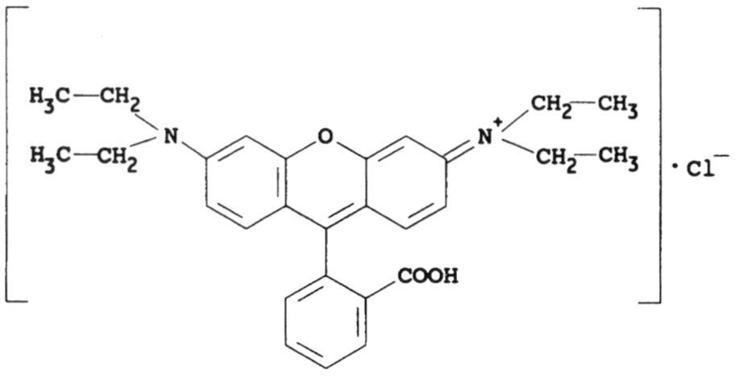

rhodamine B

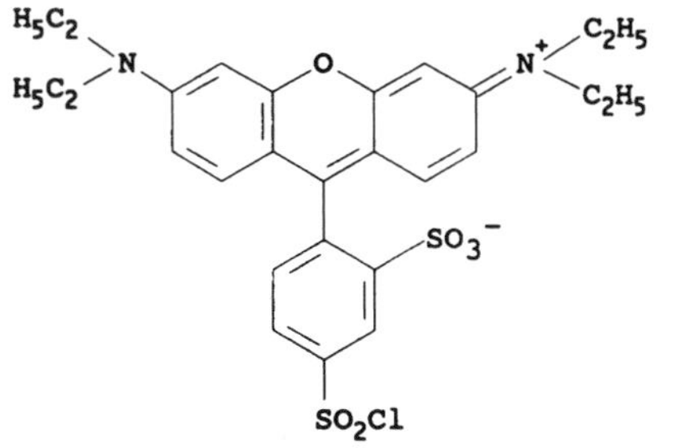

lissamine

under ultraviolet light, made by condensing phthalic, succinyl and other acid anhydrides with *m*-aminophenol, They are used as biological stains in immunofluorescence microscopy, and for photometric determinations of antimony, bismuth, cobalt, manganese and some other metals. Some specifically attach to components of mitochondrial and other membranes. Rhodamine B (basic violet, shown above) is *N*-[9-(2-carboxyphenyl)-6-(diethylamino)-3*H*-xanthen-3-ylidene]-*N*-ethylethaminium chloride. Lissamine is rhodamine B sulfonyl chloride.

Rh$_0$(D) immune globulin: a human immunoglobulin preparation that contains anti-Rh antibodies in quantities sufficient to suppress immunological reactions in Rh⁻ mothers bearing Rh⁺ fetuses (*see* **Rh factor**).

rhodopsin: visual purple; a 40K integral membrane protein composed of scotopsin and 11-*cis*-retinal, synthesized during darkness by retinal rod cells. Light decomposes it in a series of steps that culminates in liberation of scotopsin + 11-*trans*-retinal. *See* also **rhodopsin kinase, transducin, arrestin**, and **recoverin**.

rhodopsin kinase: an enzyme that contributes to termination of visual excitation in rods by catalyzing ATP-mediated phosphorylation of the protein component of light-activated rhodopsin. Phosphorylated rhodopsin then combines with arrestin, a 48K protein that competes with rhodopsin for transducin binding sites.

RhoGAM: a trade name for an anti-Rh gamma globulin; *see* **Rh$_0$ (D)**.

rhombencephalon: hindbrain; the most caudal of the three embryonic brain vesicles. It divides into the metencephalon (the precursor of the pons) and the myelencephalon, from which the medulla oblongata and cerebellum develop.

rhythm: describes phenomena that recur regularly at predictable time intervals; *see* specific types, such as **circadian**, **infradian**, and **ultradian**; and *see* also **biological clocks**.

"rhythm methods" for contraception: fertility control methods based on assumptions that the time of ovulation can be accurately predicted, and that conception cannot occur if abstinence is practiced during the time interval that begins several days before and continues until several days after the predicted time of ovulation. In the "calendar" method (which is the most widely used), the timing of previous menstrual cycles is recorded. It is then assumed that future cycles will follow the same pattern, and that ovulation will occur approximately midway between two menstrual periods. "Symptothermal" variations employ other indices, such as changes in the quality of uterine cervix mucus, or body temperature elevations attributed to progesterone secretion. The failure rate is high because the timing of ovulation is affected by many factors (*see* **paracyclic ovulation**), and because spermatozoa can survive for several days in vaginal crypts. Since abstinence is required at times when sexual interest is high, other failures follow noncompliance. According to at least some observers, using the methods increases the probability that immature oocytes or "over-ripe" gametes will engage in fertilization, with consequent higher incidences of zygote defects.

RIA: radioimmunoassay.

ribavirin: 1-β-D-ribofuranosyl-1-H-1,2,4-triazole-3-carboxamide; a synthetic, broad spectrum antiviral agent effective against influenza and several other DNA and RNA types.

ribitol: adonitol; an alcohol formed by reduction of the ribose aldehyde group, made by some flowering plants,

ribavirin

and a component of some bacterial cell walls and some flavins.

riboflavin: riboflavine; lactoflavin; vitamin B$_2$; vitamin G; 7,8-dimethyl-10-(D-*ribo*-2,3,4,5-tetrahydroxypentyl)isoalloxazine; an essential nutrient used to make FAD and FMN components of flavoproteins. Milk is a major dietary source for infants and children. The vitamin is also present in eggs and in green leafy vegetables, and small amounts occur in free form in retinas. The major signs of severe deficiency include cheilosis, dermatitis, magenta coloration of the tongue, dermatitis, and corneal vascularization.

riboflavin mononucleotide: riboflavin phosphate: flavin mononucleotide; FMN; *see* **flavin nucleotides**.

ribonucleases: RNases; enzymes that hydrolyze phosphate ester bonds of ribonucleic acids. Various types occur in pancreatic juice, lysosomes, and cell nuclei. Ribonuclease A is a 13.7K pancreatic juice endonuclease that cleaves 5′ phosphate moieties of pyrimidine nucleotides. Although most enzymes are proteins, the catalytic component of bacterial ribonuclease P is an RNA subunit (*see* **ribozymes**).

ribonucleic acid[s]: RNAs; the term usually refers to single stranded ribose polynucleotides whose synthesis in eukaryote cells is directed by DNAs. Some viruses have RNA genomes; and double-stranded RNAs can form in eukaryotes. The major nitrogenous bases are adenine, guanine, cytosine and uracil; but some RNAs contain small amounts of posttranscriptionally modified types. *Ribosomal* RNAs (rRNAs) are structural components of ribosomes, synthesized in the nucleoli of eukaryote cells via processes that require RNA polymerase I enzymes. The small subunits of eukaryote ribosomes contain an 18S form analogous to a 16S type in prokaryotes; and the large subunits have 28S and 5S RNAs analogous to prokaryote 23S and 5S molecules. Eukaryote ribosomes also contain a 5.8 species. *Messenger* RNAs (mRNAs) attach to ribosomes and direct translation. They have codons (triplets, sets of three bases), most of which hydrogen bond to specific kinds of aminoacyl *transfer* RNAs (tRNAs). Some accept more than one type of tRNA, and a few provide different kinds of signals, for example for initiation or termination of peptide chain assembly. Genes direct formation of primary transcripts with bases complementary to those of the DNA, via processes that require RNA polymerase II enzymes. The molecules are then capped at their 5′ ends, and most undergo polyadenylation at their 3′ ends before release as premessenger RNAs. Subsequent processing usually includes spliceosome-mediated excision of introns, and joining of exon sequences. Some premessenger RNAs can be spliced in more than one way, and thereby direct formation of two or more protein types. Transfer RNAs are small, cloverleaf shaped molecules that contain rare bases, such as pseudouridine and methyl cytidine. Their synthesis in eukaryote nucleoli is catalyzed by RNA polymerase III. Each bears an anticodon (a set of three bases complementary to those of an mRNA codon), a site that binds to the ribosome, and another that binds a specific kind of amino acid. A few tRNAs recognize more than one codon. *Small nuclear* ribonucleic acids (snURPs, snurps), made in nucleoli, associate with proteins to form small nuclear ribonucleoprotein particles (snRNPs) that regulate RNA processing. *Small cytoplasmic* RNAs (scRNAs) associate with specific proteins to form small cytoplasmic ribonucleoprotein particles (scRNPs).

anti-sense **ribonucleic acid[s]**: anti-sense RNAs: polyribonucleotides with nitrogenous base sequences complementary to those of messenger RNAs. By attaching to and "masking" the associated mRNAs, they can block the synthesis of a specific proteins. A few types made in small amounts by cells code for special products. Artificially constructed ones are used to study the roles of specific mRNAs and/or their associated proteins.

double-stranded **ribonucleic acids**: dsRNAs; RNAs composed of complementary nucleic acid strands. They are synthesized by viruses with RNA-directed RNA polymerases, and are potent stimulants for induction of **interferons** (*q.v.*), especially IFNβ types. Interferons, in turn, antagonize viral replication by inducing two enzymes activated by dsRNA. Protein kinase 2a attacks the α subunit of eIF2 (the factor that carries initiator tRNA to the 40S ribosomal subunit), and thereby blocks formation of new polypeptide chains. The second enzyme destroys mRNA templates.

ribonucleic acid polymerases: *see* **ribonucleic acids** and **RNA polymerases I**, **II**, and **III**.

ribonucleoproteins: RNPs; ribonucleic acid and protein complexes. Some are essential for RNA processing (*see* also **ribonucleic acids** and **ribozymes**). Others are **signal recognition proteins** (*q.v.*).

ribonucleosides: adenosine, guanosine, cytosine, uridine, and other compounds composed of nitrogenous bases covalently linked to ribose moieties.

ribonucleotides: ATP, ADP, AMP, GTP, CDP, UDP, cAMP, cGMP, FMN, and other compounds composed of covalently liked nitrogenous base, ribose, and phosphate groups. RNAs are ribonucleotide polymers.

ribonucleotide diphosphate reductases: ribonucleotide reductase; enzymes essential for DNA synthesis that convert ribonucleotides to deoxyribonucleotides.

ribophorins: two small endoplasmic reticulum membrane integral proteins, ribophorins I and II. They bind to ribosomes that are assembling peptide chains with signal sequences, and facilitate threading of the chains through the membranes, and chain entry to the endoplasmic reticulum lumen.

ribose: D-ribose; an aldohexose. It is a component of ribonucleic acids, of ATP, GTP, cAMP, FAD and other ribonucleotides, and a precursor of deoxyribose. Some foods contain it, but much of the sugar is synthesized from glucose via the hexose monophosphate shunt pathway.

ribose-5-phosphate: a pentose phosphate formed from ribulose-5-phosphate and used for ribonucleotide biosynthesis.

ribose phosphate isomerase: an enzyme that catalyzes interconversion of ribose-5-phosphate and ribulose-5-phosphate, via an enol intermediate.

ribosomal proteins: 50 or more proteins that associate with ribonucleic acids to form the structural components of **ribosomes** (*q.v.*); *see* also **ribonucleic acids**.

ribosomes: organelles composed of several kinds of ribonucleic acids and proteins, on which new proteins are assembled (*see* **translation**). Eukaryote types are 80S particles with 40S and 60S subunits. Some assemble in cytoplasm as single units that make limited quantities of proteins. Others are components of clusters (polysomes) that translate more efficiently, since a single messenger RNA molecule "read" by one member of the complex is passed directly to the next. Rough endoplasmic reticulum (RER), composed of ribosomes associated with endoplasmic reticulum membranes, is used to synthesize proteins destined for incorporation into vesicles, or into plasma and other membranes. Prokaryote ribosomes are 70S particles with 30S and 50S subunits. Most mitochondrial proteins are assembled on cytoplasmic ribosomes, but eukaryote mitochondria make a few on ribosomes that resemble prokaryotes type in composition, responses to antibiotics, and other properties.

ribozymes: ribonucleic acids that function as enzymes. They contribute to RNA processing by catalyzing the cleavage of RNA precursors that is essential for excising introns.

ribulose-5-phosphate: D-erythro-2-pentulose; a ketopentose formed in the pentose (hexose monophosphate) pathway via: 6-phosphogluconate + $NADP^+ \rightarrow$ ribulose-5-phosphate + NADPH + H^+ + CO_2, catalyzed by 6-phosphogluconate dehydrogenase. The reaction provides NADPH for anabolic reactions. The sugar phosphate can be converted to ribose-5-phosphate, xylulose-5-phosphate, or ribulose 1,5-biphosphate.

ribulose-1,5-biphosphate: a diphosphorylated pentose made from ribulose-5-phosphate + ATP. It is the intermediate in the Calvin-Benson photosynthesis cycle that reacts with carbon dioxide to yield two molecules of 3-phosphoglycerate.

ribulose biphosphate carboxylase: the most abundant chloroplast enzyme, essential for CO_2 fixation during photosynthesis. In the absence of oxygen, it catalyzes formation of 3-phosphoglycerate from CO_2 + ribulose biphosphate. In the presence of oxygen, the products are phosphoglycerate and phosphoglycolate.

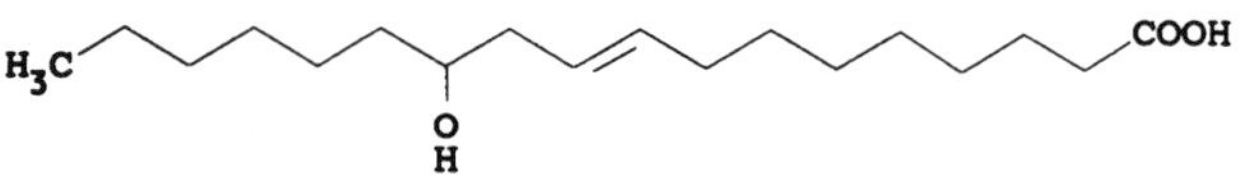

ricinoleic acid

ricin: a toxin mixture derived from the castor bean, *Ricinus communis* that contains two lectins and two hemagglutinins, used to study cell surface properties, and for its anti-cancer potency. Low doses invoke mucous membrane inflammation and hemorrhages. High levels are lethal. The major biologically active component is a 66K lectin composed of a 32K A subunit that inactivates ribosomes and a 34K type that binds to β-galactosyl moieties. *Ricinus communis* agglutinin is a less toxic 120K lectin.

ricinoleic acid: *d*-12-hydroxyoleic acid; the major component of castor oil, obtained from *Ricinus Euphorbiaceae*. It irritates the gastrointestinal tract, and is used as a cathartic. The sodium salt is a sclerosing agent. It is also spermicidal, and is a component of some contraceptive jellies.

rickets: a disease most common in infants and children, usually caused by vitamin D deficiency. The manifestations include poor bone mineralization (often associated with excessive osteoid production), bone deformities (especially in the limbs, pelvis, thoracic cage and other regions subjected to mechanical pressure) and skeletal muscle weakness. Parathyroid hormone levels are usually high, and account in part for the hypophosphatemia. Less common causes include inability to absorb the vitamin from the intestines (in individuals who do not receive adequate exposure to ultraviolet light), to convert the vitamin to calciferol hormones, and/or to respond to those hormones. A different form of rickets is caused by renal defects that impair phosphate transport. *Cf* **osteomalacia**.

Rickettsia: microorganisms that cause typhus and Rocky Mountain spotted fever, and other members of a genus of very small parasitic microorganisms. They are usually transmitted to vertebrates by lice and ticks.

rifamycins: several chemically related antibiotics obtained from *Streptomyces mediterranei* that interact with bacterial RNA polymerase beta subunits and inhibit prokaryotic (but not eukaryotic) DNA-dependent RNA synthesis by affecting transcription initiation (but not elongation). They block formation of the first phosphodiesterase bond, but permit continued synthesis of molecules in which the bond has been formed. Rifampicin (rifampin, rifamycin AMP, 5,6,9,17,19-21-hexahydroxy-23-methoxy-2,4-12,16,18,20,22-heptamethyl-8-[N-4-(4-methyl-1-piperazinyl)formimidoyl]2,7(epoxypentadeca[1,11,13]trienimino)naphthol[2,1-*b*]furan-1,11(2*H*)dione-21-acetate), shown below, is a semisynthetic derivative used to treat pulmonary tuberculosis and some other infections (including gonorrhea and leprosy in some countries), and as an investigative tool.

rigin: Gly-Gln-Pro-Arg; a peptide component of human IgG type immunoglobulin that stimulates phagocytosis.

rigor mortis: stiffening of skeletal muscle that occurs soon after death. ATP depletion and Ca^{2+} release create a condition in which actin-myosin bridges can be formed but not broken. The rigidity subsides when the proteins undergo postmortem deterioration.

rimcazole: *cis*-9-[3-93,5-dimethyl-1-piperazinyl)propyl]-9*H*-carbazole; an "antipsychotic" agent that acts on sigma type receptors (*see* **opioid receptors**).

rimorphin: dynorphin B.

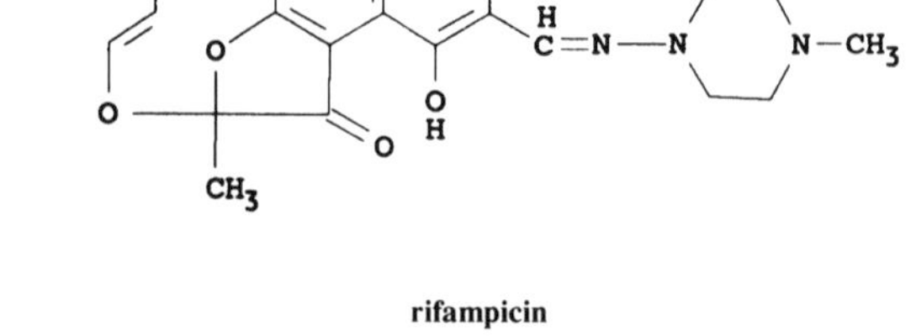

rifampicin

ring chromosomes: circular chromosomes that lack telomeres. Single ring chromosomes are normally present in prokaryotes, mitochondria, and chloroplasts. Aberrant types can form in eukaryote nuclei during meiosis.

Ringer's solution: isotonic balanced salt solutions used topically to prolong the viability of excised cells and tissues. One deciliter of the original type (*Frog* Ringer solution, isotonic for most amphibian tissues) contains 0.65g NaCl, 0.014g KCl, 0.012g $CaCl_2$, 0.02g $NaHCO_3$, and 0.001g NaH_2PO_4. Glucose, 0.2g, is sometimes added. A deciliter of *Ringer-Locke* solution for mammalian tissues and cells contains 0.9g NaCl, along with three times as much KCl, and twice as much $CaCl_2$ as the frog type. Other variants include *Ringer-Tyrode* solution which additionally contains $MgCl_2$.

ring gland: a structure in the larvae of *Drosophila* and some other Diptera, formed by fusion of the corpus cardiacum, corpus allatum, and prothoracic gland.

ring tests: qualitative tests for detecting antigens or antibodies, based on formation of precipitates at interfaces when solutions of antigens or antibodies are layered over (but not mixed with) ones that contains complementary compounds that bind to them.

Riopan: a trade name for magaldrate, a hydroxymagnesium aluminate used to counteract gastric acidity, with the approximate formula: $[Mg(OH)^+]_4[Al_2(OH)_{10}^{4-}]\cdot 2H_2O$.

rioprostil: (11α,13E)-1,11,16-trihydroxy-16-methyl-prost-13-en-9-one; a prostaglandin E_1 (PGE_1) analog used to protect the gastric mucosa in individuals taking large doses of cyclooxygenase inhibitors. *See* **misoprostol**.

ristocetin: ristomycin; a mixture of two antibacterial agents made by the actinomycete fungus, *Nocardia lurida*, ristocetins A and B. It stimulates phagocytosis and platelet aggregation. The A type is shown.

Ritalin: a trade name for the hydrochloride of methylphenidate (α-phenyl-2-piperidinacetic acid) methyl ester, an agent that usually causes central nervous system stimulation but is reported to be exert beneficial effects in hyperactive children (possibly by improving attention span).

ritanserin: 6-[2-[4-[*bis*(fluorophenyl)-methylene]-1-piperidinyl]-ethyl]-5H-thiazole[3,2-alpyr-imidin-5-one; a potent $5H_2$ type serotonin receptor antagonist that penetrates blood brain barriers.

ristocetin A

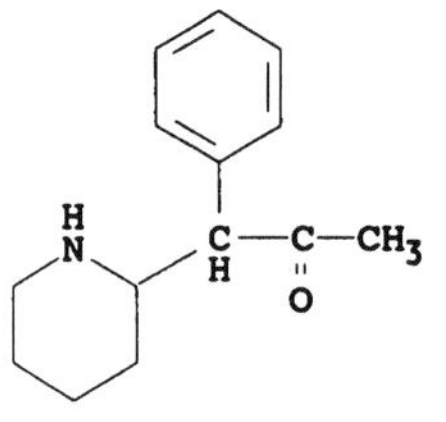

Ritalin

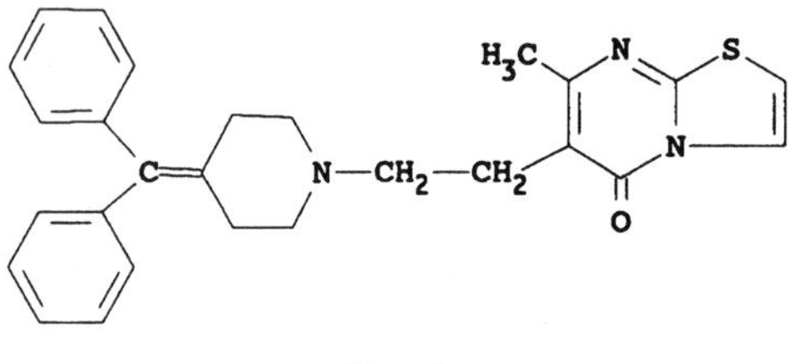

ritanserin

Ro 15-1788: flumenazil.

Ro 15-4513: ethyl-8-azido-6-dihydro-5-methyl-6-oxo-4*H*-imidazol[1,5-*a*]-[1,4]benzodiazepine-3-carboxylic acid; a partial agonist for benzodiazepine receptors that antagonizes ethyl alcohol effects and has anxiolytic properties.

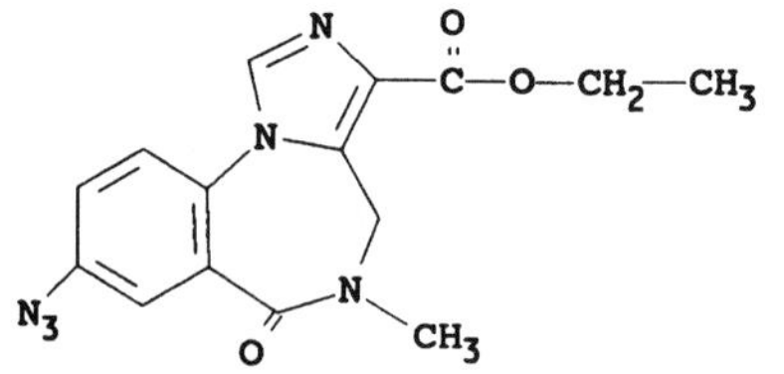

Ro 16-6491: *N*-(2-aminoethyl)-4-chlorobenzamide; the chloride is an orally effective, short-acting inhibitor of B type monoamine oxidases with no sympathomimetic properties.

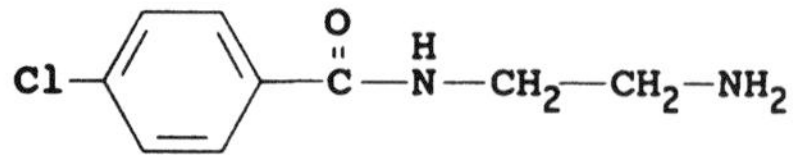

ritodrine: 4-hydroxy-α-[1-[[2-(4-hydroxyphenyl)ethyl]-amino]ethyl]benzene methanol; a β-type adrenergic receptor agonist. The hydrochloride is used to relax uterine smooth muscle and thereby delay premature labor.

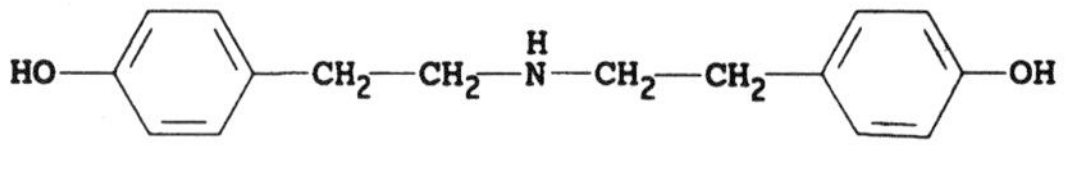

Ro 20-1724: 4-[(3-butoxy-4-methoxyphenyl)methyl]-2-imidazolidinone; a selective inhibitor of cyclic nucleotide-dependent phosphodiesterases that enhances cAMP accumulation stimulated by forskolin and other agents, but does not affect adenylate cyclase activity. It also inhibits protein kinase A and arachadonic acid mediated platelet aggregation.

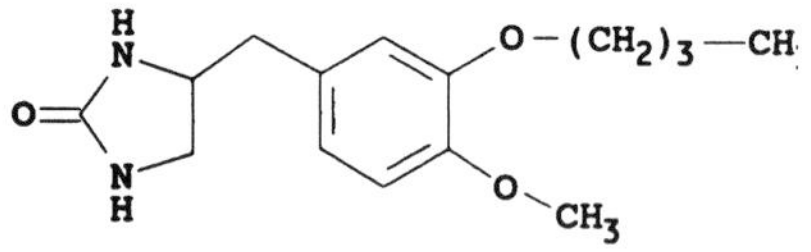

R loops: structures visible under electron microscopy, formed when messenger RNA molecules anneal to complementary segments of partially denatured DNA. Since an mRNA lacks introns, it hybridizes with only some parts of a DNA strand, distorts it, and displaces most of the other DNA strand in that region. (DNA-RNA complexes are more stable than DNA-DNA types). The structures are used to identify DNA sites that code for mRNAs, and to provide information on the locations of noncoding regions.

RO 41-0960: 2′-fluoro-3,4-dihydroxy-5-nitrobenzophenone; a specific, reversible inhibitor of catecholamine-*O*-methyltransferase (COMT).

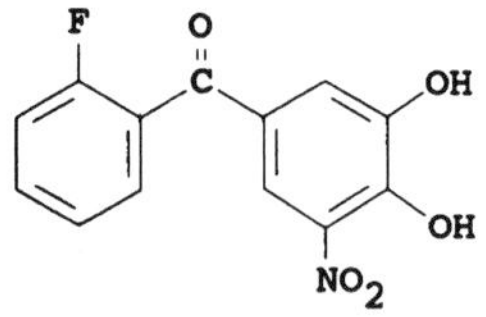

RLX: relaxin.

Rn: radon.

RNAs: *see* **ribonucleic acids**.

RNA capping: *see* **ribonucleic acids**.

RNA polymerases: ribonucleic acid polymerases; enzymes essential for assembling **ribonucleic acids** (*q.v.*) from nucleotides.

RO 41-1049: *N*-(2-aminoethyl)-5-(3-fluorophenyl)-4-thiazolecarboxamide; a selective, reversible inhibitor of A type monoamine oxidases.

RNA primer: a short RNA sequence attached by an RNA polymerase to the 5′ end of a DNA chain that serves as a template for initiating DNA replication. It is removed before DNA synthesis is completed.

RNases: ribonucleases.

RNA splicing: removal of intron segments from primary transcripts, followed by joining of exon components to form mature messenger RNAs. Many primary transcripts can be spliced in more than one way to yield two or more kinds of messengers. *See*, for example **calcitonin/CGRP gene**.

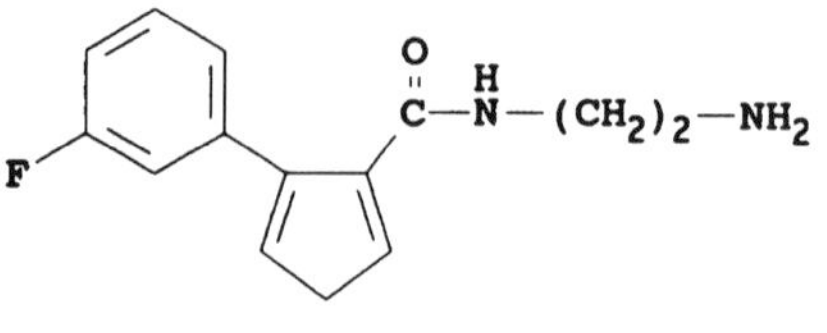

ROCC: receptor operated **calcium channels** (*q.v.*).

rod[s]: photoreceptor cells in vertebrate retinas used for scotopic vision; *see* **rhodopsin** and **transducin**. They are

RNP: ribonucleoprotein.

much more sensitive to light than **cones** (*q.v.*), but do not contain pigments for color perception, and lack neural connections required for observation of fine detail.

ROD: relative optical density.

rodent: rats, mice, guinea pigs, hamsters, squirrels, marmosets, and other mammals of the order Rodentia. All have incisor teeth adapted for gnawing or nibbling, different from those of rabbits and related species.

Roentgen: a unit of radiation exposure equivalent to 2.58 x 10^{-4} coulomb per kilogram.

Rogaine: a trade name for minoxidil.

ros: a UR2 chicken sarcoma oncogene that codes for p68$^{gag\text{-}ros}$ protein, which resembles insulin receptors and contains a tyrosine kinase domain.

ROS cells: a rat osteoblast/osteocyte type osteosarcoma cell line.

rosette: in immunology, a cluster erythrocytes surrounding a centrally located lymphocyte; *see* **E** and **EAC rosettes**.

R$_0$t: in systems in which RNA molecules hybridize with single-stranded DNAs, the RNA concentration multiplied by the incubation time. It is a measure of the amount of RNA complementary to the DNA probe.

rotamases: peptidyl-prolyl *cis-trans* isomerases; PPIs; enzymes that change the positions of protein prolyl moieties by acting on bonds between them and other amino acids. They thereby affect protein folding patterns, and appear to be essential for optimum activities of peptidyl disulfide isomerases (which catalyze formation of S-S bonds), for collagen maturation, and other functions. PPIs occur in bacterial as well as eukaryote cytoplasm; and high levels accumulate in endoplasmic reticulum lumens. Secretory forms are also made. The immunophilins bound by cyclosporins, FK506, and rapamycin are PPIs; but they suppress immune responses in other ways, at least some of which involve calcium-dependent processes and drug-immunophilin complex binding to calcineurin.

rotenone: [2*R*-(2α,6α,12α)]-1,2,12,12*a*-tetrahydro-8,9-dimethoxy-2-(1-methylethenyl)-[1]benzopyrano[3,4*b*]-furol[2,3-h][1]benzopyran-6(6*aH*)-one; an agent used to kill ectoparasites that inhibits electron transport in mitochondrial NADH:Q reductase complexes.

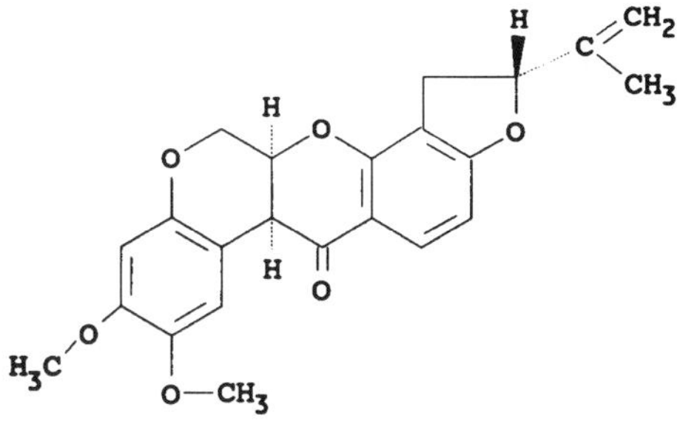

rough endoplasmic reticulum: RER: endoplasmic reticulum studded with ribosomes. It is used to synthesize proteins destined for insertion into organelles or membranes. *See* also **ribosomes** and **signal sequences**; and *cf* **smooth endoplasmic reticulum**.

rouleaux: cylindrical stacks of erythrocytes. Their rate of formation correlates with sedimentation rates, and is affected by fibrinogen and immunoglobulin concentrations.

roundworms: *Caenorhabditis elegans* (*q.v.*), several disease-causing worms, and other members of the phylum Nematoda.

Rous sarcoma virus: RSV; an avian retrovirus whose genome codes for pp60$^{v\text{-}src}$, a non-receptor protein kinase closely related to pp60$^{c\text{-}src}$ (a *c-src* proto-oncogene product that associates with plasma membranes, participates in signal transduction and contributes to cell cycle control; *see* also **SH domains**). The viral counterpart is a truncated version that transforms fibroblasts and invokes transmissible solid tumors (sarcomas) in chickens. In common with other retroviruses, it has a *gag* gene that codes for its viral capsid protein, a *pol* gene for the reverse transcriptase, and an *env* type for the protein that forms envelope spikes.

royal jelly: a nutrient mixture secreted by worker bees and consumed by the queen of a honey bee colony, and by larvae reared to develop into queens. It contains proteins, B vitamins, small amounts of Fe, Mn, Ni, Co, Cr, As, Si, Au, Hg, and Bi, and royal jelly acid (*trans*-10-hydroxy-Δ^2-decenoic acid, shown below). Purported beneficial effects on health and fertility in humans have not been substantiated.

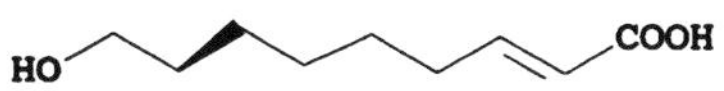

RPF: renal plasma flow.

R plasmid: an extrachromosomal DNA molecule that confers bacterial resistance to antibiotics.

rpm: revolutions per minute.

RQ: respiratory quotient.

-rrhacia: a suffix that refers to conditions of the spinal cord or cerebrospinal fluid.

-rrhexis: a suffix that denotes tearing or rupture.

rRNAs: ribosomal RNAs; *see* **ribonucleic acids**.

RSKs: receptor activated signal kinases; serine/threonine protein kinase products of *rsk* genes activated by epidermal, platelet derived, and fibroblast growth factors (EGF, PDGF, and FGFs), and by other mitogens. They contribute to signal transduction, and are components of phosphorylation cascades that control cell proliferation. Full activity requires phosphorylation on both tyrosine and serine/threonine moieties (and both protein phosphatase 1B and protein phosphatase 2A inactivate). One type, pp90^{rsk}, phosphorylates ribosomal protein S6. RSKI is a 44K protein similar to the sea star meiosis activated kinase that phosphorylates myelin basic protein and microtubule associated protein 2 (MAP-2), (but does not directly affect S6). It is partially activated by pp90^{rsk}. RSK II is a different, 42K protein with similar properties.

RSV: Rous sarcoma virus.

rT_3: reverse triiodothyronine; *see* **reverse T_3**.

RTF: resistance transfer factor, a component of R plasmids that mediates transfer to other bacteria.

Ru: ruthenium.

RU 486: 11β-dimethylaminophenyl-17α-hydroxy-17β-propynyl-19-nortestosterone; mifepristone; a synthetic steroid that binds to progesterone receptors and blocks most of the genomic actions of the steroid in humans and in other mammals with similar progesterone receptors (but not in hamsters or chickens). It is used in conjunction with a prostaglandin analog to impede implantation or interrupt pregnancy soon after implantation has occurred, to treat endometriosis, and to arrest the growth of some breast and brain cancers. Higher concentrations are potent glucocorticoid receptor antagonists useful for treating Cushing's disease and other conditions associated with glucocorticoid excess. Although special permission has been obtained for some individuals with inoperable brain tumors, general use of RU 486 has not been approved by the United States Food and Drug Administration.

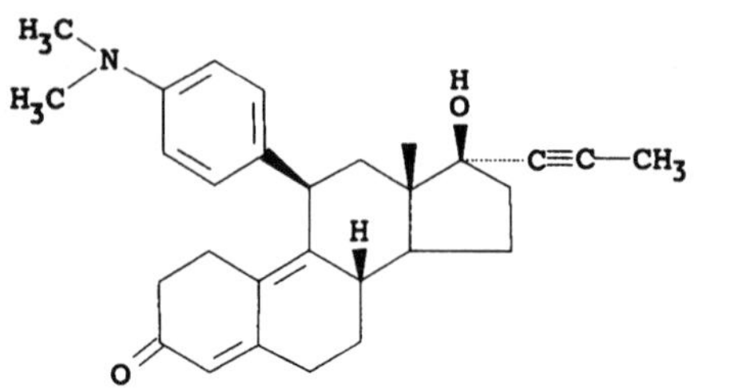

RU 2858: moxestrol.

RU 5020: promegestone.

RU 5135: 3α-hydroxy-16-imino-5β-17-aza-androstan-11-one; a potent synthetic neurosteroid.

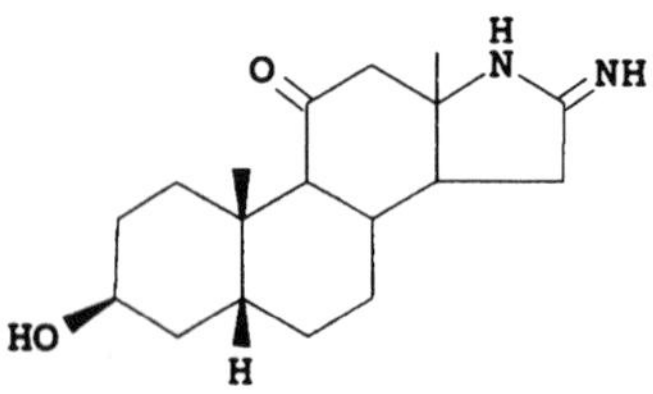

RU 26988, RU 28362: glucocorticoid receptor agonists chemically related to RU 486.

RU 38486: RU 486.

rubidium: Rb; a metallic element (atomic number 37, atomic weight 85.47), used to study potassium transport.

rubor: red coloration.

rubro-: a prefix that (1) means red, or (2) refers to the red nucleus of the midbrain.

rudiment: an early developmental form of a structure that will give rise to a component of the mature organism.

ruffled border: the appearance under electron microscopy, of cell edges with many microvilli.

ruffled edges: the appearance of motile cell surfaces with numerous small cytoplasmic projections.

ruga [**rugae**]: a fold or wrinkle.

runt disease: (1) severe pathological conditions in young individuals caused by graft-versus host disease. Growth retardation and high susceptibility to infection are usually followed by early death; (2) wasting diseases (with severely impaired lymphoid tissue development) in rodents subjected to neonatal thymectomy.

Russell bodies: spherical immunoglobulin clusters that form in normal plasma cells, and in myeloma types.

rut: a period of intense sexual activity in male animals of many species.

ruthenium: Ru; an element (atomic number 44, atomic weight 101.07), used as a catalyst for synthesizing long-chain hydrocarbons; *see* also **ruthenium red**.

ruthenium red: an ammoniated ruthenium oxychloride polycationic dye that irreversibly blocks ryanodine-sensitive and nucleotide-activated calcium ion channels, and thereby both calcium efflux from the sarcoplasmic reticulum and calcium uptake by mitochondria. It is used to study calcium transport mechanisms. The tetrahydrate is a stain for pectins and cell surface acidic glycosaminoglycans.

$$[(NH_3)_5RuO(NH_3)_5ORuNH_3)_5]Cl_6 \bullet 4H_2O$$

rutin: quercetin-3-rutinoside; 3,3′4′,5,7-pentahydroxyflavone-3-rutinoside; a flavin glycoside made by several plants, present in high concentrations in buckwheat (*Fagopyrum esculentum*), tobacco (*Nicotiana tabacum*), forsythia, pansies, and eucalyptus leaves. It is used to control capillary fragility, and to inhibit aldose reductase. Hydrolysis catalyzed by rhamnosediastase releases rutinose.

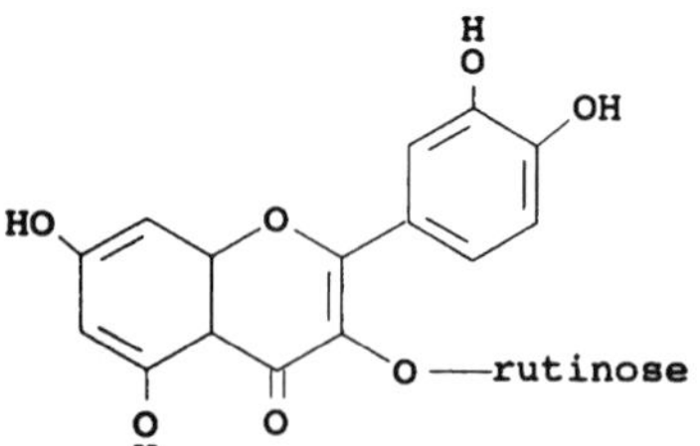

rutinose: 6-*O*-α-L-rhamnosyl-D-glucose; a disaccharide obtained from rutin.

ryanodine: 3-(1*H*-pyrrol-2-carboxylate; an alkaloid made by *Ryania speciosa* that activates a set of gap junction type calcium channel proteins ("ryanodine receptors") involved in excitation-contraction coupling in cardiac and skeletal muscle sarcoplasmic reticula (and some receptors in neurosecretory and epithelial cells),

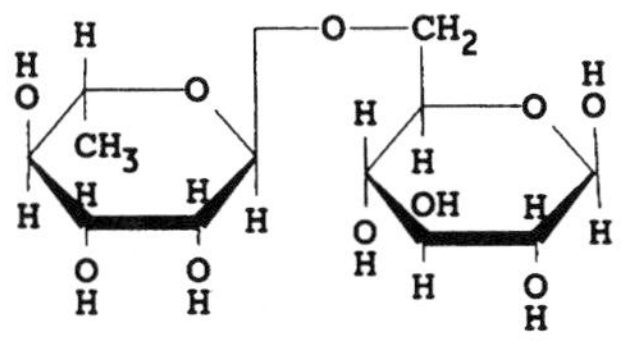

rutinose

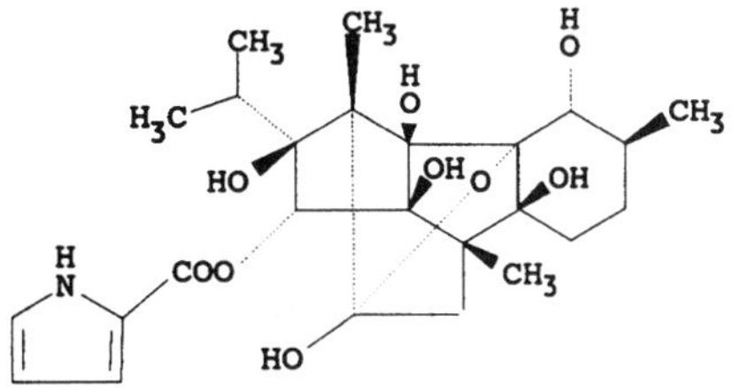

ryanodine

and promotes Ca^{2+} release. *See* also **cyclic adenosine diphosphate ribose**. It is used as an insecticide, and, although toxic, to treat some cardiac dysrhythmias. It causes sustained skeletal muscle contractures and ele-

vates metabolic rates in individuals with mutant ryanodine receptors. Some inhalant anesthetics and muscle relaxants activate those receptors and invoke malignant hyperthermia.

S

S: (1) serine; (2) sulfur; (3) left (sinister; *see* **stereoisomerism**); (4) Svedberg unit; (5) entropy unit; (6) siemens.

s: (1) standard deviation; (2) sedimentation coefficient.

Σ: Sigma; sum of; a symbol used in calculations, for example of standard deviations.

σ: sigma; (1) standard deviation; (2) a protein activated by PCPs, previously believed to be an opioid receptor.

S1: soluble 102K fragments of myosin heads and heavy meromyosin released by papain catalyzed cleavage. They display ATPase activity, bind actin, and are used to identify filaments in electron micrographs.

S2: fibrous heavy meromyosin fragments that link S1 heads to low molecular weight meromyosin molecules.

S6: proteins on the messenger RNA binding sites of eukaryote 40S ribosome subunits essential for initiating protein synthesis. They are activated, via phosphorylation, by **S6 kinases** (*q.v.*), which are, in turn activated by numerous physiological growth stimulants and oncogene products. S6 activity rises during cell cycle G1 phases, and prepares cells for entry into S phases. Some anabolic actions of insulin are mediated by S6 proteins.

S-100: a diverse group of 10-21K calcium binding proteins, soluble in saturated ammonium sulfate, made by all animal species (including protozoa) in both intracellular and secreted forms. Some are αβ heterodimers; others are αα, or ββ homodimers. All types contain acidic, basic and hydrophobic domains, and resemble calmodulin subunits in configuration (but not amino acid composition). They do not function directly as enzymes, but bind calcium and then attach to and affect the functions of other proteins. Various types are implicated as mediators of cell-type specific cell cycle progression, differentiation, cytoskeleton-plasma membrane interactions, signal transduction, and exocytosis. S-100β types (disulfide bonded β-β dimers) are made in largest amounts by neuroglial and Schwann cells, but are also secreted by pituitary cells and adipocytes. A subtype (neurite extension factor) is released to cerebrospinal fluid; and measurements of its levels are used to assess the progress of individuals with brain injuries. In humans, its synthesis is directed by chromosome # 21; and overexpression may contribute to Downs' syndrome pathology. It specifically inhibits phosphorylation of pp80 (an 87K major kinase C substrate), and is believed to modulate Ca^{2+}/inositol-mediated signal transduction. In pituitary glands, it promotes prolactin release. S-100α proteins are mostly αβ dimers, made in adipocytes and muscle cells as well as

brain. In common with S-100β, they affect microtubule assembly and depolymerization by inhibiting phosphorylation of tau protein. (Excessive tau phosphorylation has been detected in the brains of individuals with Alzheimer's disease). Other members of the group include p11 (which complexes with calpactin p36 and affects exocytosis), and calcyclin (2A9, a cell cycle regulated protein induced by growth factors, maximally expressed during cell cycle G_1 phases, and constitutively made by acute myeloid leukemia cells). Protein 18A2 is an S-100 protein induced by serum in growth arrested cells that attains maximal levels during cell cycle S phases. p9Ka, initially identified as a protein whose levels increase rapidly during mammary gland differentiation, may be the rat 18A2 homolog. MRP8, which is identical to or closely related to cystic fibrosis antigen, is made by myeloid cells, and can be detected in the sera of cystic fibrosis and rheumatoid arthritis patients. MRP14 is also made by myeloid cells and released to the blood of individuals with rheumatoid arthritis. Yet different members of the protein family include a 7K intestinal binding protein.

sabril: γ-vinyl-**GABA**.

sac: a pouch-like structure.

SAC: a B lymphocyte mitogen made by *Staphylococcus aureus*.

SAC I, SAC II: endonucleases made by *Streptomyces achromogens* that cleave, respectively, T:C bonds of GAGC/T and C:G bonds of CCGC/GG nucleotides.

saccharides: sugars and sugar polymers, including mono-, di-, tri-, oligo- and polysaccharides.

saccharin: 1,2-benzisothiazol-3-(2*H*)-one-1,1-dioxide; a compound 300-500 times as effective as cane sugar for eliciting perception of a sweet taste by humans and most other animals species. Since it does not affect blood glucose levels, and is not an energy source, it is used in place of sugar by individuals with diabetes mellitus, to lower the caloric content of foods and beverages, and in some studies of taste perception. It is also fed to control groups in experiments designed to assess effects of sugar intake on other functions. High concentrations can inhibit glucose-6-phosphatase, and are reported to induce morphine tolerance in some mutant rat strains. There is no evidence for carcinogenicity in humans. The ability of massive doses administered to rats throughout pregnancy and then to their offspring to increase the incidence of urinary bladder cancer in the progeny has been attributed to a contaminant in the preparation.

saccharin

Saccharomyces cerevisiae: *S. cerevisiae*; baker's yeast; budding yeast; a simple eukaryote microorganism used for studies of genetics, cell cycle control, and signal transduction. The functions of some small guanine nucleotide binding proteins, the controls over cell cycles, and the mechanisms for reproduction differ in some ways from those of *Schizosaccharomyces pombe*.

sacculus: a small pouch-like structure.

sacculus rotundus: a lymphoid structure near the terminal end of the rabbit ileum.

sacculus vasculosus: a vascularized organ on the floor of the third brain ventricle in some fish species. It is connected to other brain regions, and may contribute to neurohypophysial functions.

Sach's disease: *see* **Tay-Sach's disease**.

SAD: seasonal affective disorder.

*S***-adenosylmethionine**: SAM; a major methyl group donor for the synthesis of epinephrine, acetylcholine, and melatonin, for formation of catechol estrogens and catecholamine inactivation, and for other biochemical pathways, made in the reaction: methionine + ATP → SAM + Pi + P-P. Demethylation yields *S*-adenosylhomocysteine, which can be hydrolyzed to adenosine + homocysteine.

safflower oil: oil extracted from *Carthamus tinctorius* seeds. Purported beneficial effects on lipoprotein levels are attributed to its high linoleic and low saturated fatty acid content.

saffron: yellow dyes obtained from crocus stigmas. They are used to color foods, and are components of some biological stains.

safranin O: 3,7-diamino-2,8-dimethyl-5-phenylphenazinum chloride; a stain for nuclei, and for the cell walls of meristem tissue, and a counterstain for bacteria.

SAgs: *see* **superantigens**.

sagittal: (1) resembling an arrow or arrow head; (2) a median plane, or one parallel to it. A midsagittal section

safranin

separates a bilaterally symmetrical animal into right and left halves; a parasagittal one divides it into two parts of different sizes. The sagittal suture joins the left and right parietal bones of the mature skull.

salbutamol: albuterol; 2-(*tert*-butylamino)-1-(4-hydroxy-3-hydroxymethylphenyl)ethanol; a selective β$_2$-type adrenergic receptor agonist used as a bronchodilator, and to inhibit uterine contractions that threaten premature delivery.

salicylates: *salicylic acid* (2-hydroxybenzoic acid), a keratolytic compound that promotes skin desquamation, is used topically to destroys warts, with benzoic acid (in Whitfield's ointment) as a fungicide, and with other agents to treat psoriasis. *Methyl salicylate* (oil of wintergreen) is the counterirritant component of liniments used to ease muscle pains. *Sodium salicylate* and some related compounds are orally effective analgesic, antipyretic and anti-inflammatory agents used to alleviate nonvisceral pain, reduce fever, and treat rheumatoid arthritis. Most of the therapetuic and toxic effects are attributed to inhibition of prostaglandin synthesis (but *see* **nonsteroidal anti-inflammatory agents**). High concentrations exert inhibitory influences on neutrophilic leukocytes; but therapeutic doses may not be sufficient for such actions. Unlike glucocorticoids, salicylates do not suppress cytokine release or the formation of leukotrienes and some other eicosanoids. They do, however inhibit blood platelet aggregation; and daily use has been advocated for some individuals at risk for developing thrombi. Since platelets cannot synthesize new enzymes, irreversible inhibitors of prostaglandin synthesis such as acetylsalicylic acid (aspirin) are more effective than sodium salicylate and others that act reversibly. Large amounts of salicylates can diminish the contraceptive effectiveness of intrauterine devices, and slow parturition. Prolonged use of high doses leads to irritation of the gastric mucosa and can cause ulceration. The agents can also diminish renal blood flow and affect Na$^+$ and water excretion, but are less likely to cause renal damage than phenylbutazone or ibuprofen. Salicylates can additionally augment the production of adrenocortical steroids by stimulating hypothalamic neurons that secrete corticotropin releasing hormone (CRH), accelerate the clearance of iodinated thyroid hormones from blood plasma by displacing them from binding proteins, and inter-

| salicylic acid | salicylamide | sodium salicylate | aspirin | methyl-salicylate |

salicylates

fere with iodine concentration in thyroid glands. Elevation of the metabolic rate results from uncoupling of oxidative phosphorylation via mechanisms described for 2,4-dinitrophenol. Effects on the nervous system can invoke respiratory alkalosis (via direct actions on neurons that control ventilation), and tinnitus. Influences on the liver can lead to hepatomegaly, nausea, anorexia, and (in severe cases) jaundice and necrosis. In limited numbers of susceptible individuals, allergic reactions include not only skin rashes, but also bronchoconstriction and anaphylaxis. *See* also **salicylism**.

salicylism: tinnitus, nausea, headache, mental confusion, rapid pulse, hyperpnea, and other symptoms caused by high levels of **salicylates** (*q.v.*). It can occur, for example in individuals with rheumatoid arthritis who regularly ingest large amounts. The acute symptoms usually subside when the drug levels fall (but some kinds of tissue damage caused by prolonged use of high doses are not repaired).

salivary glands: digestive system glands that secrete water, mucus, salts, and other substances (including salivary amylase in many species). In mice and some other rodents, androgen-regulated cells synthesize substantial quantities of nerve growth factor (NGF), epidermal growth factor (EGF), angiotensin-II, and other hormones, and release them during some forms of stress. The glands of some snakes make highly potent toxins, some of which are used as pharmacological tools. The very large chromosomes in the glands of some insect larvae are used for genetics studies. In humans, the parotid glands are the largest of the group. They secrete watery solutions, rich in salts and amylase, and are stimulated by acetylcholine released from postganglionic fibers of the otic ganglia (which synapse with preganglionic fibers of the glossopharyngeal nerves). A parotid hormone that decreases tooth decay has been described; *see* also **parotin**. The smaller submaxillary (submandibular) glands, innervated by postganglionic fibers of the submandibular ganglia (which synapse with different branches of the glossopharyngeal nerves), produce a more viscous product, high in mucin. Viscous saliva is also made by small sublingual glands. The major inhibitory controls over watery secretion are exerted by branches of the superior cervical sympathetic ganglia. Watery solutions are also made by numerous small buccal glands that are constitutively active. Under most conditions, small amounts of saliva, continuously released, lubricate and cleanse the mouth, and are essential for speech. Dehydration and stress (which promotes catecholamine release) decrease the volume. Food and other stimuli acting on tactile as well as chemoreceptors in the mouth initiate reflexes that augment the amounts.

Pleasant odors, and thoughts of food also increase the secretion. Although mildly unpleasant food odors can inhibit, noxious agents acting on olfactory receptors are powerful stimulants. The larger volumes buffer food and other chemicals, aid in mastication, and are needed to form boluses for swallowing. Measurements of salivary Na:K ratios are used as preliminary tests for aldosterone functions.

salmine: a 6-7K protamine of salmon sperm.

Salmo: a genus that includes the Atlantic salmon, the rainbow trout, and other fishes used for food and as sources of calcitonin and other regulators.

Salmonella: a bacteria genus that includes some diarrhea causing organisms. *S.typhimurium* is used in genetics studies.

salping-: a prefix that refers to the Fallopian tubes.

salpingectomy: removal of the Fallopian tubes.

salt: (1) any product formed when an acid neutralizes a base; (2) any compound formed by the union of electronegative and electropositive ions to form electrovalent (ionic) bonds; (3) when the chemical nature is not specified, NaCl or common table salt.

salt appetite: desire to ingest, or avid ingestion of sodium chloride. It is stimulated by some physiological and pharmacological agents that lower blood and/or extracellular fluid volume, and/or the salt content of the fluids, via influences on baro- and chemoreceptors. Angiotensin II is a potent physiological factor that acts directly on receptors in the hypothalamus, and at some other sites. Although high levels of mineralocorticoids elevate both blood volume and extracellular fluid Na^+ concentrations, they also increase salt appetite, probably by lowering intracellular sodium levels.

saltation: (1) the theory that new species arise suddenly when mutations invoke large phenotypic changes; (2) sudden jerky or leaping movements, for example in individuals with Huntington's chorea; (3) abrupt jumping movements of intracellular particles; (4) saltatory conduction.

saltatory conduction: rapid passage of nerve impulses down large peripheral, myelinated axons, in which excitation travels from one node of Ranvier to the next.

saltatory replication: lateral replication of DNA segments that leads to gene amplification.

salt craving: a strong drive to ingest sodium chloride, caused, for example by diets deficient in NaCl, or by conditions such as aldosterone deficiency and renal defects that accelerate salt loss to urine. *See also* **angiotensin II**, and **salt appetite**.

salt glands: nasal and lacrimal glands of some birds and reptiles that contribute to electrolyte balance by secreting sodium chloride. In most species, the activities are stimulated by aldosterone.

salting in, salting out: techniques for separating protein components of mixtures on the basis of differences in solubilities in various concentrations of ammonium sulfate or other salts.

salt wasting: conditions in which large amounts of sodium chloride are lost to the urine. Aldosterone deficiency is a major cause. *See also* **adrenogenital syndrome** and **pseudohypoaldosteronism**.

salubrious: conducive to good health.

saluresis: increased urinary excretion of salt.

salvage compartment: the *cis*-Golgi network, which receives newly translocated proteins with **signal sequences** (*q.v.*).

salvage enzyme: HGPRT; *see* **salvage pathways**.

salvage pathways: chemical reactions in which partially degraded compounds that would otherwise be further degraded and/or excreted are recovered and converted to useful forms. The term is most commonly applied to reactions catalyzed by hypoxanthine-guanine phosphoribosyltransferase (HGPRT, salvage enzyme), in which hypoxanthine and guanine are phosphoribosylated to yield, respectively, inosine monophosphate and guanosine monophosphate.

SAM: *S*-adenosylmethionine.

sambucus nigra: a lectin from the inner bark of elder trees that binds to oligosaccharide lactose components.

Sandostatin: SMS-201-995: a trade name for octreotide.

Sanfilippo syndrome: mucopolysaccharidosis III; autosomal recessive lysosomal diseases in which synthesis of keratan sulfatase or *N*-acetyl glucosaminidase is impaired. The manifestations include mental retardation and facial deformities.

Sanger's reagent: 2,4-dinitrofluorobenzene: DNFB; a compound used in thin-layer chromatography that selectively reacts with NH_2 groups of amino acids (and ε-amino groups of lysine) to form yellow DNP compounds.

S antigens: soluble, 195K heat-stable antigens on the surfaces of *Plasmodium falciparum*.

SAP: steroidogenesis activator polypeptide.

sapogenins: several 27-carbon steroid components of plant saponins.

saponification: alkaline hydrolysis of esters to salts and free alcohols. Triacylglycerols treated with heat and alkali yield fatty acid salts (soaps) and glycerol.

saponins: plant glycosides that yield sapogenins and sugars when hydrolyzed. Low concentrations are detergents, used to solubilize membrane components and increase permeabilities. Higher ones destroy membranes and cause hemolysis.

saprophytes: heterotrophs that feed on organic components of dead and decaying organisms. Some authors reserve the term for plants that are nourished in this way, and use the terms *saprozoites* for mushrooms, bread molds, and other fungi, and *saprobes* for bacteria.

Sar: sarcosine;

SAR: systemic acquired resistance.

sarafotoxins: three cyclic 21-carbon cardiotoxic peptides chemically related to endothelins, obtained from the venom of *Actractapsis engaddensis* snakes. All are potent vasoconstrictors that act on coronary blood vessels. They also bind directly to atrial membranes and exert ionotropic effects that do not involve voltage-gated Na^+, K^+, or Ca^{2+} channels, and are not antagonized by adrenergic receptor blockers. (Intravenous injection of small amounts of either the A or B type causes lethal cardiac arrest in mice within minutes.) Additionally, they stimulate contraction of the ileum. At least some effects are related to activation of phosphodiesterases. Agents that block muscarinic, dopaminergic, α or β adrenergic, opiate, or H_1-type histaminergic receptors do not antagonize their influences on phosphoinositide hydrolysis and elevation of intracellular Ca^{2+} levels. In the structures of the A (S6a), B (S6b), and C (S6b) peptides, shown consecutively, the cysteine moieties are connected by disulfide bridges at postions $1 \rightarrow 15$ and $3 \rightarrow 11$:

Cys-Ser-Cys-Lys-Asp-Met-Thr-Asp-Lys-Glu-Cys-Leu-Asn-Phe-Cys-His-Gln-Asp-Val-Ile-Trp

Cys-Ser-Cys-Lys-Asp-Met-Thr-Asp-Lys-Glu-Cys-Leu-Tyr-Phe-Cys-His-Gln-Asp-Val-Ile-Trp

Cys-Thr-Cys-Asn-Asp-Met-Thr-Asp-Glu-Glu-Cys-Leu-Asn-Phe-Cys-His-Gln-Asp-Val-Ile-Trp

saralasin: 1-(*N*)-methylglycine-5-L-valine-8-L-alanine-angiotensin; Sar-Arg-Val-Tyr-Val-His-Pro-Ala; an angiotensin II analog used to treat some forms of hypertension. It is an angiotensin II receptor antagonist and partial agonist.

sarcoidoses: chronic, progressive diseases in which proliferation of reticuloendothelial system cells causes formation of granulomatous lesions in the skin, lungs, liver, lymph nodes, spleen, eyes, and other organs.

sarco-: a prefix that designates (1) soft tissue; (2) muscle; (3) mesodermal or mesenchymal tissue.

sarcoblast: myoblast.

sarcoid: resembling a sarcoma.

sarcolemma: the plasma membrane of a skeletal muscle cell.

sarcolysis: destruction of soft tissue.

sarcoma[s]: liposarcomas, chondrosarcomas, lymphomas, and other (usually malignant) tumors derived from immature connective tissue cells.

sarcoma virus: *see* **Rous sarcoma virus**.

sarcomere: the repeating unit of a skeletal muscle myofibril that extends from one Z line to the next.

sarcoplasm: the cytoplasm of a skeletal muscle cell.

sarcoplasmic reticulum: the endoplasmic reticulum of a muscle cell.

sarcosine: Sar: *N*-methylglycine; an amino acid in shellfish, peanuts, and some antibiotics made by fungi (including actinomycin D). Small amounts in vertebrate blood are acetylcholine degradation products. Sarcosine is incorporated into some hormone analogs (such as saralasin) to achieve resistance to endogenous peptidases.

$$HN\!-\!CH_3$$
$$H_2C\!-\!COOH$$

sarcosinemia: an autosomal recessive disease in which inadequate amounts of sarcosine dehydrogenase lead to sarcosine accumulation. The most common manifestation is a mild form of mental retardation.

sarin: isopropylmethylphosphorylfluoride; a nerve gas that irreversibly inhibits acetylcholinesterases and other enzymes whose active sites contain serine. It has been used to kill insects (by arresting ventilation), but is highly toxic to other species.

satellite: a chromosome segment connected to the rest of the chromosome by a thin filament.

satellite cells: quiescent myoblasts that persist in mature skeletal muscle and retain the ability to divide by mitosis. They are activated when muscle fibers are injured.

satellite DNA: simple sequence DNA. Light (A-T rich) and heavy (G-C rich) DNA segments with highly repetitive base sequences that can separated from the coding types by density gradient centrifugation. Some forms, present only in centromeres, contribute to chromosome alignment during mitosis and meiosis. Telomeric types protect chromosome ends against shortening during replication. *See* also *Alu* **sequences**.

satiety: satisfaction of the appetite for food. Fed laboratory animals are assumed to be experiencing satiety when they engage in behavior regarded as consistent with that state (for example, meal termination, grooming, and drowsing), and show no signs of malaise. Some observers regard the aversion invoked by force feeding as an exaggerated form of satiety.

satiety "centers": neuron clusters within the brain purported to sense nutritional states and motivate animals to limit the numbers of meals taken per day and/or the quantities consumed per meal to amounts required to maintain normal body weights. The ventromedial and paraventricular nuclei of the hypothalamus have been proposed to contain such loci; but most observers believe that control sites for such behavior are widely distributed (rather than localized to specific brain regions).

satiety factors: regulators that invoke satiety. Hormones suggested to exert such effects include cholecystokinin (CCK), calcitonin, pancreatic polypeptide, gastrin releasing peptide (GRP), and enterogastrone. Pyro-Glu-His-Gly-OH, isolated from the urine of patients with anorexia nervosa, is an additional candidate. Glucagon transiently suppresses appetite, but promotes insulin secretion. Insulin usually augments appetite by invoking hypoglycemia; but it may act directly on brain neurons to limit food intake when blood glucose levels are maintained. Several kinds of food components and their metabolites, including glucose, glycerol, and fatty acids are implicated as signals for neurons that affect the behavior.

saturated: containing the maximum amount of a substance, a term applied for example to fully hydrogenated organic molecules (with no double bonds), or to solutions that contain as much of a solute as they can hold.

saturation density: the numbers of cells that must accumulate in a given volume of culture medium to inhibit further cell proliferation. The inhibition is attributed to limited access to growth stimulants and/or nutrients, or to signals provided by neighboring cells. Transformed cells usually stop dividing at much higher densities than normal types, because they make growth factors normal cells must acquire from external sources, are insensitive to inhibitory factors, or have lost dependence on contact with substrates.

sauvagine: Asn-Asp-*p*Glu-Gly-Pro-Ile-Ser-Ile-Asp-Leu-Ser-Leu-Glu-Leu-Leu-Arg-Lys-Met-Ile-Glu-Ile-Glu-Lys-Gln-Glu-Lys-Glu-Lys-Gln-Gln-Ala-Ala-Asn-Asn-Arg-Leu-Leu-Leu-Asp-Thr-Ile-NH$_2$; a frog skin peptide chemically and biologically related to corticotropin releasing hormone (CRH). It mimics CRH effects on adrenocorticotropic hormone (ACTH) and β-endorphin secretion, and on mesenteric blood flow, and can invoke hypotension.

saxitoxin: STX; a very potent neurotoxin made by "red tide" dinoflagellates (*Gonyaulax catanella* and *Gonyaulax tamarensis*), used as a laboratory tool to block sodium channels. Mussels (for example *Mytilus californianus*), clams (such as *Saxidomus giganteus*), scallops, and some other shellfish can cause food poisoning because they eat the protozoa and accumulate the toxins.

Sb: antimony.

Sbx: a gene on the X chromosome that codes for a ubiquitin activating enzyme essential for cell cycle progression in both males and females; *cf* ***Sby***.

Sby: a segment of the Y chromosome homologous to *sbx* that may identical to *spy*. It codes for a ubiquitin activat-

saxitoxin

ing enzyme that appears to be essential for spermatogenesis. Its expression is limited to the testis, and is germ cell dependent; *see also sxr*.

SC-1: an antigen identified as the earliest marker of motor neuron differentiation.

scabies: mange; conditions in which *Sarcoptes scabiei* and related mite species cause skin rashes and itching.

scala: resembling a staircase. The *scala media* of the inner ear holds the Organ of Corti, and is filled with endolymph. The surrounding *scala tympani* and *scala vestibuli* contain perilymph.

scanning electron microscopy: SEM; techniques used to study surface properties of cells, tissues, and small organisms, in which images are formed by electrons reflected from specimen surfaces that bombard fluorescent screens. They can be used with very much larger objects than is possible with **transmission electron microscopy** (*q.v.*).

scanning tunneling microscopy: STM; versatile, high-resolution techniques that can define atomic-scale surface features. Microprobes positioned just a few angstroms away from specimens subjected to ultravacuums, maintained in liquid nitrogen or air, or immersed in media such as oil or saline, are moved along the surfaces. In one procedure, constant voltage is applied between platinum-iridium probe tips and the samples. The currents produced by electrons that tunnel across the gaps vary with the distances between the probes and the specimens, and images are generated from records of the vertical positions required to maintain constant currents. In another, high currents are generated, and tungsten probes are used to move single molecules and atoms.

SCARP: steroid and cyclic AMP regulated proteins; proteins that function optimally only when exposed to both steroid hormones and cyclic adenosine monophosphate. By activating kinase A, cAMP can phosphorylate effector molecules, or stabilize proteins induced by the steroid. The steroid can inhibit phosphodiesterases, or indirectly activate different kinases. Some "**permissive actions**" (*q.v.*) are explained by the need for one kind of regulator to prepare molecules for activation by another.

SCAT: (1) sheep cell agglutination test; (2) sickle cell anemia test.

Scatchard plots: graphs in which the concentrations of bound substances (B) are plotted along the X axis (abscissa), and the ratio of bound to free substance (B/F) along the Y axis (ordinate). They are used to distinguish specific (high affinity) from nonspecific (low affinity)

binding, for example in studies of hormone-receptor interactions.

scato-: a prefix that refers to feces.

scatter factor: motility factor; a protein secreted by fibroblasts that is similar to or identical with hepatopoietin A. It promotes dissociation and movements of epithelial cells, contributes to embryogenesis, and is implicated as a promoter of tumor invasiveness.

scavenger: a term applied to phagocytic cells that remove debris, substances that inactivate or destroy toxins, and enzymes that recover usable metabolic intermediates.

SCC: *see* **cholesterol side-chain cleavage**.

S cells: secretin secreting gastrointestinal tract cells.

S channel: a potassium ion channel of the sea snail *Aplysia punctata* regulated by serotonin. The neurotransmitter acts via a G protein to raise cAMP levels and promote kinase A-catalyzed phosphorylation of a channel protein.

SCF: (1) sertoli cell factor; *see* **inhibin**; (2) stem cell factor.

SCG: superior cervical ganglion.

Schiff bases: compounds with the general formula shown, formed by condensations of amino groups on lysyl and other moieties with aldehydes or ketones. They are intermediates in several biochemical pathways (for example formation of fructose from dihydroxyacetone + 3-phosphoglyceraldehyde), and are used for collagen cross-linking, attachment of 11-*cis*-retinal to opsins, and the biosynthesis of tryptophan by bacteria. *See also* **Schiff reagent**.

Schiff reagent: fuchsin sulfurous acid; an alkaline solu-

$$R-\overset{\overset{\displaystyle H}{|}}{C}=N-X$$

tion of basic fuchsin or pararosaniline decolorized with SO_2 that reacts with aldehyde groups on glycoproteins and other molecules and generates a pink color. It is used in the periodic acid Schiff (PAS) reaction to identify thyrotropes, gonadotropes and other cells that make large quantities of glycoproteins, in the Feulgen stain for deoxyribonucleic acids, and to stain polysaccharides.

scission: cutting, tearing, or dividing.

schistosomiasis: bilharziasis; snail fever; diseases caused by *Schistosoma mansoni* and some related helminth species that can seriously damage the liver and other organs. Blood flukes are carried by snails.

schiz-: schizo-: a prefix meaning split or divided.

schizogony: a series of rapid mitotic cell divisions with no increase in cytoplasm. Several kinds of parasites form spores in this way.

schizophrenia: loosely defined disorders in which perception of reality is distorted, and thinking processes are disrupted. Affected individuals can have delusions and hallucinations, and display bizarre behaviors. Suggested causes include abnormal patterns for neurotransmitter release and/or metabolism in the brain, receptors that are defective in structure or aberrantly distributed, and exposure to unusual forms of stress during infancy and childhood. Autopsies have revealed subnormal sizes of brain temporal lobe regions in some individuals. Some of the agents used to treat the conditions are dopamine receptor antagonists.

Schizosaccharomyces pombe: a fission yeast used for studies of genetics, reproduction, and other processes. It differs in several ways from ***Saccharomyces cerevisiae*** (*q.v.*).

Schlemm, canal of: an endothelium-lined canal that drains aqueous fluid from the anterior chamber of the eye. Obstruction of the canal causes glaucoma.

Schmidt's Syndrome: Addison's disease associated with diabetes mellitus and/or chronic thyroiditis, more prevalent in females than in males. Some individuals also have other autoimmune disorders such as pernicious anemia, vitiligo, or infertility.

Schutz-Dale reaction: contraction of isolated uterine or intestinal strips in response to antigens. It is attributed to histamine release.

Schwann cells: non-neuronal cells that wind around peripheral nerve axons and secrete myelin. They have receptors for nerve growth factor (NGF) and other regulators. In neuropathies associated with diabetes mellitus, Schwann cell swelling has been attributed to accumulation of sorbitol (which draws in water by osmosis).

Schwartzman reaction: *see* **Shwartzman reaction**.

SCI: a glycoprotein of the immunoglobulin superfamily on neuron cell surfaces. It is used as a marker for the earliest stages of motor neuron differentiation.

SCID: severe combined immunodeficiency disease.

SCID mice: a mutant BALB/17 strain with an autosomal recessive defect that impairs synthesis of a lymphocyte-specific DNA recombinase which acts on hematopoietic stem cells, and is essential for development of B and T lymphocytes. The animals have normal granulocyte and natural killer cell numbers, but cannot mount cellular immunity responses. Although most do not make immunoglobulins, a few acquire the ability late in life. SCID mice are used to study immune system functions, and as transplant hosts.

scillarenin: 3β-14-dihydroxybufa-4,20-trienolide; one of several digitalis-like cardiotonic steroids made by sea onions (sea leaks, squill) of the genus *Urginea*, used to treat some forms of myocardial insufficiency. Scillaren is a mixture of related glycosides.

scintillation counter: *see* **liquid scintillation counter**.

scission: splitting, dividing, cutting, or tearing, a term applied to biological entities and chemical reactions.

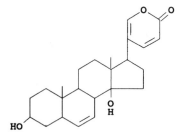

scillarenin

sclera: the outer, fibrous tunic of the eye that covers four fifths of the eyeball, is continuous anteriorly with the cornea and posteriorly with the optic nerve sheath, and provides attachment sites for the external ocular muscles that move the eyeball.

sclero-: a prefix meaning hard or hardening.

scleromeres: dense, mesenchymatous masses around notochords that contribute to the development of vertebrae.

scleroproteins: insoluble fibrous proteins, such as collagens and keratins. Most perform structural functions.

sclerosis: hardening.

SCN: suprachiasmatic nucleus.

SCO: subcommissural organs.

scolex: the anterior end of a tapeworm, used for attaching to the host intestine.

scopolamine: 6,7-epoxytropine tropate; hyoscine; an alkaloid made by *Datura metel*, *Scopola carniolica*, *Atropa belladonna*, *Hyoscyamus niger*, and some other *Solanaceae* species. It is a muscarinic type acetylcholine receptor antagonist used for preanesthetic sedation, to achieve mydriasis, and to prevent motion sickness. The peripheral actions are similar to those of atropine, but scopolamine more rapidly penetrates the blood-brain barrier, can cause euphoria and amnesia, and more commonly invokes hallucinations and delirium when presented in high dosage.

scorbutic: pertaining to scurvy.

scoto-: a prefix meaning darkness.

scotoma: an area of blindness or impaired vision, usually caused by localized retinal damage.

scotophase: the dark period of a light/dark cycle.

scotophobin: Ser-Asp-Asn-Asn-Glu-Glu-Gly-Lys-Ser-Ala-Glu-Glu-Gly-Gly-Tyr-NH$_2$; a peptide that accumulates in the brains of rats with acquired fear of darkness, and invokes dark-avoidance when injected into untrained mice.

scotopic vision: vision in dim light, mediated by rod type photoreceptors; *see* **rods**.

scotopsin: the protein component of rhodopsin.

scototropism: movement away from light.

scRNAs: small cytoplasmic ribonucleic acids.

scrapie: a disease most common in sheep, believed to be caused by a prion that acts on nervous tissue. After a long latent period, the animals develop tremors, scrape against objects to relieve severe itching, and eventually die of spongiform encephalitis.

scratch tests: allergy tests for IgE type immunoglobulin on mast cells. In sensitized individuals, histamine release leads to rapid development of a flare or wheal when a drop of aqueous solution containing an offending antigen is applied to abraded skin.

scrotum: a sac-like extra-abdominal structure of most mammalian males that develops from the embryonic genital folds. It houses the testes and epididymides, and provides an environment favorable for sperm maturation and storage. As blood passes through the pampiniform plexus, it is cooled, and arteriolar pulses are dampened to provide a smooth, steady flow. In species that possess the structure, cryptorchism is believed to cause loss of fertility because spermatozoa are damaged by the higher abdominal temperatures. Elephants and whales are among the few animal types that do not form the structures.

scurvy: a condition caused by vitamin C deficiency; *see* **ascorbic acid**.

SD, S.D.: standard deviation.

SD-25: Tyr^2-D-Met-(O)-Gly-N-Me-Phe-ol; a μ-type opioid receptor agonist.

SDA: specific dynamic action.

SDE: specific dynamic effect.

SDH: steroid dehydrogenase; *see* 3β-, 11β- and other **hydroxysteroid dehydrogenases**.

SDS: sodium dodecylsulfate.

SDS-PAGE: sodium dodecylsulfate polyacrylamide gel electrophoresis; *see* **electrophoresis**.

Se: selenium.

S.E.: standard error.

sea urchins: spiny skinned Echinoderms used for studies of fertilization, embryonic development, cell cycle control, and histone production.

seborrhea: copious production of sebum.

sebum: sebaceous gland secretions. They contain triacylglycerols, waxes, squalene, and cell debris. The glands are stimulated by androgens.

sec: seconds.

secobarbital sodium: Seconal sodium; 5-allyl-5-(1-methylbutyl)malonylurea sodium salt; a short-acting sedative and hypnotic used for preanesthetic medication, and to induce hypnotic states for psychiatric examinations.

secondary endocrinopathy: hormone dysfunction initiated by factors other than a primary endocrine gland disease which leads to secretion of excessive or insufficient amounts of the regulator. For example, a renal defect that impairs phosphate excretion can cause 1,25-dihydroxyvitamin D$_3$ deficiency, since high inorganic phosphate inhibits the 25-hydroxycholecaliferol 1α-hydroxylase enzyme.

secondary follicle: an ovarian follicle that has acquired several layers of granulosa cells surrounded by a theca, in which the oocyte has undergone some growth. It can advance to the vesicular stage and serve as an estrogen-secreting cohort, or complete maturation to the preovulatory stage. *Cf* **primordial**, **primary**, and **preovulatory follicle**.

secondary immune response: anamnestic response; a rapid immune system reaction to an antigen to which the system has been previously exposed, mediated by memory cells.

secondary immunodeficiencies: impaired immune system responses in an individual in whom B and/or T lymphocytes have matured. The causes include infections, toxins, and neoplastic diseases.

secondary lysosomes: intracellular vesicles formed by fusion of phagosomes with lysosomes. After digestion of the components is completed, the remnants are transiently retained as residual bodies.

secondary oocyte: a large cell with two complete copies of one set of alleles, formed (along with a first polar body) when a primary oocyte completes meiosis I. It enters meiosis II and is arrested at the metaphase stage at the time of ovulation. After fertilization, it completes meiosis II and gives off a second polar body.

secondary set rejection: accelerated rejection of a second graft by an individual sensitized to the antigens by previous exposure to a first graft of similar tissue.

secondary sex characteristics: adult male or female phenotypic features that do not directly affect reproduction, but can contribute to sexual attractiveness and choice of mates. Examples include the beard, moustache, and skeletal muscle development in men, the mammary glands in women, the mane of the male lion, and the plumage of the peacock. Gonadal hormones are the major stimulants for maturation of most of the structures, but gonadotropins and other regulators contribute to some.

secondary sex ratio: *see* **sex ratio**.

secondary spermatocytes: two secondary spermatocytes form when a primary spermatocyte completes meiosis I. Each contains two copies of a single set of alleles. When a secondary spermatocyte completes meiosis II, two haploid spermatids are formed.

secondary structure of proteins: *see* **proteins**.

second law of thermodynamics: a concept stated in several ways: (1) a process that proceeds spontaneously leads to an increase in entropy; (2) a process proceeds spontaneously in the direction that maximizes entropy; (3) the entropy of a system and its surroundings increases until equilibrium is attained; (4) when one form of energy is transformed to another, some energy becomes unavailable for useful work; (5) $\Delta G = \Delta H - T\Delta S$, where ΔG is the change in free energy (energy available for useful work), ΔH is the change in enthalpy (a measure of heat transfer), T is the absolute temperature, and ΔS is the change in entropy.

second messenger hypothesis: a concept most commonly applied to amine, peptide, protein, and glycoprotein hormones and neurotransmitters that initiate responses by binding to receptors on cell surfaces. The hormone (first messenger) promotes generation of second messengers (such as cAMP, cGMP, diacylglycerols, inositol phosphates, or nitric oxide) that mediate the subsequent events. In most cases, transducers couple interactions between hormone-receptor complexes and enzymes that catalyze messenger generation. *See* also **G proteins**. Second messengers can also be generated by hormones that rapidly cross plasma membranes.

second polar body: a small cell with very little cytoplasm, formed when a secondary oocyte completes meiosis II. It carries away excess DNA, and soon disintegrates. Some sex differentiation disorders are caused by adherence of a surviving polar body to a fertilized oocyte. In rare cases, the polar body is fertilized.

secosteroids: calciferols and other steroid-like molecules with one or more open rings.

secretagogues: agents that stimulate secretion.

secretin: species-specific hormones chemically related to glucagon, vasoactive intestinal peptide (VIP), and glucose dependent insulinotropic peptide (GIP). Partially digested proteins, and acids produced by the stomach are major stimulants for their release by cells of the duodenum and jejunum. Secretin promotes bile flow, augments the water and salt content of pancreatic juice, and opposes some gastrin effects. The human hormone has the amino acid sequence: His-Ser-Asp-Gly-Thr-Phe-Thr-Ser-Glu-Leu-Ser-Arg-Leu-Arg-Glu-Gly-Ala-Arg-Leu-Gln-Arg-Leu-Leu-Gln-Gly-Leu-Val-NH$_2$.

secretion: cell release of synthesized and/or stored products, usually to body fluids. *See* also **apocrine**, **holocrine**, **merocrine** secretion and **exocytosis**; and *cf* **excretion**.

secretogranins: acidic glycoproteins in the granules of many kinds of neurons and endocrine cells, including types I and II which are identical with chromogranins A

and B, respectively. They are co-secreted with hormones and neurotransmitters. Some are implicated as modulators of endocrine system functions.

secretory component of IgA: a 75K polypeptide in tears, bile, colostrum, and some other exocrine gland products, usually complexed with IgA immunoglobulins. It is believed to function as a receptor that facilitates IgA secretion, and to protect immunoglobulins against enzymatic degradation.

secretory granules: membrane-bound organelles that store hormones or other products, and release them by exocytosis.

secretory protein 1; SP-1: *see* **chromogranin A**.

sedatives: usually (1) mild central nervous system depressants that do not necessarily invoke sleep or analgesia; (2) a term applied to regulators that depress specific functions, as in cardiac or gastric sedative. *Cf* **tranquilizers** and **hypnotics**.

sedimentation: settling of particles suspended in a fluid. The rates can be accelerated by centrifugation.

sedimentation coefficient: s; the sedimentation velocity per unit of centrifugal field force, usually expressed in Svedberg units.

sedimentation equilibrium: ultracentrifugation techniques for separating proteins on the basis of densities. Gradients are created in centrifuge tubes by layering gradually decreasing concentrations of a non-reactive solvent (such as sucrose) in centrifuge tubes, and adding the protein mixtures to the tops. The position of a protein after a balance between sedimentation and diffusion is established with low speed ultracentrifugation under standardized conditions provides information on its size. When other factors are determined, such as frictional coefficients (*f*), which vary with molecular shape, the molecular weight can be estimated. However, **sedimentation velocity** procedures (*q.v.*) are usually preferred for weight determinations.

sedimentation rate: a term usually applied to settling rates for erythrocytes in freshly drawn blood samples treated with anticoagulants. Factors that affect them include the relative numbers, sizes, and shapes of the cells. High albumin concentrations retard sedimentation, whereas high fibrinogen accelerates.

sedimentation velocity: the rate at which suspended particles sediment in liquids when strong centrifugal fields are applied. It varies directly with the force of the centrifugal field, $\omega^2 x$ (in which ω is the velocity of rotation in radians per second and x the radius of the axis of rotation), and inversely with the density of the liquid. When frictional coefficients and other factors are determined, the molecular weights of the particles can be calculated. The relationship between the frictional coefficient f (which depends on molecular shape) and the diffusion coefficient D (in square centimeters per second) is defined by the equation: $D = RT/f$, in which R is the gas constant and T the absolute temperature. The molecular weight M (in grams per mole) = sRT/D(1-$\overline{v}$)ρ, where s is the sedimentation constant, $\overline{v}$ the partial specific volume in milliliters per gram, and ρ the density in grams per milliliter of solvent.

sedoheptulose: a 7-carbon ketose initially identified in *Sedum* plants. D-Sedoheptulose-7-phosphate is an intermediate the hexose monophosphate pathway. In the Calvin-Benson pathway. it is made in the reaction catalyzed by a transketolase: ribose-5-phosphate + xylulose-5-phosphate → sedoheptulose-7-phosphate + glyceraldehyde-3-phosphate. A transaldolase catalyzes its reaction with glyceraldehyde-3-phosphate to yield one molecule each of erythrose-4-phosphate and fructose-6-phosphate.

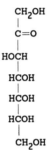

seed: (1) a mature plant ovule that contains an embryo in an arrested state of development, and (usually) also food reserves. Plant seeds are important sources of oils; (2) a spermatozoan; (3) to inoculate with microorganisms; (4) to initiate a process (such as mineralization) by introducing a specific factor.

segmentation: (1) cleavage; (2) division of body parts (or their embryonic precursors) into similar sections, arranged in parallel; (3) ring-like contractions of intestine circular muscle that transiently create constricted regions.

segregation: (1) separation of allelic genes during meiosis; (2) progressive restriction of differentiation potentials in various regions of a developing embryo.

Seldane: a trade name for terfenadine.

selectins: LEC-CAMs; a family of calcium-dependent mammalian glycoprotein lectins on vascular system cells whose members play essential roles in cell to cell and cell to matrix adhesions and interactions; *see* also **CD62 (PADGEM)** and **ELAM-1**. L-selectin on leukocytes recognizes specific endothelial cell ligands with heparin-like chains. It mediates trafficking of lymphocytes by binding to sialylated sulfated ligands on high endothelial cell venules (HEVs) of lymph nodes, and participates in the migration of neutrophils and monocytes through other epithelia. P- and E-selectins are inducible receptors that recognize specific sialylated fucosylated ligands on leukocytes and contribute to migration of the cells to sites of inflammation and injury.

selegiline: deprenyl.

selenium: Se; a nonmetallic element (molecular number 34, molecular weight 78.96). It is an essential trace element, and a component of the active site of glutathione peroxidase. Se is believed to protect against erythrocyte fragility, liver necrosis, some forms of muscular dystrophy, and other conditions in which oxidants such as hydrogen peroxide can cause tissue damage. [75]Se is used for metabolic and transport studies. Selenocysteine is a component of some transfer RNAs and bacterial enzymes; and selenomethionine is made by bacteria.

self-antigens: substances that invoke immune responses within the individuals that make them. Severe autoimmune reactions rarely occur because most immature cells that come in contact with self-antigens against which more mature cells react are destroyed during fetal life. The diseases can be initiated by over-reactive cells that persist, by release of self-antigens from injured tissues of the kinds not normally encountered (because they are sequestered), or by exposure to foreign antigens that closely resemble native types.

self-assembly: spontaneous joining of small components to form larger ones. The term can refer to nucleic acid strands, or to more complex structures such as microtubules.

self-fertilization: a form of reproduction in which ova are fertilized by sperm produced within the same organism. The strategy is employed by tapeworms, some deep-sea fishes, and some other organisms that have limited contact with other members of the same species. The related process in plants is self-pollination. Cross-fertilization is more common among naturally occurring hermaphrodites such as earthworms, in which gonads and their ducts are arranged in ways that do not permit self-fertilization.

"selfish" DNA: "junk" DNA; DNA regions that replicate but are not transcribed. Although no functions have been identified for some of the base sequences, certain types are known to contribute to nucleic acid processing and/or chromosome stabilization. Others may mediate evolutionary changes.

self recognition: immune system cell recognition of autoantigens.

self stimulation: techniques used to determine the loci of "pleasure", "aversion", or "addiction" "centers" in laboratory animals, and to study the effects of factors such as food deprivation, force-feeding and neurotransmitters on motivation and behavior. *See* **"pleasure centers"**. Externally applied patches laden with pharmaceutical preparations that can be rubbed to accelerate drug release, are among the devices used to alleviate addictions and other problems in humans.

self tolerance: failure to mount an immunological reaction against an autoantigen.

sella turcica: a depression in the sphenoid bone that houses the hypophysis in many species.

SEM: scanning electron microscopy.

S.E.M.: S.E; standard error of the mean; *see* **standard error**.

semeiotic: pertaining to signs or symptoms of disease.

semen: the mixture of **seminal fluid** (*q.v.*) and spermatozoa that is ejaculated.

semialdehydes: compounds related to dicarboxylic acids, in which one of the carboxyl groups has been reduced to an aldehyde.

$$R_1 - \overset{\overset{\displaystyle H}{|}}{C} = O$$
$$R_2 - COOH$$

semiconservative replication: the major mechanism for DNA replication, in which each DNA strand directs formation of a complementary one, and each daughter cell receives one old (parental) and one newly synthesized (complementary) DNA strand.

semidecussation: incomplete crossing, a term usually applied to nerve fiber tracts.

semidominance: *see* **incomplete dominance.**

seminal fluid: a mixture of fluids secreted by male accessory reproductive organs, and released in the ejaculate; *see* also **seminal vesicles** and **prostate gland**. The fluid, which is essential for sperm transport, contains nutrients, buffers, several kinds of prostaglandins, other hormones, antigens, lubricants, and enzymes. Various components affect sperm viability, capacitation, and coagulation. *Cf* **semen**.

seminal plasma inhibin: *see* **inhibins.**

seminal plasmin: a 5.4K enzyme in seminal fluid that contacts sperm at the time of ejaculation, inhibits sperm motility and acrosome reactions, and can also block RNA synthesis. It does not directly bind calcium, but slows Ca^{2+} uptake and calmodulin actions. Antiseminalplasmin opposes its effects.

seminal vesicles: accessory reproductive organs of most male mammals that (along with prostate glands) make most of the seminal fluid. In addition to water, the secretory products include prostaglandins (some of which assist sperm transport through female reproductive tracts of animals with large uteri by stimulating smooth muscle), fructose (a major energy source for sperm), acid and alkaline phosphatases, nucleases, and other enzymes. The cells also take up and destroy abnormal and deteriorating spermatozoa. Dihydrotestosterone promotes seminal vesicle growth and maturation, and maintains the functions.

seminiferous growth factor: SGF; a 15.7K acidic peptide made in large amounts by prepubertal Sertoli cells, and in smaller ones by mature types. It is believed to function as an autocrine or paracrine stimulant and mitogen, and to contribute to the regulation of spermatogenesis. Unlike several other factors made by the cells, its production does not appear to be dependent on follicle stimulating hormone (FSH).

seminiferous tubules: long, hollow, tortuous tubules of mature testes in which spermatozoa are produced. In addition to spermatogonia, spermatocytes, spermatids, and spermatozoa, they have Sertoli and myoid cells.

seminomas: usually, malignant testicular neoplasms derived from embryonic primordial germ cells. The term is also applied to ovarian tumors derived from female embryonic gonads; but those types are more commonly called ovarian dysgerminomas (or ovarian seminomas).

semiochemicals: pheromones and other biologically active agents released to the environment.

semipermeable membranes: selectively permeable membranes; membranes that permit free diffusion of some substances, but not of others. All cell membranes are permeable to water, oxygen, carbon dioxide, nitric oxide, some other gases, and to many lipid soluble compounds. The ones in most cell types limit uptake of Na^+, Ca^{2+}, and many other ions (which enter via specific channels), and of glucose and other nutrients (whose entry is facilitated by carriers); but there are important regional differences. Glucose freely enters hepatic cells, some renal tubule cells permit rapid diffusion of Na^+ and Cl^-, and specific permeabilities of some types are regulated by hormones.

Sendai virus: Parainfluenza virus type I. Ultraviolet light-inactivated virus is used for cell fusion studies.

senescence: processes associated with normal aging. Most cell types go through developmental stages during which they proliferate and then differentiate. The kinds that continue to divide after attaining maturity eventually lose this ability and ultimately deteriorate, mostly because repair mechanisms become inefficient. Types unable to replace defective components (such as erythrocytes and spermatozoa) are short-lived. Observations on immortalized cells fused to normal ones are consistent with the concept that specific genes contribute to the controls. but external factors such as access to growth factors are also important; and high glucocorticoid levels hasten senescence of some types. In epidermis, terminal differentiation and senescence are accelerated by nutrient and oxygen deprivation, when newly formed cells displace older ones from positions near dermal blood vessels. Chemical and mechanical injury cause deterioration of cells that line digestive tract lumens. In corpora lutea and at some other sites, "programmed" degeneration follows a predictable time course; *see* also **apoptosis**. Neurons and skeletal muscle fibers are among the non-proliferating kinds that survive for long time-periods. *See* also **progeria**.

senescent cell antigen: a 62K protein on the surfaces of senescent erythrocytes, immunologically similar to band III. It binds an autoantibody recognized by Kupffer cell Fc receptors.

senility: deterioration or pathology associated with aging.

senktide: *Suc*-Asp-Phe-*Me*Phe-Gly-Leu-Met-NH$_2$; a selective agonist for B and N type substance P receptors.

sense codons: sets of three messenger RNA bases that recognize transfer RNA anticodons.

sense strand: a DNA strand that is transcribed. Some segments of complementary "anti-sense" strands are also transcribed.

sensitization: induction of a heightened state of responsivity.

sensory neurons: neurons that communicate with receptors and transmit information to the central nervous system. Most of the cell bodies reside in dorsal root ganglia; but some are in the brain. *Cf* **motor** and **internuncial neurons**.

Sephacryl, Sephadex: trade names for beads used in filtration columns, composed of covalently cross-linked dextrose gels.

sepsis: serious conditions caused by circulating microorganisms and/or their toxic products.

septal: referring to a septum.

septi-: a prefix meaning seven.

septic shock: circulatory failure initiated by microorganisms and/or their products. Endotoxin is a major mediator.

septum: (1) a dividing wall, usually composed of connective tissue; (2) the tissue that separates the first and second cerebral ventricles.

sequence homology: usually describes proteins with common sets of identical or very similar amino acid sequences, often derived from the same ancestral molecule. Although many homologous proteins perform similar functions, small differences in amino acid compositions profoundly affect the biological properties of a few.

SER: smooth endoplasmic reticulum.

serine: ser; S; 2-amino-3-hydroxypropionic acid; a nonessential glucogenic amino acid, a component of many peptides and most proteins (*see* also **serine proteases**), a major acceptor of phosphate groups for reactions catalyzed by kinases A, C and G and other enzymes, and a precursor of ethanolamine and choline, glycine, cysteine and pyruvate. Although present in most foods, much of it is synthesized via reactions in which 3-phosphoglycerate (from glycolysis) is oxidized by NAD^+ to 3-phosphopyruvate, and the product accepts an amino group from glutamate to form 3-phosphoserine. A phosphatase then liberates the free amino acid.

$$HO-CH_2-\overset{\overset{\displaystyle NH_2}{|}}{\underset{\underset{\displaystyle H}{|}}{C}}-COOH$$

serine dehydratase: serine-threonine dehydratase; serine deaminase; an enzyme that converts serine to pyruvate + NH_4+ via an enol intermediate (dehydroalanine) which is hydrolyzed to the end products. Threonine dehydratase catalyzes a similar conversion of threonine to α-ketoglutarate + NH_4+.

serine proteases: trypsin, chymotrypsin, elastase, plasmin, thrombin, kallikrein, subtilisins, some enzymes involved in complement activation and acrosome reactions,

$$CH_2=\overset{\overset{\displaystyle NH_2}{|}}{C}-COOH$$

dehydroalanine

and other proteolytic types whose active sites contain serine, histidine, and aspartatic acid.

serine protease inhibitors: SERPINs; anti-thrombin, anti-trypsin, pepstatin, and other inhibitors of serine proteases.

seromucoid: an obsolete term for circulating α_1-acidic glycoprotein.

seronegative: describes serum that lacks antibodies directed against a specific antigen.

serosa: tunica serosa; a membrane composed mostly of serous cells; *see* **serous membranes**.

serosal surface: the cell surface farthest from the lumen of a hollow structure, and closest to the blood vessels.

serotherapy: administration of sera with specific kinds of antibodies, to convey passive immunity.

serotonin: 5-HT; 5-hydroxytryptamine; a hormone, neurotransmitter, and precursor of melatonin, 5-methoxytryptophol, and other biologically active derivatives, made by bacteria, plants, and invertebrate as well as vertebrates. The major sites for biosynthesis in mammalian central nervous systems are the raphe nuclei, from which neurons project to the cerebral cortex, limbic system components (especially hippocampus), basal ganglia, and hypothalamus. The rate-limiting reaction, catalyzed by **tryptophan hydroxylase** (*q.v.*), yields 5-hydroxytryptophan (5-HTP) which is rapidly decarboxylated to serotonin. Since the levels of blood tryptophan are lower than those of most amino acids, precursor availability can affect the amounts synthesized; and exogenous 5-HTP accelerates serotonin formation. Much of the serotonin in pineal glands is rapidly acted on by *N*-acetyltransferase, a rate-limiting enzyme for melatonin synthesis in many species. Hydroxyindol-*O*-methyltransferase (HIOMT) then converts *N*-acetylserotonin to melatonin. Similar reactions proceed in Harderian glands, and to some extent in vertebrate retinas. Serotonin effects are short-lived if release does not continue, because the amine is taken up by serotoninergic neuron terminals and sequestered in synaptic vesicles. Monoamine oxidases initiate degradation of unsequestered 5-HT (mostly to 5-hydroxyindole acetic acid). The amine is also taken up by dopaminergic and catecholaminergic nerve endings; and some indirect effects are accomplished by displacing catecholamines from synaptic vesicles, or by competing with them for monoamine oxidases. Centrally produced serotonin affects mood, appetite, sleep-wake cycles, and other body rhythms in humans (and aggression, sexual activity and other behaviors in laboratory animals). Migraine headaches, sleep disorders, some forms of psychic depression, and some other kinds of brain dysfunction are attributed to production of inappropriate amounts of serotonin and its metabolites, or to abnormal secretory rhythms. Several anxiolytic, antidepressant, and appetite suppressing agents elevate the levels by promoting its release, inhibiting its uptake by nerve endings, or slowing its degradation. Deranged metabolic pathways can lead to production of metabolites that invoke hallucinations or damage brain tissue. Serotonin also contributes to the control of blood pressure, body temperature, and skeletal muscle functions, in part by affecting the release of acetylcholine, other neurotransmitters, and renin. Influences on the the release of adrenocorticotropic hormone (ACTH), β-endorphin, growth hormone, prolactin, luteinizing hormone (LH), vasopressin, oxytocin, and gonadotropins are neurally mediated, whereas other endocrine system effects are accomplished via paracrine mechanisms within pituitary glands. Peripherally, serotonin is made by gastrointestinal tract myenteric plexus neurons, where it affects smooth muscle contraction. It is also enters the bloodstream, and is taken up by, stored in, and released from blood platelets; and it contributes to hemostasis, blood coagulation, inflammation, and pain perception. Additionally, serotonin can synergize with fibroblast growth factors (FGFs) and other mitotic stimulants, and is tumorigenic for some cell types. Direct effects on several kinds of receptors variously affect the activities of adenylate cyclases, phospholipases, and membrane channels for calcium, chloride, and potassium.

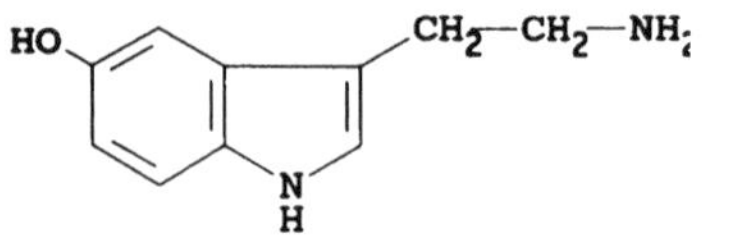

HO — ... — CH_2—CH_2—NH_2 ... N H

2-methyl-**serotonin**: a $5HT_3$ type serotonin receptor agonist.

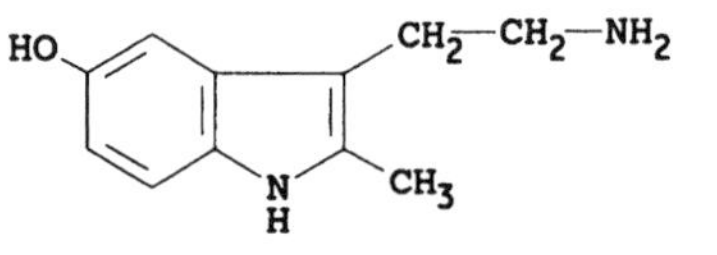

HO — ... — CH_2—CH_2—NH_2 ... N H CH_3

serotoninergic: describes (1) neurons that synthesize and release serotonin; (2) serotonin effects.

serotonin receptors: at least six classes of cell surface molecules, with multiple subtypes that bind serotonin with high affinity and mediate its actions. Classification has proven difficult because of overlapping direct functions, serotonin-mediated release of and interactions with other regulators, the presence of two or more receptor types on the same cell, and observations that receptor subtypes with similar ligand-binding properties can invoke different responses in one cell type as compared with another. Some effects of ligand binding are cited:

$5HT_{1A}$: inhibits adenylate cyclase, closes K^+ but opens voltage-dependent Ca^{2+} channels, stimulates release of adrenocorticotropic hormone, β-endorphin and dopamine, and hyperpolarizes some cell types. Some anxiolytic agents act on these receptors.

$5HT_{1B}$: inhibits adenylate cyclase, promotes prolactin release, activates phospholipase C isozymes, opens some K^+ channels, synergizes with fibroblast growth factor and to a lesser extent with epidermal growth factor and insulin to promote growth and mitogenesis; stimulates smooth muscle. Some 1B types are autoreceptors.

$5HT_{1C}$: activates phospholipase C and promotes phosphatidylinositol hydrolysis; acts on Cl^- channels; promotes release of vasopressin and prolactin; stimulates smooth muscle contraction, affects skeletal muscle, and can synergize with growth factors to promote transformation of some cell types. Although the affinities for some pharmacological agents resemble those of other $5HT_1$ subtypes, the physiolological properties more closely resemble those of the $5HT_2$ class. High receptor concentrations are present in the choroid plexuses and salivary glands of some species.

$5HT_{1D}$: affects Ca^{2+}, Na^+ and K^+ transport; (The receptors may be channel components that do not interact with G proteins.) Some 1D types inhibit adenylate cyclases, and at least some are autoreceptors.

$5HT_2$: activates phospholipase C, kinase C, and inositol-phosphate generation; augments eicosanoid production and the release of adrenocorticotropic hormone, β-endorphin, and prolactin; promotes vasoconstriction. A $5-HT_{2B}$ subtype mediates blood platelet aggregation.

$5HT_3$: affects sensory nerve endings (including ones involved in pain perception); contributes to inflammation. Cerebral cortex types affect sleep and mood, and also sexual activity in laboratory animals.

$5HT_4$: unlike most other types, augments adenylate cyclase activity.

serous cells: exocrine cells that secrete watery solutions which serve as lubricants.

serous membranes: double membranes composed mostly of serous cells. The visceral layers adhere closely to internal organs, and are separated by small amounts of fluid from parietal layers that line cavities. Examples include pericardium, pleura, peritoneum, and tunica vaginalis testis.

SERPIN: serine protease inhibitor.

serrated: having notched or saw-toothed edges.

Sertoli cells: sustentacular cells; nurse cells; non-germinal cells that comprise the bulk of the seminiferous tubules. Mature types have tight junctions that enclose compartments in which specialized fluids support secondary spermatocyte maturation and spermiogenesis; and they participate actively in spermiation. The functions are regulated by follicle stimulating hormone (FSH) which induces androgen binding proteins, inhibin, and other factors, testosterone taken up from interstital cells (which is converted to dihydrotestosterone, estradiol and other steroids), and to some extent by luteinizing hormone.

Testis determining antigen initiates Sertoli cell differentiation in young embryos. Soon after they associate with gonocytes, the cells secrete Müllerian duct inhibitor (MDI). FSH is the major regulator of subsequent growth and proliferation. Adult types acquire resistance to the growth-promoting effects, but respond again if gonadotropin deprivation causes testicular atrophy.

Sertoli cell factor: SCF; *see* **inhibins** and **seminiferous growth factor**.

serum: the liquid that separates from formed elements when blood clots; *cf* **plasma**. It contains nutrients and growth factors that support the survival and proliferation of many kinds of cultured cells (*see* **serum response elements**), but only minute amounts of prothrombin, fibrinogen, and other coagulation proteins. *See* also **immune** and **antilymphocytic serum**.

serum albumin: the major circulating blood protein, made in and secreted by hepatocytes. It is essential for maintaining oncotic pressure; and it binds fatty acids, many hormones and other blood components. *See* **albumins**.

serum amyloid A: a 20K serum stress protein; *see* **amyloid**.

serum response elements: SREs; DNA segments of many genes that bind serum components, and also numerous growth factors and oncogene products. They direct the synthesis of G_o phase proteins essential for progression to S phases, and mediate other effects of growth stimulants.

serum sickness: immune complex diseases (hypersensitivity responses) that develop when large amounts of foreign proteins are introduced into the bloodstream (for example during serotherapy, or when incompatible blood is infused). The manifestations can include fever, joint pains, skin rashes, and hematuria. Tissue injury is caused mostly by antigen-antibody complex mediated complement fixation, and neutrophil activation.

serum thymic factor: thymulin.

sesame oil: oil extracted from *Sesamum indicum* seeds and used as a lubricant, a solvent for hormone preparations, a flavoring agent, and a component of oleomargarines. The major triacylglyceride fatty acids are oleic, stearic, palmitic, myristic, and linoleic.

seta: a bristle or bristle-like hair.

set point: the level around which a regulated system is adjusted, for example the optimum concentration of calcium ions in blood, or the optimum body temperature under a given set of conditions.

sevenless: a *Drosophila* gene that directs photoreceptor development.

seven up: a *Drosophila* gene whose product is homologous to mammalian COUP-TF.

severe combined immunodeficiency: SCID; conditions in which T lymphocyte maturation is impaired, insufficient numbers of B lymphocytes are made, and B cells do not effectively response to most foreign molecules. Affected individuals cannot cope with infections easily resisted by normal ones. The causes include genetic defects that limit or block the production of adenosine deaminase or purine nucleoside phosphorylase. *See* also **SCID mice** and **acquired immune deficiency syndrome.**

severin: a 45K *Dictostelium* cytoskeleton protein chemically and biologically related to gelsolin, that promotes Ca^{2+}-dependent F actin cleavage.

sex: a term that can refer to gender, phenotype, chromosomes that differ in males as compared with females, hormones that affect reproduction, or behavior related to reproduction, such as mounting and intromission in males, and proceptivity and receptivity in females. Under normal conditions, chromosomal, gonadal, phenotypic, hormonal, and behavioral sex all conform to a pattern characteristic of just one gender; but *see* **hermaphroditism, pseudohermaphroditism, gender role**, and **gender preference**. *See* also **sex chromosomes, gametes**, and **gonads**.

sex assignment: a decision concerning gender, usually made at the time of birth, and usually on the basis of phenotype. When the external genitalia appear normal, male and female designations are routinely assigned without consideration of sex chromosome patterns. An infant with ambiguous structures but a well-developed phallus is most commonly accepted as male; and androgens may be administered to promote further masculinization. Otherwise, surgery and other procedures may be used to accentuate the female phenotype. *See* also **pseudohermaphroditism, feminizing testis**, 5α-**reductase** deficiency, and **adrenogenital syndrome**.

sex attractants: pheromones released by mature animals of one gender that attract members of the opposite gender of the same species, and stimulate behaviors that lead to insemination. The most widely studied types are made by female insects that fly. *See* also **pheromones, androstenone** and **copulin**.

sex cells: gametes and their precursors; in higher animals, spermatozoa or oocytes.

sex chromatin: (1) the components of sex chromosomes in a cell or organism (for example of X and Y types in mammals, or W and Z types in birds); (2) *see* **Barr body**.

sex chromosomes: chromosome sets that differ in males as compared with females. In mammals and many other vertebrates, a typical female diploid cell contains two of the X type, and a normal haploid ovum contains one X. In males of the same species, the diploid cell has one X and one Y, and a spermatozoan contains either an X or a Y. In birds and some other vertebrates, a female diploid cell has one W and one Z sex chromosome, whereas the male counterpart has two of the Z type. The X chromosomes in most mammals account for something like 5% of the total genome, and they code for many factors unrelated to reproduction. At least one is essential for survival. Y chromosomes are smaller, but affect functions such as spermatogenesis and growth of long bones, as well as **sex determination** (*q.v.*). At least 19 autosomes in humans contribute to reproductive system functions (including steroid hormone production). *See also* **sex linked inheritance**.

sex conditioned: describes a phenotype feature (such as larynx size, plumage color, or hepatocyte enzyme pattern) characteristic of one gender.

sex determination: mechanisms whereby an individual acquires the gonad type characteristic of one gender of the species. In mammals, differentiation along male-type patterns is initiated by a **testis determining antigen** (*q.v.*) whose synthesis is directed by a Y chromosome gene. If the product is not made in sufficient amounts at the right time, indifferent gonads differentiate into ovaries or ovary-like structures. Later, the gonads direct development of accessory reproductive structures and secondary sex characteristics. *See* **Müllerian duct inhibitor** and gonadal steroids.

sex differentiation: usually, changes in cells of indifferent gonads that lead to formation of embryonic testes or fetal ovaries. The term can additionally refer to other developmental changes associated with acquisition of phenotypic sex.

sexduction: in bacteria, transfer of a fragment of genetic material associated with a sex factor from one organism to another.

sex factor: fertility factor; *see* **F factor**.

sex hormones: a term loosely applied to regulators such as estrogens and androgens made in gonads, and (less commonly) to other hormones that affect reproduction.

sex hormone binding globulin: SHBG: *see* **sex steroid binding globulin**.

sex limited: a phenotype feature normally expressed in members of just one gender of a species. The genetic information can be carried by an autosome.

sex-linked inheritance: in mammals, transmission of X chromosomes genes. The typical female somatic cell contains two X chromosomes. If one carries a defective gene, but the associated trait is recessive, a mother can appear phenotypically normal. She is said to be a carrier, because there is a 50% probability that she will pass the defect to a son or daughter. Sons that receive the defect express it (since a typical male somatic cell has just one X chromosome, which is maternally derived). Daughters express it only when they also inherit a defective gene from the father. A father with the defective trait transmits it to all of his daughters (but not to his sons, who inherited their X chromosomes from their mothers). X chromosomes contain genes that affect color vision, production of some blood coagulation factors, and many important enzymes.

sex pili: filamentous projections on the surfaces of some bacteria that mediate adhesion, and are used in conjugation.

sex preference: gender preference; the gender type to which a member of a species is attracted. *See* **homosexual** and **heterosexual**.

sex ratio: the relative numbers of males and females in a population. *Primary* sex ratio refers to the relative numbers at the time of conception, and *secondary* to the numbers that survive to the time of birth. In humans, the secondary ratio is approximately 106:100. The ratio for zygotes is higher, but more male than female embryos and fetuses die.

sex reversal: a change to gonadal sex functions of the opposite gender. It occurs regularly in some species, and is associated with changes in phenotypic, hormonal, behavioral sex (*see* sequential **hermaphroditism**). In a tank of female coral fishes of some species, one individual often assumes male characteristics, and can release gametes that fertilize those of the remaining females. Newly hatched fishes of other species treated with gonadal steroids can be converted to types that express all of the characteristics of the sex opposite to the type specified by the chromosome pattern; and in some other ectothermic vertebrates, the temperature of the surrounding water is a major factor for sex determination. Phenotypic development in the embryos and young fetus of mammals (including humans) are influenced by gonadal steroids and other prenatal factors (*see* **adrenogenital syndrome** and **freemartin**). However, after the critical period for sex differentiation is passed, although gonadotropin releasing hormone patterns are affected, and sterility can be invoked, the most obvious influences of the hormones are exerted on accessory reproductive organs and secondary sex characteristics. Voluntary "sex changes" cannot be completed without surgery, and cannot accomplish formation of different kinds of gametes.

sex steroid binding globulin: SSBG; sex hormone binding globulin, SHBG: testosterone-estrogen binding proteins, TeBP; 84K species specific plasma glycoproteins composed of two kinds of subunits, one of which is glycosylated. They avidly, but reversibly bind gonadal steroids in a noncovalent manner, and assist their transport through the bloodstream. Most observers believe that the hormones must dissociate from the proteins before entering target cells. SSBGs may therefore provide mechanisms for retaining readily recruitable sources of active hormones in the bloodstream, and for protecting target cells when steroid concentrations rapidly rise to excessive levels. Since they display higher affinities for testosterone than for estradiol, they may additionally protect females against excessive androgen when androgen:estrogen ratios rise. However, it has also been proposed that cell membranes contain SSBG receptors that mediate hormone uptake. In humans and some other species, estrogens and thyroid hormones stimulate hepatic production and secretion of the proteins, whereas androgens inhibit.

sex vesicle: germinal vesicle.

sexual dimorphism: phenotypic features that distinguish male from female members of a species. The term can refer to externally visible reproductive organs which are obviously different in most animal types, and to secondary sex characteristics (which include, for example the mane of the male lion and the plumage of the peacock). It has also been applied to gender differences in other characteristics such as brain morphology, liver and kidney enzymes, hormone secretion patterns, and receptor numbers and distributions. Phenotypic differences are not obvious in some animal types, such as hyenas (in which females undergo prenatal masculinization), and bald eagles. In nonhuman species, marked dimorphism has been linked with behavioral patterns for mating, care of the young, and other interactions among individuals, but not with reproductive efficiency.

sexual interest: libido.

sexual precocity: *see* **precocious and pseudoprecocious puberty**.

sexual reproduction: production of new individuals of a species via mechanisms that involve fertilization, and transmission of genetic components from two parents to the progeny; In higher organisms, it requires gametogenesis. *Cf* **asexual reproduction**.

sexual selection: evolutionary theories that relate changes in a species to genetic factors transmitted by males. The selection can result from male:male interactions in which weaker animals are driven from territories or prevented from mating, or from female preferences for male characteristics such as body size, aggressiveness, plumage and song quality in birds, or antler length in deer.

SF: (1) Sertoli factor; (2) sulfation factor.

SFO: subfornical organ.

SGF: seminiferous growth factor.

SGOT: serum glutamic acid-oxaloacetic acid transaminase; aspartate aminotransferase; mitochondrial and cytoplasmic enzymes that catalyze: aspartate + α-ketoglutarate $\rightarrow$ oxaloacetate + glutamate. The enzymes leak from injured cells; and serum levels are used to assess the damage.

SGPT: serum glutamate-pyruvate transaminase; alanine aminotransferase; an enzyme that catalyzes: alanine + α-ketoglutarate $\rightarrow$ pyruvate + glutamate. The levels are high in some forms of liver disease, and in infectious mononucleosis; *cf* **SGOT**.

shadow casting: coating specimens for electron microscopy with metals, to accentuate contrasts.

sham feeding: procedures used to distinguish behaviors, hormone release patterns, salivation and other events initiated neurally by food intake, from ones related to changes in blood composition. The animals are permitted to eat, but gastric or intestinal fistulas (or other devices) prevent them from absorbing nutrients.

sham injection: "control" animal groups are often injected with vehicles used to dissolve agents given to experimental groups, to distinguish nonspecific reactions to injections (that can involve restraint, pain, irritation and localized increases in fluid volume), from the more specific effects of the test agents.

sham operation: procedures such as anesthesia and incisions, performed on "control" animals, to distinguish the effects of nonspecific stress and trauma from ones caused by ablation of structures or other surgical manipulations.

SHBG: sex steroid binding globulin.

SH domains: src homology domains; protein segments with amino acid sequences similar to sequences of the $pp^{c\text{-}src}$ proto-oncogene product. Receptors for epidermal growth factor, platelet derived growth factor, insulin, and some other growth stimulants autophosphorylate tyrosine residues of their cytoplasmic regions when activated by their ligands. SH2 domains (approximately 100-amino acid noncatalytic segments, present in one or more copies in phospholipase Cγ isozymes, inositol-3-phosphate kinase, GTPase activating proteins, some phosphatases, and some oncogene proteins) recognize the phosphotyrosines, and complex with those receptors. The SH2-containing proteins are then directly phosphorylated (without the need for second messengers). The activated products detach, to exert influences on nuclear, cytoskeletal, or other targets, form signal transfer particles that mediate translocations of cytoplasmic components, or in other ways contribute to signal transduction pathways. (Regulators at cell surfaces can thereby communicate with cell interiors, and can affect transcription and other processes.) SH3 domains occur in many of the same proteins, and in others that do not have SH2 types. They bind microtubular and other cytoskeletal proteins, and provide signals that affect cell shape and organelle organization. Some are directly implicated as mediators of transformation initiated by oncogenes.

shearing: breaking DNAs or other large molecules by subjecting them to mechanical stress, in electrically powered blenders or other devices.

Sheehan's syndrome: postpartum necrosis of the pituitary gland, usually with severe adenohypophysial hormone deficiencies.

shell gland: a specialized component of the bird oviduct in which egg shells are made. Its development and functions are controlled by gonadal steroids, and are influenced by calcitonin and other mineral metabolism regulators.

shell membranes: non-cellular protective coatings on the surfaces of marsupial blastocysts that prolong survival and block implantation during diapause.

Shigella: a genus of *Escherichia* bacteria whose members invade intestinal cells and cause bacillary dysentery.

shikimic acid {**shikimate**}: 3,4,5-trihydroxy-1-cyclohexene-1-carboxylic acid; a precursor for bacterial and plant cell synthesis of phenylalanine, tyrosine, and tryptophan.

shingles: an infectious disease caused by *Varicella zoster* virus. The same organism causes chicken pox.

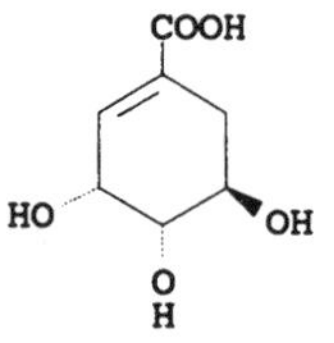

shikimic acid

shock: usually, circulatory collapse. The causes include toxins, blood loss, anaphylactic reactions, prolonged general anesthesia, and intestinal manipulation during surgery.

short day: describes (1) photoperiod-sensitive responses that occur during exposure to fewer than twelve hours of light per day; (2) organisms in which some processes are activated by short days, for example plants that produce flowers in autumn or winter.

short feedback loops: negative feedback systems in which regulators travel short distances to their target cells. Hypothalamic releasing hormone controls over adenohypophysial functions provide an obvious example. Both the release factors, and the hormones made by the target cells are transported via hypothalamo-hypophysial portal blood vessels. *Cf* **ultra-short** and **long feedback loops**.

Shwartzman phenomenon: Schwartzman reaction; hemorrhagic lesions invoked by endotoxin injection, usually in rabbits. A localized skin reaction develops at the site of an intradermal injection if the same toxin is subsequently administered intravenously. A second intravenous injection some time later can cause renal tubular necrosis and hemorrhagic lesions in the lungs, liver, kidneys, or other organs.

Si: silicon.

SIADH: syndrome of inappropriate ADH secretion.

sialagogues: agents that stimulate saliva flow.

sialic acid: a term than can refer specifically to *N*-acetyl-muraminic acid (shown below), or to all nonulosaminic acids (sugar amines with nine or more carbon atoms and their *N*- or *O*- acetylated derivatives). They are components of mucoproteins, glycosaminoglycans, glycoproteins, and glycolipids that confer viscosity, affect configurations, and protect proteins against rapid enzymatic degradation. Mucins and erythropoietins contain large amounts.

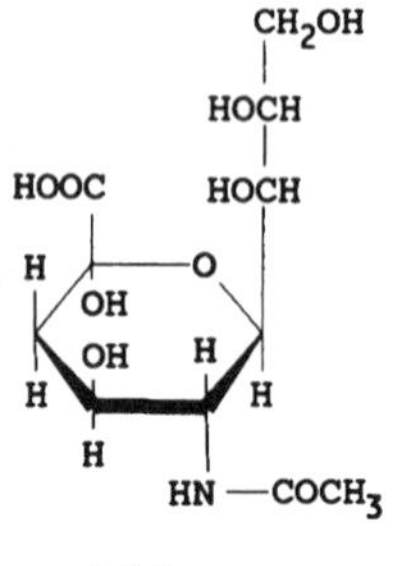

sialidase: *see* **neuraminidase**.

sialoadenectomy: removal of the salivary glands.

sialoglycoproteins: glycoproteins with one or more sialic acid moieties.

sialophorins: 115K glycoproteins similar to rat leukosialins, on the surfaces of human lymphocytes and monocytes, and related 135K glycoproteins on neutrophilic leukocytes and platelets. *See* **CD43**.

sialyltransferases: enzymes that catalyze addition of sialic acid moieties to glycolipids and glycoproteins. High levels are present in synaptic regions.

sib: sibling.

Siberian hamster: Djungarian hamster; *Phodopus sungorus*; a small rodent used to study pineal gland functions. *See also* **hamsters** and **pineal**.

siblings: brothers and sisters; all of the progeny a common set of parents, including twins, triplets, and ones of different ages.

sibling species: species reproductively isolated from each other that are very similar or morphologically identical.

sickle cell anemia: a serious, potentially lethal autosomal codominant disease in which individuals homozygous for the mutation make large quantities of hemoglobin S (which contains an abnormal globin). The cells assume sickle-like and filamentous forms when oxygen tensions fall only slightly below the usual levels, and then clump and occlude blood vessels. *See also* **sickle cell trait**.

sickle cell trait: a condition in heterozygotes in which limited amounts of hemoglobin S are made (*see* **Sickle cell anemia**). Affected individuals can remain symptom-free if oxygen tensions do not fall drastically below normal levels. They are resistant to malaria infection.

SICM: scanning ion conductance microscope.

side-chain cleavage: SCC; *see* **cholesterol side-chain cleavage**.

side-effects: responses invoked by pharmacological agents other than the ones for which the substances are administered. Most chemicals exert such effects; and most of the responses are regarded as undesirable.

sidero-: a prefix meaning iron.

siderocyte: a mature erythrocyte that contains iron granules.

siderophilin: *see* **transferrin**.

SIDS: sudden infant death syndrome.

siemens: S; the reciprocal of ohm; a unit of conductance. Values for cell membrane conductance are usually expressed in picosieman (pS) units. Most are in the range of $1\text{-}150 \times 10^{-12}$S (1-150pS).

SIFs: small intensely fluorescent cells.

Sigma: Σ; sum of; a symbol used, for example in standard deviation calculations, where $\Sigma(y\text{-}\bar{y})^2$ = the sum of the squares of the deviations from the mean.

sigma: σ; (1) standard deviation; (2) the σ receptor (which binds phencyclidine); *see* also **opioid receptors**.

sigma factor: σ factor; a noncatalytic peptide component of *Escherichia coli* RNA polymerase that recognizes DNA binding sites and contributes to transcription initiation.

sigmoid: S-shaped. In many systems, a plot of dose along the X axis and response along the Y yields a sigmoid curve. A straight line can usually be obtained by converting the dosage to logarithmic form.

sigmoidoscope: a device used to examine the sigmoid colon.

sign: an objective indication of disease; *cf* **symptom**.

signal hypothesis: the strongly supported concept that translation of a protein destined for incorporation into a secretory granule, lysosome or other vesicle, or insertion into a membrane begins with formation of a **signal sequence** (*q.v.*) that mediates attachment of the ribosome on which it is synthesized to the endoplasmic reticulum membrane, and is required for subsequent transport of the peptide chain to the endoplasmic reticulum lumen for completion of tranlsation and processing of the finished protein.

signaling pheromones: a term usually applied to pheromones made by animals with well developed brains that act rapidly on the nervous systems of recipients and affect behavior (which can vary with the context in which the stimulus is presented). *Releaser pheromone* is used for compounds made by insects and other invertebrates that invoke stereotyped behavioral responses. *Cf* **primer pheromones**.

signal peptidases: enzymes that cleave **signal sequences** (*q.v.*).

signal recognition particle: SRP; a 325K ribonucleoprotein composed of a 300-nucleotide (7S) RNA molecule and six polypeptide chains. It binds to the signal sequence on a growing peptide chain, transiently arrests chain elongation, and assists delivery of the ribosome and its attached peptide chain to the endoplasmic reticulum membrane. It then binds to a signal recognition receptor, but dissociates from it when the the ribosome has been properly positioned.

signal recognition receptor: an integral endoplasmic reticulum membrane protein adjacent to sets of two ribophorins. After binding a signal recognition particle that has attached to the signal sequence of a nascent peptide chain, it assists in positioning of the ribosome on the endoplasmic reticulum membrane. The peptide chain is then transported to the endoplasmic reticulum lumen.

signal sequence: leader sequence; a 13-36 amino acid sequence at the *N*-terminal of a partially synthesized protein that will be incorporated into a secretory, lysosomal or other vesicle, or inserted into a membrane. It binds to a signal recognition particle which directs the ribosome to a receptor on the endoplasmic reticulum membrane. After the peptide chain is threaded through the membrane, translation resumes, and (in most cases)

the signal sequence is cleaved by a signal peptidase. (Therefore, pre sequences of most hormones and other proteins cannot be recovered from intact cells, but can be obtained when translation is accomplished in cell free systems that lack the peptidase.) All known signal sequences have at least one positively charged moiety, a set of 10-15 hydrophobic amino acids (with varying amounts of phenylalanine, valine, leucine, isoleucine and alanine) at the center, and a more polar region that precedes the cleavage site. Albumins and a few other proteins destined for secretion, and some that are inserted into cell membranes, lack the *N*-terminal sequences described but have "internal signal sequences" that perform the same functions and are retained by the mature molecules. Proteins that lack both *N*-terminal and internal sequence are released to the cytoplasm.

signal transduction: transmission of messages from cell surfaces to cell effector sites, mediated by ligand binding to plasma membrane receptors. Most processes involve G proteins or other transducers, and the generation of second messengers; but for some, transmission is accomplished via direct influences on ion channels, or on cytoskeletal components. *See* also **SH domains**.

signet ring cells: (1) enlarged gonadotropes with eccentric nuclei, formed in the pituitary glands of some species when gonadectomy (or some other factor) impairs negative feedback controls over gonadotropin secretion; (2) adipocytes in which large quantities of centrally located lipid have displaced the living components, so that the cytoplasm forms a narrow peripheral ring, and the nucleus bulges at one end; (3) any cell type in which matter produced by the cell accumulates centrally, displaces the cytoplasm, and causes the nucleus to bulge at one surface, for example a mucin-laden cell.

significance: *see* **statistical significance**.

silencer sequence: a promoter region that interacts with a repressor protein.

silent allele: a DNA segment that resembles a gene, but does not code for a detectable product or perform a known function.

silent mutation: a DNA change that does not affect the phenotype.

silica: silicon dioxide; a mineral used to make cuvettes. The crystalline (but not amorphous) forms cause silicosis if inhaled over long time periods. Silica gels are dry, granular forms of silicic acid used as dehydrating agents and absorbents.

silicates: anions that contain SiO_44- and related radicals, and their salts.

silicon: Si; a nonmetallic trace element (atomic number 14, atomic weight 28.086). Minute amounts may be required for normal bone development. Sand (silicon dioxide) and silica gels are chemically inert substances used in thin-layer chromatography and other laboratory procedures. Carborundum (an abrasive) is silicon carbide.

silicones: organic compounds in which some or all of the carbons are replaced by silicon atoms. Polymers with repeating units of the general type —O—Si-R, in which R is an alkyl group, are used as lubricants and resins. *See* also **simethicones**.

silicosis: pneumoconiosis, caused by inhaling silica quartz or related substances, prevalent in individuals who work in quarries, or as stone cutters. Nodules that form in the lungs impair gas exchange and increase susceptibility to tuberculosis infection.

silk: the cocoon filament spun by fifth instar *Bombyx mori* (silkworm) larvae. Fibroin is the major protein.

silver: Ag; a metallic element (atomic number 47, atomic weight 107.87). It has no known function in animals. Metallic silver displays low chemical reactivity under biological conditions in vertebrates, and is used in dentistry. Silver salts are germicidal; and Ag is a component of some antibacterial and antifungal agents. Silver salts used in photography and chemical analyses can irritate the skin and mucous membranes. High concentrations damage tissues, and are used to remove warts.

simethicones: purified mixtures of silicones and siloxane polymers used to absorb gastrointestinal tract gas.

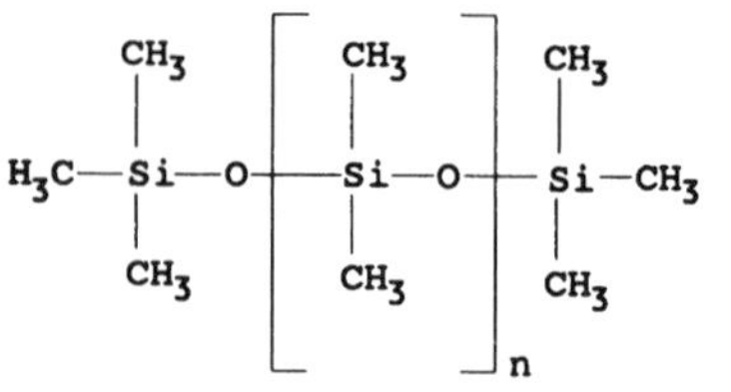

n = 200 – 350

simian: pertaining to, derived from, or characteristic of apes and monkeys.

simian virus 40: SV40; a small *Papovaviridae* virus whose genome is a circular DNA duplex with 5243 base-pairs that replicates in and lyses the cells of permissive (simian) hosts. In mice and other nonpermissive hosts, it can stably integrate into various genome sites, transform small numbers of cells, and promote tumor formation. The genome contains an early region that codes for an 81K large T antigen (made soon after infection and essential for initiation of DNA replication, transformation, and other effects), and a 20K small T antigen (also made early, via differential splicing of the same messenger RNA). The genome additionally contains a "late region" that promotes host synthesis of three capsid proteins, VP1, VP2, and VP3.

Simmonds disease: panhypopituitarism; severe deficiency of all adenohypophysial (and in some cases also neurohypophysial) hormones that is not caused by a pituitary gland tumor.

simple sequence DNA: satellite DNA.

simplesse: a protein obtained from whey, and used as a low-calorie fat substitute.

simvastatin: synvinolin.

SINE: short interspersed nuclear elements; small DNA segments located between regions that direct RNA synthesis.

single photon sensitivity: describes retinal rods in which a single photon can promote the closing of hundreds of cation-specific membrane channels.

single stranded DNA: ssDNA; long deoxyribonucleotide polymers (including the genomes of some viruses) that are not hydrogen bonded to complementary strands. Eukaryote ssDNAs can be prepared by denaturing double stranded molecules with heat (or other means), and then rapidly cooling the mixtures to prevent re-association. The products hybridize with complementary DNAs or RNAs.

singlet oxygen: an energized but uncharged form of oxygen, produced in chemical reactions initiated by activated neutrophilic leukocytes. Since it is highly reactive and cytotoxic, it can contribute to tissue damage during inflammatory responses.

sinistral: left, a term used for the left side of a molecule (*see* **stereoisomerism**) or the left side of the body.

sino-atrial node: sinu-atrial node; S-A node; cardiac pacemaker; primary cardiac pacemaker; a small U-shaped band of specialized muscle in the right atrium, close to the entrance site of the superior vena cava, that initiates and controls cardiac cycles by providing stimuli for atrial muscle. The cells are the most excitable of all cardiac types. After a short delay, the signals are picked up by atrioventricular (A-V) node cells and transmitted to ventricular Purkinje fibers.

sinus: (1) a hollow space or cavity, which may contain fluid; (2) a curve.

Sipple's syndrome: an inherited variant form of multiple endocrine neoplasia (MEN type II), in which medullary carcinomas of the thyroid gland are often associated with pheochromocytomas, and in some cases with parathyroid adenomas and/or neurofibromas.

sister chromatids: two identical chromosomes, formed when DNA replicates prior to cell division. They are joined by a centromere.

site specific mutagenesis: *in vitro* procedures that alter DNA molecules at specific loci. They are used to define the functions of the associated nucleotide sequences, or to invoke specific kinds of changes.

sitosterols: plant sterols chemically related to vitamin D, including β-sitosterol (sitosterin; 24β-ethyl)-Δ^5-cholesten-3β-ol; stigmasten-5-en-3-ol), extracted from wheat germ and corn oils, and γ-sitosterol, (24S)-stigmast-5-en-3β-ol) from soy bean oil (shown below), both of which are used to lower blood cholesterol levels. α_1-sitosterol is 4-methylstigmasta-7-, 24(28)-dien-3-ol.

sitotaxis: movement of an organism in the direction of a food stimulus.

sitotherapy: food therapy.

γ-sitosterol

SITS: 4-acetamido-4′-isothiocyano-2,2′disulfonic acid stilbene; a fluorescent agent used to block $Na^+/HCO_3^-/Cl^-$ ion exchange channels, and as an erythrocyte membrane marker. It that does not cross plasma membranes.

Sjogren's syndrome: an autoimmune disease that can be initiated by a graft vs host reaction (for example in an individual with a bone marrow transplant) in which several kinds of autoantibodies are produced, and lymphocytes infiltrate into the lacrimal and salivary glands, and sometimes also into joints. The manifestations can include keratoconjunctivitis, xerostomia, and rheumatoid-arthritis like symptoms.

skatol: 3-methyl-$1H$-indole; a malodorous tryptophan degradation component of feces, made by bacteria that colonize the intestine.

skeletal muscle: the major muscle type of vertebrates, composed of very long, multinucleate cells (fibers) with numerous mitochondria, thick filaments composed mostly of myosin and thin filaments that contain actin, tropomyosin, and troponins. In common with cardiac muscle, it is striated; but unlike cardiac muscle, it is under voluntary control and contracts under physiological conditions only when stimulated by acetylcholine released from motor nerve endings. It contains insulin-sensitive glucose transport carriers, and is a major contributor to blood glucose homeostasis and other metabolic functions, and a major site for heat generation. *Red* fibers, which are rich in myoglobin, contract more slowly than glycogen-rich *white* fibers, and are more resistant to fatigue. *See* also **sliding filament theory**, and **MyoD**.

skeleton: usually, (1) rigid or semi-hard structures that support and protect body parts, including the *exoskeletons* of arthropods, echinoderms and molluscs, the cartilaginous *endoskeletons* of elasmobranchs, and the bony endoskeletons of other vertebrates. The vertebrate *axial* skeleton includes the cranium, spinal column, and ribs, and the *appendicular* component comprises bones and associated structures that support limbs (and also wings and fins), and serve as levers for movement. The skeletons of most vertebrates house hematopoietic tissue and are major contributors to calcium and phosphorus homeostasis; (2) a term used with modifiers for non-mineralized connective tissue and other body components that provide support, as in cardiac skeleton; *see* also **cytoskeleton**; (3) in chemistry, a linear component of a compound that has side-chains, such as the carbon chain of a sugar or fatty acid.

SKF 525A: an agent used to inhibit cytochrome P-450 enzymes, including types used for eicosanoid synthesis.

SKF 10047: *N*-**allylnormetazocine** (*q.v.*).

SKF 91488: 4-(*N*,*N*-dimethylamino)butylisothiourea; an inhibitor of histamine-*N*-methyltransferase.

SKF 12185: 2-(*p*-aminophenyl)-2-phenylethylamine; an agent used to inhibit steroid 11β-hydroxylation.

SKF 104353: a leukotriene LTD$_4$ receptor antagonist.

SKF 38393: **feneldopam** (*q.v.*).

skin: an outer covering. The vertebrate type, composed of **dermis** and **epidermis** (*q.v.*), protects against ultraviolet radiation, mechanical injury, water loss, changes in environmental temperature, and some chemicals. The cells also contribute to water and electrolyte balance, body temperature control, immune system functions (*see* **keratinocytes**), vitamin D synthesis, and other functions. They produce and respond to autocrine factors (including parathyroid hormone-like polypeptide), and are affected by many hormones. Regulators of skin cell differentiation, proliferation, and functions include epidermal growth factor (EGF), transforming growth factors (TGFs), and retinoids. The skins of many poikilothermic vertebrates are sources of numerous biologically active peptides, including thyrotropin releasing hormone and tachykinins.

S6 kinases: at least two enzyme types, S6KI (pp70^{S6K}) and SKII (pp90^{S6K}), that contribute to translation initiation by catalyzing phosphorylation of ribosomal protein S-6, and additionally act on other substrates involved in protein synthesis and cell proliferation. They are directly activated by S6 kinase kinases, and are end-components of cascades initiated by insulin and other anabolic hormones.

S6 kinase kinases: RSKKI (44K), RSKKII (42K), and other enzymes that catalyze phosphorylation (and thereby activation) of S6 kinases. The also phosphorylate microtubule associated protein-2, myelin basic protein, and some other substrates, but do not act directly on S6. The kinase kinases are, in turn, activated by kinase C isozymes and other kinases, some of which are components of cascades initiated by insulin and other growth factors. Full activity requires phosphorylation on both tyrosine and serine-threonine moieties; and both protein phosphatase 1B, and protein phosphatase 2A inactivate.

SKSD: a mixture of streptodornase and streptokinase.

SLE: systemic lupus erythematosus.

sleep: naturally occurring periods of decreased central nervous system activity associated with loss of consciousness, low reticular activating system firing, and characteristic changes in electroencephalogram patterns, in which perception of external stimuli is diminished, but from which arousal is easily achieved. *See also* **slow wave sleep** and **rapid eye movement sleep**; and *cf* **torpor** and **coma**. Prostaglandin D_2 (PGD_2) is implicated as a major sleep-inducing factor, whose effects are antagonized by PGEs; but *see* also **sleep peptides** and **serotonin**. Although patterns for secretion of growth hormone and other regulators are related to sleep stages, the control mechanisms have not been elucidated.

sleep peptides: several small molecules identified in brain tissue, and implicated as factors that induce sleep, including δ-sleep inducing peptide, H_2N-Trp-Ala-Gly-Gly-Asp-Ser-Gly-Glu, and some muramyl types.

SLF: steel ligand factor; *see* **stem cell factor**.

SLI: somatostatin-like immunoreactivity.

sliding filament theory: the accepted model for skeletal muscle contraction, in which shortening of sarcomeres is accomplished by formation of actin-myosin cross bridges that mediate sliding of thin (actin) filaments over thick (myosin) filaments. When acetylcholine released from motor nerves opens Na^+ ion channels and promotes muscle fiber depolarization, the excitation is transmitted along T tubules. This leads to release of Ca^{2+} from the sarcoplasmic reticulum. By binding to and changing the configuration of troponin C (with secondary effects on tropomyosin), Ca^{2+} unmasks actin binding sites for myosin, and permits cross bridge formation. Activation of thick filament ATPase then releases energy required for both cross bridge changes that mediate sliding, and the subsequent severing of cross bridges essential for relaxation. *See also* **myosin**.

slime molds: organisms of the order *Myxomycetes*. When food is abundant, *Dictostelium discoideum* forms single, independently functioning ameba-like cells. Nutrient deprivation leads to generation of cAMP, which promotes cell aggregation and organization into multicellular organisms (slugs). The species is used to study signal transduction, cell to cell adhesion, cell differentiation,

chemotaxis, motility, and factors that influence development.

slow reacting substance of anaphylaxis: SRS-A; leukotrienes C_4, D_4, and E_4. The term was initially applied to uncharacterized substances released from guinea pig lungs exposed to cobra venom that invoked many of the symptoms of anaphylaxis, and could be assayed by their ability contract guinea pig ileum.

slow virus: (1) a member of the *Lentivirinae* group; (2) any virus whose manifestations develop after a long latent period, for example the agent that causes scrapie, and possibly also one involved in Paget's disease. Prions are now believed to cause Creutzfeldt-Jacob disease and some other disorders initially attributed to infection by slow viruses.

slow wave sleep: SWS; sleep stages during which electroencephalogram waves are slow and of high voltage, autonomic system activity is depressed but regular, and skeletal muscles can contract, but no rapid eye movements occur; *cf* **rapid eye movement** (REM) **sleep**. SWS can account for 80% of total sleep time in normal human adults.

slp: sex limited protein of mice; an androgen inducible, nonhemolytic product of the C4A complement gene, usually expressed only in males.

slugs: several kinds of soft-bodied terrestrial and aquatic invertebrates, including some nematodes and molluscs. A few are intermediate vectors for parasites that live at different life cycle stages in humans. *See also* **slime molds**.

SM-A: somatomedin-A; *see* **somatomedins** and **insulin-like growth factor II**.

small cytoplasmic ribonucleic acids: scRNAs; *see* **ribonucleic acids** and **small cytoplasmic ribonucleoprotein particles**:

small cytoplasmic ribonucleoprotein particles: scURPs, scurps: cytoplasmic particles composed of small RNAs and specific proteins that contribute to translation controls, but do not code for amino acids; *see* for example **signal recognition particles**.

small G proteins: approximately 21K proteins that bind to guanine nucleotides and possess GTPase activity. They contribute to signal transduction and the control of cell proliferation, and activate adenylate cyclase in some yeasts. *See* **GTP binding proteins**. (For larger, trimeric proteins that function as transducers, *see* **G proteins**.)

small intensely fluorescent cells; SIFs; dopaminergic neurons in carotid and aortic bodies, and in superior cervical and other autonomic ganglia (including ones in the lungs, kidneys, and intestines).

small intestine: enteron; the part of the gastrointestinal tract that extends from the pyloric orifice to the ileocecal valve, and includes the duodenum, ileum, and jejunum. It receives partially digested nutrients from the stomach, as well as pancreatic juice, and bile, and is the major site for nutrient absorption. Various cell types secrete digestive enzymes, hormones, and neurotransmitters.

small nuclear ribonucleic acids: snRNAs; *see* **ribonucleic acids** and **small nuclear ribonucleoprotein particles.**

small nuclear ribonucleoprotein particles: snURPs, snurps; particular components of splicosomes, composed of small nuclear RNAs (*see* **U RNAs**) and specific proteins.

small nucleolar ribonucleic acids: snoRNAs; components of ribonucleoprotein particles in nucleoli that participate in the processing of ribosomal RNAs.

small T antigen: *see* **simian virus 40.**

SM-B: somatomedin B; *see* **somatomedins.**

SM-C: somatomedin C; *see* **somatomedins** and **insulin-like growth factor I.**

SMDA: serologically detectable male antigen; the protein product of a gene in the *sxr* region of the short arm of the Y chromosome (made only in males); *see* **sxr**.

"smell brain": *see* **rhinencephalon.**

smgs: small G stimulants; several proteins that accelerate GTP binding to small G (guanine nucleotide binding) proteins. Smg p25A may be identical with rab3 protein.

smooth endoplasmic reticulum: SER; a continuous system of membrane-enclosed sacs and tubules that communicates with the plasma membrane and nucleus, and is associated at some sites with rough (ribosome studded) endoplasmic reticulum. The configurations, sizes, and activities vary with the cell types and with metabolic factors, and are affected by endogenous regulators and pharmacological agents. At various sites, it holds enzymes for cholesterol, phospholipid, and ceramide synthesis, and for P-450 dependent processes that include drug detoxification as well as steroid metabolism. It processes some proteins, delivers products (in vesicles that bud from its membranes) to the Golgi apparatus, and contributes to calcium homeostasis and responses to hormones and neurotransmitters by taking up, sequestering, and releasing Ca^{2+}. The membranes are complex and extensive in somatotropes, hepatocytes, adrenocortical, and other cells that secrete large quantities of proteins and/or lipids; *see* also **sarcoplasmic reticulum.**

smooth muscle: muscle that does not contain the orderly arrangements of thick and thin filaments characteristic of skeletal and cardiac types, and therefore appears "smooth" (not striated) when viewed under a high power light microscope. It is most abundant in the gastrointestinal tract, in large arteries and arterioles, and in the uterus. Smaller amounts are in the spleen, testis, ovary, and elsewhere; and many organs contain myoepithelial cells that share some of the properties. At most sites, smooth muscle undergoes spontaneous contraction and relaxation, with both phases slower than those of skeletal types; but it is responsive to mechanical stimuli, and to hormones, neurotransmitters, and other chemicals. Circularly arranged smooth muscle groups (sphincters) reduce the diameters of lumens and elongate tubular structures, whereas longitudinally arranged groups en-

large the lumens and shorten the tubes. Some specialized types (for example in the eyes) react more rapidly than the others, and are under predominantly neural control The activities are involuntary, but some can be manipulated by biofeedback techniques.

SMS-201-995: octreotide.

sn: in chemistry, a prefix that defines stereoisomer derivatives of glycerol and related compounds. For example, the L isomer of *sn*-3-glycerophosphate has the phosphate group attached to the third carbon. The numbers are reversed for D-glycerol derivatives.

Sn: tin.

SNAP: *S*-nitroso-*N*-penicillamine; an agent that promotes vasodilation by releasing nitric oxide.

SNAPs: soluble NAF attachment proteins. *N*-maleimide sensitive fusion protein (NSF) is a soluble factor that attaches to Golgi membranes and triggers the membrane fusion essential for directed transport of uncoated vesicles that hold newly translocated proteins. The binding is stabilized when α-SNAP (35K) or β-SNAP (36K) attaches to one of its ATP domains, and γ-SNAP (39K) to the other.

Snell-Bagg mouse: a mutant strain in which homozygotes (dw/dw) have small thymus glands, impaired cell-mediated immunity, and a Pit-1 defect that causes growth hormone deficiency and dwarfism.

snoRNAs: small nucleolar ribonucleic acids.

snRNAs: small nuclear ribonucleic acids.

S1 nuclease: an endonuclease made by *Aspergillus oryzae* that selectively degrades single-stranded DNAs to 5′phosphoryl mono- and oligonucleotides. It also open loops that form at 3′ends of complementary DNA strands (cDNAs) synthesized from messenger RNAs and then treated with enzymes that destroy the RNAs.

snURPs: snurps; small nuclear ribonucleoprotein particles.

social hormones: regulators released externally by one organism that act on another. The term is sometimes restricted to pheromones that affect social organization; but it can refer to kairomones, allomones, and synomones.

SOD: superoxide dismutase.

sodium: Na; a metallic element (atomic number 11, atomic weight 22.990). Na^+ is the major extracellular fluid cation, a component of the most important blood buffer system ($NaHCO_3$/$HHCO_3$), and a regulator of plasma membrane Na^+/K^+-ATPases. It diffuses across endothelial cell plasma membranes, but enters most other cell types primarily through regulated **sodium ion channels** (*q.v.*). Since the channels are closed most of the time, high extracellular Na^+ draws water from cells (whereas low levels cause water-logging). The problems are averted under physiological conditions by compensatory changes in blood and extracellular fluid volumes that maintain isotoninc levels. (Extracellular Na^+ is therefore a primary regulator of extracellular fluid volume). The high extracellular levels are also major factors for establishing **polarization** (*q.v.*) and for mounting action potentials. Aldosterone, natriuretic peptides, and other hormones control the amounts excreted to the urine, and also affect Na^+ transport across plasma membranes. Vasopressin acts mostly indirectly (by augmenting water retention). Although extracellular Cl^- ions follow Na^+ movements at many sites, Ca^{2+}/Na^+ and Na^+/H^+ exchange systems and Na^+/K^+-ATPases specifically affect Na^+. Several growth factors elevate cytoplasmic pH by activating Na^+/H^+ exchange. Sodium ions are cotransported with some amino acids, and with phosphate at some sites; and they bind to carriers for active glucose transport. [24]Na^+, with a half-life of 15 hours, emits β and γ radiation, and is used to study sodium transport, extracellular fluid volume, and circulation time.

sodium channels: structures composed of integral membrane proteins that permit rapid exchanges of Na^+ between extracellular fluids and cells. They are closed in most "resting" cell types, but open in response to appropriate stimuli. The small pore sizes may explain the limited ability of K^+ ions to pass through; but Li^+ is admitted, and some other ions enter in small amounts. Nicotinic type acetylcholine receptors on skeletal muscle, some neurons, and some other cell types have 5 subunits (2 α and one each of the β, γ, and δ types). Acetylcholine binds to α subunits, and invokes conformational changes that open receptor-activated types. Na^+ entry then depolarizes postsynaptic membranes. For a brief time period, Na^+ buildup within the cells transiently enhances channel opening, but soon afterward the channels revert spontaneously to the closed state. Depolarizations by other stimuli (some of which act on different ions) open voltage gated channels. In retinal rods, Na^+ channels are maintained in a partially opened states during darkness by cGMP (which binds directly to them). Light acting on rhodopsin initiates a train of events (*see* **transducin**) that leads to activation of a phosphodiesterase, cGMP hydrolysis to GMP, and closing of Na^+ channels.

sodium chloride: NaCl; table salt; the major dietary source of both **sodium** and **chloride** (*q.v.*). In many (but not all) biological systems, Na^+ and Cl^- move in parallel. For example, active transport of Na^+ by intestinal and renal proximal convoluted tubule cells invokes passive transport of Cl^-; and active transport of Cl^- in the Henle loops causes passive movement of Na^+. NaCl is the major constituent of Ringer's, Locke's and some other fluids used to bathe tissues.

sodium dodecylsulfate: SDS; sodium laurel sulfate; an agent that disrupts noncovalent bonds within proteins. Since reduction of disulfide bonds permits proteins to assume random coil configurations, molecular weights obtained with SDS-PAGE electrophoresis procedures can differ from those obtained by ultracentrifugation of undenatured proteins.

sodium etidronate: *see* **disodium etidronate**.

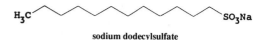

sodium dodecylsulfate

sodium-potassium ATPases: Na^+/K^+-ATPases: enzymes that use energy liberated by ATP hydrolysis to drive Na^+: K^+ exchanges against concentration gradients. Most cell types maintain resting potentials and accomplish repolarization by extruding Na^+ and taking up K^+. Proximal convoluted tubule enzymes control interstitial fluid volume, pH, and sodium content (and contribute to excretion of excess K^+) by recovering Na^+ from glomerular filtrates. Aldosterone is a major inducer and activator in more distal parts of the nephron and at other sites; and the effects of triiodothyronine (T_3) on some cell types are components of its calorigenic actions. Natriuretic hormones inhibit.

sodium sensors: cells that respond specifically to changes in Na^+ concentrations. It has been suggested that they contribute directly to the control of vasopressin secretion, and to renin release indirectly. In contrast, osmoreceptors are affected by many agents that alter total solute concentrations.

soft agar: a semisolid seaweed preparation used as a culture medium. Many transformed eukaryotic cell types are anchorage-independent, and can proliferate in soft agar layered over a more solid medium. In contrast, most normal types require direct contact with solid substrates.

solenoids: coils; *see* **nucleosomes**.

solid phase synthesis: techniques for synthesizing nucleic acids, proteins, and other large polymers, in which monomers are added sequentially to growing chains linked to solid supports that position unfinished molecules for subsequent reactions. Reagents that establish linkages at each step of the synthesis are washed away, along with unused units just added, and are replaced by solutions that contain the next monomer.

solubility product: K_s; a value that defines the tendency of a compound poorly soluble in water to precipitate under a given set of conditions. For a substance that separates into one cation, B^+ and one anion, A^-, and is in equilibrium with the precipitate, AB, $K_s = [B^+] \cdot [A^-]/[AB]$. Since the value of AB is close to one, the simpler form, $K_s = [B^+] \cdot [A^-]$ is used. Although it does not conform to the chemical definition, the term "solubility product" is also applied to the product of the calcium and phosphate concentrations in blood plasma. Since the blood plasma of healthy human adults contains approximately 10 mg Ca and 5 mg P per deciliter, the normal value is around 50. Very high products are associated with increased risks for metastatic calcification, and very low ones with defective bone mineralization. However, factors such as the concentrations of albumin and other plasma proteins, of anions such as citrate and bicarbonate (all of which bind Ca^{2+}), and the relative amounts of calcium as compared with phosphate, affect the availability of free Ca^{2+} ion, the tendencies for precipitation in soft tissues, and the effects on mineralization.

solute: the dispersed phase of a mixture; *see* **solutions** and *cf* **solvent**.

solutions: mixtures composed of continuous (solvent) and homogeneously dispersed (solute) phases. Although most commonly applied to solids dispersed in water, solutions can be mixtures of liquids dissolved in other liquids, or of gases dissolved in liquids. *True* solutions, with homogenously dispersed small solvent particles, are transparent, but can be colored (since light rays pass through freely, but are refracted by some solutes.) *Colloidal* solutions have larger, charged solute particles that remain dispersed because of mutual repulsions. They scatter light, and are translucent (cloudy). Polysaccharides and proteins with hydrophilic groups usually form colloidal solutions. *Cf* **suspensions**.

solvent: the continuous phase of a mixture; *cf* **solute**. Water is the major solvent for hydrophilic compounds. Benzene, acetone, and ether are commonly used commercial types for hydrophobic compounds. Alcohols dissolve many compounds of both groups.

soma: (1) perikaryon; the part of a neuron that surrounds the nucleus; (2) the perinuclear region of any cell type; (3) body components other than germ cells; (4) the axial part of the body (all parts except limbs or other appendages); (5) the body, as distinct from the mind.

somatic cells: body cells. Most are diploid. *Cf* **germ cells**.

somatic mutations: mutations that arise in somatic cells. They can be transmitted via mitosis to similar daughter cells within the same individual, but are not incorporated into gametes; *cf* **germ line mutations**. Some invoke transformation and tumorigenesis.

somatocrinin: *see* **growth hormone releasing hormone**.

somatodendritic synapse: a site of functional communication between the dendrite of one neuron and the perikaryon of another.

somatoliberin: growth hormone releasing hormone.

somatomammotropes: somatomammotrophs; mammosomatotropes; acidophilic adenohypophysial cells that secrete both growth hormone and prolactin. Some fetal and neonatal types later become somatotropes; others continue to make both GH and PRL.

somatomammotropins: placental lactogens.

somatomedins: a term initially used for uncharacterized peptides induced by growth hormone that mediate many GH effects on bone and cartilage. Somatomedin C types, the major ones that affect those tissues, and the ones most dependent on GH for induction, are now more commonly called insulin-like growth factor I (IGF-I). Somatomedin As, formerly known as multiplication stimulating activity (MSA) are now called insulin-like growth factor II (IGF-II). Somatomedin Bs are acidic peptides of similar size that are mitogenic for some cell types. Since they do not stimulate bone and cartilage growth, and their synthesis is not strongly growth hormone dependent, they are no longer regarded as a "true" somatomedins.

somatomedins A, **B**, and **C**: *see* **somatomedins**.

somatomegaly: gigantism.

somatostatins: SS; somatotropin release inhibitory factor; SRIF: peptides synthesized in the hypothalamus, extra-hypothalamic brain, retina, spinal cord, gastrointestinal tract, pancreatic islets, thyroid gland, and pituitary gland, and at other sites, named for the inhibitory effects on growth hormone (somatotropin) secretion. They also inhibit the secretion of glucagon, prolactin, adrenocorticotropic hormone (ACTH), thyrotropic hormone (TSH), several gastrointestinal hormones (especially gastrins), calcitonin, parathyroid hormone (PTH), and renin; and high concentrations additionally affect insulin. In the gastrointestinal tract, they depress motility and slow food absorption; and in the kidney they oppose vasopressin-mediated water retention. The most widely reported influences on the brain are stimulatory. Exogenous SS decreases sleep time, facilitates arousal, and antagonizes the effects of some central nervous system depressants. Large doses can invoke stereotypic behaviors, muscle tremors, muscle rigidity, and seizures in laboratory animals. In many cell types, they lower adenylate cyclase activity, and also antagonize the effects of cAMP (at least in part via influences on cytoplasmic Ca^{2+} levels). They also inhibit the growth of some tumors. Factors that promote SS release include growth hormone releasing hormone, IGF-I, dietary glucose, fatty acids, some amino acids, gastrin, secretin, cholecystokinin (CCK), epinephrine, acetylcholine, and melatonin. Inhibitors include substance P and metenkephalin. Several isohormones differ in sizes and the abilities to act on various cell types; and there is evidence for the existence of more than one kind of receptor. The most widely distributed form (with S-S bonds connecting the cysteine moieties) is somatostatin-14 (SS-14): Ala-Gly-Cys-Lys-Asn-Phe-Phe-Trp-Lys-Thr-Phe-Thr-Ser-Cys. Somatostatin-28 (SS-28), with 14 additional *N*-terminal amino acids (Ser-Ala-Asn-Ser-Asn-Pro-Ala-Met-Ala-Pro-Arg-Glu-Arg-Lys- in the porcine type), is also called prosomatostatin, since it can be cleaved to SS-14; but it acts directly on some receptors. SS has limited clinical value because it is rapidly degraded. Longer-lived analogs, such as **octreotide** (*q.v.*) are used to suppress hormone secretion in some individuals with vipomas, gastric ulcers, and other diseases. Inadequate SS release may contribute to some forms of diabetes mellitus.

somatostatinomas: malignant D cell tumors that secrete excessive amounts of somatostatin. The manifestations can include hypoglycemia and impaired gastrointestinal tract functions.

somatotropes: somatotrophs; acidophilic adenohypophysial cells that secrete growth hormone, but not prolactin; *cf* **somatomammotropes**.

somatotropin: growth hormone.

somatotropin release inhibitory factor; SRIF: *see* **somatostatins**.

somatotype: body type; *see* **ectomorph**, **endomorph**, and **mesomorph**.

somesthesia: body sense; sense of muscle and joint position.

somnambulism: sleep walking. It can occur during slow wave (but not REM) sleep.

somni-: a prefix meaning sleep.

somnifacient: (1) hypnotic; soporific; sleep inducing; (2) an agent that induces sleep.

somnolence: drowsiness, a term most commonly applied to abnormal conditions in which alertness is impaired and there is an exaggerated tendency to fall asleep.

Somogyi phenomenon: nocturnal hyperglycemia in patients with diabetes mellitus who take large doses of insulin. Insulin invokes hypoglycemia, which leads to excessive secretion of glucocorticoids, epinephrine, growth hormone, and other regulators that raise blood glucose levels and assume importance as insulin levels decline.

SON: supraoptic nuclei.

sonic: related to, or affected by sound.

soporific: (1) sleep inducing; (2) an agent that induces sleep.

sorbefacient: an agent that promotes absorption.

sorbic acid: 2,4-hexadienoic acid; an agent used to inhibit the growth of fungi in foods, obtained from the lactone, parasorbic acid in mountain ash (*Sorbus aucuparia*).

$$H_3C - \overset{H}{\underset{}{C}} = \overset{H}{\underset{}{C}} - \overset{H}{\underset{}{C}} = \overset{H}{\underset{}{C}} - COOH$$

sorbinil: (*S*)-6-fluoro-2,3-dihydrospiro[4*H*-1-benzopyran-4,4'-imidazolidine]-2',5'-dione; an agent that inhibits aldose reductase, and thereby formation of **sorbitol** (*q.v.*). It can protect against formation of osmotically induced cataracts and a form of neuropathy that develops in individuals with diabetes mellitus.

sorbitol: D-glucitol; a sugar alcohol in berries, cherries, plums, pears, apples, seaweed and algae. Since small amounts are rapidly converted to fructose, it is isocaloric with that sugar, and with glucose. "Sugarless" foods that contain it are therefore not "low calorie" nutrients. It is claimed, however, that such foods can be used more freely by individuals with diabetes mellitus, since they do not rapidly raise blood sugar levels, and that "sugarless chewing gums" with sorbitol cause less tooth decay than those made with glucose or sucrose. The sorbitol seminal vesicles release to seminal fluid is a major source of fructose for spermatozoa. In eye lens and some other cell types that do not have insulin-regulated transport systems, hyperglycemia causes glucose to be taken up more rapidly than it can be phosphorylated by hexokinase. Aldose reductase reduces the excess to sorbitol via: glucose + NADH + H⁺ → sorbitol + NAD⁺. Since sorbitol does not readily diffuse across plasma membranes, it accumulates in the cells, osmotically draws water, and can cause cataract formation.

$$
\begin{array}{c}
CH_2OH \\
| \\
HCOH \\
| \\
HOCH \\
| \\
HCOH \\
| \\
HCOH \\
| \\
CH_2OH
\end{array}
$$

Sos: a *Drosophila* gene that directs development, named *Sos* (*son of sevenless*) because it is expressed after the *sevenless* gene. The yeast counterpart is *cdc25*. Mammalian mSoS is a component of phosphorylation cascades activated by factors that link events initiated at plasma membranes to changes in nucleic acid functions. In unstimulated cells, the protein complexes with a growth factor receptor binding protein, GRB2. When receptors for epidermal growth factor (EGF) and some other mitogens bind their ligands and undergo autophosphorylation, and in the presence of some other tyrosine kinases, phosphorylated products bind GRB2 in a manner that leads to release of Sos. Free Sos accelerates GTP exchange for GDP on Ras proteins, and Ras-GTP activates Raf-1 (a protein kinase that undergoes and is activated by autophosphorylation). Raf-1, in turn, activates MAP kinases that act on myc, jun, ets, and other transcription factors.

SOS response: reactions to DNA damage in *E.coli* initiated by cleavage of lex A protein, which normally functions as a repressor. The cells then make large quantities of recA (a protease and recombinase), and other proteins that mediate DNA repair.

sotalol: 4'-[1-hydroxy-2-(isopropylamino)ethyl]methanesulfonamide; a β-type adrenergic receptor antagonist used to treat some forms of angina, dysrhythmia, and hypertension.

Southern blotting: techniques for separating and analyzing DNA fragments, in which segments released by endonucleases are separated by agarose gel electrophoresis and transferred to nitrocellulose sheets. Radioactively labeled DNAs with complementary bases are then used as probes to identify the fragments; *cf* **Northern blotting**.

sow: an adult female swine.

soybean trypsin inhibitor: ST1; STB1; a 21K enzyme obtained from soybeans that binds irreversibly to trypsin, and also inhibits some other serine proteases.

SP: substance P.

SP1: SP1 transcription factor: a 95-105K eukaryote protein that binds to GC (guanine-cytidine) boxes, and is essential for transcription of genes that contain such promoters.

SP-1: secretory protein-1; chromogranin A.

SP₁: pregnancy specific glycoprotein.

SP-A, SP-B, SP-C, SP-D: *see* **SP proteins**.

hSP: human spasmolytic protein; *see* **trefoil proteins**.

spacer DNA: nontranscribing DNA segments of eukaryotic and some viral genes, most of which contain highly repetitive base sequences. Some may contribute to chromosome alignment during cell division.

SPARC: a 43K cysteine-rich, acidic glycoprotein chemically related to or identical with osteonectin, made in embryonic endoderm, and in the central nervous system, bone, endothelium, fibroblasts, smooth muscle, and testicular Sertoli and interstitial cells. It is secreted by some cell types, and is a component of testicular fluid. SPARC binds calcium, copper, and iron, and inhibits hydroxyapatite formation. The proposed functions include metallic ion transport and sequestration.

spare receptors: receptors present in numbers that exceed those required for maximal responses. They can augment sensitivities to low hormone concentrations by increasing the probability that binding will occur, and can assure continuous availability of receptors when occupied ones are internalized by endocytosis. In some cases, very high ligand concentrations invoke pharmacological responses by binding to spare receptors.

sparganum: a plerocercoid tapeworm larva of the order Pseudophyllidea that matures in some fishes. *See* **plerocercoid factor**.

sparsomycin A: tubercidin; 7-β-D-ribofuranosyl-7*H*-pyrrolo[2,3-d]pyrimidin-4-amine; an antibiotic made by *Streptomyces sparsogenes*, used to treat tuberculosis and some other bacterial infections, and as a fungicide and antineoplastic agent. It binds to large ribosomal subunits, and inhibits peptide bond formation in eukaryotic and prokaryotic cells.

spasms: involuntary, often prolonged, muscle contractions.

spasmolytic: describes agents or processes that relax spasms.

spasticity: exaggerated muscle tone and reflex responsivity, with resistance to passive stretching, usually associated with increased alpha and gamma motor neuron excitability. Damaged upper motor neurons, and cor-

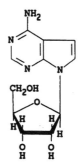

sparsomycin A

ticospinal tract lesions can cause spastic paralysis, whereas damaged lower motor neurons cause flaccid paralysis.

spatial summation: augmentation of a response by recruitment of additional responding elements. The term can refer to activation of a high threshold postsynaptic neuron by several presynaptic ones, strong contraction of a skeletal muscle accomplished by activation of several motor units, or a common response to two or more humoral regulators that act via different mechanisms.

spawn: to deposit eggs.

spay: to remove the ovaries, a term usually applied to domesticated animals.

speciation: splitting of an ancestral species into new groups that coexist but differ genetically and phenotypically; *cf* **species selection** and **species transformation**.

species: usually, (1) a genus subdivision composed of individuals who share certain phenotypic characteristics, and whose genomes are sufficiently similar to permit creation of viable progeny, but who differ significantly from other members of the genus. A species can be subdivided into strains on the basis of differences in alleles that can affect anatomical as well as immunological, biochemical, and other attributes, but not the ability to interbreed. The term is useful for most animals, but not easily applied to plants, in which hybridization is common; (2) a group of very similar proteins or other large molecules.

species selection: an evolutionary process in which certain kinds of organisms (species) survive, as related ones become extinct.

species specificity: characteristic of, or effective for a single species. Some regulators unique to a species act only in the animals of origin. Human growth hormone closely fits the definition, since its composition differs from that of other species, and only human and primate growth hormones act on human receptors (which are also species specific). In contrast, species specific insulins made by fishes, cows, pigs, and others invoke similar responses when injected into humans and other mammals.

species transformation: conversion of one species type to another.

specific activity: the ratio of the numbers of radioactive to the numbers of nonradioactive atoms or molecules of the same kind. It can be expressed as numbers of radioactive atoms per million stable ones, but a more common measure is radioactivity per unit weight or volume (for example curies per mole, or microcuries per ml.).

specific dynamic action: SDA; specific dynamic effect; SDE: the extent to which metabolic rate is elevated above basal levels by metabolism of nutrients, usually expressed as % of basal level. It does not include energy exchanges related to ingestion or digestion. When fed (or otherwise administered) to fasted subjects, proteins and amino acids raise the rate by approximately 30%, whereas the values for carbohydrates and lipids are closer to 10%. SDA is used to determine the numbers of food calories required to maintain stable body weights when the basal metabolic rates are known (and adjustments are made for energy expenditure related to skeletal muscle and other activities).

specific dynamic effect: SDE; specific dynamic action.

specific immune suppression: loss of the ability to respond to just one kind of antigen (or to a group of very closely related ones), usually because of effects invoked by previous exposure to the same antigen.

specificity: restricted to a one kind of structure, function, or chemical entity. Some agents display cell or tissue type specificity (act on only certain cell or tissue types). Receptors are said to bind their ligands with high specificity, since they have little or no affinity for different kinds of ligands; and most enzymes have limited substrate specificities. *See* also **species specificity**.

spectrin: the major protein of the erythrocyte plasma membrane skeleton. It forms dimeric flexible rods approximately 100 nm in length, each composed of a 260K α chain and a 225K β chain wound around each other to form a helix. Both chains contain repeating 160-amino acid units. Spectrin binds to actin filaments; and protein 4.1 links spectrin-actin complexes to glycophorin. It also indirectly affects ion channels by binding to ankyrin.

spectrotype: the pattern of bands on an isoelectric focusing gel. The patterns are used to identify the protein types.

"speed": a street term for methamphetamine preparations.

speract: Gly-Phe-Asp-Leu-Asn-Gly-Gly-Gly-Val-Gly; a species specific peptide on the surfaces of eggs of the sea urchin *Strongylocentrotus purpuratas* that functions as a sperm attractant and activator. Its effects are similar to those described for **resact** (*q.v.*), but the peptide made by one species does not bind to the receptors for the other.

speract receptor: a 77K glycoprotein on the surfaces of sea urchin sperm that binds speract. The sperm is then activated via processes mediated by guanylate cyclase.

spergualin: an antibiotic made by *Bacillus latrosporus* with immunosuppressant and antitumor properties. Deoxysperagualin, a more potent, long-acting analog, 1-amio-19-guanidine-11-hydroxy-4,9,12-triazanonadecane-10,13-dione, induces transplant tolerance, suppresses autoimmune diseases, protects against delayed-type hypersensitivity, diminishes inflammatory reactions, and synergizes with cyclosporine A and antithymocyte globulin. It binds tightly to heat shock proteins hsp70 and hsp90, and exerts its influences on the functions of macrophages as well as on B lymphocytes and both CD4$^+$ and CD8$^+$ T cells. The observed effects include marked diminution of superoxide generation and lysosomal enzyme release by macrophages, interference with the functions of anigen presenting cells, inhibition of *oct-2* and *NF-KB* activation, suppression of lymphocyte proliferation, and decreased antibody production.

sperm: (1) a single spermatozoan or sperm cell; (2) many spermatozoa.

spermacrasia: abnormally low numbers of sperm in ejaculates.

spermagglutination: clumping of sperm, a process normally initiated by seminal fluid components following ejaculation.

spermateliosis: spermiogenesis.

spermatheca: an organ of a female (or of a hermaphrodite) that receives and stores spermatozoa. In some species, a single insemination is used for successive fertilizations.

spermatic tubules: seminiferous tubules.

sperqualin

deoxysperqualin

spermatid: one of two small, round, haploid cells formed when a secondary spermatocyte completes meiosis. Spermiogenesis is the process that converts it to an immature spermatozoan.

spermatocides: spermicides; agents that kill spermatozoa. Some types are used in barrier-type contraceptive preparations such as vaginal jellies, foams, and suppositories.

spermatocoele: spermatocele; a cyst in the scrotum that contains spermatozoa, formed when seminiferous tubules are partially obstructed.

spermatocytes: *primary* spermatocytes are diploid germinal cells that differentiate from spermatogonia. When they complete maturation, and then meiosis I, each gives rise to two secondary spermatocytes. The members of a pair differ in chromosomal makeup, since each carries two copies of a single set of alleles (and either two X or two Y chromosomes). Each secondary spermatocyte then gives rise (via meiosis II) to two haploid spermatids.

spermatocytogenesis: differentiation of primary spermatocytes from spermatogonia.

spermatogenesis: usually, formation of spermatids from spermatogonia via processes that include spermatocytogenesis and both stages of meiosis. Some authors include spermiogenesis. Differentiation begins in the peripheral regions of seminiferous tubules, but completion of meiosis requires a special environment provided by **Sertoli cells** (*q.v.*).

spermatogonia: diploid germinal cells of the testis that differentiate from gonocytes. The ones formed in embryos divide rapidly by mitosis for a brief period, and then become quiescent until puberty onset. Several adult types have been described, including "stem cells" that remain quiescent but resist several kinds of injury and can provide new populations when other types are destroyed. A second set divides rapidly to provide new spermatogonia. Some of the progeny go through several maturational stages, become primary spermatocytes, and subsequently acquire the ability to divide by meiosis.

spermatolysins; spermolysins: agents that destroy sperm plasma membranes. Naturally occurring types are used to break down degenerating and dead sperm. Synthetic ones are components of some barrier type contraceptive preparations.

spermatophytes: higher plants, including gymnosperms (which form pollen tubes and seeds), and angiosperms (flowering plants).

spermatozoan [**spermatozoa**]: a mature male gamete. In mammals, the ones that contain a Y chromosome are smaller and more motile than X types. *See* **sperm** and **spermiogenesis**.

sperm capacitation: the final stage in the preparation of spermatozoa for acrosome reactions. It usually proceeds in the uterus or oviduct, and involves changes in the cell surfaces, and the release of enzymes. Stimulation by oocyte factors has been suggested. Estrogens promote secretion of oviductal and uterine fluids favorable for sperm survival and capacitation around the time of ovulation. During luteal phases, progesterone regulated fluids retard the reactions. Capacitated sperm that do not fertilize deteriorate with 24-48 hours. Seminal fluid contains factors that protect against premature capacitation. According to some observers, it also contains decapacitation factors.

spermiation: extrusion of fully formed spermatozoa from Sertoli cells, along with some testicular fluid. The cells then enter the rete testes and commence their journey to the epididymis for further maturation. Adenohypophysial gonadotropins are the physiological stimulants. The "frog" test for pregnancy is based on the ability of human chorionic gonadotropin (hCG) in urine to promote spermiation in amphibians.

spermicide: spermatocide.

spermidine: N-(3-aminopropyl)-1,4-butanediamine; a polybasic amine, synthesized from putrescine + S-(5-adenosyl)-3-methylmercaptopropylamine via a reaction catalyzed by an aminopropyl transferase. Spermidine binds to nucleic acids, and is believed to contribute to stabilization of DNAs, messenger RNAs, and transfer RNAs. The highest concentrations are found in sperm, but the amine also mediates some actions of prolactin and other regulators on protein synthesis in different cell types; and it potentiates NMDA actions on ion channels. It is also the direct precursor of **spermine** (*q.v.*). *See* also **polyamines**.

spermine: N,N'-bis(3-aminopropyl)-1,4-butanediamine; a polybasic amine made by spermine condensation with S-(5-adenosyl)-3-methylmercaptopropylamine. It is a component of ribosomes and some viruses; and the high

NH_2
|
$(CH_2)_3$
|
CH_2-NH_2

putrescine

NH_2
|
$(CH_2)_3$
|
NH
|
$(CH_2)_3$
|
CH_2-NH_2

spermidine

NH_2
|
$(CH_2)_3$
|
NH
|
$(CH_2)_3$
|
NH
|
$(CH_2)_2$
|
CH_2-NH_2

spermine

levels in sperm permit its use as a marker for semen. In common with spermidine, it binds to and stabilizes nucleic acids, and additionally stabilizes some liver enzymes. Spermine and related **polyamines** (*q.v.*) appear to be essential for initiation of cell proliferation, and for some differentiation processes. They augment the activities of some phosphatases, inhibit some protein kinases, and regulate Ca^{2+} cycling across mitochondrial membranes. Their synthesis in prostate glands and release to seminal fluids are androgen dependent. In immature testes, polyamines contribute to maturation, and in more mature ones they inhibit the binding of follicle stimulating hormone (FSH) to its receptors. Binding sites have also been identified in intestinal mucosa.

spermiogenesis: spermatid maturation to spermatozoa. The processes are androgen dependent, and are accomplished when the germinal cells are embedded in Sertoli cells. The spermatid loses much of its cytoplasm, and the nucleus condenses to form a head composed mostly of DNA and associated proteins. The acrosome (which develops from the Golgi region) holds enzymes essential for the acrosome reaction and penetration of oocyte membranes. The midpiece is composed mostly of mitochondria. Special proteins are synthesized and incorporated into a long tail. Sperm leaving the testes appear morphologically mature, but have not yet acquired the ability to swim or engage in fertilization.

SPG1: Sertoli cell glycoprotein 1; a glycoprotein chemically related to SPG2, made by Sertoli cells and believed to deliver lipids to developing spermatozoa and/or regulate the lipid content of the sperm plasma membrane.

SPG2: Sertoli cell glycoprotein 2; a glycoprotein made by Sertoli cells that is incorporated into sperm plasma membranes.

S phase: the stage of a cell cycle during which DNA is synthesized. It is preceded by G_1 and followed by M (mitosis or meiosis).

spherocytes: spherical erythrocytes, made by individuals with some genetic defects or acquired hemolytic diseases, and in ones with severe burns who receive transfusions of normal blood. They are more fragile than the usual kinds of red cells (which are biconcave disks).

spheroidin: tetrodotoxin.

spherophysine: *N*-(4-aminobutyl)-*N*-(3-methyl-2-butenyl)guanidine; a ganglionic blocking agent obtained from *Swaisona salsula* and some other Central Asiatic legumes.

sphincter: a ring of smooth muscle that surrounds a cavity. Contraction narrows or closes the orifice.

sphinganine: 3-dihydrosphingosine; *see* **sphingosine**.

3-dehydro-**sphinganine**: an alcohol used for sphingomyelin biosynthesis. A pyridoxal-dependent enzyme catalyzes its formation from palmitoyl-coenzyme A + serine, and an NADPH-dependent enzyme converts it to 3-dihydrosphinganine. *See* **sphingosine**.

3-dihydro-**sphinganine**: a component of sphingolipids, made from 3-dehydrosphingosine via reaction catalyzed by an NADPH-dependent reductase. *See* **sphingosine**.

4-**sphingenine**: sphingosine.

sphingolipids: ceramides, cerebrosides, sphingomyelins, gangliosides, and other lipids that contain sphingosine, present in cell membranes, with highest levels in nervous tissue.

sphingolipidoses: several inherited diseases in which sphingolipids accumulate because the production of degrading enzymes is impaired; *see* also **sphingomyelinase**.

sphingomyelinase: an enzyme that cleaves phosphorylcholine from sphingomyelin and releases sphingosine. In Niemann-Pick disease, impaired synthesis leads to sphingomyelin accumulation in the brain, spleen and liver.

sphingomyelins: phospholipids in which a sphingosine moiety is covalently linked to the first carbon of glycerol, a long chain fatty acid to the second, and phosphorylcholine to the third. Lignoceric and nervonic acids are the most abundant fatty acids, but some molecules contain stearic or palmitic acid. Sphingomyelins are major components of myelin sheaths.

sphingomyelin synthase: phosphatidylcholine:ceramide transferase; an enzyme that catalyzes reactions in which acylated sphingosines combine with CDP-choline to yield CMP and sphingomyelins; *see* **sphingosine**.

sphingosine: 4-sphingenine; 2-amino-4-octadecene-1,3-diol; an alcohol component of gangliosides and other sphingolipids. When released by hydrolysis, it binds directly to regulatory domains of kinase C isozymes, calmodulin kinases, and some other enzymes, and blocks their activation. The biosynthesis begins with a reaction in which serine combines with palmitoyl-CoA to yield 3-dehydrosphinganine + CO_2 + CoA. The product is reduced by NADPH + H^+ to 4-dihydrosphingosine, which is then oxidized by FAD to sphingosine (4-sphingenine). Sphingosine combines with long-chain fatty acyl-CoAs to form ceramides (*N*-acyl-sphingosines) which, in turn react with CDP-choline (cytidine diphosphate choline) or in some cases CDP-ethanolamine to form sphingomyelins + CMP, or with uridine diphosphate sugars (most commonly UDP-galactose) to yield cerebrosides. When sulfated on sugar moieties, they become sulfatides. Gangliosides are more complex molecules made by sequential additions of sugars to cerebrosides.

3-dihydro-**sphingosine**: sphinganine; (2*S*,3*R*)-2-aminooctadecane-1,3-diol; an alcohol component of some sphingolipids, formed from 3-dehydrosphinganine in a reaction catalyzed by an NADPH-dependent reductase. An FAD-dependent reductase converts it to **sphingosine** (*q.v.*).

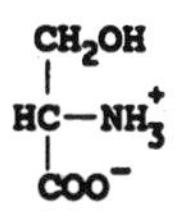

serine

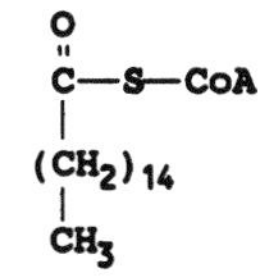

CH_2OH
$HC-NH_3^+$
COO^-

palmitolyl-CoA

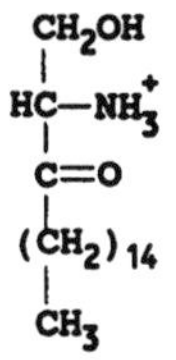

O
$C-S-CoA$
$(CH_2)_{14}$
CH_3

3-dehydro-sphinganine

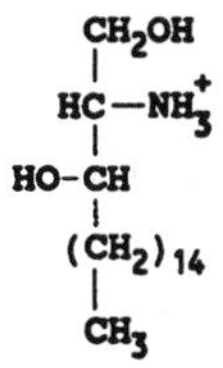

CH_2OH
$HC-NH_3^+$
$C=O$
$(CH_2)_{14}$
CH_3

3-dihydro-sphingosine

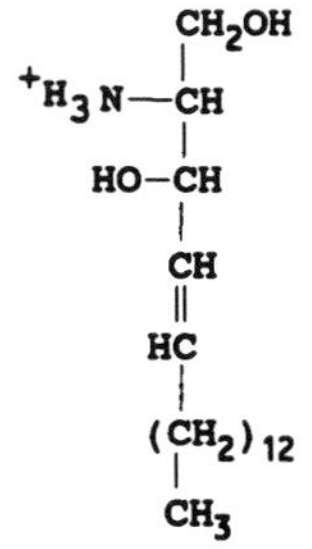

CH_2OH
$HC-NH_3^+$
$HO-CH$
$(CH_2)_{14}$
CH_3

sphingosine

CH_2OH
$^+H_3N-CH$
$HO-CH$
CH
HC
$(CH_2)_{12}$
CH_3

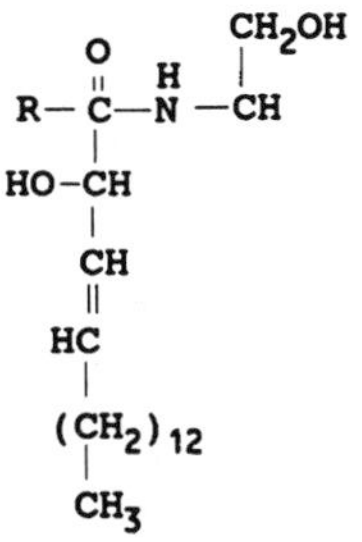

N-acyl-sphingosine (ceramides)

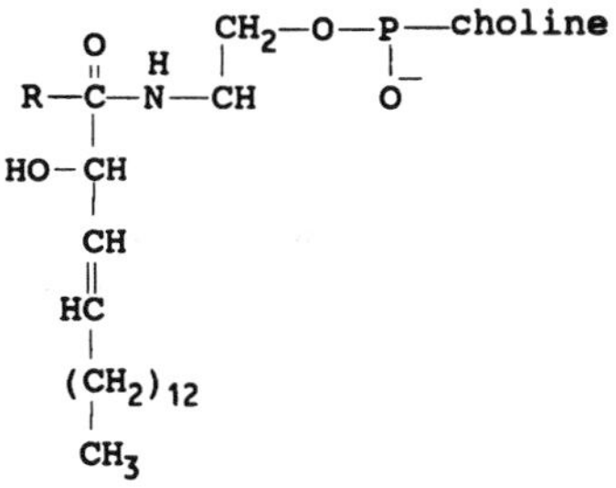

$O \quad H \quad CH_2OH$
$R-C-N-CH$
$HO-CH$
CH
HC
$(CH_2)_{12}$
CH_3

sphingomyelin

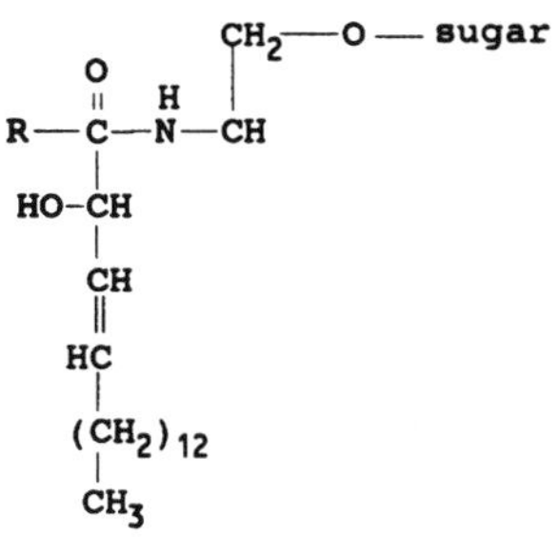

$O \quad H \quad CH_2-O-P-choline$
$R-C-N-CH \quad O^-$
$HO-CH$
CH
HC
$(CH_2)_{12}$
CH_3

cerebroside

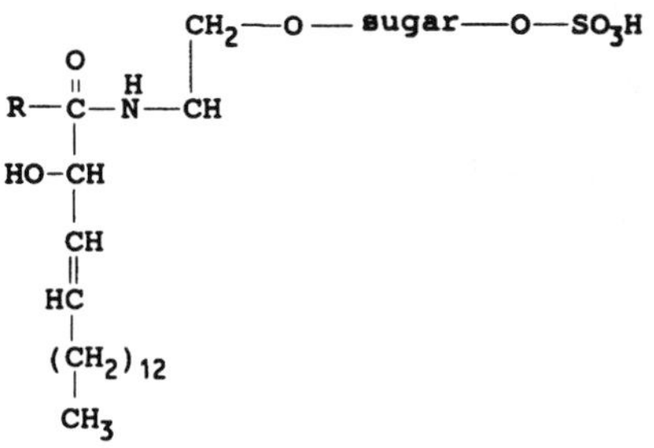

$\qquad CH_2-O-sugar$
$O \quad H$
$R-C-N-CH$
$HO-CH$
CH
HC
$(CH_2)_{12}$
CH_3

sulfatides

$\qquad CH_2-O-sugar-O-SO_3H$
$O \quad H$
$R-C-N-CH$
$HO-CH$
CH
HC
$(CH_2)_{12}$
CH_3

sphygmo-: a prefix meaning pulse.

sphygmodynamometers: instruments for measuring pulse force.

sphygmomanometers: instruments for measuring blood pressure. In the most common type, an inflatable cuff connected to a rubber bulb and a manometer is placed around the upper arm, and air is pumped into the bulb until the pressure in the cuff exceeds the pressure in the brachial artery. At this point, no blood flows past the occluded site, and no sound is heard. When the pressure is then gradually lowered to just below that of the systolic pressure, a sharp tapping sound is detected. The sounds change with continued lowering of the cuff pressure; and the diastolic reading is taken at the point where they become muffled.

spike: (1) a rapid change in the electrical activity of a neuron, usually of brief duration, and usually associated with passage of a nerve impulse; (2) a sharp-angled upward deflection on a densitometric or other tracing.

spina: a thornlike projection.

spina bifida: birth defects that affect formation of one or more vertebrae. In the most common type, one or more of the posterior vertebral arches in the lumbar and/or sacral region is incomplete. In another, some vertebral bodies in the thoracic and/or abdominal regions are affected. The spinal cord can herniate at the defect sites, and may or may not be covered with skin and subcutaneous tissue. Associated nervous system damage is related to the amount of nervous tissue exposed, and the pressure exerted on spinal cord segments. The consequences vary from mild urinary function disturbances to severe mental retardation and paralysis. These and other neural tube defects are associated with high α-fetoprotein levels. Very small imperfections that are difficult to detect externally do not cause problems. Folic acid supplements taken by mothers during pregnancy are said to decrease the incidence.

spinal ganglion: dorsal root ganglion.

spinal nucleus of the cavernosus: an androgen-regulated neuron cluster in the spinal cord essential for intromission and ejaculation.

spindle: (1) microtubule fibers and associated proteins that form during mitosis or meiosis, and direct chromosome alignment and movements. Long polar fibers extend from organizing centers at each cell pole to the equator (*see* also **centrioles**), where they interdigitate with fibers from the opposite pole. Short astral fibers with free ends radiate from the poles. Some authors include kinetochore fibers that attach to chromosome centromeres; (2) a wave form of constant frequency but varying amplitude in an electroencephalogram. *See* also **spindle organ**.

spindle attachment region: centromere.

spindle organ; a typical skeletal muscle is composed mostly of large (extrafusal) fibers that contract in response to acetylcholine released by large (alpha type) motor neurons. A spindle organ is a slender structure within the muscle, attached to the same tendons, that contains a centrally located stretch receptor. Small, *intrafusal* muscle fibers, which connect the stretch receptor to the tendon ends, are innervated by fine gamma motor fibers. When the intrafusal fibers contract, they activate the stretch receptor by drawing its ends toward the tendons. This initiates a reflex that leads to contraction of the large, extrafusal muscle fibers. The receptor is also activated mechanically, if the extrafusal fibers elongate. When contraction of the large fibers is initiated by messages transmitted from pyramidal tract neurons to alpha fibers, the gamma fibers are also stimulated. If the muscle contraction is sufficient for its purpose, the spindle is shortened (inactivated). However, if the contraction of the large fibers is inadequate, the gamma neurons stretch the spindle receptors, and reflexly augment extafusal fiber contraction. The spindle organs can thereby maintain muscle tone and augment the effects of motor nerve stimulation. *See* also **stretch reflexes**.

spinnbarkeit: the tendency for uterine cervical mucus to form threads when stretched between two glass slides (or coverslips). Estrogens, which attain highest levels around the time of ovulation, promote formation of an elastic, viscous mucus that displays the property. Progesterone secreted during luteal phases facilitates formation of secretions that lack those characteristcs. The observations have been used by women with low fertility to estimate the time periods during which there is the greatest probability that coitus will lead to conception. *See* also **"rhythm methods" for contraception**.

spiperone: spriroperidol; 8-[4-(4-fluorophenyl)-4-oxobutyl]-1-phenyl-1,3,8-triazaspirol[4,5]decan-4-one; a $5HT_{1A}$ type serotonin receptor antagonist. It is a potent neuroleptic that blocks haloperidol binding to D_2 dopamine and serotonin receptors, and is also used as a D_2 antagonist.

spiracles: respiratory apertures, used by arthropods to take up air, and by cartilaginous fishes to take up water.

spiral cleavage: a type of embryonic development in annelids, molluscs, and some other invertebrates, in which small displacements of cleavage planes generate corkscrew-like structures.

spirochetes: nonflagellated bacteria of the *Spirochaetaceae* family that move through viscous fluids by corkscrew flexing of their bodies. Some survive for many years, and invoke symptoms after long latent periods. The group includes *Treponema pallidum* (which causes syphilis), other pathogenic *Treponema* and *Leptospira* organisms, and some nonpathogenic forms.

spirometers: instruments for measuring inspired and expired air volumes.

spironolactone: Aldactone A; 7-(acetylthio)-17-hydroxy-3-oxo-pregn-4-ene-21-carboxylic acid γ-lactone; an orally effective aldosterone receptor antagonist, used to promote diuresis and antagonize other effects of excess hormone. It can invoke hyponatremia and hyperkalemia, and indirectly elevate angiotensin II levels. High concentrations slow testosterone synthesis by inhibiting 17α-hydroxylase and 17,20 lyase enzymes, and testosterone conversion to dihydrotestosterone by inhibiting 5α-reductase. They are also testosterone receptor antagonists, and can augment estrogen synthesis by increasing aromatase activity. The "side-effects" are undesirable in men, but have been used to treat hirsutism in women.

spiroperidol: spiperone.

splanchnic: pertaining to the viscera.

spleen: the largest lymphatic system organ. It contains germinal centers in which B lymphocytes proliferate, macrophages that ingest and process antigens, and regions that house several kinds of T lymphocytes; and the regulators it produces include thymopoietin and splenins. The spleen also removes debris and degenerating cells from the blood that circulates through it, serves as a reservoir for erythrocytes (which can be recruited during exercise or after a hemorrhage), and retains the capacity for erythropoiesis when bone marrow function is inadequate.

splenin: two species specific peptides made by spleen cells that are chemically and biologically related to thymopoietin. The amino acid sequence for human splenin A is shown with asterisks that mark moieties different from those of thymopoietin: Gly-Leu-Pro-Lys-Glu-Val-Pro-Ala-Val-Leu-Thr-Lys-Gln-Lys-Leu-Lys-Ser-Glu-Leu-Val-Ala-Asn-Asn*-Val-Thr-Leu-Pro-Ala-Gly-Glu-Met-Arg-Lys-Ala*-Val-Tyr-Val-Glu-Leu-Tyr-Leu-Gln-Ser*-Leu-Thr-Ala-Glu*-His. Some splenin A actions have been linked with elevation of cyclic guanosine 3′,5′-monophosphate (cGMP) levels. Both splenin A and splenin B augment capillary permeability. The B type additionally prolongs bleeding time.

spliceosomes: 60S complexes composed of small nuclear ribonucleoprotein particles (snURPs) and messenger RNA precursors. U4, U5, and U6 contribute to splice-osome assembly. U1, U2, and U5 snURPs catalyze removal of mRNA precursor introns, and joining of exons to form mature messenger molecules.

splicing: splitting; usually, excision of premessenger RNA introns, followed by joining of the exons to produce mature mRNAs.

split genes: genes that contain both exons and introns. Most eukaryote genes are of this type. Some transcripts undergo differential splicing to yield two or more different messenger RNAs; *see*, for example **calcitonin/CGRP genes**.

split tolerance: inability to react to some, but not to other allogeneic antigens.

spondyl-, spondylo-: prefixes meaning vertebra or vertebral.

spondylosis: usually, noninflammatory degenerative diseases of the spine associated with osteoarthritis.

spongioblasts: (1) glioblasts; embryonic neural tube cell precursors of astrocytes and oligodendrocytes; (2) embryonic retinal cells that gives rise to sustentacular fibers.

spongiocytes: lipid-laden adrenocortical cells.

spontaneous ovulators: animals in which ovarian cycles are endogenously controlled, and mating stimuli are not required for ovulation. *See* also **ovarian cycles**, and *cf* **induced ovulators**.

spores: (1) dehydrated bacterial cells with low metabolic activity, formed under adverse conditions. They are resistant to heat, cold, drying, environmental toxins, radiation, and nutrient deprivation; (2) haploid plant or fungus cells produced by meiosis; (3) fungus cells that detach from the parents, and can germinate. They form new haploid individuals, or function as gametes.

sporophyte: the diploid generation of the life cycle of a plant. In simpler plants such as club mosses, the more prominent haploid gametophyte produces both male and female gametes (without further reduction division). After fertilization, sporophytes develop at the tips of the gametophyte and gives rise (via meiosis) to haploid spores which germinate to form the gametophytes of the next generation. In higher plants, the sporophytes are the large, long-lived structures with roots, stem, leaves, and flowers. The ovules and stamens of the flowers are the reproductive organs that produce haploid male and female gametes. After fertilization the seeds germinate to produce the next spermatophyte generation.

S protein: an old term for vitronectin.

SP proteins: surfactin associated proteins; SAPs; proteins synthesized by type II pulmonary epithelial cells that are essential for establishing and maintaining surfactant films (which protect against alveolar collapse during expiration by lowering surface tension at air-liquid interfaces). The three major types, SP-A, SP-B, and SP-C, are encoded by separate genes on different chromosomes, and are differentially regulated. A fourth (SP-D) type has also been identified. The proteins are stored in lamellated organelles, and released by exocytosis. SP-A is the largest and most abundant type, composed of 28-36K monomers structurally similar to complement protein C1q, that form 640K hexameric triple helix aggregates. The monomers undergo extensive posttranslational processing that includes hydroxylation, carboxylation, sulfation, *N*-acetylation, glycosylation, and addition of sialic acid groups. They bind calcium, sugars, and lipids, promote calcium-dependent surfactant lipid aggregation, accelerate surface film formation and spreading, and control the amount of surfactant that accumulates by regulating lipid endocytosis and recycling. SP-A additionally contributes to tubular myelin formation. Since it also activates alveolar macrophages, it is believed to protect against infection and perform other immunological functions. PS-A synthesis begins late in fetal life, and can then be detected in amniotic fluid. It is likely that inhibitors, which probably include transforming growth factor β (TGFβ), block its formation at earlier times. High insulin levels also inhibit. Epidermal growth factor (EGF) and cAMP stimulate its production. Glucocorticoids also stimulate, both alone and in synergy with cAMP and triiodothyronine (T$_3$); and fetuses subjected to stress make larger amounts. However, high glucocorticoid levels destabilize the messenger RNA. In contrast, glucocorticoids exert only stimulatory influences on SP-B and SP-C, both of which are made by younger fetuses. SP-B is a hydrophobic protein composed of 7-8K monomers that aggregate to 18K forms. SP-C, which is also hydrophobic, is composed of 5K monomers that dimerize. Both B and C type proteins enhance surfactant film formation, but inhibit phospholipid synthesis.

sprue: two diseases in which intestinal absorption is impaired. The nontropical type (*celiac disease*) is caused by an inherited defect that invokes hypersensitivity to wheat gluten and some other grain components. *Tropical sprue* is caused by a microorganism.

spy: a gene on the short arm of the mouse Y chromosome essential for spermatogenesis. It may be identical with *sby*. *See* **sxr**.

SQ: subcutaneous.

SQ 22536: an agent used to inhibit adenylate cyclase enzymes.

SQ 29548: a thromboxane TXA$_2$ receptor antagonist.

squalene: 2,6,10,15,19,23-hexamethyl-2,6,10,14,18,22-tetracosa hexane; a plant and animal hydrocarbon,

SQ 29548

present in high concentrations in shark liver oils and in smaller ones in yeasts, olive oils, and wheat germ oils. It is an intermediate in the pathway for biosynthesis of cholesterol and related compounds from acetyl-coenzyme A, formed in the reaction: 2 farnesyl-pyrophosphate + NADPH → squalene + NADP$^+$ + 2 P—P + H$^+$. Squalene undergoes cyclization to lanosterol, via reactions that use O$_2$ and NADPH, in which a squalene epoxide is a short-lived reactive intermediate. It is bactericidal, and is used as a lubricant, surface-active agent, and lipid solvent.

squalene monooxygenase: an enzyme that converts squalene to squalene epoxide.

squamous: scale-like.

squill: sea onion; sea leak; white squill; the leaves and bulbs of *Urginea maritima*. It contains several substances used as expectorants and emetics, as well as digitalis-like cardiotonic glycosides. *Red* squill (*Urginea indica*) is a rat poison that invokes cardiac arrest.

SR: steroid hormone-receptor complex. The complexes form when **steroid hormones** (*q.v.*) bind to their receptors.

SR*: activated steroid-hormone complex; an acronym applied to receptors that have bound their ligands, and have completed the changes that facilitate avid binding to steroid response elements.

Sr: strontium.

SR 95103: a phenylaminopyridazine derivative of gamma aminobutyric acid, used as a GABA$_A$ type receptor antagonist.

SRBC: sheep red blood cells.

SRBC Rc: sheep red blood cell receptor; ERc; T11; *see* **CD2**.

src: a family of plasma membrane-associated 55-62K nonreceptor tyrosine kinases that includes pp60^{v-src} made by the Rous sarcoma virus, and the products of *yes*, *fgr*, *fyn*, *hck*, *lck*, and *lyn*, genes, all of which affect growth and differentiation and can invoke transformation. They lack transmembrane domains, but some, anchored by lipids to the bilayers, have peripheral extensions. The relatively low potency of the 60K product of the normal cellular proto-oncogene, *c-src* is attributed in part to rapid covalent inactivation by endogenous enzymes. *See* also **SH domains** and **mitogen activated kinases**.

SRE: (1) steroid response element; (2) serum response element.

SRF: somatotropin release factor; *see* **growth hormone releasing hormone**.

SRIF: somatotropin release inhibitory factor; *see* **somatostatins**.

SRIH: somatotropin release inhibiting hormone; *see* **somatostatins**.

SRP: signal recognition particle.

SRS-A: slow reacting substance of anaphylaxis.

SRY: a 14-kilobase region on the human Y chromosome that codes for **testis determining factor** (*q.v.*). *Sry* is the analogous region in the mouse.

sry: a gene on the short arm of the mouse Y chromosome that may be identical with *Tdy* (*q.v.*).

SS: somatostatin.

ss: single stranded, as in ssDNA.

SSBG: sex steroid binding globulin.

Ss protein: a hemolytic protein whose formation is directed by the C4B component of the mouse complement locus.

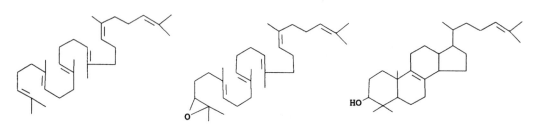

farnesyl pyrophosphate

squalene   squalene epoxide   lanosterol

676

stable isotope: an element that does not spontaneously decompose and emit energy; *cf* **radioactive isotope**. The term is often applied to a form with more (or fewer) neutrons than a more common type with the same numbers of protons and electrons.

stallion: an adult male horse, donkey, or zebra, or an adult male of a related species.

standard conditions: (1) 0° Centigrade and 760 mm atmospheric pressure, when used without qualification for gas measurements, or 0° Centigrade with reactants present in 1 molar concentrations; (2) a specified set of conditions maintained throughout an experiment.

standard deviation: SD; s; the square root of the variance, a statistical measure of the dispersion of data values around their mean, based on the assumption that the parameters follow normal distributions. Sigma (σ) is the theoretical value for the total population from which the samples are drawn. The variance $= \Sigma(y-\bar{y})^2/n\text{-}1$, where y values are the measurements, $\bar{y}$ is the mean, and n = the number of measurements. It is usually calculated as: $\Sigma[y^2 - (\Sigma y)^2]/n\text{-}1)$. In a normal distribution, 68.26% of the measurements fall within the range of $\bar{y} = \pm \sigma$, 95.46% within $\bar{y}= \pm 2\sigma$, and 99.73% within $\bar{y} = \pm 3\sigma$. The mean and SD are used in various ways to compare populations, for example to determine the probability that experimental animals differ significantly from controls, if animals on treatment A differ from those on treatment B to a greater extent than could occur by chance (*see* also **Student's *t* test**), or if a population displays a greater range of variation for one parameter than for another.

standard error of the mean: S.E; a statistical measure for determining the probability that the mean value for a set of measurements is a reliable measure of the mean for the entire population from which the samples were drawn (the mean that would be obtained if an infinite number of subjects could be tested in the same way). It is calculated as $s/\sqrt{n}$ (the standard deviation divided by the square root of the number of measurements). Standard errors are also calculated for other statistical measurements.

standard free energy: G_0 ; a parameter used to measure changes in **free energy** (*q.v.*), represented at pH 7 as G'_0, and expressed in Calories per mole. For a reaction of the general type $A + B \rightleftarrows C + D$, at a pressure of one atmosphere, the change in free energy, $\Delta G, = G'_0 + RT \ln_e$ [C]·[D]/[A]·[B], where R = the gas constant, T = the absolute temperature, $\ln_e$ is the natural logarithm, and [A], [B], [C], and [D] are the reactant concentrations in moles per liter. A negative value for ΔG indicates that the reaction can proceed spontaneously, whereas a positive one means energy from another source is required to drive it in that direction.

Stannius corpuscles: corpuscles of Stannius; bilateral glands attached to the kidneys of bony fishes, initially believed to secrete adrenocortical-like steroids. One cell type makes hypocalcin (a hormone that lowers extracellular Ca^{2+} levels), and another secretes a peptide that regulates the monovalent cation metabolism.

stanolone: 4-dihydrotestosterone; androlone; Anabolex; a synthetic androgen receptor agonist used for its anabolic effects, and for treating some forms of breast cancer.

stanozolol: stanozol; 17-methyl-2′*H*-androst-2-eno[3,2-c]-pyrazol-17-ol; a synthetic androgen used for its anabolic actions, and for treating some forms of anemia.

Staphylococcus: a genus of nonmotile, gram negative bacteria that includes strains which cause skin infections, food poisoning, toxic shock syndrome, and other diseases. The organisms make coagulase, staphylokinase, hyaluronidase, lipase type toxins, and enterotoxins A, B, C, and D. *See* also **superantigens** and **α-toxin**.

staphylokinase: a plasminogen activator made by *Staphylococci*.

starch: water-insoluble polysaccharides composed of two glucose polymers, amylose (a linear glycan with 1 → 4 glycosidic linkages), and amylopectin (a branching molecule that also has 1 → 6 linkages). Starch is the major storage carbohydrate of plants. It accounts for much of the carbohydrate content of foods, and is rapidly degraded to glucose by digestive system enzymes. Its demulcent and astringent properties contribute to the effectiveness of some preparations for controlling diarrhea; and it serves as an emollient and absorbant in dusting powders. Additionally, it is used for determinations of iodine (which generates a blue color) and other chemicals, and in electrophoresis.

start: the G1 → S transition of a **cell cycle** (*q.v.*). Cells that reach this stage can progress to M without external supplies of essential amino acids.

start codon: AUG; a triplet (set of three ribonucleotides) that codes for the methionine incorporated into the complex that initiates translation on eukaryote ribosomes (and for *f*-methionine with comparable functions in prokaryotes).

stasis: cessation or slowing of movement, for example of blood through a vessel, or of partially digested food through the gastrointestinal tract lumen.

statistical significance: a judgment concerning the relationship one measurable parameter to another, based on probability calculations. For example, if two groups of laboratory animals are randomly selected from a population (theoretically comprising all animals of that kind), members of one group are treated with a pharmacological agent, those of the other receive a similarly administered placebo, and a parameter that may be affected by the agent is measured in all animals, the probability that the agent invokes a change can be tested. One procedure is calculation of a *t* value (*see* **Student's *t* test**) whose magnitude varies directly with the difference between the means, and with the numbers of individuals tested, and is inversely related to the range of variations within the test groups. The probability, P, that differences as great as (or greater than) the ones observed could be obtained simply by "sampling error" is then determined by consulting tables constructed from theoretical normal distributions. A P value of <0.001 signifies a probability of less than 1 in 1000. For most studies, this indicates that the differences between the drug and placebo treated animals are real, and are said to be *highly significant*. For values that are >0.001 but <0.01, >0.01 but <0.05, and >.05, respectively, the terms *statistically significant*, *probably significant*, and *not statistically significant* are often applied. However, there are studies for which less stringent judgments are made. (For example, <0.02 may be accepted as highly significant.) P values are also used for correlation and other statistical assessments.

statoconia: otoliths; statoliths; minute particles in the utricles and saccules of vertebrate inner ears, composed of calcium carbonate and protein suspended in gelatinous matrices. Associated stereocilia and kinetocila that project into the matrices are stimulated when changes in head position act via gravitational forces to alter statoconium orientation.

statocysts: invertebrate vesicles analogous to vertebrate saccules and utricles, used for perception of body orientation. They contain statoliths composed of sand, calcium carbonate crystals, or other hard substances.

statoliths: sand grains, calcium carbonate crystals, or other hard particle components of statoconia or stratocysts.

status: a condition or severe attack, as in status asthmaticus or status epilepticus.

status thymicolymphaticus: an obsolete term formerly applied to infants with "enlarged" thymus glands and other lymphatic system organs. The thymus gland was believed to exert sufficient pressure on the respiratory tract to suffocate, and thereby cause sudden infant death syndrome (SIDS).

staurosporine: an antibiotic obtained from *Streptomyces*. It is a potent inhibitor of kinase C isozymes, and of collagen and ADP (but not thrombin) induced platelet aggregation.

STD: sexually transmitted disease.

stearates: soaps (such as Na-stearate) obtained by neutralizing stearic acid with NaOH, KOH, or other inorganic bases.

stearic acid {**stearate**}: octadecanoic acid; a long-chain saturated fatty. It is a major component of fat depot and animal food triacylglycerols, and is contained in some phospholipids, sphingolipids, and other lipids.

stearin: tristearin; a triacylglycerol with three stearic acid moieties.

stearo-, steato-: a prefix meaning fat.

steatomas: sebaceous gland tumors.

steatopygia: accumulation of large amounts of adipose tissue in the buttocks. The tendency can be inherited, and is prevalent among African pygmies.

steatorrhea: excessive fat in the feces, usually caused by impaired intestinal absorption of lipids. *See* also **sprue**.

steel locus: *Sl*; a gene on chromosome 10 of the mouse that directs formation of steel cell factor; *see* **stem cell factor**.

Stein-Levinthal Syndrome: *see* **polycystic ovary disease**.

stellate: star-shaped.

stem: the main axis of a structure. For animal types, *see* for example **brain stem** and **infundibular stem**.

stem cell[s]: in animals, usually (1) hematopoietic stem cells in bone marrow, or other pluripotent kinds that give rise to two or more differentiated types; (2) immature quiescent cells (for example some spermatogonia) that

stearic acid

678

persist in mature individuals, but resume mitosis and replenish populations when a tissue has been damaged.

stem cell factor: SCF: stem cell growth factor; *c-kit* ligand; KL; mast cell growth factor; MGF; a mammalian growth regulator, initially named Steel factor when identified as a product of the mouse Steel locus. It is a heavily glycosylated protein with both *O*- and *N*-linked carbohydrate groups, synthesized as a transmembrane component (and present in that form on some cell types), but also processed to smaller (30-36K) soluble forms. SCF is an essential regulator of the proliferation and differentiation of hematopoietic, germinal, and pigment cell precursors; and it promotes development and migration of neural crest derivatives, gonocytes, and some other cell types. It also contributes to the functions of differentiated cells. SCF is expressed first in the embryonic yolk sac, then in the liver, and soon afterward in developing bone (in which it stimulates osteogenesis), in lung, kidneys, ovaries, testes, and dorsal root ganglia. Most of its effects require binding of soluble forms to receptors whose formation is directed by *c-kit* (*q.v.*); but membrane-bound SCF may serve as a receptor for extracellular matrix components. In addition to acting directly on some cell types, it synergizes with interleukin-7, erythropoietin, granulocyte-macrophage colony stimulating factor (GM-CSF), and other regulators.

stenbolone: stenobolone; 17β-hydroxy-2-methyl-5α-androstan-1-en-3-one; a synthetic androgen receptor agonist, used for its anabolic effects.

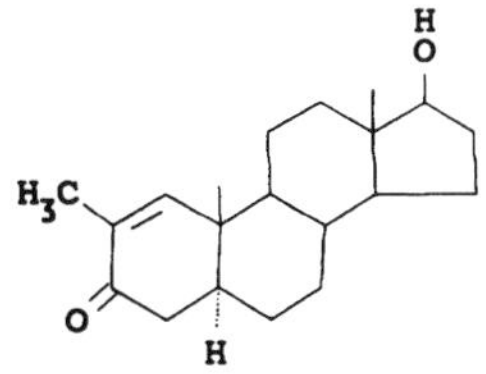

stenohaline: describes fish species that cannot tolerate marked variations in environmental salinity; *cf* **euryhaline**.

stenosis: narrowing or constriction.

sterco-: a prefix meaning feces.

stercobilin: *l*-urobilin; a bile pigment derivative that accounts for much of the brown color of feces. It is a

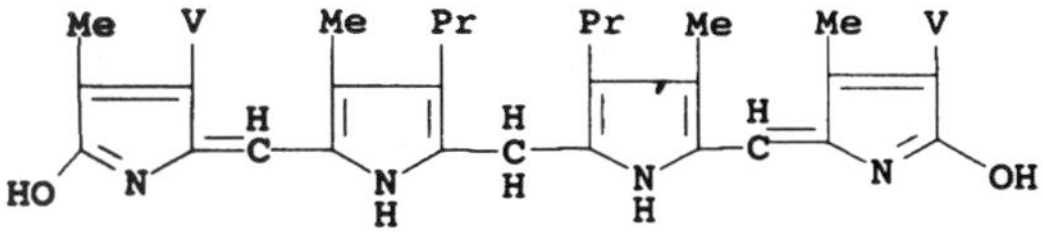

bilirubin

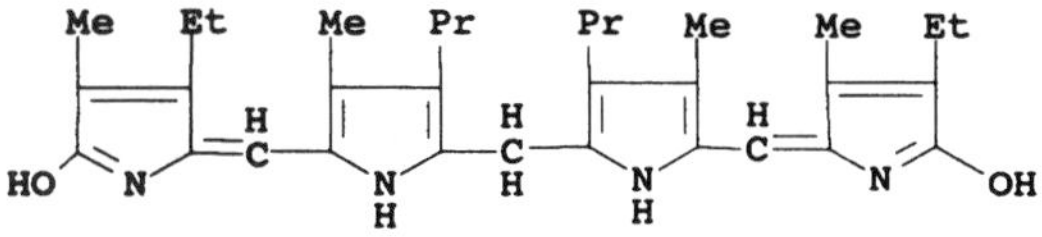

mesobilirubin

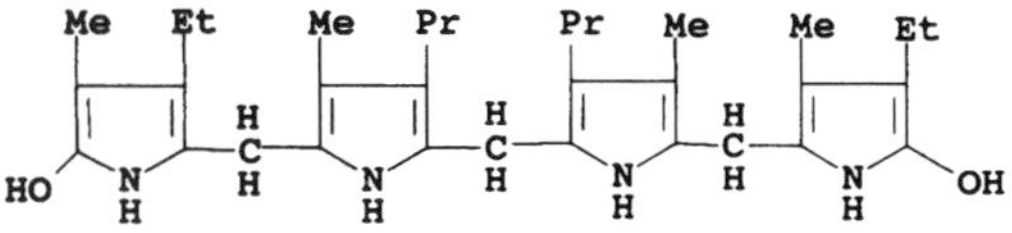

mesobilirubinogen

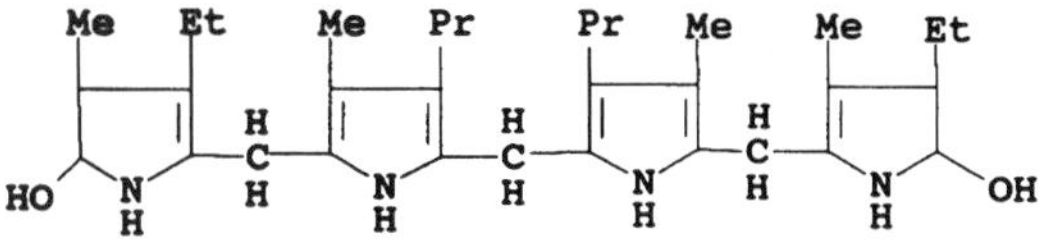

stercobilinogen

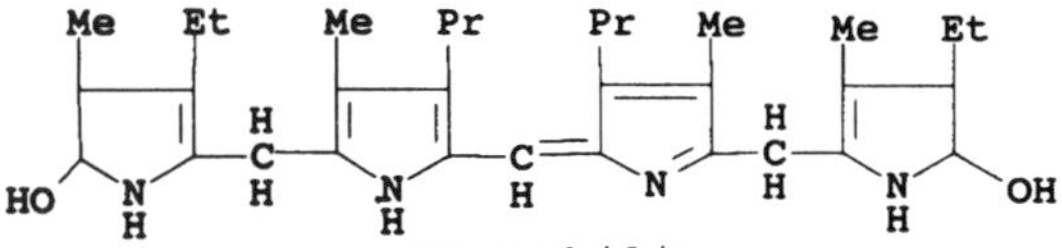

stercobilin

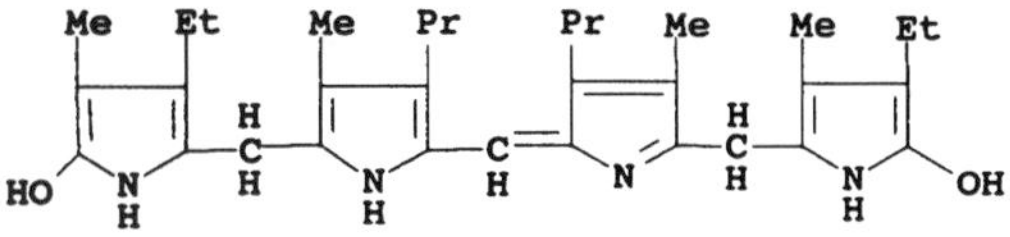

urobilin

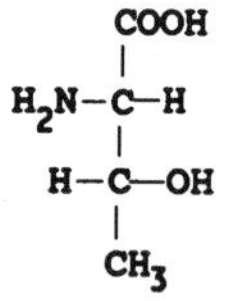

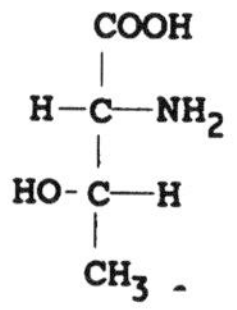

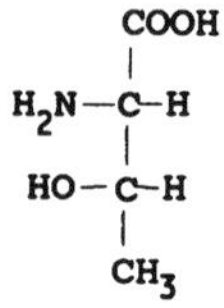

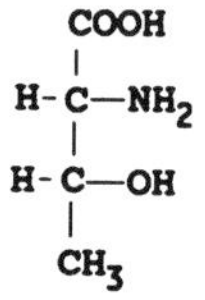

L-threonine   D-threonine   L-allothreonine   D-allothreonine

stereoisomers

reduction product of stercobilinogen, which is derived (via mesobilirubin and mesobilirubinogen intermediates) from bilirubin.

stereognosis: recognition of size, shape, and texture.

stereoisomers: compounds with identical overall compositions, but different arrangements of atoms around one or more asymmetric carbon atoms. The differences can profoundly affect the biological and pharmacological properties, since most enzymes and receptors interact with just one form. When there is a single asymmetric carbon atom, the D and L isomers are mirror images. Usually, they rotate the plane of polarized light in opposite directions when dissolved in water. The prefix allo- distinguishes one set of mirror images from the other when four diastereoisomers form from molecules with two asymmetric carbons, as in D and L threonine, plus D and L allothreonine. *See also* **stereoisomerism**.

stereoisomerism: molecular asymmetry; chirality; "handedness". In the system used for amino acids, the structure is represented with the carboxyl group of the carbon chain at the top. If a designated functional group (for example NH_2) projects to the left, the molecule is said to be left-handed and is designated L. The upper case letter refers to levo. An L compound is not necessary levorotary. (Lower case letters d and l are used for optical rotation). Two alanine enantiomorphs (mirror image forms) are shown. Most naturally occurring amino acids are L, and most natural sugars are D types. The spatial rotations of certain kinds of molecules are restricted by chemical groups such as C=O. If two chemical groups attached to them are in the same plane, the molecule is said to have a *cis* configuration; in different planes, the configuration is *trans*. Maleic acid and fumaric acid are *cis-trans* isomers. As shown for cystine, other arrangements are possible for compounds with other covalent linkages. For **steroids** (*q.v.*), the rings are thought of as parallel to the plane of the paper. Substitutions on carbon atoms that project above the plane are designated β and represented by solid lines. Those projecting below the plane are α, with broken lines. In a different system the substitutions on an asymmetric carbon are assigned "priorities" a, b, c, and d according to atomic weights (a for highest, d for lowest). If substitutions a, b, and c are oriented in a clockwise direction, the molecule is R (rectus); if counterclockwise, S (sinister). Some structures that appear symmetrical when represented on paper are not recognized as such by enzymes, and these are said to possess prochirality. One example is citric acid.

stereopsis: use of binocular vision to discern depth and three-dimensional structures.

stereospecific: displaying selectivity for stereoisomers, a term usually applied to enzymes or substrates, but also used for chemical reactions that do not require enzymes.

stereospecific number: *see sn*.

stereotaxy: use of instruments to guide three-dimensional positioning of electrodes, knife blades, or other devices, usually within the brain.

stereotropism: movement of an organism or part of it with respect to a solid object. It can be positive (toward) or negative (away from the object).

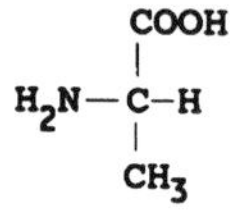

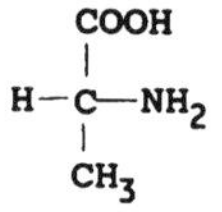

L-alanine   D-alanine

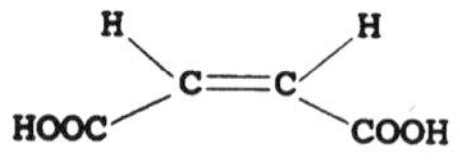

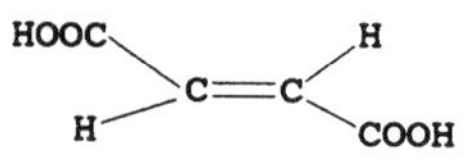

maleic acid (*cis*)   fumaric acid (*trans*)

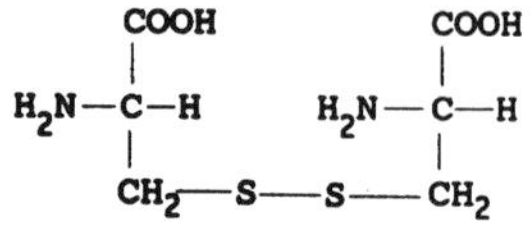

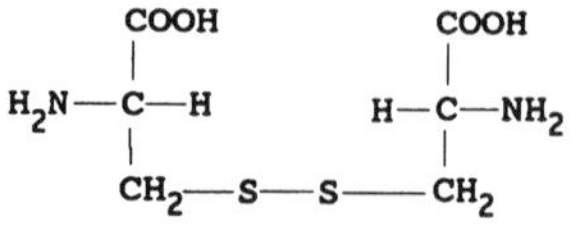

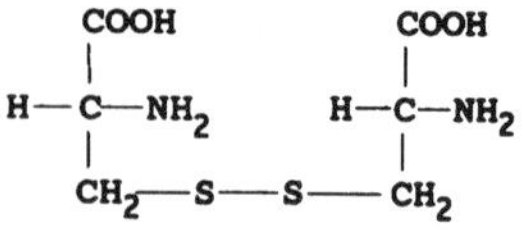

L-cysteine   meso-cysteine   D-cysteine

stereoisomerism

680

stereotyped behavior: invariable, reproducible responses unrelated to learning or memory, a term applied for example to the changes invoked by insect pheromones, and by agents such as dopamine applied to specific brain loci of other animal types.

sterilization: (1) destruction or elimination of all microorganisms; (2) surgical removal or destruction of organs required for reproduction, for example gonadectomy, vasectomy, or salpingectomy.

steroids: compounds related to cyclopentanoperhydrophenanthrene, which has one five-membered, and three six-membered rings. The numbering system for the carbon atoms and the letters assigned to the rings are shown. Most steroids made by living organisms have one or more double bonds, a methyl group (carbon 18) attached at position 13, and alcoholic and/or ketone groups. Several types have additional side-chains. The group includes cholesterol and bile acids, as well as **steroid hormones** (*q.v.*). Vitamin D and related calciferols, with one open ring, are called *secosteroids*. See also **anabolic steroids**.

steroid binding globulins: SSBGs: usually, plasma proteins that bind steroids with high affinities, but differ from hormone receptors; *see* for example **sex steroid binding globulin**. Some species do not have circulating SSBGs, but make chemically related intracellular androgen binding proteins.

steroid dehydrogenases: enzymes that remove hydrogen atoms from steroids, and thereby create unsaturated bonds. They are named for their sites of action; *see* for example 3β- and 17β- **hydroxysteroid dehydrogenases**, and *cf* **hydroxylases**.

steroid hormones: androgens, estrogens, glucocorticoids, mineralocorticoids, progestins, and all other hormones with steroid-type structures; *see* specific types. The term is usually extended to calciferols (*secosteroids*, with related structures and similar biological properties). The best known actions are initiated by binding to intracellular **steroid hormone receptors** (*q.v.*); but a few are exerted directly on plasma membranes.

steroid hormone receptors: the term usually refers to intracellular glycoproteins that bind steroid hormones with high affinities and specificities and mediate their actions. They are members of a superfamily that includes receptors for triiodothyronine (T_3), retinoids, peroxisome proliferators, and some other regulators. When unoccupied, most are components of 8-9S complexes with heat shock and other proteins that block their abilities to interact with chromatin components (and are implicated in other functions such as modification of ligand affinities and protection against enzymatic degradation). Most of the binding proteins are released when the ligands bind. Hormone-receptor complexes then undergo "activation" which includes configurational changes that facilitate dimerization, binding to chromatin, and interactions with **steroid response elements** (*q.v.*). The changes usually include phosphorylations at specific sites. The response elements mediate both stimulatory and inhibitory influences on transcription of limited numbers of gene types. Some of the resulting changes in protein synthesis are detected within an hour; but influences on cell proliferation can require up to 48 hours to develop. However, steroid hormones also act rapidly on some cell types, even when bound to plasma globulins, and when protein synthesis is inhibited by pharmacological agents. For example, adrenal corticosteroids affect the firing rates of hippocampal neurons, and progesterone invokes germinal vesicle breakdown in amphibian oocytes. Some rapid effects are attributed to nonspecific modification of membrane bilayers. Influences on the functions of receptors for oxytocin, gamma-aminobutyric acid (GABA), and other regulators may be related to changes in membrane fluidity. Plasma membrane components that bind steroid hormones with high affinities and specificities have also been described, some of which appear to be chemically related to the intracellular types. *See* also specific kinds of receptors.

steroid hydroxylases: steroid monooxygenases.

steroid monooxygenases: steroid hydroxylases; mixed function oxygenases that catalyze formation of alcoholic side chains on the carbon atoms of steroids at specific sites. *See*, for example 3β-, 11-β-, 17α- and 21-**hydroxylases**.

steroid reductases: enzymes that catalyze addition of hydrogen atoms to steroid molecules, and thereby convert unsaturated to saturated bonds. *See*, for example 5α- and 20α-**reductases**.

steroidogenesis: biosynthesis of steroid hormones.

steroidogenesis activator polypeptide: SAP; *H*-Ile-Val-Gln-Pro-Ile-Ile-Ser-Lys-Leu-Tyr-Gly-Ser-Gly-Gly-Pro-Pro-Pro-Thr-Gly-Glu-Glu-Asp-Thr-Asp-Glu-Lys-Lys-Asp-Glu-Leu-OH; an acidic, hydrophobic protein, initially isolated from a Leydig cell tumor, that promotes dose-dependent acceleration of cholesterol side-chain cleavage, possibly by facilitating cholesterol redistribution within mitochondria. It displays marked amino acid homology with, and may be cleaved from the *C*-terminal region of the 78K heat shock protein GRP78. SAP synthesis is stimulated by gonadotropins.

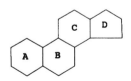

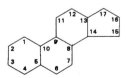

steroids

steroidogenic factor 1: SF-1; a factor that regulates transcription of genes that code for steroid hydroxylases, coordinates expression of the enzymes in adrenocortical cells, and promotes aromatase expression in gonads. It appears to be the mouse homolog of the *Drosophila fushi tarazu factor 1* (a regulator of homeobox expression during development). Since no ligand is known, it has been classified as an orphan receptor.

sterols: steroids with one or more alcoholic side-chains. Examples include cholesterol and ergosterol, as well as many steroid hormones.

sterol carrier protein-2: SCP2; a widely distributed basic 13.5K microsomal protein, homologous with IgG type immunoglobulin variable domains, that serves as an essential noncatalytic factor for conversion of lanosterol to cholesterol. It is identical to a protein that promotes cholesterol transfer from lipid droplets to mitochondria and accelerates side-chain cleavage activity. SCP2 is most abundant in the liver, but is also made in the adrenal cortex, ovaries, and testes. Although constitutively expressed, its synthesis is augmented by adrenocorticotropic hormone (ACTH).

stethoscopes: devices for amplifying and conducting sounds to the ears of observers.

STH: somatotropic hormone; somatotrophin; *see* **growth hormone**.

sticky ends: short single-stranded DNA fragments produced by the actions of restriction endonucleases. They bond to other fragments generated by the same enzymes, and are used to construct artificial DNAs.

stigma: (1) a small, bulging region on the surface of the ovary from which a secondary oocyte and its surrounding cumulus cells exit during ovulation; (2) a distinguishing mark or aberration that can be used for identification or diagnosis; (3) a spot.

stigmasterol: 3β-hydroxy-24-ethyl-$\Delta^{5,22}$-cholestadiene; a steroid chemically related to cholesterol, obtained from soy, cacao, and calabar beans, and from other plants. It is used in the industrial manufacture of biologically active steroids.

stigmata: (1) plural of stigma; (2) the characteristic signs of an illness.

stilalgin: mephenesin.

stilbestrol: *see* **diethylstilbestrol**.

stibium: antimony.

stimulus: any change in the internal or external environment. An *effective* stimulus invokes a biological response. It must be of a quality (for example chemical, photic, osmotic, or mechanical) sensed by the cell, and of sufficient intensity and duration. A *threshold* (*minimal*) stimulus has the least intensity and/or duration capable of initiating a response. A single smaller (*subthreshold, subliminal*) stimulus of the right quality is not effective, but does invoke a transient, localized (rapidly dissipated) change that augments cell excitability. Several subthreshold stimuli presented in rapid succession can summate to achieve threshold. Some cell types react on an all-or-none basis. (Stronger stimuli achieve no greater effects than those of threshold level.) In other cells types, graded changes are achieved with stronger stimuli. A *maximal* stimulus then elicits the greatest response obtainable from the system. A *supramaximal* stimulus (stronger than maximal) usually does nothing more, if it is not of a damaging intensity.

stimulus response coupling: the linking of changes invoked by effective stimuli to cellular responses, for example stimulus-contraction or stimulus-secretion coupling.

STM: scanning tunneling microscopy.

stoichiometry: determination of atomic weights of elements, the proportions in which they combine, and the weight changes that result from chemical reactions.

stoma [stomata]: a small opening or pore.

stomach: in addition to serving as the major storage site for undigested and partially digested food, the stomach contains cells that secrete hydrochloric acid, pepsinogen, and other factors that contribute to digestion, intrinsic factor, and regulators for other cell types, such as gastrin and histamine.

stomatitis: inflammation of the oral mucosa.

stomodeum: a depression in the head ectoderm of an embryo that contains the progenitors of the mouth and related structures.

stop codons: termination codons; messenger RNA triplets UAA, UGA, or UAG. They are not recognized by transfer RNA anticodons, but bind release factors (proteins RF1 and RF2) that activate peptidyltransferases. Those enzymes terminate translation by hydrolyzing bonds between nascent polypeptide chains and tRNAs at ribosomal P sites.

storm: a sudden exacerbation of symptoms.

STP: standard temperature and pressure; *see* **standard conditions**.

strain: a subpopulation within a species. Many purebred mouse strains are used for histocompatibility studies; and mutant types such as *db/db* and *ob/ob* are models for metabolic diseases (*see* also **mouse**). Nonmutant rat strains used in laboratory studies include Long-Evans, Wistar, Sprague-Dawley, and Fischer.

stramonium: Jimson weed; thorn apple; the dried leaves of *Datura stramonium*. Its components include atropine, scopolamine, and hyoscyamine.

stratified: in layers, as in stratified epithelium.

stratum [**strata**]: a layer.

stratum basale: (1) the deepest layer of a stratified epithelium. In skin epidermis, it is the component of the stratum germinativum that rests on a basement membrane, closest to underlying dermal blood vessels. In endometrium it contains the lower (blind) ends of uterine glands, and undergoes minimal changes during uterine cycles.

stratum compactum: the dense layer of endometrial cells that contains the necks of the uterine glands. It is a component of the stratum functionale.

stratum corneum: the outer, keratinized layers of dry, stratified epithelium. The stratum corneum *epidermidis* is the part of the skin that contains the remnants of dead cells (which desquamate). The stratum corneum *ungues* is the horny layer of fingernail.

stratum functionale: the stratum compactum and stratum spongiosum of the endometrium. The layers build up during early phases of uterine cycles and slough off during late luteal and menstrual phases.

stratum germinativum: the innermost cells of a stratified epithelium in which mitoses occur and precursors of outer layer cells are made. The skin Malpighian layer comprises stratum basale plus stratum spinosum.

stratum granulosum: (1) the concentric layers of epithelial cells that surround the oocyte of a secondary or more mature ovarian follicle and support oocyte survival and development (*cf* **pregranulosa**). The cells take up, synthesize, metabolize, and secrete steroid hormones (especially estrogens), and they make inhibin, oocyte maturation inhibitor, activins, and factors that affect follicle stimulating hormone (FSH) actions and luteinization. The major direct stimulants of their growth and activities are FSH and estrogens; but several autocrine factors have been identified. Luteinizing hormone (LH) indirectly affects their functions by promoting androgen secretion in theca cells; (2) the granular layer of the skin epidermis, located just above (superficial to) the stratum spinosum.

stratum spinosum: *see* **prickly cells**.

streak gonads: ovaries or testes that have never completed development, or ones that have deteriorated and been replaced by scar tissue to the point where they are devoid of germinal cells. They are commonly found in individuals with Turner's and Klinefelter's syndromes.

strepogenin: chick growth factor S; a peptide mixture that stimulates the growth of some microorganisms, obtained by partially hydrolyzing liver, flour, yeast, and other naturally occurring substances.

streptavidin: a bacterial protein with high affinity for avidin, used to label immunoglobulins and nucleotides.

strepto-: a prefix meaning curved or twisted.

streptococcins: bacteriocins released by streptococci.

Streptococcus: a genus of chain-forming gram positive cocci that includes *S. pyogenes*, *S. pneumoniae*, and others that cause human diseases. The toxins released include hemolysins and subtilisins.

streptodornase: an enzyme made by hemolytic streptococci that degrades deoxyribonucleoproteins. Bacteria use it to decrease pus viscosity, and thereby facilitate their motility. Clinical preparations are used alone to destroy pus and other debris, and in combination with **streptokinase** *(q.v.)*.

streptokinase: Streptococcal fibrinolysin; plasminokinase; two enzymes (A and B), released by *Streptococcus pyogenes* that activate tissue plasminogen and degrade fibrinogen and fibrin. They are used to both avert and retard intravascular coagulation and remove small clots, and in combination with streptodornase to remove clotted blood, pus, and other debris. (The enzymes are not true kinases.)

streptokinase-streptodornase: varidase; *see* **streptokinase**.

streptoleukocidin: an exotoxin released by some *Streptomyces* strains that promotes leukocyte degranulation, and can kill the cells.

streptolydigin: portamycin; an enzyme made by *Streptomyces lydicus* that binds to bacterial RNA polymerases and blocks peptide chain elongation.

streptolydigin

683

streptolysins: Streptolysin O is a 68K thiol-activated hemolysin inactivated by oxygen. The molecules aggregate, bind to cholesterol, and form plasma membrane channels that permit free passage of water, ions, and small molecules. It also augments a secretory processes in neutrophilic leukocytes but inhibits motility, and is directly cardiotoxic in laboratory animals. Its ability to stimulate production of specific antibodies is used in the diagnosis of infectious diseases. Streptolysin S is a smaller, oxygen-stable peptide that promotes hemolysis and exerts toxic effects on leukocytes and some other cell types, and on blood platelets.

Streptomyces: a large genus of actinomycetes that includes many soil-dwelling organisms. Antibiotics derived from them include tetracycline and chloramphenicol, as well as streptomycins.

streptomycins: several basic trisaccharide antibiotics obtained from *Streptomyces griseus* and related strains that inhibit translation initiation, and can cause misreading of prokaryote messenger RNAs by interfering with aminoacyl-tRNA binding to ribosomes. They also affect eukaryote mitochondrial (but not cytoplasmic) ribosomes, and are used to treat tularemia, tuberculosis, plague, brucellosis, and some other infections, and to maintain sterility in cell culture media. Streptomycin A (also called streptomycin) is *O*-2-deoxy-2-(methylamino)-α-L-glucopyranosyl-(1→2)-*O*-5-deoxy-3-C-formyl-α-L-lyxofuranosyl-(1→4)-*N*,*N*′-bis(aminoiminomethyl)-D-streptamine (shown below). Streptomycin B is mannosidostreptomycin.

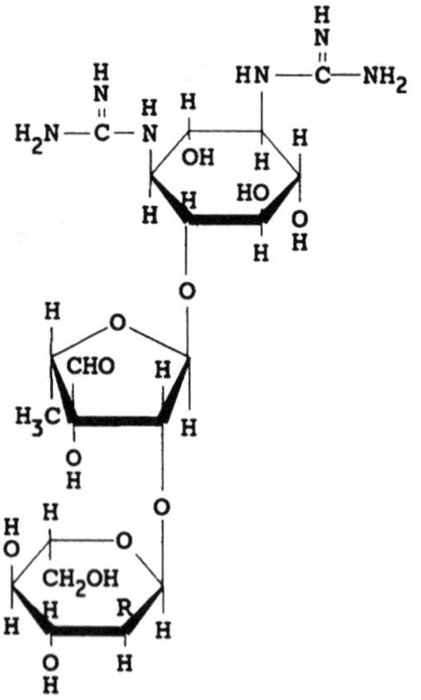

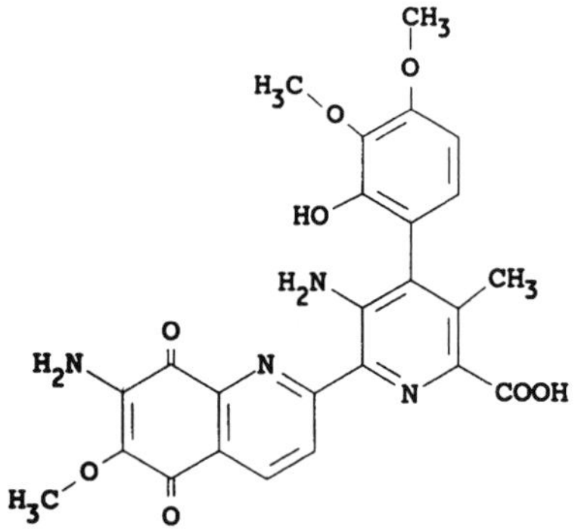

streptonigrin

streptonigrin: Nigrin; bruneomycin; 5-amino-6-(7-amino-5,8-dihydro-6-methoxy-5.8-dioxo-2-quninolyl)-4-(2-hydroxy-3,4-dimethoxyphenyl)-3-methyl-2-pyridine-carboxylic acid; an antibiotic made by *Streptomyces flocculus* that causes chromosomal breakage. It is used to arrest the growth of some neoplasms.

streptozotocin: streptozocin; STZ; 2-deoxy-2-(3-methyl-3-nitrosoureido)-D-glucopyranose; an antibiotic, antineoplastic, and potentially carcinogenic agent derived from *Streptomyces achromogenese* that depletes cell NAD$^+$ stores by promoting ADP-ribosylation. Small amounts decrease insulin release; *see* **cyclic adenosine diphosphate ribose**. Larger ones injure pancreatic islet β-cells, and are used to invoke insulin deficiency in laboratory animals. The extent of damage is more easily controlled than with alloxan, since it is dose related. Moreover, animals can be studied during the recovery phase that follows drug withdrawal. Some of the effects are exerted on the immune system. Streptozotocin is used clinically to treat islet cell tumors, gastrinomas, and some other hormone-secreting tumors, and is effective against some gram negative bacteria.

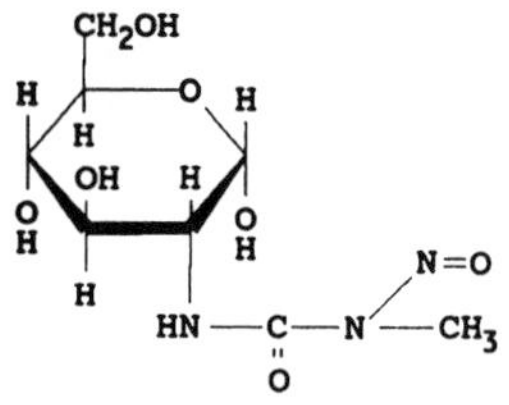

stress: any adverse condition that does not rapidly cause death. "*Nonspecific*" types include excessively hot or cold environments, immobilization, electric shock, loud noises, trauma, anesthesia, hypoxia, hemorrhage, food and/or water deprivation, and impediments to food intake such as heavy weights on food cups. The responses to adverse conditions usually include increased secretion of glucocorticoids, catecholamines, and other hormones. In many kinds of studies, attempts are made to eliminate variables attributable to nonspecific stress by subjecting control animals to procedures such as sham operation, injection of vehicles for drugs given to experimental groups, and pair feeding.

stress fibers: long bundles of microfilaments prominent in quiescent fibroblasts but also present in non-muscle cells, composed of actin and some tropomyosin, cross-linked by filamen. Most occur in parallel arrays in the cytoplasm adjacent to the plasma membrane, where they connect plasma membrane components with nearby cytoskeletal structures; but some extend the full lengths of the cells. They provide strength and resiliency, and facilitate both attachments to extracellular matrices and cell spreading along surfaces. The fibers can contract in the presence of ATP, but disintegrate in cells that become motile or assume globular forms.

stress proteins: several proteins synthesized in large amounts when cells are exposed to adverse conditions such as high environmental temperatures and glucose deprivation. Some are made constitutively in small amounts by non-stressed cells, whereas others are not detectable under favorable conditions. *See* also **heat shock** and **glucose regulated proteins**.

stretch reflexes: responses inititated by activation of the stretch receptors of **spindle organs** (*q.v.*). They maintain skeletal muscle tone, can enhance the contraction of the large fibers of the muscle, and contribute to the abilities to maintain posture and to hold and lift weights. The tendon ("knee-jerk") and some other reflexes are invoked to test neurological functions.

stria [striae]: a streak, stripe, line, or band-like structure.

stria medullaris: several nerve fiber bundles in the brain. The *striae medullaris thalami* are bilateral bands that originate in the amygdaloid nuclei, hippocampus, olfactory tubercles, preoptic, and other forebrain structures and terminate mostly in the habenula nuclei.

striated muscle: **skeletal** and **cardiac muscle** (*q.v.*), in which orderly arrangements of thick (myosin) and thin (actin, tropomyosin and troponin) filaments impart a banded appearance visible under high-power light microscopy; *cf* **smooth muscle**.

stria terminalis: bilateral bands of nerve fibers that form the borders between the thalamus and the caudate nuclei and mediate communication among amygdaloid, septal and hypothalamic neuron groups.

stringent response: in bacteria, cessation of transfer RNA and ribosome synthesis in response to poor growth conditions.

stroma: (1) non-parenchymal components of animal organs that can contain reticular fibers or reserve cells and provide support, compartmentalize, or supply humoral factors, but do not perform the major functions associated with those structures. Examples include adipose tissue components that do not store triacylglycerols, and bone marrow constituents that create environments conducive for hematopoietic cell proliferation and differentiation. Some ovarian stroma cells make steroid hormones; (2) the semifluid phase of a chloroplast that contains enzymes for the dark reactions of photosynthesis; (3) the mitochondrial matrix.

stromelysin: a protein secreted by fibroblasts and some other cell types that degrades fibronectin, laminins, elastin, immunoglobulins, other proteins, and proteoglycans. Its production is regulated coordinately with that of collagenase. Tumor-promoting phorbol esters are among the agents that augment its synthesis.

Strongylocentrotus purpuratus: a sea-urchin species used for studies of genetics, development and fertilization.

strontium, Sr: a metallic element (atomic number 38, atomic weight 87.62). Since its behavior resembles that of calcium, the stable and radioactive forms are used to study calcium transport and metabolism.

strophanthin: a mixture of digitalis-like glycosides derived from *Strophanthus kombé* initially used as an arrow poison, and now as a myocardial stimulant. Strophanthidin (shown) is 3,5,14-trihydroxy-19-oxo-card-20(22)-enolide.

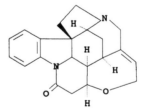

structural genes: DNA segments that direct the synthesis of messenger RNAs; *cf* **regulatory genes**.

structural proteins: proteins that contribute to the shapes and structures of cells and tissues.

strychnine: an alkaloid made by *Strychnos noxvomica* and related species. It is a powerful stimulant for all parts of the central nervous system that enhances perception, exaggerates reflexes, and invokes rigidity and convulsions by blocking reciprocal inhibition of antagonistic muscles. The major effects are attributed to competition with glycine for excitatory amino acid receptor sites. Although dangerous, minute amounts are sometimes administered for their stimulatory properties. Strychnine is also a component of some rat poisons.

Student's *t* test: a procedure for evaulating the statistical significance of differences between mean values of normally distributed parameters. In a study of two experimental groups of equal size, the *t* value can be estimated by substracting the smaller mean value from the larger one and dividing the difference by the square root of the sum of the two standard errors. A table that relates *t* values for sample sizes to **P values** (*q.v.*) then provides information on the probability that differences as great (or greater) can be attributed to random sampling error (*see* **statistical significance**).

STX: saxitoxin.

styramate: 1-phenyl-1,2-ethaneiol 2-carbamate; a muscle relaxant with properties similar to those described for mephenesin.

styramate

STZ: streptozotocin.

SU 4885: metyrapone.

SU 8000: 3-(chloro-3-methyl-2-indenyl)pyridine: an agent that blocks aldosterone synthesis by inhibiting the steroid 18-hydroxylase that converts cortisol to 18-OH-cortisol. High levels also inhibit the 17α-hydroxylase required for androgen and estrogen biosynthesis.

SU 9055: 2-methyl-1,2,-di-3-pyridyl-1-propanone-3-(1,2,3,4,-tetrahydro-1-oxo-2-naphthyl)-pyridine; an agent that blocks conversion of 18-OH-cortisol to aldosterone.

subacute: describes conditions that progress more rapidly than chronic, and more slowly than acute disorders.

subarachnoid space: the region between the arachnoid and pia mater brain meninges. It contains cerebrospinal fluid which can be aspirated for diagnosis, and into which anesthetics, antibiotics, and other substances can be injected.

subcommissural organs: SCO; circumventricular organs derived from ependymal cells that line the third ventricle of the brain. They facilitate exchanges of molecules and ions between blood and cerebrospinal fluid, secrete regulators, and give rise to some pineal gland components.

subculture: a secondary culture, obtained by transferring cells from a stock (or primary culture) to fresh media.

subfornical organs: SFO; circumventricular organs located near the fornix. They have angiotensin II receptors and contribute to regulation of vasopressin secretion. Although clearly involved in thirst perception and the control of drinking behavior, the concept that they are major sites for such functions has been questioned.

subiculum: (1) an underlying or supporting structure; (2) *subiculum cornu ammonis*, the superior portion of the parahippocampal gyrus adjacent to the hippocampal fissure and contiguous with the horn of Ammon. It is a component of the limbic system.

sublimation: (1) passage from a solid to a vapor state, with no intermediate liquid phase; (2) subconscious

shunting of an instinct or drive to an acceptable channel of expression.

subliminal: subthreshold; *see* **stimulus**.

subluxation: partial displacement of joint surfaces.

submaxillary: below the upper jaw bone. Mouse submaxillary (submandibular) salivary glands produce large quantities of nerve growth factor (NGF), epidermal growth factor (EGF), and other regulators. *See* also **salivary glands**.

submaximal: *see* **stimulus**.

submicroscopic: not visible under high power light microscopy.

substance B: a neuromodulator made in the brain that reverses presynaptic inhibition of acetylcholine release.

substance K: SK; *see* **neurokinin β**.

substance P: SP; Arg-Pro-Lys-Pro-Gln-Gln-Phe-Phe-Gly-Leu-Met-NH$_2$; a tachykinin chemically related to neurotensin and somatostatin. It is widely distributed throughout the brain and spinal cord, and is released from nerve endings in the gastrointestinal tract and at other peripheral sites. Substantial amounts are made by some tumor cells. Although a potent stimulant of gastrointestinal tract smooth muscle, it promotes vasodilation. SP also increases the secretion of corticotropin releasing, growth and luteinizing hormones (CRH, GH, and LH), and of prolactin, insulin, glucagon, histamine, and other regulators; and it stimulates salivation. It augments microvascular permeability and is implicated as a mediator of nociception and inflammation (but can under some conditions invoke analgesia). It also promotes T lymphocyte proliferation, and exerts other effects on the immune system. Exogenous SP is reported to protect against formation of amyloid deposits in brains.

substantia gelatinosa: usually, Rolando's gelatinous substance; gelatinous substance of the spinal cord; lamina II or lamina II plus lamina III; the viscous, semisolid region of the spinal cord that contains small neurons involved in transmission of pain signals. The *substantia gelatinosa centralis*, composed mostly of neuroglial cells, surrounds the spinal cord central canal.

substantia nigra: a pigmented region of the midbrain, rich in dopamine and gamma aminobutyric acid. It communicates with the basal ganglia and contributes to the control of voluntary muscle contraction.

substrate: (1) a chemical to which an enzyme binds, and on which it exerts its actions; (2) substratum.

substratum [substrata]: an underlying layer (for example of cells, or of matter on which cells are cultured); also called substrate (definition 2).

subtilin: a pentacyclic, 32-amino acid polypeptide antibiotic made by *Bacillus subtilis* that contains some rare amino acids (lanthionine, β-methyl-lanthionine, D-alanine, dehydroalanine, and dehydrobutyramine), but no methionine, and is effective against gram positive bacteria, tubercle bacilli, and some other microorganisms. It is a serine protease, used for studies of protein structure, and as a food preservative.

subtilisins: alkaline serine proteases made by *Bacillus licheniformins* that act on native and denatured proteins, and are inhibited by aprotinin.

subtilysin: a hemolytic surfactant made by *Bacillus subtilis*, composed of a cyclic heptapeptide covalently linked to a long-chain hydroxy-fatty acid.

subunit: a defined component of a larger entity, such as a polypeptide chain of a dimeric or multimeric protein, or a tubulin component of a microtubule.

suc-1: a *Saccharomyces pombe* gene that codes for p13^{suc1}, a subunit of p34^{cdc2} (*see* **MPF**). A similar protein is made by eukaryotes.

succinic acid {**succinate**}: butanedioic acid; an intermediate in the Krebs Cycle, formed from succinyl-coenzyme A and converted to malate (*see* **succinic dehydrogenase**). It is also a gamma aminobutyric acid (GABA) degradation product.

$$CH_2-COOH$$
$$|$$
$$CH_2-COOH$$

succinic dehydrogenase: a mitochondrial enzyme of the Krebs cycle that catalyzes: succinate + FAD → malate + FADH$_2$. It is induced by triiodothyronine (T$_3$) and some other hormones, and is used as a mitochondrial marker in cell fractionation studies.

succinylcholine chloride: Anectine; 2,2'-[(1,4-dioxo-1,4-butanediyl)bis[*N,N,N*-trimethyl-ethanaminium] dichloride; an agent used with anesthetics to promote skeletal muscle relaxation during surgery and electroshock therapy. It acts on neuromuscular junction receptors, augments permeability to both Na$^+$ and K$^+$, and transiently depolarizes and stimulates (but soon afterward invokes long-term neurotransmission block). Succinylcholine iodide and succinyl bromide have similar properties.

succinyl coenzyme A: a Krebs cycle intermediate formed in the reaction catalyzed by the α-ketoglutarate dehydrogenase complex: α-ketoglutarate + NAD$^+$ + CoA→succinyl-CoA. A substrate-linked phosphorylation is coupled to the next step of the cycle, catalyzed by succinyl synthetase: succinyl-CoA + GDP + Pi → succinate + Co A + GTP. Succinyl-Co A also reacts with glycine to form δ-aminolevulinic acid, a porphyrin precursor.

succus: a fluid secretion.

$$HOOC-CH_2-CH_2-\overset{\overset{\displaystyle O}{\|}}{C}-S-CoA$$

succinyl coenzyme A

suckling: (1) drawing milk from a mammary gland; *see* **suckling reflex**; (2) describes a breast-fed infant mammal, or the maternal act of feeding the infant.

suckling reflex: responses initiated in the mother when a suckling infant stimulates nerve endings in the nipple region that communicate with hypothalamic neurons. Oxytocin (OT) released from magnocellular nuclei promotes release of preformed milk by stimulating contraction of mammary gland myoepithelial cells. It also protects the mother against postpartum hemorrhage by directly stimulating uterine muscle; and it later promotes physiological involution of the uterus. In at least some species, it additionally contributes to maternal behavior; and in a few it is involved in the initiation of lactational diapause. OT release can also be stimulated by factors associated with lactation (for example the cry of an infant). The odor of young pups is effective in most species; and in dairy cows, OT is released in response to the sight of a milking machine. The largest amounts of OT are secreted during the early stages of lactation. After the function is well established, nerve stimulation alone can promote milk ejection. Some forms of stress inhibit. The prolactin release from the adenohypophysis initiated by suckling is attributed to increased production of a **prolactin releasing factor** (*q.v.*). Prolactin stimulates the synthesis of milk components; and it, too affects behavior in many species. It additionally exerts variable inhibitory influences on gonadotropin release. The time period during which it contributes to lactational suppression of fertility is prolonged in marginally nourished mothers.

sucralfate: Carafate; Ulcerban; a viscous sucrose octakis (hydrogen sulfate) aluminum polymer used to treat gastric ulcers. It coats the gastric mucosa, adheres to ulcer cavities, diminishes gastric acidity and pepsin hydrolysis, and may additionally stimulate prostaglandin synthesis. In the structure shown, R = —SO$_3$[Al$_2$(OH)$_5$].

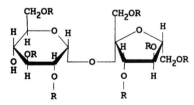

sucrase: an intestinal cell enzyme that hydrolytically cleaves sucrose to glucose + fructose.

sucrose: α-D-glucopyranosyl-β-D-fructofuranoside; table sugar; cane sugar; beet sugar; a major food disaccharide that does not diffuse across plasma membranes. It is digested to glucose + fructose, but is chemically stable in biological preparations and *in vitro* systems that lack the enzyme. It is used for its osmotic properties, and as inert solute for density gradient centrifugation.

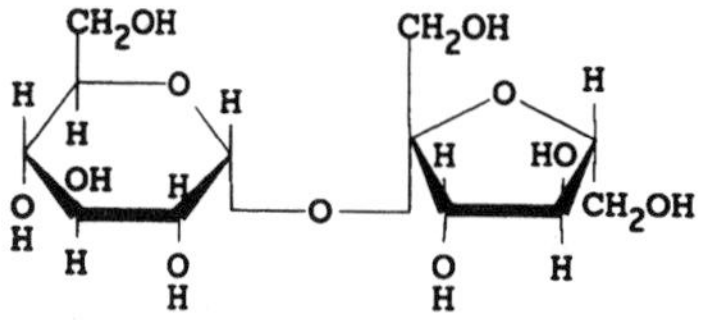

sucrose

sucrose gradient centrifugation: *see* **sedimentation equilibrium.**

Sudan dyes: several hydrophobic azo dyes used to stain lipids, including Sudan I {solvent yellow 14; 1-phenyl-azo-2-naphthol}; Sudan II {solvent orange 7; 1-(2,4-dimethylphenylazo)-2-naphthol}; Sudan III {solvent red 23; 1-[4-(phenylazo)phenylazo]-2-naphthol}; Sudan IV {scarlet red; solvent red 24; 1-[2-methyl-4-(2-methyl-phenylazo)phenylazo]-2-naphthol}; and Sudan Orange G {4-(phenylresorcinol)}. Sudan Black B (fat black BH) is also used to define the Golgi apparatus, and to stain leukocyte granules, and some microorganisms.

sudden infant death syndrome: SIDS; conditions in which apparently healthy infants die, usually while sleeping. An old concept that enlarged thymus glands cause suffocation has been discarded. Currently proposed causes include autonomic nervous system defects that affect breathing reflexes, and fulminating infections that proceed too rapidly for clinical detection.

sudorific: (1) sweat-promoting (2) an agent that increases sweating.

sugars: water-soluble compounds, sweet to the taste, that contain hydrogen atoms and alcoholic groups covalently bonded to carbon chains and aldehyde or ketone groups that are free or components of glycoside linkages. *Monosaccharides* (single sugars) have free reducing groups, and cannot be hydrolyzed to smaller sugar units.

Glucose, the major kind in living organisms, is used directly as a fuel, stored in the form of glycogen in animals (and starch in plants), and incorporated into numerous proteins and lipids. Other widely distributed monosaccharides include deoxyribose (in DNAs), ribose (in RNAs, ATP, cAMP, and other compounds), and fructose (in many fruits). Galactose, mannose, fucose and others are constituents of many large molecules, including glycoproteins and glycolipids. *Disaccharides* (double sugars) are composed of two monosaccharide moieties linked by glycoside bonds. Sucrose (table sugar, glucose + fructose) is a nonreducing type present as such in many foods, lactose (glucose + galactose) is the major milk sugar, and maltose (glucose + glucose) is formed during starch and glycogen digestion. Larger molecules include *trisaccharides, tetrasaccharides,* and *oligosaccharides.*

suicide: self-destruction; for cell suicide, *see* **apoptosis.** *See also* **suicide inhibitors.**

suicide inhibitors: agents that irreversibly block the actions of enzymes, by destroying them, binding tightly to and occluding the active sites, or permanently changing the configurations. *Cf* **competitive** and **noncompetitive inhibitors.**

sulcus: a groove or furrow.

sulfactin: dimercaprol; 1,2,-dithioglycerol; *see* **BAL.**

sulfadiazine: 2-sulfanilamidopyrimidine; an orally effective **sulfa drug** (*q.v.*) that is rapidly absorbed and can enter the cerebrospinal fluid. It is used alone (both orally and topically), systemically in combination with other sulfonamides, and with trimethoprim (which inhibits microbial dihydrofolate reductase).

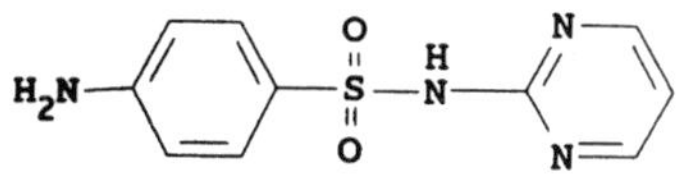

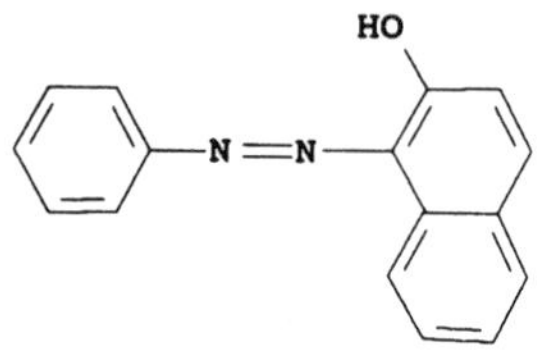

Sudan I

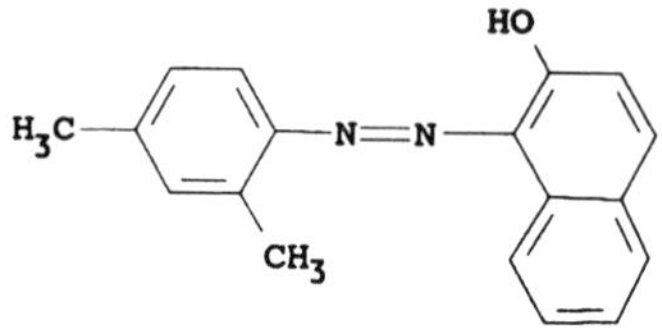

Sudan II

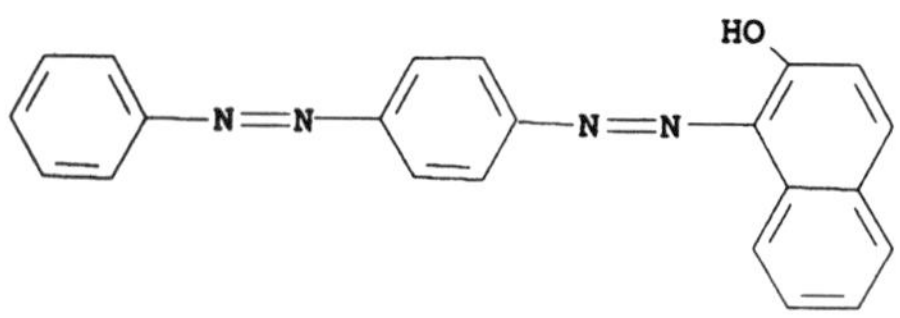

Sudan III

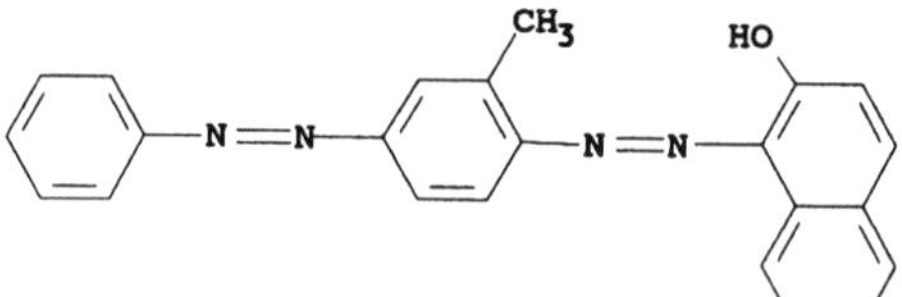

Sudan IV

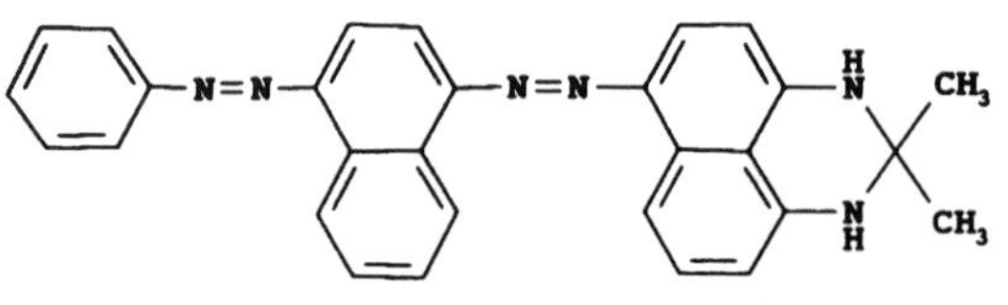

Sudan Black B

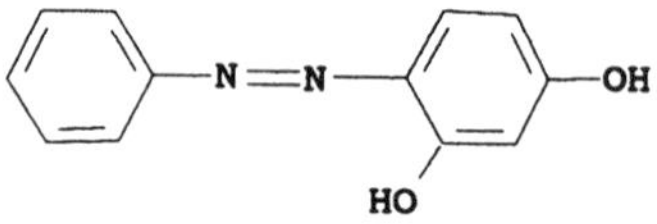

Sudan Orange G

Sudan dyes

688

sulfa drugs: sulfadiazine, sulfamerazine, sulfisoxazole, sulfapyrazine, and other bacteriostatic agents related to sulfonamide. They kill microorganisms by competing with paraaminobenzoic acid (PABA), the dihydropteroate synthase substrate used to make folic acid. (Humans and sulfa-resistant bacteria require preformed folic acid). Three rapidly absorbed types are often used in combination, to lessen the amount of any one kind needed, and thereby the tendency to precipitate in renal tubules and at other sites. Poorly absorbed types are more suitable for treating gastrointestinal tract infections. They can invoke allergic reactions and hematopoietic dysfunction in susceptible individuals; and some inhibit thyroid gland functions.

sulfaguanidine: 4-amino-N-[aminoiminomethyl]benzene sulfonamide; a sulfa drug that is poorly absorbed when taken orally, used mostly to treat intestinal infections. It is more toxic that some other types when it enters the bloodstream, and a more potent inhibitor of thyroid gland functions.

sulfamerazine: sulfamethyldiazine; a **sulfa drug** (*q.v.*) more rapidly absorbed than some of the others, and less likely to precipitate in kidney tubules. Its toxicity is similar to those of sulfadiazine and related compounds.

sulfanilamide: *p*-aminobenzenesulfonamide; the first "sulfa" type antibacterial agent. It has been replaced by sulfadiazine, sulfamerazine, sulfathiazole, and other derivatives.

sulfatases: enzymes that cleave sulfate groups from organic molecules. Some act on steroid hormones, and are indirectly regulated by them. Others are needed for the metabolism of sulfatides and other sulfolipids. *See also* **sulfokinases**.

sulfate: the SO_4^{2-} ion, or a compound that contains it. The S ion is hexavalent. Most sulfur released when amino acids and sulfur-containing lipids are degraded is excreted to urine as inorganic sulfate.

sulfatides: esters composed of sulfated sugars and long-chain fatty acid moieties, abundant in brain myelin; *see* **sphingosine**. They are degraded to galactocerebrosides in reactions catalyzed by cerebroside sulfate sulfatase. Metachromatic leukodystrophies are among the diseases caused by inability to make enough of the enzyme.

sulfation factor: SF; sulfomedin; an obsolete term for insulin-like growth factor I (IGF-I). The name derives from its ability to promote sulfate incorporation into cartilage proteoglycans.

sulfenic acids: compounds with one or more —S—OH groups.

sulfhydryl: —SH, a component of many peptides and proteins with cysteine and/or methionine moieties; *see* **sulfhydryl agents**.

sulfhydryl agents: glutathione, 1,4-dithiothreitol, β-mercaptoethanol, penicillamine, cysteamine and other SH-containing compounds. They maintain the sulfhydryl (—SH) groups of organic molecules by blocking oxidation to disulfides (—S—S—), combine with heavy metals, and reduce hydrogen peroxide to water via reactions of the general type: 2 R—SH + H—O—OH → R—S—S—R + 2 H₂O. They are used to preserve proteins (including enzymes whose active sites contain the groups), protect against some forms of radiation damage, treat cystinuria and heavy metal poisoning, and cleave protein disulfide bonds for analytical procedures.

sulfides: S^{2-} ions, H_2S, FeS and other small compounds that contain divalent S, and compounds with thioether linkages.

sulfinic acids: compounds that contain the chemical group —S—OH.

sulfites: SO_3^{2-} ions, and compounds that contain quadrivalent S.

sulfisoxazole: Gantrisin; 3,4-dimethyl-5-sulfanilamidoisoxazole; a rapidly absorbed, rapidly excreted **sulfa drug** (*q.v.*), more water-soluble than most other types. It is used to treat urinary tract infections.

sulfobromophthalein: bromosulfophthalein; BSP; 3,3'-(4,5,6,7-tetrabromo-3-oxo-1(3H)-isobenzofuranylidene)-*bis*[6-hydroxybenzenesulfonic acid]; a dye taken up by the liver and excreted to bile. It is used to evaluate hepatic function and biliary obstruction.

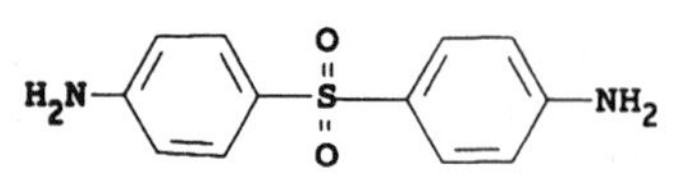

dapsone

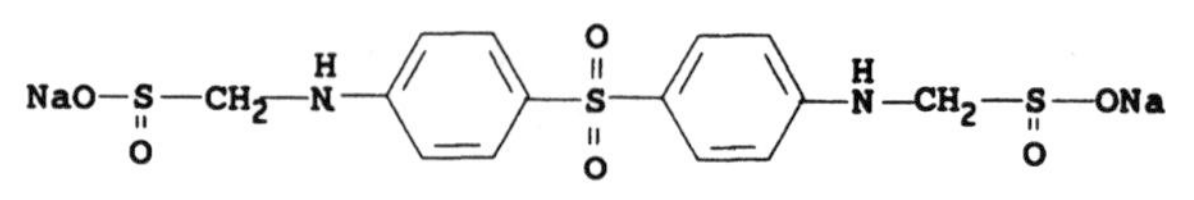

sulfoxone sodium

sulfokinases: enzymes most abundant in the gonads, adrenal cortex, liver, and placenta that add sulfate groups to steroid hormones and other compounds. Sulfation alters the biological activities, increases polarity, and contributes to storage, transport, and excretion. Phosphoadenosine phosphosulfate is the major cellular sulfate donor.

sulfolipids: sulfatides and other lipids with polar heads that contain sulfate groups, present in largest amounts in nervous tissue and chloroplasts.

sulfones: dapsone (4,4′-diaminodiphenylsulfone), sulfoxone sodium, and related compounds used to control leprosy. The bacteriostatic mechanism is similar to those of sulfa drugs (but most sulfonamides used for other purposes are ineffective against the organisms).

sulfonylureas: tolbutamide, acetohexamide, tolazamide, chlorpropamide, and chemically related oral hypoglycemic agents. Since the actions depend in part on stimulation of insulin secretion (by increasing β cell sensitivity to glucose), they are effective only in individuals with functioning islet tissue; cf **biguanides**. They additionally augment insulin receptor numbers, enhance the antilipolytic effects of the hormone, and exert other actions, but are toxic. More effective, better tolerated successors include glipizide and **glibenclamide** (q.v.).

sulfoximine: the phosphate group binds to and thereby inhibits γ-glutamylcysteine synthetase and glutathione synthetase (essential for glutathione synthesis), and glutamine synthetase. Sulfoxamine is used as a laboratory tool. It is formed from methionine in a process for bleaching flour; and inhalation of large amounts can invoke convulsions.

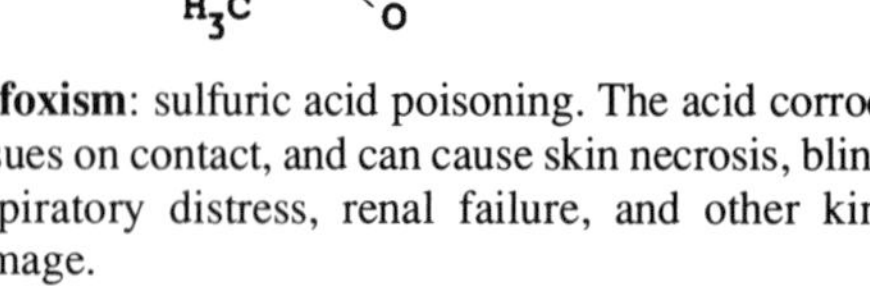

sulfoxism: sulfuric acid poisoning. The acid corrodes all tissues on contact, and can cause skin necrosis, blindness, respiratory distress, renal failure, and other kinds of damage.

sulfoxone sodium: *see* **sulfones**.

sulfur, S: a nonmetallic element (atomic number 16, atomic weight 32.064). It is a component of cysteine, cystine, methionine, glutathione, adrenodoxin and other iron-sulfur compounds, steroid sulfates, sulfolipids, and glycosaminoglycans. The active sites of several enzymes contain —SH groups. SO_4^{2-} is the major anion type in biological fluids. Radioactive isotopes used to investigate the functions include ^{35}S and [38]S, with half-lives of 84.7 days and 2.87 hours, respectively.

sulindac: *cis*-5-fluoro-2-methyl-1-[*p*-(methylsulfinyl)benzylidene]indene-3-acetic acid; an agent chemically related to indomethacin, used to treat rheumatoid arthritis and other inflammatory disorders. It is slowly oxidized to a sulfone which is, in turn reduced to a sulfide derivative that inhibits cyclooxygenases. Although purported to be less irritating to gastric mucosa than indomethacin (since the gut is not directly exposed to the active metabolite when the compound is ingested), it invokes the kinds of toxicities described for other nonsteroidal anti-inflammatory agents.

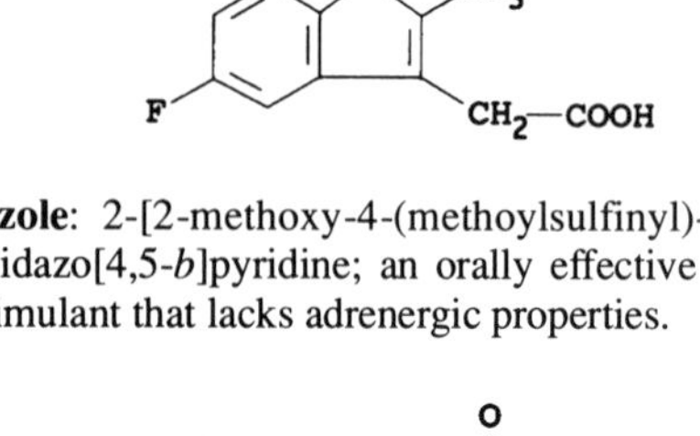

sulmazole: 2-[2-methoxy-4-(methoylsulfinyl)-phenyl]-1*H*-imidazo[4,5-*b*]pyridine; an orally effective myocardial stimulant that lacks adrenergic properties.

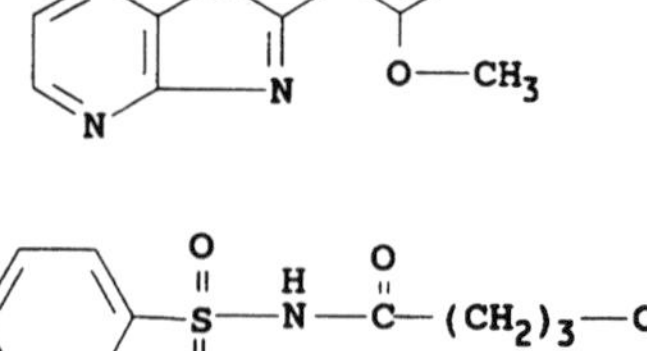

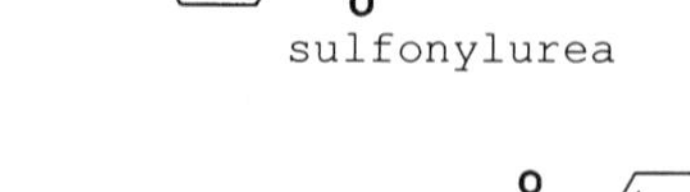

sulfonylurea

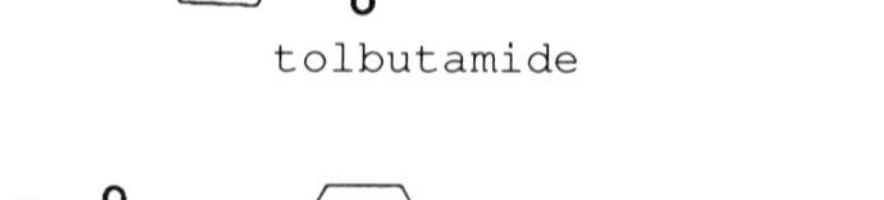

tolbutamide

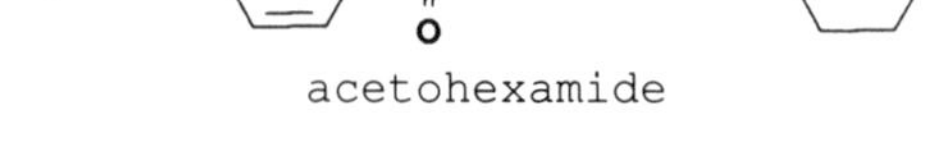

acetohexamide

sulmepride: 5-(aminosulfonyl)-2-methoxy-*N*-[(1-me-thyl-2-pyrrolidinyl)methyl]benzamide; a sulpiride analog used as a neuroleptic. It is reported to block only presynaptic dopaminergic receptors.

sulpiride: 5-(aminosulfonyl)-*N*-[(1-ethyl-2-pyrrolidinyl)-methyl]-2-methoxybenzamide; a D_2-type dopamine receptor antagonist, used as an antidepressant and "antipsychotic" agent.

sumatriptan: 3-[2-(dimethylamino)ethyl]-*N*-methyl-1*H*-indole-5-methanesulfonamide; a selective $5HT_1$ type serotonin receptor agonist used to treat migraine headaches.

summation: *see* **additive effects, spatial summation,** and **temporal summation.**

superantigens: *Staphylococcus* enterotoxins, some Mycobacterial toxins, and other substances that invoke massive immune responses by acting on large numbers of T lymphocyte subsets (as many as 1 in 5, in contrast to more conventional antigen types that affect more like 1 in 10,000). By binding directly to outer surfaces of class II MHC proteins, they bypass the requirement for processing by antigen presenting cells. Superantigen/ MHC complexes then interact with β chain variable ($V_β$) regions of T cell receptors (different from the grooves that bind conventional antigens), and also with some other TCR regions. Although various types affect only certain $V_β$ species, the target molecules are present on large numbers of T cells, most of which are not directly involved in protection against the offending agent. The major consequences are attributed to massive release of interleukin-2, interferon γ, and other cytokines via signal transduction mechanisms that do not require helper type (T_H) cells, CD4, or accelerated phosphatidylinositol hydrolysis and elevation of cytosolic Ca^{2+} levels. In addition to T lymphocyte proliferation, the excessive amounts of cytokine invoke numerous systemic effects (and can cause nausea, vomiting, malaise, fever, gastric pain, diarrhea, and hypotension). *Staphylococcus* enterotoxins are the major causes of food poisoning. One type (TSST) initiates toxic shock syndrome. Disruption of T cell functions can impair responses to infectious agents and aberrant cell types, initiate autoimmune diseases, and (depending on the timing, cell types affected, cytokine levels, and other factors) either impair or stimulate antibody production by B cells. Roles in destruction of helper type T cells in individuals with AIDS have also been suggested. Some superantigens (MIs) encoded by mouse genomes derive from mammary tumor viruses. Other regions of mammalian genomes code for small amounts of superantigens expressed in tissue-restricted ways. Ones on B lymphocytes in embryonic thymus glands are implicated as regulators of T cell repertoires.

supercoiling: usually, coiling of a circular DNA duplex around its own axis (positive if clockwise, and negative if counterclockwise); *see* also **topoisomerases** and **nucleosomes**.

supercooled: describes substances that are liquid at or below their usual freezing points.

superfamily: in molecular biology, families are groups of very closely related entities, such as insulins made by various species or the genes that direct their synthesis. Superfamilies are composed of related families, for example (1) genes derived from a common ancestral precursor that has undergone species or cell type specific changes during the course of evolution. (Growth hormone, prolactin, and placental lactogen genes belong to a superfamily); (2) proteins or peptides derived from a common ancester that differ somewhat from each other, for example the group that includes secretin, vasoactive intestinal peptide (VIP), and glucose-dependent insulinotropic peptide (GIP); (3) compounds whose members share common structural features and/or amino acid sequences, but do not necessarily perform comparable functions, such as integrins and immunoglobulins. Although they bind different ligands, the structurally related receptors for retinoids, triiodothyronine, and steroid hormones are members of a superfamily.

superfecundation: fertilization, after a single ovulation, of more than the usual numbers of oocytes.

superfemale: (1) a poorly chosen term for female mammals with more than two X (but no Y) chromosomes. The imbalance in women is often associated with mental

sumatriptan

retardation, and in some cases with circulatory system defects. Some individuals are sterile. (2) in *Drosophila*, the female phenotype associated with an X chromosome: autosome ratio greater than 1. The flies have low viability, and are more commonly called metafemales.

superfetation: (1) formation of larger numbers of fetuses than can be accommodated by the uterus and carried through the gestation period; (2) fertilization of a second oocyte released when an embryo or fetus is undergoing prenatal development.

superfusion: continuous replacement of surrounding fluids in a culture system.

supergene: a chromosome segment (with one or more genes) that is protected against crossing-over during meiosis.

superinduction: formation of larger quantities of messenger RNAs than usually occurs in response to a positive regulator. Protein synthesis inhibitors presented with a stimulant can block formation of enzymes or other factors that would otherwise destabilize or degrade the mRNAs.

superior: (1) above. The head is superior to the neck in upright species, but can be anterior in tetrapods; (2) better.

superior cervical ganglia: SCG: bilateral sympathetic system ganglia that receive inputs from the suprachiasmatic nuclei, make functional connections with retinohypothalamic tracts, and send axons to the pineal gland and other structures that control biological rhythms. The postganglionic neurons release norepinephrine which (among other things) acts via cAMP to accelerate melatonin synthesis by augmenting *N*-acetyltransferase activity.

supermarket diet: *see* **cafeteria diet**.

superovulation: release of more secondary oocytes that is characteristic for the species. It is deliberately invoked with gonadotropins or other agents, to increase the probability of conception in women with low fertility, or to acquire large numbers of oocytes for *in vitro* fertilization.

superoxides: compounds that contain the superoxide free radical (O_2^-), made by activated neutrophilic leukocytes, and in some oxidative reactions in other cell types. Excessive amounts can cause severe tissue damage.

superoxide dismutases: SOD; metalloenzymes that protect against superoxide toxicity by converting superoxide radicals to hydrogen peroxide. Most eukaryote cytosol types contain copper or zinc. Mitochondrial enzymes contain manganese. Bacterial dismutases have manganese or iron.

suppression: (1) inhibition of nerve impulse transmission; (2) inhibition of vision in one eye during binocular vision; (3) conscious repression of a thought or action; (4) restoration of normal messenger RNA translation after a frame-shift mutation. *See* also **repression**.

suppressor cells: usually, lymphocytes that protect against overactivity of the immune system. Some investigators believe that specific types mediate the functions, and that impaired control contributes to autoimmune and other diseases. Others question the existence of specific cell types that perform such functions. The ones implicated include a subpopulation of CD^{8+} T lymphocytes (T_S cells) that differs from cytotoxic (T_C) types in that the cells express CD28 and secrete interleukin-4 (but not interferons, interleukin-2, and other mediators made T_C cells). Small subsets of B lymphocytes and suppressor type macrophages may contribute.

suppressor mutation: one mutation that counteracts the effects of another.

suppuration: pus formation.

suprachiasmatic nuclei: SCN; bilateral neuron clusters in the hypothalamus, located above the optic chiasmata. They display intrinsic oscillatory activity, release many regulators, communicate with other hypothalamic regions and with the pineal gland, receive inputs from other sources, and are implicated as biological clocks that generate several biological rhythms. They can function autonomously; but inputs from retinal photoreceptors (via retinohypothalamic tracts) are required for synchronization with photoperiods. In some infant mammals and older members of a few vertebrate species, they receive and respond to light stimuli that enter the skull but do not pass through the retinas.

supraliminal stimulus: a less than maximal **stimulus** (*q.v.*), of greater intensity and/or longer duration than a threshold quantity.

supramaximal stimulus: a **stimulus** (*q.v.*) of greater strength and/or intensity than one capable of eliciting a maximal response. In most cases, it invokes no greater response; but very high intensities can damage cells.

Supranol, Suprol: trade names for suprofen.

suprarenal: (1) situated above the kidney; (2) an old term for adrenal glands.

supraoptic nuclei: SON: bilateral neuron clusters located above the optic chiasmata that contain magnocellular neurons which synthesize vasopressin, oxytocin, and their associated neurophysins and send them down long hypothalamo-hypophysial nerve tract axons to neural lobes for storage and subsequent release to the systemic blood. Paraventricular and some other neurons make the same hormones; and other kinds of regulators originate in the SON. Osmoreceptors, pressoreceptors, thermoreceptors, and several hormones (including angiotensin II and atrial natriuretic peptides) control vasopressin release. Estrogens are major stimulants for oxytocin-secreting cells.

supravital staining: staining of cells that have been removed from a living organism; *cf* **intravital staining**.

suprofen: Suprol; Supranol; α-methyl-4-(2-thienylcarbonyl)benzeneacetic acid; a nonsteroidal anti-inflammatory, antipyretic agent with analgesic properties that acts in part by inhibiting prostaglandin synthesis. It can exert toxic effects on the kidneys.

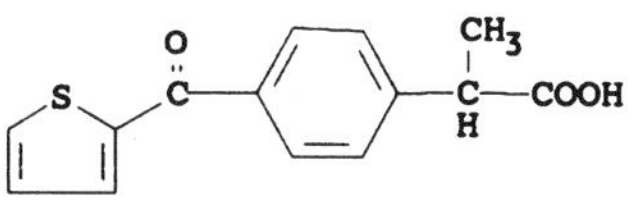

suprofen

suramin sodium: 8,8′-[carbonyl*bis*[imino-3,1-phenyl-enecarbonylimino(4-methyl-3,1-phenylene)carbonylimino]]*bis*-1,3,5-naphthalenetrisulfonic acid hexasodium; an agent that inhibits some reverse transcriptases, and binds to complement factor C3b. It is used to treat *Trypanosome* and roundworm infestations, but is not effective against acquired immune deficiency syndrome (AIDS) viruses. In addition to fatigue and skin rashes, it can invoke neurological, gastrointestinal, hepatic, and hematopoietic, and other problems, and often causes nausea. Large doses are used to destroy adrenal glands in laboratory animals.

surface tension: the cohesive force generated by the greater attraction of components of a liquid for each other than for other substances (liquid or gas) in contact with its surface. It minimizes the surface area of the fluid, and decreases the tendency for mixing with the other substance. The surface of water (or of a dilute aqueous solution) exposed to air behaves like a stretched membrane that can support small dust particles, some insects, and other light objects. *See* also **surfactants**.

surfactants: (1) soaps, detergents, phospholipids, and other amphipathic substances that lower surface tension. Some (for example nonoxynol) are components of barrier type contraceptives used by women; (2) complexes composed of lecithin, sphingomyelins, and proteins made by type II cells of pulmonary alveoli and respiratory passages that protect against alveolar collapse during expiration by lowering surface tension at pulmonary fluid/air interfaces. Their induction by glucocorticoids begins shortly before completion of the gestation period in human fetuses. (The cells do not respond at earlier times.) Inability to make pulmonary surfactant is a major cause of respiratory distress and death in premature infants. *See* also **SP proteins**.

surfactin: a 1034K peptide-lipid made by *Bacillus subtilis* that inhibits protein denaturation and blood coagulation, but accelerates fibrinolysis.

surrogate mothers: *see* **embryo transfer**.

Sus: a genus that includes domestic pigs and some wild hogs.

suspensions: dispersions of undissolved, fine particles in liquids that settle out under the force of gravity when left undisturbed. Examples include mixtures of fine sand or starch and water (dispersed by shaking). Since the particles block passage of light rays, suspensions are opaque; *cf* **colloidal solutions**.

sustained action mechanism: describes effects of substances that must be presented for extended time periods to elicit certain responses, although no intermediate changes during the latent period are apparent. The influences of estradiol on cell proliferation are not achieved with a single presentation of shorter acting estriol, which binds to the same receptors; but repeated administraiton of estriol is effective. *Cf* **domino effect**.

sustentacular cells: supporting cells; *see* **Sertoli cells**.

suture: (1) to sew; (2) a stitch; (3) a ridge or similar marking where two anatomical structures have fused; (4) an immovable, or slightly moveable joint, initially fibrous but usually partially or totally replaced by bone.

SV40: *see* **simian virus 40**.

Svedberg unit: a unit equivalent to 10^{-13} seconds; *see* **sedimentation coefficient**.

SVG: sauvagine.

swainsonine: 8α,β-indolizidine-1α,2α,8β-triol; an alkaloid made by the fungus *Swainsona canescens* that impairs protein *N*-glycosylation by inhibiting Golgi mannosidases that trim excess mannose groups.

swine: domesticated breeds of *Sus scrofa* species, used for studies of ovarian, circulatory, integumentary, and other functions.

switch region: a DNA recombination site; *see* **class switching**.

SWS: slow wave sleep.

sxr: a segment on the short arm of the Y chromosome named for its ability to cause sex reversal in female mice. The human counterpart is *SXR*; and analogous base se-

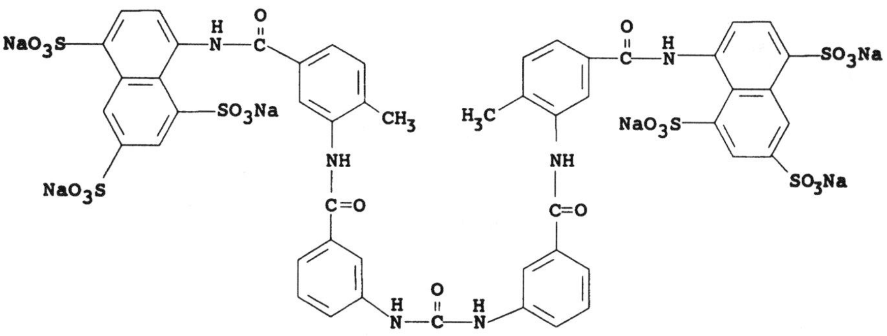

suramin sodium

quences are present in other mammals. The component initially described, now called *sxr^a*, contains *Tdy* (testis determining Y component, the gene that initiates masculinization of male embryos), *Hya* (which directs synthesis of H-Y antigen), *spy* (a gene required for survival and proliferation of spermatogonia that may be identical with *sby*), *zf1* and *zf2* (which code for two zinc finger proteins of unknown function), and genes that direct formation of SMDA, a serologically identified protein made only by males). *Sxr* can replicate and attach to the pseudoautosomal region of the Y chromosome (the segment that pairs with the X chromosome during meiosis). XY mice with the extra segment are phenotypically normal, fertile males that transmit the duplicated segment to all of their male, and half their female progeny. Most XX females that acquire the gene (XX*sxr* females) through inheritance or by transfection, develop into sterile, phenotypic males that express *Tdy*, *Hya*, *Zf1*, and *Zf2*, but not *spy* (which is germ cell dependent). It has been suggested that they cannot support spermatogenesis because two X chromones block progression of prespermatogonia to meiosis-competent spermatogonia. However, most females that have just one X chromosome and acquire the segment (XO*sxr* females) also develop into sterile males. One possibility is that the gene functions only when correctly positioned on a Y chromosome. Some XX*sxr* and XO*sxr* mice become hermaphrodites, possibly because the extra gene is inactivated on some X chromosomes. *Sxr'* is a deletion variant that may be identical with *sxr^b*. It includes *Tdy*, and invokes the male phenotype in XX mice, but lacks the *Hya* and SMDA coding segments. A different variant, *scr''* contains the *Hya*, reacquired during crossing over at meiosis.

SXR: the human counterpart of the *sxr* gene. The *Tdy* component codes for a protein that differs by 27 amino acid moieties from the mouse product, and is ineffective for masculinizing XX mice when transfected. It has been identified in XX men, but is deleted in XY women.

symbiosis: (1) living together; close associations between two different kinds of organisms, including *mutualism* (in which both types benefit), *commensalism* (in which one benefits and the other is not affected), *parasitism* (beneficial to one but harmful to the other), *amensalism* (detrimental to one but without effect on the other), and *synnecrosis* (damaging to both); (2) in psychiatry, any of several kinds of interrelationships between two individuals.

sympathectomy: removal of, or disruption of the functions of the sympathetic nervous system. Total surgical sympathectomy is virtually impossible to perform. Agents that inhibit enzymes required for catecholamine synthesis are used to achieve **"chemical" sympathectomy** (*q.v.*). **Immunosympathectomy** (*q.v.*) is accomplished with antibodies directed against substances such as nerve growth factor (NGF) that are essential for sympathetic nervous system development and/or functions.

sympathetic nervous system: the branch of the autonomic nervous system with presynaptic perikarya in the thoracic and lumber regions of the spinal cord. Most neurons extend short axons to postsynaptic types in ganglia near the spinal cord. The major neurotransmitter released by postganglionic neurons is norepinephrine. The system is most active during times of physical exertion, stress, and exposure to cold environments. *Cf* **parasympathetic nervous system**.

sympathin: before the chemical structures and functions of catecholamines were defined, it was proposed that some sympathetic nervous system neurons release an excitatory neurotransmitter (*sympathin E*), whereas others release an inhibitory one (*sympathin I*). The concept was abandoned when it was recognized that differential responses depend on the kinds of target cell receptors activated, and that epinephrine can excite some cell types but inhibit others. *See also* **adrenergic receptors**.

sympatric: describes species whose areas of distribution coincide or overlap.

symphysis pubis: the joint between the pubic bones. It usually consists mostly of fibrocartilage; but relaxin promotes replacement of some cartilage by fibrous connective tissue and other changes that loosen the joint in preparation for parturition.

symport: processes in which transport of one substance across a membrane is linked to simultaneous transport of another in the same direction. Usually, Na^+ ions travel passively down their concentration gradient, as the other component (for example an amino acid) goes against its gradient. *Cf* counterport.

symptom: usually, a subjective indication of disease; *cf* **sign**.

symptothermal "rhythm" methods: modifications of the "rhythm method" for contraception in which the time of ovulation is estimated from externally visible indicators such as the quality of the mucus secreted by uterine cervix glands and/or body temperature changes at the time of awakening. They were introduced to reduce the numbers of "failures" experienced by users of "calendar" methods, but have not proven more effective.

synalbumin: an unidentified blood component proposed to interfere with insulin actions.

synapse: a functional connection between a neuron and either another neuron or an effector organ (muscle fiber or gland). Most synapses are chemical, with communication accomplished via presynaptic release of neurotransmitters that travel across small spaces (clefts) and act on postsynaptic receptors. Limited numbers are electrical. Although most neuronal synapses are axodendritic (axon of one to dendrites of the other), a few are dendrodendritic (dendrite to dendrite), axoaxonic, (axon to axon), or axosomatic (axon to perikaryon). Some authors additionally apply the term to gap junctions and other sites of cell: cell communication.

synapsins: 67-80K nerve terminal proteins that contribute to synaptic vesicle and synapse formation and the control of neurotransmitter release (but not to neurite outgrowth). Dephosphorylated forms bind to microtubules and position vesicles for exocytosis. They detach when neurotransmitters promote calcium-calmodulin kinase II and kinase A mediated phosphorylation. Synapsins Ia and Ib, derived via differential splicing of a single messenger RNA, display strong homology with erythrocyte protein 4.1. They are larger and more abundant than synapsins IIa and IIb, whose formation is directed by a different gene.

synapsis: association of homologous chromosomes during meiosis; tetrad formation.

synaptene: the stage of meiosis during which homologous chromosomes begin to form tetrads. (Preparations are made during late leptotene). The pairing is completed during zygotene, and persists through pachytene (during which crossing over occurs). Desynapsis proceeds during diplotene.

synaptic cleft: the minute space between the terminals of a presynaptic neuron and the receptor components of a postsynaptic neuron or neuromuscular junction, into which neurotransmitters are released. Acetylcholinesterase is released to cholinergic types.

synaptic delay: the time interval between initiation of a presynaptic neuron action potential and the response of a postsynaptic neuron or other target cell. Synaptic transmission is slower than electrical communication, because time is required for exocytosis (neurotransmitter release from presynaptic nerve terminals), messenger diffusion across the synaptic cleft, and neurotransmitter binding to target cell receptors.

synaptic vesicles: small membrane-bound vesicles that take up, store and release neurotransmitters. Some regulators are chemically processed within the vesicles.

synaptophysins: integral membrane proteins of presynaptic neuron and neuroendocrine vesicles that contribute to exocytosis by facilitating fusion of vesicle and plasma membranes. They are used as markers for neuroendocrine cells.

synaptosomes: vesicles that form in brain or spinal cord homogenates when broken membranes spontaneously reseal. Since they take up, hold, and release neurotransmitters, and are osmotically active, they are used to study neurotransmitter functions.

synchorial: describes siblings that develop in a common chorionic sac.

synchronous cell population: a population in which all cells enter mitosis at the same time. It can be achieved by shaking cells from a culture dish into a new medium, or exposing them briefly to a mitotic poison such as colchicine. The techniques are used to study chromosomes and cell cycle regulators. Because of individual differences in cell responsivities, synchrony is rarely complete, and is lost after a few cycles.

syncope: fainting; transient loss of consciousness, caused by insufficient blood flow through the cerebral cortex.

syncytiotrophoblast: the trophoblast layer that forms along the superficial surface of the cytotrophoblast. The cells are multinucleate, with indistinct boundaries. They secrete chorionic gonadotropins, placental lactogens, and

other regulators, and make estradiol dehydrogenase (which converts estradiol to estrone), and aromatase.

syncytium: a large cell with two or more nuclei, formed by fusion of two or more smaller ones. Examples include skeletal muscle fibers, macrophages, and syncytiotrophoblast cells.

syndesmochorial: describes a type of **placenta** *(q.v.)*.

syndesmosis: a fibrous joint.

syndrome: the signs, symptoms, and other characteristics of a disease.

syndrome of inappropriate ADH secretion: SIADH; conditions in which more vasopressin is secreted than is appropriate for the state of hydration. Although edema does not usually develop, and blood volume can be maintained within the normal range, water is retained, plasma Na$^+$ levels are subnormal, and the extracellular fluid volume expands. The causes include head injuries that affect transmission of regulatory signals to vasopressin secreting cells, tumor cell products, and some pharmacological agents.

syndyphalin: H$_2$N-Tyr-D-Met(SO)-Gly-*N*-methylphenethylamide; a metenkephalin analog used as a specific ligand for μ-type opioid receptors.

synemin: a 230K protein that cross-links vimentin filaments.

synephrine: 1-(4-hydroxyphenyl)-2-methylaminoethanol; a catecholamine made in very small amounts under normal conditions, and in larger ones when metabolism is disrupted (for example by monoamine oxidase inhibitors). It is a false transmitter that acts on α-type adrenergic receptors. Synthetic preparations are used for their vasopressor activity.

syneresis: contraction of a gel, with release of fluid.

synergism: cooperation; describes (1) coordinated activity of two or more similar entities to achieve a higher level of a common function than can be accomplished with one component acting alone, such as contraction of two or more muscle groups to accomomplish a movement, control posture, or hold a weight; (2) the additive effects of different agents that invoke the same kind of response. The term *potentiation* is usually applied when the combined effects of maximal doses exceed the sums of those obtained with either agent acting alone.

syngamy: union of gametes; *see* **fertilization**.

syngeneic: having identical phenotypes.

synlactin: a mitogen similar to an insulin-like growth factor, induced in the liver by prolactin. It augments prolactin stimulation of casein synthesis and other processes in mammary glands, but is not effective when presented alone.

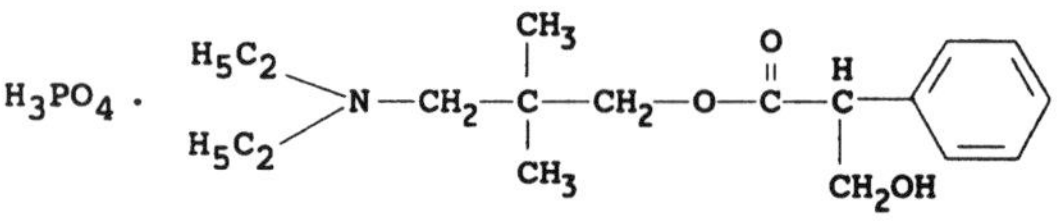

Syntropan

synnecrosis: *see* **symbiosis.**

synomone: an ectohormone beneficial to both the donor and the recipient; *cf* **allomone.**

synovial: resembling egg-white, a term applied to the fluid in the cavities of moveable joints.

synovial fluid: the fluid in moveable joints. It serves lubricant and nutritive functions, and is a site of inflammation in some forms of arthritis.

synthases, synthetases: enzymes that catalyze formation of large molecules from smaller ones; *see* for example **fatty acid**, **citrate**, and **glycogen synthase.**

Synthroid: a trade name for levothyroxine.

syntide: Pro-Leu-Ala-Arg-Thr-Leu-ser-Val-Ala-Gly-Leu-Pro-Gly-Lys-Lys; a synthetic substrate for calmodulin-dependent protein kinases.

Syntropan: a trade name for amprotropine phosphate, α-(hydroxymethyl)-benzeneacetic acid 3-(diethylamino)-2,2-dimethylpropyl ester phosphate, an anticholinergic agent with atropine-like properties, used mostly to alleviate intestinal muscle spasms.

syntropic: converging; pointing to, or leading in the same direction.

syntropy: describes the unlikelihood that certain kinds of diseases (such as sickle cell trait and malaria) will occur in the same individual.

synvinolin: simvastatin; 1,2,3,7,8,8a-hexahydro-3,7-dimethyl-8-[2-(tetrahydro-4-hydroxy-6-oxo-2*H*-pyran-2-yl]-1-napthalenyl ester; an inhibitor of HMG-CoA (hydroxymethylglutaryl-coenzyme A) reductase with properties and uses similar to those of **mevinolin** (*q.v.*).

syringo-: a prefix for a duct or passageway; *see* also **syrinx.**

syrinx: (1) a fistula; (2) a pathological tube-shaped cavity within the brain or spinal cord; (3) a bird vocal organ. The plural, syringes, is seldom used, because of possible confusion with syringe (the double barreled device used to inject and withdraw fluids).

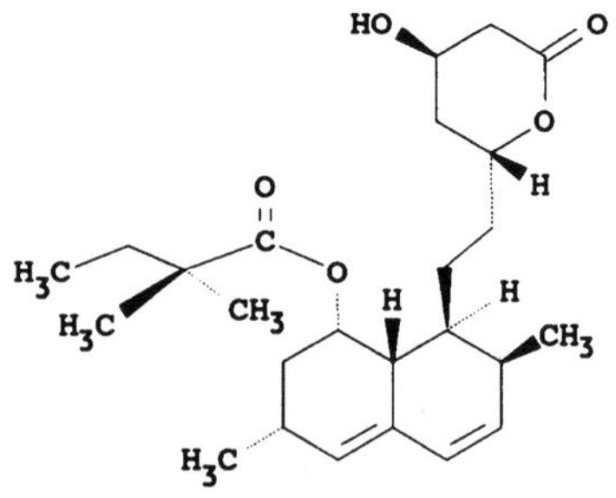

synvinolin

system: in anatomy and physiology, a set of organs that performs a common function, as in circulatory, respiratory, or reproductive system.

systematics: taxonomy.

systemic bloodstream: the blood that circulates through all large vessels, and through capillaries that supply most body cells. The term excludes specialized compartments, such as the hypothalamo-hypophysial, the hepatic, and the renal portal systems.

systemic lupus erythematosus: SLE; autoimmune diseases in which autoantibodies against nuclear components are made. The symptoms, which vary among individuals and tend to wax and wane, usually include inflammation of joints and other organs, hypersensitivity to heat and cold, and skin rashes (which can assume butterfly-like or "wolf-like" patterns around the nose). The incidence is approximately ten times higher in women than in men. *See also* **lupus erythematosus** and **lupus erythematosus cells.**

systemin: an 18-amino acid peptide made by injured tomato leaves, and also induced by abscisic acid, α-methyl jasmonate, and some other plant hormones. In addition to roles in protection against microorganisms, it appears to be involved in signal transduction, and may perform metabolic functions.

systole: the contraction phase of a cardiac cycle, a term applied to both atria and ventricles; *cf* **diastole.**

T

T: (1) threonine; (2) thymine; (3) thymidine; (4) transmittance.

t: (1) time; (2) temperature; (3) *see t test*.

τ: Greek letter tau; *see* **tau proteins**.

T1: *see* **CD5**.

T4: (1) *see* **CD4**; (2) *see* **T4 phage**.

T6: *see* **CD1**.

T8: *see* **CD8**.

T11: *see* **CD2**.

T_0: thyronine.

T_1: **monoiodothyronine** (*q.v.*); MIT; *see also* **thyronines**.

T_2: **diiodothyronine** (*q.v.*); DIT; *see also* **thyronines**.

T_3: triiodothyronine.

T_4: tetraiodothyronine; *see* **thyroxine**.

t/2, $t_{1/2}$: half-life; the time theoretically required for a 50% change, for example for half the radioactive atoms in a sample to disintegrate, or for half the molecules of a specific kind to disappear from circulating blood.

T-1824: Evans blue.

TA: triamcinolone acetamide.

Ta: tantalum.

TAA: tumor associated antigens.

tabes: melting, liquefaction, or disintegration. *Tabes dorsalis* is a form of neurosyphilis in which posterior spinal nerve roots deteriorate and perception of kinesthetic, pain, and other stimuli is impaired.

tabun: dimethylamidoethoxyphosphoryl cyanide; an extremely potent acetylcholinesterase inhibitor absorbed through the skin and eyes, and by inhalation. It was developed for chemical warfare, and is too toxic for other uses.

Tac: CD25; T cell activation receptor; the low-affinity p55 subunit of the interleukin-2β receptor. Anti-Tac is a mouse monoclonal antibody that blocks T cell activation by that cytokine by inhibiting IL-2 binding.

Tac promoters: hybrid molecules constructed from parts of *E. coli trp* and *lac* promoters, used mostly because the functions are easily controlled. *Trp* (the tryptophan synthesis operon) can be induced with 3β-indoleacrylic acid. Allolactose (formed from lactose in high lactose media) increases the activity of *lac* (the lactose operon) by binding to the *lac* repressor and promoting its dissociation from the operon.

TACE: a trade term for chlorotrianisene.

tachistoscopes: devices that flash light or test patterns for very brief time periods. They are used to study visual perception and corpus callosum functions.

tachy-: a prefix meaning rapid.

tachycardia: rapid heart rate.

tachykinins: substance P, neurokinins, neuromedins, kassinin, eledoisin, physalaemin and other small peptides made by neurons and other neural crest derivatives, and by cells of vertebrate gastrointestinal tracts, amphibian skin, and invertebrate salivary glands. All are potent smooth muscle stimulants with common *C*-terminal amino acid sequences of the general type: Phe-X-Gly-Leu-Met-NH_2, where X is either an aromatic or a branched-chain aliphatic amino acid moiety. Receptors have been identified in arterioles, venules, joints, and both longitudinal and circular gastrointestinal tract muscle. Premessenger RNAs encoded by a single mammalian gene undergo alternate splicing to yield three different preprotachykinins (A or α, B or β, and γ). Some of the precursors are transported to peripheral terminals and released to effector organs in which enzymes release the active peptides. Tachykinins contribute to inflammation, immune system functions, and the release of digestive system hormones; and some affect drinking and other behaviors. The ones made in dorsal root ganglia mediate nociception by transmitting messages to the central nervous system.

tachykinin receptors: three kinds of proteins that mediate tachykinin actions by interacting with G proteins. The NK_1 type preferentially binds substance P. NK_2 displays high affinity for neurokinin A (NKA), and NK_3 for neurokinin B (NKB). Types 1 and 3 are present in the brain. A form of type 2 in the stomach differs from one in urinary bladder. Additional receptors that do not interact with G proteins have also been described.

tachyphylaxis: progressive decrease in responsiveness to an agent that is presented repeatedly at short intervals, or continuously. *See also* **desensitization** and *cf* **down regulation**.

tachysterol: (6*E*,22*E*)-9,10-secoergosta-5(10),6,8,22-tetraen-3-ol; a secosteroid obtained by irradiating ergosterol; *see* **dihydrotachysterol**.

tacrine: 1,2,3,4-tetrahydro-9-acridinamine; a long-acting acetylcholinesterase inhibitor, used to stimulate breathing and to counteract the effects of excessive amounts of curare. It enters the brain, but there are conflicting reports concerning beneficial effects on memory in individuals with early symptoms of Alzheimer's disease.

Tagamet: a trade name for cimetidine.

taipoxin: a 46.2K component of the venom of *Oxyuranus scutellatus scutellatus* snakes that acts presynaptically to inhibit acetylcholine release and invokes degeneration of myotube and muscle satellite cells.

talin: (1) a 215K cytoskeleton protein that binds to cytoplasmic domains of fibronectin receptors, and to vinculin, and indirectly affects actin filaments. It is present in the plasma membranes of cytotoxic lymphocytes, where it may protect those cells against self-destruction; (2) Talin is a trade name for a mixture of plant peptides (thaumatins) under investigation for use as artificial sweeteners.

talipes: a term used with qualifiers to designate various kinds of foot deformities.

TAME: *N*α-*p*-tosyl arginine methyl ester; an artificial substrate for assays of plasmin, trypsin, thrombin, and other compounds that is resistant to chymotrypsin, and unaffected by soybean trypsin inhibitor. It facilitates formation of kallidin-α$_2$-macroglobulin complexes.

tamoxifen: 2-[4-(1,2-diphenyl-1-butenyl)phenoxy]-*N*,*N*-dimethylethanamine; a nonsteroidal agent that interacts directly with estrogen receptors, and is slowly converted to 4-hydroxytamoxifen (which binds with higher affinity) and other metabolites. Depending on the species, dosage, and target organ, it is an estrogen receptor antagonist, agonist, or mixed agonist-antagonist. In humans and some others, high concentrations oppose estrogen mediated mitogenesis, are used to treat some breast and uterine cancers, and are under investigation for prophylactic use in women at high risk for developing the cancers (for example ones with close relatives who have the disease). However, high concentrations of cAMP are among the factors that cause it to function as an agonist. Low doses exert favorable, estrogen-like influences on bone in women with some forms of osteoporosis, and may additionally confer beneficial cardiovascular effects. Although said to be less toxic than steroidal estrogens administered for such purposes, the side effects can include nausea, hot flashes, menstrual irregularities, and vaginal bleeding in postmenopausal women, and also hypercalcemia and many of the undesirable consequences described for oral contraceptives. In mice, tamoxifen is a potent estrogen agonist for reproductive system cells, but an antagonist at some other sites. Tissue specific differences in responses (for example in liver as compared with oviduct) have also been described for chickens. Tamoxifen binding to other proteins accounts for some actions that are not opposed by estrogens. Kinase C is one of the proposed targets.

tanacytes: tanycytes; ependymal cells that border the cerebral ventricles and facilitate exchange of substances between blood and cerebrospinal fluid.

tandem repeats: identical or very similar DNA segments arranged sequentially along chromosomes.

tannic acids: several substances obtained from the barks of oak, sumac, and other trees, and used as astringents. Representative carbohydrate-containing and flavonol types are shown.

tantalum: Ta; a metallic element (atomic number 73, atomic weight 180.95). Since it is malleable and noncorrosive, it is used in dentistry, surgical wires, disks, and prostheses.

T antigens: proteins made by oncogenic viruses that regulate viral DNA replication and transcription. *Large* (80K) T antigens invade the nucleus, integrate randomly into host genomes, invoke transformation, and kill permissive host cells. Nonpermissive cells can be permanently transformed; but some eject the foreign DNA and revert to normal growth. **Simian virus 40** (*q.v.*) makes a second, cytoplasmic 20K *small* T antigen. Polyoma viruses make an additional 45K *middle* T antigen

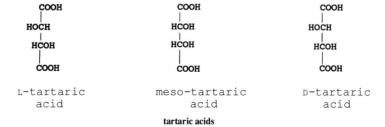

tannic acids

that localizes to plasma membranes and can activate pp60$^{c\text{-}src}$ and pp62$^{c\text{-}yes}$ tyrosine kinases, phosphatidy-linositol kinase-3, and other enzymes.

Tapazole: a trade name for methimazole.

tapeworms: several parasitic Cestode flatworms (including mostly segmented, but also some nonsegmented species). Many inhabit the intestines of specific mammalian animal types, grow rapidly, and deprive the hosts of nutrients. The adult forms are hermaphrodites that reproduce by self-fertilization.

tapeworm larvae growth factor: *see* **plerocercoid growth factor**.

TAPS: 4-[Tris(hydroxymethyl)methylamino]-1-propane sulfonic acid; a zwitterion type physiological buffer.

Taq polymerase: a heat-stable DNA polymerase made by the hot spring bacteria, *Thermus aquaticus*. It is used for polymerase chain reactions.

TAR: transactivation response site; a human immunotropic (HIV) virus nucleic acid segment located immediately downstream from the transcription initiation site, in the 5′ long-terminal repeat region. It binds tat protein, and is essential for tat stimulation of transcription and translation. Although formerly believed to activate the enzyme, it appears to block double-stranded RNA activation of the interferon-induced protein kinase, DAI

(dsI, p68, dsRNA-activated inhibitor of protein synthesis), and to thereby protect the virus against host defense mechanisms. The activated enzyme inhibits protein synthesis by catalyzing phosphorylation of eukaryotic initiation factor eIF2.

tardive: describes conditions manifested long after the initial exposure to a causative agent.

tardive dyskinesia: a neurological disorder that impairs extrapyramidal system function. It develops in some individuals after long-term therapy with "antipsychotic" agents that block dopamine receptors. The major symptoms include involuntary, stereotyped movements which disappear during sleep. Although they resemble some described for Parkinson's disease, they abate in many individuals when the therapy is terminated.

target cells: cells that possess receptors for, and can respond to one or more hormones, neurotransmitters, or other agents.

target organs: organs that contain target cells.

tartaric acids: 2,3-dihydroxybutanedioic acids. The L isomer is the most common form, and is used in food preparation and other industries.

tartrate resistant acid phosphatase: TRAP; purple phosphatase: an enzyme made by osteoclasts that contributes to bone resorption. It is used as a marker for those cells.

TAT: (1) tyrosine aminotransferase; (2) T.A.T.

T.A.T: TAT; thematic apperception test; a psychological diagnostic tool. The subject is presented with pictures

```
        COOH                    COOH                    COOH
         |                       |                       |
       HOCH                     HCOH                    HOCH
         |                       |                       |
       HCOH                     HCOH                    HCOH
         |                       |                       |
        COOH                    COOH                    COOH

    L-tartaric            meso-tartaric            D-tartaric
      acid                    acid                   acid
```

tartaric acids

699

that can be interpreted in more than one way, and is asked to explain them.

Tat: tat; an 86-amino acid *trans*-activating protein made by human immunotropic (HIV) viruses that binds to mediates the effects of TAR viral RNA and protein synthesis.

TATA box: Hogness box; Goldberg-Hogness box; short DNA segments located upstream from the transcription initiation site, with TATAAAA or very similar nucleotide sequences analogous to the prokaryote Pribnow (TATAAT) box. It is the promoter component that binds and positions RNA polymerase II for most eukaryotic genes.

tau proteins: τ proteins; 40-60K proteins that bind to and stabilize microtubule polymers, and also bind to ribosomes and nucleoli. High levels of phosphorylated tau accumulate in the brains of individuals with Alzheimer's disease and Down's syndrome. S-100 inhibits the phosphorylation.

taurine: 2-aminoethane sulfonic acid; a sulfonic β-amino acid (in which S replaces the carboxyl C). It is by far the most abundant *free* amino acid in vertebrates, and can be concentrated by all cell types. Because of their bulk, myocytes hold the most; but cell: extracellular fluid concentration ratios are in the neighborhood of 400:1 for photoreceptors, 500:1 in brain, and up to 7000:1 for some tumor cells. High concentrations are present in human (but not bovine) milk, and in many marine invertebrates and red algae. At physiological pH, taurine is a strongly hydrophilic zwitterion that does not diffuse across membrane phospholipid bilayers, but is transported by systems specific for β-amino acids. It contributes to membrane composition, fluidity and stabilization, to ionic movements across internal as well as plasma membranes (including light-sensitive chloride fluxes in retinal rod cells), and to intracellular and extracellular osmoregulation. It is also a neuromodulator that affects the release of and responses to gamma aminobutyric acid (GABA), catecholamines, opioids, and other neurotransmitters, and is involved in functions as diverse as myocardial contraction, carbohydrate metabolism, energy storage, cell proliferation and cerebellum maturation. In pineal glands and suprachiasmatic nuclei, it contributes to the control of body rhythms. Various effects are mediated via influences on adenylate cyclases, protein kinases, phosphodiesterases, and other enzymes. Ad-

ditionally, taurine is an antioxidant; and it enhances the detergent properties of bile salts.

taurocholic acid: *N*-chololyltaurine. Sodium taurocholate is the major bile salt for most mammals.

tautomerism: reversible shifting of protons between keto and enol isomers (as in the interconversion of phosphoenol pyruvate and pyruvate, and of amino and imino acids). An adenine tautomer can cause mutation during DNA replication by pairing with cytosine (rather than with thymine).

tax: a nuclear protein made by human T-cell leukemia virus HTLV-I. It is a *trans*-activator that invokes transformation and accelerates transcription of fos, interleukin-2, the α subunit of the IL-2 receptor, and several other cellular genes.

taxis: oriented movement towards or away from a stimulus.

taxol: 5β-20-epoxy, 1,2α,4,7β,10β,138α–hexahydroxytax-11-en-9-one-4,10-diacetate 2-benzoate with (2*R*,3*S*)-*N*-benzoyl-3-phenylisoserine; an alkaloid from bark of the Pacific yew tree, *Taxus brevifolia* that binds to microtubules and blocks depolymerization, facilitates ATP-independent microtubule assembly, and inhibits mitosis progression after the spindle has formed. It is used to treat some leukemias and neoplastic tumors resistant to other agents, and as a laboratory tool. Since the trees are scarce, and only minute amounts can be obtained from the bark, other methods for obtaining the drug are being developed. Taxol synthesis has recently been accomplished.

taxonomy: classification of organisms. Older systems were based mostly on morphological features. Newer ones consider evolutionary relationships and biochemical components.

Tay-Sachs disease: a rare, severe inherited lipoidosis in which impaired ability to synthesize hexosaminidase leads to the accumulation of ganglioside GM$_2$ in the nervous system. The symptoms, which first appear 3-6 months after birth, include loss of vision, seizures, and poor muscle tone. Most victims die before the age of 5 years.

taurocholic acid

taxol

T4 bacteriophage: a complex DNA bacteriophage that infects *Escherichia coli*. It is used as a tool in molecular biology. *See* **T4 phage**.

TBG: thyronine binding globulin; thyroxine binding globulin.

TBPA: thyronine binding prealbumin; *see* **transthyretin**.

Tc: technetium.

TCA: (1) trichloroacetic acid; (2) tricyclic antidepressant; (3) tricarboxylic acid.

TCBD: *see* **TCCD**.

TCCD: TCDBD; dioxin; 2,3,7,8-tetrachlorodibenzo-*p*-dioxin; an extremely potent toxin formed in some industrial processes. The anorexia, weight loss, vascular lesions, liver damage, and other effects of Agent Orange are attributed to its release. It induces aryl hydrocarbon hydroxylase (a microsomal P450 monooxygenase), and is carcinogenic.

T_C cells: cytotoxic T lymphocytes; *see* **T lymphocytes**.

T cells: T lymphocytes.

3T3 cells: several easily cultured fibroblast cell lines used to study factors that promote differentiation, and the effects of oncogenes and mutations.

T cell activation receptor: the low-affinity interleukin-2 receptor on activated T lymphocytes; *see* **Tac**.

T cell chemotactic polypeptide: T cell chemotactic factor; TCF; NAP-1; an 8K protein that activates T lymphocytes and polymorphonuclear leukocytes. *See* **neutrophil activating protein-1**.

T cell growth factor: TCGF; when used without qualification, interleukin-2 (T cell growth factor-1). T cell growth factor-2 is interleukin-4.

T cell leukemia viruses: T cell lymphoma viruses. HTLV-1 is a retrovirus that causes some forms of leukemia in humans, and is implicated in the etiology of multiple sclerosis. Cells transformed by it do not require interleukin-2. In addition to *gag*, *pol*, and *env*, its genome codes for **tax** *(q.v.)*. HTLV-II is a related retrovirus initially identified in individuals with hairy cell leukemia.

T cell receptors: TCR; TcR; glycoproteins of the immunoglobulin superfamily expressed on T cell surfaces, noncovalently linked to CD3 complexes. They recognize major histocompatibility complex (MHC) proteins, usually in association with processed antigens. The most common types are αβ dimers; but subpopulations that accumulate in gastrointestinal tract and skin and perform special functions are γδ types. Some of the latter may not require maturation in the thymus gland; but there is also evidence that thymocytes can initially express the γδ molecules and later replace them by αβ types.

T cell replacement factor: thymocyte-dependent growth factor; TDGF: *see* **interleukin-5**. The acronym TRF is not used by endocrinologists because of possible confusion with thyrotropin release factor.

T cell rosettes: E rosettes; erythrocyte rosettes; clusters of sheep erythrocytes around T lymphocytes, bound to them via CD2 (T11). The binding has been used to identify T cells in mixed lymphocyte populations.

TCF: T cell chemotactic factor.

TCGF: *see* **T cell growth factor** and **interleukin-2**.

T3 complex: CD3; a complex of three proteins physically associated with T lymphocyte antigen receptors.

[³H]TCP: [3]H*N*-[1-(2-thienylcyclohexyl]piperidine; a phencyclidine analog used to identify PCP receptors.

TCR: TcR; T lymphocyte receptor.

TCT: thyrocalcitonin; an old name for calcitonin.

TDA: (1) TSH displacing antibody; (2) testis determining antigen.

T_D cells: T lymphocytes that mediate delayed hypersensitivity; *see* **T lymphocytes**.

T-dependent antigens: antigens made by B lymphocytes only in the presence of factors made by activated helper type T lymphocytes.

Tdf: *Tdy*; a Y chromosome gene that codes for a DNA binding protein essential for initiating masculinization in mouse embryos. Analogous genes have been identified in other mammals. *See* **testis determining genes**.

TDF: the human counterpart of the mouse *Tdf* gene; *see* **testis determining factor**.

TDGF: TCGF; thymocyte-dependent growth factor: *see* **interleukin-2**.

Tdt: terminal deoxynucleotidyl transferase.

TEA: tetraethylammonium.

TeBG: testosterone-estrogen binding globulin.

tebutate: tertiary butyl acetate; a solvent used in chromatography.

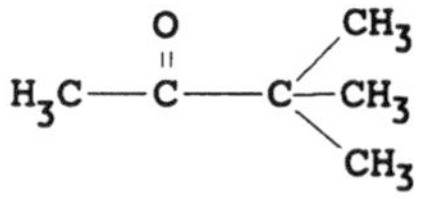

technetium: Tc: a metallic element (atomic number 43); a uranium fission product that can be produced artificially from molybdenum, with chemical properties intermediate between those of manganese and rhenium. No stable isotopes are known, but some forms have very long half-lives. Ones with shorter half-lives are used as radioactive imaging agents. For example, albumin aggregates of ^{99}Tc, ^{99m}Tc etidronate (a stannous chloride chelate), and TcO$_4^-$ (pertechnetate) are used, respectively, for lung, for bone, and for brain, thyroid, salivary gland, stomach, heart and joint scans.

tectum: (1) the corpora quadrigemina and closely associated components of the midbrain dorsal to the cerebral aqueduct; (2) any roof-like structure.

Teflon: a trade name for tetrafluoroethane homopolymer (polytetrafluoroethylene). It is used for test tubes and other laboratory items, and as an inert coating for syringes.

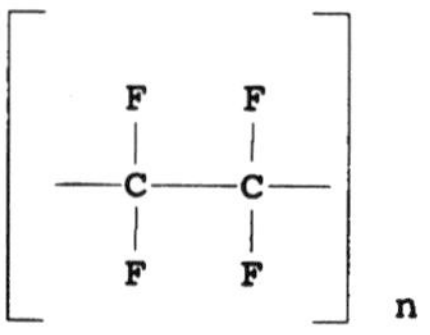

tegmentum: usually, (1) the part of the midbrain between the tectum (definition 1) and the crus cerebri, that contains the red nucleus. It merges with the tegmentum of the pons and subthalamus; (2) a covering structure.

tegument: a covering or enveloping structure.

teichoic acids: acidic polymers with numerous phosphodiester linkages, made by gram positive bacteria. The types in cell membranes contain alanyl and glycosyl-substituted polyglycerol phosphate chains. Cell wall types, which contain polyribitol phosphate chains, are more diverse and account for 10-50% of the dry weights of the walls. In the structures shown, R represents glycosyl groups.

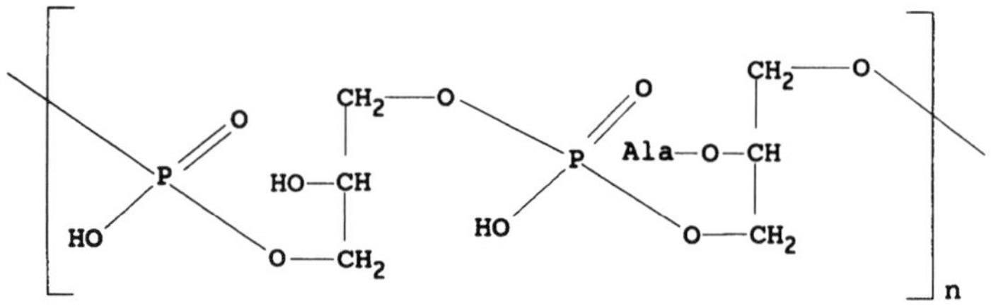

membrane types

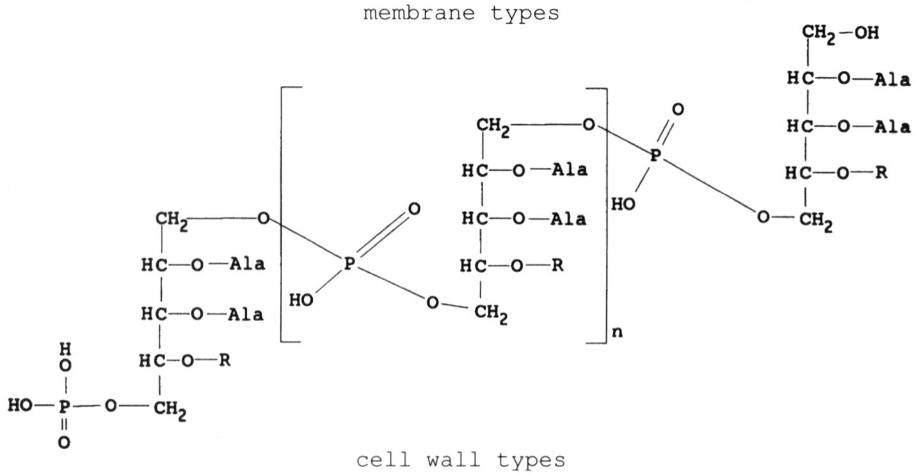

cell wall types

teichoic acids

tektin: an intermediate filament protein component of the walls shared by A and B microtubule doublets.

tela-: a prefix meaning web or woven.

telangiectasis: spider-like lesions in skin and/or mucous membranes formed by permanently dilated small blood vessels.

tele-: telo-: a prefix meaning (1) end; (2) distant.

teleceptor; teloreceptor: a structure specialized for perception of light, sound, or other stimuli that originate in the external environment; *cf* **interoceptor**.

telencephalon: the largest component of the forebrain. It includes the cerebral hemispheres and lateral ventricles (but not the thalamus).

telenzepine: 4,9-dihydro-3-methyl-[(4-methyl-1-piperazinyl)acetyl]-10*H*-thieno[3,4-*b*][1,5]benzodiazepin-10-one; a very potent muscarinic receptor antagonist with highest affinity for M_1 subtypes, especially effective for inhibiting hydrochloric acid production in the stomach.

teleocalcins: 40-50K species specific glycopeptides with disulfide bonds made by Stannius corpuscles of bony fishes, that inhibit calcium transport.

telocentric: describes one-armed replicating chromosomes with terminally located "centromeres".

telodendrons: teleodendrons: fine neuron terminal branches.

telogen: the resting phase of a hair growth cycle; *cf* **anagen**.

telolecithal: describes egg cells or oocytes with yolk concentrated in the vegetal hemispheres.

telomeres: 2-20 kilobase sequences with tandemly repeated TTAGGG base sequences on the extreme ends of chromosomes. They contribute to genetic stability by enabling transcription of base sequences located near the chromosome ends, blocking DNA exonuclease catalyzed degradation, and preventing end-to-end chromosome fusion.

telopeptides: linear peptides located at the ends of helical proteins.

telophase: the final stage of cell division, during which new nuclear membranes form. It is usually, but not necessarily associated with cytokinesis.

telepheron: a hypothetical regulator that attracts gonocytes to indifferent gonads.

teloreceptor: teleceptor.

TEM: (1) triethylenemelamine; (2) transmission electron microscopy.

temperature sensitive mutants: variant forms of bacteria (or other organisms) that can either survive and function only when maintained in a restricted ("permissive") range of environmental temperatures, or overtly display their mutant characteristics only within a restricted temperature range.

template: a mold or pattern, for example a DNA strand that directs synthesis of nucleic acid molecules with complementary bases. Template RNA is messenger RNA (which directs amino acid alignment).

tenascin: myotendinous antigen; glioma mesenchymal extracellular matrix antigen; J1 glycoprotein; an extracellular adhesive glycoprotein composed of six disulfide-linked peptide chains; *see* also **cytotactin**. It is most abundant in embryonic tissues, but is also made by neuroglia cells, and is implicated as a mediator of tissue repair following inflammation. It decreases monocyte adhesion to fibronectin and suppresses some immune system responses. Since tenascin accumulates in the stromas of malignant mammary gland tumors, it is used as a marker for such cells.

tendon[s]: dense connective tissue cords that attach muscles to bone periosteum.

tendon organs: Golgi tendon organs; small structures within tendons or junctions between muscles and tendons that are activated when tendons are stretched. They initiate reflexes that inhibit contraction of the associated muscles.

tendon reflex: *see* **tendon organs**.

Tenormin: a trade name for atenolol.

Tensilon: a trade name for edrophonium chloride.

TEPA: triethylenephosphoramide.

TEPP: tetraethyl pyrophosphate.

teprotide: *p*Glu-Trp-Pro-Arg-Pro-Gln-Ile-Pro-Pro; an angiotensin converting enzyme (ACE, kininogen II) inhibitor used to treat some forms of hypertension. It blocks kallidin degradation as well as angiotensin I conversion to angiotensin II.

teratogenic: capable of causing gross developmental abnormalities.

teratomas: malignant neoplasms that contain pluripotential embryonal carcinoma cells. Most types have three or more different kinds of tissues, none of which occur normally at that site, or cells derived from all three embryonic germ layers.

terazosin: 1-(4-amino-6,7-dimethoxy-2-quinazolinyl)-4-[(tetrahydro-2-furanyl)carbonyl]piperazine; a water soluble, long-acting α_1-type adrenergic receptor antagonist with properties similar to those described for prazosin.

terbutaline: 1-(3,5-dihydroxyphenyl)-2-(*tert*-butylamino) ethanol; a β_2-type adrenergic receptor agonist used as a bronchodilator. It also relaxes uterine smooth muscle,

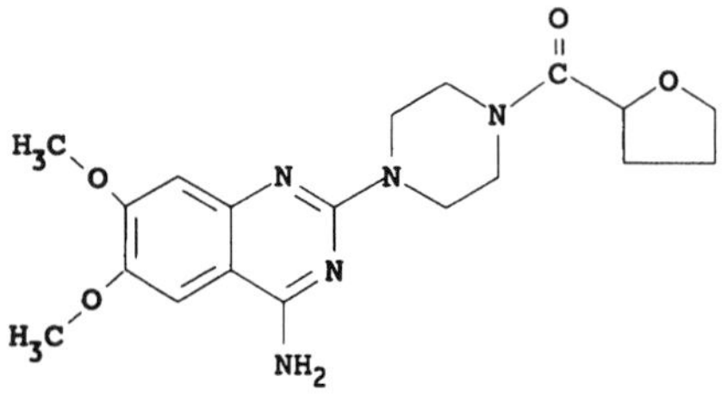

terazosin

and has been administered to protect against premature parturition. Although it can delay birth for a limited time period, during which interventions such as glucocorticoid administration (to promote surfactant production) can be accomplished, it has not proven effective for long-term delay.

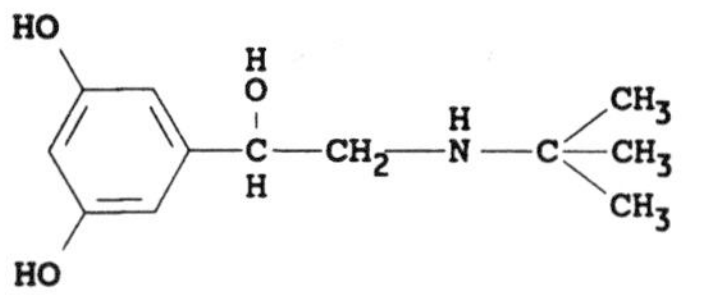

terbutaline

terconazole: triaconazole; *cis*-1-[4-[[2-(2,4-dichloro-phenyl)-2-(1*H*-1,2,4-triazol-1-ylmethyl)-1,3-dioxolan-4-yl]methoxy]phenyl]-4-(1-methylethyl)piperazine; an antifungal agent that inhibits sterol 14-methylase (a microsomal P-450 enzyme essential for ergosterol synthesis).

terfenadine: Seldane; α-[4-(1,1-dimethylethyl)phenyl]-4-(hydroxydiphenylmethyl)-1-piperidinebutanol; an H_1-type histamine receptor antagonist that does not invoke drowsiness.

terguride: *N,N*-dimethyl-*N'*-[(8α)-6-methylergolin-8-yl] urea; a D_1-type dopamine receptor agonist with properties similar to those of lisuride. It is used to treat hyperprolactinemia and acromegaly, and is under investigation for possible beneficial effects in Parkinson's and Huntington diseases.

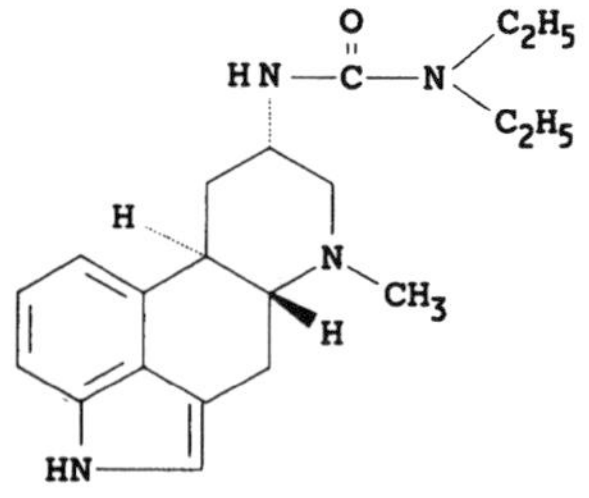

teriparatide acetate: an acetic acid ester of the first 34 amino acids of parathyroid hormone, used to distinguish between hypoparathyroidism (in which blood Ca^{2+}, urinary cAMP, and urinary phosphate rise in response to the agent) from pseudohypoparathyroidsm, and is under investigation for the treatment of osteoporosis.

terlipressin: Glypressin; 1-triglycyl-8-lysine vasopressin; a lysine vasopressin analog that is metabolized to lysine vasopressin. It contracts vascular smooth muscle and is used to control esophageal and uterine bleeding. The cysteines in the structure shown are linked by an S-S bond: Gly-Gly-Gly-Cys-Tyr-Phe-Gln-Asn-Cys-Pro-Lys-Gly-NH2

terminal cisternae: continuous sarcoplasmic reticulum membrane channels that surround skeletal muscle myofibril Z disks and adjacent T tubules. They store Ca^{2+}, and release it when the cells are stimulated.

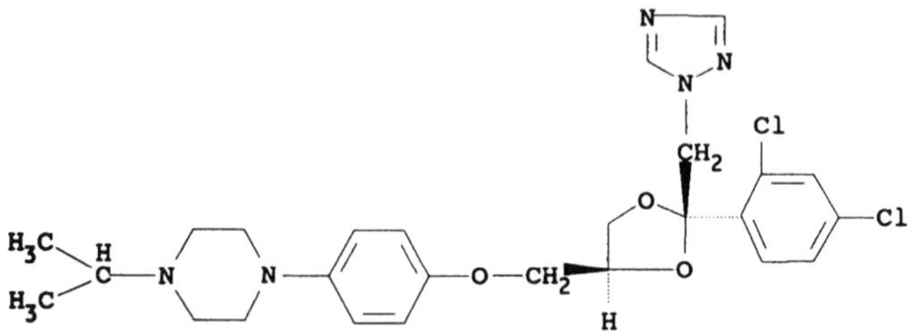

terconazole

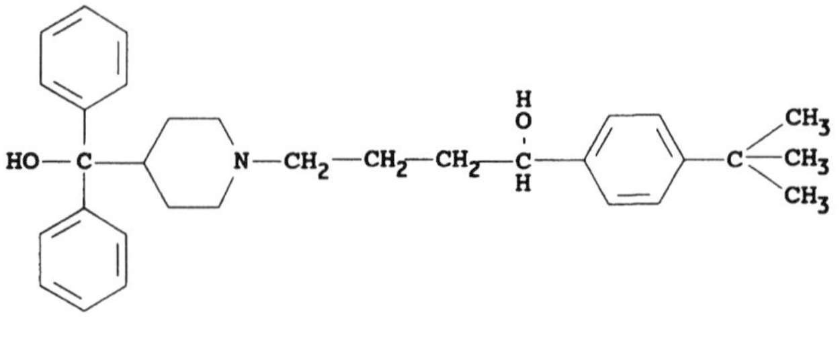

terfenadine

terminal deoxynucleotidyl transferase: Tdt; a template-independent enzyme that catalyzes addition of deoxynucleoside-triphosphates to the 3′—OH ends of DNA molecules and their fragments. It is expressed by some hematopoietic precursor bone marrow cells, by immature B lymphocytes at the stage when heavy chain immunoglobulin joint regions are formed, and by most cortical thymocytes (in which it is believed to be essential for acquisition of receptor specificity). The numbers of Tdt⁺ bone marrow cells increase in individuals with acute lymphocytic and some other forms of leukemia. The enzyme is used as a marker for immature lymphocytes, and to create cohesive ends for constructing recombinant DNAs that can be cloned.

terminally differentiated: describes cells that have achieved their highest levels of specialization. Most kinds lose their capacity for proliferation; and many physiological and pharmacological agents that accelerate the maturation inhibit proliferation. Some acquire features that lead to senescence; but skeletal muscle cells and neurons are among the long-lived types.

terminal webs: intermediate filament networks in the cortical regions of intestinal epithelial cells that anchor the parallel bands of microvilli actin filaments, and similar filament networks that occur elsewhere, for example in desmosomes.

termination codons: stop codons; UAA, UGA, and UAG; RNA triplets that terminate translation (usually when all the required amino acids have been assembled). In eukaryotes, they are recognized by a 56.5K termination factor that facilitates peptide release from the ribosome. In prokaryotes, the codons (ochre, amber, and opal) are recognized by three bacterial proteins. Some mutant transfer RNAs, and some factors made under conditions of nutrient deprivation can overcome the effects of the signals.

terodiline: 4,4-diphenyl-2-(*tert*-butylamino)butane; a vasodilator that blocks some Ca^{2+}-mediated, and some muscarinic type acetylcholine-mediated actions. It is used to treat urinary incontinence, and angina pectoris.

terofenamate: 2-[(2,6-dichloro-3-methylphenyl)-amino] benzoic acid ethoxymethyl ester; a nonsteroidal anti-inflammatory agent, used mostly in individuals who do not respond to or are allergic to other NSAIDs.

terpenes: unsaturated hydrocarbons composed of isoprene units, with formulas for monoterpenes, diterpenes, and sesquiterpenes of $C_{10}H_{16}$, $C_{15}H_{24}$, and $C_{20}H_{32}$, respectively. Large amounts are made by plant cells, and are components of many resins and oils. Animal types include squalene. Dolichol and retinoic acid are terpene derivatives. Several types are toxic when ingested or applied to the skin. Pinene and limonene can injure skin. Thujone and camphor are among the kinds that stimulate the central nervous system. Eucalyptus is a mild irritant used in some expectorant cough preparations. In common with camomile (a component of some teas), it can depress the central nervous system and irritate the kidneys and urinary bladder.

terpin: 4-hydroxy-α-α-4-trimethylcyclohexane methanol; a synthetic terpene derivative. It is a mild irritant, and a component of some expectorant cough preparations.

tertiary structure of proteins: *see* **proteins**.

Teslac: a trade name for testolactone.

test cross: procedures for defining the genotypes of individuals who express dominant phenotypes for one or more genes. If they are homozygous for the dominant trait, all matings with homozygous recessives yield heterozygous progeny that also display the dominant phenotypes. If all of the parents are heterozygous, the probability that progeny will display the recessive form is 1 in 4.

testes: *see* **testis**.

testibumin: A Sertoli cell protein chemically related to albumin and α-fetoprotein, induced by follicle stimulating hormone (FSH) and testosterone. In rodents, the levels are highest at puberty onset.

testicular feminization: a sex differentiation disorder caused by androgen receptor defects that block the ability to respond to testosterone and dihydrotestosterone. Individuals with male-type sex chromosomes have testes, but acquire female type external genitalia and secondary sex characteristics. Although Wolffian ducts do not develop, and external reproductive organs do not undergo virilization, Müllerian ducts usually degenerate (since responses to Müllerian duct inhibitor are retained). When gonadotropin levels rise at puberty, testicular androgen secretion accelerates, and aromatization provides estrogens in amounts sufficient to promote mammary gland maturation and acquisition of other female secondary sex characteristics.

testicular fluid: fluid produced by Sertoli cells and secreted into seminiferous tubule lumens. It facilitates transport of immature spermatozoa to the epididymides, and carries androgens, androgen binding protein, and other regulators.

testins: two related proteins made by Sertoli cells of testes that contain germinal cells. *See* also **testis determining genes**.

testis [testes]: testicle; the male gonad. The vertebrate components include seminiferous tubules with Sertoli and germinal cells (spermatogonia, spermatocytes, and immature spermatozoa), interstitial (Leydig) cells that secrete testosterone, and contractile myoid cells that contribute to humoral controls.

testis determining antigen: TDA; testis determining factor; Tdf; *see* **testis determining genes**.

testis determining factor: Tdf; *see* **testis determining genes**.

testis determining genes: DNA segments on Y chromosomes that initiate masculinization of mammalian embryos. A 14 kilobase region known as *SRY* (*TDF*) in humans, and *sry* (*Tdy*) in mice, codes for a species specific DNA binding protein that acts on gonadal ridge somatic cells, which then differentiate to pre-Sertoli types, associate with prespermatogonia, and align to form primitive spermatic cords. The genes are believed to serve as genetic switches that turn on other (autosome and/or X chromosome) genes required to complete the differentiation and then maintain reproductive system functions. In XY mice, sry protein can be detected for approximately 1.5 days, during the time that immediately precedes organization of indifferent gonads to embryonic testes. Its expression is not dependent on the presence of germinal cells (and can occur in animals with Steel and White spotting gene mutations.) The genes are never expressed in normal females, or in any mature male structure other than the testes. Mutant XY mice that lack *sry* develop into phenotypic females, whereas some transgenic XX animals that carry *sry* acquire testes and normal male phenotypes; *see* **sxr**. Human *SRY* does not invoke sex reversal in mice, probably because the protein contains a 27 amino acid segment different from the mouse type. It has been been identified in XX men; and *SRY* deletions occur in XY women. Older concepts that the genes code for H-Y antigen or for the zinc-finger proteins Zfy-1 and Zfy-2 have been discarded.

testolactone: Teslac; Fludestrin; D-homo-17α-oxandrosta-1,4-diene,3,17-dione; an aromatase inhibitor used to lower estrogen levels in women with breast cancer, and as a laboratory tool.

testonolactone: testolactone.

testosterone: T; the major gonadal steroid made by testicular interstitial cells. It acts directly on Wolffian ducts, skeletal muscle, and a few other structures, and may exert some special influences on the testes. However, reduction to 5α-dihydrotestosterone (DHT) is essential for the effects of physiological levels on most target organs. Other metabolites used at special sites include androstanediols and 5β-dihydrotestosterone. In addition to supporting spermatogenesis, androgens promote maturation of accessory reproductive organs and secondary sex characteristics, and maintain the functions of the adult system. They also exert anabolic influences on skeletal muscle, bone, visceral organs, sebaceous glands, hair follicles and other structures, stimulate libido in both males and females, and exert negative feedback control over LH and GnRH secretion. In at least some species, they promote aggression, territorial behavior, and pheromone production. Although human behavior is controlled by many non-hormonal factors, physiological androgen levels impart a sense of well-being; and the large amounts of anabolic steroids used illicitly by some atheletes do invoke aggression and other psychological effects. LH stimulates androgen production in ovaries, and small amounts circulate in women; but most ovarian testosterone is rapidly aromatized to estrogens. Testosterone secretion is constitutive in embryos. The cells soon acquire receptors, and make larger amounts in response to chorionic gonadotropin (hCG). When the adenohypophysis and circulatory systems mature sufficiently, LH becomes the major stimulant, and this continues throughout postnatal life. *See* also **adrenal androgens**.

5α-dihydro-testosterone: DHT; the major biologically active testosterone metabolite; *see* **testosterone**.

5β-dihydro-testosterone: a testosterone metabolite that stimulates hematopoiesis.

testosterone binding globulin: *see* **testosterone-estrogen binding protein**.

testosterone-estrogen binding protein: TeBG; sex hormone binding globulin; SHBG; a 95K plasma β-globulin secreted by the liver that binds gonadal steroids. The amino acid sequences are similar to those of androgen binding proteins (ABPs). Estrogens and thyroid hormones stimulate, whereas androgens inhibit the production. In addition to facilitating steroid transport through the bloodstream, TeBG serves as a readily recruitable source of temporarily inactive hormone, and as a buffer against sudden changes in the content of circulating free hormone. It also slows steroid degradation. Since its affinity is greater for testosterone and dihydrotestosterone than for estradiol, it may protect females against excessive androgen.

tetanus: (1) lock-jaw; the tonic muscle contractions, exaggerated reflexes, and in some cases convulsions caused by activated tetanus toxin; (2) sustained muscle contraction without twitching that can occur when high intensity stimuli are delivered at intervals too short to permit relaxation; *cf* **clonus**. (The muscle fibers soon fatigue if the stimulation is continued. Under physiological conditions, muscle contraction is sustained by successive activation of motor units, so that some fibers relax as others work.)

tetanus toxin: a potent neurotoxin released by *Clostridium tetani* (an anaerobic organism that proliferates in infected wounds). After activation by cleavage to 100K heavy and 50K light chains, the heavy chains bind to disialogangliosides and form membrane pores. The toxin is taken by motor neurons (via retrograde transport), and acts presynaptically as an inhibitor of glycine release that causes tetanus (definition 1).

tetany: exaggerated neuromuscular excitability that can progress to tremors, muscle spasms, and convulsions, usually caused by hypocalcemia (for example in parathyroid hormone deficiency states).

tetrabenazine: 1,3,4,6,7,11b-hexahydro-9,10-dimethoxy-3-(2-methylpropyl)-2*H*-benzoquinolizin-2-one; an inhibitor of catecholamine uptake by synaptic vesicles and secretory granules. Since enzymes rapidly degrade molecules that are not sequestered, it slowly depletes catecholamine stores, and is used a as a tranquilizer.

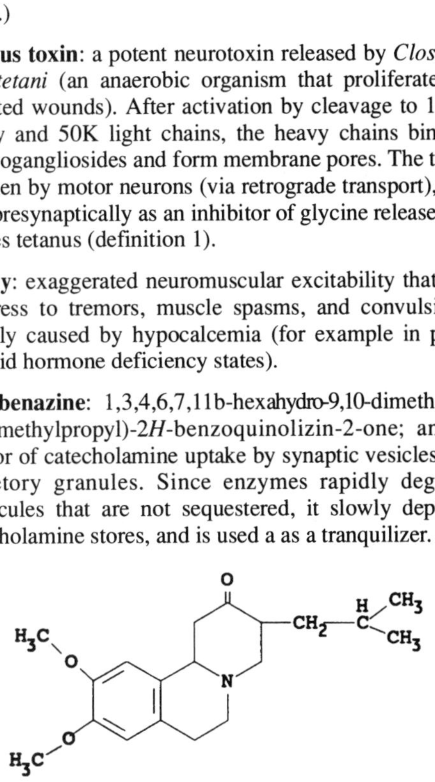

TETRAC: tetraiodothyroacetic acid.

tetracyclines: broad spectrum antibacterial, antirickettsial, and antiamebic compounds made by *Streptomyces* species that block protein synthesis by interfering with aminoacyl-tRNA binding to ribosome A sites. The term can refer specifically to 4-(dimethyl-amino)-1,4,4a,

5,5a,6,11,12a-octahydro-3,6,10,12,12a-pentahydroxy-6-methyl-1-11-dioxo-2-naphthacenecarboxamide (shown below). Since tetracycline attaches to regions of bone mineralization and fluoresces, the rate of new bone growth can be estimated from the distance between two fluorescent sites when two doses, separated by a specified time interval, are administered.

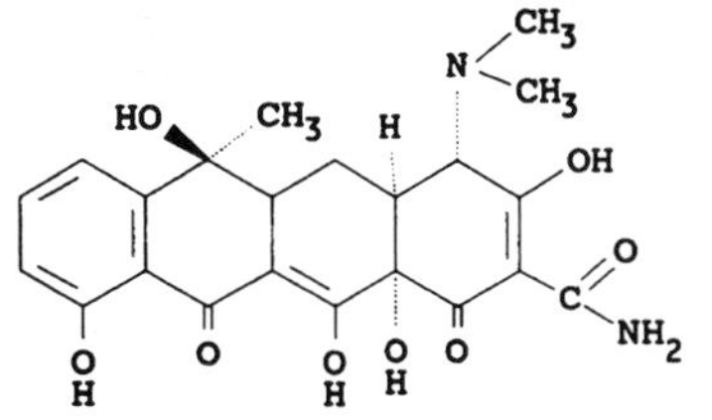

tetrad: the structure formed when homologous chromosomes pair during synapsis, composed of four chromatids, two for each member of the allele pair.

tetraethylammonium: TEA; Etamon; a monovalent cation that blocks voltage-gated potassium channels. The chloride and other derivatives inhibit transmission in autonomic ganglia.

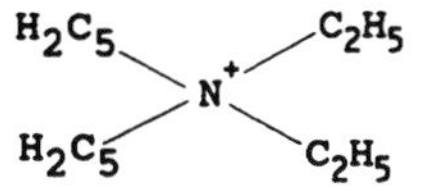

tetraethylpyrophosphate: TEPP: a potent, irreversible inhibitor of acetylcholinesterases.

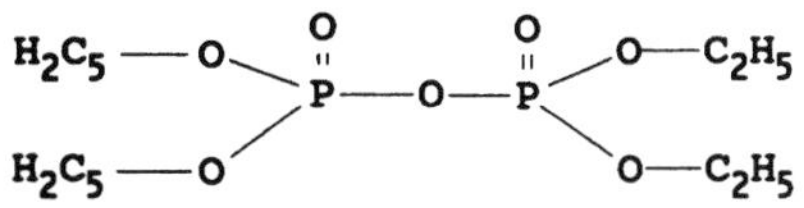

tetrahydrobiopterin: *see* **dihydrobiopterin**.

tetrahydrocannabinol: tetrahydro-6,6,9-trimethyl-3-pentyl-6*H*-dibenzo[b,d]pyran-1-ol. The Δ^1-3,4-*trans* isomer, Δ^9-THC is the active component of marihuana. *See* tetrahydro-**cannabinols**.

tetrahydrocortisol: 3α,17α, 21-trihydroxy-5β-pregnane-11, 20-dione; a cortisol degradation product made mostly from another degradation product, 5β-dihydrocortisol, and converted to cortol. The *allo* isomer (tetrahydro-F) made from 5α-dihydrocortisol is converted to *allo*-cortol.

tetrahydrocortisone: 3α,17α,21-trihydroxy-5β-pregnane-11,20-dione; a cortisone degradation product made from 5-β-dihydrocortisone and convertible to a cortolone. The *allo* isomer (tetrahydro-E) is made from 5α-dihydrocortisone.

tetrahydrofolic acid {**tetrahydrofolate**}: *see* **folic acid**.

Tetrahymena pyriformis: an easily cultured ciliated protozoan that adapts to a wide range of environmental conditions. It is used for studies of palindrome formation, gene amplification, RNA processing, evolution, and protozoan nutrition.

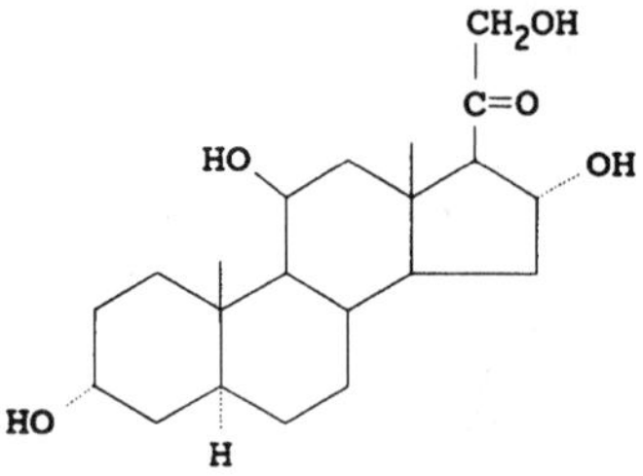

3α-tetrahydrocortisol

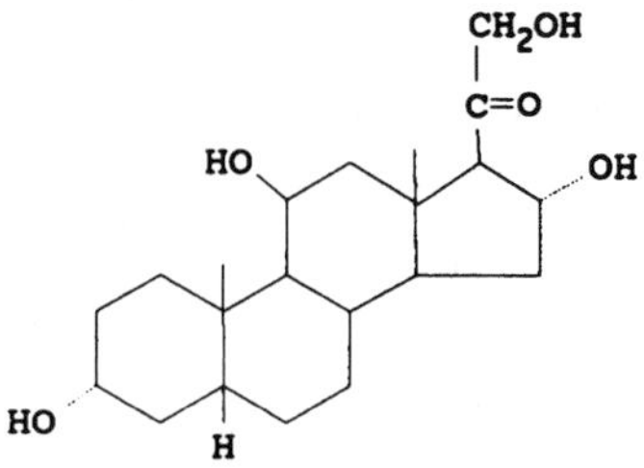

allo-tetrahydrocortisol

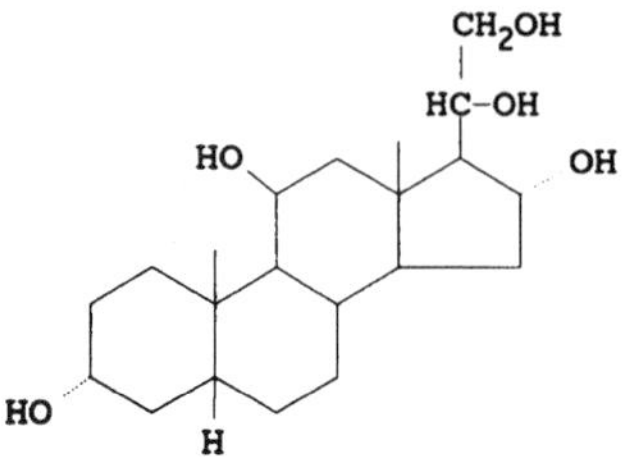

cortol

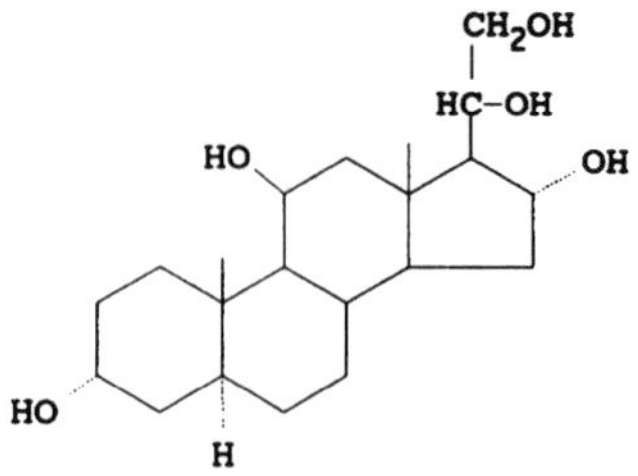

allo-cortol

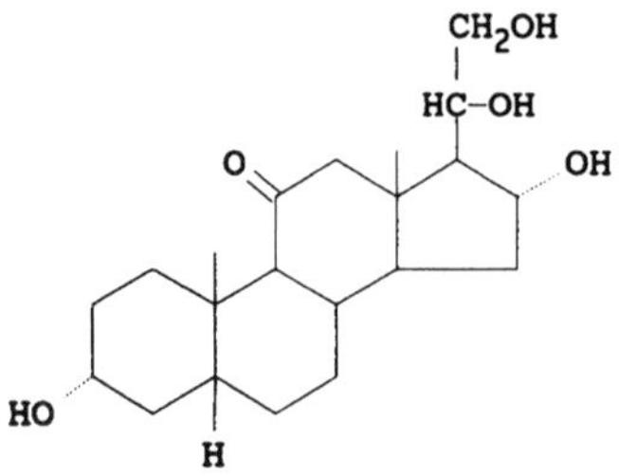

tetrahydrocortisone

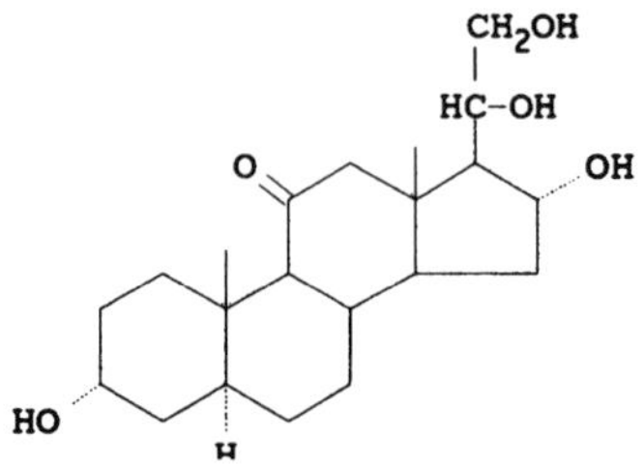

allo-tetrahydrocortisone

tetraiodothyroacetic acid: TETRAC; a thyroid hormone metabolite less potent than triiodothyroacetic acid.

tetraiodothyronine: T_4; *see* **thyroxine**.

4,5,6,7-tetrahydroisoxazolo[4,5-*c*-]-pyridin-3-ol: an inhibitor of neuronal gamma aminoisobutyric acid (GABA) uptake.

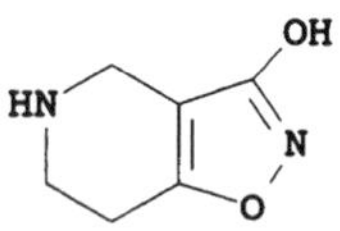

tetrakis: having four substitutions, as in tetrakis inositolphosphate (with four phosphate groups).

tetramer: an entity composed of four parts (usually a protein with four peptide chains).

tetraploid: having four complete sets of haploid chromosomes.

tetrapods: four-footed animals, a term usually applied to mammals, amphibians, and some reptiles.

tetrasomy: the presence of four homologous chromosomes of one type (two more than the number usually present in a diploid cell).

tetrazepam: 7-chloro-5-(1-cyclohexen-1-yl)-1,3-dihydro-1-methyl-2*H*-1,4-benzodiazepin-2-one; a **diazepine** *(q.v.)* used as a muscle relaxant.

tetrazolium blue: BT; 3,3′-dianisol-*bis*-[4,4′-(3,5-diphenyl)tetrazolium chloride; a dye used to study oxidation-reduction reactions, and as a stain for bacteria and molds.

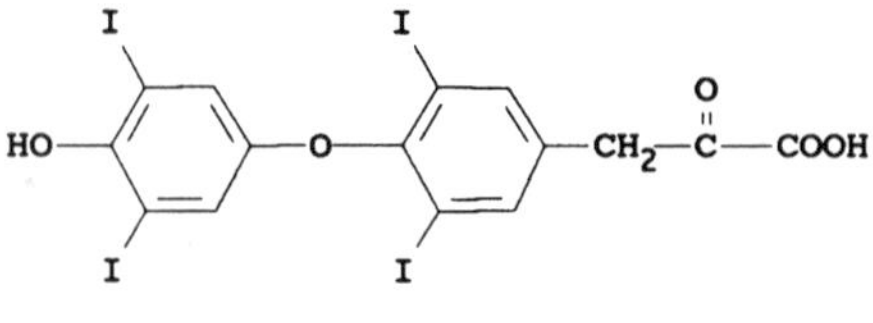

tetraiodothyroacetic acid

tetrazepam

tetrodotoxin: TTX; macrotoxin; fugu toxin; octahydro-12-(hydroxymethyl)-2-imino-5,9:7,10a-dimethano-10a*H*-[1,3]dioxocino[6,5-d]pyrimidine-4,7,10,11,12-pentol;a toxin in the liver, skin, and ovaries of the Japanese puffer fish of the *Tetraodontoidea* family, and in the California newt, *Taricha torosa*. It specifically blocks voltage-gated sodium channels, and can be used to determine the numbers of such channels per cell. If ingested, it can rapidly invoke malaise, convulsions, and respiratory paralysis.

TF: (1) thymidine factor; (2) transcription factor; (3) transfer factor.

TF I, TF II, TF III: *see* **transcription factors**.

***Tfm* mutants**: rodent strains with androgen receptor defects, in which animals with male-type sex chromosomes acquire female phenotypes.

TFP: trifluoperazine.

TG: thioguanine.

TGF-α: *see* **transforming growth factor-α**.

TGF-β: *see* **transforming growth factor-β**.

Th: thorium.

thalamus: the largest component of the diencephalon. It surrounds the upper two thirds of the third brain ventricle, contains neurons that make many kinds of regulators, relays information from photic, auditory, gustatory, tactile and skeletal muscle receptors to the telencephalon, and contributes to coordination of skeletal muscle movements.

thalassemia: several hereditary forms of anemia caused by deletion or partial inactivation of one or more genes that direct globin subunit synthesis. The symptoms vary inversely with the amounts of normal hemoglobin made. *Thalassemia major* (Mediterranean anemia, Cooley's anemia), in which two β-globin defects are inherited, causes severe growth retardation and bone defects, and is usually fatal before the time of puberty.

thalidomide: 3-phthalimidoglutarimide; an agent formerly used as a sedative and hypnotic, and to control the nausea and vomiting associated with pregnancy. Although apparently harmless when tested in small laboratory animals, it severely impairs organogenesis in humans. Phocomelia is the most common defect in infants whose mothers took the drug during days 20 to 36 of pregnancy. Others include malformations of the face and internal organs. Thalidomide is, however an effective immunosuppressant that can prevent rejection of bone marrow transplants in nonpregnant recipients; and its anti-inflammatory properties appear to be useful for treating leprosy.

thallium: Tl; a metallic element (atomic number 81, atomic weight 204.37), toxic and potentially carcinogenic in low concentrations. [210]TlCl is used in radiology.

thanat-: thanato-; a prefix meaning death.

thapsigargin: a naturally occurring tumor-promoting sesquiterpene lactone that enters cells, inhibits endoplasmic reticulum Ca^{2+}-ATPases in hepatic and several other cell types, and elevates cytoplasmic Ca^{2+} by promoting inositol-phosphate independent discharge of the ions. The secondary effects include stimulation of arachidonic acid metabolism in macrophages, histamine discharge

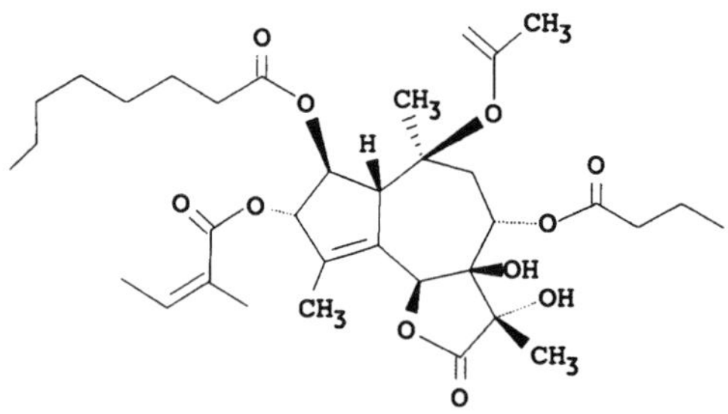

thapsigargin

from mast cells, and blood platelet aggregtion. It is less potent for the cardiac muscle sarcoplasmic reticulum enzyme, and does not act on the Ca^{2+}-ATPases of skeletal muscle sarcoplasmic reticulum or plasma membranes, on Mg^{2+}-ATPases, or on kinase C. It is used as a probe for intracellular Ca^{2+} storage and release processes.

T_H cells: helper-type **T lymphocytes** (*q.v.*). Two subsets (T_{H1} and T_{H2}) have been described.

Δ^9-THC: *see* tetrahydro-**cannabinol**.

THE: *allo*-tetrahydrocortisol.

thebaine: dimethylmorphine; 6,7,8,14-tetrahydro-4,5-epoxy-3,6,-dimethoxy-17-methylmorphinan; an opium alkaloid that can invoke convulsions and strychnine-like muscle spasms when used as in analgesic dosages. Brain cells make minute amounts and can convert it to morphine.

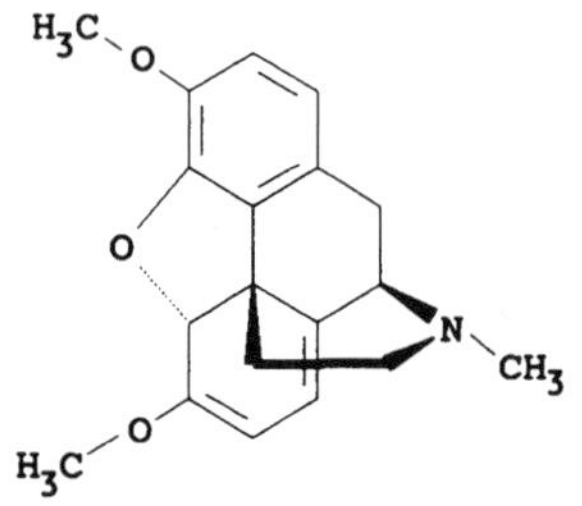

theca: a sheath.

theca externa: an external sheath. The term usually refers to the outer theca layers of ovarian follicles; *see* **theca folliculi** and *cf* **theca interna**.

theca folliculi: the theca interna and theca externa of a vesicular ovarian follicle.

theca interna: an internal sheath; usually, the cell layer closest to the stratum granulosum of an ovarian follicle that carries blood vessels, contributes to steroid hormone production, and is surrounded by the theca externa.

thelarche: the beginning of breast development at puberty.

thelium [thelia]: nipple.

thenyldiamine hydrochloride: *N,N*-dimethyl-*N'*-2-pyridinyl-*N'*-(3-thienylmethyl)-1,2-ethanediamine hydrochloride; an H_1-type histamine receptor antagonist used for preoperative sedation, analgesia potentiation, and control of postoperative nausea.

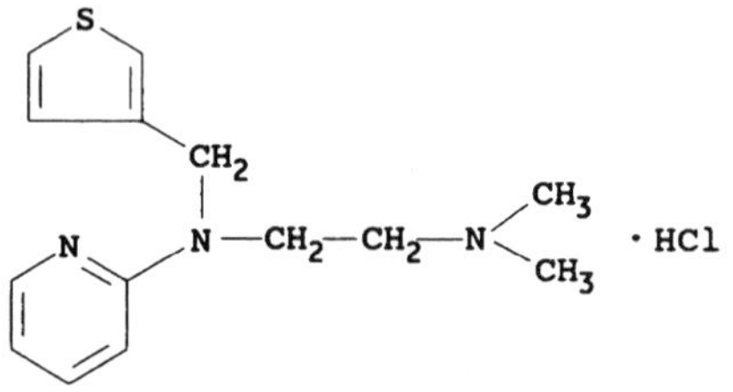

theobromine: 3,7-dimethylxanthine; an alkaloid in cacao beans (and chocolate), and in smaller amounts in cola nuts and tea. It inhibits cAMP-phosphodiesterases, stimulates smooth muscle contraction, and is used as a diuretic, cardiac stimulant, and vasodilator.

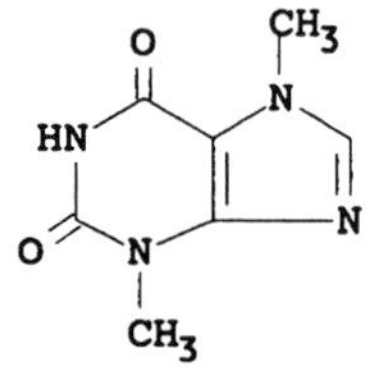

theofibrate: 2-(4-chlorophenoxy)-2-methylpropanoic acid 2-(1,2,3,6-tetrahydro-1,3-dimethyl-2,6-dioxo-7*H*-purin- 7-yl)ethyl ester; a clofibrate derivative that inhibits platelet aggregation and lowers lipoprotein levels.

theophylline: 1,3-dimethylxanthine; an alkaloid in tea leaves that inhibits cAMP-phosphodiesterases and affects intracellular calcium translocation. Its anti-inflammatory properties are attributed to adenosine receptor antagonism. It is a more potent central nervous system stimulant than theobromine, but less effective than caffeine. Several preparations are used as diuretics, vasodilators, cardiac stimulants, and smooth muscle relaxants.

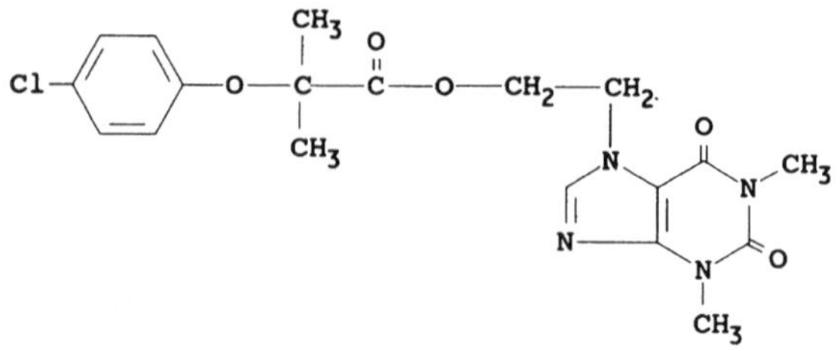

theofibrate

theophylline

theory: a set of concepts used to explain a process or phenomenon, usually established after hypotheses have been investigated.

thermodynamics: the quantitative study of factors that govern conversion of one form of energy to another, the availability of energy for work, and the direction of heat flow. *See* **first**, **second**, and **third laws** of thermodynamics.

thermogenesis: heat production; calorigenesis.

thermogenic drinking: increased water intake in response to warm environmental temperatures.

thermogenin: a 64K homodimeric inner mitochondrial membrane protein, abundant in brown adipose tissue that mediates the major form of nonshivering thermogenesis, contributes to arousal from hibernation, and may play roles in control of body weight and fat content. It binds guanosine diphosphate (GDP), augments proton and chloride conductance, and elevates metabolic rates by dissipating proton gradients and uncoupling oxidative phosphorylation. Norepinephrine and other regulators rapidly increase its affinity for GDP and mediate early responses to cold. Slowly developing, long-term acclimation depends more on thyroid hormone-mediated increases in mitochondrial thermogenin content.

thermography: techniques in which infrared cameras record heat radiation and body surface temperatures, used to obtain information on cancer cell locations and activity levels.

thermolysin: a 37.5K zinc and glutamate-containing neutral proteolytic enzyme made by *Bacillus thermoproteolyticus*, with properties similar to those of enkephalinases. It cleaves peptide bonds formed with amino groups of aliphatic and phenylalanine moieties, and is used to define amino acid sequences.

thermophilic: heat-loving; describes microorganisms that grow optimallly at temperatures of 50°-70°C.

thermoregulation: body temperature control.

thermotaxis: movement in response to a temperature gradient, positive when toward a heat source and negative in the opposite direction.

theta: the Greek letter θ.

theta antigen: a cell surface marker on most thymocytes and peripheral T lymphocytes.

THF: (1) tetrahydrofolate; (2) thymic humoral factor.

thiaminase: an enzyme in raw fish that degrades thiamine to pyrimidine and thiazole end products, used

for nutrition studies. Large amounts can cause thiamine deficiency in humans on vitamin deficient diets.

thiamine: thiamin; vitamin B_1; antineuritic vitamin; antiberiberi factor; 3-[(4-amino-2-methyl-4-pyrimidinal)methyl]-5-(2-hydroxyethyl)-4-methylazonium; a vitamin B complex component required to make **thiamine pyrophosphate** (*q.v.*). "Dry" beri-beri is a defiency disease characterized by poor appetite, rapid weight loss, skeletal muscle weakness, enlargement of the heart, peripheral neuritis, sensory defects, anxiety, mental confusion, and, in some cases, hallucinations. In "wet" beri-beri, the weight loss is less easily detected because of edema. Vitamin supplements contain it in the form of chlorides or nitrates.

thiamine

thiamine hydrochloride hydrochloride

thiamine pyrophosphate: TPP: co-carboxylase; a coenzyme synthesized from thiamine and ATP. It is a component of complexes that convert pyruvate to acetyl-CoA and α-ketoglutarate to succinyl-CoA, and oxidize other keto-acids. It is also required for the transketolase reactions of hexose monophosphate and photosynthesis pathways. The highly reactive second carbon atom of the thiazole ring (indicated by an asterisk) gives up a proton to form a carbanion, and the neighboring nitrogen atom stabilizes the ionic shift. When linked to the decarboxylase component of the pyruvate dehydrogenase complex (PD), the carbanion reacts directly with the carbonyl group of pyruvate, which takes up the proton. The complex then rearranges electrons to form a linkage that destabilizes the carboxyl group of the pyruvate, and CO_2 is ejected, leaving behind a hydroxyethyl-TPP intermediate. The same dehydrogenase transfers the hydroxyethyl group to the lipoic acid component of lipoamide (a co-factor linked by a lysyl nitrogen moiety to the transacylase of the pyruvate dehydrogenase complex). An acetyllipoamide derivative is formed, and thiamine-PP is released. The transacylase then transfers the acetyl group to coenzyme A to yield a dihydrolipoic acid derivative + acetyl-CoA. Finally, the lipoamide is restored to its oxidized form via a reaction catalyzed by the dehydrogenase of the enzyme complex that uses NAD^+.

thiamphenicol: D-threo-2,2-dichloro-*N*-[β-hydroxy-α-(hydroxymethyl)-*p*-methylsulfonyl)-phenethyl]acet-

thiamine pyrophosphate

thiamine-PP-pyruvate intermediate

α-hydroxy derivative

lipoamide

acetyl-lipoamide group

dihydrolipoamide group

amide; an antibiotic that inhibits mitochondrial oxidation and exerts therapeutic effects similar to those described for chloramphenicol, but does not cause aplastic anemia.

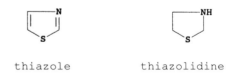

thiazole   thiazolidine

thick filaments: usually, the thick filaments of skeletal muscle myofibrils, composed mostly of **myosin** (*q.v.*). They form cross-bridges with **thin filaments** (*q.v.*) when myosin binds to actin.

thiazides: **chlorothiazide** (*q.v.*), and related benzothiadiazenesulfonamide derivatives used as diuretics.

thigmo-: a prefix meaning touch.

thigmotropic: responding (positively or negatively) to mechanical stimulation.

thiazoles: compounds with 5-membered rings that contain sulfur and nitrogen atoms. Hydrogenated derivatives are thiazolidines.

thin filaments: usually, the thin filaments of skeletal muscle myofibrils. They contain actin, tropomyosin, and troponins. When a skeletal muscle is stimulated, the Ca^{2+} released binds to and changes the configuration of troponin C. Tropomyosin is thereby displaced from the myosin binding sites, and forms cross bridges with myosin. *See* also **sliding filament theory**.

thin layer chromatography: *see* **chromatography**.

thiobarbital: 5,5-diethyl-2-thiobarbituric acid; a short-acting central nervous system depressant with properties similar to those of other barbiturates. It displaces thyroxine from binding sites on plasma proteins, disrupts hepatic metabolism of many compounds, and can interfere with thyroid hormone function.

thioctic acid: α-lipoic acid.

thiocyanate: (1) any compound of the general type R—S—C≡N; (2) the —S—C=N⁻ ion. It competes with iodide for transport, promotes iodide extrusion form thyroid gland cells, and thereby interferes with thyroxine biosynthesis. Some thiocyanates are present in cigarette smoke, and small amounts are made from cysteine-rich foods such as cabbage and kale. Since it can invoke histotoxic anemia, its use as a vasodilator has been discontinued.

thioesters: compounds of the general types shown. Some are high energy intermediates in biochemical pathways (for example for oxidation of glyceraldehyde-3-phosphate in glycolysis). Similar linkages anchor some proteins to membrane lipids; *see* also **prenylation**.

5-D-**thioglucose**: a glucose analog that inhibits glucose transport and glucose-mediated insulin release by competing for the carrier. It kills some neoplastic cells, is a reversible inhibitor of spermatogenesis, and is used as a laboratory tool for studying the effects of hypoglycemia and other aspects of carbohydrate metabolism.

thioglycolic acid: mercaptoacetic acid (*see* also **mercaptoethanol**); an agent that breaks disulfide bonds and combines with metals. Combinations with bismuth and other metals are components of some medications. Ammonium salts are the active ingredients of permanent wave and hair-stretching lotions; and calcium salts are used as depilatories. Thioglycolates are sensitive reagents for detecting iron, silver, molybdenum, and tin. They also protect tryptophan in amino acid analyses, and are used in the preparation of some bacteriological media, but have been replaced by different agents for denaturing proteins for electrophoresis and other investigative purposes.

$$HS—CH_2—COOH$$

thioguanine: TG; 2-aminopurine-6-thiol, a guanine analog that disrupts DNA synthesis by interfering with purine and ribonucleotide synthesis. It is used to treat acute granulocytic, acute lymphocytic, and chronic granulocytic leukemias.

thiokinases: acyl-CoA synthases; enzymes that catalyze reactions in which addition of —SH groups is coupled to ATP hydrolysis. Fatty acid "activation", fatty acid + ATP + HS—CoA → fatty-acyl—CoA + AMP + P-P, is catalyzed by fatty acid thiokinase.

thiokinin: a rat $α_1$-type acute phase protein chemically related to T kininogen, made in the liver and secreted to the bloodstream. It may be identical with $α_2$-cysteine protease inhibitor.

thiolases: enzymes with —SH groups that catalyze reactions in which acetyl-coenzyme A is used to cleave compounds with —C—S— bonds. β-ketothiolases of fatty acid oxidation cycles catalyze reactions of the general type: fatty-acyl-CoA (with *n* carbon atoms) + HS-CoA → fatty acyl-CoA (*n*-2 carbons) + acetyl-CoA.

thiol proteases: chymotrypsin, papain, and other proteolytic enzymes whose catalytic sites contain cysteine.

thioneine: ergothioneine; erythrothionine; thiolhistidinebetaine; an amine initially identified in ergot (*Claviceps purpurea*) but also made by *Neurospora crassa* and other fungi. Healthy mammals synthesize small amounts from histidine in liver, kidneys, and some other organs, release it to blood, semen, and urine, and accumulate it in erythrocytes. Some neoplasms make large amounts.

thionine: 3,7-diamino-5-phenothiazinium; a dye used to stain chromatin, Nissl granules, and mucins.

thionine

thiopanic acid: pantoyl taurine; a compound that competes with pantothenic acid, used to inhibit the growth of bacteria.

thiopental sodium: pentothal sodium; thionembutal; 5-ethyl-5-(1-methylbutyl)-2-thiobarbituric acid; a very short-acting compound chemically similar to **thiobarbital** (*q.v.*). It is used intravenously for induction of anesthesia and transient relaxation, and in psychiatry. Large amounts inhibit sympathetic nervous system neurons and can cause serious hypotension and respiratory depression.

thioperamide: *N*-cyclohexyl-4-I(imidazol-4-yl)-1-piperidinecarbothioamide; a competitive H$_3$ type histamine receptor antagonist, used for its central actions.

thioperazine: thioproperazine; 3-dimethylsulfamoyl-10-[3-(4-methylpiperazino)propyl]phenothiazine; a phenothiazine used as an analeptic, and to control emesis.

thioredoxins: ubiquitous acidic proteins with disulfide isomerase activity, made by T4 phage, bacteria and other small organisms, and by higher animals. Most contain around 108 amino acids. They participate in numerous hydrogen, electron, and phosphate transfer reactions, reduce disulfide bonds, donate electrons for ribonucleotide reductase (which converts ribonucleotides to deoxyribonucleotides), and reactivate denatured ribonucleotides. The dithiol groups oxidized in the reactions are restored by thioredoxin reductase, a flavoprotein enzyme that transfers electrons and hydrogen from NADH + H$^+$.

thioridazine: Mellaril; 10-[2-(1-methyl-2-piperidyl-)-ethyl]-2-(methylthio)phenothiazine; an orally effective D$_2$ type dopamine receptor antagonist, used as a sedative

and "antipsychotic" agent. High concentrations can cause hypotension.

thiostatin: an acute phase α$_1$ macroglobulin.

thiostrepton: a sulfur-containing polypeptide antibiotic made by *Streptomyces azureus* that inhibits protein synthesis in prokaryotes by blocking attachment of elongation factor EFTu and translocase EF-G to ribosomes.

thio substituted amino acids: amino acid analogs in which sulfur atoms replace some oxygens. Many compete with endogenous counterparts, and are used as antagonists in metabolic studies. Compounds labelled with radioactive S are convenient markers.

thiosulfates: compounds of the general type R—S$_2$O$_3$. Some are reagents, used for example in iodine determinations.

thiosulfate sulfurtransferase: rhodanase; a hepatic enzyme that can protect against cyanide accumulation by catalyzing reactions of the general type: R—S—SO$_3$ + X—C≡N → R—S—C≡N + X—SO$_3$.

thiothixene: *N,N*-dimethyl-9-[3-(4-methyl-1-piperazinyl)propylidene]-2-(dimethylsulfonamido)thioxanthene; a thioxanthene type "antipsychotic" agent that acts on dopamine receptors. It invokes less sedation than chlorprothixene, but is equipotent for effects on the extrapyramidal system, and on blood pressure.

thiouracils: 2-mercapto-4-hydroxypyrimidine (2-thiouracil, shown), and its methyl and propyl derivatives. The compounds block iodide oxidation and incorporation into thyroglobulins by inhibiting thyroid gland peroxidase enzymes, and are used to treat some forms of hyperthyroidism. Since they impair negative feedback control over thyroid stimulating hormone (TSH) secretion, they are goitrogens. Some members of the group additionally inhibit thyroxine conversion to triiodothyronine. The

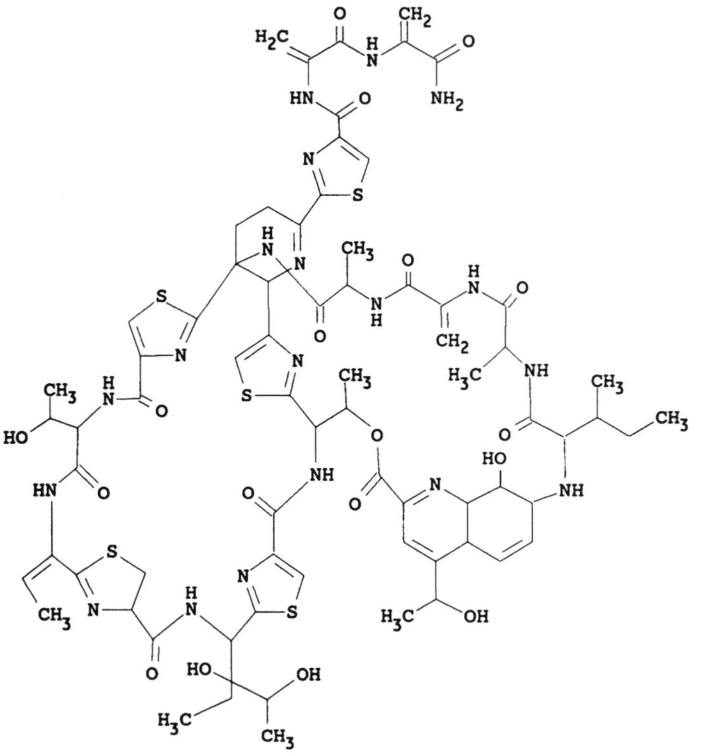

thiostrepton

toxic effects include allergic skin reactions and bone marrow dysfunction. *See* also **propylthiourcil**.

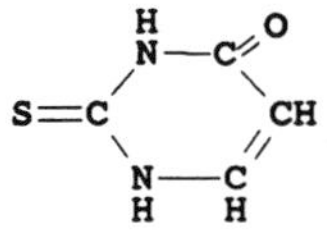

2-thiouracil

thiourea: thiocarbamide; an agent formerly used to inhibit thyroxine synthesis, but replaced by thiouracils, methimazole, and others that exert fewer side effects.

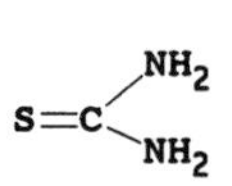

thioxanthene: dibenzthiopyran. The term *thioxanthenes* refers to a group of dopamine receptor antagonists (including thiothixene and chlorprothixene), used as "antipsychotic" agents, that are chemically related to phenothiazines but have the dibenzothiopyran group shown (in which a carbon substitutes for a nitrogen atom).

THIP: 4,5,6,7-tetrahydroisoxazolo[5,4-*c*]pyridin-3(2*H*)-one; a GABA$_A$ type gamma aminobutyric acid receptor antagonist.

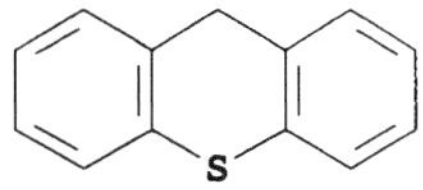

thioxanthene

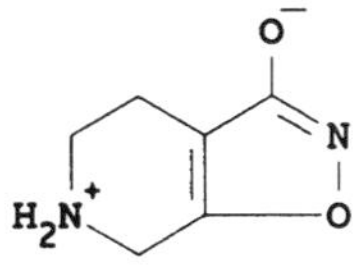

THIP

third eye: a light-sensitive component of the pineal complex of some lizards not involved in visual perception, but believed to contribute to thermoregulation.

third eyelid: nictitating membrane.

third factor: describes an uncharacterized regulator different from aldosterone and vasopressin that contributes to the control of renal water and electrolyte excretion. It is used synonymously with natriuretic hormone by some authors. *See* also **atrial peptides**.

third law of thermodynamics: at a temperature of absolute zero (0°K), molecules become motionless and zero entropy is attained.

third polar body: *see* **polar bodies**.

thixotropic: describes gels that reversibly liquefy when shaken.

thoracic duct: the major efferent lymphatic duct. It collects lymph from the left side of the body and delivers it to the left subclavian vein.

thorax: chest; the part of the trunk between the neck and the abdomen that contains the heart, lungs, trachea, bronchi, thymus gland, and the largest blood vessels.

Thorazine: a trade name for chlorpromazine hydrochloride.

thorium: Th; a radioactive, radio-opaque metallic element (atomic number 90, atomic weight 232.04) with a half-life of 1.4×10^{10} years, used in roentgenography.

threonine: Thr; T; 2-amino-3-hydroxybutyric acid; an essential amino acid, metabolizable to isoleucine, α-ketobutyrate, and pyruvate. It is a component of many proteins, and an acceptor of phosphate groups for reactions catalyzed by several protein kinases.

threonine dehydratase: a pyridoxal dependent enzyme that converts threonine to α-ketobutyrate + NH_4+, so named because a dehydration step precedes the deamination. The products can be metabolized to isoleucine.

threonyl-seryl-lysine: TSL; a pineal gland tripeptide implicated as a regulator of gonadotropin secretion.

threshold stimulus: liminal stimulus; a stimulus of just sufficient intensity and duration to elicit a response; *see* also **stimulus**.

thrombasthenia: several conditions in which platelet aggregation is defective. Glanzmann's disease is attributed to an autosomally inherited mutation that impairs synthesis of integrin IIb/IIIa.

thrombin: a 34K dimeric, vitamin K-dependent trypsin-like serine protease in blood and lymph that plays essential roles in hemostasis, contributes to inflammation, and is implicated in the etiology of atherosclerosis. It generates fibrin by cleaving fibrinogen arginine-lysine bonds, promotes platelet aggregation, stimulates the release of serotonin, platelet derived and transforming growth factors (PDGF and TGFβ), and other mediators, activates phospholipases and kinase C isozymes, augments inositol phosphate, eicosanoid, and cGMP synthesis, and has chemotactic potency. Thrombin also promotes mitogenesis in fibroblasts and accelerates proliferation of smooth muscle cells of injured blood vessels, but can inhibit neurite growth. Its precursor, prothrombin, is made in and secreted by the liver; *see* also **coagulation**.

thrombocytes: blood platelets; cells derived from megakaryocytes that contribute to hemostasis and blood coagulation. Mediators released include platelet derived and transforming growth factors (PDGF and TGF-β). *See* **platelets** and items that follow it.

thrombocytopenia: inadequate numbers of circulating thrombocytes, a major cause of blood coagulation defects.

thrombocytopenic purpura: severe thrombocytopenia with bleeding into the skin. A primary form is caused by autoimmune destruction of blood platelets. Secondary types can involve coating of platelets with antibodies directed against foreign agents that leads to complement-mediated killing.

thromboembolism: clogging of a blood vessel by a thrombus that has been transported via the bloodstream from its initial site of formation.

thrombogenic: promoting blood clot formation.

β-thromboglobulin: a platelet basic protein digestion product that interacts with that protein and contributes to hemostasis.

thrombokinase: (1) Xa; activated Factor X of the blood coagulation cascade, a serine protease that converts prothrombin to thrombin; (2) thromboplastin.

thrombokinesis: blood clot formation.

thrombokinin: thromboplastin.

thrombolamban: a 22K microsomal protein of blood platelets that may be identical with rap-1. It is antigenically related to Ras p21 proteins, and is a kinase A substrate. The concept that it regulates a Ca^{2+}-ATPase and promotes Ca^{2+} uptake by microsomal vesicles has been discarded.

Thrombolysin : a trade name for plasmin.

thrombolysis: dissolution of intravascular blood clots.

thrombomodulin: TM; a 100K receptor on endothelial cell luminal surfaces that binds thrombin and serves as a cofactor for protein C activation. It may protect against intravascular clotting.

thrombophlebitis: thrombosis-associated inflammation of a vein.

thromboplastin: thrombokinin; blood coagulation factor III; a term used for several substances released from damaged cell surfaces, including an integral membrane glycoprotein and some lipoproteins that contain phosphatidylethanolamine, phosphatidylserine, or phosphatidylcholine. They act in conjunction with Ca^{2+} to initiate blood coagulation.

thrombopoietin: a growth factor made by bone marrow cells that promotes megakaryocyte differentiation and blood platelet formation.

thrombosis: formation, presence of, or growth of thrombi.

thrombospondin: glycoprotein G; thrombin-sensitive protein; TSP; a 450K extracellular adhesion molecule secreted by platelets that stabilizes platelet aggregation.

Platelet derived growth factor (PDGF) stimulates its synthesis.

thromboxanes: TXs: 20-carbon lipids synthesized from prostaglandin endoperoxides (PGHs) in platelets and leukocytes, and in cells of the lungs, spleen, kidneys, brain and other organs. Although short-lived, they are potent stimulants for platelet aggregation, platelet release of serotonin and ADP, and smooth muscle contraction (especially in bronchioles and parts of the vascular system). They contribute to inflammation, and are implicated in the etiology of vascular lesions, angina, stroke, hypertension, asthma, renal damage, and gastric ulcers. However, they may also exert negative feedback control over arachidonic acid release. Thrombin, collagen, epinephrine, and other regulators stimulate their production. Some actions may be mediated via cyclic guanosine 3′5′-monophosphate (cGMP) and/or elevation of cytosol Ca^{2+} levels. *See* specific types.

thromboxane A$_2$: TXA$_2$; [1S-[1α,3α(1E,3R),4β(Z), 5α]]-7-[3-(3-hydroxy-1-octenyl)-2,6-dioxabicyclo[3.1.1]-hept-4-yl]-5-heptenoic acid; a 20-carbon lipid synthesized from prostaglandin endoperoxide PGH$_2$. It is rapidly and spontaneously converted to thromboxane B$_2$ (TXB$_2$), which mediates most or all of the effects.

thromboxane B$_2$: TXB$_2$; [2R-2α(1E,3S),3β(Z)-4β-6α]]-7-tetrahydro-4,6-dihydroxy2-(3-hydroxy-1-octenyl)-2H-pyran-3-yl]-heptenoic acid; a 20-carbon lipid rapidly formed from thromboxane A$_2$ that accounts for most thromboxane effects.

thrombus [thrombi]: a blood clot.

thujone: 4-methyl-1-(1-methylethyl)bicyclo[3.1.0]-hexan-3-one; a terpene component of many aromatic oils. High concentrations can invoke convulsions.

Thy-1: in mice, two closely related 19K cell surface glycoproteins expressed on all T (but not B) lymphocytes, all T cell precursors (including ones in bone marrow and embryonic liver), and on dendritic cells. They are the smallest known members of the immunoglobulin superfamily, and are anchored to the membranes by glycosylated phospholipids. The resemblances to CD7 include derivation from genes that lack TATA boxes, expression before the appearance of CD2, CD3, and other thymocyte markers, distribution, and ability to elevate cytosol Ca^{2+} levels. Their roles in T cell activation may involve associations with CD45 (which also binds T cell receptor complexes). In humans, very few mature T cells express Thy-1; but the glycoproteins are abundant in the central nervous system and may contribute to brain development. The ones that appear on astrocytes after axonal growth is completed are proposed to stabilize neuronal connections and suppress axonal regrowth after injury. According to some observers, Thy-1 interacts with growth factors via signaling mechanisms similar to those described for T cells. However, others have suggested that the astrocyte ligand differs from lymphocyte Thy-1. The antigens are also present on peripheral sympathetic neurons, fibroblasts, kidney cells and other cell types, but are never expressed by olfactory neurons (which retain the ability to grow into the central nervous system).

Thy-1-DEC cells: *see* **dendritic cells**.

thylakentrin: an obsolete term for follicle stimulating hormone (FSH).

thylakoids: disk-like sacs within chloroplasts composed of membranes that surround fluid-filled spaces and hold the energy-generating systems. Grana typically contain stacks of five to thirty thylakoids.

thymectomy: removal of the thymus gland. It can alleviate certain autoimmune disorders, and is performed in some humans with myasthenia gravis. Neonatal thymectomy in rodents impairs maturation of the cellular immunity system and invokes a wasting syndrome; and it impairs ovarian development in animals that survive the condition.

-thymia: a suffix that refers to a mental or emotional condition, as in cyclothymia.

thymic humoral factor: THF; an acidic, heat-stable 31-amino acid peptide identified in bovine thymus glands and blood. It promotes thymocyte differentiation and proliferation and enhances T lymphocyte responses to mitogens.

thymidine: usually (1) thymine-2-deoxyriboside (deoxythymidine), a nucleoside used directly (and in the salvage pathway) for DNA synthesis; *see* **thymidine kinase**. The rate of radioactively labeled thymidine uptake is used as an indicator of DNA synthesis (although some factors dissociate uptake form incorporation); (2) thymine-2-riboside; small amounts occur in ribosomal and transfer RNAs, and are believed to be made via posttranscriptional methylation of uracil.

thymidine factor; TF; an obsolete term for insulin-like growth factor-I (IGF-I), based on its ability to promote thymidine incorporation into cartilage DNA.

thymidine kinase: an enzyme of the salvage pathway for DNA biosynthesis that catalyzes: thymidine + ATP →

thymidine

thymidine-5-phosphate + ADP. Several hormones promote synthesis of the enzyme.

thymin: *see* **thymopoietins.**

thymine: T; 5-methyluracil; a DNA pyrimidine base (*see* also **thymidine.**) Ultraviolet radiation can cause formation of thymine dimers.

thymocytes: thymus gland cells that originate from bone marrow lymphocytic precursor cells. Some undergo maturation to **T lymphocytes** (*q.v.*), but many die within the gland.

thymocyte dependent growth factor: TDGF; *see* **interleukin-2.**

thymol blue: thymolsulfonphthalein; 4,4′-(3*H*-2,1-benzoxathiol-3-ylidene)bis[5-methyl-2-(1-methylethyl)phenol] *S*,*S*-dioxide; an indicator that is red at pH 1.2, yellow at 2.8-8.0, and blue at 9.6.

thymoleptics: agents that elevate mood in individuals with psychic depression, mania, and other serious affective disorders, but do not invoke similar effects (or euphoria) in persons classified as "normal". The group includes tricyclic antidepressants, monoamine oxidase inhibitors, and lithium.

thymolytic: promoting thymus gland involution or atrophy.

thymopoietins: Tpos; species specific peptides chemically related to splenin, formerly known as thymins or nucleosins. They are made by thymus gland epithelial cells, skin keratinocytes, and some spleen and lymph node cells. In addition to promoting prothymocyte differentiation and T lymphocyte maturation, Tpos act on corticotropes, bind to and change the configurations of nicotinic type acetylcholine receptors in skeletal muscle and Torpedo electric organs, desensitize those receptors, block neuromuscular transmission, and also affect calcium channels in a manner that appears to be unrelated to receptor binding. They are implicated in the etiology of myasthenia gravis; and thymectomy ameliorates the symptoms in some individuals. Some TP effects have been linked with cGMP generation. Two 49-amino acid peptides (bovine thymopoietins I and II) with different *N*-terminals but a common thymopoietin pentapeptide have been identified in cattle. The human type (hTPo) has 48 amino acid moieties, with the sequence: Gly-Leu-Pro-Lys-Glu-Val-Pro-Ala-Val-Leu-Thr-Lys-Gln-Lys-Leu-Lys-Ser-Glu-Leu-Val-Ala-Asn-Gly-Val-Thr-Leu-Pro-Ala-Gly-Glu-Met-Arg-Lys-Asp-Val-Tyr-Val-Glu-Leu-Tyr-Leu-Gln-His-Leu-Thr-Ala-Leu-His.

thymopoietin pentapeptide: thymopoietin(32-36); Arg-Lys-Asp-Val-Tyr; a thymopoietin fragment that retains the biological activity of the larger peptides.

thymosins: several peptides initially identified in thymus gland extracts that promote maturation of T lymphocyte-dependent components of the immune system. Fraction 5 contains a mixture of heat-stable 1K-15K peptides with isoelectric points in the 4.0-7.0 range. Thymosin α_1 (made and secreted by thymus epithelial cells) is reported to restore the immune functions of thymectomized mice, and to be useful for treating some human immunodeficiencies and cancers. The form obtained from rats and cattle has the amino acid sequence: *Ac*Ser-Asp-Ala-Ala-Val-Asp-Thr-Ser-Ser-Glu-Ile-Thr-Thr-Lys-Asp-Leu-Lys-Glu-Lys-Lys-Glu-Val-Val-Glu-Glu-Ala-Glu-Asn. Related peptides, including des-(25-28)-thymosin-α_1 (which lacks four of the amino acids), and an α_{11} type (with a seven moietiy *C*-terminal extension) have been identified. A 113-amino acid prothymosin α may be the true hormone, as well as the precursor of several biologically active fragments. Thymosin β_1 (polypeptide β_1) was initially believed to be thymus gland specific; but although it acts on some T lymphocyte lineage cells, it is now known to be closely related to ubiquitin. Thymosin β_4, which promotes maturation of prothymocytes and T lymphocytes but may not be secreted, has the sequence *Ac*Ser-Asp-Lys-Pro-Asp-Met-Ala-Glu-Ile-Glu-Lys-Phe-Asp-Lys-Ser-Lys-Leu-Lys-Lys-Thr-Glu-Thr-Gln-Glu-Lys-Asn-Pro-Leu-Pro-Ser-Lys-Gly-Thr-Ile-Glu-Gln-Glu-Lys-Gln-Ala-Glu-Ser. Thymosin β_3 may be a proteolytic fragment of the β_4 peptide. Little is known about a thymosin β_{10} peptide associated with the β_4. Some thymosin effects appear to be mediated via cGMP.

thymosin α_1, thymosin α_{11}: *see* **thymosins.**

thymosin β_1: a peptide initially believed to be a thymus gland hormone, but now known to be similar to or identical with ubiquitin. See **thymosins.**

thymosins β_3, β_4, and β_{10}: *see* **thymosins.**

thymostatin: an approximately 2K heat-stable thymus gland glycopeptide that inhibits incorporation of labeled nucleosides into DNAs and RNAs of lymphocytes and some other cell types, and is reported to oppose some other thymosin effects.

thymosterin: a lipid component of thymus gland extracts implicated as a contributor to T lymphocyte formation and maturation.

thymotaxin: a peptide made by thymus gland epithelial cells that promotes migration of Thy-1$^+$ prethymocytes to the gland.

thymulin: facteur serum thymique; FTS; serum thymic factor: Glx-Ala-Lys-Ser-Glx-Gly-Gly-Ser-Asn; a thymus gland hormone active only when associated with zinc. It is believed to promote proliferation and differentiation of T lymphocyte precursor cells.

thymus dependent antigens: antigens that stimulate B lymphocyte responses only in the presence of activated T lymphocytes (which release cytokines). Most small antigens are of this type.

thymus gland: a bilaterally symmetrical lympho-epithelial organ in all vertebrates except cyclostomes that provides an environment for proliferation, differentiation, and selection of T lymphocyte precursor cells, and secretes several hormones (*see*, for example **thymulin** and **thymosins**). In addition to essential roles in cellular immunity, it affects differentiation of the ovaries, adenohypophysis, and other organs. The cells have receptors for androgens, estrogens, glucocorticoids, growth hormone, prolactin, and other regulators. Dysfunctions are believed to contribute to autoimmune diseases. Stress, food deprivation, and other factors associated with high glucocorticoid levels promote reversible shrinking (involution) of the gland. During normal aging, the thymus size decreases, as active cells are replaced by lipid-rich connective tissue.

thymus independent antigens: antigens to which B lymphocytes respond by producing specific antibodies, even when no T lymphocytes are present. Examples include bacterial lipopolysaccharides, some protein polymers, and other bivalent or multivalent types.

thymus protein: an uncharacterized component of thymus gland extracts implicated as a regulator of T lymphocyte functions.

thymus replacing factor: interleukin-5. The acronym TRF is now seldom used, because of possible confusion with thyrotropin releasing factor.

thyralbumin: a thyroid gland protein chemically related to and probably derived from blood albumins. Its functions have not been established; *cf* **thyroxine binding prealbumin**.

thyrocalcitonin: TCT; a name initially given to calcitonin when its origin in thyroid glands was discovered. The term is still used by some authors.

thyrocalcitonin release factor: a proposed regulator of calcitonin secretion made by thyroid gland follicular cells. Its existence has not been confirmed.

thyroglobulins: TGbs; 650-660K glycoproteins synthesized by thyroid gland follicular cells and secreted to the lumens, where they undergo maturation that includes peptide chain cross-linking, iodination on tyrosyl moieties, and a coupling reaction that leads to formation of iodothyronyl moieties. The products are taken up by follicular cells via endocytosis, incorporated into phagolysosomes, and subjected to proteolysis which releases thyroxine (T_4), along with some triiodothyronine (T_3) and small amounts of monoiodo- and diiodo-tyrosines. Minute quantities of iodinated thyroglobulins exit via lymphatic vessels and enter the bloodstream. There are species variations in TGb composition; and some regulators (especially thyroid stimulating hormone, TSH) affect the carbohydrate content.

thyroidectomy cells: enlarged thyrotropes that form when negative feedback controls normally exerted by thyroid hormones are impaired, for example in thyroxine deficiency states, after thyroidectomy, or when conversion of thyroxine to triiodothyronine in the pituitary gland is inhibited. They usually synthesize and store large amounts of thyroid stimulating hormone (TSH).

thyroid glands: organs in all vertebrates that synthesize thyroxine (T_4) and triiodothyronine (T_3). Mammalian glands also contain parafollicular cells that secrete calcitonin. In most species they are bilateral structures joined by an isthmus, located in the neck region. In many, the capsules enclose the parathyroid glands (but some animal types have parathyroid glands at other sites). Thyroid stimulating hormone (TSH) is the major stimulant for follicle growth and iodinated hormone secretion. Several other regulators appear to exert mostly fine controls.

thyroid hormone[s]: although the thyroid glands of many species secrete other regulators (for example calcitonin in most mammals), the term usually refers to the thyroxine (T_4) and **triiodothyronine** (T_3, *q.v.*), made by the follicular cells.

thyroid hormone receptors: the major types are nuclear proteins that bind triiodothyronine (T_3) to form complexes that attach to thyroid response elements (TREs) and affect gene transcription. They resemble the receptors for steroid hormones, calciferols, and retinoic acid, but are somewhat smaller than the steroid kinds, and do not bind heat shock protein 90. *See* also **triiodothyronine receptors** and c-erbA. Different kinds of receptors that do not affect genome functions on plasma membranes, mitochondria and other intracellular components have been described.

thyroiditis: inflammation of the thyroid glands. It can be associated with hyperthyroidism during early stages; but follicular cell deterioration soon follows. Although some forms are initiated by infections, Hashimoto's thyroiditis is an autoimmune disease. Inflamed glands can release antigens that are normally sequestered. Some antibodies made against them impair thyroid gland functions.

thyroid peroxidase: TPO; a membrane-associated enzyme in thyroid glands that catalyzes oxidation of iodide and incorporation of the product into thyroglobulin tyrosyl moieties. Some autoimmune thyroid disorders are attributed to production of antibodies directed against the enzyme. The activity is inhibited by goitrogens. Thyroid stimulating hormone (TSH) is the major inducer. Other stimulants include insulin-like growth factor-I.

thyroid response elements: TREs; DNA segments on genes that code for growth hormone, malic enzyme, α-myosin, and many other substances whose transcription is regulated by triiodothyronine (T_3). They resemble response elements for steroid hormones, calciferols, retinoic acid, and some proto-oncogene products; and they interact with receptors for those molecules as well as with thyroid hormone-receptor complexes and some other kinds of heterodimeric proteins. *See* also c-**erbA**.

thyroid stimulating antibodies: several immunoglobulins that bind to and activate thyroid stimulating hormone (TSH) receptors on thyroid glands. They are made in large amounts by some individuals with autoimmune hyperthyroidism. *See* also **Graves' disease** and **long acting thyroid stimulator** (LATS).

thyroid stimulating hormone: TSH; thyrotropin; thyrotrophin: species-specific 28.3K glycoprotein hormones secreted by thyrotropes that promote thyroid gland growth, iodide uptake, thyroglobulin synthesis and iodination, endocytosis, and the release of iodinated thyroid hormones. They are heterodimers with α subunits similar to or identical with gonadotropin α subunits, plus β subunits unique to TSH secreting cells in the adenohypophysis. Thyrotropin releasing hormone (TRH) is the major stimulant. Thyrotropes take up T_4 and convert it to T_3, the major negative regulator that acts mostly by decreasing the numbers of TRH receptors and otherwise diminishing the sensitivity to TRH. A closely related glycoprotein is made in the placenta.

thyroid storm: acute, severe thyrotoxicosis. A major problem is tachycardia that impairs filling of the heart ventricles during diastole. *See* **triiodothyronine**.

thyroliberin: thyrotropin releasing hormone.

thyronine, T_o: *O*-(4-hydroxyphenyl)-tyrosine; one of several thyroid hormone degradation products; *see* **iodothyronines**.

thyronine binding globulin: thyroxine binding globulin; TBG; 63K plasma glycoproteins secreted by the liver that in humans usually associates reversibly with 70-77% of circulating thyroxine (T_4) and triiodothyronine (T_3), along with some diiodo- and monoiodothyronines. Although believed to facilitate thyroid hormone transport through body fluids, genetic defects that impair its synthesis do not consistently affect the hormone functions. Estrogens augment TBG production in primates. Factors that decrease it include stress, glucocorticoids, androgens, and high levels of growth hormone. Salicylates and some other pharmacological agents decrease the binding affinity. *Cf* **transthyretin**.

thyrotoxicosis: severe hyperthyroidism. *See* **triiodothyronine** and **Graves' disease**.

thyrotropes: thyrotrophs; basophilic adenohypophysial cells that synthesize and secrete thyroid stimulating hormone. Thyrotropin releasing hormone (TRH) maintains their morphologies and stimulates their activities. Thyroxine (T_4), taken up from the bloodstream and converted to triiodothyronine (T_3) exerts negative feedback controls. *See* also **Pit-1**.

thyrotropin: thyrotrophin; TSH; *See* **thyroid stimulating hormone**.

thyrotropin release factor: thyrotrophin releasing factor; TRF; a term for **thyrotropin releasing hormone** (TRH, *q.v.*), introduced before the chemical structure was known, and still used by some authors.

thyrotropin releasing hormone: thyrotrophin releasing hormone; TRH; thyroliberin; *pyro*-Glu-His-Pro-NH$_2$; a hormone, neurotransmitter and neuromodulator initially identified as the major hypothalamic factor that maintains thyrotrope structure and functions and promotes the release of thyroid stimulating hormone (TSH). Thyrotropes, in turn exert the major negative feedback controls by taking up thyroxine (T_4) from the bloodstream and converting to triiodothyronine (T_3), which decreases the numbers of TRH receptors. Hypothalamic TRH can also stimulate prolactin synthesis and release, but the physiological importance of this effect is not known. Although TRH levels can rise during suckling, there is no concomitant increase in TSH release. TRH additionally affects ACTH secretion in some individuals with Cushing's syndrome, and growth hormone release in some with acromegaly, liver disorders, and anorexia nervosa. More TRH is made outside of than within the hypothalamus, with highest levels in the gastrointestinal tracts of mammals and the skins of amphibians. It is additionally synthesized in extra-hypothalamic brain, spinal cord, pineal gland, pancreatic islet delta cells, and at other sites not involved in TSH secretion. It affects mood, sleep and motor behavior, and body temperature, and contributes to the control of food intake and gastrointestinal tract functions, stimulates the heart, and exerts influences on blood vessel smooth muscle. In ectotherms it is a regulator of melanocyte stimulating hormone (α-MSH) secretion. Some effects have been linked with influences on catecholamine metabolism, on the distribution of the various catecholamine receptor types, or on somatostatin release.

thyroxine: T_4; 3,5,3'5'-tetraiodothyronine; the major hormone secreted by thyroid gland follicular cells. It must be converted to **triiodothyronine** (*q.v.*) to act on receptors in most (possibly all) target cells. Excess T_4 is degraded to reverse triiodothyronine (rT_3), which displays little or no biological activity, and to thyronines with fewer iodine atoms.

thyroxine binding prealbumin: TBPA: an old term for transthyretin.

thyroxine

Ti: (1) thallium; (2) a dimeric component of T lymphocyte receptors that binds antibodies and determines immunological specificity.

TIA-1: a protein implicated as a direct mediator of Tc cell toxicity.

tiaprost: 7-[3,5-dihydroxy-2-[3-hydroxy-4-(3-thienyloxy)-1-butenyl]cyclopentyl]-5-heptanoic acid; a prostaglandin analog used for its luteolytic activity.

tight junctions: zona occludens; specialized structures on the apical surfaces of adjacent epithelial cells that block intercellular passage of water and small dissolved substances, and permit the buildup of high electrical resistance. They are formed by interlocking molecules produced by both apposing cells. In most cases the two plasma membranes are fused at some sites.

tiglic acid: *trans*-2,3-dimethylacrylic acid; (*E*)-2-methylbutenoic acid; a compound made by parasitic intestinal roundworms, and a component of many plant oil esters. It forms a thioester with coenzyme A that is used in leucine metabolism. It also binds to and protects alcoholic groups, and is used in the perfume industry, in flavoring agents, and to break emulsions.

tigloidine: 3-β-tigloyloxytropane; an alkaloid made by *Solanaceae* species. It is a central nervous system depressant with anticholinergic properties that can alleviate symptoms in some individuals with Parkinson's disease.

TIL: tumor infiltrating lymphocytes.

timolol: 1-[(1,1-dimethylethyl)amino]-3-[[4-morpholinyl-1,2,5-thiadiazol-3-yl]oxy]-2-propanol; a nonselective β-adrenergic receptor blocking agent used to alleviate some forms of hypertension and to treat glaucoma.

TIMP: thioinosinic acid; an endogenous tissue nucleotide that inhibits metalloproteinases and suppresses tumor growth.

tin: Sn; a metallic element (atomic number 50, atomic weight 118.69). Although there are indications that animals require trace amounts, no biological functions have been established.

tiotidine: an H₂-type histamine receptor antagonist with properties similar to those of ranitidine.

Ti plasmid: a tumor-inducing plasmid of *Agrobacterium tumefaciens* that causes crown gall disease in plants. Plants produce phenolic compounds at wound sites that facilitate entry of microorganisms. A 20 kb segment of the plasmid DNA (T-DNA) then integrates into the host genome, and it stimulates production of opines on which the bacteria feed, and also of auxin and cytokinins that support growth of the tumor. Ti plasmids are efficient vectors for introducing foreign DNA into broad-leafed plants. They are used to study transformation, and can improve the food value and crop yields of a few types.

tissues: aggregations of similar (or of embryologically related) cells and their extracellular products whose components collectively perform common functions. Examples include connective, epithelial, nervous, and muscle tissues. *Cf* **organs.**

tissue CRF: the name given to an uncharacterized circulating factor released during prolonged stress that promotes secretion of adrenocorticotropic hormone (ACTH) in animals with lesions that remove the major sources of hypothalamic corticotropin releasing hormone (CRH). It may be an interleukin. Its release in inhibited by high glucocorticoid levels.

tissue culture: initially, maintaining explanted tissues in culture media. The term is now applied more commonly to the growth of cells in culture media.

tissue factor: (1) blood coagulation factor III; tissue thromboplastin; (2) a term variously applied to uncharacterized components that contribute to the actions of one or more regulators.

tissue plasminogen activator: t-PA; TPA; fibrinokinase; a 527 amino acid (70K) serine protease that converts plasminogen to plasmin and thereby promotes fibrinolysis. The enzyme activity is very low in the absence of fibrin. *See* **plasminogen activators.**

tissue typing: determination of major histocompatibility complex (MHC) antigen types expressed on cell surfaces (usually of grafts) to predict the probability of acceptance or rejection by host tissues.

titer: (1) the quantity of one reagent required to react with a specified amount of another; (2) the reciprocal of the highest dilution (usually of an antigen or antibody) that invokes a reaction.

titin: an approximately 2500K flexible protein that forms elastic networks. In skeletal muscle it links thick filaments to Z discs and confers passive elasticity.

tk: thymidine kinase.

T kinin: isoleucyl-seryl-bradykinin; *see* **kallikreins.**

T kininogen: a low molecular weight, kallikrein-resistant kinin precursor chemically related to α-microtubule associated protein.

TKT: **tyrosine transketolase**: TAT; *see* **tyrosine aminotransferase.**

Tl: thallium.

TL antigens: mouse thymus leukemia antigens; surface glycoproteins expressed on some leukemia cells, some prothymocytes, and a subset of cortisone-sensitive thymocytes in the gland medulla (at least some of which lose the antigen during maturation). They are disulfide bonded tetramers composed of two 45K and two 12K chains.

TLCK: Nα-*p*-tosyl-L-lysine chloromethylketone; 1-chloro-3-tosylamido-7-amino-2-heptanone hydrochloride; an agent used to inhibit papain, trypsin, and the activities of T lymphocytes.

T lymphocyte: thymus-dependent lymphocytes that mediate cellular immunity and transplant rejection, and contribute to autoimmune diseases. They derive from prethymocytes (which appear in the embryonic liver

TLCK

before production shifts to bone marrow). Most "home" to the thymus gland cortex in which they proliferate. Limited numbers pass through prothymocyte and thymocyte stages, migrate to the medulla, and finally leave as T cells that travel via the bloodstream to the lymph nodes, spleen, and other sites. A selection process in the thymic cortex eliminates most immature cells capable of reacting against self antigens. Most medullary thymocytes express surface antigens different from those of cortical types (*see* **CD antigens**), and also differ in other ways that include sensitivities to glucocorticoids and other regulators. All T lymphocytes possess TCR (CD3) receptors essential for recognizing specific antigen types (but *see* also **superantigens**). Ones with α and β type subunits predominate in lymphatic tissues. γδ types populate the skin, the mucosa of the gastrointestinal and respiratory tracts, the lungs, and a few other sites; and it has been suggested that some of those derive from prethymocyte subsets that mature outside the thymus under the influence of factors released by the gland. T_C (*cytotoxic*) lymphocytes are CD4$^-$CD8$^+$ (display CD8, but not CD4 surface antigens). They recognize foreign peptides that have been processed by antigen presenting cells and displayed to them in conjunction with class I type major histocompatibility (MHC) antigens. T_C cells attach to virus-infected, tumor, incompatible transplant, and other cell types they recognize as foreign, and destroy them directly by producing perforins. T_H (*helper*) lymphocytes, which are mostly CD4$^+$8$^-$, recognize processed peptides presented in conjuction with class II MHC antigens. They secrete lymphokines (including interleukins 2, 3, and 5, interferon γ, and granulocyte-macrophage colony stimulating factors (GM-CSF) that affect other lymphocytes, including B types. Subsets have been described for some species, including T_{H1} types that secrete interleukin-2 and acquire interleukin-2 receptors when activated, and T_{H2} cells that secrete interleukin-4 and are insensitive to interleukin-2. Some authors distinguish between helper cells that affect B lymphocytes and those that regulate T lymphocyte functions; but such dichotomies have been questioned, at least for some species. The relationships of T_C and T_H lymphocytes to inducer types are not clear. Many (but not all) observers recognize the existence of T_S (*suppressor*) lymphocytes, at least some of which are CD4$^-$CD8$^+$ but distinguishable by other markers from T_C cells. They are said to protect against potentially toxic effects of overactive immune system processes and against development of autoimmune diseases. T_D cells are classified on the basis of function (roles in delayed hypersensitivity), and appear to be mostly helper types. At least some cells pass through a double-negative (CD4$^-$CD8$^-$ prethymocyte) stage before acquiring typical surface antigens; but some mature pulmonary $\gamma\delta$ T cells are also CD4$^-$CD8$^-$. A CD4$^+$CD8$^+$ intermediary stage has also been described.

T lymphocyte chemotactic factor: T cell chemotactic factor; TCF; *see* **neutrophilin**.

T lymphocyte receptors: TCRs; TcRs; immunoglobulin-like cell surface components on T lymphocytes that confer antigen specificity. They recognize specific kinds of peptides that have been processed by antigen presenting cells and displayed along with major histocompatibility complex (MHC) antigens. The most abundant type has a 40-43K α subunit linked by a disulfide bond to a 40-55K β type. but populations in the gastrointestinal tract, skin and lungs contain δ and γ subunits. The TcR associates with a CD3 glycoprotein that is essential (but not sufficient) for antigen recognition. *See* also **T lymphocytes**.

T$_m$: tubular maximum; the maximum rate for active transport of a solute across kidney tubule epithelium. The solutes are taken up from glomerular filtrates and transferred to capillary blood. Under normal conditions the glucose T$_m$ is sufficient for recovery of all the sugar that enters the filtrate. In hyperglycemic states the rate of glucose presentation exceeds the T$_m$, and glucose that cannot be reabsorbed enters the urine.

TM: thrombomodulin.

TM-3 cells: a mouse cell line derived from testicular Leydig cells.

TMA: tetramethylammonium.

TMB-8: 8-(*N,N*-dimethylamino)octyl-3,4,5-trimethoxybenzoate hydrochloride; an agent that inhibits Ca^{2+} release from intracellular sequestration sites.

TMV: tobacco mosaic virus.

TNFs: *see* **tumor necrosis factors α and β**.

TO: tryptophan oxidase.

tobacco: the dried leaves of *Nicotiana tabacum*. In addition to **nicotine** (the major alkaloid, *q.v.*), tobacco smoke contains among other things carbon monoxide (recently recognized as an endogenous regulator of neuron functions), nitrogen oxides, volatile carbohydrates, nitrosamines, and nitriles. Although the motivation to smoke is widely attributed to the central actions of nicotine, other chemical components (and factors such as aromas, and the physical handling of cigarettes, cigars or pipes) probably contribute. Some of the chemicals are carcinogenic when repeatedly applied to the shaved skins of laboratory animals, and some enhance the effects of other carcinogens. However, although smoke also irritates the respiratory tract, is ciliotoxic, and affects immune system functions, attempts to invoke lung cancers by exposing animals to high levels of smoke have been generally unsuccessful. Chewing tobaccos irritate mucous membranes and their use is associated with high risk for developing cancers of the mouth. The plants are used for studies of phytohormones and viruses.

tobacco mosaic virus: TMV; the first plant virus isolated, and the major cause of tobacco leaf disease. The single-stranded RNA core of approximately 6400 nucleotides is surrounded by a protein coat with 2130 158-amino acid subunits. Since it can reform from separated subunits, it is used to study macromolecule self-assembly.

tobramycin: *O*-3-amino-3-deoxy-α-D-glucopyranosyl-(1→6)-*O*-[2,6-diamino-2,3,6-trideoxy-α-D-ribohexopyranosyl-(1→4)-2-deoxy-D-streptamine; an aminoglucoside antibiotic made by *Streptomyces tenebrarius* that kills *Pseudomonas* bacteria. It is chemically related to and exerts actions similar to those described for gentamycin.

tocainide: 2-amino-*N*-(2,6-dimethylphenyl)propanamide; an orally effective agent that directly affects electrical activity in the heart and can alleviate ventricular dysrhythmias in some individuals refractory to other agents. It also inhibits leukocyte motility. The side effects can include dizziness, nausea, vomiting, and severe bone marrow depression.

TMB-8

tocinoic acid: MRF; melanocyte release factor; the ring component of oxytocin. It can be cleaved from OT by endogenous enzymes. MRF is a purported stimulant for secretion of α-melanocyte stimulating hormone (α-MSH), and a precursor of linear MIF-II (Cys-Tyr-Ile-Gln-Asn-OH), which inhibits.

toco-: a prefix meaning birth.

tocolysins: agents that block the mounting of organized uterine contractions, and thereby protect against premature onset of labor.

tocopherols: the term **vitamin E** (*q.v.*) usually refers to α-tocopherol [(3,4-dihydro-2,5,7,8-tetramethyl-2-(4,8,12-trimethyltridecyl)-2H-1-benzopyran-6-ol)]. Chemically and biologically related plant terpenes include β-tocopherol (3,4-dihydro-2,5,8-trimethyl-2-(4,8,12-trimethyltridecyl)-2H-1-benzopyran-6-ol), and also γ, δ, ε, ζ₁, ζ₂, and η types.

tolazamide: N-(p-toluenesulfonyl)-N'-hexamethyleniminourea; a sulfonylurea type oral hypoglycemic agent.

tolazoline: Priscol; Priscoline; 2-benzyl-2-imidazoline; an orally effective, short acting smooth muscle relaxant used to treat vasospasm. Although classified as an α₁-type adrenergic receptor blocker, it also acts directly on vascular muscle, inhibits responses to serotonin, and exerts histamine-like and parasympathomimetic effects. It can also stimulate the heart and raise blood pressure, in part by blocking α₂ type receptors.

tolbutamide: Orinase; N-(sulfonyl-p-methylbenzene)-N'-butylurea; a sulfonylurea type **oral hypoglycemic agent** (*q.v.*).

Tolectin: a trade name for tolmetin.

tolerance: (1) insensitivity to a hormone, neurotransmitter, other substance, or condition to which different members of the species normally respond, or to which the individual has responded at an earlier time; (2) failure to respond to one or more specific antigen types. Under normal conditions, tolerance to most *self-antigens* develops during fetal life. Afterward, a single very large dose of a foreign antigen, or a very small one, followed over an extended time period by a series of gradually increasing concentrations, can invoke insensitivity to types that previously elicited responses.

tolerogens: agents that invoke immunological tolerance.

Tollens reagent: a mixture that contains silver nitrate, sodium hydroxide, and ammonia. It is used as an oxidizing agent and to characterize sugars, aldehydes, and hydrazides.

tolmetin: Tolectin; 1-methyl-5-(4-methylbenzoyl)-1H-pyrrole-2-acetic acid; an eicosanoid synthesis inhibitor used for its anti-inflammatory, antipyretic, and analgesic properties.

tolonium chloride: toluidine blue O; 3-amino-7-dimethylamino-2-methylphenazathionium chloride; a basic dye that stains nuclei, used to identify mast cells and to delineate oral and cervical neoplasms. Its hemostatic properties are attributed to heparin antagonism.

toloxatone: 5-(hydroxymethyl)-3-(3-methylphenyl)-2-oxazolidinone; a competitive inhibitor of A-type monoamine oxidases, used as an antidepressant.

toluene: methylbenzene; phenylmethane; an organic solvent used in chromatography and industrial processes. High concentrations invoke narcosis; and prolonged exposure to the vapors can cause liver damage.

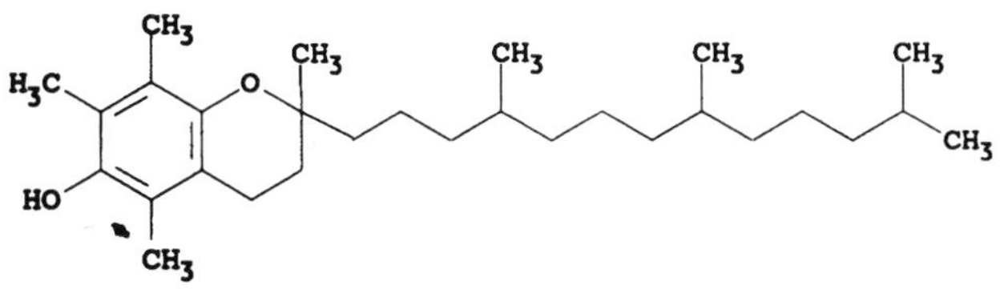

α-tocopherol

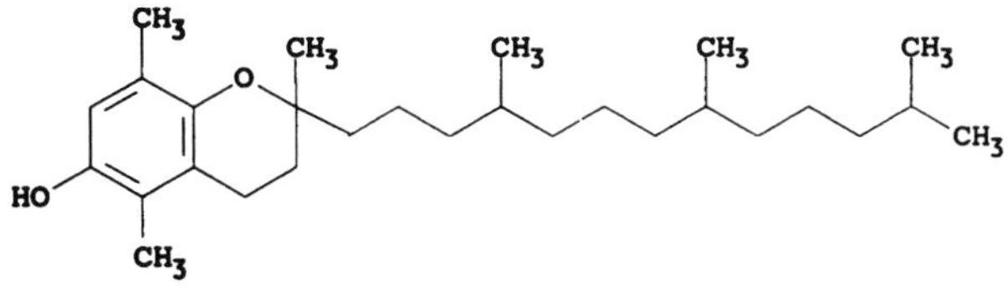

β-tocopherol

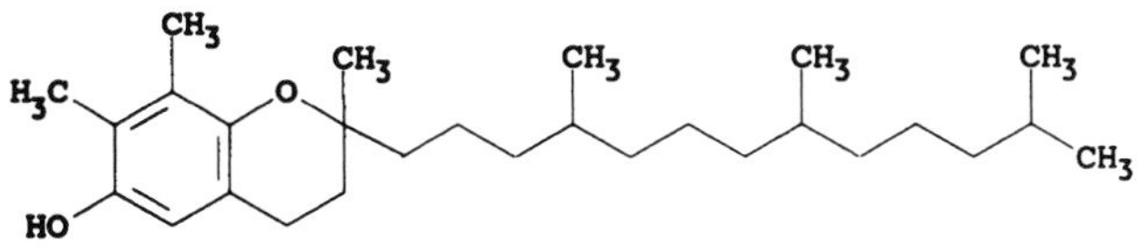

γ-tocopherol

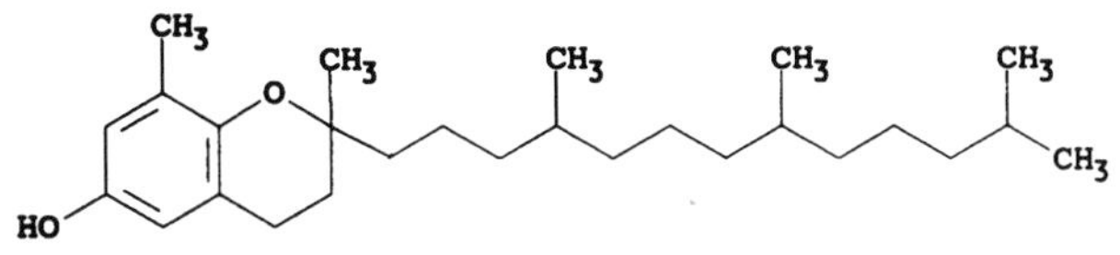

δ-tocopherol

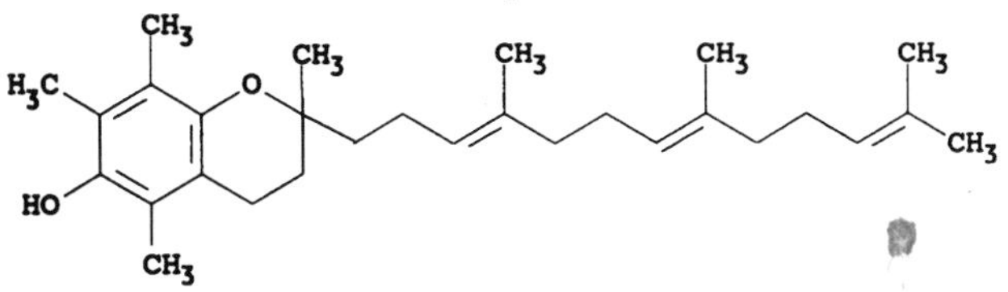

ξ₁-tocopherol

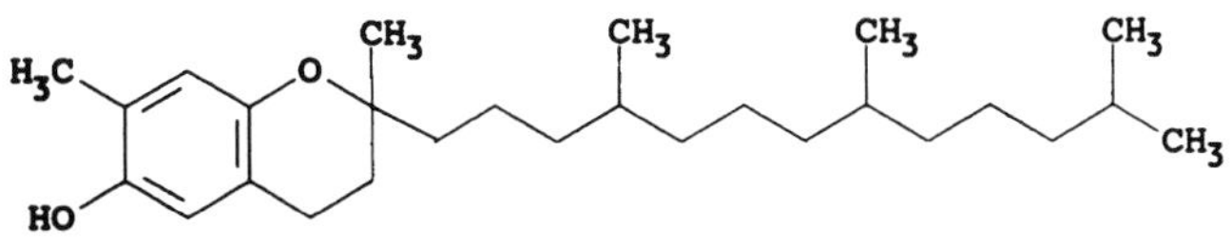

η-tocopherol

tocopherols

toluidine blue: tolonium chloride.

tomography: several techniques for constructing images of internal organs, based on differences in density or other properties that affect the transmission of X-rays or gamma rays. For CAT (CT) scanning (computer assisted tomography, computerized axial tomography), the intensities of beams that emerge when X-rays are sent through tissues in many planes are measured with scintillation counters and recorded on electronic disks. Computers are then used to analyze the patterns and construct images. Positron emission tomography (PET scanning) is based on differences in use of glucose (or other physiological substances). Positron emitting isotopes are incorporated into the compounds, and gamma ray paths through the tissues are measured.

tone: usually, (1) the normal state of skeletal muscle tension, maintained by the activities of motor nerves and muscle spindle organs; (2) any continuous level of normal activity.

tonic: (1) describes a prolonged activity, such as contraction or secretion, that can be continuous or repeated frequently on a regular basis, or prolonged presentation of an agent or stimulus; (2) an agent administered to improve function.

tonicity: (1) a state of tone or tension; (2) *see* **isotonic**, **hypertonic** and **hypotonic**.

tonins: serine proteases that cleave His—Phe bonds and generate angiotensin II directly from renin substrates via reactions that do not require angiotensin converting enzyme (and are not affected by ACE inhibitors). They can also convert angiotensin I (A-I) to A-II.

tonofibrils: tonofilament bundles. They provide cytoskeletal support for some epithelial cells, and strengthen tissues by binding one cell to another.

tonofilaments: intermediate filaments of cytoskeletons and desmosomes composed mostly of keratins.

tonsils: lymphoid tissue nodules embedded in the mucous membranes of the upper digestive tract. They protect against the entry of infectious agents, and are sites for B lymphocyte proliferation and antibody production.

Töpfer's test: a now obsolete titration procedure for measuring gastric acidity, in which dimethylazobenzene is used as the indicator.

topical: restricted (or applied) to a surface, or to a circumscribed area.

topo-: a prefix meaning (1) place or region; (2) localized.

topobiology: the study of position-dependent regulation of cell behavior and morphogenesis.

topoisomerases: enzymes that change DNA coiling by catalyzing strand breakage and resealing. Topoisomerase I affects one strand of the duplex, whereas topoisomerase II acts on both strands.

Torpedo fish: electric rays of the *Torpedo* genus. The cholinergically innervated electrocytes of *T. californicus* electric organs have 1000 times as many nicotinic receptors as mammalian skeletal muscle cells, and are used to study those receptors. *T. marmorata* electrolyte syncytia are used for dystrophin studies.

torpor: a depressed metabolic state usually associated with low body temperature, from which arousal can be achieved only with stimuli stronger than those required to interrupt normal sleep; *cf* **hibernation** and **coma**. Bears and some other large animals that do not go into true hibernation enter this state during the winter months; and torpor can be invoked in many species by subjecting the animals to cold environmental temperatures and/or long photoperiods. Central nervous system damage can lead to development of an abnormal state of torpor in humans and other mammals.

torr: 1 torr is the pressure exerted by a column of mercury 1mm high at standard gravity and 0°C.

tosyl-: the chemical group *p*-toluene-sulfonyl-, used for affinity labeling and enzyme function studies. It binds to amino acids and to compounds with some other reactive groups. TLCK (*Nα-p*-tosyl-L-lysine chloromethylketone) and TPCK (tosyl-L-phenylalanine chloromethylketone) somewhat resemble natural substrates for proteolytic enzymes, bind with high specificity to the active sites, additionally bind to nearby chemical groups, and block the enzyme activities.

tosyl

*N*α-**tosyl-**L-arginine methyl ester hydrochoride: *see* **TAME**.

tosyl-lysyl-chloromethylketone: *see* **TLCK**.

tosyl-L-phenylalanine ketone: *see* **TPCK**.

totipotent: describes (1) zygotes or other entities capable of giving rise to all cell types of more mature organisms of the species; (2) hematopoietic or other stem cell types that can differentiate into any of the morphologically distinguishable progeny associated with the tissue type; (3) entities with the potential for performing or acquiring the ability to perform all of the functions associated with the tissue type.

toxemia: poisonous substances in circulating blood, usually of the kinds contained within and/or released by pathogenic microorganisms; *see* also **toxemia of pregnancy**.

toxemia of pregnancy: eclampsia; disorders that develop in some women during pregnancy (or in some cases soon after parturition) characterized by hypertension, edema, proteinuria, and often also seizures. Usually, exaggerated responses to angiotensin II can be demonstrated; but circulating aldosterone and potassium ion levels are often in the ranges found during normal pregnancies. It has been suggested that as yet unidentified placental factors contribute to the etiology.

toxin: (1) a substance made by members of one species that is poisonous to another; (2) any poison.

α-toxin: a 34K protein made by *Staphylococcus aureus* that promotes formation of small plasma membrane channels which permit free diffusion of small molecules and ions, but block passage of macromolecules. Large amounts kill the target cells. Low concentrations are used in laboratory studies to permeabilize plasma membranes.

T-2 toxin: 4β-15-diacetoxy-3α-hydroxy-8a-[13-methyl-butyryloxy]-12,13-epoxytrichothec-9-ene; an extremely potent poison made by the fungus, *Fusarium sporotrichoides* that inhibits both initiation and termination of protein synthesis.

toxin II: three chemically similar approximately 4.9K peptides derived from *Anemonia sulcata* that act on Na^+ channels and block neuromuscular transmission and cardiac function. One type has the amino acid sequence H-Gly-Ile-Pro-Cys-Leu-Cys-Asp-Ser-Asp-Gly-Pro-Ser-Trp-His-Asn-Cys-Lys-Lys-His-Gly-Pro-Thr-Ile-Gly-Trp-Cys-Cys-Lys-Gln-OH.

toxoid: a nonpoisonous substance derived from a toxin that retains the antigenic properties of the parent substance, for example a vaccine that contains a modified bacterial exotoxin.

TP: tryptophan pyrrolase; *see* **tryptophan oxidase**.

TPA: (1) 12-*O*-tetradecanoyl-phorbol-13-acetate (shown below), a phorbol ester component of croton oil. It is a diacylglycerol analog that augments calcium-dependent activation of protein kinase C isozymes and promotes tumor growth; (2) t-PA, tissue plasminogen activator.

TPCK: tosyl-L-phenylalanine chloromethylketone; L-1-(*p*-toluenesulfonyl)-aminopentyl-chloromethylketone; an agent used to irreversibly inhibit chymotrypsin.

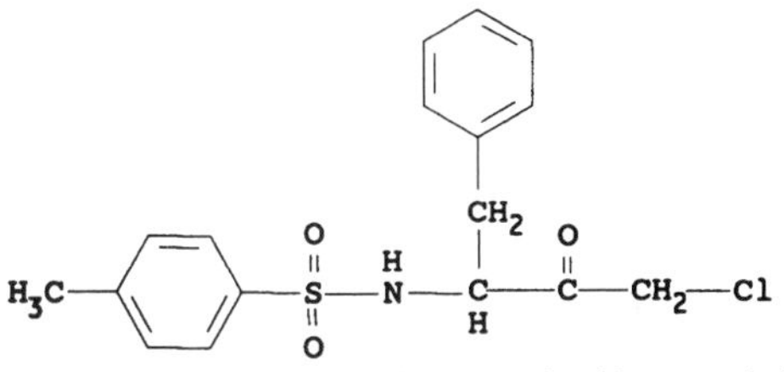

T4 phage: T4 bacteriophage; a double-stranded DNA virus with approximately 165 genes, many of which have been studied in detail. Fibers on the long tail bind to specific sites on *E. coli* membranes, ATP-driven contraction propels the nucleotide core into the host cell, and soon afterward most DNA, RNA, and protein synthesis is directed by viral genes.

TPN, TPNH: oxidized and reduced forms of triphosphopyridine nucleotide, now more commonly called NADP and NADPH.

Tpo: thymopoietin.

TPO: thyroid peroxidase.

T:P ratio: the ratio of the iodide concentration in the thyroid gland to its concentration in blood plasma, a measure of the ability of thyroid gland follicular cells to concentrate the ion. The values for healthy human adults are in the general range of 20:1 to 25:1, but can exceed 250:1 when iodine deficiency severely impairs thyroxine (T_4) synthesis, and thereby the negative feedback control over thyroid stimulating hormone (TSH) levels.

TPP: thiamine pyrophosphate.

trabecula [trabeculae]: a connective tissue strand that anchors or supports.

trabecular bone: spongy bone. It is lighter, less resistant to fracture, and metabolically more active than dense bone; and much of it houses bone marrow. At some sites, it forms first and is then replaced by the dense type.

trace elements: Cr, Mn, Cu, Zn, Se, and some other chemical elements required in very small amounts to maintain normal cell functions. Most are enzyme components or activators.

tracer doses: usually, minute quantities of radioactive isotopes employed as markers for biochemical reactions or physiological processes such as membrane transport. Tracer amounts of ^{131}I are used to monitor iodide uptake and release by thyroid glands. The amounts administered do not disrupt functions or cause significant damage.

tract: (1) a set of contiguous structures arranged in series that collectively performs a common function, as in gastrointestinal or urinary tract; (2) a bundle of nerve fibers that extends from one defined region to another, as in corticospinal, or hypothalamo-hypophysial nerve tract.

trailer: a set of untranslated bases at the 3′ end of a messenger RNA.

tranquilizers: agents used to alleviate anxiety. They invoke less central nervous system depression than hypnotics and most sedatives.

trans-: a prefix that (1) means through, across, beyond, as in transport, or transmit; (2) refers to a change in structure and/or function, or to a process by which the change occurs, as in transformation; (3) describes enzymes that transfer chemical groups from one compound to another, as in transaminase or transketolase, or non-enzyme compounds that move molecules or ions from one site to another, as in transferrin; (4) describes mechanisms for transferring genetic components, as in transfection; (6) is used when one compound directs formation of another, as in transcription or translation, and

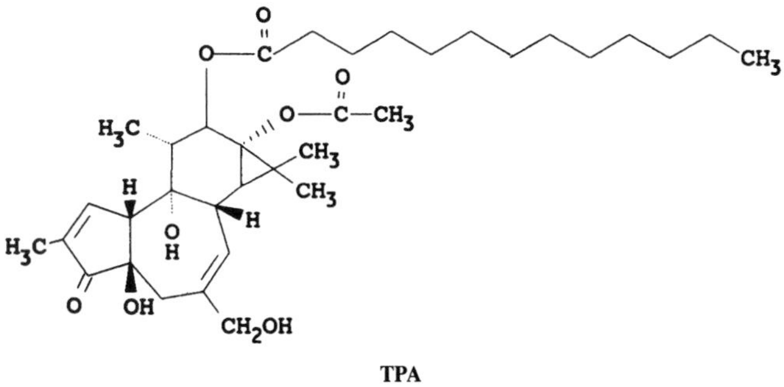

TPA

$$(1) \quad R_1\text{—}\overset{\displaystyle O}{\overset{\|}{C}}\text{—}\overset{H}{\overset{|}{N}}\text{—}R_2 \;+\; X\text{—COOH} \;\longrightarrow\; R_1\text{—COOH} \;+\; X\text{—}\overset{\displaystyle O}{\overset{\|}{C}}\text{—}\overset{H}{\overset{|}{N}}\text{—}R_2$$

$$(2) \quad R_1\text{—}\overset{\displaystyle O}{\overset{\|}{C}}\text{—}\overset{H}{\overset{|}{N}}\text{—}R_2 \;+\; H_2N\text{—}X \;\longrightarrow\; R_1\text{—}\overset{\displaystyle O}{\overset{\|}{C}}\text{—}\overset{H}{\overset{|}{N}}\text{—}X \;+\; H_2N\text{—}R_2$$

$$(3) \quad R\text{—}\overset{\displaystyle O}{\overset{\|}{C}}\text{—}NH_2 \;+\; H_2N\text{—}X \;\longrightarrow\; R\text{—}\overset{\displaystyle O}{\overset{\|}{C}}\text{—}\underset{H}{\overset{|}{N}}\text{—}X \;+\; NH_4^+$$

transamidases

for enzymes that catalyze such processes, as in transcriptase. *See also* **trans-**.

trans-: a prefix (1) for chemical groups that extend in different directions from a carbon chain, as in *trans*-retinaldehyde; *cf cis*; *see also* **stereoisomerism**; (2) that describes the effects of one compound on the properites of another, as in *trans*-activation.

transacetylases: enzymes that catalyze acetyl group transfers, usually to coenzyme A or from acetyl-CoA. One example is the dihydrolipoyl transacetylase of the pyruvate dehydrogenase complex.

transacylases: acyltransferases; enzymes that transfer acyl groups from one compound to another. For example, acylcarnitine transferase catalyzes: acetyl-CoA + carnitine → acylcarnitine + coenzyme-A.

transaldolase: an enzyme of the hexose monophosphate pathway that catalyzes transfers of 3-carbon units. In the reaction: sedoheptulose-7-phosphate + glyceraldehyde-3-P → erythrose-4-phosphate + fructose-6-P, a 3-carbon unit is removed from a 7-carbon sugar (converting it to a 4-carbon derivative), and is added to glyceraldehyde (which has 3 carbons) to form the 6-carbon fructose-P.

transactivation: *trans*-activation; processes by which a component of one molecule interacts with and augments the activity of another. For example, a transcription factor that binds to a DNA segment can facilitate transcription by changing the DNA configuration. *Cf cis* **activation**.

transamidases: amidotransferases; enzymes that catalyze reactions in which amide groups are transferred from one compound to another (as in reactions 1 and 2), or react with amino groups to crosslink or form large molecules from smaller ones (reaction 3). When thrombin converts factor XIII of the blood coagulation cascade to factor XIIIa, a transglutamidase (fibrin-stabilizing factor) strengthens blood clots by forming lysine-glutamine cross-linkages in fibrin. Different transglutamidases cross-link hormone receptors and facilitate endocytosis. *Cf* **transaminases**.

transaminases: enzymes that transfer amino groups from one compound to another, usually from an amino acid or amine to a keto acid. Most types require a pyridoxal phosphate cofactor. Some are used for gluconeogenesis and ureagenesis. Glutamic-oxaloacetate transaminase catalyzes: glutamate + oxaloacetate → α-ketoglutarate + aspartate. Since the enzyme leaks from injured cells, serum levels (SGOT) are used as indicators of muscle damage in patients with myocardial infarcts.

transcalciferin: DBP; *see* **vitamin D binding proteins**.

transcarboxylases: enzymes that catalyze transfers of COO⁻ moieties; *see* for example **acetyl CoA** and **pyruvate carboxylases**.

transcobalamins: transcobalamin II is a 35K protein secreted by the liver that binds vitamin B_{12}, is taken up with the vitamin via endocytosis, and is essential for absorption of that vitamin. Transcobalamin I (120K) and transcobalamin III bind to vitamin metabolites and contribute to their excretion to bile. The term *R proteins* is also used because the compounds move rapidly in electrophoresis fields.

transcortin: corticosteroid binding globulin.

transcript: a nucleic acid molecule whose formation is directed by a template with complementary bases. Most transcripts are RNAs, and most templates DNAs; but *see* **reverse transcriptases**. Premessenger RNAs are primary transcripts that require posttranscriptional processing to functioning messenger RNAs. *See also* **transcription**.

transcriptases: (1) RNA polymerases; (2) *see* **reverse transcriptases**.

transcription: although some viruses use RNA templates, and eukaryotes make some **reverse transcriptases** (*q.v.*) most transcription is DNA-directed. It begins with formation of a protein complex essential for attaching an RNA polymerase to a promotor site on the DNA. The polymerase then facilitates unwinding of a region of the double helix, linking an ATP or GTP to the start site on one strand, and sequential additions of other nucleo-

$$R_1\text{—}\overset{\displaystyle O}{\overset{\|}{C}}\text{—COOH} \;+\; R_2\text{—}\underset{H}{\overset{NH_2}{\overset{|}{C}}}\text{—COOH} \;\rightleftharpoons\; R_1\text{—}\underset{H}{\overset{NH_2}{\overset{|}{C}}}\text{—COOH} \;+\; R_2\text{—}\overset{\displaystyle O}{\overset{\|}{C}}\text{—COOH}$$

transaminases

tides with bases complementary to those of the template to the 3′ end of the growing ribonucleotide chain. The processes are complex, and require several **transcription factors** (*q.v.*).

transcription factors: TFs; proteins that interact with DNA templates and mediate transcription. The *general* types, essential for initiation are known in eukaryotes under names that begin with TF, followed by Roman numbers that refer to the polymerase type with which they interact (TFI, TFII, and TFIII, respectively, for polymerases I, II, and III). A letter that designates the type can follow, as in TFIID. RNA polymerase II catalyzes assembly of premessenger RNAs. Most genes that use it contain TATA boxes; and transcription begins with the binding of TFIID (a multimeric protein, also known as TATA factor) to the TATA sequence. TFIIA facilitates the binding, and enters into formation of a DA complex (TFIID + TFIIA bound to the TATA sequence). TFIIB (bridge factor) then binds to form a DAB complex, the recognition site for RNA polymerase II. TFIIF (a heterodimer with 30K and 74K subunits identical to RAP30 and RAP 74, respectively) binds to the RNA II polymerase and promotes its association with the DAB complex. Correct positioning and initiation requires association of TFIIE (a 56K and 34K dimer), and TFIIH with the complex. After performing its function at the initiation site, the RNA polymerase II dissociates from the complex and moves along the DNA to the next position, a process accompanied by dissociation of TFIIE and TFIIH. After completion of one round of premessenger RNA synthesis, TFIIE and TFIIH direct positioning of the enzyme for the next round. TFII also contributes to transcription initiation for genes that do not contain TATA boxes. CTF binds CAAT boxes, and SP1 binds CG boxes. TFIIIA, a zinc-containing protein, TFIIIB and TFIIIC are essential for the actions of RNA polymerase III, which catalyzes 5S RNA (and tRNA) synthesis. In prokaryotes, σ factors are the major regulators of RNA polymerase positioning and RNA synthesis initiation. *Specific* transcription factors act upstream as activators or repressors of limited numbers of genes; *see*, for example **AP-1**, **CREB**, **NF-kB**, and **Oct-1**. Additional specific types include receptors for steroid, thyroid, and other hormones that bind DNA after forming complexes with their ligands, and some proto-oncogene products.

transcription unit: a DNA segment that extends from the initiation site for formation of a primary RNA transcript to the termination site. Most eukaryote units contain several exons and introns.

transcriptional control: regulation of the rates for synthesis of specific kinds of proteins, exerted at the level of premessenger RNA formation; *cf* **posttranscriptional**, **translational**, and **posttranslational controls**.

transcuprein: a plasma protein different from ceruloplasmin that binds to and facilitates copper transport.

transcytosis: unidirectional transport into and across the cytoplasm. The term can describe movements of a substance that enters the plasma membrane at one surface of a polarized cell and is extruded from the opposite side, or to endocytosis and intracellular transport to processing sites.

transdifferentiation: conversion of one specialized cell type to another specialized cell type; *cf* **differentiation**. *Transmodulation* is used for functional changes in normal tissues, such as osteoblast conversion to osteocytes.

transducers: (1) devices, cell components, or cells that convert one form of energy to another. Various receptor types convert photic, mechanical or chemical stimuli to electrical signals; (2) cell components that link stimulation with cell responses, such as G proteins that couple hormone-receptor binding to enzyme activation.

transducins: G_Ts; retinal G proteins that participate in visual perception. In rods, which contain G_{T1} types with α_{T1} subunits, cyclic guanosine-3′5′-monophosphate (cGMP) maintains a "dark current" by promoting partial depolarization of the cells. It stabilizes Na^+ channels in states that permit inward "Na^+ leak". When light-activated rhodopsin associates with $G_{\alpha T1}$, the α subunit exchanges GTP for GDP, and the β and γ subunits are released. The α_1-GTP then causes dissociation of the catalytic component of a cGMP phosphodiesterase from its inhibitory subunit, and cGMP hydrolysis leads to closing of the ion channels. *See also* **rhodopsin kinase** and **arrestin**. In cones, G_{T2} (with α_{T2} subunits) is believed to perform comparable roles.

transduction: (1) viral-mediated transfer of nucleic acids from one organism to another, for example bacteriophage-directed transfer of DNA from one bacterium to another, or retroviral transfer of oncogenes; (2) processes accomplished by transducers.

transfection: insertion of foreign DNAs that integrate into host cell genomes.

transferases: phosphotransferases, sulfotransferases, aminotransferases, and other enzymes that catalyze exchanges of phosphate, sulfate, amino, methyl, and other chemical groups between donor and acceptor molecules.

transfer factors: TFs; lymphokines made by sensitized T cells that can confer cellular immunity or invoke delayed-type hypersensitivity when injected into other individuals.

transferrin[s]: siderophilin; several closely related species-specific metal binding β-globulins that interact with **transferrin receptors** (*q.v.*). They are the major iron transport proteins, essential for normal distribution of that metal. Their abilities to bind copper, manganese, vanadium and some other metals *in vitro* may not be physiologically relevant; but roles in chromium, magnesium, and zinc metabolism have been suggested. The major mature form in human blood plasma (approximately 80K when fully glycosylated) has 678 amino acid moieties and two Fe^{3+} binding sites. One site may preferentially deliver iron to erythrocyte precursors, and the other to various other cell types. Roles in transport across the blood-brain barrier have also been described. Hepatocytes synthesize the apoprotein, and much of the iron comes from hepatic reticuloendothelial cells. The form in the mucosa of the small intestine arrives via the bile. It contributes to absorption of dietary iron, and is released to the lumen when intestinal cells are shed. Ovotransferrins, testicular types made by Sertoli cells, and forms in fibroblasts, brain, and elsewhere are believed to act locally. Their production is controlled at specific sites by follicle stimulating hormone (FSH), insulin, and other hormones. High iron concentrations exert negative feedback controls over synthesis of the messenger RNA, whereas the estrogen levels attained during pregnancy or oral contraceptive use stimulate. Transferrins are mitogens and/or progression factors for some cell types, probably because they deliver the iron needed to make cytochromes and other essential compounds. (The apoprotein alone is ineffective). Transferrins can also contribute to defenses against infection by binding iron that would otherwise be taken up by microorganisms. Interleukin-2 blocks release of the iron. Lactoferrins of milk, saliva, tears, gastric juice, bronchial secretions, and leukocytes, melanoferrins of pigment cells, and some other glycoproteins are chemically related to the others, but they do not interact with the same receptors.

transferrin receptors: widely distributed dimeric proteins that bind **transferrins** *(q.v.)* and mediate iron uptake, but do not bind apotransferrin. Most are approximately 180K transmembrane glycoproteins composed of disulfide-linked 90K monomers, expressed in largest numbers on reticulocytes and some tumor cells, and in smaller ones on pachytene spermatocytes, Sertoli, ovarian follicular, and other cell types. The receptors reside in coated pits. After binding transferrin, they are taken up by endocytosis. Clathrin coated vesicles transport the molecules to cell interiors, shed their clathrin coats, and become acidified endosomes in which the iron dissociates from the proteins. The endosomes then fuse with CURL (compartment for uncoupling of receptors from ligands) vesicles that release iron for binding to intracellular ferritins. Both receptor and apoferritin molecules are recycled to plasma membranes. High concentrations of iron inhibit receptor synthesis.

transfer RNAs: tRNAs; twenty or more small (approximately 25K) ribonucleic acids essential for protein synthesis. Each molecule has an attachment site for a specific kind of amino acid, a corresponding anticodon that recognizes a complementary messenger RNA codon, and a ribosomal attachment site. (A few types can bind two or more kinds amino acids). The molecules are phosphorylated at their 5′ ends, and contain unusual bases (including methylated and dimethylated derivatives of the more common kinds).

transformation: cell changes that include conversion to states in which normal inhibitory controls over growth and replication are impaired or lost, usually associated with altered morphology and surface properties and accelerated proliferation rates. The changes can be invoked by infection with oncogenic viruses, artificial insertion of foreign nucleic acids, some chemicals, and radiation. Excessive levels of some hormones promote similar changes, but these can usually be reversed during early stages.

When injected into normal animals, some transformed cell types cause cancers.

transforming growth factors: TGFs; two classes of peptides initially identified in transformed cells and believed to be essential for maintaining the transformed state. They are made by virtually all somatic cell types (except erythrocytes), and appear to play major roles in normal development and numerous functions by acting directly on receptors and/or affecting the actions of other regulators. *See* **transforming growth factor-α** and **transforming growth factor-β**.

transforming growth factor α: TGF-α; several closely related species specific single chain peptides made by both normal and many transformed cell types, and also induced by oncogenes. Pro-TGFαs are cleaved to 17K linear glycoproteins that undergo secondary proteolysis to yield 15K (approximately 70 amino acid) membrane-bound, and 6K, 50-amino acid soluble derivatives, both of which are biologically active. Soluble human TGF-α has the amino acid sequence: H_2N-Val-Val-Ser-His-Phe-Asn-Asp-Cys-Pro-Asp-Ser-His-Thr-Gln-Phe-Cys-Phe-His-Gly-Thr-Cys-Arg-Phe-Leu-Val-Gln-Glu-Asp-Lys-Pro-Ala-Cys-Val-Cys-His-Ser-Gly-Tyr-Val-Gly-Ala-Arg-Cys-Glu-His-Ala-Asp-Leu-Leu-Ala-OH. It (and related forms in other species) display approximately 80% amino acid homology with epidermal growth factor (EGF). The hormones bind to EGF receptors, mimic many EGF effects (such as activation of receptor tyrosine kinases and of kinase C isozymes, stimulation of *c-myc* synthesis, and influences on plasma membrane Na^+/H^+ transport). However, although they appear to act only on cells with EGF receptors, the potencies and/or time courses differ at many sites; and different tissue distributions suggest the existence of special receptors for soluble types. Membrane-bound TGF-α binds to EGF receptors on neighboring cells and mediates juxtacrine adhesion and signal transduction. TGF-αs expressed on morulas are implicated in morula to blastocyst transitions, zona pellucida shedding, and blastocyst activation. Several influences on development of older embryos and fetuses have been described; and stimulation of angiogenesis and mitogenesis in epithelial and some other cell types is consistent with roles in wound healing and tissue regeneration. TGF-αs also accelerate bone resorption and decrease collagen and alkaline phosphatase synthesis in osteoblasts, and affect steroidogenesis in gonads and responses to gonadotropins. Additionally, they are made by lactotropes and may play paracrine roles in the adenohypophysis. Anterior hypothalamic injury in rats leads to increased production in neuroglial cells, and it is proposed that TGF-α then stimulates prostaglandin release and consequent increases in gonadotropin releasing hormone (GnRH) secretion that account for the precocious puberty which often follows. Unregulated activity at other sites may contribute to development of psoriasis, some forms of breast cancer, and some malignancy associated hypercalcemias. Although chemically unrelated to TGF-βs, they mimic some actions of those peptides; but they antagonize others. For example, whereas TGFαs stimulate liver growth, TGF-β_1 mediates the apoptosis that protects against hypertrophy.

transforming growth factor β: TGF-β; a family of peptides chemically related to activins, inhibins, Müllerian duct inhibitor, bone morphogenetic proteins, osteogenin, *Drosophila* pentaplegic gene product, and *Xenopus* Vg-1. Five subtypes (TGF-β1, β-2, β-3, β-4, and β-5) have been identified. Although all are chemically similar, heat and acid stable, approximately 25K, 112-amino acid dimers composed of disulfide-linked glycopeptide subunits, the isoforms are products of separate genes and derive from precursors with *N*-terminal regions that vary in composition and size. They are secreted in latent forms that require processing for biological activity. Plasmin and some other enzymes promote the activation, and parathyroid hormone can "unmask" TGF-β receptors. α_2-Macroglobulin binds to and inactivates TGF-β_1s, and has weaker effects on other subtypes. All nucleated cell types make at least one isoform; and blood platelets are especially rich sources. The kinds vary with the cell types and are differentially regulated. For example, estrogens specifically induce the β_1 type in bone. This effect may be related to the ability of those steroids to protect against osteoporosis; but bone morphogenetic protein 2-B (BMP-2B) also induces the peptide, and in its presence TGF-β_1 not only stimulates osteoprogenitor cell proliferation and osteoblast differentiation and promotes bone remodeling, but also recruits and activates monocytic cells that contribute to bone matrix production, acts on chondrocytes to induce type II collagen and cartilage-specific proteoglycans, and stimulates fibronectin formation by fibroblasts. It also synergizes with osteoinductive factor. Roles in immunosuppression, influences on the secretion of several hormones, and interactions with interleukins, bombesin, platelet-derived growth factor (PDGF), vasopressin, and insulin-like growth factor-I (IGF-I) have also been described. Since TGF-βs facilitate differentiation of a wide variety of cell types, and inhibit proliferation in some, they may protect against the development of malignancies. They also inhibit the release of follicle stimulating hormone (FSH) and antagonize adrenocorticotropic hormone (ACTH) stimulation of cholesterol conversion to pregnenolone (but do not lower cAMP levels in pituitary glands). Although the actions of all forms are qualitatively similar, up to 100-fold differences in potencies for various effects are known. For example, the β_1 and β_3 isoforms are much more potent than TGF-β_2 for inhibiting proliferation of endothelial and some hematopoietic cells and endothelial cell migration. The β_3 isotype is also a very efficient

mesoderm inducer in *Xenopus*, but the β_1 type is inactive (and only high concentrations of β_2 type are effective). Seemingly contradictory reports of TGF actions are probably related to differentiation states and microenvironments. For example, when myoblasts are maintained in mitogen-rich environments, TGFβ-1 suppresses *myc* synthesis and slows G_1 to S cell cycle progression. This may explain its ability to facilitate differentiation. In contrast, when myoblasts proliferate slowly in mitogen-poor media, the same peptide can inhibit myotube formation and the expression of myogenin and other specific proteins, and antagonize the effects of Myo-D. The observations suggest regulatory roles in both development and repair.

transforming factor-β receptors: cell components that bind to and mediate the actions of TGF-βs. Unlike receptors described for **TGF-α** (*q.v.*), they lack intrinsic tyrosine kinase activity. Three widely distributed kinds bind all TGF-β isoforms but have little affinity for related peptides: Type I (53K glycoproteins that function in signal transduction), Type II (83K proteins with similar properties), and Type III (110-120K betaglycans whose functions have not been established). A 60K Type IV has been identified only in the adenohypophysis, and is the only type known to additionally bind activins, inhibins, and other peptides related to TGF-βs.

transfusion: transfer of blood or other fluids from one individual to another.

transgenic: containing genetic material from other species. Transgenic animals can be produced by injecting DNA into zygotes or very young embryos, treating cells with factors that affect the membranes and permit uptake of processed DNAs, or infecting cells with some viruses. Molecules that incorporate into the genome are transmitted to progeny. Transfection is used to produce large quantities of specific kinds of molecules (such as growth hormones and insulin-like growth factors), to study the effects of overproduction, and to identify the importance of mutations at specific sites.

transglutaminases: enzymes that catalyze reactions of the general type shown. *See* also **transamidases**.

trans-Golgi network: TGN; a complex of membranes, vesicles, and tubules near the *trans* phase of the Golgi apparatus, formerly known as GERL. It is a site for formation of clathrin-coated vesicles, for sorting substances destined for secretion, transport to the plasma membrane, or entry into lysosomes, and for vesicle discharge.

transhydrogenases: enzymes that catalyze reversible transfers of hydrogen atoms and electrons, usually via cofactors such as NAD^+/NADH and $NADP^+$/NADPH.

$$\text{—Glu—} \overset{\overset{\text{O}}{\|}}{\text{C}} \text{—NH}_2 \; + \; \text{H}_2\text{N—R} \; \longrightarrow \; \text{—Glu—} \overset{\overset{\text{O}}{\|}}{\text{C}} \text{—} \overset{\overset{\text{H}}{}}{\text{N}} \text{—R} \; + \; \text{—NH}_2$$

transglutaminases

transin: (1) a protease whose activity rises during early G1 phases of cell cycles; (2) a protease secreted by some malignant cells that acts on extracellular matrix components and may contribute to metastasis.

transitional elements: (1) specialized regions of rough endoplasmic reticulum in which membranes of vesicles that transport proteins and other substances to the cisternae of the Golgi apparatus originate; (2) eight groups of metallic elements with incomplete, unstable inner electron orbits. Each type can acquire more than one valence value and form colored ions. The group includes scandium, yttrium, lanthanum, actinium, zirconium, tungsten, rhenium, and titanium, as well as chromium, vanadium, manganese, molybdenum, and other "trace" metals found in living organisms.

transitional epithelium: epithelium of the kind in urinary bladder, with cells of diverse sizes and shapes arranged in a manner that permits accommodation to fluid accumulation with no increase in pressure.

transkaryotic implantation: insertion of a nucleus with altered DNA into a cell other than the one from which it was taken.

transketolase: an enzyme of the hexose monophosphate pathway that catalyzes transfers of 2-carbon units, as in the reaction: ribulose-4-phosphate + xylulose-5-phosphate $\rightarrow$ sedoheptulose-7-P + glyceraldehyde-3-P, in which two 5-carbon compounds react to yield one 7-carbon and one 3-carbon product; *cf* **transaldolase**.

translation: RNA-directed protein synthesis on ribosomes. It begins with formation of an initiation complex and requires several enzymes as well as initiation, elongation, termination, and other factors, energy sources, and transfer RNAs. *See* also **ribosomes, A** and **P sites**, and **messenger RNAs**.

translation acceleration factor: an uncharacterized factor released by mitochondria of triiodothyronine (T_3)-treated cells that accelerates translation.

translational control: regulation of the rate of formation of specific kinds of proteins at the level of protein synthesis; *cf* **transcriptional** and **posttranslational controls**.

translation factors: substances other than amino acids, nucleic acids, and ribosomal proteins that are essential for and/or affect the rates of protein synthesis. *See* **initiation** and **elongation factors**.

translocases: *see* **elongation factors**.

translocation: movement from one site to another, for example of (1) substances across plasma or organelle membranes; (2) nascent peptide chains from P to A sites on ribosomes; (3) steroid-receptor complexes from the cytoplasm to the nucleus; (4) genes (or other DNA segments) from one chromosome site to another on the same chromosome (intrachromosomal translocation) or to a different, often nonhomologous chromosome (interchromosomal translocation). *Reciprocal translocations* are exchanges of DNA segments between two chromosomes. All of the described nucleic acid processes involve DNA breakage and resealing.

transmembrane proteins: proteins that span membranes, with ends that project from the surfaces. Plasma membrane receptors for many hormones extend ligand binding sites towards extracellular fluids, and have intracellular components that interact with cytoplasmic and/or cytoskeletal elements.

transmission electron microscopy: TEM; techniques for visualizing cell components in which electron beams focused by grids are passed through specimens to form images on fluorescent screens and/or photographic plates. They permit visualization of entities too small for examination under light microscopy. However, since the sections must be very thin, only minute amounts of material can be observed at any one time. Moreover, the processing techniques, and the need for examination under vacuums distorts some structures. *See* also **shadow casting**, and *cf* **scanning electron microscopy**.

transmittance: T; the ratio of the quantity of light transmitted through a test solution to the quantity transmitted by the solvent or another reference solution.

transmodulation: modification by one hormone of the properties of receptors for another; *cf* **modulation**.

transmutation: conversion of one kind of element to another during radioactive decay.

transpiration: (1) loss of water vapor from leaf surfaces. Most of the water is transported upward from the roots and is released from stomata; (2) insensible perspiration in animals; (3) passage of water across lung epithelium, and formation of water vapor in respiratory passages.

transplant: a graft; a tissue or organ removed from one part of the body and inserted into another part of the same body or into another individual.

transplantation antigens: transplantation associated antigens; TSTAs; antigens expressed on graft cell surfaces that can initiate immunological rejection if perceived as foreign by the host. Their synthesis is directed by histocompatibility genes.

transplant rejection: immune system mediated destruction of tissues or organs that contain substances perceived as foreign. *See* also **cellular immunity** and **T lymphocytes**.

transport maximum: *see* **Tm**.

transposable elements: small DNA segments that can move from one chromosome to another; *see* also **transposon**.

transposase: an enzyme required for insertion of a transposon.

transposon: a short, highly mobile transposable element (typically around 1000 base pairs in length) that can insert into chromosomes at numerous sites. It includes a transposase, and often also elements required for mobility. The base sequences at the two ends are identical but oriented in opposite directions. One copy is retained at the initial site, and others can be synthesized at acceptor (insertion) sites. Transposons are believed to mediate the DNA amplification associated with multiple drug resistance, and are suspected of contributing to some cancers.

transsexual: describes an individual who identifies with a gender that does not agree with his (or her) phenotype, or one who has undergone changes to increase resemblance to members of the other gender.

transthyretin: TBPA; thyroxine binding prealbumin; species specific 55K plasma proteins secreted by liver cells that bind approximately 20% of circulating thyroxine (but have little affinity for triiodothyronine). Each molecule is a homotetramer of 127-amino acid subunits with one high and one lower affinity binding site for T_4. TBPAs associate with equal numbers of retinol binding protein molecules, and may thereby protect RBPs against loss to the urine. The complexes are stabilized by retinol (but not by thyroxine). Since TBPAs additionally bind to DNAs, other functions have been proposed. Androgens and glucocorticoids are among the factors that accelerate TBPA synthesis, whereas estrogens lower the levels.

transudate: a fluid (usually clear and low in protein content) passed through a membrane or extruded from a tissue; *cf* **exudate**.

transverse tubules: T tubules; small tubular invaginations of skeletal muscle plasma membranes that contribute to excitation-contraction coupling by mediating rapid transmission of stimulatory signals. The external faces are exposed to extracellular fluids, and the internal ones contact sarcoplasmic reticula at the Z disks.

transvestite: an individual who dresses in clothing of the opposite sex, often for sexual gratification (but differs from a transsexual). Transvestites are more commonly heterosexual than homosexual.

tranylcypromine: *trans*-2-phenylcyclopropanamine; a monoamine oxidase inhibitor used as an antidepressant and to treat narcolepsy. It additionally affects some other enzymes and exerts actions unrelated to MAO inhibition. The toxic effects can include hyperthermia, disturbances in blood pressure regulation, hallucinations, and convulsions.

TRAP: (1) tartrate resistant acid phosphatase; (2) thyroid receptor auxiliary protein.

Trasylol: a trade name for aprotinin.

TRE: thyroid response element.

trefoil peptides: small proteins with common structural features that confer resistance to degradation by proteolytic enzymes. They contribute to control of epithelial cell proliferation and differentiation and to maintenance of mucosal membrane integrity. Each molecule has three intra-chain peptide loops established by disulfide bonds. Intestinal trefoil factors (ITFs) are 81-amino acid types made by goblet cells and secreted to viscoepithelial coats that overly mucosal surfaces. They activate adenylate cyclases, and promote healing after mucosal injury. Increased amounts are made by individuals with peptic ulcers and inflammatory bowel disease. Porcine pancreatic spasmolytic polypeptide (PSP) and its human counterpart (hSP), made in large amounts by exocrine pancreas, additionally affect intestinal motility and gastric acidity. An estrogen responsive type, pS2 protein initially identified in breast cancers, is also made by gastric mucosa and in inflamed exocrine pancreatic tissue. *Xenopus* spasmolysin is a related amphibian skin protein.

trehalose: α-D-glucopyranosyl-α-D-glucopyranoside; a sugar made by many invertebrates, plants, fungi, and bacteria.

Trematodes: a genus of flatworms that includes parasitic flukes.

tremorine: 1,4-dipyrrolidino-2-butyne; it is converted to oxotremorine, a potent muscarinic acetylcholine receptor agonist that enters the brain and acts on basal ganglion receptors, and is used to invoke a Parkinson-like syndrome in laboratory animals.

trenbolone: trienolone; 17-hydroxyestra-4,9,11-trien-3-one; a synthetic androgen used for its anabolic actions. *See* **anabolic steroids**.

trephone: a hypothetical substance said to promote mitosis and repair when released by injured cells; *cf* **chalone**.

tretinoin: all-*trans*-retinoic acid.

TRF: (1) thyrotropin release factor; (2) an old acronym for T cell replacing factor, now known as interleukin-5.

TRH: thyrotropin releasing hormone.

TRIAC: triiodothyroacetic acid.

triacylglycerols: triglycerides; fats; molecules composed of three fatty acid moieties linked by ester bonds to glycerol carbon atoms, and digested to the components by lipases. Most kinds stored in adipocytes contain stearic, palmitic, oleic, and other long-chain fatty acids. Tributyrate is a short-chain type in some dairy foods. Synthesis from the components requires fatty acyl coenzyme As and glycerol-3-phosphate (which is derived from dihydroxyacetone phosphate). Since two high energy phosphate bonds from ATP are required to make each fatty acyl CoA from a fatty acid, and the glycerol-phosphate is derived from an early step in glycolysis (when two ATP have been converted to ADP), fatty acid cycles in which triacylglycerols are degraded and resynthesized generate large quantities of heat (liberated from ATP hydrolysis). They may thereby contribute to calorigenic responses to cold environments. Insulin is the primary stimulant for lipogenesis. *See* also **triacylglycerol lipases**.

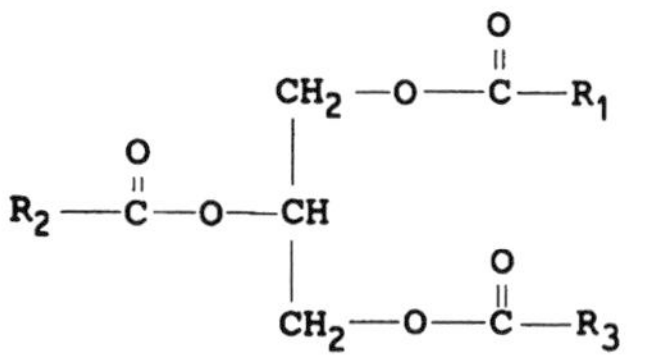

triacylglycerol lipases: triglyceride lipases; enzymes that initiate lipolysis by converting triacylglycerols to diacylglycerols (substrates for diacylglycerol lipases) plus free fatty acids. Catecholamines activate hormone-sensitive types by promoting kinase A-mediated phosphorylation. *Cf* **lipoprotein lipases**.

triads: structures in skeletal muscle fibers that contribute to excitation-contraction coupling, each composed of three transverse tubules and the sarcoplasmic reticulum components with which they associate.

triamcinolone: 9-fluoro-11β-16α,17,21-tetrahydroxy-pregna-1,4-diene; a potent synthetic glucocorticoid with negligible mineralocorticoid activity, used for its anti-inflammatory properties.

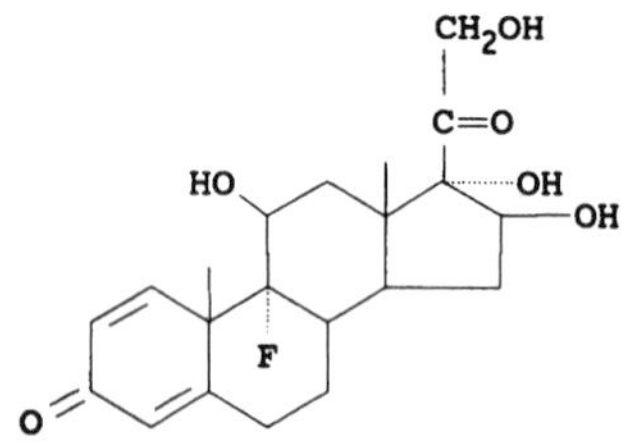

triamterene: 6-phenyl-2,4,7-pteridinetriamine; an orally effective diuretic that has been used to treat hypertension. Although initially believed to act as an aldosterone receptor antagonist, it promotes Na⁺ and Cl⁻ excretion in adrenalectomized animals, and does not affect potassium retention.

triazolam: Halcyon; 8-chloro-6-(2-chlorophenyl)-1-methyl-4*H*[1,2,4]triazolo[4,3-*a*][1,4]benzodiazepine; a benzodiazepine type sedative and hypnotic.

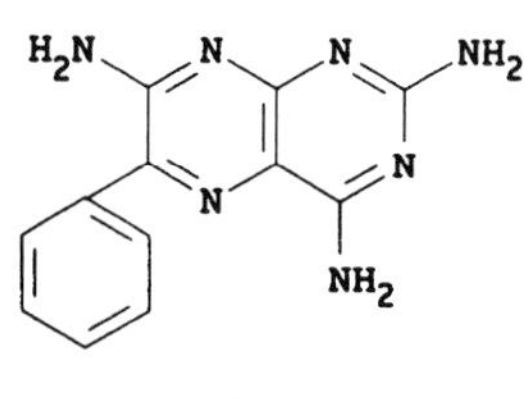

triamterene

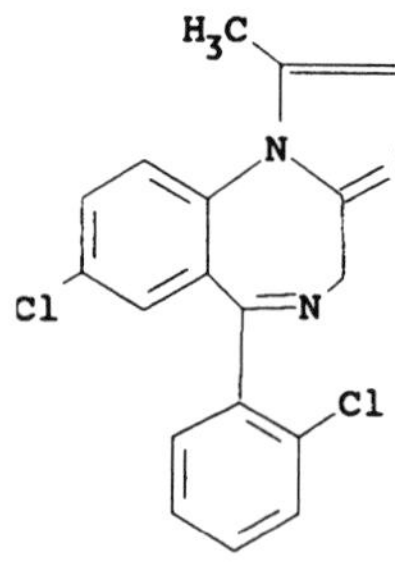

triazolam

3-amino-1,2,4-**triazole**: an agent used to inhibit catalases.

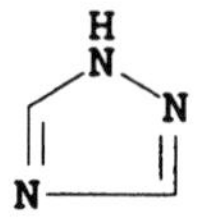

tributyrin: glyceryl tributyrate; a triacylglycerol component of butter and some other dairy foods with short-chain fatty acids.

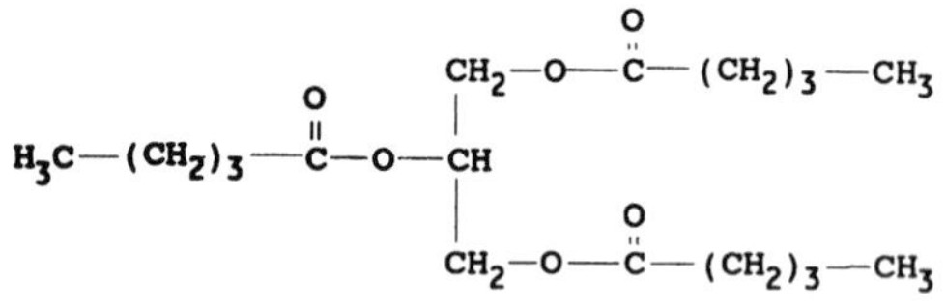

tricaine: Metacaine; ethyl *m*-aminobenzoate methanesulfonate; an agent used to anesthetize fish.

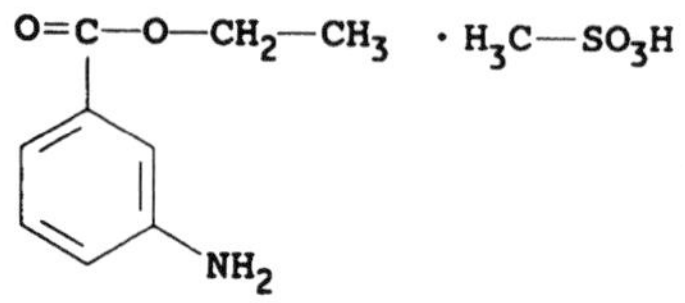

tricarboxylic acid: any acid with three carboxyl groups; *see* for example **citric acid**.

tricarboxylic acid cycle: citric acid cycle; Krebs cycle: a series of reactions in mitochondria that begins with condensation of acetyl-coenzyme A (obtained from glucose, fatty acids and other fuels) with oxaloacetate (present in the organelles) to form citric acid, and ends with generation of new molecules of oxaloacetate. It is the major pathway for oxidation of acetyl-CoA, and for reduction of coenzymes that are sent to electron transport chains for oxidative phosphorylation. The overall effects are: acetyl-CoA + 3 NAD⁺ + FAD + GDP + Pi + 2 HOH → 2 CO₂ + CoA-SH + 3 NADH + 3 H⁺ + FADH₂ + GTP.

Enzymes that catalyze the reactions are indicated by numbers in brackets. The cycle also generates α-ketoglutarate, malate, and other intermediates used for different purposes.

acetyl-CoA + oxaloacetate → citrate; [1]

citrate + HOH → *cis*-aconitate; aconitate + HOH → isocitrate; [2]

isocitrate + NAD^+ → α-ketoglutarate+$NADH+H^+$ + CO_2; [3]

α-ketoglutarate + NAD^+ + CoA → succinyl-CoA + $NADH + H^+ + CO_2$;[4]

succinyl-CoA + Pi + GDP → succinate + GTP + CoA; [5]

succinate + FAD → fumarate + $FADH_2$; [6]

fumarate + HOH → malate; [7]

malate + NAD^+ → oxaloacetate + $NADH + H^+$; [8]

[1] = citrate synthase; [2] = aconitase; [3] = isocitric dehydrogenase; [4] = α-ketodehydrogenase; [5] = succinyl-CoA synthase; [6] = succinic dehydrogenase; [7] = fumarase; [8] = malate dehydrogenase.

Trichinella: a genus of parasitic nematodes that can live in humans, hogs, rats, mice, cats, and some other species, and cause trichinosis. Immature forms encyst in muscle fibers, and are ingested with infected meat (usually pork). When released during digestion, they penetrate the mucosa of the small intestine, in which they complete maturation and mate. Young larvae released to the bloodstream settle in skeletal muscle, grow rapidly, and encyst. Their movements and waste products invoke inflammation, eosinophilia, and degeneration of the enclosing muscle fibers.

trichloroacetic acid: TCA; a reagent used to precipitate proteins, fix tissues for some histological studies, and remove calcium from solutions. Its corrosive properties are used to destroy warts and some moles.

trichloroethanol: a chloral hydrate metabolite that mediates most of the hypnotic and sedative effects of the parent compound.

tricho-: a prefix meaning hair or hair-like.

trichocysts: rod-shaped structures arranged radially below the pellicles of *Paramecia* and other ciliated protozoa, and discharged as filaments in response to chemical or mechanical stimuli. The proposed functions include assistance in trapping prey, defense against predators, and anchoring during feeding.

trichomes: hair cells on the surfaces of plant leaves, stems, petioles, and sepals.

Trichomonas: a genus of flagellate protozoa. *T. buccalis* co-exists with pyogenic organisms in infected gums but may not be pathogenic. *T. vaginalis* causes disease when it infects the vagina, urethra, and possibly also the prostate gland.

trichrome pigments: chromatophore pigments chemically related to melanins that impart bright coloration to feathers and other epidermal derivatives.

tricyclamol chloride: procyclidine; 1-(3-cyclohexyl-3-hydroxy-3-phenylpropyl)-1-methylpyrrolidinium hydrochloride; a muscarinic type acetylcholine receptor antagonist used to inhibit gastrointestinal tract motility and gastric acid secretion.

tricyclic antidepressants: amitriptyline, chlortryptiline, desipramine, and related agents with three fused carbon rings that are used to alleviate some forms of psychic depression, compulsive behaviors, and phobias (but can invoke psychic depression in healthy humans). They potentiate the effects of catecholamines, serotonin, and other endogenous amines by inhibiting their uptake across neuron plasma membranes, and additionally antagonize some acetylcholine actions.

tridihexethyl iodide: γ-cyclohexyl-*N,N,N*-triethyl-γ-hydroxybenzenepropanaminium iodide; an acetylcholine receptor antagonist used to relieve intestinal spasms. It was initially called Pathilon, but that name is now applied to the chloride which has replaced it.

triethylenemelamine: TEM; tetramine; 2,4,6-triethylenimino-1,3,5-triazine; a nitrogen mustard type cytotoxic agent used to treat some chronic (but not acute) leukemias.

triethylenephosphoramide: TEPA; 1,1′,1″-phosphinyli-dynetrisaziridine; a nitrogen mustard used to treat some urinary bladder, breast and ovary cancers, and some lymphomas.

trifluoperazine: TFP; 2-trifluoromethyl-10-[3′-(1-methyl-4-piperazinyl)propyl]phenothiazine; a phenothiazine type "antipsychotic" agent employed to a limited extent in individuals with nonpsychotic anxiety, but more toxic than some other agents. The undesirable effects include drowsiness and impaired mental functions, increased prolactin secretion, altered responses to vasopressin, and changes in insulin secretion. Since it is a dopamine antagonist, prolonged use can invoke tardive dyskinesia. Susceptible individuals also develop autonomic instability and hyperpyrexia; and some Stelazine (TFP hydrochloride) preparations contain substances that can invoke allergic reactions. TFP is used as a laboratory tool that effectively but nonspecifically interferes with calmodulin actions and affects cyclic nucleotide phosphodiesterase activity. It also binds to and alters the properties of plasma membrane constituents.

trifluoromethane sulfonic acid: a very strong acid used to release O- and N-linked oligosaccharides from peptide chains.

trifluperidol: 4′-fluoro-4-[4-hydroxy-4-(α,α.α-trifluoro-m-tolyl)piperidino]butyrophenone; a phenothiazine type tranquilizer used to treat mania.

triflupromazine: N,N-dimethyl-2-(trifluoromethyl)-10H-phenothiazine-10-propanamine; a tranquilizer used to control emesis.

trigeminal: having three roots or origins, a term usually applied to the fifth (and largest) pair of cranial nerves. The dendrites carry pain and other messages from the face, teeth, mouth, and nasal cavity. The axons include motor fibers to muscles used for chewing.

triglycerides: true fats; see **triacylglycerols**.

triglyceride lipases: triacylglycerol lipases.

trihexphenidyl hydrochloride: Aparkane; Parkinsan; Artilan; Tsiklodol; α-cyclohexyl-α-phenyl-1-piperidine-propanol hydrochloride; an anticholinergic agent used to treat Parkinsonism.

triiodothyroacetic acid: TRIAC; a triiodothyronine (T_3) metabolite. Although less potent than T_3, it acts on the same receptors. Since it does not bind with high affinity to circulating TBG (thryonine binding globulin), it acts more rapidly in some systems.

triiodothyronine; T_3; 3,5,3′-triiodothyronine: the major iodinated thyroid hormone. Small amounts are synthesized in and secreted directly by thyroid gland follicular cells; but most circulating T_3 is formed from T_4 (**thyroxine**, q.v.) taken up by hepatic and other cell types; see also **deiodinases**. Thyroid stimulating hormone (TSH) promotes thyroid gland growth, and acts in conjunction with growth factors to stimulate cell proliferation. It accelerates iodine uptake and thyroglobulin formation, affects thyroglobulin glycosylation, and promotes T_4 release as well as synthesis. Thyrotropin releasing hormone (TRH) maintains the thyrotropes that make TSH; and T_4 taken up from the bloodstream and converted to T_3 exerts negative feedback control over TSH, mostly by diminishing the numbers of TRH receptors. The absolute amounts of T_3 directly secreted by thyroid glands, and the T_3:T_4 ratios increase when iodide deficiency or other conditions elevate TSH levels. Small amounts of T_3 are excreted to the bile. Larger ones are degraded to diiodothyronines, monoiodothyronines and other metabolites. The best known actions of T_3 are me-

trifluperidol

diated via nuclear **triiodothyronine receptors** (*q.v.*) that bind to **thyroid response elements** and affect the functions of many genes. They are major regulators of somatic growth and cell differentiation that act directly and also affect the secretion and functions of other hormones. They accelerate oxygen consumption in skeletal muscle and several other cell types and thereby elevate basal metabolic rates and maintain body temperatures. They also affect the metabolism of carbohydrates, proteins, lipids, and nucleic acids, augment sensitivities to catecholamines and modulate the numbers of receptor subset types, exert profound influences on the circulatory system, and are essential for normal somatic growth and maturation of the skeletal, reproductive, and central nervous systems. Several effects become apparent after very long latent periods, and involve formation of new organelles. Full development of calorigenic stimulation can require four weeks in humans. Different kinds of receptors that mediate early influences are present in mitochondria, plasma membranes, and possibly also other cell components; and some influences are exerted on erythrocytes (which lack nuclei and mitochondria). *See* also **hyperthyroidism, hypothyroidism, cretinism,** and **reverse T₃.**

reverse **triiodothyronine**: rT₃; *see* **reverse T₃.**

triiodothyronine receptors: molecules that interact with triiodothyronine and mediate its actions. The major types are nuclear proteins encoded by α and β type *c-erbA* genes (*q.v.*) that undergo differential processing to yield several subtypes with cell-specific distributions. When bound to T₃ they exert mostly stimulatory influences on the transcription of numerous genes; but unbound receptors can function as repressors. Nuclear T₃ receptors are members of a superfamily of ligand-binding transcription factors that includes receptors for steroid hormones, calciferols, retinoids, and peroxisome proliferators, and for other regulators. In addition to direct influences on specific DNA base sequences, the various receptor types interact in several ways with each other and with recep-

tors for other members of the superfamily. Different kinds of receptors are on plasma membranes, mitochondria, and other cell components.

trilostane: 4,5-epoxy-17-hydroxy-3-oxoandrostane-2-carbonitrile; a glucocorticoid receptor antagonist used to treat Cushing's syndrome. It also blocks pregnenolone conversion to progesterone.

trimer: a molecule composed of three subunits, usually three peptide chains.

trimester: a three month period. For some purposes, human pregnancy is divided into first, second and third trimesters.

trimethadione: 3,5,5-trimethyl-2,4-oxazolidine-dione; a ganglionic blocking agent. It has been used to control epilepsy, but the side effects include sedation, blurring of vision, and dermatitis. It can invoke severe blood dyscrasias, hepatitis, and nephrosis; and it increases the incidence of stillbirths and birth defects when taken by pregnant women.

trimethaphan camsylate: 4,6-dibenzyl-5-oxo-1-thia-4,6-diazatricyclo[6.3.O.O]undecanium (+)-β-camphor-sulfonate; a ganglionic blocking agent used in special cases to control hypertension and autonomic hyper-reflexia.

trimethoprim: 2,4-diamino-5-(3,4,5-trimethoxybenzyl) pyrimidine; an agent that enhances the antibacterial effectiveness of sulfonamides by inhibiting prokaryote dihydrofolate reductases.

trimethaphan camsylate

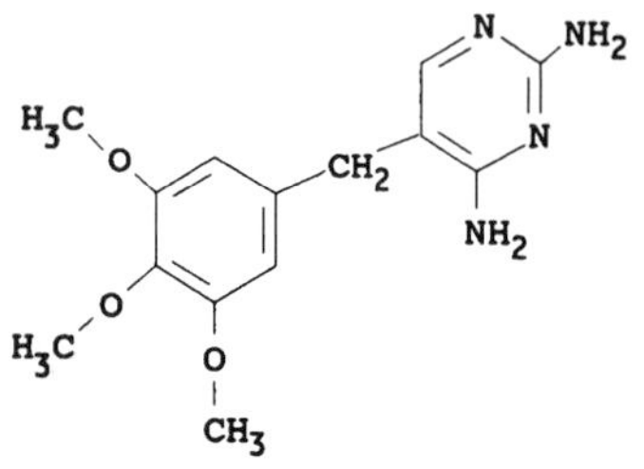

trimethoprim

trimethylamine: *N,N*-dimethylmethanamine; a degradation product of choline and some other organic molecules, identified in plants, fish, menstrual blood and urine.

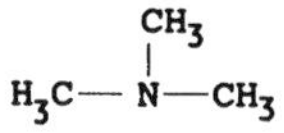

trimethylamine oxide: a compound made by some elasmobranch fishes that contributes to maintenance of blood osmotic pressure.

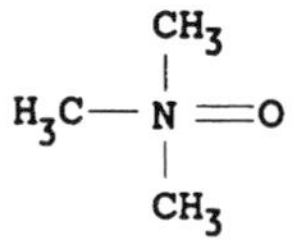

triolein: glyceryl trioleinate; a triacylglycerol composed of 1 glycerol and 3 oleate moieties.

trioses: three-carbon sugars, for example glyceraldehyde or dihydroxyacetone.

triose kinases: enzymes that transfer phosphate groups from ATP to triose sugars. One type mediates glyceraldehyde entry into the glycolysis pathway.

triose phosphate isomerase: an enzyme of the glycolytic pathway that catalyzes interconversion of glyceraldehyde-3-phosphate and dihydroxyacetone phosphate.

trioxsalen: 6-hydroxy-β-2,7-trimethyl-5-benzofuranacrylic acid δ-lactone; 4,5′8-trimethylpsoralen; an agent used to promote pigmentation in vitiliginous skin, protect against excessive ultraviolet radiation, and facilitate skin

tanning. It is reported to enhance sunlight mediated cell growth, proliferation, and differentiation, as well as tyrosine hydroxylase activity in melanocytes.

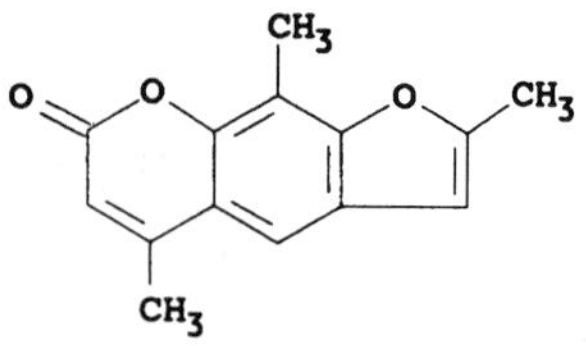

tripalmitin: glyceryl tripalmitate; a triacylglycerol composed of 1 glycerol and 3 palmitate moieties.

tripamide: 3-(aminosulfonyl)-4-chloro-*N*-(octahydro-4, 7-methano-2*H*-isoindol-2-yl)benzamide; a sulfonamide derivative that directly dilates peripheral blood vessels. It is used for its diuretic and antihypertensive effects.

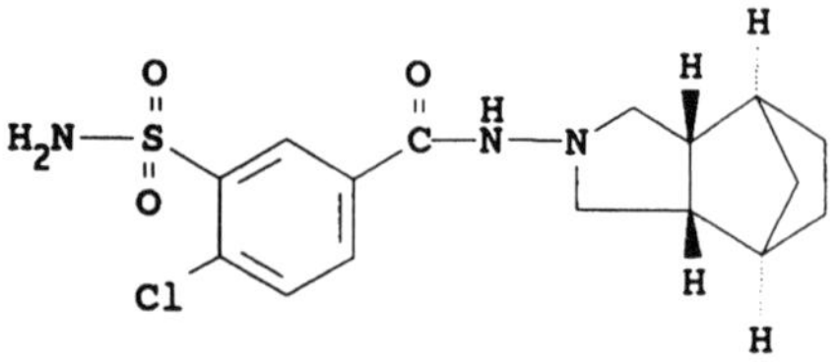

triparanol: MER-29; 4-chloro-α-[4-[2-(diethylamino)-ethoxy]phenyl]-α-(4-methylphenyl)benzene ethanol; an agent that inhibits cholesterol biosynthesis but is too toxic for use as an antilipemic in humans. It can cause cataracts, impotence, and baldness.

tripelennamine: Pyribenzamine, PBZ; β-dimethylaminoethyl-2-pyridylaminotoluene; an H_1 type histamine receptor antagonist with minimal effects on the central nervous system.

triple response: a skin reaction to histamine that includes localized reddening, warmth, and wheal formation.

triplets: sets of three, for example three messenger RNA bases that code for a specific amino acid type, or three siblings that develop during a single gestation.

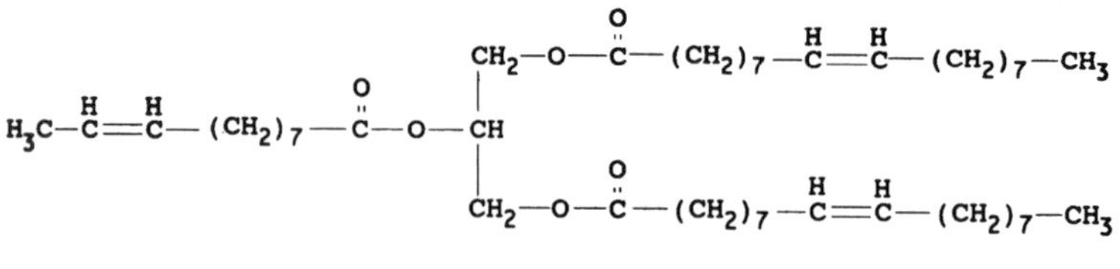

triolein

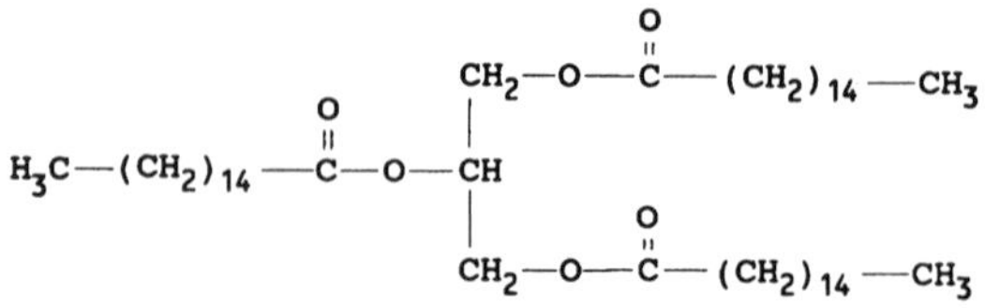

tripalmitin

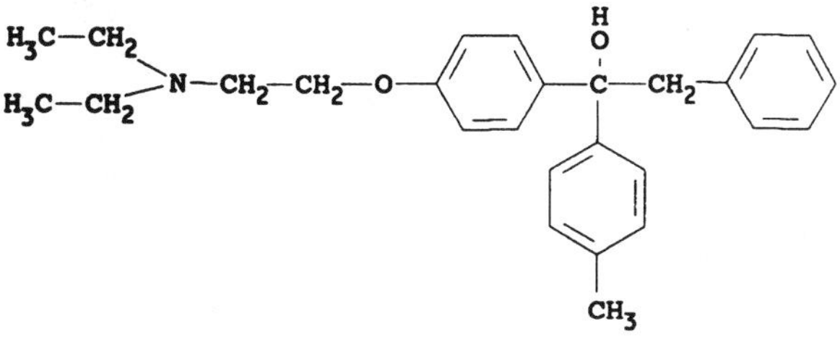

triparanol

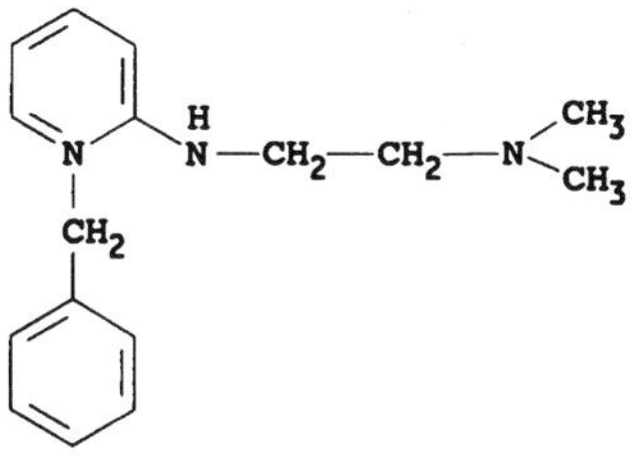

tripelenamine

triploid: having three complete sets of haploid chromosomes.

triptorelin: 6-D-tryptophan-LRH; 6-oxoPro-His-Trp-Ser-Tyr-D-Trp-Leu-Arg-Prop-Gly-NH₂; a gonadotropin releasing hormone (GnRH) analog. It is a potent receptor antagonist, used to treat prostatic carcinomas.

TRIS: tromethamine; tris(hydroxymethyl)aminomethane; 2-amino-2-hydroxymethyl-1,3-propane diol; a buffer used *in vitro* to maintain pHs greater than 8, and as an emulsifying agent.

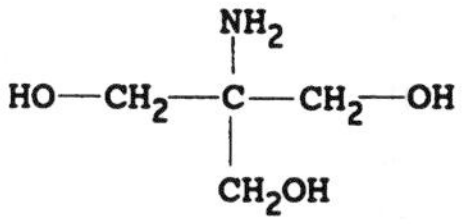

triskelion: a three-legged structure formed by three peptide chains. Clathrin triskelions assemble into basket-like networks.

trisomy: the presence of an extra chromosome of one type in otherwise diploid cells, a condition that usually originates during gametogenesis (*see* **nondisjunction**) and can cause fetal defects. Some individuals with Down's syndrome have three copies of chromosome 21. Others have an extra segment on the long arm of that chromosome.

tristearin: glyceryl tristearate; a triacylglycerol composed of one glycerol and three stearate moieties.

tritium: ^{3}[H]; a long-lived radioactive hydrogen isotope used to label thymidine, amino acids, steroids, and other molecules in metabolic studies, in radioautography, and for its effects on microtubules.

Triton N: nonoxynol.

Triton X: Triton X-100; octoxynol; octylphenoxy polyethoxyethanol; a nonionic detergent and emulsifying agent that increases membrane permeability and is used in some spermatocides. *See* also **polyethylene *p-t*-octyl phenol**.

trk: a gene expressed by cells responsive to **nerve growth factor** (*q.v.*) that can no longer divide. Some thyroid gland carcinoma cells have DNA rearrangements.

tRNAs: transfer ribonucleic acids.

Trolox: 6-hydroxy-2,5,7,8-tetramethylchroman-2-carboxylic acid; a tocopherol derivative used for its antioxidant properties.

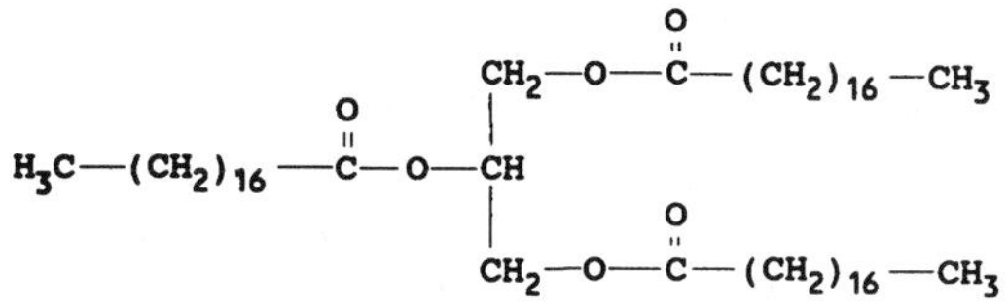

tristearin

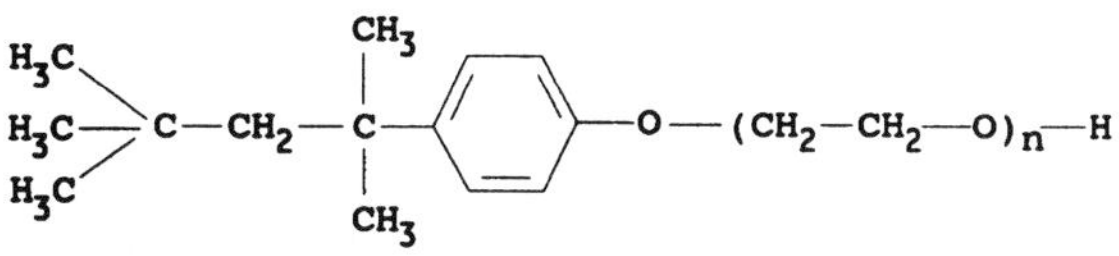

Triton X

-trope: a suffix meaning going towards, used for cells whose secretory products travel to specific target cell types, as in gonadotrope.

troph: both the prefix (troph-, as in trophoblast), and the suffix (-troph, as in gonadotroph) are used for entities that nourish and/or stimulate.

trophectoderm: trophoblast.

trophic: promoting nourishment or growth. It is also used as a suffix (-trophic), as in somatotrophic or adrenocorticotrophic hormone.

trophoblast: trophectoderm; the outer layer of the blastocyst and the cytotrophoblast and syncytiotrophoblast that develop from it. It participates in formation of the chorion, functions in implantation and nourishment of the conceptus, and secretes chorionic gonadotropin and other regulators.

trophoblastomas: choriocarcinomas; malignant tumors derived from trophoblastic tissues.

trophoblast protein-1: ovine pregnancy factor; an interferon-α (IFNα) subtype made by pregnant ewes.

tropic: going towards. It can be used as a suffix, as in thigmotropic or gonadotropic.

-tropin: a suffix for agents that go towards a structure, as in thyrotropin.

tropism: turning, bending, or growth toward a stimulus, often used as a suffix, as in phototropism.

tropocollagen: (1) collagen; (2) an intermediate in the pathway for collagen biosynthesis, formed when procollagen undergoes limited proteolysis.

tropomyosin: a rigid, rod-shaped protein of skeletal muscle thin filaments, composed of two identical 248 amino acid chains that entwine to form a coiled coil. It wraps around actin molecules, stabilizes and strengthens the filaments, and covers the binding sites for myosin in unstimulated cells. *See* also **troponins**.

troponins: 78K complexes composed of three skeletal muscle thin filament proteins. Troponin T (30K) binds tropomyosin, and troponin I (30K) binds actin. Troponin C (18K) is a calmodulin-like protein that attaches to both troponin I and troponin T. When cell stimulation leads to release of Ca^{2+} from the sarcoplasmic reticulum, each troponin C molecule binds four of the ions and undergoes a conformational change. Consequently, troponin I is displaced from actin, and tropomyosin is shifted away from the myosin binding sites on actin. This permits the forma-

tion of cross-bridges, and the myosin ATPase activation essential for contraction.

Trousseau's sign: flexion of the fingers at metacarpophalangeal joints and extension of the thumb, a response invoked in hypocalcemic subjects when arterioles that supply the forearm are occluded. It is used as an indicator of parathyroid hormone deficiency.

Trp: tryptophan.

TRPM-2: testosterone repressed protein messenger; clusterin; a protein in prostate tissue undergoing regression after androgen withdrawal, used as a marker for apoptosis.

trypan blue: sodium ditolyl-diazo*bis*-8-amino-1-naphthol-3,6-disulfonate; a dye excluded by living but not dead cells, used to test cell viability.

Trypanosomes: a genus of protozoa that includes members of the *brucei* group carried by tsetse flies.

trypsin: serine proteases that cleave peptide bonds on the *C*-terminal sides of arginine and lysine moieties. Pancreatic acinar cells secrete **trypsinogen** (*q.v.*). After conversion to trypsin it acts directly on food proteins and partially digested products delivered to the small intestine, autocatalytically activates additional trypsinogen molecules, and also activates chymotrypsinogen, procarboxypeptidase, and proelastases. Trypsins of various species are used as to study enzyme actions, cleave renin substrates *in vitro*, and partially hydrolyze other proteins. Low concentrations activate some cell surface receptors in the absence of their hormone ligands; but high levels destroy receptors.

trypsin inhibitors: several proteins that bind to trypsin active sites, inhibit the enzymes, and thereby protect against excessive proteolysis. A 6K type made by pancreatic acinar cells limits trypsinogen conversion to trypsin. α₁-Antitrypsin (α-1-antiproteinase), a 53K plasma protein, inhibits elastase and protects against potential cell injury by enzymes released from neutrophilic leukocytes. Soybean trypsin inhibitor is a laboratory tool.

trypsinogen: a proenzyme (zymogen) secreted by exocrine pancreas acinar cells. Cleavage of a single peptide bond yields active trypsin. The reaction is initiated by enterokinin, an enteropeptidase released from the cells of the small intestine. Soon after small amounts are formed, trypsin becomes the major zymogen activator.

tryptamine: 1*H*-indole-3-ethanamine; a tryptophan decarboxylation product formed in small amounts in pineal glands and other sites of serotonin synthesis. It is metabo-

trypan blue

lized to dimethyltryptamine and other biologically active amines, some of which are hallucinogens; and it can affect catecholamine metabolism by competing with the amines for monoamine oxidases. Its major degradation product is indole acetic acid (IAA).

5-methyl-*N,N*-dimethyl-tryptamine: a serotonin receptor antagonist. (Dimethyl tryptamine is a hallucinogen in the leaves of *Prestonia amazonica* that animals also make in minute amounts from tryptamine.)

5-hydroxy-tryptamine: serotonin.

tryptophan: Trp; W; 2-amino-3-indolylpropanoic acid; an essential amino acid, a component of many proteins, and the precursor of serotonin, melatonin, other hormones, and niacin; *see* also **tryptophan hydroxylase** and **tryptophan monooxygenase**. The blood levels undergo diet-related circadian variations. Since the concentrations are lower than those of most amino acids, they can be rate-limiting for the synthesis of proteins (*see* **tryptophan oxidase**) and for serotonin and related amines. Although released from most protein foods, ingestion of additional amounts has been advocated for ameliorating psychic depression, affective diseases, schizophrenia, insomnia, premenstrual syndrome, chronic pain, and behavioral disorders. Some individuals taking large quantities made by a *Bacillus amyloliquefaciens* strain developed an eosinophil myalgia syndrome (EMS) characterized by severe muscle pain and profound eosinophilia (up to 6,000 cells per cubic milliliter of peripheral blood), often accompanied by arthralgias, muscle weakness and fatigue, headache, skin rashes, cough, peripheral edema, fever, and paresthesia. Cytotoxic eosinophilic granule products, and high transforming growth factor-β1 (TGFβ1), type IV collagen, and fibronectin concentrations in the affected tissues, and elevated serum aldolase levels (a marker of muscle injury) have also been found. Pathological findings consistent with abnormal immune system activity include lymphocyte infiltration into dermis, fascia, and skeletal muscle. Although some individuals have recovered after discontinuing tryptophan use, others remain ill; and a few have died. The syndrome has been attributed to the presence of contaminants in the tryptophan preparations. The ones most commonly implicated include 3-phenylamino-L-tryptophan, and 1,1′-ethylidene *bis*-tryptophan. However, toxic levels of tryptophan itself, and of its endogenous metabolites, may contribute.

tryptophan

1,1′-ethylidene *bis*-tryptophan: a contaminant of tryptophan preparations made by bacteria, implicated as a cause of eosinophil myalgia syndrome; *see* **tryptophan**.

5,7-dihydroxy-tryptophan: a neurotoxin that selectively destroys serotoninergic neurons.

5-hydroxy-tryptophan: 5-HTP; an intermediate in the pathway for tryptophan conversion to serotonin and other biologically active amines, formed in a rate-limiting reaction catalyzed by tryptophan hydroxylase. Oral administration can accelerate synthesis of the amines.

tryptophan dioxygenase: *see* **tryptophan oxidase**.

tryptophan hydroxylase: an enzyme induced by neurotransmitters and inhibited by high levels of phenylalanine that converts tryptophan to 5-hydroxy-tryptophan (the rate-limiting step for serotonin biosynthesis). The reaction uses molecular oxygen and requires a pteridine cofactor.

tryptophan oxidase: TO; tryptophan pyrrolase; TP; tryptophan 2,3-dioxygenase; **indoleamine 2,3-dioxygenase** (*q.v.*); an enzyme that converts tryptophan to formylkynurenine. Its synthesis in liver cells is augmented by glucocorticoids, glucagon and tryptophan loading, and is decreased by growth hormone. Metabolites derived from the product include alanine, acetyl coenzyme A, and glucose precursors. *See* also **carcinoid syndrome**. High levels deplete tryptophan stores. Since synthesis of proteins that contain it cannot proceed, tryopphan deficieny increases the availability of other amino acids for gluconeogenesis.

tryptophan pyrrolase: TP; tryptophan oxidase.

tryptophol: 3-indolethanol; a tryptophan metabolite; *see* 5-hydroxy- and 5-methoxy-**tryptophol**.

5-hydroxy-tryptophol: a tryptophan metabolite made in pineal glands. According to some observers, it is a pineal hormone that decreases gonadotropin release.

5-methoxy-tryptophol: a tryptophan metabolite made in pineal glands. It is a proposed inhibitor of gonadotropin releasing hormone (GnRH) secretion that contributes to regulation of seasonal reproduction patterns.

O-acetyl-5-hydroxy-**tryptophol**, *O*-acetyl-5-methoxy-**tryprophol**: sertonin and melatonin degradation products.

tryptorelin: triptorelin; 6D-tryptophan-LRH; a highly potent gonadotropin releasing hormone analog and agonist, used to decrease reproductive system hormone secretion by desensitizing gonadotropes to GnRH.

TSAs: tumor specific antigens.

TSAbs: thyroid stimulating antibodies; immunoglobulins that bind to thyroid stimulating hormone (TSH) receptors on thyroid gland follicular cells and mimic the hormone actions. They are made by some individuals with autoimmune forms of hyperthyroidism.

TSBAbs: thyroid stimulating hormone blocking antibodies made by some people with autoimmune forms of hypothyroidism. They compete with thyroid stimulating hormone (TSH) for binding to receptors on thyroid glands.

T_S **cells**: suppressor type T lymphocytes.

T:S ratio: the ratio of the iodine concentration in the thyroid gland to the iodine concentration in blood serum; *see* **T:P ratio**.

TSH: thyroid stimulating hormone.

O-acetyl-5-hydroxy-
tryptophol

TSH displacing antibodies: TDAs; immunoglobulins that compete with TSH for binding to receptors on thyroid glands. Some stimulate, whereas others inhibit thyroid gland functions.

TSL: threonyl-seryl-lysine.

ts mutants: temperature sensitive mutants.

TSP: thrombin-sensitive protein; *see* **thrombospondin**.

tst-1: a protein made in testes; *see* **POU-III**.

TSTAs: transplantation associated antigens.

t **test**: *see* **Student's *t* test**.

T tubules: *see* **transverse tubules**.

TTX: tetrodotoxin.

tuber: a rounded projection.

tubercidin: 7-deaza-adenosine; sparsamycin A; an antibacterial, antifungal, and antineoplastic agent made by *Streptomyces tubercidus* that causes misreading of genetic codes and can inhibit peptide chain elongation. Although toxic, it is used to arrest tuberculosis.

tuber cinereum: a mass of grey matter that forms part of the floor of the third ventricle of the brain and is continuous with the infundibular stalk. In primates it contains the lateral tuberal and tuberomammillary nuclei.

tubercle: a small nodule.

tuberculin: a mixture of mostly protein components of *Mycobacterium* cultures filtrates; *see* **tuberculin test**.

tuberculin test: a procedure in which tuberculin is injected intradermally and the injection site is later examined for a delayed hypersensitivity reaction. A positive test can indicate that a cell-mediated immunity response has been mounted against *Mycobacterium* species; but other antigens can affect it.

O-acetyl-5-methoxy-
tryptophol

tuberculosis: infectious diseases caused by *Mycobacterium* species. They most commonly affect the lungs, but can destroy adrenal glands and other organs.

tuberoinfundibular tracts: fine nerve tracts that originate in the arcuate, ventromedial, dorsomedial, and other hypothalamic nuclei and course through the median eminence. They receive projections from the anterior periventricular, retrochiasmatic and posterior regions of the hypothalamus, the amygdala, the thalamus, and other brain components, and extend most of their axons toward capillaries of the hypothalamo-hypophysial portal system. The neurons release dopamine, gonadotropin releasing hormone (GnRH), and other regulators of adenohypophysial cell functions.

tubocurarine: an alkaloid in the stems and bark of *Chondodendron tomentosum*, initially used as an arrow poison to paralyze animals but keep them alive during transport; *see* **tubocurarine chloride**.

tubocurarine chloride: 7′,12′-dihydroxy-6,6′-dimethoxy-2,2′,2′-trimethyltubocuraranium chloride. The *d*-(+) isomer (Intocostrin) is an acetylcholine receptor antagonist that acts almost exclusively on skeletal muscle neuromuscular junctions in the concentrations generally employed. It is used as a muscle relaxant, and for the diagnosis of myasthenia gravis.

tubulins: the major components of microtubules. They are heterodimers, composed of similar α and β 50-55K subunits. Several growth factors affect their properties.

tubuloglomerular feedback: intrarenal control systems in which signals from nephron tubules transmitted to glomeruli of the same nephrons adjust glomerular filtration rates. Angiotensin II is implicated as the major mediator.

tuftsin: Thr-Lys-Pro-Arg; a peptide cleaved from leukokinin that enhances phagocytosis by macrophages. It is also mitogenic, chemotactic and bactericidal.

tularemia: an infections disease of rabbits and some rodents caused by *Pasteurella tularensis*. It can be transmitted by contact to humans.

tumescence: swelling.

tumor: (1) a swelling; (2) an abnormal clump of cells formed in response to injury, or when negative controls over cell division are defective. *Benign* tumors remain localized and are usually encapsulated; *malignant* ones can metastasize.

tumor associated antigens: TAAs; antigens made in substantial amounts by tumor cells and expressed on their surfaces or in nuclei. Normal cells make smaller or undetectable amounts. *See* also **tumor specific antigens**.

tumor necrosis factors: TNFs; a term that can refer specifically to tumor necrosis factor-α (TNFα), or to both TNFα and tumor necrosis factor β (TNFβ). The two kinds of species-specific peptides display overlapping biological properties, the genes that direct their synthesis reside on the same chromosome, and there is coordinate control in some cell types. Both TNFα and TNFβ interact with interleukins 1 and 6, interferons, and other regulators, stimulate production of interleukin-1, prostaglandin E_2 (PGE$_2$), and collagenases, and inhibit lipogenic gene expression in adipocytes; and both mediate numerous components of immunological and inflammatory responses, some aspects of which can be deleterious. They also contribute to the control of normal cell proliferation and differentiation, exert some antitumor effects, kill some virus infected cells, and invoke limited apoptosis in neuroglial and a few other types. Receptors that bind both TNFα and TNFβ have been identified on all nucleated somatic cell types. However, the α and β types display only 30% amino acid homology with each other, and their production is differentially regulated at some sites. TNFs also associate with a 200K protein distinct from their receptors that seems to be essential for the cytotoxic effects. Although some TNF receptors resemble CD40 and others nerve growth factor receptors, neither of those proteins binds TNFs.

tumor necrosis factor-α: TNFα; cachectin; species specific single chain proteins that tend to form dimers, trimers, and oligomers. The human and mouse types, with 157 and 156 amino acid subunits, respectively, are made in largest amounts by activated macrophages. Other sources include normal endothelial, neuroglial, and some tumor cells. The most prevalent mature forms appear to be 50K trimers that undergo pH-dependent conformational changes and can, under acid conditions insert into membranes and increase Na^+ permeability. When present in appropriate amounts, they contribute to body defense mechanisms by augmenting several components of inflammatory reactions, including neutrophilic leukocyte adhesion and degranulation, phagocytosis, fever, and eosinophil activation (which contributes to parasite killing). They also protect against the growth of some tumor types and can promote leukemia cell maturation. They additionally accelerate blood coagulation and fibroblast proliferation, and may thereby exert beneficial effects when tissues are injured. Endotoxin (LPS) stimulates the release of large amounts. TNFαs mediate many LPS effects but additionally act in other ways (both beneficial and deleterious) to affect responses to infections. Certain influences of high levels on the liver such as accelerated glycogenolysis are believed to provide energy to cope with infections; but only some of the effects on lipid metabolism fit the pattern. TNFαs very rapidly elevate the concentrations of circulating tri-acylglycerols, and more slowly augment very low density lipoprotein (VLDL) levels. A major mechanism is stimulation of citrate synthesis, with consequent activation of acetyl-CoA carboxylase (the rate limiting enzyme for fatty acid synthesis). TNFαs also accelerate lipolysis in some (but not all) adipose tissue. However, the availability of fatty acids for general tissue use is limited by inhibition of lipoprotein lipases. High VLDL levels may contribute to body defenses, since the particles bind and inactivate retroviruses (and in other ways counteract LPS toxicity). The term *cachectin* refers to the catabolic ("wasting") effects, which include depletion of adipocyte triacylglycerol stores and of body proteins. An early component is appetite suppression, but this influence usually subsides with time. TNFαs also induce collagenases that promote bone resorption, elevate the metabolic rate, and invoke diarrhea, lactacidosis, and hypotension. Additional effects include activation of a neutral sphingomyelinase, with consequent lowering of sphingomyelin and elevation of ceramide levels. (Sphingomyelins are precursors of sphingosines, which activate kinase C isozymes and several other enzymes, and ceramides act directly on some protein kinases). Although they preferentially attack tumor and virus-infected cells, high levels of TNFα are cytotoxic for normal types; and excessive amounts are believed to mediate injury associated with rheumatoid arthritis and multiple sclerosis. When the peptides are administered in therapeutic doses to inhibit cancer growth, they can invoke nausea, malaise, headache, chills, fever, myalgia, anorexia, leukocytosis, tachycardia, hypotension, and severe hemorrhagic necrosis. Some actions are directly mediated via specific receptors (which also bind TNFβ peptides), whereas others have been linked with the release of PGE_2, and/or interactions with interleukins 1 and 6, platelet activating factor (PAF), interferons, granulocyte-monocyte colony stimulating factor (GM-CSF), adrenocorticotropic hormone (ACTH), ceramides, insulin and other mediators. Glucocorticoid inhibition of TNFα release accounts for some steroid-mediated anti-inflammatory effects.

tumor necrosis factor-β: TNFβ; lymphotoxin, LT; species specific 18-19K lymphokines released by mitogen-activated cytotoxic (T_c) lymphocytes that display limited homologies to tumor necrosis factor-α peptides (*q.v.*). Several subtypes (β1, β2, β3, β4, *and* β5) exert similar effects on some (but not all) target organs, in part via interactions with the same receptors and secondary release of other mediators. The term *lymphotoxin* refers mostly to their ability to promote DNA fragmentation in some cell types. They augment vascular permeability and collagenase activity, but accelerate fibroblast proliferation, and are angiogenic and procoagulant. They also promote glycogenolysis in the liver. The proteins made in pituitary glands promote release of prolactin, adrenocorticotropic, follicle stimulating, and luteinizing hormones (PRL, ACTH, FSH, and LH).

tumor promoters: usually, agents that augment the effects of carcinogens but cannot cause tumor formation when presented alone; *see* also **phorbols**. Some directly accelerate cell proliferation (and thereby increase the probability that mutations will occur); others act on cells that have been altered by other agents, or synergize with growth factors.

tumor specific antigens: TSAs: antigens on the surfaces of specific kinds of tumor cells that are not detected on normal cell types.

tumor suppressor genes: DNA segments that code for factors that limit cell proliferation, and thereby protect against development of some forms of cancer. At least some contribute to recognition of mutations, and then arrest cell division until repairs are made. Most appear to act as dominant genes; and the presence of a single normal allele can be sufficient to provide the protection. When one allele is defective or deleted, mutation of the remaining functional allele in just a few cells can lead to tumorigenesis. DCC is a 190K transmembrane protein coded for by normal human chromosome #18, named for its failure to be expressed in some colon cancer cells. *NF-1* codes for neurofibrin (NF-1), a protein believed to modify *ras*-mediated mitogenic signals by augmenting GTPase activity. Mutations have been found in neurofibromas and are implicated in their etiology; *see* also **von Recklinghausen neurofibromatosis. p53** (*q.v.*) is the product of another gene believed to interact with small GTP binding proteins, and to diminish radiation-induced damage. Loss of the activity of both alleles appears to be the direct cause of **Lee-Fraumeni syndrome** (*q.v.*). However, it has been suggested that the p53 proteins promote apoptosis primarily in cells that have differentiated to states in which they are incapable of division. *See* also *Rb*, **retinoblastoma**, and **WT-1**.

tunica: usually, a covering membrane composed of connective tissue.

tunica adventitia: the outermost coat of all blood vessels except capillaries, composed mostly of connective tissue. It provides mechanical protection and carries blood vessels that supply vascular tissue. The width varies with vessel size.

tunica intima: the innermost coat of all blood vessels except capillaries, composed of endothelium that rests on a basement membrane surrounded by some connective tissue. The luminal component provides a smooth surface that protects circulating erythrocytes and blood platelets against mechanical injury; and the connective tissue protects against contact between blood constituents and collagens and other tunica media layer proteins that can initiate processes which lead to the development of atherosclerotic lesions. *See* also **endothelial cells**.

tunica media: the middle layer of arteriole, artery, venule and vein walls, composed mostly of smooth muscle. Contraction and relaxation of arteriolar smooth muscle selectively shunts blood towards (and away from) specific regions, and contributes in major ways to regulation of diastolic blood pressure. Elastic tissue in larger vessels modulates pulse pressure; *see* also **resistance** and **capacitance vessels**.

tunicamycin: a family of nucleoside antibiotics derived from *Streptomyces lysosuperificus*. The members vary in

tunicamycin

side-chain lengths, but all contain uracil, *N*-acetyl-glucosamine, an 11-carbon aminodialdose (tunicamine), and a fatty acid. By inhibiting *N*-acetylglucosamine binding to dolichol phosphate, they block the first step for formation of core (asparagine-linked) oligosaccharides of glycoproteins, and affect intracellular protein transport, cell morphology and adhesion, and also impair fibronectin production.

tunica serosa: the outermost coat of a visceral structure, usually composed of mesothelium and some fibrous connective tissue. *See* also **serous membranes**.

tunica vaginalis: the tunica serosa of the testis and epididymis.

turgor: in plants, the pressure that builds up when cells take up water by osmosis, and the surrounding rigid cell walls resist expansion. (It accounts for the "crispness" of celery and other vegetables.) In animals, the normal fullness of a capillary.

Turner's syndrome: sex differentiation disorders usually associated with X chromosome defects or deletions. The most common type occurs in individuals with XO (45X) patterns who present as phenotypic, but poorly developed, sterile females of short stature, with streak gonads. Most afflicted individuals additionally display one or more of the following: webbed neck, facial deformity, shield-shaped chest, cardiac and/or renal defects, cubitus valgus, and some mental retardation. In some cases two X chromosomes are present, but one is defective; and in a few the problem is X/XXX mosaicism. Noonan's syndrome is attributed to an autosomal dominant defect that can occur in males as well as females, in which only some cells lack X chromosome genes. Individuals with normal Y, but defective X chromosomes are phenotypic males, but can have any or all of the described somatic abnormalities, as well as mental retardation. Unlike humans, mice with XO chromosome patterns can be fertile and normal in appearance. They tend to have short life-spans.

turnover number: the numbers of substrate molecules converted to products per minute by one molecule of an enzyme under standardized conditions which include saturating concentrations of substrate.

Tween 80: a trade name for polysorbate 80.

twins: two offspring produced during the same pregnancy. *Monozygotic* twins develop from the same fertilized oocyte, are usually genetically identical, and can be *monoamniotic*. *Dizygotic* (nonidentical) twins develop from two separately fertilized oocytes. They differ genetically, and, in humans, acquire separate placentas that do not communicate; *cf* **freemartin**.

TX: (1) thyroidectomy; (2) tetrodotoxin; (3) thromboxane.

TXA$_2$, TXB$_2$: *see* **thromboxanes**.

Tylenol: a trade name for acetaminophen.

Tyndall effect: Tyndall phenomenon; the cloudy appearance of a gas or liquid when suspended particles scatter a transverse beam of light sent through it.

Tyr: tyrosine.

tyramine: a tyrosine decarboxylation product in red wine, cheese, beer, chocolate, and some other foods, believed to cause migraine headaches in susceptible individuals. Intestinal cells make small amounts from tyrosine; and low concentrations are present in the caudate nuclei, hypothalamus, other brain regions, spinal cord, heart, kidneys, and blood vessels. Monoamine oxidase inhibitors and other factors that alter neurotransmitter metabolism can cause much larger amounts to accumulate. Tyramine does not act directly on specific receptors, but displaces norepinephrine and other amines from secretory vesicles. It can be metabolized to octopamine, phenylethylamine, dopamine, and other biologically active amines.

Tyrode's solution: a modified Locke's solution used to irrigate the peritoneum, and to maintain mammalian tissues *in vitro*. A liter contains 1 gram each of glucose and NaHCO$_3$, and 8.0, 0.2, 0.2, 0.1, and 0.5 grams, respectively, of NaCl, KCl, CaCl$_2$, MgCl$_2$, and Na$_2$HPO$_4$.

tyrosinases: tyrosine-3-monooxygenases; copper dependent enzymes that convert tyrosine to dihydroxyphenylalanine (DOPA) in melanin synthesizing cells (*cf* **tyrosine hydroxylase** and **tyrosine aminotransferase**).

The largest amounts are made in skin and skin derivatives; and genetic defects that impair their synthesis lead to albinism. Low levels are present in neural and other tissues. A temperature-sensitive isotype accounts for the dark coloration of the ear tips and other cool regions of Siamese cats.

tyrosine: Tyr; Y; a glucogenic and ketogenic amino acid obtained directly from food and also synthesized from phenylalanine. It is a precursor of dopamine, norepinephrine, epinephrine, iodinated thyroid hormones, and melanins, and can be metabolized to octopamine and tyramine. It is also a constituent of many proteins, and a phosphate acceptor for tyrosine kinase reactions. Since the concentrations of tyrosine in body fluids are lower than those of most amino acids, they can be rate-limiting for protein synthesis (*see* also **tyrosine aminotransferase**). Genetically transmitted tyrosine metabolism disorders include tyrosinemias and tyrosinosis.

tyrosine aminotransferase: TAT; tyrosine transketolase; TKT; tyrosine transaminase; a hepatic enzyme that catalyzes: tyrosine + α-ketoglutarate → 4-hydroxyphenylpyruvate + glutamate. The 4-hydroxyphenylpyruvate is then usually metabolized via homogentisate to 4-maleylacetoacetate, which yields both fumarate and acetoacetate. Deficiency of the enzyme that metabolizes homogentisate leads to development of alkaptonuria. Glucocorticoid inhibition of protein synthesis and stimulation of gluconeogenesis is accomplished in part via TAT induction and consequent tyrosine depletion. *See* also **tyrosinosis** and **tryptophan oxidase**.

tyrosine hydroxylase: a rate-limiting enzyme for catecholamine biosynthesis that requires a pteridine cofactor to convert tyrosine to dihydroxyphenylalanine (DOPA), made in neurons and adrenomedullary cells; *cf* **tyrosinase**. The major inducer is nerve growth factor (NGF). Others include glucocorticoids and acetylcholine; and cyclic adenosine 3′5′-monophosphate (cAMP) in-

creases the activity. High norepinephrine levels exert negative feedback control.

tyrosine kinases: enzymes that catalyze phosphorylations of specific tyrosyl moieties on many proteins. The receptors for insulin, for insulin-like, epidermal, and platelet-derived growth factors (IGF-I, EGF, and PDGF), and several other regulators of cell proliferation are transmembrane proteins with cytoplasmic domains that contain latent enzyme components. When ligand binding activates the enzymes, the receptors undergo autophosphorylation, and then affect the activities of other cell components, including some serine-threonine kinases. Some of the target proteins require either tyrosine or serine/threonine phosphorylation, whereas others must undergo both kinds of covalent modifications to achieve full activity. Different tyrosine kinases (including numerous oncogene products) are activated in other ways; *see* **SH domains**. Tyrosine phosphorylation is essential for lymphocyte activation and many other processes. When deregulated, it contributes to cell transformation.

tyrosinemia: several inherited disorders in which tyrosine aminotransferase (TAT) deficiency leads to tyrosine accumulation in the bloodstream. The organs affected include the brain, liver, gastrointestinal tract, kidneys, skin, and eyes.

tyrosine phosphatases: enzymes that catalyze removal of phosphate groups from protein tyrosyl moieties; *see* also **protein phosphatases**. They counteract the effects of tyrosine kinases on cell proliferation, protect against tumorigenesis, and contribute to some processes that can be regarded as degenerative (such as Müllerian duct atrophy). The levels rise in some cell types when active phases of proliferation are completed, and they contribute to contact inhibition of growth. Some have extracellular domains that resemble those of cell adhesion molecules.

tyrosine transaminase: tyrosine aminotransferase.

tyrosine transketolase: TKT; *see* **tyrosine aminotransferase**.

tyrosinosis: a form of tyrosinemia; *see* **tyrosine aminotransferase**.

U

U: (1) uracil; (2) uridine; (3) uranium.

U, U. unit (as in international or USP unit).

U-0521: propiophenone.

U-46619: 9,11-methanoepoxy-PGH$_2$; a thromboxane A$_2$ receptor agonist.

U-50488: *trans*-3,4-dichloro-*N*-methyl-*N*-2(1-pyrrolidin-yl)cyclohexyl benzeneactamide; a selective agonist for κ-type opioid receptors.

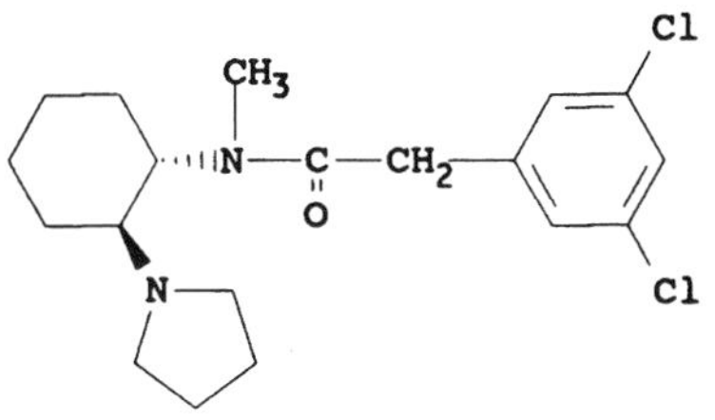

U-69593: (5α,7α.8β)-*N*-methyl-*N*-[7-(1-pyrrolidinyl)-1-oxaspiro[4,5]dec-8-yl]-benzacetamide; a selective antagonist for κ-type opioid receptors.

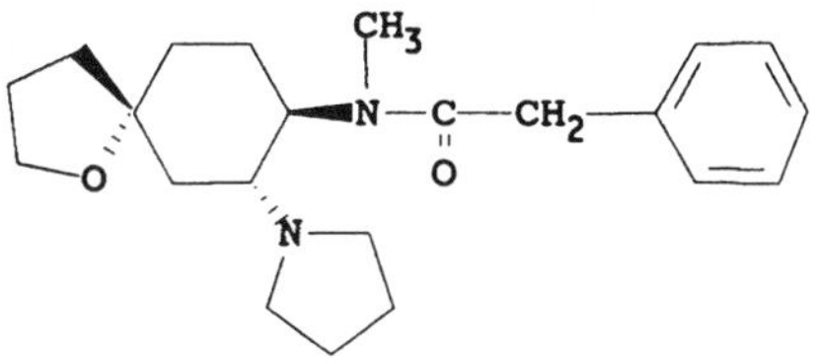

U-73122: 1-[6-[[(17β)-3-methoxyestra-1,3,5(10)-trien-17-yl]amino]hexyl]-1*H*-pyrrole-2,5-dione; an aminosteroid that inhibits phospholipases A$_2$ and C and generation of inositol$_{1,4,5}$-triphosphate (IP$_3$) by interfering with G protein-mediated transduction (but not with adenylate cyclase activation). It blocks Ca^{2+}-mediated responses to cholecystokinin and acetylcholine in pancreatic acinar cells, thyrotropin releasing hormone stimulation of growth hormone secreting cells, and phospholipase C dependent responses of blood platelets and polymorphonuclear leukocytes.

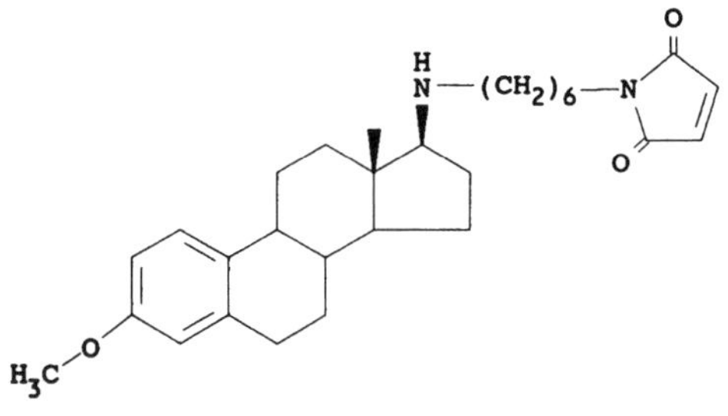

UB: ultimobranchial body.

Ub: ubiquitin.

ubenimex: *see* **bestatin**.

ubiquinols: reduced **ubiquinones** (*q.v.*) that function in electron transport and protect some lipoproteins and other molecules against oxidative damage.

ubiquinones; 2,3-dimethoxy-5-methylbenzoquinones; coenzyme Q$_{10}$ (the major mammalian type) and other oxidized forms of coenzyme Q with 1 to 12 terpene side-chains (indicated by n in the structure shown). Naturally occurring types are mobile lipid components of mitochondrial electron transport chains. Transfer of one electron and one hydrogen from reduced flavine mononucleotide (FMNH$_2$) converts a ubiquinone to a free radical (semiquinone), which then forms a ubiquinol (QH$_2$) by accepting a second electron and hydrogen atom. The electrons are then transferred to a cytochrome b, and the hydrogen atoms to molecular oxygen. Triiodothyronine augments Q$_{10}$ synthesis. Some synthetic derivatives are used to treat cardiovascular diseases.

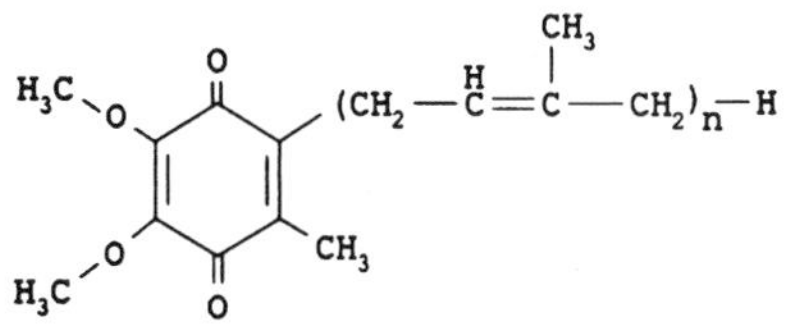

ubiquitins: Ub; 76-amino acid stress proteins in all eukaryote cells (and closely related molecules in prokaryotes) that form conjugates with ribosomal proteins, histones 2A and 2B, actins, neurofibrillary tangles, many enzymes, T lymphocyte homing receptors, receptors for platelet derived growth factors, growth hormones, and other cell proteins. Usually, the *C*-terminal lysyl moieties of several ubiquitinins attach to, and thereby affect affect the conformation and stability of a target molecule. (Molecules ending in methionine, glycine, alanine, serine, threonine, and valine are stabilized, whereas those with arginine, lysine, leucine, phenylalanine, or aspartic acid are rapidly degraded.) One function is preparation of proteins that are foreign to the cell, damaged, or present in excessive amounts for ATP-mediated, nonlysosomal degradation. Cells are thereby protected against accumulation of oncogene products, proteins improperly formed because of transcriptional and/or translational errors, and substances that were made in large amounts for a situation which no longer prevails. Another is selective shielding of certain protein types against degradation, an activity that assumes special importance in stressed cells whose survival would be threatened by loss of those molecules. By affecting their half-lives, ubiquitins maintain the correct proportions of various enzymes and other protein species. They contribute to cell cycle progression by associating with histones during interphase and preventing chromosome condensation (by inhibiting close packing of nucleosomes), dissociating during prophase, and reassociating when mitosis is completed, and by attaching to cyclins and inactive **MPF** (*q.v.*). During translation they maintain the three dimensional configurations required for correct establishment of covalent linkages. They also contribute to DNA repair, filament assembly, and cell surface recognition. E_1-SH (ubiquitin activating enzyme) is a dimeric protein with 110K subunits and terminal —SH groups that initiates the processes by reacting with ATP and forming thioester bonds with the *C*-terminal glycine of Ub: Ub—COOH + E_1—SH + ATP → Ub—CO—S—E_1 + AMP + PP. E_2 (with several 16-20K isoforms) then replaces the first enzyme: Ub—CO—S—E_1 + E_2—SH → Ub—CO—S—E_2 + E_1—SH. Finally, a third enzyme, E_3 (ubiquitin-protein ligase) catalyzes conjugation to a lysyl moiety of the target protein: Ub—CO—S—E_2 + protein → Ub—CO—NH—Lys—Protein + E_2—SH.

ubiquitous RNAs: *see* **URNAs**.

udders: organs of cattle, goats, and other ungulates with two or more mammary glands.

UDP: uridine-5′-diphosphate.

UDPG: uridine diphosphate glucose.

UDP-galactose: uridine diphosphate-galactose.

UDP-glucosamine: uridine diphosphate-glucosamine.

UK 14,304: 5-bromo-*N*-(4,5-dihydro-1*H*-imidazol-2-yl)-6-qunioxalinamine; an α_2 type adrenergic receptor agonist.

UK 37,248: dazoxiben.

ulapulides: macrolides with three contiguous oxazoles in 28-membered rings, made by some nudibranchs and sponges and used to defend against predators. They kill some fungi and some kinds of leukemia cells. The structure of ulapulide A is shown.

ultimobranchial bodies: UBs: innervated, calcitonin-secreting organs that develop from branchial pouches in submammalian vertebrates. In mammals, the calcitonin cells are incorporated into thyroid glands.

ultracentrifugation: *see* **centrifugation**.

ultradian: have a periodicity shorter than one day; *cf* **circadian** and **infradian**. Many hormones (including ones said to have circadian patterns) are released in regularly recurring pulses at hourly or other intervals.

ultrafiltration: separation of very small particles from surrounding solvents by passing the mixtures through semipermeable membranes with minute pores. Ultrafilters can trap colloidal particles, separate viruses from bacteria, and free T_3 and T_4 from protein-bound forms. Most capillary membranes function as ultrafilters that permit passage of water and small solutes but retain most proteins. The fluid that enters nephron Bowman's capsules is an ultrafiltrate of blood plasma.

ultramicroscopic: not discernible under ordinary light microscopy. By sending light rays through the sides of the specimens, dark field microscopes (ultramicroscopes) permit visualization of somewhat smaller entities as bright objects against dark backgrounds.

ultramicrotomes: instruments for cutting ultrathin tissue sections for electron microscopy. Some have units that rapidly freeze specimens and thereby avoid problems caused by chemical fixation.

ultrared: infrared; describes heat rays (with wavelengths longer than those at the red end of the visible spectrum).

ultrashort feedback loops: control pathways in which regulators travel very short distances to their target sites. When large amounts of certain hormones are released to extracellular spaces, some molecules enter the cells of origin and inhibit additional hormone synthesis. *See* also

ulapulides A

autocrine, **paracrine**, and **intracrine**, and *cf* **short feed-back loops**.

ultrasonography: use of sound waves of with frequencies above the range detectable by human ears (usually greater than 500 kilocycles per second) to generate images on fluorescent screens. The amount of heat generated varies with the acoustical resistance of the target. Differences in reflection at tissue interfaces can be used to diagnose some tumor types, and to visualize fetuses without inflicting the kinds of damage caused by X-rays. Ultrasound waves can also be focused to destroy calculi and pathologic tissue.

ultrastructure: fine structure; usually, morphological features visible under electron microscopy.

ultraviolet: describes light rays with wavelengths shorter than those at the violet end of the visible spectrum. Sunlight can include near (300-400 nm) and far (200-300 nm) types.

ultraviruses: viruses small enough to pass through the pores of an ultrafilter.

UM 1072: a benzomorphan with mixed opiate receptor agonist and antagonist properties.

umbelliferone: 7-hydroxycoumarin, a major coumarin metabolite made by animals and some plants. It is used in sunscreen lotions and creams, as a blood-brain barrier probe, and as a fluorescent pH indicator.

umbilicus: navel; the structure that marks the former placenta attachment site.

UMP: uridine 5′-monophosphate.

Unc-86: a protein similar to rat brain protein Brn-3 that contributes to development in *Caenorhabditis elegans*. Its synthesis is directed by a POU-IV gene.

uncinate: hook shaped.

unconditioned: describes responses that do not depend on prior learning or experience.

uncoupling: dissociation of processes that are usually linked, such as bone resorption with new bone formation, coenzyme oxidation with ATP synthesis in mitochondria, or hormone-binding with cell responses.

uncoupling agents: factors that dissociate processes which are usually linked; *see* for example **dinitrophenol** and **thermogenin**.

uncus: the curved rostral end of the parahippocampal gyrus, on the inferomedial aspect of the temporal lobe of the cerebral hemisphere just above the amygdaloid nucleus.

undecylenic acid: 10-undecenoic acid; a fatty acid made in small amounts by sweat glands. It is prepared commercially from ricinoleic acid and used as a topical fungicide.

$$CH_2 = \overset{\overset{\displaystyle H}{|}}{C} - (CH_2)_8 - COOH$$

undecylenic acid

ungulates: hoofed mammals. The subgroups are *Perissodactyla*, which includes horses, zebras, and others with odd numbers of toes, and *Artiodactyla* (cattle and sheep, with even numbers).

unilaminar: having a single layer.

uniovular twins: monozygotic twins; *see* **twins**.

unipolar: describes (1) a neuron with a single process that divides into axon and dendrite branches; (2) mood disorders characterized by depressive, but no manic (or manic, with no depressive) episodes; (3) a kind of lead used to study electrical changes in the heart or brain.

unipotent: capable of developing into just one kind of structure; *cf* **totipotent**.

unit: (1) a group of anatomic entities (such as a motor nerve and the muscle fibers it innervates), or a group of interacting individuals; (2) a defined quantity used as a reference standard such as the amount of a hormone that elicits a defined quantitative response under specified conditions. International, USP, mouse, or other qualifying terms can be applied.

univalent: having one combining site. The term can describe ions such as Na^+ or Cl^-, or antibodies.

unoccupied receptors: receptors that have not bound their ligands; *see* **spare receptors**.

unprimed: not previously activated; in immunology, not exposed to an antigen that affects the response. In endocrinology, the term can describe target organs that have not been exposed to regulators that augment the numbers of receptors; *see* also **upregulation**.

unsaturated: containing less than the maximum amount, such as a solution in which more of the same kind of solute can dissolve, or an organic compound with double or triple bonds that can incorporate additional hydrogen atoms.

uperolein: a tachykinin related to substance P, identified in bullfrog and carp retinas.

upregulation: induction of larger numbers of receptors. For example, estradiol stimulates formation of additional estrogen receptors in some cell types, and progesterone receptors in others; *cf* **downregulation**.

upstream: (1) located toward the 3′ end of a nucleic acid molecule (away from the transcription start site); *cf* **downstream**; (2) located closer to the *C*-terminal of a peptide or protein (away from the translation start site).

uracil: U; 2,4-dioxopyrimidine; the nitrogen base of uridine, uridine nucleotides, uridine diphosphate glucose (UDPG) and related compounds, and a component of ribonucleic acids. It hydrogen bonds to adenine during transcription. *See* also **thiouracil**, **propylthiouracil**, and **uracil mustard**.

uracil

uracil mustard: uramustine; 5-[di(β-chloroethyl)amino] uracil; an orally effective antineoplastic agent that binds to DNA bases, alters DNA structure, and is teratogenic.

uranium: U; a radioactive element (atomic number 92, atomic weight 238.029). It occurs in the earth of some regions, along with two other radioactive isotopes with mass numbers 234 and 235. Eleven other radioactive isotopes are known. The radioactivity emitted is used to kill some cancer cells. The chloride and nitrate salts are used in analytical chemistry and for industrial purposes.

urapidil: 6-[[3-[4-(o-methyoxyphenyl)-1-piperazinyl] propyl]-amino]-1,3-dimethyluracil; a selective, orally effective α_1-type adrenergic receptor antagonist, chemically different from most other types, that is used to lower blood pressure.

urates: uric acid salts or ions.

urate oxidase: uricase.

urea: carbamide; the metabolic waste product that in most mammals and some other vertebrates accounts for most of the circulating nonprotein nitrogen, and for approximately 90% of urinary nitrogen. It is made mostly in the liver, where glucagon, glucocorticoids, and other factors that accelerate protein degradation and/or gluconeogenesis increase its production. By removing amino groups that could otherwise be converted to ammonium ions and enter the bloodstream, ureagenesis protects against toxicity. Minute amounts are made in the central nervous system, mostly from purines. In humans and most other mammals, urea is is rapidly excreted by the kidneys; and urea clearance tests are used to assess renal function. Since it is osmotically active, it draws water to the urine. Small amounts in renal interstitial fluids contribute to mechanisms for controlling water balance. Exogenous urea is used as a diuretic to reduce some forms of edema, and also to lower intracranial pressure in preparation for surgery. Since it diffuses across most plasma membranes and can be taken up by erythrocytes, sugars are added to intravenous preparations to maintain isotonicity and prevent hemolysis. Although concentra-

tions twice as high as normal levels are well tolerated, toxic amounts slowly penetrate blood-brain barriers, and can damage the membranes of erythrocytes, neurons, and some other cell types; *see* **uremia**. Topical preparations moisten dry skin, and the disinfectant properties are used to promote healing of infected wounds. Urea has also been observed to increase the effectiveness of sulfonamides. Ruminants and some plants synthesize amino acids form urea (a component of some fertilizers). Strong solutions are used *in vitro* to denature proteins, hold them in solution, and expose chemical moieties masked in the native molecules.

urea cycle: the major pathway for urea biosynthesis, called a cycle because ornithine is used and then regenerated. The enzymes for the reactions are indicated by numbers in brackets:

$NH_4^+ + CO_2 + ATP \rightarrow$ carbamoylphosphate + 2 ADP + Pi; [1]

carbamoyl phosphate + ornithine $\rightarrow$ citrulline; [2]

citrulline + aspartate + ATP $\rightarrow$ arginosuccinate + AMP + Pi; [3]

arginosuccinate $\rightarrow$ arginine + fumarate; [4]

arginine + HOH $\rightarrow$ ornithine + urea: [5]

[1] = carbamoyl phosphate synthetase; [2] = ornithine transcarbamoylase; [3] = arginosuccinate synthetase; [4] = arginosuccinase; [5] = arginase.

Fumarate can enter the tricarboxylic acid cycle; and both ornithine and arginine are polyamine precursors.

ureagenesis: urea formation; *see* **urea** and **urea cycle**.

urease: urea aminohydrolase; a 489K enzyme made by some plants, invertebrates, yeasts, and algae, and obtained commercially from the jack bean, *Canavalia ensiformis*). It hydrolyzes urea to ammonium carbonate (which decomposes to carbon dioxide and ammonia) and is used to determine urea concentrations in body fluids.

uremia: abnormally high blood urea concentrations, usually caused by renal dysfunctions that impair excretion. Since **urea** (*q.v.*) is the major nitrogenous waste in mammals, and uremia is usually associated with retention of creatinine and other metabolic waste products, the term is often used synonymously with azotemia. Glucocorticoids, glucagon, and other factors that promote proteolysis and/or gluconeogenesis accelerate urea production; but healthy kidneys usually maintain the blood levels within normal ranges. Although concentrations two or three times higher are often well tolerated, very high urea levels are toxic. Some effects, such as nausea, vomiting, itching, pericarditis, and pulmonary edema are attributed to them directly. The conditions that cause uremia often simultaneously invoke acidosis, hyperphosphatemia, hyperkalemia, and other metabolic imbalances.

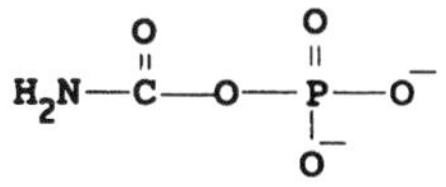

$$H_2N-C(=O)-O-P(=O)(O^-)-O^-$$

carbamoyl phosphate

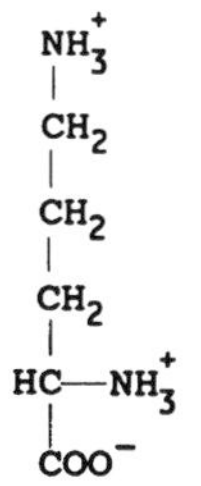

$$\overset{+}{N}H_3-CH_2-CH_2-CH_2-\overset{|}{C}H(\overset{+}{N}H_3)-COO^-$$

ornithine

$$HN-C(=O)-NH_2,\ CH_2-CH_2-CH_2-\overset{|}{C}H(\overset{+}{N}H_3)-COO^-$$

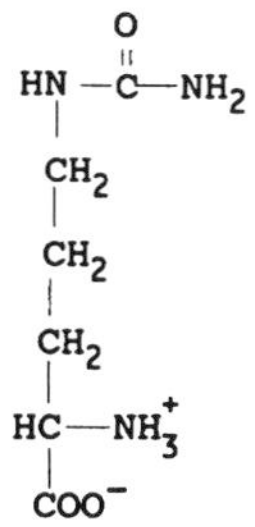

citrulline

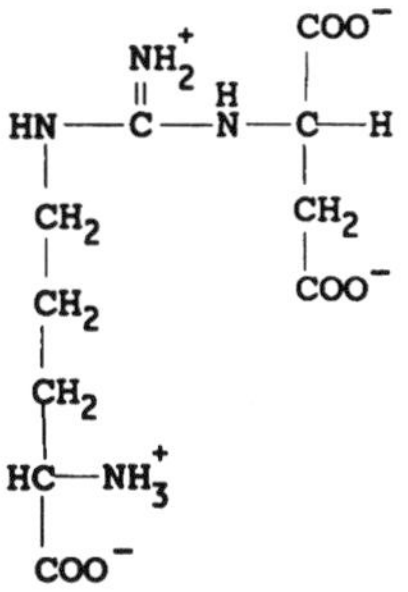

arginosuccinate

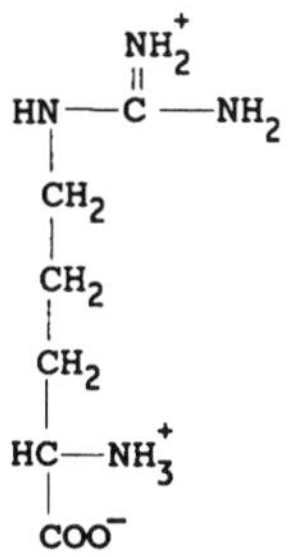

arginine

urea cycle

ureotelic: describes animals in which urea is the major nitrogenous waste product; *cf* **uricotelic**.

-uresis: a suffix used with qualifiers to designate increased urinary excretion of specific substances, as in natriuresis, kaluresis, chloruresis, and diuresis.

ureters: fine, bilateral, fibromuscular tubes that convey urine from the renal pelvises to the urinary bladder in mammals and some other vertebrates, and to the cloaca in species that do not possess urinary bladders.

urethan: urethane; ethyl carbamate; an agent that invokes narcosis in many species, but has only mild hypnotic effects in humans. It is used as an anesthetic in amphibians and fishes, but has been largely replaced by barbiturates in veterinary medicine. Since it depresses bone marrow functions, it is effective for treating some lymphatic and myeloid leukemias and plasma cell myelomas, but is mutagenic and hepatotoxic.

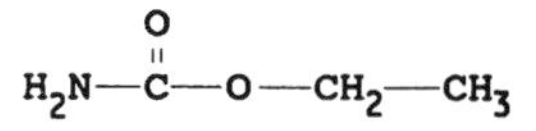

$$H_2N-C(=O)-O-CH_2-CH_3$$

urethra: the canal that extends from the internal urethral orifice at the neck of the urinary bladder to the external urethral orifice. In female mammals, it is short (~ 4 cm in women), passes behind the symphysis pubis, opens into the vestibule of the vagina below the clitoris, and transports only urine. In males it passes through the prostate gland (where present) and the corpus spongiosum of the penis, opens at the tip of the glans penis, and additionally conveys semen.

urethral folds: urogenital folds.

urethral orifices: the openings at the two ends of the urethra. The internal orifice at the neck of the urinary bladder is regulated by autonomic innervation to the smooth muscle sphincter. The external orifice is below the clitoris in females, and at the tip of the glans penis in males. Voluntary control of the muscles that surround it is acquired (by learning) during early childhood.

URI: upper respiratory tract infection.

uric acid: 8-hydroxyxanthine; 7,9-dihydro-$1H$-purine-2,6,8($3H$)-trione; the major waste product of nucleic acid metabolism in humans and some other mammals, the major nitrogenous waste in birds and some reptiles, and a component of iridophore white pigments. It is poorly soluble in water, but usually present in concentrations that dissolve in the blood and urine of species in which urea is the major nitrogenous waste. However, urates can deposit in joints (*see* **gout**) or in ureters when metabolic defects augment its synthesis and/or slow its degradation, or when pathological processes change the tissue composition. In uricotelic species, precipitation is not a problem because the ureters lead into a cloaca in which urine is concentrated, and from which it is eliminated through a wide opening as a semisolid paste. Uric acid is oxidized to allantoin in many mammals (but not in humans). It is used for some purposes as an anti-oxidant.

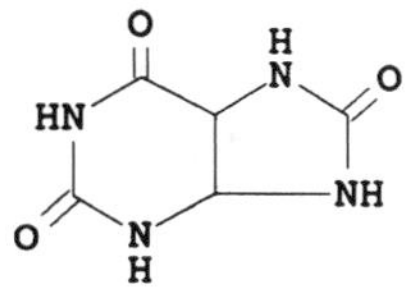

uricase; urate oxidase: a copper-dependent hepatic enzyme made by most mammals (but not primates) that catalyzes oxidation of uric acid to allantoin. It is used for measuring uric acid concentrations.

uridine diphosphate-galactose

uricemia: hyperuricemia; uricacidemia; excessively high blood concentrations of uric acid. A major cause is inability to make adequate amounts of hypoxanthine phosphoribosyltransferase (HPRT).

uricosuric: a condition or agent that accelerates urinary excretion of uric acid.

uricotelic: describes species that excrete uric acid as the major nitrogenous waste product. Birds and some reptiles are uricotelic. *Cf* **ureotelic**.

uridine: uracil riboside; 1-β-ribofuranosyluracil; a nucleoside derived from nucleic acids; *see also* **uridine triphosphate** and **uridine diphosphate glucose**.

uridine 5′-diphosphate: UDP; a nucleotide composed of uracil, ribose, and phosphate; *see* **uridine triphosphate** and **uridine diphosphate glucose**.

uridine diphosphate-galactose: UDP-galactose: uracil-phosphate-phosphate-galactose; *see* **uridine diphosphate glucose**.

uridine diphosphate-glucosamine: UDP-glucosamine: uracil-phosphate-phosphate-glucoseamine; *see* **uridine diphosphate glucose**.

uridine diphosphate glucose: UDPG; co-galactoisomerase; uracil-phosphate-phosphate-glucose; a coenzyme for several metabolic pathways. Glycogen synthesis begins with the reaction catalyzed by a uridyltransferase: glucose-1-phosphate + UTP → UDPG + P-P. The glucose component of UDPG is then transferred to the end of a glycogen chain, and UDP is released. Galactowaldenase catalyzes: UDPG ⇄ UDP-galactose, and thereby interconversion of glucose-1-phosphate and galactose-1-phosphate. UDPG is also used to make uridine diphosphate-glucosamine, an intermediate in the pathway for glycosaminoglycan biosynthesis.

uridine 5′-monophosphate: UMP; uridylic acid; uracil-ribose-phosphate; a nucleotide that can be phosphorylated to **uridine 5′-triphosphate** (*q.v.*).

uridine 5′-triphosphate: UTP; uracil-ribose-phosphate-phosphate-phosphate; a nucleotide used for RNA synthesis. It releases energy in the reactions: UTP → UDP + Pi, and UTP → UMP + P-P, and is a precursor of uridine diphosphate glucose, uridine diphosphate-galactose, and uridine diphosphate-glucosamine.

uridylic acid: uridine 5′-monophosphate.

uridyltransferases: enzymes that catalyze reactions of the general type: UTP + X-P → UDPX + P-P; *see* **uridine diphosphate glucose.**

uridine diphosphate glucose

uridine diphosphate glucose

uridine 5′-triphosphate

urinary bladder: an organ in mammals and many other vertebrates (but not birds) that receives and stores urine delivered by the ureters and releases it via an external orifice. It has transitional epithelium that accommodates to changing volumes while maintaining almost constant pressure until filling exceeds a threshold level. In human adults, stretch receptors activated when the bladder contains around 400 ml of fluid initiate a micturition reflex mediated by parasympathetic nerves from the sacral spinal cord. The smooth muscles of the walls then contract, and the internal urethral sphincter relaxes. In infants, the external sphincter then relaxes and urine is released. Conscious control over the external sphincter is learned during early childhood. Messages descending from the cerebral cortex can arrest the reflex, but it is repeatedly initiated at decreasing intervals as pressure builds in the bladder. In terrestrial frogs and some other animals, the urinary bladder serves as reservoir from which water and electrolytes can be recovered via processes regulated by mineralocorticoids and hypothalamic nonapeptide hormones. Some limited exchange of water and electrolytes also proceeds in mammalian bladders. In birds and other vertebrates that lack the organs, ureters deliver urine to cloacas, in which concentration and other changes can occur.

urination: micturition; discharge of urine. *See* **urinary bladder**, and *cf* **uropoiesis**.

urine: a fluid made in the **kidneys** (*q.v.*), released to the ureters, and delivered for storage and subsequent release to the urinary bladder in some species (including eutherian mammals), or to the cloaca in birds and some other vertebrates. Since urine formation is the major mechanism for removing metabolic wastes and adjusting water and electrolyte metabolism to changing needs, the volume, composition, and appearance vary with the species and with factors such as diet, fluid intake, and water loss via different channels. There are also species variations in urine processing in the bladder and cloaca. Under ordinary conditions, a typical adult human excretes one to two liters of yellowish fluid per day that contains around 25 to 35 grams of urea, 1.5 grams of creatinine, 0.5 grams of uric acid, 15 grams of sodium chloride, smaller quantities of several other salts, and some pigments, ketones, amino acids, hormone degradation products, and other substances. Representative values for other inorganic components include 3.5 g of potassium, 2.5 g each of sulfate and phosphate, 0.3 g of calcium, and 0.1 g of magnesium. The ammonium and bicarbonate levels can vary over a wide range. In some species, urine is also an important source of pheromones. Vasopressin promotes water conservation, and thereby exerts major direct controls over the volume; but other determinants include mineralocorticoids that augment potassium and hydrogen excretion (but promote sodium and bicarbonate retention), parathyroid hormone which (among other things) increases urinary phosphate content, and natriuretic peptides. Many regulators indirectly affect the volume and composition, including insulin which protects against glucose loss, glucocorticoids which increase the nitrogen content, and factors that influence blood pressure and glomerular filtration and renal blood flow. Many of the same regulators function in other vertebrates, but arginine vasotocin and related nonapeptides exert the major controls over volume, mostly by affecting renal blood flow and glomerular filtration rates.

U1, U2, U4, U5, U6 RNAs: ubiquitous RNA components of small nuclear ribonucleoproteins (snRNPs), and of spliceosomes, composed, respectively, of 165, 185, 145, 116, and 106 nucleotides. They contribute to spliceosome assembly and premessenger RNA processing. U1 RNA, the most abundant type, contains a base sequence complementary to 5′ splice sites of premessenger RNAs, and it protects those nucleotide regions against digestion. U2 RNA binds to premessenger RNA branch sites.

U1-, U2-, U4-, U5-, U6-snRNPs: small nuclear ribonucleoprotein particle components of spliceosomes, named for their U RNA content.

urobilins: brown, linear tetrapyrrole pigments excreted mostly to the feces. Bacteria that colonize the large intestines make them from bile pigments. Small amounts are absorbed into the bloodstream and excreted to the urine. *See* for example **stercobilin**.

urobilinogen: stercobilinogen.

urocanic acid: 4-imidazoleacrylic acid; a histidine deamination product.

urochromes: urinary pigments derived from urobilins.

urodilatin: a 32-amino acid peptide excreted to urine, composed of an *N*-terminal H_2N-Thr-Ala-Pro-Arg- sequence linked to the 28 amino acid form of atrial natriuretic peptide. It acts on ANP receptors in kidney collecting ducts.

urogastrones: peptides related to epidermal growth factor (EGF), in saliva, submaxillary glands, and Brunner's glands, and released to urine in larger amounts in pregnant as compared with nonpregnant mammals. They inhibit gastrin and hydrochloric acid secretion, exert trophic effects on gastric mucosa, and can protect against development of peptic and duodenal ulcers in a manner not antagonized by secretin (which inhibits the trophic effects of gastrins). In the amino acid sequence for human β-urogastrone shown, S-S bonds connect the cysteine moieties at positions 6 → 20, 14 → 31, and 33 → 42: Asn-Ser-Asp-Ser-Gly-Cys-Pro-Leu-Ser-His-Asp-Gly-Tyr-Cys-Leu-His-Asp-Gly-Val-Cys-Met-Tyr-Ile-Glu-Ala-Leu-Asp-Lys-Tyr-Ala-Cys-Asn-Cys-Val-Val-Gly-Tyr-Ile-Gly-Glu-Arg-Cys-Gln-Tyr-Arg-Asp-Leu-Lys-Trp-Trp-Glu-Leu-Arg. γ-urogastrone lacks the terminal arginine moiety.

urogenital folds: urethral folds; embryonic structures that develop into labia minora in female mammals, and into the penile urethra in males.

urogenital sinus: an embryonic structure that gives rise to most of the vagina in females, and to the prostate gland in males. The 5α-reductase activity (essential for formation of the 5α-dihydrotestosterone that promotes male-type differentiation) is increased by testosterone.

urogenital swellings: embryonic structures that fuse to form the scrotum in males, and give rise to the labia majora in females.

urokinases: species specific serine proteases in blood and urine that convert plasminogen to both high (50K) and low (30K) molecular weight plasmins. The enzymes are administered for their thrombolytic activities. Renal kallikreins cleave pro-urokinases to their active forms.

urolithiasis: formation of calculi ("stones") in the urinary tract, usually because the urine is strongly alkaline or contains excessive quantities of calcium salts, oxalates, and/or other poorly soluble compounds.

uromodulin: an 85K urinary glycoprotein excreted by pregnant women that inhibits interleukin-1 stimulation of T lymphocyte proliferation. It may be an immunosuppressant that contributes to protection against rejection of conceptuses.

uronic acids: sugar derivatives in which the $-CH_2OH$ groups farthest from the reducing ends have been oxidized to carboxyls. They are made when UDP-sugars (*see* **uridine-diphosphate glucose**) are oxidized by NAD^+-dependent dehydrogenases. Glucuronic, galacturonic, iduronic, and some others are used for glycosaminoglycan synthesis. Hepatic enzymes conjugate many kinds of molecules with glucuronic acid to form products that are more hydrophilic than the parent substances, and therefore more easily excreted to the urine.

uropepsins: pepsins made in the stomach that are excreted to the urine. They cleave renal kininogens and release met-kallidin. Although the levels are low, uropepsin concentrations in urine are used as indices of gastric function.

urophysins: peptide components of urophysis hormone precursors that are co-secreted with urotensins.

urophysis: a neurosecretory structure at the caudal end of the spinal cord of bony and some cartilaginous fishes. It releases hormones that affect blood pressure and electrolyte balance; *see* **urotensins**.

uropoiesis: urine formation; *cf* **urination**.

uropods: uropodia; cytoplasmic projections on the surfaces of activated cytotoxic (T_C) lymphocytes used for attachment to target cells. They may additionally contribute to other surface-related processes.

uroporphyrins: brownish-red protoporphyrin derivatives excreted in the urine and feces. Excessive amounts accumulate in individuals with liver diseases and pernicious anemia and deposit in bones and teeth, and in soft tissues (including skin, in which they invoke lesions and photosensitivity). Porphobilinogen, derived from δ-aminolevulinic acid via reactions catalyzed by uroporphyrinogen synthetase, is converted to uroporphyrinogen III (shown). It can be decarboxylated to coproporphyrinogen III.

urotensins: hormones secreted by the urophysis; *see* **urotensins I, II, III**, and **IV**.

urotensin I: a urophysial hormone chemically related to corticotropin releasing hormone (CRH) and sauvagine. When administered to mammals, it stimulates the release of adrenocorticotropic hormone (ACTH) and lowers blood pressure by dilating mesenteric blood vessels. In fishes it stimulates smooth muscle contraction and augments calcium excretion. Teleost urotensin I is: Asn-Asp-Asp-Pro-Pro-Ile-Ser-Ile-Asp-Leu-Thr-Phe-His-Leu-Leu-Arg-Asn-Met-Ile-Glu-Met-Ala-Arg-Ile-Glu-Asn-Glu-Arg-Glu-Gln-Ala-Gly-Leu-Asn-Arg-Lys-Tyr-Leu-Asp-Glu-Val-NH_2.

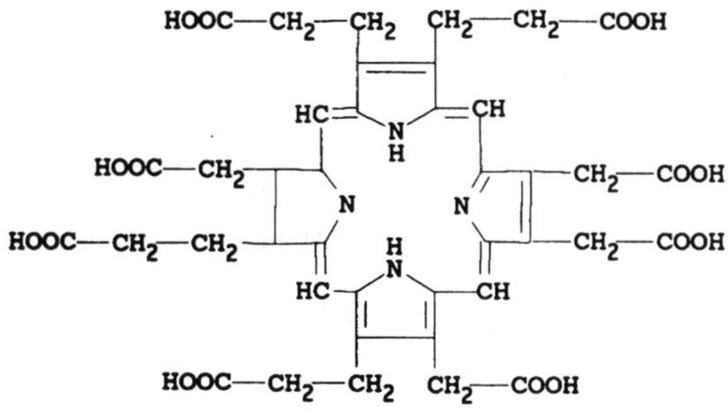

HOOC—CH₂—CH₂ CH₂—CH₂—COOH

uroporphyrins

urotensin II: a urophysial hormone chemically related to somatostatin-14. It promotes oxytocin-like stimulation of smooth muscle and affects prolactin release and sodium metabolism in fishes. In the teleost urotensin sequence shown, the two cysteine moieties are linked by an S-S bond: Ala-Gly-Thr-Ala-Asp-Cys-Phe-Trp-Lys-Tyr-Cys-Val.

urotensin III: an uncharacterized peptide hormone believed to be secreted by the urophysis and to contribute to control of water and electrolyte balance.

urotensin IV: a urophysial hormone that may be identical with arginine vasotocin.

Urotropin: a trade name for methenamine.

ursodiol: $3\alpha,7\beta$-dioxycholanic acid; ursodeoxycholic acid; a bile acid made by humans and some other species. Actigall is the trade name for a preparation used to protect against gallstone formation.

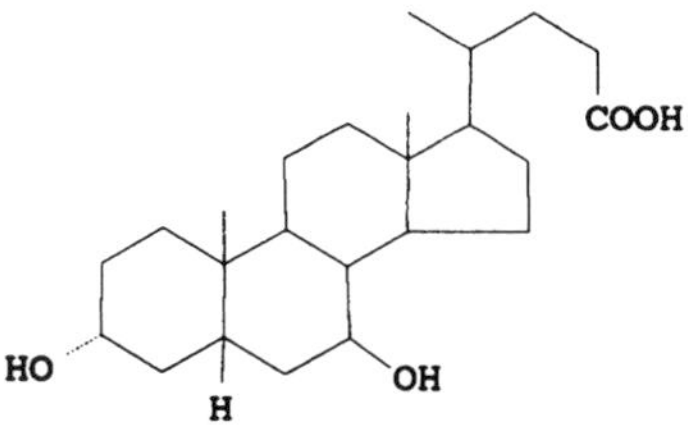

urticaria: skin reactions invoked in sensitive individuals by irritants, insect bites, allergens and other stimuli. Histamine, the major mediator, augments dermal capillary permeability and causes erythema, itching, rash, and often also localized edema and wheal formation.

urushiol: major components of poison ivy (*Toxicodendron radicans*), poison oak (*T. diversilobum*) and some other plants that cause allergic reactions, used to desensitize susceptible individuals. They are mixtures of pentadecadienyl catechol derivatives. In the structure shown, R can be $(CH_2)_{14}$—CH_3, or $(CH_2)_7$—CH=CH— followed by $(CH_2)_5$—CH_3, CH_2—CH=CH$(CH_2)_2$—CH_3, CH_2—CH=CH—CH=CH—CH_3, or CH_2—CH=CH-CH_2—CH=CH_2.

UsnRNPs: small nuclear ribonucleoprotein particles that contain U RNAs. They are spliceosome components.

USP: United States Pharmacopeia, a legally recognized compendium of standards for therapeutic agents, and of tests for determining the strength, quality, and purity.

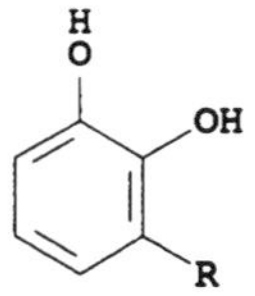

urushiol

uterine: derived from, or characteristic of the uterus.

uterine cervix: the distal end of the uterus that projects into the vagina through which spermatozoa enter and neonates are expelled. Close to the time of ovulation, estrogens stimulate cervical gland production of watery fluids that facilitate sperm survival, motility, and entry into the uterine cavity. During luteal phases of ovarian cycles, progesterone promotes formation of viscous fluids that are hostile to sperm.

uterine "milk": fluids secreted by endometrial cells during pregnancy in some mammalian species. They provide nutrients for, and prolong the survival of preimplantation blastocysts. Progesterone is a major stimulant for their production.

uterine specific protein: the creatine kinase isoform made by uterine cells.

uterine tubes: oviducts; *see* **Fallopian tubes**.

uteroferrin: purple protein: an iron-transporting protein with phosphatase activity secreted by the endometrium of the pregnant sow.

uteroglobins: blastokinins; homodimeric glycoproteins with 70-amino acid subunits secreted by endometrial cells of pregnant mammals. They bind steroid hormones for presentation to conceptuses, inhibit phospholipase A_2 enzymes, and may contribute to protection against immunological rejection.

uterotropic: going toward, or stimulatory to the uterus.

uterus [uteri]: hollow female reproductive organs specialized in mammals for implantation, nurturing of conceptuses, and parturition. They are bifurcated in most mammalian species that produce large litters (and in a few there are two cervices). During the follicular phases of ovarian cycles, estrogens stimulate proliferation of superficial endometrial cells and induce progesterone receptors. During luteal phases progesterone promotes specializations and antagonizes some estrogen effects. When appropriately prepared by prolonged exposure first to estrogen and then to progesterone, followed by a brief second exposure to estrogen, the endometrium becomes receptive to blastocysts. If conception does not occur, corpora lutea degenerate and superficial endometrial cells slough before a new cycle begins. In some species, hormones made by the uterus contribute to luteolysis during the late luteal phases of ovarian cycles. If conception does occur, implantation begins soon after blastocysts arrive in the uterus. The endometrium participates in implantation and later contributes to formation of the placenta. The high levels of estrogens secreted during pregnancy stimulate growth and strengthening of myometrial smooth muscle, and promote contractions. In some species progesterone is the major regulator that blocks the mounting of organized activity which could lead to premature expulsion of the conceptuses; but relaxin is more important in others. Prostaglandins are major initiators of contractions that lead to parturition. Since blood oxytocin levels do not rise substantially until after parturition has begun, and since parturition can occur when release of that hormone from the neuro-hypophysis is blocked, it has been stated that it functions primarily in expulsion of the placenta and in maintaining postpartum contractions. However, both oxytocin levels in the uterus and oxytocin receptors increase before that time; and that hormone is now accorded additional roles.

uterus-derived growth factors: peptides related to fibroblast growth factors that contribute to uterine growth.

UTP: uridine triphosphate.

UTRs: untranslated regions; ribonucleic acid (RNA) segments that do not direct protein synthesis but contribute to the control mechanisms.

UV: uvomorulin.

uvomorulin: UV: E-cadherin; a 120K cell surface glycoprotein identified on mouse blastocysts and embryos, and on embryonal carcinoma cells. *See* **cadherins**.

V

V: (1) valine; (2) vanadium; (3) volt; (4) variance.

V: (1) velocity; (2) volume; (3) voltage.

v-: a prefix for viral, as in *v-erb B*.

V₁, V₂, V₃: *see* **vasopressin receptors**.

vaccenic acid: 11-octadecenoic acid. The *cis* isomer, present in butter and some other dairy products, is reported to promote growth in laboratory animals. The *trans* isomer predominates in bacterial lipids.

vaccine: a suspension of modified or dead microorganisms used to induce active immunity against those and related antigens.

vacuolar ATPases: electrogenic H^+/ATPases that function as proton pumps for lysosomes, chromaffin granules, and other acidic vesicles. They differ chemically from mitochondrial and plasma membrane H^+/ATPases, and are not inhibited by agents that affect those enzymes. Roles in prehormone processing, molecular packaging, receptor-mediated endocytosis, and receptor-ligand dissociation have been described.

vacuoles: lysosomes, food vacuoles, water vacuoles, and other small membrane enclosed cavities.

vagi: vagus nerves.

vagina: usually (1) the fibromuscular female accessory reproductive organ that develops from the urogenital sinus through which neonates pass during parturition. It receives the penis during copulation and is the site for insemination in most species. The epithelium undergoes estrogen and progesterone-mediated cyclic changes during ovarian cycles in most mammals; *see* also **vaginal smears** and **uterine cervix**. Estrogens promote proliferation of vaginal mucosa cells and formation of acidic vaginal fluids that protect against infections. Progesterone facilitates secretion of a mucus-rich fluid that impedes sperm movements and thereby decreases the probability that "overripe" (deteriorating) oocytes will be fertilized. Vaginal crypts of some species store sperm. In guinea pigs and a few others, vaginal membranes block sperm entry to the uterus during much of ovarian cycle

and undergo estrogen-dependent opening shortly before the time of ovulation. Spermatocides and some other chemicals are absorbed across the vaginal epithelium and delivered to underlying blood vessels; (2) a sheath-like structure.

vaginal rings: devices inserted into the vagina to block conception. Some contain spermatocides, progestins that affect vaginal fluid composition, and/or copper (which impedes fertilization).

vaginal smears: preparations of cells and associated components of vaginal mucosa surfaces, usually obtained by gently scraping the tissue with saline-moistened cotton swabs and transferring the materials to liquids on glass slides. They are examined under light microscopy directly or after staining, to obtain information on ovarian cycle phases or detect cancerous and precancerous cells. Cycle-associated changes are obvious in laboratory rats and mice. During the early follicular phase (proestrus) the mucosa is thin, and the smears contain small, nucleated epithelial cells along with leukocytes that enter via diapedesis. As the time of ovulation approaches (estrus) the mucosa contains many layers of epithelial cells, the most superficial of which become keratinized, die, and slough off. The smears are then crowded with enlarged, cornified cell remnants. Following ovulation (metestrus), mucus shreds appear along with fewer cornified cells, some nucleated epithelial cells, and limited numbers of leukocytes. Towards the end of the luteal phase, when there is comparative quiescence (diestrus), small epithelial cells, leukocytes, mucins, and debris appear. Similar, but less well-defined changes in vaginal smears are associated with ovarian cycles in women and other primates.

vagotomy: usually, surgical sectioning of vagus nerves to disrupt the associated functions. "Chemical vagotomy" can be accomplished with acetylcholine receptor antagonists, and with toxins that damage the cells.

vagotonia: excessive dominance of vagal (parasympathetic) over sympathetic nervous system control.

vagotropic: affecting the vagus nerves.

cis: $\quad H_3C—(CH_2)_5—\overset{\overset{H}{|}}{C}=\overset{\overset{H}{|}}{C}—(CH_2)_9—COOH$

trans: $\quad H_3C—(CH_2)_5—CH$
$\qquad\qquad\qquad\qquad ||$
$\qquad\qquad\qquad HC—(CH_2)_9—COOH$

vaccenic acid

vago-vagal reflexes: unconditioned responses (including some respiratory reflexes) in which both afferent and efferent impulses travel along vagus nerve branches.

vagus nerves: the tenth pair of cranial nerves. They mediate many functions of the **parasympathetic nervous system** (*q.v.*) via afferent and efferent branches that affect the cardiovascular, respiratory, digestive, excretory, reproductive, and endocrine systems. Stimulation leads to increased secretion of insulin and several other hormones, slowing and weakening of myocardial contraction, vasodilation, increased gastrointestinal secretory activity and motility, and other effects.

Val: valine.

valence: (1) the number of sites on an atom available for binding to other atoms, a property related to the numbers of electrons on the outermost energy shell; (2) the number of antigen binding sites on an antibody.

valeric acid: pentanoic acid; a minor component of foods, used for fuel and for formation of pyruvic acid. Small amounts are made during β-oxidation of longer chained fatty acids with uneven numbers of carbon atoms. Conjugates of steroids and other compounds are long-acting because hydrolysis is slow. Although the odor is unpleasant, valeric acid is used in the perfume industry.

$$H_3C - CH_2 - CH_2 - CH_2 - COOH$$

valgus: twisted; bent outward; a term used in conjunction with others to describe deformities in which structures are bent away from the midline of the body, as in cubitus or talipes valgus; *cf* **varus**.

validity: the extent to which a measurement or test relates to the parameter it is designed to measure; *cf* **precision**.

valine: Val; V; α-aminoisovaleric acid; an essential, branched chain hydrophobic, glucogenic amino acid in most proteins and especially abundant in collagen and other fibrous types. Valine aminotransferase deaminates it to α-ketoisovaleric acid, and an α-keto dehydrogenase converts the product to isobutyryl-CoA. Additional reactions that proceed via methylacrylyl-CoA, β-hydroxyisobutyryl-CoA, methylmalonate semialdehyde, propionyl-CoA, and methylmalonyl-CoA intermediates yield the tricarboxylic acid cycle component, succinyl-CoA. Maple syrup disease, in which valine and related amino acids accumulate, is caused by genetic defects that block the synthesis or activity of the α-keto dehydrogenase. Valine also accumulates when valine aminotransferase activity is subnormal. Different defects lead to accumulation of methylmalonyl-CoA by affecting methylmalonyl-CoA mutase activity. Locomotor dysfunction is the major manifestation of valine deficiency.

valinol: 2-amino-3-methylbutanol; an agent used to inhibit protein synthesis.

valinomycin: a cyclododecadepeptide ionophore antibiotic made by *Streptomyces fulvissimus* composed of 3 molecules each of L-valine, D-α-hydroxyisovaleric acid, D-valine, and L-lactic acid, linked to form a 36-membered ring. It is effective against *Mycobacterium tuberculosis*, kills some roundworms, and is used as an insecticide. The actions include acceleration of K^+ (and Rb^+) transport across membranes and indirect influences on Na^+, Ca^{2+}, and H^+ metabolism. It impairs oxidative phosphorylation by increasing the K^+ permeability of mitochondrial membranes, thereby discharges electrical gradients across the membranes, and consequently increases the activities of proton pumps.

Valisone: a trade name for β-methasone valerate.

valitocin: a neurohypophysial peptide made by sharks. It is chemically and biologically related to oxytocin, but less potent in mammalian bioassay systems. The cysteine moieites are joined by an S-S bond in the sequence: Cys-Tyr-Ile-Gln-Asn-Cys-Pro-Val-Gly-NH₂.

Valium: a trade name for diazepam.

valosin: Val-Gln-Tyr-Pro-Val-Glu-His-Pro-Asp-Lys-Phe-Leu-Lys-Phe-Gly-Met-Thr-Pro-Ser-Lys-Gly-Val-Leu-Phe-Tyr-NH₂; a peptide in porcine small intestine that retards motility and stimulates the secretion of gastrin, pancreatic polypeptide, and exocrine pancreas proteins. Precursors have been identified in adrenal medulla and cortex, in heart and liver, and in several parts of the central nervous system. However, since the precursor lacks the kinds of peptide bonds usually cleaved by converting enzymes, it has been suggested that it is not processed under physiological conditions, and that the valosin in tissue extracts is produced artifactually.

valproic acid: 2-propylvaleric acid. It inhibits repetitive neuron firing and promotes gamma aminobutyric acid (GABA) accumulation, but is not a sedative. The salts are used to treat petit mal epilepsy.

$$H_3C-CH_2-CH_2$$
$$\overset{H}{\underset{}{C}}-COOH$$
$$H_3C-CH_2-CH_2$$

valyl-glycyl-aspartyl-glutamic acid: VGAG; a peptide that stimulates eosinophil chemotaxis.

valyl-glycyl-seryl-glutamic acid: VGSG; a peptide with properties similar to those of valyl-glycyl-aspartyl-glutamic acid.

VAMP: vincristine, methotrexate, 6-mercaptopurine, and prednisone, a drug combination used to treat some forms of cancer.

vanadium, V: a metallic element (atomic number 23, atomic weight 50.942), required in trace amounts. Orthovanadate inhibition of several kinds of phosphatases may account for most of the biological effects (but V can displace P in some reactions). Vanadium salts augment insulin receptor tyrosine kinase activity and exert some insulin-like actions; and deficiencies may contribute to the etiology of certain forms of diabetes mellitus. They also inhibit components of some Na^+/K^+-ATPases and calcium pumps, and of enzymes required for glucose metabolism and the actions of Müllerian duct inhibitor. Microtubule enzymes are sensitive to low concentrations. High levels can accelerate DNA synthesis and mitogenesis in fibroblasts and enhance the effects of some transforming factors. Toxic amounts irritate conjunctival and respiratory tract epithelia and can cause blood dyscrasias. V is a cofactor for bacterial nitrate reductases that convert atmospheric nitrogen to ammonium ions. Vanadate is used *in vitro* to stabilize steroid hormone receptor complexes.

Vandenbergh effect: the stimulatory effects of pheromones in the urine of adult male mice and some other rodents on reproductive system maturation in young females of the same species.

Van den Bergh's test: a procedure for measuring water-soluble, conjugated "posthepatic" bilirubin in serum, based on formation of a colored product when the molecules react with paradimethylaminobenzaldehyde.

van der Waals force: a weak attractive force between the electrons of one atom and the nucleus of another. Over a limited range the magnitude varies inversely with the distance; but atoms close enough for outer electron shells to overlap repel each other. Attractive and repulsive forces balance when the distance between two atomic species is equal to the van der Waals radius characteristic for the atomic types.

van der Waals radius: the distance between atoms at which the attractive and repulsive forces are equivalent in magnitude; *see* **van der Waals forces**.

Van Dyke protein: an obsolete term for hypothalamic neurophysins.

vanillyl mandelic acid: VMA; 3-hydroxy-4-methoxy mandelic acid; a common degradation product of peripheral norepinephrine and epinephrine metabolism, formed in reactions catalyzed by catechol-*O*-methyl-transferase (COMT) and monoamine oxidases (MAOs). Approximately one-third of the norepinephrine and epinephrine secreted by the adrenal medulla is excreted to urine in this form.

$$H_3C_{\diagdown}O \quad \text{(ring)} \quad \overset{H}{\underset{H}{\overset{O}{C}}}-COOH$$
$$HO$$

vanishing testis syndrome: sex differentiation disorders in which testes of individuals with XY chromosome patterns undergo prenatal atrophy. The effects on the accessory reproductive organs and external genitalia vary with the developmental stage at which atrophy occurs.

van't Hoff equation: a mathematical expression of the effects of temperature on the behavior of dissolved molecules and ions. The form $\pi = CRT$, in which C = the solute concentration in equivalents/liter, T = the absolute temperature, and R = the gas constant (0.82 liter atmospheres per degree per mole) is used to calculate π, the osmotic pressure (in osmoles/liter) at an atmospheric pressure of 760 mm Hg. The effect of temperature on the equilibrium constant of a reaction is defined by $\ln K = C - \Delta H/RT$, where $\ln K$ is the log of the equilibrium constant, C is an integration constant, ΔH is the heat of the reaction (in calories/mole), T is the temperature, and R is the gas constant (1.98 calories/mole/degree).

variable: a parameter that can have many values. *Independent* variables (such as ages of children or concentrations of pharmacological agents) are selected, and their relationships to *dependent* variables (for example weights of children in the first case and cellular responses in the second) are measured.

variable domain: a component of a specific kind of immunoglobulin light or heavy chain that can differ from related immunoglobulin components within the same individual.

variable region: V segment; the *N*-terminal portion of a variable domain that binds a specific antigen type (or a set of closely related antigens).

variance: V; a statistical measure of population distribution, obtained by determining the differences of all measured values (y) from the mean value ($\bar{y}$), squaring the differences, adding them, and dividing the sum by the degrees of freedom (one less than the total numbers of measurements, n): $V = \Sigma(y-\bar{y})^2/n-1$. The **standard deviation** (*q.v.*) is the square root of the variance.

variant: a cell, individual, or other entity that differs from most other members of the population.

Varicella zoster: type 3 human *Herpes simplex* virus, which causes smallpox and shingles.

varices: plural of varix.

varicocele: abnormally dilated spermatic cord veins, usually painful, and usually associated with oligospermia.

varicosities of neurons: enlarged autonomic system nerve terminals with synaptic vesicles.

Varidase: a trade name for a preparation of streptokinase plus streptodornase.

varix [**varices**]: a mass of distended, usually tortuous blood or lymphatic vessels.

varus: bent or twisted inward, a term used in conjunction with modifiers to describe deformities in which structures are bent toward the midline of the body; *cf* **valgus**.

vas [**vasa**]: a vessel or tube; it can be used as a prefix as in vasodilation, or with qualifiers, as in vasa recta.

vasa recta: long capillary loops with hairpin turns that run parallel to descending and ascending Henle loop limbs. Slow blood flow through the vessels and countercurrent exchanges with interstitial fluids contribute to maintenance of the high osmotic pressure within the renal medulla essential for vasopressin mediated water conservation.

vascular: relating to, or containing blood vessels.

vascular endothelial growth factor: *see* **VEGF**.

vascularization: growth of new blood vessels in a tissue, organ, or tumor.

vascular permeability factor: VPF: a 40K dimeric glycoprotein similar to the B subunit of platelet derived growth factor (PDGF) that augments blood vessel permeability, accelerates blood flow to the myometrium, and suppresses uterine muscle contractility.

vasculitis: inflammation of a blood vessel, usually with necrosis.

vasculotropin: *see* **VEGF**.

vas deferens [**vasa deferentia**]: ductus deferens; a muscular tube on each side of the body that originates in the epididymis. The two tubes join seminal vesicle ducts to form the ejaculatory duct from which spermatozoa and seminal fluid are transported to the urethra. The tubes derive from embryonic mesonephric ducts, and require testosterone for differentiation. Dihydrotestosterone is then needed for further growth and maturation, and for maintaining the morphology and functions of the mature structures. Opioid peptides acting on κ (and possibly also δ) type receptors contribute to the control of contractility.

vasectomy: usually, ligation of (or insertion of plugs or valves into) the vasa deferentia to block sperm delivery to the ejaculate. The procedures can damage the blood testis barrier and invoke immune system dysfunction and testicular cell damage in some species.

vasoactive: affecting vascular smooth muscle.

vasoactive intestinal peptide; VIP; widely distributed species-specific peptides chemically related to glucose dependent insulinotropic peptide (GIP), secretin, glucagon, growth hormone releasing hormone (GRH), corticotropin releasing hormone (CRH), sauvagine, PACAP (pituitary adenylate cyclase activating protein), and helodermin, that function at various sites as neurotransmitters, neuromodulators, and hormones. They are cleaved from proteins that are also precursors for PHM (peptide histidine methionine) in humans, and PHI (peptide histidine isoleucine) of other species. The form made by humans, rats, pigs, and cows has the amino acid sequence: His-Ser-Asp-Ala-Val-Phe-Thr-Asp-Asn-Tyr-Thr-Arg-Leu-Arg-Lys-Gln-Met-Ala-Val-Lys-Lys-Tyr-Leu-Asn- Ser-Ile-Leu-Asn-NH$_2$. Large amounts are synthesized in several brain regions, including the cerebral cortex, the suprachiasmatic, arcuate, paraventricular, periventricular and magnocellular nuclei, and the median eminence region of the hypothalamus. VIP is also secreted by autonomic system, motor, and sensory neurons, and is made in the adrenal medulla and pineal glands, and in Harderian glands of some species. Substantial amounts are made by H cells of the small intestine; and the peptide is distributed throughout the gastrointestinal tract, including the esophagus and rectum. The peptide is also made in pituitary and thyroid glands, and in both male and female genitourinary tracts and gonads; and APUD-derived tumors release large amounts (*see* **VIPomas**.) Receptors are also very widely distributed. Although some direct effects are mediated by them, there are complex interactions with many other regulators. VIP is co-released with PHM or PHI at some sites, and those peptides act on VIP receptors. It is also co-synthesized and co-secreted at other sites with acetylcholine, norepinephrine, NPY (neuropeptide Y), substance P, opioid peptides, CGRP, calcitonin, corticotropin releasing hormone, neurotensin, cholecystokinin (CCK) and gamma aminobutyric acid (GABA). Some effects involve interactions with receptors for secretin and glucagon, potentiation of catecholamine actions, and influences on acetylcholine affinity for muscarinic receptors. Stimuli that promote its release include acetylcholine (from vagus nerve endings) and agents that generate cAMP or activate kinase C. Somatostatin is a major inhibitor; and VIP antagonizes SS actions at some sites. Some effects are opposed by NPY. Since it is neurotropic, VIP may contribute to nervous system development. Centrally, it participates in the control of sleep-wake cycles, stimulates oxytocin synthesis, affects vasopressin release, and is a potent prolactin releasing hormone that may function during lactation and a potentiator of CRH effects on adrenocorticotropic hormone (ACTH) secretion. Circulating VIP relaxes vascular smooth muscle and lowers blood pressure, in part by antagonizing the effects of stimulants. Peripheral effects on the endocrine system include stimulation of insulin release; and control of thyroid hormone function is consistent with its formation in both thyrotropes and thyroid gland cells. There are numerous influences on exocrine glands. VIP stimulates water and electrolyte transport in the intestine and exocrine pancreas, augments amylase production, and promotes bile flow, but antagonizes histamine and gastrin stimulation of hydrochloric acid formation. It also acts on salivary, sweat, lachrymal, tracheal and mammary glands. In the reproductive system it relaxes uterine muscle and Fallopian tube sphincters, increases blood flow to the endometrium, and is implicated as a regulator of ovarian and testicular differentiation and establishment of steroidogenic competence. In granulosa cells it augments $P450_{scc}$ synthesis and enhances the effects of estrogens and progesterone. It is also believed to contribute (probably via vasodilation) to erection of the penis. In the immune system receptors have been identified on T and B lymphocytes and on IgA-secreting plasma cells; and observed effects include inhibition of cell proliferation and IgA secretion, with accelerated lymphocyte homing to Peyer's patches. The peptide additionally stimulates glycogenolysis and lipolysis in the liver, and is reported to accelerate bone resorption. Many actions have been linked with activation of adenylate cyclase; but some are antagonized by high cAMP levels.

vasoconstriction: contraction of vascular smooth muscle. Localized effects confined to areterioles and precapillary sphincters decrease blood flow to affected regions, and thereby shunt it to other areas. For example more blood is sent to skeletal muscles and less to viscera during exercise, whereas the gastrointestinal tract receives increased amounts after food intake. Generalized contraction of arterial and arteriolar muscle raises diastolic blood pressure; and contraction of venous smooth muscle hastens return of blood to the heart. Stimulants include norepinephrine, angiotensin-II, endothelins, vasopressins, and some eicosanoids. Most act selectively on some vascular beds without affecting others.

vasodilation: relaxation of vascular smooth muscle. Localized dilation improves blood flow to specific regions. Generalized relaxation of arteriolar muscle lowers systemic blood pressure; and dilation of veins slows return of blood to the heart. Nitric oxide is a major regulator; but atrial natriuretic peptides, prostacyclins, and others act at various sites.

vasopressins: mammalian hormones chemically and biologically related to the vasotocin made by most other vertebrates (and to a lesser extent to oxytocin, mesotocin, and other hypothalamic nonapeptide hormones). The terms vasopressin and anti-diuretic hormone are often used synonymously with **arginine vasopressin** (AVP, *q.v.*). However, lysine vasopressin (LVP) in which a lysyl moiety replaces the arginyl moiety exerts virtually identical effects, except that it is slightly less potent on a molecule for molecule basis. It is made by domestic pigs and a strain of Peruvian mice; and both AVP and LVP have been identified in hippopotamuses and peccaries. Most circulating vasopressin is synthesized in the supraoptic and paraventricular nuclei and associated neuron clusters of the hypothalamus and is sent via long hypothalamo-hypophysial nerve tract axons to the neural lobe, in which it is stored in vesicles for subsequent release to the bloodstream. The prohormones (propressophysins) additionally yield vasopressin neurophysin and a C-terminal glycopeptide for which no function has

been established. The best known actions are exerted on renal collecting ducts, where the hormones augment the water permeability of plasma membranes on the luminal surfaces, and thereby facilitate return of water to the bloodstream. The effects are mediated via cAMP which promotes translocation of cytoplasmic vesicles to plasma membranes, where they insert and function as water channels. The actions are antagonized by prostaglandin $F_{2\alpha}$ ($PGF_{2\alpha}$). Failure to secrete or respond to the regulator leads to the development of **diabetes insipidus** (*q.v.*). It can be treated with preparations of LVP and related agents administered intranasally. Some influences are also exerted on electrolyte transport; and excessive amounts can invoke hyponatremia as well as hypervolemia and edema. AVP exerts other effects by acting on different **vasopressin receptors** (*q.v.*), at least some of which involve elevation of cytoplamic Ca^{2+}. High concentrations stimulate smooth muscle in some vascular beds. Influences on brain regions involved in the blood pressure controls, facilitation of baroreceptor reflexes, and modulation of atrial natriuretic peptide secretion, as well as effects on water retention contribute to the hypertensive effects of high levels; but AVP is also involved in a negative feedback loop in which angiotensin promotes AVP secretion and AVP inhibits renin release. Exogenous AVP is used to elevate blood pressure in individuals with circulatory shock secondary to prolonged anesthesia, and its ability to constrict esophageal vessels is useful during surgery in that region. High hormone levels also stimulate gastrointestinal smooth muscle; and the "side-effects" of peptides used to treat diabetes insipidus can include nausea and pain. It is used to restore tone to muscles of the large intestine that have reacted unfavorably to prolonged manipulation during surgery. Some vasopressin is released along with oxytocin during parturition, and its stimulatory effects on uterine muscle may contribute to the delivery. At other sites vasopressin potentiates corticotropin releasing hormone (CRH) stimulation of adrenocorticotropic hormone (ACTH) secretion and can also lower body temperature. Although the circulating hormone can stimulate steroidogenesis and affect steroid metabolism in the adrenal cortex and gonads, more important effects may be exerted by locally produced AVP at both sites. The peptide made in the extrahypothalamic brain contributes to learning and long-term memory, affects avoidance behavior in laboratory animals, and is reported to exert beneficial effects in some forms of amnesia. (Administration to individuals with Alzheimer's disease has been advocated.) Pharmacological amounts promote glycogenolysis in the liver via mechanisms different from those exerted by glucagon. The effects may assume importance during severe hypoglycemia. AVP can also accelerate proliferation of some cell types. It acts on the thymus gland and can mimic the effects of interleukin-2 on interferon-γ production. The stimuli for release from the neural lobe include high blood osmotic pressure, low blood volume, hypotension, exposure to hot environments, and messages received from nociceptors; and large amounts are secreted during some forms of stress. Both stimulatory and inhibitory effects of opioid peptides within the neural lobe have been described. Atrial naturiuretic peptides inhibit AVP release, and some negative feedback control is exerted by glucocorticoids. *See also* **Brattleboro rats.**

vasopressin neurophysin: pressophysin; nicotine stimulated neurophysin; NSN; a 10K peptide cleaved from propressophysin, the precursor of vasopressin. It is co-secreted with the hormone and may contribute to vasopressin stability and packaging within magnocellular neurons. However, although effects of high levels on lipid mobilization and some other processes have been described, no physiological functions have been established. Responses to vasopressin alone appear to be identical with those to vasopressin administered in combination with the neurophysin.

vasopressin receptors: molecules that bind to and mediate the actions of vasopressins. Activation of the V_1 type transiently elevates cytoplasmic Ca^{2+}, probably via generation of inositol phosphates, and mediates the influences on smooth muscle, glycogenolysis, and lipolysis. The V_2 type in kidney collecting ducts accelerates cAMP generation and accounts for the effects on water conservation. A V_3 type in the brain appears to be required for the influences on learning and memory.

Vasotec: a trade name for enalapril maleate.

vasotocin: arginine vasotocin; AVT; a neurohyophysial peptide made in substantial amounts by most nonmammalian vertebrates. It is cyclic nonapeptide structurally similar to **arginine vasopressin** (*q.v.*) but with the amino acid sequence Cys-Tyr-Phe-Gln-Asn-Cys-Pro-Arg-Gly-NH_2, and biological properties that more closely resemble those of oxytocin. It is cleaved from a prohormone that also yields AVT-neurophysin. Although the hormone exerts only weak vasopressin-like effects on mammalian kidneys, it promotes water conservation in vertebrates that lack Henle loops by slowing renal blood flow and diminishing glomerular filtration. It also contributes to blood pressure controls, and is a potent stimulant for oviduct smooth muscle in birds and reptiles. It augments the release of adrenocorticotropic hormone (ACTH) in fishes and acts on the salt glands of some species. Mature mammals use mostly vasopressins and oxytocin, respectively, to promote water conservation and uterine contraction; but fetuses make AVT, and the peptide affects water transport across amniotic membranes. Small amounts are made postnatally in suprachiasmatic nuclei and pineal glands where contributions to the control of some circadian rhythms have been suggested.

vasotonin: an old term for an uncharacterized factor released by blood platelets that stimulates vascular smooth muscle, now believed to be serotonin.

Vasoxyl: a trade name for methoxamine hydrochloride.

VCAMs: cell adhesion molecules on high venule endothelial cells.

V cells: an old term for adenohypophysial corticotropes.

VDR: DR; *see* **vitamin D receptors.**

VDRE: DRE; *see* **vitamin D response elements.**

vector: (1) a carrier; an individual who harbors an infectious pathogen and can transfer it to other members of the species but does not display disease symptoms; (2) a phenotypically normal individual with a recessive defect that can be transmitted to progeny; (3) an arthropod or other animal that supports part of the life cycle of a disease producing organism and passes the organism to hosts of other species in which it continues maturation and/or reproduces; (4) a plasmid or viral chromosome with one or more nucleic acid fragments foreign to a host that can incorporate into a host genome. It usually replicates autonomously, but its activity can be regulated by host factors; (5) a quantity having direction as well as magnitude.

vecuronium bromide: 1-[3,17-*bis*-(acetyloxy)-2-(1-piperidinyl)androstan-16-yl]-1-methyl-piperidinium bromide; a nonpolarizing neuromuscular blocking agent that exerts curare-like effects. It is used as a muscle relaxant.

vegan: an individual who does not eat any foods of animal origin; *cf* **vegetarian.**

vegetal hemisphere: the part of a telolecithal egg that contains most of the yolk and is farthest from the nucleus. It is usually more heavily pigmented than the animal hemisphere and may be separated from it by a marginal zone. Amphibian vegetal pole cells give rise to midgut and hindgut components and release regulators similar to or identical with fibroblast growth factors and/or int-2 that provide signals for mesoderm induction in animal pole derivatives.

vegetal pole: the end of a telolecithal egg farthest from the nucleus; *see* **vegetal hemisphere.**

vecuronium bromide

vegetative: describes (1) involuntary activities, especially ones controlled by the autonomic nervous system; (2) individuals with brain injuries or defects who cannot consciously perceive or engage in voluntary activities; (3) nutritional and growth processes (as opposed to reproductive and cognitive functions); (4) the growth phases of spore forming organisms and plant sporophyte generations; (5) the noninfective stage during which a phage genome replicates and directs host synthesis of substances that establish and sustain the infection.

vegetative reproduction: asexual reproduction such as budding in yeasts, or growth of a new plant from a stem or shoot.

VEGF: vascular endothelium growth factor; vasculotropin; a 46K dimeric protein similar to vascular permeability factor that contributes to angiogenesis, but differs from fibroblast and platelet derived growth factors (FGFs and PDGF) in that it does not affect the growth of fibroblasts, keratinocytes, adrenocortical cells, corneal endothelium, or lens epithelium. A circulating form is secreted by mononuclear leukocytes and macrophages. VEGF made by adenohypophysial folliculo-stellate cells may be a paracrine regulator of pituitary hormone secretion, ion transport within the gland, and localized angiogenesis. Direct contributions to the development of estrogen-induced pituitary gland tumors have been suggested.

vehicle: (1) a substance used to dissolve or suspend an agent (for injection or other use); (2) a vector, definitions 1-4.

veiled cells: interdigitating lymph node cells.

vein: (1) in animals a vessel that receives blood from venules or smaller veins and transports it directly, or via larger veins to the heart; *cf* **artery**. The blood oxygen content is low in sytemic veins and high in those of the pulmonary tree; (2) in plants a branching vascular bundle continuous with a stem stele that passes through a petiole and conducts fluids to a leaf. It contains xylem and phloem cells

venation: the distribution and arrangement of veins.

venereal: (1) sexual or erotic; (2) describes infections disseminated via sexual contact or intercourse.

venesection: phlebotomy; venipuncture.

venipuncture: insertion of a needle into a vein, usually to draw blood or to inject substances directly into the bloodstream.

venoms: secretions released by plants, insects, amphibians, reptiles, or other organisms that are poisonous to other species. Many types obtained from saliva, skin glands and other sources contain components that act on neurons or neurotransmitter receptors, and are used as pharmacological tools.

ventral: pertaining to or situated on the abdominal side; *cf* **dorsal**. It is roughly equivalent to anterior in humans and other upright species, and to inferior in quadrupeds, snakes, and fishes.

ventral lobe of the hypophysis: a component of cartilaginous fish pituitary glands believed to derive from the pars tuberalis.

ventromedial nuclei: VMN; bilateral hypothalamic neuron clusters that contribute to the control of growth hormone, insulin, and possibly also glucagon, thyrotropin (TSH), and gonadotropin secretion, of some autonomic nervous system functions (including gastric emptying) and of food intake and circadian rhythms. The concept that they contain "**satiety centers**" (*q.v.*) has been modified.

venule: a small vessel that receives blood from capillaries or smaller venules; *cf* **arterioles** and *see* also **vein**. Most venules transport the blood to larger venules or veins, but *see* **portal systems**.

verapamil: 5-[(3,4-dimethoxyphenethyl)methylamino]-2-(3,4-dimethoxyphenyl)-2-isopropylvaleronitrile; an agent that blocks both T and L type Ca^{2+} channels, affects Na^+ transport, and lowers blood pressure. It exerts negative chronotropic, dromotropic, and inotropic effects on the heart and is used both orally and intravenously to dilate coronary vessels, and to treat some forms of tachycardia. It is a less potent vasodilator than dihydropyridines.

veratridine: 3-veratroylveracevine; a toxic alkaloid obtained from the seeds of *Veratrum album* and *Schoenocaulon officinale*, and a component of **veratrine** (*q.v.*). It promotes depolarization, and is used as a laboratory tool.

veratrine: a mixture of alkaloids obtained from the seeds of *Schoenocaulon officinale* that includes **veratridine** (*q.v.*) and also cevine, cevadine, and sabadine. The compounds irritate mucous membranes and have been used

verapamil

veratridine

as emetics (to promote elimination of poisons), and as topical counterirritants to treat neuralgias and arthritis.

veratrum: a mixture of **alkaloids** obtained from *Veratrum viride* and *Veratrum album* that includes jervine, cevadine, germine, veratralbine, and veratroidine. It was once used for its emetic, parasiticidal, and antihypertensive properties, but has been replaced by less toxic agents.

v-erbA: an oncogene related to ***c-erbA*** (*q.v.*), made by the E-S4 avian erythroblastosis virus. It codes for protein $p75^{gag\text{-}erbA}$.

v-erbB: an oncogene related to ***c-erbB*** (*q.v.*), made by E-Sw avian erythroblastosis virus. It codes for protein $p72^{erbB}$.

vermiform: worm-like.

vermin: animals regarded as pests, or as a competitors for food supplies or territory.

Verner-Morrison syndrome: *see* **VIPidoma**.

vernix: the cheese-like material on skin surfaces of near-term fetuses and newborn infants, composed mostly of desquamated epithelium and sebum.

veronal buffer: a barbital buffer used to prepare fixatives for electron microscopy.

verrucosity: a wart-like protuberance.

versene: EDTA; *see* **ethylenediaminetetraacetic acid**.

vertebral lime sacs: paravertebral lime sacs; amphibian organs that store calcium. The functions are regulated by calcitonin, parathyroid hormone, and prolactin.

vertical evolution: formation of new species from ancestral types via gradual changes in successive generations.

vertical transmission: passage of genetic information from an individual to progeny, or from a parent cell to its daughters; *cf* **horizontal transmission**.

vertigo: giddiness; dizziness; whirling or turning sensations. Toxins and other stimuli can invoke it in normal subjects. Chronic conditions that arise spontaneously are usually caused by internal ear dysfunctions; but gastrointestinal tract and other diseases, and factors that impede blood flow to the brain can activate receptors involved in the sensations.

very high density lipoproteins: VLDLs; *see* **lipoproteins**.

very late antigens: VLAs; plasma membrane glycoproteins of the integrin superfamily with common 130K (β1 type) beta subunits that mediate cell adhesion to extracellular matrix proteins, contribute to antigen recognition and signal transduction, and play critical roles in T lymphocyte migration. Their abilities to undergo regulated activation (mediated in part via ligand binding) and inactivation appear to be crucial for the attachment and detachment essential for migration and localization. Each subtype has its a specific kind of α subunit noncovalently linked to the β_1. The α component affects the binding properties and functions; and subtle differences among members within a subtype have been described. The name was introduced when it was observed that VLA-1 and VLA-2 are not detected until approximately two weeks after T cell activation; but it is now applied to at least ten different kinds of molecules, some of which are expressed at earlier times. Several are made in larger amounts by memory, as compared with naive T cells (ones that have not been exposed to the specific antigens). VLA-1 ($\alpha_1\beta_1$ integrin) with a 120K α subunit, and VLA-2 ($\alpha_2\beta_2$ integrin) with a 165K α, are T cell activation antigens. Both bind to collagens and laminin (LN) but use different attachment sites. VLA-1 is also expressed on fibroblasts and smooth muscle cells, and VLA1$^+$ cells are present in lower respiratory tract epithelium, and in synovial fluids of individuals with rheumatoid arthritis. VLA-2 is similar to or identical with platelet protein Ia/IIb. It is expressed on a subset of CD8$^+$ lymphocytes in individuals with acquired immunodeficiency syndrome (AIDS). VLA-3 ($\alpha_3\beta_1$ integrin) is abundant on some cultured T lymphocyte clones, but is expressed in very small amounts on resting T cells. It, too has binding sites for collagens and LN but additionally binds fibronectin (FN) and epiligrin (an epithelial cell basement membrane protein). VLA-4 ($\alpha_4\beta_1$ integrin), with a 150K subunit, binds to FN and is expressed on all lymphocytes (including B types for which it may be the only FN receptor) and on natural killer (NK) cells and monocytes. It additionally binds the cell adhesion molecule, VCAM-1. Although it is just one of many compounds that binds FN, VLA-5 has also been called the FN receptor. It, and VLA-6 (which binds to LN) are expressed on resting CD^{4+} cells; and memory types have three to four times as much of them and of VLA-3 proteins as naive cells.

very long chain fatty acids: VLCFA: fatty acids with more than 20 carbons such as hexacosanoate. They are catabolized primarily in peroxisomes via reactions similar to those described for β-oxidation of shorter fatty acids in mitochondria.

very low density lipoproteins: VLDLs: *see* **lipoproteins**.

L(-)-**vesamicol**: (-)-2-(4-phenylpiperidino)cyclohexanol; a nonocompetitive inhibitor of acetylcholine transport that acts on the inner surfaces of vesicle membranes and blocks accumulation of the neurotransmitter.

vesicle: usually a membrane-enclosed organelle that contains a fluid or semifluid substance.

vesicular follicle: an ovarian follicle that has acquired theca layers and a stratum granulosum with fluid-filled vesicles which contain estrogen and other regulators. Several follicles of this kind develop during a typical human ovarian cycle, but only one matures to the preovulatory stage. The others serve for a time as estrogen-secreting cohorts that soon undergo atresia. Many follicles simultaneously complete maturation in species that produce large litters. The incidences of nonidentical twin and triplet births provide some indication of the frequency in humans; but it is not uncommon for one or more embryos to die at an early stage of development. "Fertility drugs" that elevate follicle stimulating hormone (FSH) levels increase the numbers that mature, and thereby the incidence of multiple human births.

vesiculase: a protein synthesized by rodent coagulating glands that clots semen. Copulation plugs thus formed block loss of spermatozoa from female reproductive tracts.

vestibule: (1) an entry site; (2) a cavity that leads into another cavity; (3) vestibulum.

vestibulum: the central part of the bony labyrinth of the inner ear that houses the saccule and utricle.

vestigial: describes incompletely developed or atrophic structures morphologically related to functional ones in ancestral species, or regulators that no longer function but resemble ones used by ancestral species.

vestigial hormones: hormones identified in, but not known to perform functions in a given species, although made and used by species lower on the phylogenetic scale. It has been suggested that they are "evolutionary carryovers" retained because they are harmless. Some hormones initially classified as vestigial have been shown to exert effects in "higher" animals, at least under special conditions.

VGAG: valyl-glycyl-aspartyl-glutamic acid.

V genes: major histocompatibility complex (MHC) DNA segments that code for the first 95-100 amino acid moieties of light and heavy immunoglobulin chain and T lymphocyte receptor variable regions. (J gene segments code for the remaining components of immunoglobulin chain variable regions and T cell receptor β and δ chains.)

Vgl: a vegetal hemisphere signal released from endoderm that affects embryonic mesoderm commitment and enhances induction mediated by fibroblast growth factors and related regulators. It is a member of the transforming growth factor-β superfamily, named TGFβ2 to distinguish it from the more common TGFβ1.

VGSG: valyl-glycyl-seryl-glutamic acid.

V$_H$: the variable region of an immunoglobulin heavy chain.

viable: capable of survival, a term applied to cells, and to fetuses sufficiently mature to survive outside the uterus.

viability test: determination of the numbers of surviving organisms of a species or cell type relative to others, under specified conditions. *See* also **trypan blue**.

Vibrio cholerae: the bacterium that causes cholera; *see* **cholera toxin**.

VIC: vasoactive intestinal contractor; endothelin β; *see* **endothelins**.

Vicia faba: a bean plant with cells that contain six large chromosomes, used for cytogenetics studies.

vicinal: near or neighboring, a term applied to chemical groups of compounds.

vidarabine: ara-A; adenine arabinoside; 9-β-D-arabinofuranosyladenine monohydrate; an antiviral agent made by *Streptomyces antibioticus* that is phosphorylated by both host and virus-induced thymidine kinases. It inhibits viral DNA polymerases to a greater extent than host types, is effective against some *Herpes* strains, and is potentially useful as an anticancer agent.

vif: virion infectivity factor.

villi: plural of villus.

villikinin: a peptide component of intestinal extracts and human blood plasma that differs chemically from established gastrointestinal hormones. It stimulates lymph flow and the pumping activity of intestinal villi.

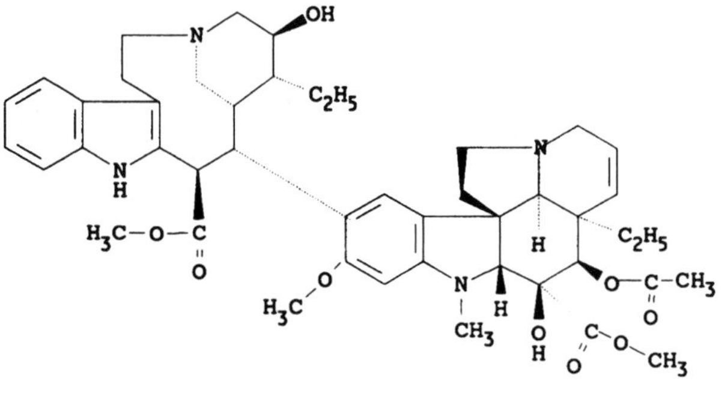

vinblastine

villin: a 95K protein of intestinal microvilli that cross-links actin filaments at low Ca^{2+} concentrations, but can sever long filaments at micromolar levels. It also binds to actin fragments and blocks filament elongation.

villus [**villi**]: (1) any finger-like projection; (2) one of many multicellular protrusions of the luminal wall of the small intestine lumen that contributes to nutrient absorption into blood and lymph; *see* also **lacteal**, and *cf* **microvillus**; (3) a finger-like projection on the surface of the chorion.

vimentin: an insoluble, 53K intermediate filament protein of fibroblasts, endothelium, leukocytes, neuroglia, some smooth muscle, and some other cell types. It accumulates in focal contacts where microfilaments anchor to plasma membranes, binds to desmin in smooth muscle, is associated with a 50K acidic protein in glial cells, and affects morphology and motility. Vimentin is a substrate for kinases A and C; and phosphorylation promotes disassembly of vimentin filaments. Insulin enhances phosphorylation in insulinomas, and follicle stimulating hormone (FSH) exerts similar effects in Sertoli cells. Proteins that bind vimentin to microtubules may control its distribution.

vinblastine: vincaleukoblastine; an antineoplastic alkaloid derived from *Vinca rosea*, chemically and biologically related to vincristine. By binding to tubulin and blocking microtubule polymerization, it arrests mitosis in metaphase and affects phagocytosis and other functions.

vinca alkaloids: mitotic poisons obtained from the Madagascar periwinkle, *Vinca rosea*. *See* **vinblastine and vincristine**.

vincristine: 22-oxo-vincaleukoblastine; an alkaloid derived from *Vinca rosea* chemically related to vinblastine. Although it exerts similar effects on microtubules and suppresses tumor growth, there are some differences in clinical responses; and cross-resistance does not develop. Both agents are used to block spindle formation and facilitate collection of cells in metaphase, and to study microtubule-dependent transport.

vinculin: a 130K intermediate filament protein chemically related to gelsolin. It binds talin, anchors actin filaments to inner surfaces of plasma membranes, is a component of adhesion plaques that link adjacent cells, and is implicated as a mediator of cell adhesion to extracellular matrix components. Some kinases, including ones activated by platelet derived growth factor (PDGF) and pp60[v-src] promote its phosphorylation and may thereby destabilize actin filament linkages, affect cell morphology (permit rounding), loosen intercellular associations, and facilitate metastasis of transformed cells.

vinculum: a slender connecting band or fold.

vinyl: the chemical group $H_2C=CH-$.

viosterol: ergocalciferol.

VIP: vasoactive intestinal peptide.

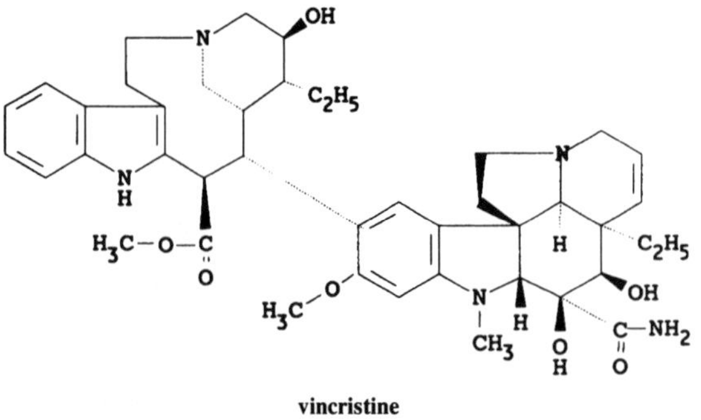

vincristine

viper: any venomous snake of Viperidae family.

VIPidomas: vipomas: tumors that secrete **vasoactive intestinal peptide** (*q.v.*) and other biologically active substances. The symptoms include watery diarrhea, hypokalemia, impaired gastric acid production, accelerated glycogenolysis, and disturbances in calcium metabolism.

vipomas: VIPidomas.

viral: pertaining to or caused by viruses.

virilization: acquisition of male phenotypic characteristics by females. In women it can include growth of hair on the face and trunk, clitoromegaly, increased skeletal muscle development, and enlargement of the larynx with deepening of the voice. In this context the term is sometimes used synonymously with masculinization. In rodents and some other laboratory animals, masculinization refers to maturation of brain regions that support male-type sexual behavior; *cf* **defeminization**.

virion: a structurally complete virus; *cf* **viroid**.

viroid: a single-stranded infectious RNA particle not enclosed by proteins; *cf* **virion**. Viroids can replicate to form double-stranded RNAs and activate dsRNA protein kinases; but they do not encode polypeptides. Some cause plant diseases.

virulence: pathogenicity of infectious agents; ability to cause disease.

virulent phages: phages that promote lysis in host microorganisms.

virus: an ultramicroscopic entity capable of autonomous replication when it infects a host cell, composed of a nucleic acid molecule (RNA or DNA) surrounded by a protein coat (capsid) which may in turn be enclosed by a lipid envelope.

virus receptor: a host cell plasma membrane component to which a virus attaches before injecting its nucleic acid into the cell.

viscera: plural of viscus; a term that refers to internal organs.

viscus [viscera]: (1) any soft internal organ; (2) an internal organ regulated by the autonomic nervous system.

visinin: 28K calbindin.

vision: usually, conscious perception of photic stimuli that act on the retina which involves transmission of messages along primary optic tracts, through the thalamus, to the cerebral cortex. The term can also encompass associated processes required for interpretation of the stimuli, and ones such as lens accommodation and adjustment of pupil size that require the accessory optic tracts and their connections to the midbrain. However, it is not used for effects of light stimuli relayed via the retinohypothalamic tracts to the hypothalamus and pineal gland that mediate synchronization of circadian and seasonal rhythms with changes in photoperiods.

vital: pertaining to, characteristic of, or essential for life.

vital red: brilliant red; ditolyldiazo-3,6-disulfo-β-naphthylamine-β-naphthylamine-6-sulfonic acid sodium salt; a dye used for blood volume determinations.

vital staining: staining of living cells with dyes such as Janus green or methylene blue; *cf* **supravital staining**.

vitamin: an organic nutrient required in very small amounts by an organism that cannot synthesize it; *see* specific types. Food is the major source; but some vitamins are obtained primarily from microorganisms that reside in gastrointestinal tracts. The term is also used for dietary components such as choline that are required for optimal function but can be made in small amounts, and for a few other substances that can be synthesized only under special conditions (such as vitamin D which most animals cannot make without exposure to ultraviolet light). It has been incorrectly applied to some agents not known to exert physiological actions; *see*, for example **vitamin B$_{15}$**. Most vitamin B complex types are used to make coenzymes. These and vitamin C are water-soluble. Some lipid-soluble vitamins (including vitamins A and D) are prohormones.

vitamin A: usually, vitamin A$_1$; *see* **retinol**.

vitamin A$_1$: vitamin A alcohol; the predominant form of vitamin A in vertebrates; *see* **retinol**.

vital red

Vitamin A$_2$: 3,4-didehydroretinal; the major form of vitamin A made by fresh-water fishes and stored in their livers. It combines with an opsin to form the visual pigment porphyropsin.

vitamin A aldehyde: *see* **retinal**.

vitamin A receptors: *see* **retinoic acid receptors**.

vitamin B$_1$: thiamine.

vitamin B$_2$: vitamin G; *see* **riboflavin**.

vitamin B$_3$: usually, niacinamide. The term is also used for niacin and pantothenic acid. Niacinamide is also called vitamin B$_5$ and vitamin PP.

vitamin B$_4$: *see* **adenine**.

vitamin B$_5$: usually pantothenic acid. The term is also used for niacinamide; *see* also **vitamin B$_3$** and **vitamin B$_x$**.

vitamin B$_6$: pyridoxine, pyridoxal, or pyridoxamine.

vitamin B$_{10}$: an obsolete term for a factor that supports growth and feathering in chickens, now believed to be folic acid or a related compound.

vitamin B$_{11}$: an uncharacterized growth factor said to act in conjunction with vitamin B$_{10}$.

vitamin B$_{12}$: cyanocobalamin.

vitamin B$_{13}$: orotic acid.

vitamin B$_{15}$: pangamic acid; an uncharacterized mixture of variable composition derived from fruit seeds and purported to confer beneficial effects in schizophrenia, alcoholism, indigestion, cardiovascular disease, and other disorders. Calcium gluconate is a major component of most preparations. No therapeutic or toxic effects have been established.

vitamin B$_{17}$: laetrile; *see* **amygdalin**.

vitamin B$_c$: a polyglutamate derivative of folic acid.

vitamin B$_x$: (1) pantothenic acid; (2) *o*-aminobenzoic acid.

vitamin B complex: a mixture of B-type vitamins. The term is used for extracts of yeast and other naturally occurring substances that contain variable amounts of the compounds, and for others prepared from known quantities of the constituents. Folic acid is usually not included because it can mask some vitamin B$_{12}$ deficiency symptoms; but that vitamin is now believed to protect against some birth defects.

vitamin B$_t$: carnitine.

vitamin C: antiscorbutic vitamin; *see* **ascorbic acid**.

vitamin D: antirachitic vitamin; usually ergocalciferol or cholecalciferol.

vitamin D$_1$: a mixture of approximately equimolecular quantities of lumisterol and ergocalciferol. The term is seldom used, since most vitamin D preparations contain ergocalciferol or cholecalciferol.

vitamin D$_2$: ergocalciferol; the major form of vitamin D obtained by irradiating ergosterol and some other plant precursors. Small amounts are present in some fish oils.

vitamin D$_3$: the form of vitamin D made by most animal species; *see* **calciferol**.

vitamin D receptors: VDR; DR; Vitamin D is not known to act directly on target organs. Vitamins D$_2$ and D$_3$ are rapidly converted in the liver to 25-hydroxy-ergocalciferol, and 25-hydroxy-cholecalciferol, respectively. Those are major storage and transport forms that are not believed to interact with specific receptors when present in physiological concentrations. The kidneys contain a 1α-hydroxylase that converts the compounds to their 1,25-dihydroxy derivatives; and small amounts of the enzyme are made in other tissues. 1,25-dihydroxy-**cholecalciferol** (*q.v.*) also known as calcitriol, 1,25-dihydroxyvitamin D$_3$ and 1,25-D, is the major ligand for vitamin D receptors. The same receptors interact with synthetic 1α-dihydroxyvitamin D and to a lesser extent with some vitamin D metabolites such as 1,24,25-trihydroxyvitamin D. The existence of somewhat different types for 24,25-dihydroxy-**cholecalciferol** (*q.v.*) and some other metabolites has been suggested. In humans and many other species, ergocalciferol is an effective vitamin supplement, since its 1,25-hydroxy derivative acts on calcitriol receptors; but that secosteroid is very rapidly degraded by chickens, some monkeys, and some other species. Although direct effects on plasma membranes can be detected within 20 minutes after administration, the major actions of calciferols involve binding to 50-60K proteins called calcitriol (or vitamin D) receptors that reside in target cell nuclei. The proteins are members of a superfamily that includes receptors for glucocorticoids, mineralocorticoids, androgens, estrogens, triiodothyronine, retinoids, peroxisome proliferators, and some other ligands. They most closely resemble the thyroid hormone types. In common with the others, the ligand-bound receptors form dimers that bind to **vitamin D response elements** (*q.v.*). Homodimers are effective, but heterodimers also form; and interactions with retinoic acid receptors are known to affect the functions. Ligand binding promotes protein kinase C$_b$ and casein kinase II mediated phosphorylation of serine residues that seems to be essential for response element mediated effects. Accessory proteins are also required.

vitamin D response elements: VDRE; DRE; DNA components that bind dimers formed when 1,25-dihydroxycalciferols associate with their receptors, and also bind heterodimers composed of two different ligands, each bound to its associated member of the steroid-thyroid hormone receptor superfamily. They mediate the influences on transcription of specific gene types; *see* 1,25-didhyroxy **cholecalciferol**.

vitamin E: α-**tocopherol** *(q.v.)*; antisterility vitamin; 3,4-dihydro-2,5,7,8-tetramethyl-2-(4,8,12-trimethyltridecyl)-2*H*-1-benzopyran-6-ol; a vitamin in wheat germ and the seeds of several other plants, and in some leafy vegetables. It is a major lipid-soluble antioxidant that interacts with selenium and stabilizes unsaturated fatty acids and phospholipids. The requirements and effects vary with the species. Deficiency symptoms in some include sterility, skeletal muscle degeneration, and impaired hematopoiesis.

vitamin F: essential fatty acids.

vitamin G: riboflavin.

vitamin H: biotin.

vitamin K: lipid-soluble naphthoquinones and related compounds essential for the biosynthesis of osteocalcin, prothrombin and some other blood coagulation factors, and for some proteins with different functions that contain γ-carboxyglutamate moieties. *See* specific protein types.

vitamin K$_1$: phytomenadione; phylloquinone; antihemorrhagic vitamin; 2-methyl-3-phytyl-1,4-naphthoquinone; *see* also **vitamin K**.

vitamin K$_2$: menaquinones; 2-methyl-3-*all trans*-polyprenyl-1-4-naphthoquinones; members of the vitamin K family with side chains that can contain one to thirteen carbon atoms. Most have seven, eight, or nine. *See* **vitamin K**.

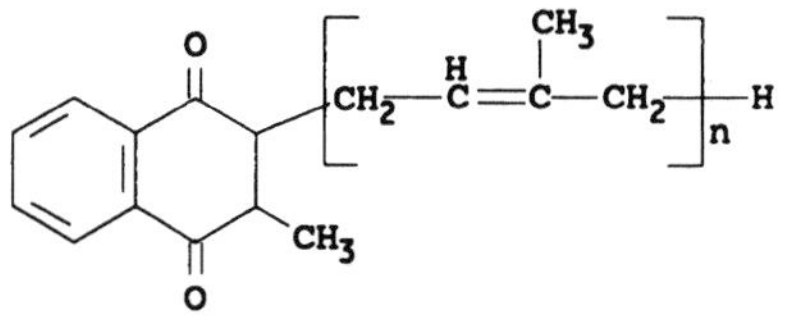

vitamin K$_5$: 4-amino-2-methyl-1-naphthol.

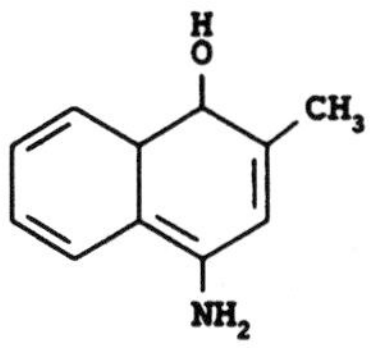

vitamin K$_6$: 2-methyl-1,4-diaminonaphthaline.

vitamin K$_7$: 3-methyl-4-amino-1-naphthol.

vitamin L: vitamins L$_1$, L$_2$ and other undefined substances purported to be essential for lactation.

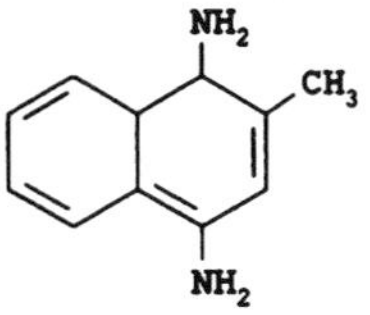

vitamin K$_6$

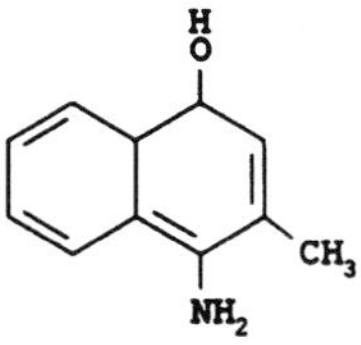

vitamin K$_7$

vitamin L$_1$: vitamin B$_x$; *o*-aminobenzoic acid; anthranilic acid; a compound purported to be essential for lactation. The cadmium salt is used as an ascaricide in veterinary medicine.

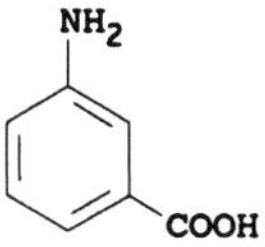

vitamin L$_2$: 7-[tetrahydro-3,4-dihyroxy-5-(methylmercaptoethyl)-2-furyl]adenine; *see* **vitamin L**.

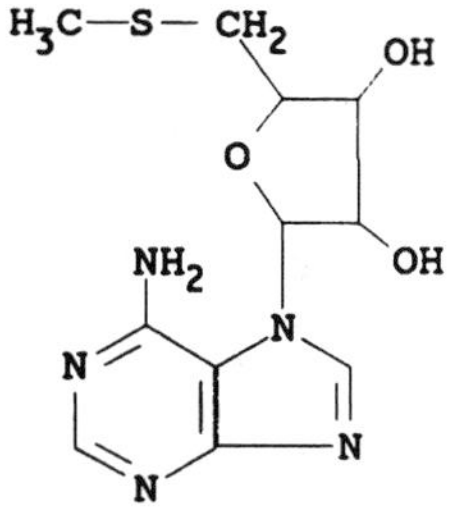

vitamin M: folic acid.

vitamin P: bioflavonoids; citrus flavonoids; mixtures of substances derived from citrus fruits, currants, and some other plant foods that contribute to the maintenance of normal capillary permeability and protect against fragility.

vitamin PP: niacinamide.

vitamin T: termitin; torutilin; tegotin; a mixture of substances initially obtained from termites but also made by yeasts, said to exert favorable influences on intermediary metabolism. It may contain several of the known vitamins and growth factors.

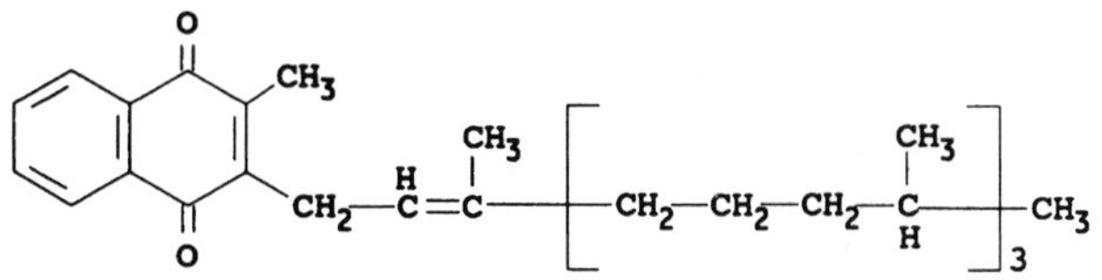

vitamin K$_1$

vitamin U: (3-amino-3-carboxypropyl)dimethyl sulfonium chloride; methylmethioniesulfonium chloride; MMSC; antiulcer vitamin; a component of leafy vegetables that is used to treat some gastric disorders. Its status as a vitamin has not been established.

vitellin: phosphatidylcholine, or phosphatidylcholine associated with egg yolk proteins.

vitelline membrane: the membrane that surrounds a mature oocyte or ovum.

vitellogenin: an estrogen-dependent protein secreted by the livers of adult female submam-malian vertebrates. It accumulates in oocytes in which it is cleaved to lipovitellin and phosvitin.

vitellus: egg yolk.

vitiligo: a disorder characterized by patchy loss of skin pigmentation in which melanocytes lose their ability to make melanins and later disappear from the affected sites. In at least some cases it is an autoimmune disease.

vitronectin: VN; S protein; serum spreading factor; approximately 70K heterodimeric extracellular matrix adhesion glycoprotein members of the β_3 subfamily of integrins. They have RGD (Arg-Gly-Asp) sequences recognized by platelet glycoprotein IIb/IIIa, by related receptors on endothelial cells, and by some other receptors, as well as domains that bind heparin and other molecules. The major vitronectin receptor, VLA-4 which resembles the fibronectin receptor, is a glycoprotein with 150K α and 115K β subunits. VN binds to talin and tensin but does not directly attach to actin. It is believed to contribute to wound healing, cell proliferation, and apoptosis.

viviparous: live-bearing; describes species in which females nurture embryos within their reproductive tracts and give birth to living young that can survive without protective coats and stored nutrients; cf **oviparous** and **ovoviviparous**.

vivisection: performance of surgery on living (usually anesthetized) animals.

vivo: occurring in, or conducted in living animals.

vixen: a female fox.

V_K: the variable region of an immunoglobulin kappa chain.

V_L: the variable region of an immunoglobulin light chain.

VLAs: *see* **very late antigens**.

VLCFA: very long chain fatty acids.

VLCFA-CoA synthetase: very long chain fatty acid-CoA synthetase; a peroxisomal enzyme that catalyzes the first step in the β-oxidation of very long chain fatty acids. Deficiency leads to accumulation of the fatty acids with consequent deleterious effects on central nervous system myelination and on adrenocortical function. *See* also **adrenoleukodystrophy**.

VLDLs: very low density lipoproteins; *see* **lipoproteins**.

V leads: unipolar connecting wires used in electrocardiography to record electrical differences between exploring electrodes placed on the chest (from precordial leads) or on the arms and left foot, and indifferent electrodes.

VMA: vanillyl mandelic acid.

V_{max}: the maximum rate for an enzyme-controlled reaction. When the substrate concentration is not a limiting factor, V_{max} usually varies directly with the quantity of active enzyme.

VMN: ventromedial nucleus.

vol: v; volume.

voles: fieldmice; small short-tailed short-limbed mouselike rodents of *Microtus* and related genera. They are used for studies of pineal gland and reproductive system functions.

volt: V; a unit of electrical potential; the electromotive force that will cause a current of 1 ampere to flow through a conductor against a resistance of one ohm. One volt x one ampere = 1 watt of power. Electrical potentials across plasma membranes are measured in millivolts (mv). For many cell types in the "resting" (unstimulated) state, they are approximately -70 mv (with the inside negative relative to the outer surface). Depolarization abolishes the potential difference or renders it less negative.

voltage: electromotive force or potential difference, measured in volts.

voltage clamping: application of electric currents to hold plasma membrane potentials at constant voltages. The procedures are used to study the effects of factors that act on ion channels.

voltage-gated channels: ion channels whose operation is regulated by changes in plasma membrane potentials; *cf* **receptor operated channels**.

vomeronasal organ: Jacobson's organ; a sensory structure in or near the nasal septum that senses environmental chemicals of low volatility which are sniffed or ingested. It is functionally associated with the accessory olfactory system and relays pheromone signals to the hypothalamus (but is not involved in conscious perception of odors).

Von Gierke's disease: an autosomal recessive disorder in which insufficient glucose-6-phosphatase is made, glycogenolysis is impaired, and excessive amounts of glycogen accumulate in the liver and at other sites. The manifestations include hypoglycemia, growth retardation, and gout.

Von Recklinghausen's disease: neurofibromatosis; *see* **Recklinghausen's disease**. Von Recklinghausen's disease of bone is **osteitis fibrosa cystica** (*q.v.*).

Von Recklinghausen's disease of bone: Recklinghausen's disease of bone: **osteitis fibrosa cystica** (*q.v.*).

Von Willebrand disease: several dseases caused by autosomal defects that impair synthesis of von Willebrand factor. The manifestations, which are most severe in those homozygous for the trait include prolonged bleeding time, reduced blood platelet adhesiveness, and hemorrhages in mucosal tissues.

Von Willebrand Factor: vWF: a plasma glycoprotein synthesized in and secreted by endothelial cells and megakaryocytes and released from thrombin-activated platelets. It circulates as 1000K to 12,000K multimers complexed to coagulation factor VIII. By binding to cell surfaces, it mediates platelet attachment to basement membranes, formation of platelet plugs at sites of vascular injury, and other platelet functions.

VPF: vascular permeability factor.

V_1, V_2 receptor[s]: *see* vasopressin receptors.

V region: the variable region of an immunoglobulin chain or T lymphocyte receptor.

V segment: the variable region of an antibody.

vulva: the region that includes the labia majora, labia minora, vaginal vestibule, and vaginal orifice of the female mammal external genitalia.

v/v: volume for volume; volume of solute per volume of solvent.

vWF: von Willebrand Factor.

W

W: (1) tryptophan; (2) tungsten; (3) watt.

W-5: *N*-(6-aminohexyl-1-naphthalene)sulfonamide hydrochloride; an agent used to inhibit calcium-dependent functions mediated by calmodulins.

O=S—N(H)—(CH₂)₆—NH₂ ·HCl

W-7: *N*-(6-aminohexyl)-5-chloro-1-naphthalanesulfonamide hydrochloride; an agent that inhibits calmodulin with greater specificity than W-5 and is a potent relaxant for vascular smooth muscle.

Cl
O=S—N(H)—(CH₂)₆—NH₂ ·HCl

W-12, **W-13**: *N*-6-amino-butyl analogs of W-5 and W-6, respectively, used to inhibit calmodulin actions.

wallerian degeneration: the retrograde disintegration of peripheral nerve axons that precedes axon repair.

waltzer: a mutation in a mouse strain that impairs neurological functions. Homozygotes display circling and head-shaking behavior, and are deaf.

Warburg apparatus: a device for manometric measurement of gases consumed or liberated by small quantities of tissues contained within vessels immersed in temperature controlled baths. It is used mostly for O_2 consumption and CO_2 production rates.

warfarin: 4-hydroxy-3-(3-oxo-1-phenylbutyl)-2*H*-benzyopyran-2-one; *see* **coumadin**.

warm antibodies: antibodies that react more strongly at 37°C than at lower temperatures. Most are IgG type immunoglobulins. *Cf* **cold agglutinins**.

wart: a benign keratotic tumor, usually caused by a *Papillomavirus*.

Wassermann test: a serological test for syphilis based on complement fixation that involves reactions between a cardiolipin and test sera components. It is not specific for *Treponema pallidum*. False-positive reactions can occur in individuals immunized against some other microorganisms.

wasting disease: cachexia; chronic conditions characterized by growth arrest, weight loss, and morbidity that often lead to early death. *See* also **runt disease** and **thymectomy**.

water deprivation test: a procedure sometimes used when vasopressin deficiency is suspected, to test the ability to produce hyperosmotic urine. *Cf* **water tolerance tests**.

water intoxication: conditions in which electrolyte imbalance is caused by retention of relatively more water than sodium chloride. Although urine volume can be adjusted to a wide range of fluid intakes, there is a limit to the extent to which urine can be diluted. Severe psychogenic drinking or ingestion of very large quantities of beer but little food can slowly "wash out" electrolytes. Other causes include secretion of more vasopressin than is appropriate for the extracellular fluid salt content, continued polydipsia in an individual undergoing treatment for diabetes insipidus, overuse of some kinds of diuretics, circulatory system defects, protein deficiency (or loss) that leads to development of edema,

O=S—N(H)—(CH₂)₄—NH₂ ·HCl

W-12

Cl
O=S—N(H)—(CH₂)₄—NH₂ ·HCl

W-13

aldosterone deficiency, glucocorticoid deficiency, and some kinds of renal defects. Hyponatremia usually provides a stimulus for secretion of aldosterone (which promotes sodium retention), but the effects can be over-ridden by hypervolemia. Cells take up excessive amounts of water when blood and extracellular fluid electrolyte levels fall below the normal range. The effects on brain neurons invoke headaches, lethargy, and somnolence and in severe cases convulsion and coma and ultimately death. Prolonged, severe hyponatremia can also cause hemolysis.

water tolerance tests: procedures in which the time required to excrete an administered water load is measured. They were once used to test for adrenocortical insufficiency (in which the time is prolonged) but have been superseded by more dependable, less dangerous methods; *see* also **water intoxication**.

Watson-Crick model: the model for the most common (B) form of DNA, in which two antiparallel deoxyribonucleic acid chains with hydrogen bonds between complementary bases form a right-handed double helix. *Cf* **Z DNA**.

watt: W; a unit of electrical power, equivalent to one volt-ampere.

wavelengths: for phenomena with periodic peaks and troughs, the distances between points at the same phases of consecutive cycles. Absorption spectra for radiation in the visible, ultraviolet, or infrared range are used in chemical analyses; *see* also **light**. Measurements are also made for sound and other forms of stimuli that affect cells.

waxes: cholesterol, cerumen, sebum components, and other hydrophobic substances that are solid or semisolid at room temperature. Many are long-chain alcohol esters of long-chain fatty acids. Commonly used types include paraffin, beeswax (composed mostly of cerotic acid and myricin), and synthetic resin mixtures used in dentistry.

WBC: white blood cells.

W chromosome: the sex chromosome in female birds and some other female submammalian vertebrates that carries genes for sex determination and codes for H-Y antigen and some other proteins. In those species the normal female is the heterozygous sex (has one W and one Z chromosome) whereas the male has two Z types; and animals that lack W genes develop as males. (In contrast, female mammals are XX and males XY. The "default" condition is then female, expressed in individuals that lack Y chromosomes.)

WDHA syndrome: Verner Morrison syndrome: watery diarrhea, achlorhydria, and hypokalemia.

weak molecular interactions: easily formed, easily disrupted associations that are neither electrovalent nor covalent; *see* **hydrogen bonds** and **Van der Waals forces**.

weal: wheal.

Wellbutrin: a trade name for bupropion.

Wermer's syndrome: multiple endocrine neoplasia, type I; MEN-1; disorders characterized by hyperparathyroidism often in combination with pancreatic islet and/or pituitary gland tumors that may or may not secrete excessive quantities of hormones. Associated manifestations can include carcinoid tumors, adrenocortical hyperplasia, and thyroid gland dysfunction.

Werner's syndrome: an inherited disease in which premature aging is associated with short stature and often also with vascular disease, testicular atrophy and diabetes mellitus. It is usually fatal before the age of 50. Fibroblasts have blunted sensitivities to fibroblast and platelet derived growth factors (FGFs and PDGF) and prematurely lose the ability to divide.

western blotting: techniques for transferring proteins separated on agarose gels by electrophoresis to nitrocellulose filter paper or other supports; *cf* **Southern** and **northern blotting**.

wether: a gonadectomized lamb.

WGA: wheat-germ agglutinin.

W gene: *wg*; *D-wnt-1*; the *wingless* gene (*q.v.*) of *Drosophila*; *see* **wnt genes**.

Wharton's ducts: tubules that transport saliva from submandibular glands to mouth cavities.

Wharton's jelly: the hyaluronic acid-rich glycosaminoglycan of umbilical cords.

wheal: localized edematous swelling of the skin; *see* **wheal and flare response**.

wheal and flare response: triple skin response; localized erythema, heat, and wheal formation, a component of allergic reactions mediated mostly by histamine release.

wheat-germ agglutinin: WGA; a plant lectin obtained from *Triticum vulgaris* that binds *N*-acetylglucosaminyl and neuraminic acid moieties of di- and oligosaccharides. It is used to study glycoprotein structures and some immune system functions, and in affinity chromatography.

whelp: an unweaned puppy.

whey: the lipid-free fluid that separates from coagulated milk. It contains lactose and many proteins, including immunoglobulins and some albumin, but no casein. β-lactalbumin is the major type in cow's milk; but that protein is not present in the fluid of humans and most other mammals.

white blood cells: leukocytes. Healthy human adults have 5-10,000 per cubic millimeter of circulating blood, approximately 52-64% of which are neutrophils (polymorphonuclear leukocytes). The two other granular types are eosinophils (1-3%) and basophils (1%). The "nongranular" white cells are lymphocytes (25-33%) and monocytes (3-9). *See* also specific types.

white matter: nervous system components composed mostly of myelinated nerve fibers; *cf* **gray matter**.

white muscle: fast-twitch type skeletal muscle. It is rich in glycogen and mitochondria (but not myoglobin), and fatigues more rapidly than **red muscle** (*q.v.*).

white rami: myelinated preganglionic nerve fiber bundles that connect the spinal cord with the paravertebral sympathetic ganglia.

white spotting locus: *see* **W locus**.

Whitten effect: induction of regular ovarian cycles in female mice and some other rodents whose cycles have become lengthened, irregular, or arrested following confinement in group cages in the absence of males, by introduction of an adult male of the species (or of a pheromone in adult male urine).

WHO: world health organization.

wild type: naturally occurring; not mutated. The term usually describes an allele type regarded as normal for the species; *cf* **feral**.

S(-)-5-fluoro-**willardine**: *S*(-)-α-amino-5-fluoro-3,4-dihydro-2,4-dioxo-1(2*H*)-pyrimidinepropanoic acid; an AMP/kainate type excitatory amino acid agonist.

Willis, circle of: a circular blood vessel arrangement in the brain, formed by cerebral artery branches of the left and right internal carotid arteries and the anterior and posterior communicating arteries.

Wilms tumors: nephromas; nephroblastomas; malignant kidney tumors that develop early in life, contain embryonic-type cells, and usually cause death during early childhood. They are attributed to deletion of both alleles on the short arms of human chromosome 11 that code for tumor suppressor WT-1, a zinc finger protein that binds to GCGGGGGCG DNA base sequences, negatively regulates blastema proliferation in the kidneys, protects against overexpression of insulin-like growth factor-II (IGF-II), and facilitates cell differentiation.

Wilson' disease: an autosomal recessive disorder in which copper excretion to the bile and incorporation into ceruloplasmin are impaired, and the liver and brain are damaged by copper accumulation.

WIN 22,005: urokinase.

WIN 62,577: 17β-hydroxy-17α-ethynyl-Δ⁴-androstanol-[3,2-*b*]pyrimido[1,2-*a*]benzimidaole; an NK-1 type tachykinin receptor antagonist.

wingless: *Dwnt-1*; *D-int-1*;a *Drosophila* segment polarity gene essential for normal embryonic development. It codes for a 468-amino acid protein, the fruit fly homolog of the mammalian *wnt-1* gene product (with 370 amino acids). *See* also *wnt* **genes**.

Wiskott-Aldrich syndrome: a condition characterized by the presence of small, irregularly shaped platelets,

WIN 62,577

increased susceptibility to infections, and the tendency to develop eczema. It is caused by a defect in the gene that codes for an ultraviolet ray induced endonuclease required for repair of damaged DNA. At least some cases involve cellular immunity defects that include CD43 deficiency.

witch's milk: a milk-like fluid released by the mammary glands of neonates. During fetal life the glands transiently mature in response to the high levels of estrogens, progesterone, prolactin and other pregnancy-associated hormones, and become responsive to the oxytocin secreted shortly before and during parturition. The glands regress soon after birth.

W locus: white spotting locus; a DNA segment identified in mice as the *kit* proto-oncogene that codes for a protein with tyrosine kinase activity and functions as the Steel factor receptor; *see* **stem cell factor**. It is required for normal development of embryonic precursors of melanocytes, hematopoietic cells, and germ cells. Factors that impair production of stem cell factor invoke defects that closely resemble those of W locus mutations.

wnt **genes**: *wingless* genes; at least eleven genes essential for normal *Drosophila* development, and their related mammalian counterparts. When it was recognized that *int-1*, *int-2*, and *int-3* (*q.v.*) code for very different proteins, and are related only by their ability to integrate into mouse mammary tumor viruses, and that *int-1* is the mammalian homolog of the *Drosophila wingless* gene, it was suggested that the genes be renamed. The terms *Dwnt-1*, *Xwnt-1*, and *WNT-1* now apply, respectively to homologous genes in *Drosophila*, *Xenopus* and humans. *Wnt-2* is the proposed new name for a mouse gene formerly known as *irp*. *WNT-2* is its human counterpart. The members of the *wnt* gene family (which includes *Wnt* genes 3, 3A, r, 5A, 5B, 6, 7A, and 7B) are not tightly linked.

wobble hypothesis: the concept that movements of the third nitrogenous base of a messenger RNA codon permit pairing with more than kind of transfer RNA anticodon.

Wolffian body: mesonephros.

Wolffian ducts: mesonephric ducts; bilateral embryonic and fetal organs of male vertebrates that undergo androgen-dependent development in males and give rise to male-type accessory reproductive organs (including epididymides, vasa deferentia, and seminal vesicles). The structures degenerate in normal female embryos because their gonads do not release sufficient androgen to promote the development.

Wolff-Chaikoff effect: decreased iodine incorporation into thyroglobulin caused by excess iodine in thyroid glands. It has been attributed to the formation of complexes composed of iodide and oxidative products of iodine metabolism. High levels of triiodothyronine (T_3) can directly inhibit iodide uptake and concentration.

Wolman disease: an inherited disorder in which synthesis of lysosomal lipase is impaired.

working hypothesis: a concept based on tentative interpretations of limited amounts of information that is used to design experiments. If consistently supported by data, it can advance to a **theory** (*q.v.*).

worm factor: plerocercoid factor.

wound healing: repair of injured tissue that involves cell migration and proliferation and usually also angiogenesis. Fibroblast and transforming growth factors (FGFs and TGFs) and histamine are among the agents that stimulate. Glucocorticoids and some others inhibit. According to some observers, chalone production is suppressed.

WR 2721: 2,2-(3-aminopropylamino)-ethylphosphorothionic acid; an agent used to inhibit parathyroid hormone secretion.

Wright stain: a mixture of eosin and methylene blue in methanol used to stain blood smears for differential counts.

W substance: Hogben substance of whitening; a component of pituitary gland extracts that promotes melanin concentration in some cell types. It differs from melatonin but may be related to melanin concentrating hormone.

wt: weight.

Wulzen, cone of: an epithelial cell mass derived from Rathke's pouch in the pituitary glands of sheep and some other mammals.

w/v: weight per unit volume.

w/w: weight per unit weight.

WZ: the sex chromosome pattern for female birds and some other female submammalian vertebrates. Males of those species have two Z sex chromosomes.

X: (1) a symbol for an unknown entity such as an as yet unidentified amino acid or other component of a compound; (2) a symbol for an independent variable; *see* also **x** and **X axis**; (3) *see* **X chromosome**.

x: (1) a symbol for the value of an independent variable. When the upper case X is used for such variables, x = X−$\overline{X}$; (2) in genetics, crossed with as in A ♂ x B ♀ .

$\overline{X}$ or $\bar{x}$: the arithmetic mean for the independent variable of a study or population; *cf* $\overline{y}$.

X.: *Xenopus*.

X-: a prefix used for *Xenopus levis* genes, as in *X-wnt-1*.

Xanax: a trade name for alprazolam.

xanth-, **xantho-**: prefixes for yellow, as in xanthine and xanthophore.

xanthine: (1) 3,7-dihydro-1-*H*-purine-2,6-dione (shown below); a metabolite formed by oxidizing hypoxanthine or hydrolyzing guanine, that can be converted to uric acid; (2) any purine chemically related to xanthine; *see*, for example **caffeine**, **theophylline**, **theobromine** and **methylisobutylxanthine**.

xanthine oxidase: an iron and molybdenum containing enzyme that converts hypoxanthine and xanthines to uric acid.

xanthinuria: a rare autosomal recessive disorder in which xanthine oxidase deficiency leads to excretion of large quantities of xanthine and formation of xanthine calculi.

xanthocyte: a cell that makes substantial quantities of xanthine.

xanthomatosis: an inherited metabolic defect that leads to the formation of lipid nodules, usually in subcutaneous fat, skin, and tendons.

xanthophores: carotene-containing chromatophores that impart yellowish coloration.

xanthopsin: all-*trans* retinal.

xanthophyll: vegetable lutein; β-ε-carotene-3,3′-diol; a yellow pigment devoid of vitamin A potency, most abundant in plant leaves but also present in egg yolk and blood plasma.

xanthopterin: 2-amino-4,6-pteridinedione; a butterfly wing pigment that arrests the growth of some animal tumors. Yeasts convert it to folic acid.

xanthurenic acid: 4,8-dihydroxyquinaldic acid; a tryptophan metabolite excreted to urine. Large amounts are made by pyridoxine-deficient animals.

X:A ratio: the ratio of X sex chromosomes to autosomes. In *Drosophila*, in which the Y chromosome does not determine male morphology or mating behavior but is required for spermatogenesis, the value is 0.5 for normal males and 1.0 for normal females. The X chromosome does not directly affect testicular development. When the ratio is 1.0, *sis-a* and *sis-b* (sisterless a and b) genes act in conjunction with a maternally derived *da* (daughterless) gene to initiate female type splicing of *Sxl* (sex lethal) gene transcripts by acting on an early promoter. A protein product then directs other female-specific kinds of transcript processing by acting on a late promoter, and cascades which lead to female type development are initiated. The male *Sxl* gene is transcribed, but the RNA has a translation terminating exon that blocks formation of the proteins. The sex difference has been linked with the presence of a single *sis* gene in males.

xanthophyll

X axis: abscissa; the horizontal line along which values for an independent variable are plotted; *cf* **Y axis**.

X cells: (1) pituitary gland cells of bony fishes believed to secrete adrenocorticotropic hormone; (2) vertebrate pancreatic and gastrointestinal tract F cells that secrete pancreatic polypeptide.

X chromosome: (1) a sex chromosome of mammals, many other vertebrates, and some invertebrates (but *cf* **W chromosome**). Normal females of species in which Y chromosomes initiate male type sex differentiation have two Xs, and in most both are needed for normal development and fertility. (Mice and some other mammals with a single X chromosome but no Y can be produce oocytes.) Normal males have one X and one Y chromosome. In mammals, the X chromosome is much larger than the Y, and it codes for many proteins essential for survival, only some of which affect reproduction. The human type accounts for more than 5% of the total DNA, and carries several thousand genes (*see* also **Turner's syndrome, X chromosome inactivation**, and **X-linked inheritance**). Some fishes and other nonmammalian vertebrates with XX/XY patterns can survive without an X chromosome because their Y chromosomes are large and carry the essential genes. Sex determining patterns are different for many invertebrates that have X and Y genes; *see* **X:A ratio**.

X chromosome inactivation; in female mammals with XX sex chromosome patterns, a substantial portion of one X chromosome is transcriptionally inactive during most of the life-span; *see* also **Barr body**. The inactivation is attributed to DNA hypomethylation. For many cell types there appears to be random selection of the one affected, but once established all progeny of that cell inactivate the same chromosome. In most species both X chromosomes function during gametogenesis and the earliest developmental stages; but *see* **X chromosome** and **XO**, and *see* also **Turner's syndrome**.

xeno-: a prefix meaning foreign, as in xenograft.

xenobiotic: not occurring in nature, a term usually applied to chemical compounds, especially ones that are not biodegradable.

xenogeneic: xenogenic; heterologous.

xenogenic: heterologous; having foreign genetic elements.

xenografts: grafts (*q.v.*) that are genetically foreign to the host. They usually derive from different species.

xenoparasites: parasites that can thrive in hosts with weakened resistance, but not in healthy members of the same species.

xenopsin: p-Glu-Gly-Lys-Arg-Pro-Trp-Ile-Leu-OH: an amphibian peptide biologically related to neurotensin.

Xenopus levis: the South African clawed toad. The male is used in "frog" tests for pregnancy. Xenopus oocytes are used to study cell cycle control, fertilization, embryonic development, and RNA metabolism. They support replication and transcription of many kinds of foreign genes inserted with appropriate promotors.

Xenopus spasmolysin: a frog skin polypeptide; *see* **trefoil proteins**.

xenorexia: pica; craving for and/or ingestion of substances not usually eaten by the species.

xenotope: an antigenic determinant on a molecule foreign to the organism, usually on the surface of a cell of another species.

xenotropic: describes viruses that can integrate into host genomes of one species, but usually infect those of another.

xero-: a prefix meaning dry, as in xerophthalmia.

xeroderma pigmentosa: several rare autosomal recessive disorders in which the skin is easily damaged by ultraviolet light. The consequences include atrophy, pigmentation changes, and high risk for development of skin cancers. *See* also **ERCC genes**.

xerophthalmia: desiccation of the conjunctiva and cornea that can lead to lead to blindness. The causes include severe vitamin A deficiency and autoimmune diseases.

xiphoid: sword-shaped.

Xiphophorus: a genus of small freshwater fishes that includes *X. maculatus* (the platyfish), and *X. helleri* (the swordtail). The animals are used for studies of genetics, development, behavior, endocrine system functions, pigmentation, and tumorigenesis, because of their small sizes, short life-spans, bright colors, obvious sexual dimorphisms, genetic patterns, the ease with which sexual differentiation can be manipulated, and other features. Tu^+R^+ wild type swordtails carry both Tu (tumor producing) and R genes (ones that code for the melanoma receptor kinase, Xmrk). When mated with Tu^-R^- homozygotes, nonhomologous recombinations lead to production of some Tu^+R^- progeny that develop melanomas.

Xiphosura: an arthropod order that includes horseshoe crabs.

X-linked: occurring on or transmitted via an X-chromosome; *see* **sex-linked inheritance**.

X-linked inheritance: *see* **sex-linked inheritance**.

Xmrk: a receptor protein kinase made by swordtail fishes; see **Xiphophorus**.

XO: the chromosome pattern in individuals of species in which normal females have two X chromosomes and males have one X and one Y. The second X is usually lost by nondisjunction during gametogenesis. In humans the XO/45 pattern, in which the autosome number is normal, is the most common aberration that causes **Turner's syndrome** (*q.v.*). Although the defect increases the incidence of prenatal mortality, many XO humans survive and most develop into phenotypic females that are sterile, suffer varying degrees of mental retardation, and have numerous somatic defects. In some other mammals X chromosomes carrier fewer essential genes; and XO mice are among the types that appear morphologically normal and can produce viable progeny.

X organ: a structure in the eyestalk complex of some crustaceans that communicates with the sinus gland and serves as the source of molt inhibiting hormone. The medulla terminalis and medulla externa ganglionic X-organs, and the sensory pore X-organ (which has a sensory papilla) are neural derivatives. The neurohemal sinus gland stores and releases the hormone. *See* also **Y organ**.

X pacemaker: one of the biological clocks in the brain, implicated as a major regulator of glucocorticoid, core body temperature, and potassium metabolism circadian rhythms, and of rapid eye movement sleep; *cf* **Y pacemaker**.

X-rays: Roentgen rays; electromagnetic radiation produced when high velocity electrons from a hot cathode bombard an anode. Deflection patterns transmitted to photographic plates or fluorescent screens are related to the sizes and distributions of certain atom types within the specimens. They are used in dentistry and medicine (*see* also **computer axial tomography**), and to provide information on crystalline and molecular structures. X-rays easily penetrate soft tissues and can cause mutations. Since rapidly dividing cells are especially susceptible to injury, damaging doses are used clinically to destroy malignant types. X-rays can also inactivate antigens on tissues that will be grafted; and irradiation can safely protect many foods against spoilage with little or no change in nutritive value. Laboratory uses include destruction of thymus glands and bone marrow cells to study hematopoietic and immune system functions, and of germinal cells for studies of reproduction.

XX: the normal sex chromosome pattern for females of mammalian and some other vertebrate groups in which normal males have one X and one Y chromosome. *See* **X chromosomes**.

XXX: the most common abnormal sex chromosome pattern of mammalian "**superfemales**" *(q.v.)*. (Others include XXXX). The condition in humans is often associated with mild mental retardation and other defects.

XXXY, XXXYY, XXYY: examples of abnormal sex chromosome patterns identified in humans. The extra chromosomes can derive from primary and/or secondary oocytes (*see* **nondisjunction**), from polar bodies that adhere to oocytes, or from sperm that penetrate already fertilized oocytes. All of the patterns are associated with defects the most common of which is mental retardation. If the **Y chromosome** *(q.v.)* is complete, affected individuals have male phenotypes but can be sterile.

XXY: the abnormal sex chromosome pattern most commonly associated with **Klinefelter's disease** *(q.v.)*. The extra X chromosome derives from the fertilizing sperm.

xylan: a plant polysaccharide composed of xylose moieties.

xylitol: *xylo*-pentane-1,2,3,4,5-pentol; a sugar alcohol isocaloric with glucose, with the sweetening potency of fructose. It is used in noncariogenic chewing gums and candies. A dehydrogenase catalyzes its oxidation to xylulose, and a kinase promotes formation of xylulose-5-phosphate which enters the hexose monophosphate (pentose) pathway.

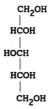

xylo-: a prefix meaning wood.

xylose: α-xylose; wood sugar; the 3-epimer of ribose. It is the major component of xylan and of some plant glycosides. The α-D form is shown.

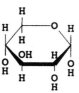

xylulose: threo-pentulose; a kinase catalyzes phosphorylation of the D form to xylulose-5-phosphate, an intermediate in the hexose monophosphate pathway. The L form (shown below) can be converted to the D via the intermediate, xylitol.

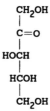

XYY: an abnormal sex chromosome pattern that occurs in human males. The most common manifestations include tall stature and mild mental retardation. The ability of some affected individuals to enjoy totally normal function is attributed to transcriptional inactivation of the extra X chromosome. Although XYY fishes are more aggressive than their normal XY counterparts, the concept that the pattern predisposes to aberrant behavior in men has not been supported.

X zone: a large component of the fetal adrenal cortex in which dehydroepiandrosterone-sulfate and related steroid hormones are synthesized. It rapidly undergoes atrophy shortly after birth in most mammals, but may provide precursor cells for the mature zona fasciculata. A related region persists in guinea pigs.

Y

Y: (1) tyrosine; (2) yttrium. *See* also **y**, **Y axis** and **Y chromosome**.

y: a symbol for a dependent variable. If the upper case Y is used, y = Y - $\overline{Y}$; *see* also **Y axis**.

$\overline{y}$ or **$\overline{Y}$**: the mean value for a set of dependent variables.

Y-1 cells: a cell line derived from an adrenocortical tumor, used to study steroidogenesis.

Y axis: ordinate; the vertical line along which values of dependent variables are plotted; *cf* **X axis**.

Yb: ytterbium.

Y chromosomes: in most mammals and in some other vertebrates, males have one Y and one X sex chromosome (and females have two X types). The Y chromosome is usually much smaller than the X but carries pseudoautosomal regions that pair with X segments during meiosis and mitosis, and genes essential for testis differentiation and spermatogenesis; *see* **testis determining antigen** and **H-Y antigen**, and *see* also **XYY**. In fishes and some other nonmammalian vertebrates Y chromosomes are comparatively large and carry genes that support survival of animals that lack X types. Y chromosomes do not determine testis development in *Drosophila* and many other invertebrates, but are needed for spermatogenesis; *see* **X:A ratio**.

yeasts: an imprecise term for many kinds of saprophytic, carbohydrate fermenting fungi, but most commonly used for sac fungi (members of the class Ascomycetes) which are also called "true" yeasts. *Saccharomyces cerevisiae*, a budding type, is the organism in Baker's yeast that generates carbon dioxide to raise dough and the one in Brewer's yeast that makes ethyl alcohol. Brewer's yeast is also a major commercial source of B complex vitamins, and of glycolytic enzymes. Its metabolism, G protein functions, reproductive patterns, and mechanisms for controlling cell cycles differ from those of *Schizosaccharomyces pombe* (fission yeast). Both types are widely used for genetics, cell cycle, pheromone, oncogene, signal transduction, intermediary metabolism, and other biological studies. Deuteromycetes have been called false or imperfect yeasts because of their reproduction patterns. The class includes *Candida albicans*, *C.tropicalis*, *Torulopsis glabrata* and other species that cause diseases in humans.

yellow body: corpus luteum. The term is appropriate for women and many other vertebrates, but the structures are not yellow in all species.

yes: a Y73 sarcoma retrovirus oncogene that directs formation of p90$^{gag-yes}$, the precursor of a 62K member of the *src* tyrosine kinase family.

Y hormone: *see* **ecdysone**.

yin-yang hypothesis: the concept that optimum levels of some functions are maintained by reciprocal changes in the levels of two regulators that exert opposing effects. The idea that cAMP and cGMP act in this way is no longer accepted.

YISGR: Tyr-Iso-Glu-Ser-Arg-; a component of laminins and some other proteins that participates directly in cell adhesion.

α-yohimbine: rauwolscine; coryanthidine; 17α-hydroxyyohimban-16-carboxylic acid; an alkaloid from the barks of *Coryanthe johimbe*, *Rauwolfia canescens* and related species used as an α$_2$-type adrenergic receptor antagonist that affects the release of growth hormone and other regulators. According to folklore, it is an aphrodisiac.

yolk: the lipid-rich nutrients stored in an oocyte or ovum that support embryonic (and in some cases fetal) development, or the structure that contains those substances.

yolk sac: the *primitive* yolk sac is the exocelomic remnant of the blastocoele cavity, visible during the second week post-conception in humans after the embryo has formed ectoderm and endoderm. It is very small and short-lived in mammals, but contains nutrients important for early development of some other vertebrates. By the end of the second week, human and most other mammalian embryos acquire a smaller endoderm-lined *secondary* yolk sac which is the source of hemopoietic stem cells and gonocytes. Portions of it contribute to formation of the embryonic digestive tube. Most of the other cells become nonfunctioning placenta components.

Y organ: the crustacean homolog of the insect prothoracic gland, located in the antennae or in maxillary segments. It produces molting hormone which is essential for proecdysis. The activity is inhibited by a regulator released from the sinus gland; *see* **X organ**.

"Y" pacemaker: a biological clock in the brain implicated as the major regulator of growth hormone, skin temperature, and calcium metabolism circadian rhythms, and of slow wave sleep. *Cf* **"X" pacemaker**.

Y protein: a heat shock protein in estrogen-responsive cells that binds to estrogen receptors.

ytterbium: Yb; a rare earth metallic element (atomic number 60, atomic weight 173.04).

yttrium, **Y**: a rare earth metallic element (atomic number 39, atomic weight 88.96).

YY: *see* **peptide YY**.

Z

Z: a symbol for (1) an amino acid component of a protein if it is not known whether the position is occupied by glutamic acid or glutamine, or when either can occur at that locus; (2) atomic number; (3) ionic charge number; (4) impedance.

Zadine: a trade name for azatadine.

Zantac: a trade name for ranitidine.

Z chromosomes: sex chromosomes of birds and of some other nonmammalian vertebrates. Normal males have two (are ZZ), whereas normal females have one plus a W chromosome (are WZ). They direct formation of several kinds of proteins some of which are essential for survival, but do not perform functions comparable to those of mammalian Y types.

Z-disc: the region of a skeletal muscle sarcomere that contains α-actinin, into which thin filaments insert. It appears in electron micrographs as a fine (Z) line that bisects thin filaments.

Z-DNA: a left-handed helix form of DNA with a single groove, assumed when purine and pyrimidine nucleotides, especially $(CG)_n$ sequences alternate. It reverts easily to B-DNA, but is stable when the cytidine bases are methylated.

Zea Mays: maize; Indian corn; many varieties of a monocotyledonous plant, including *saccharata* (sweet, the fruit of which is consumed by humans), *amylacea* (flour), *indentata* (field), and *everta* (popcorn). Most commercial types are hybrids selected for vigor and uniformity. The photosynthesis reactions differ from those of most other plants. Because of transposable elements and inherited pigment patterns, they are used for genetics studies. *See also* **zein** and **zeism**.

zearalenone: 3,4,5,6,9,10-hexahydro-14,16-dihydroxy-3-methyl-1*H*-2-benzoxacyclotetradecin-1,7(8*H*)-dione; an estrogenic resorcyclic lactone obtained from the *Gibberella zeae* fungus. It is used to promote growth in domesticated animals.

zeatin: *trans*-6-(4-hydroxy-3-methylbutyl-2-enyl)-aminopurine; the most potent cytokinin known, named for its initial identification in corn kernels. It promotes linear

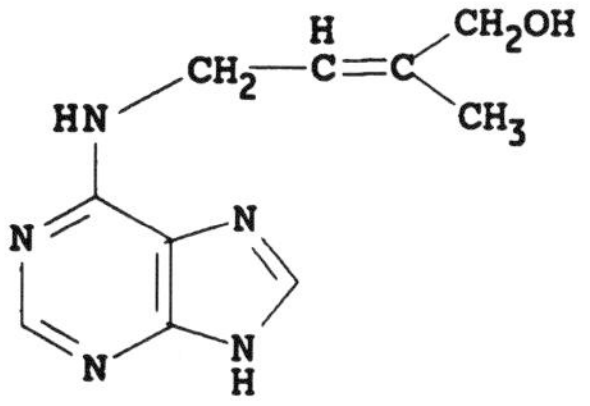

zearalenone

growth but acts in conjunction with auxins to inhibit mitosis in lateral shoots.

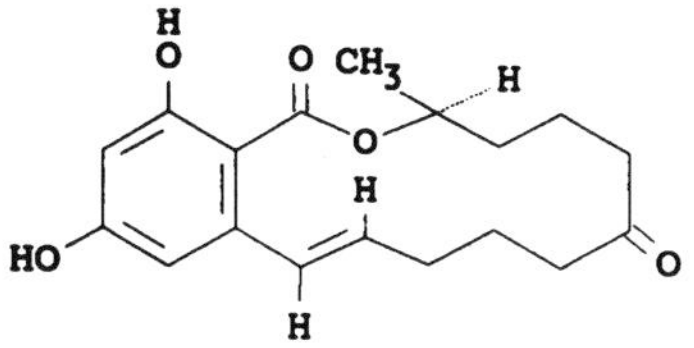

zeaxanthin: β,β-carotene-3,3'-diol; the major pigment of yellow corn and a component of many other plant pigments.

zein: the major proteins of the edible portions of corn plants. They are mostly 38K prolamines, classified as "incomplete" nutrients because they do not contain lysine or tryptophan. *See* **zeism**.

zeism: pellagra and other nutritional disorders that develop in humans whose major source of protein is zein.

Zeitgeber: a photoperiod or other factor that synchronizes (but does not generate) one or more biological rhythms.

Zellweger syndrome: a lethal autosomal recessive disease attributed to mutations in the gene that directs formation of peroxisome assembly factor-1 (PAF-1). The consequences include inability to assemble catalase-containing peroxisomes, impaired synthesis of plasmalogens, and inadequate β-oxidation of very long chain fatty acids. The major manifestations are severe neurological abnormalities, dysmorphic features, hepatomegaly, and renal cysts.

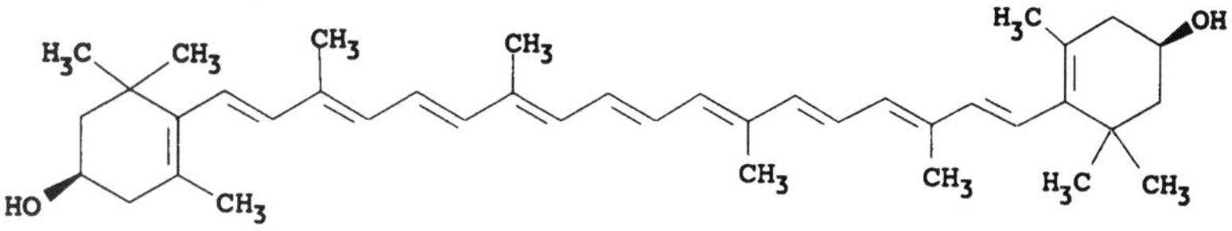

zeaxanthin

zeolites: mixtures of crystalline hydrated alkali aluminum silicates, used as molecular sieves, adsorbents, drying agents, dispersing agents, and cation exchangers.

zeranol: 3,4,5,6,7,8,9,10,11,12-decahydro-7,14-16-trihydroxy-3-methyl-1*H*-2-benzoxacyclotetradecin-1-one; a compound prepared from zearalenone used to stimulate growth in cattle.

zero order reactions: chemical reactions whose velocities are not affected by addition of more substrate; *cf* **first order reactions**.

Zestril: a trade name for lisinopril.

zeta: ζ; the sixth letter of the Greek alphabet. *See* **zeta potential**.

zeta cell: an adenohypophysial cell type identified under light microscopy. The term usually refers to melanotropes but has been applied to corticotropes with small secretory granules, chromophobes, and "neutrophils".

zeta potential: the electrokinetic potential that develops between a thin layer of fluid that adheres to a membrane or macromolecule surface and the surrounding fluid. It affects erythrocyte sedimentation rates, electrophoretic mobilities, and agglutination, and can be calculated from measurements of the velocities of particles moving in electrical fields.

ZFX: a human X chromosome gene that codes for a zinc finger protein similar to the product of the **ZFY** gene on the Y chromosomes (*q.v.*). Unlike most other X chromosome genes, it does not undergo inactivation. *Zfx* is a related mouse gene.

ZFY: a gene located in the vicinity of the sex determining region of the human Y chromosome that codes for a zinc-finger protein similar to the *ZFX* product. The concept that it is directly involved in sex determination has been discarded. Mice make two biologically related proteins, Zfy-1 and Zfy-2; *see also* ***sxr***.

zidovudine: 3′-azido-2′-deoxythymidine; azidothymidine; AZT; Retrovir; a thymidine analog used to prolong survival and suppress opportunistic infections in individuals with acquired immunodeficiency disease (AIDS). It inhibits reverse transcriptases and terminates viral peptide chain synthesis. Since it also directly inhibits erythropoiesis and myelopoiesis, it can invoke anemia and leukopenia. Additional undesirable side-effects can include nausea, malaise, headache, and insomnia.

ZIFT: zygote intrafallopian tube transfer; a technique used for couples with fertility problems, in which oocytes freshly fertilized *in vitro* are inserted into the Fallopian tubes; *see also* **GIFT**.

zidovudine

zimeldine: 3-(4-bromophenyl)-*N*-*N*-dimethyl-3-(3-pyridinyl)-2-propen-1-amine; an anti-depressant that inhibits neuronal uptake of serotonin.

zinc, Zn: an element (atomic number 30, atomic weight 65.38) required in trace amounts. It is a component of thymulin, gustin, zinc-finger proteins and other biologically important molecules, and a cofactor for or component of carboxypeptidase A, carbonic anhydrase, DNA polymerases, RNA polymerases, some aldolases, endoplasmic reticulum proteases that cleave signal sequences, and some other enzymes. It scavenges free radicals, induces metallothioneins, and synergizes with taurine to protect retinas against potential damage by excess retinol. Zinc also complexes with proinsulin and insulin in pancreatic islets (and is a component of insulin preparations). In the adenohypophysis, it complexes with growth hormone, promotes dimer formation, and may in that way contribute to hormone storage and to protection of nearby receptors against excessive stimulation. Its ability to enhance insulin-like growth factor induction probably accounts for some of its inhibitory influences on growth hormone secretion. Additionally, it contributes to hPL (human prolactin, somatomammotropin) binding to its receptors and seems to be essential for achieving functional configurations of receptors for androgens, 1,25-dihydroxyvitamin D and other hormones. In the cerebral cortex, it binds to NMDA (*N*-methyl-D-asparate) receptors and antagonizes some effects of glutamate and aspartate; and it modulates the actions of GABA (gamma aminobutyric acid) and glycine. Rodent mothers deprived of zinc during pregnancy deliver fetuses with several kinds of severe deformities. In humans, postnatal deficiency can cause skin ulcers, depress appetite, affect hair growth, and impair immune system functions. The carbonate is used as a nutritional supplement. Zinc oxide is a component of topical ointments, lotions, and powders used to protect skin and promote healing in individuals with acne, eczema, and surface wounds, and as a styptic, astringent, and deodorant. In veterinary medicine, the oxide is employed as an antiseptic and emetic, and the chloride to promote healing of ulcers. The undecate kills lice and the undecylate is an anti-fungicide. Several salts are used for industrial purposes, as chemical reagents, and as components of cosmetics, toothpastes, and mouthwashes. [65]Zn emits positrons and γ rays and has a half-life of 9.2 hours.

zinc fingers: components of many proteins, composed of two pairs of cysteinyl (or one pair of cysteinyl and one pair of histidinyl) moieties that chelate zinc. The group includes receptors for steroid hormones, calciferols, triiodothyronine, and retinoic acid. Ligand-occupied receptors form DNA-binding dimers that regulate gene transcription. In the diagram, broken lines represent chains of specific kinds of amino acids, Xs indicate the positions of chelating cysteine moieties, and Ys show positions that can be occupied by either cysteinyl or histidinyl residues. The following effects are observed with "finger-swap" studies, in which hybrid molecules are constructed by removing the ligand binding domain from the receptor component that contains the zinc-finger, and then linking a ligand-binding domain for a different kind of receptor:

native receptor for ligand A + ligand A → A type effects

native receptor for ligand B + ligand B → B type effects

receptor with B finger and A-binding site + ligand A → B type effects

Some zinc finger protein heterodimers without ligands compete with occupied receptors for DNA binding.

zirconium: Zr; a corrosion-resistant metallic element (atomic number 40, atomic weight 91.22).

ZK 98734: an agent similar to RU-486, currently under investigation for use as a progesterone receptor antagonist.

Z-line: *see* **Z disk**.

Zn: zinc.

Zollinger-Ellison syndrome: a condition in which excessive gastrin secretion leads to production of large quantities of hydrochloric acid and invokes peptic ulcer formation. The usual cause is a non-islet cell pancreatic tumor (gastrinoma), often associated with an islet cell tumor that does not release excessive quantities of insulin.

zona (**zonae**): an encircling region, zone or belt.

zona fasciculata: the region of the mammalian adrenal cortex between the **zona glomerulosa** (*q.v.*) and the zona reticularis, named for the cord-like (fascicular) cell arrangement in many species. It is usually the largest component of the mature adrenal cortex and the major site for glucocorticoid production. Adrenocorticotropic hormone (ACTH) maintains the size, structure and functions by stimulating cell growth and differentiation, enzyme synthesis, and hormone production, and by indirectly augmenting blood flow to the region. Although it can directly inhibit mitosis, ACTH may facilitate proliferative responses to fibroblast and other growth factors.

zona glomerulosa: the region of the mammalian adrenal cortex between the capsule and the zona fasciculata, in which aldosterone is synthesized. The cells of many species are arranged in whorls (glomeruli). Angiotensin II is the major stimulant for hormone production. Adrenocorticotropic hormone (ACTH) can acutely augment aldosterone synthesis (at least in part by acting on the zona fasciculata to increase the supply of precursors); but the long-range effects are mostly inhibitory. The effects of **adrenal demedullation** (*q.v.*) and *in vitro* studies which indicate that ACTH modulates glomerulosa cells to fasciculata types that lack the enzymes required for aldosterone production are consistent with the concept that new adrenocortical cells originate in this zone.

zona incerta: a thin band of gray matter and fine nerve fibers dorsal and medial to the subthalamic nucleus that receives afferent inputs from the precentral cerebral cortex and globus pallidus.

zona intermedia: describes the melanotrope containing region of adenohypophysis in some species.

zonal centrifugation: rate-zonal centrifugation; techniques for separating proteins of different molecular weights by centrifuging them at high speeds for brief time periods in tubes that contain layers of fluids of gradually increasing densities.

zona pellucida: ZP; a clear noncellular layer on the surface of an oocyte, zygote, or blastocyst secreted by stratum granulosa cells. It contains components essential for fertilization and the events that immediately follow; *see* **ZP1**, **ZP2**, and **ZP3**. After fertilization, the ZP is

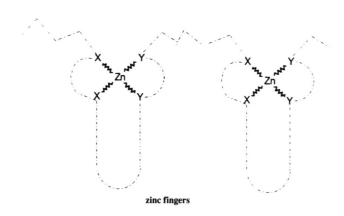

zinc fingers

believed to protect very young blastocysts against ectopic and premature uterine implantation. *See* also **hatching**.

zona pellucida proteins: species specific zona pellucida glycoproteins that contribute to fertilization and the events that soon follow. **ZP1, ZP2,** and **ZP3** (*q.v.*) are present in the relative amounts 1:10:10. Antibodies directed against them are under investigation for use as interceptives.

zona radiata: zona pellucida; *cf* **corona radiata**.

zona reaction: changes in the surface of a fertilized secondary oocyte initiated by the **cortical reaction** (*q.v.*). They provide more effective and more persistent protection against the entry of additional spermatozoa. *See* also **ZP3**.

zona reticularis. the innermost zone of the adrenal cortex, adjacent to the adrenal medulla, named for the network-like (reticular) arrangement of the cells. It is usually smaller than the zona fasciculata in mature glands and less responsive to adrenocorticotropic hormone (ACTH). Although believed to secrete adrenal androgens and some glucocorticoids, the functions have not been fully defined. According to one hypothesis, the cells perform special functions that involve interactions with both the z. fasciculata and the adrenal medulla. Another is that aging z. fasciculata cells migrate to it and die there. (An adrenal cortex with all three components can regenerate from z. glomerulosa but not z. reticularis cells if implanted into adrenalectomized animals.)

zona tuberalis: the pituitary gland pars tuberalis of some species.

zonula, zonule: a small, usually circular zone.

zonula adherens: desmosome.

zona occludens: tight junction.

zonule: zonula.

zoo-: a prefix meaning animal.

zooecdysones: ecdysones made by animals, a term used to distinguish them from related plant phytoecdysones.

zoogenous: produced by, or originating in animals.

zoogonous: viviparous.

zoonosis: a disease of other animal species that can affect humans.

zoosperm: spermatozoan.

zootic: pertaining to animals other than humans.

Zovirax: a trade name for acyclovir.

ZP: zona pellucida.

ZP1: an acidic, 200K glycoprotein synthesized by oocytes that links ZP2 with ZP3 and interconnects zona pellucida actin filaments.

ZP2: 120K species specific sulfated heterodimeric glycoproteins that (along with ZP3) border zona pellucida actin filaments. They do not bind acrosome-intact sperm, but do attach to a sperm component after ZP3 initiates acrosome reactions. A serine protease released by the cortical reaction that follows fertilization converts ZP2 to $ZP2_f$, and this leads to hardening of the zona pellucida. The reaction may contribute to protection of oocytes against entry of additional spermatozoa, and blastocysts against ectopic and premature implantation.

ZP3: an acidic 83K species-specific heterodimeric glycoprotein that, with ZP2 borders zona pellucida actin filaments. It contains carbohydrate groups that serve as receptors for spermatozoa, and it initiates acrosome reactions. Antibodies directed against it block fertilization. A glycosidase released from cortical granules during the zona reaction that follows fertilization promotes its conversion to $ZP3_f$, a form that does not bind additional sperm.

ZPG: zero population growth; describes populations in which birth rates are approximately equivalent to death rates.

Zr: Zirconium.

Z score: a measure of the similarity in amino acid composition of one protein to another, relative to its similarity to a third protein (usually selected because it is not believed to perform a comparable function). The scores are used to trace evolutionary changes and set up hypotheses. However, although some closely related proteins (for example insulins from various species) exert similar effects in many animal types, highly homologous kinds can be biologically dissimilar. Moreover, some proteins that differ markedly in amino acid make-up but have similar three-dimensional configurations exert similar actions.

Zuckerkandl, organs of: Zuckerkandl glands; para-aortic bodies; aggregates of chromaffin cells and blood capillaries near the inferior mesenteric arteries that secrete catecholamines and contain chemoreceptors sensitive to changes in oxygen tension.

Zucker rats: *fa/fa* rats; a rat strain used for endocrine and metabolic studies. Juvenile homozygotes acquire high parasympathetic and subnormal sympathetic tone and display low energy expenditure at an early age. They soon become hyperphagic and hyperinsulinemic and rapidly develop obesity associated with high plasma triacylglycerol levels, high lipoprotein lipase activity, and metabolic defects in brown adipose when fed the same kind of food as their lean counterparts. Unstressed animals of both sexes have high circulating adrenocorticotropic hormone (ACTH) and high morning corticosterone levels and exaggerated ACTH and glucocorticoid responses to stress. Males also have high glucocorticoid levels in the evenings. Adrenalectomy attenuates most of the defects.

zuclomiphene: the *cis* form of **clomiphene** (*q.v.*), a mixed estrogen receptor agonist/antagonist.

zwitterions: compounds that carry both positive and negative charges. Since amino groups can accept protons (as NH_3^+) and carboxyl groups can ionize (as COO^-), many amino acids are zwitterions in the physiological pH range.

zygo-: a prefix meaning joining or pairing, as in zygotene.

zygonema: the chromatin thread that forms during the zygotene stage of meiosis.

-zygosity: a suffix that refers to the genetic nature of a zygote, as in homozygosity (having two identical alleles for a trait), or dizygosity (a term used when twins develop from different zygotes).

zygote: usually (1) the diploid cell that forms soon after an oocyte is fertilized; (2) a very young embryo.

zygotene: the stage of meiosis I in which chromosomes pair. It is preceded by leptotene and followed by pachytene.

zymase: a cell-free yeast extract that contains the fermentation enzymes.

zymo-: a prefix meaning (1) enzyme; (2) fermentation.

zymogens: proenzymes.

zymogen granules: granules that contain proenzymes, a term usually applied to the types in the exocrine pancreas.

zymosan: a complex polysaccharide from dried yeast cell walls. It is used to activate complement.

ZZ: the sex chromosome pattern for male birds and for males of some other submammalian vertebrate groups. Females of those species are **WZ**; *see* also **W chromosome**.